# GYNECOLOGIC ONCOLOGY

# GYNECOLOGIC ONCOLOGY

**Second Edition**

*Editors*

## Robert C. Knapp, M.D.

William H. Baker Professor of Gynecology
Harvard Medical School
Prior Director of Gynecology and Gynecologic Oncology
Brigham and Women's Hospital and Dana Farber Cancer Institute
Boston, Massachusetts

## Ross S. Berkowitz, M.D.

Professor of Obstetrics, Gynecology, and Reproductive Biology
Harvard Medical School
Director of Gynecology and Gynecologic Oncology
Brigham and Women's Hospital and Dana Farber Cancer Institute
Co-Director, New England Trophoblastic Disease Center
Boston, Massachusetts

**McGraw-Hill, Inc.** *Health Professions Division*

New York   St. Louis   San Francisco   Auckland   Bogotá   Caracas   Lisbon   London   Madrid
Mexico   Milan   Montreal   New Delhi   Paris   San Juan   Singapore   Sydney   Tokyo   Toronto

This book is dedicated to our wives,
**Miriam H. Knapp** and
**Ellen R. Golding,** Ph.D., whose support,
patience, and inspiration have been
immeasurable and invaluable.

GYNECOLOGIC ONCOLOGY
**Second Edition**

Copyright © 1993 by McGraw-Hill, Inc. All rights reserved.
Formerly published and copyright © 1986, Macmillan Publishing Company, a division of Macmillan, Inc. All rights reserved. Printed in the United States of America. Except as permitted under the United States Copyright Act of 1976, no part of this publication may be reproduced or distributed in any form or by any means, or stored in a data base or retrieval system, without the prior written permission of the publisher.

1 2 3 4 5 6 7 8 9 0   HALHAL   9 8 7 6 5 4 3 2

ISBN 0-07-105403-0

This book was set in Sabon by Ruttle, Shaw & Wetherill, Inc. The editors were Jane E. Pennington and Lester A. Sheinis; the production supervisor was Richard C. Ruzycka; the project supervision was by Tage Publishing Service, Inc.; the cover designer was Marsha Cohen/Parallelogram. Arcata Graphics/ Halliday was printer and binder.

**Library of Congress Cataloging-in-Publication Data**

Gynecologic oncology / [edited] by Robert C. Knapp and Ross
   S. Berkowitz.—2d ed.
      p.        cm.
   Includes bibliographical references and index.
   ISBN 0-07-105403-0
   1. Generative organs. Female—Cancer.    I. Knapp,
Robert C.    II. Berkowitz, Ross Stuart.
   [DNLM: 1. Genital Neoplasms, Female. WP 145 G994]
RC280.G5G885   1992
616.99'465—dc20
DNLM/DLC
for Library of Congress                        91-46673
                                    CIP

# Contents

## UNIT I
### Basic Science Aspects

# UNIT II
## Sites

# UNIT III
## Management of Complications of Disease and Treatment

# UNIT IV
## Supportive Care of the Cancer Patient

# Contributors

**Karen H. Antman, M.D.** [13]
Associate Professor of Medicine, Harvard Medical School, Dana Farber Cancer Institute, Boston, Massachusetts

**Robert C. Bast, Jr., M.D.** [4]
Professor of Medicine, Director of Duke Comprehensive Cancer Center, Duke University Medical Center, Durham, North Carolina

**James A. Belli, M.D.** [6]
Professor and Chairman Radiation Therapy Department, John Sealy Centennial Chair in Radiation Therapy, President of Radiation Research Society, University of Texas Medical Branch Hospitals at Galveston, Galveston, Texas

**Jonathan S. Berek, M.D.** [19, 22]
Professor and Vice-Chair, Chief of Gynecology, Director, Gynecologic Oncology, Department of Obstetrics and Gynecology, UCLA School of Medicine, Jonsson Comprehensive Cancer Center, Los Angeles, California

**Ross S. Berkowitz, M.D.** [17]
Professor of Obstetrics, Gynecology, and Reproductive Biology, Harvard Medical School, Director of Gynecology and Gynecologic Oncology, Brigham and Women's Hospital and Dana Farber Cancer Institute, Co-Director, New England Trophoblastic Disease Center, Boston, Massachusetts

**Michael A. Bookman, M.D.** [4]
Associate Member, Department of Medical Oncology, Fox Chase Cancer Center, Philadelphia, Pennsylvania

**David Borsook, M.D., Ph.D.** [24]
Instructor in Anesthesia, Harvard Medical School, Assistant Anesthetist, Department of Anesthesia, Massachusetts General Hospital, Boston, Massachusetts

**Edward J. Callahan, Ph.D.** [25]
Professor of Psychology, Director of Behavioral Science Education, Department of Family Practice, University of California Medical Center at Davis, Sacramento, California

**Judith Campisi, Ph.D.** [1]
Senior Scientist, Division of Cell and Molecular Biology, Lawrence Berkeley Laboratories, University of California, Berkeley, California

**Daniel B. Carr, M.D.** [24]
Associate Professor of Anesthesiology and Medicine (Endocrinology), Harvard Medical School, Director, Division of Pain Management, Department of Anesthesia, Massachusetts General Hospital, Boston, Massachusetts

**Lee M. Chin, D.Sc.** [7]
Assistant Professor of Radiation Therapy, Harvard Medical School, Chief Clinical Physicist, Joint Center of Radiation Therapy, Boston, Massachusetts

**Kevin A. Craig, B.A.** [14]
Department of Medical and Scientific Communications, Roswell Park Cancer Institute, Buffalo, New York

**Daniel W. Cramer, M.D., Sc.D.** [8]
Associate Professor of Obstetrics, Gynecology, and Reproductive Biology, Harvard Medical School, Brigham and Women's Hospital, Boston, Massachusetts

**William T. Creasman, M.D.** [12]
Sims Hester Professor and Chairman, Department of Obstetrics and Gynecology, Medical University of South Carolina, Charleston, South Carolina

**Christopher P. Crum, M.D.** [10]
Associate Professor of Pathology, Harvard Medical School, Director, Women's and Perinatal Pathology, Brigham and Women's Hospital, Boston, Massachusetts

**Gary L. Eddy, M.D.** [12]
Associate Professor, Department of Obstetrics and Gynecology, Medical University of South Carolina, Charleston, South Carolina

**James Fanning, D.O.** [14]
Senior Fellow, Department of Gynecologic Oncology, Roswell Park Cancer Institute, Buffalo, New York

**Howard J. Fingert, M.D.** [1]
Assistant Professor of Medicine, Division of Hematology/Oncology, Department of Biomedical Research, St. Elizabeth's Hospital, Tufts University School of Medicine, Boston, Massachusetts

**Emil Frei III, M.D.** [2]
Richard and Susan Smith Professor of Medicine, Harvard Medical School, Physician-in-Chief, Emeritus and Chief of Division of Cancer Pharmacology, Dana Farber Cancer Institute, Boston, Massachusetts

The numbers in brackets following the contributors' names refer to the chapters written or co-written by the contributors.

**Gideon Goldman, M.D.  [20]**
Research Fellow, Department of Surgery, Harvard Medical School, Brigham and Women's Hospital, Boston, Massachusetts

**Donald P. Goldstein, M.D.  [17]**
Assistant Clinical Professor of Obstetrics, Gynecology and Reproductive Biology, Harvard Medical School, Director, New England Trophoblastic Disease Center, Boston, Massachusetts

**Neville F. Hacker, M.B.B.S.  [19, 22]**
Director, Gynaecological Cancer Centre, Royal Hospital for Women, Paddington, New South Wales, Australia

**Sharon A. Hamilton, Ph.D.  [25]**
Boca Raton Psychotherapy Center, Boca Raton, Florida

**Herbert B. Hechtman, M.D.  [20]**
Professor of Surgery, Harvard Medical School and Massachusetts Institute of Technology, Division of Health Science Technology, Senior Surgeon, Brigham and Women's Hospital, Boston, Massachusetts

**Arthur L. Herbst, M.D.  [16]**
Joseph B. DeLee Distinguished Service Professor, Obstetrics and Gynecology, University of Chicago, Chairman, Department of Obstetrics and Gynecology, University of Chicago Hospitals and Clinics, Chicago, Illinois

**Robert V. Higgins, M.D.  [11]**
Assistant Professor, Department of Obstetrics and Gynecology, University of Kentucky Medical Center, Lexington, Kentucky

**Anthony E. Howes, M.D., Ph.D.  [7]**
Associate Professor of Radiation Therapy, Harvard Medical School, Section Chief of Radiation Oncology, Brigham and Women's Hospital, Joint Center for Radiation Therapy, Boston, Massachusetts

**Gary P. Kearney, M.D.  [18]**
Clinical Assistant Professor of Surgery, Harvard Medical School, Associate Surgeon, Brigham and Women's Hospital, Boston, Massachusetts

**Robert C. Knapp, M.D.  [4]**
William H. Baker Professor of Gynecology, Harvard Medical School, Prior Director of Gynecology and Gynecologic Oncology, Brigham and Women's Hospital and Dana Farber Cancer Institute, Boston, Massachusetts

**Leo D. Lagasse, M.D.  [19, 22]**
Professor Emeritus of Obstetrics and Gynecology, Director, Gynecologic Oncology, Cedars-Sinai Medical Center, Los Angeles, California

**Philip T. Lavin, Ph.D.  [9]**
Associate Clinical Professor of Surgery (Biostatistics), Harvard Medical School, Boston Biostatistics Research Foundation, Inc., Newton Upper Falls, Massachusetts

**Maureen MacBurney, MS, RD, CNSD  [23]**
Director, Nutrition Support Services, Brigham and Women's Hospital, Boston, Massachusetts

**Donnamarie Maguire, RN  [23]**
Nutrition Support Services, Brigham and Women's Hospital, Boston, Massachusetts

**George W. Morley, M.D.  [15]**
Norman F. Miller, Professor of Gynecology, Department of Obstetrics and Gynecology, University of Michigan Medical Center, Ann Arbor, Michigan

**Donald R. Nicholas, Ph.D.  [25]**
Professor of Psychology, Department of Counseling Psychology, Ball State University, Muncie, Indiana

**Arthur B. Pardee, Ph.D.  [1]**
Professor of Biological Chemistry and Molecular Pharmacology, Harvard Medical School, Chief, Division of Cell Growth and Regulation, Dana Farber Cancer Institute, Boston, Massachusetts

**Robert E. Pawlicki, Ph.D.  [25]**
Professor of Psychology, Department of Anesthesiology, Director, Behavioral Medicine/Medical Center, University of Cincinnati, Cincinnati, Ohio

**William P. Peters, M.D.  [2]**
Associate Professor of Medicine, Director of Bone Marrow Transplantation Program, Duke University Medical Center, Durham, North Carolina

**M. Steven Piver, M.D.  [14]**
Chief, Department of Gynecologic Oncology, Clinical Professor of Gynecology, Director, Gilda Radner Familial Ovarian Cancer Registry, Roswell Park Cancer Institute, Buffalo, New York

**Edward Podczaski, M.D.  [16]**
Assistant Professor of Obstetrics and Gynecology, Division of Gynecologic Oncology, The Milton S. Hershey Medical Center, The Pennsylvania State University, Hershey, Pennsylvania

**Deborah E. Powell, M.D.  [11]**
Professor and Chairman, Department of Pathology, University of Kentucky Medical Center, Lexington, Kentucky

**Ellen E. Sheets, M.D.  [3]**
Assistant Professor of Obstetrics, Gynecology and Reproductive Biology, Division of Gynecologic Oncology, Harvard Medical School, Brigham and Women's Hospital, Boston, Massachusetts

**Peyton T. Taylor, Jr., M.D.  [10]**
Director, Division of Gynecologic Oncology, Richard N. and Louise R. Crockett Professor of Obstetrics and Gynecology, University of Virginia, Charlottesville, Virginia

**Sabah S. Tumeh, M.D.  [18]**
Associate Professor of Radiology, Harvard Medical School, Department of Radiology, Brigham and Women's Hospital, Boston, Massachusetts

**Ruth Tuomala, M.D.  [21]**
Assistant Professor, Department of Obstetrics, Gynecology and Reproductive Biology, Harvard Medical School, Director of Infectious Diseases in Obstetrics and Gynecology, Brigham and Women's Hospital, Boston, Massachusetts

**John R. van Nagell, Jr., M.D.  [11]**
American Cancer Society Professor of Clinical Oncology, Director, Division of Gynecologic Oncology, Department of Obstetrics and Gynecology, University of Kentucky Medical Center, Lexington, Kentucky

**Richard Welbourn, M.D.** [20]
Research Fellow, Department of Surgery, Harvard Medical School, Brigham and Women's Hospital, Boston, Massachusetts

**Douglas W. Wilmore, M.D.** [23]
Frank Sawyer Professor of Surgery, Department of Surgery, Harvard Medical School, Medical Director, Nutrition Support Services, Brigham and Women's Hospital, Boston, Massachusetts

**Robert C. Young, M.D.** [5]
President, Fox Chase Cancer Center, Philadelphia, Pennsylvania

# Preface

Since the first edition of this book was published, interest in malignancy of the female reproductive system has grown profoundly. The recent focus on genetics, growth factors, viruses, and monoclonal antibodies in human cancer, as well as new concepts in cancer management, have vastly increased the breadth of scientific knowledge, requiring a shift in emphasis in gynecologic oncology as it is now taught.

In this second edition we have sought to emphasize newer areas of productive investigation and also to point out gaps in our knowledge. Accordingly, in Unit I, the chapters dealing with basic science have been expanded, and a new chapter by Dr. Philip Lavin on the statistical aspects of gynecologic oncology has been included.

Although this volume contains new information regarding the basic science of gynecologic malignancy, we have not neglected the expansion of clinical knowledge. Every chapter dealing with the specific sites has been carefully revised and brought up to date. We are particularly grateful to the authors new to this edition who have provided comprehensive chapters on cancer of the cervix, uterine corpus, and ovary and on nutritional support and the management of pain: Dr. J. R. van Nagell, Jr., Dr. R. V. Higgins, and Dr. D. E. Powell; Dr.

William T. Creasman and Dr. Gary L. Eddy; Dr. M. Steven Piver, Dr. James Fanning, and Mr. Kevin A. Craig; Maureen MacBurney, RD, MS, and Donnamarie Maguire, RN, BSN; Dr. Douglas W. Wilmore; and Dr. David Borsook and Dr. Daniel B. Carr.

As more information on cervical intraepithelial lesions has come to light, we felt a separate chapter was needed to discuss this topic, and this has been provided in a scholarly manner by Dr. Christopher P. Crum and Dr. Peyton T. Taylor.

Considerable time and effort have been devoted to maintaining the most current bibliographies, which we consider of particular importance both as a stimulus to the beginner and as background for the scholar in this specialty. Although most of the references are recent, older titles were retained when they represented either classics or the best available data. A sincere attempt has been made to avoid insularity and to include significant foreign references.

Once more we are particularly grateful to Ms. Diane Q. Forti for skillfully editing the manuscripts. We also thank the medical students, residents, and fellows whose relentless search for knowledge stimulated our decision to revise this text.

# UNIT I

# Basic Science Aspects

# Chapter 1 | Molecular Biology and Biochemistry of Cancer

*Howard J. Fingert*  *Judith Campisi*
*Arthur B. Pardee*

## INTRODUCTION: CELL BIOLOGY

The basic cell biology and biochemistry of normal cells and of cancer cells are exceedingly similar. Cancer cells differ from normal due to aberrant regulation. Tumor cells generally contain the same biomolecules necessary for survival, proliferation, and expression of many cell type–specific functions. However, failure to modulate these functions properly leads to an altered phenotype and cancer.

Three cellular functions—growth, differentiation, and chromosome stability—tend to be inappropriately regulated in a tumor. First, the normal controls for cellular proliferation are relaxed. This is a necessary but often insufficient requirement for tumor formation. Second, differentiation can be distorted; the tumor cells may be blocked at a particular stage of differentiation, or they may differentiate into an inappropriate or abnormal cell type. Third, chromosomal organization may be destabilized such that variant cells arise with high frequency. Some variants may have an increased growth advantage; others may be resistant to killing by chemotherapeutic drugs or radiation.

Clearly, before an understanding of tumorigenesis is achieved, it will be necessary to understand how these three functions are controlled in normal cells.

## NEOPLASIA

### In Vivo Studies

**Kinetic Properties of Normal versus Tumor Cells** A fundamental property that distinguishes cancer from normal tissues is "neoplasia," which can be defined as "relatively autonomous growth of malignant cells in the normal host" (Pitot, 1981). The relative autonomy of cancer cell growth is a key concept: cancer cells do not grow free of all restraints, but they do increase in size and cell number in a manner that is relatively uncontrolled compared with their normal counterparts.

Laboratory techniques developed in the last few decades have improved our understanding of fundamental growth properties in cancer cell populations. In addition, the growth properties of neoplastic and normal cells have been compared. Most studies of neoplastic cell growth have utilized transplantable animal tumors or human cancer cells in culture. Numerous problems prevent the direct analysis of cancer growth in humans, including intraneoplastic diversity (Nicolson, 1982; Heppner and Miller, 1989), mixtures of normal and tumor cells in biopsy samples, and variations in tumor growth properties over time. Despite these drawbacks, experimental methods have also been designed to examine the growth properties of human cancer cell populations in experimental animals and in culture (Foulds, 1975; Fingert, 1987). Such studies have helped to answer fundamental biologic questions about how cancers grow. They provide direction for investigations of the key subcellular and molecular mechanisms of neoplasia, which will be reviewed later in this chapter.

In terms of population kinetics, the growth of any tissue or mass depends on three major parameters: (1) the rate of individual cell division; (2) the growth fraction of the cell population; and (3) cell loss from the growing population through differentiation, cell death, or other means of attrition. Normal cells reach a steady-state of growth that provides a balanced economy for the body as a whole. Each organ maintains tight controls over the growth rate, growth fraction, and cell loss. In normal tissues, physiologic stimuli can alter these parameters, leading to increased cell proliferation, but growth will cease when the stimulus is withdrawn or a new steady-state is achieved.

Cancer cells do not maintain proper controls with respect to these growth parameters (i.e., growth rate, growth fraction, and cell loss). Because some noncancerous tissues can grow faster than cancers under physiologic conditions, it is not simply rapid growth at a single time and place that distinguishes neoplasia. Rather, it is the overall change in growth regulation that characterizes neoplasia, especially the increased growth fraction that is not balanced by cell loss.

When biopsy samples from normal, inflammatory, and neoplastic lesions of the cervix, vocal cord or pharynx were analyzed to determine the rate and degree of cell proliferation, some of the inflammatory tissues were found to grow over 10 times faster than cancer in a discrete time and place. Noncancerous tissues cease to grow rapidly when healing is complete, unlike the neoplastic tissues, which continue to grow over time (Fabrikant and Cherry, 1969; Fakuda, 1990). In some respects, cancers can be thought of as "wounds that do not heal."

Most studies with animal tumors or human biopsy specimens indicate that the rate of cell division—i.e., *the doubling time of individual cells* ($T_c$)—is the least important parameter distinguishing cancer from normal cells. Many neoplastic cells divide at about the same rate as their normal counterparts, and most cancer cells divide much more slowly than cells in some normal, rapidly dividing tissues, such as intestine or bone marrow (Hellman and DeVita, 1982).

Autoradiography has been a useful tool for measuring growth rates of cell populations in vitro and in vivo. This technique identifies growing cells according to their uptake of radioactive precursors for DNA synthesis, such as tritiated thymidine. Samples of these tissues are then treated with photographic emulsion and developing agents. Black granules form over the nuclei of cells that have utilized the radioactive precursor and gone through DNA replication and cell division. In a similar technique, cells are exposed to bromo-deoxyuridine (BrdU), which is selectively utilized by cells in the DNA-synthetic phase. Subsequently, the cell population is stained with an identifiable antibody that binds only BrdU-containing cells (Fakuda, 1990). This is a sensitive assay for the number of cells that are cycling through DNA synthesis (the S phase of the cell cycle).

The *labeling index* (LI) is the ratio of labeled cells to total cells as measured in autoradiographic preparations of various tissues. This technique provides a relatively simple method for estimating proliferative rates and growth fractions of cancerous or normal cells. Many tumor cells in vivo are in a dormant, nondividing state (Wheelock et al, 1981). The average time for cell division within the growing population ($T_c$) can be estimated by taking multiple samples over time and counting the percentage of cells that are labeled at mitosis. Exposure to radioactive thymidine also provides a method for estimating the length of the cell cycle and the duration of the phases of the cell cycle—i.e., $G_1$, S, $G_2$, and M (Fig. 1-1).

When autoradiographic techniques were applied to biopsy samples of ovarian and endometrial cancers, a mean cell division time ($T_c$) of about 4 to 5 days was observed. Similar studies with other human cancers revealed a wide range of mean LI (3 to 40%) and $T_c$ (1 to 10 days) (Hellman and DeVita, 1982). Estimated mean values of LI and $T_c$ for gynecologic neoplasms as well as for some of the most rapidly proliferating normal tissues are listed in Table 1-1. Table 1-2 summarizes the mean LI from various solid tumors compared with normal tissues of similar histologic type.

Several conclusions can be drawn from the data in Tables 1-1 and 1-2. First, the rate of cell division, or

**TABLE 1-1   Growth Parameters of Gynecologic Neoplasms and Normal Tissues**

| Cell Type | Labeling Index (%) | Estimated Average Cell Doubling Time (Days) |
|---|---|---|
| Ovarian carcinoma, pleural fluid | 18 | 5 |
| Ovarian carcinoma, pleural fluid | 20 | 5 |
| Ovarian carcinoma, pleural fluid | 3 | — |
| Ovarian carcinoma, ascites | 18 | — |
| Endometrial carcinoma, ascites | 11 | 4.6 |
| Squamous cell carcinoma of the cervix | 13 | — |
| Squamous cell carcinoma of the cervix | 40 | — |
| Normal intestinal crypts | 12-18 | 1-2 |
| Normal bone marrow, myeloblasts | 32-75 | 0.7-1.1 |

*Source:* Data compiled from Clarkson et al, 1965; Bennington, 1969; and Tannock, 1978.

$T_c$, is not a major determinant of tumor growth, since many cancer cells grow at a slower $T_c$ than some normal tissues, including the intestinal mucosa and bone marrow. When comparisons have been possible between neoplastic and normal cells of the same histologic type (e.g., leukemia and normal bone marrow), it is also apparent that the $T_c$ of cancer cells can be the same as, or longer than, that of normal cells. Second, the LI and growth fraction are the parameters that commonly distinguish cancer from normal tissues of the same histologic type. Third, decreased cell loss is an important parameter in many neoplasms: cancerous tissues increase in size faster than bone marrow or intestinal mucosa, even though the $T_c$ and growth fractions predict slower growth of the tumors compared with the normal tissues. However, these normal tissues balance high proliferative rates against tremendous cell loss through exfoliation or differentiation into nondividing cells.

Growth rates of individual tumors in vivo also demonstrate the importance of LI and the growth fraction. Analysis of these data requires a clear distinction between the rate of cell division ($T_c$) and the *doubling time of the tumor mass* ($T_d$). $T_c$ refers to the time of cell division, i.e., the time required for an average cell to go through one complete cell division and return to the same phase of the cell cycle. Since autoradiography can identify radioactive thymidine-labeled cells as they pass through the DNA-replicative (S) phase of the cell cycle and into mitosis, $T_c$ is often measured by the "intermitotic time" between two consecutive mitoses. In contrast, $T_d$ is the estimated time needed to double the size of an entire tumor mass as measured by calipers,

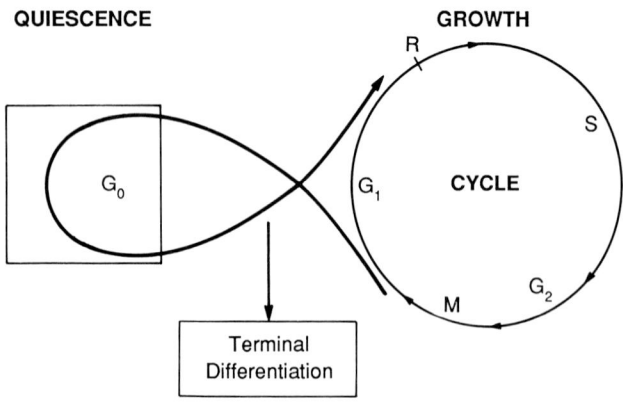

FIGURE 1-1   Mammalian cell cycle.

TABLE 1-2  Labeling Indices of Human Neoplasms and Histologically Related Normal Tissues

| Cell Type | Labeling Index* (%) | Reference |
|---|---|---|
| Cervix, carcinoma in situ | Range, 18-27 Average, 23 | Fettig and Sievers (1966) |
| Cervix, normal epithelium | Range, 4-8 Average, 6 | |
| Breast, ductal carcinoma in situ | 5.5 | Meyer (1981) |
| Breast, normal duct | 0.7 | |
| Nasopharynx, squamous cell carcinoma | 16.2 | Fabrikant and Cherry (1969) |
| Nasopharynx, normal epithelium | 2.5 | |
| Melanoma, malignant | 12.8 | Meyer (1981) |
| Nevus, benign | 0.3 | |

*Interstudy comparisons are difficult owing to differences in autoradiography techniques.

x-rays, and the like. $T_d$ is usually much longer than $T_c$ owing to cell loss, changes in the growth rate over time, and a less than 100% growth fraction. For example, a $T_c$ of about 2 to 3 days was measured in one tumor of the head and neck, and this same tumor had a $T_d$ of 21 days during the same period of measurement (Bresciani et al, 1974).

The growth fraction appears to correlate inversely with the overall $T_d$ of solid tumors—i.e., an increased growth fraction corresponds to a shorter $T_d$ and a faster growth of tumor mass. This was first demonstrated in animal tumors, which can be measured more frequently than can most human cancers (Table 1-3). A close correlation between increased LI and decreased $T_d$ has also been observed in studies of human cancers; however, methodologic differences among various laboratories present many problems in such comparisons (Meyer, 1981). A correlation between histologic grade and LI has been observed in many solid tumors, including sarcoma, lymphoma, bladder, and breast cancer. Some of these data demonstrate that LI can be an independent determinant of prognosis, especially in breast cancer, primary brain neoplasms, chronic lymphocytic leukemia, and myeloma (Meyer, 1981).

Similar to LI, the *S index* is another measure of the proliferative capacity of tumor cells. The S index employs DNA flow cytometry to measure the percentage of cells in the DNA-synthetic phase of the cell cycle (S-phase fraction). In patients with breast cancer, negative lymph nodes, and diploid tumors, a high S fraction was found to be an independent predictor of poor prognosis (Clark et al, 1989). Similar correlations have been seen in ovarian cancer. Survival in both early (stages 1 and 2) and late (stages 3 and 4) ovarian cancer was significantly worse in patients with diploid tumors when the tumor cells demonstrated a high S index (Kallioniemi et al, 1988).

***Growth Kinetics and Mechanisms of Neoplasia*** Analysis of growth parameters in cancer provides direction for more basic investigations into the mechanisms of neoplasia at the cellular, subcellular, and molecular levels. From the previous discussion, it is evident that the increased growth fraction of cancer cells is a key property distinguishing most neoplasms from normal tissues. At the level of a single cell, one process that determines the growth fraction is the initiation of cell division from a nongrowing state—i.e., the process of entering the S phase from a quiescent state in which DNA replication is inactive.

Most normal tissues, such as brain or liver, contain nondividing but viable cells that are metabolically very active. This "nongrowing state" has been designated $G_0$ to represent cells that are out of the proliferative cycle (Fig. 1-1). $G_0$ cells have the same quantity of DNA as $G_1$ cells, but they do not share the identical biologic functions of $G_1$ cells, which are committed to biochemical processes necessary for cell division. In normal tissues, $G_0$ cells enter $G_1$ and the division cycle in response to local stimuli, systemic hormones, or growth factors

TABLE 1-3  Correlation Between Growth Fraction and Mass Doubling Time ($T_d$) in Experimental Tumors

| Tumor | Cell Doubling Time ($T_c$) (hr) | Growth Fraction (%) | Mass Doubling Time ($T_d$) (days) |
|---|---|---|---|
| L1210 (mouse) | 12.8 | 86 | 0.5 |
| B16 (mouse) | 20.0 | 55 | 1.9 |
| LL (mouse) | 19.0 | 38 | 2.9 |
| DMBA (rat) | 18.0 | 10 | 7.4 |

*Source:* Goldin A, et al: Historical development and current strategy of the National Cancer Institute Drug Development Program (Chap 5). In DeVita VT Jr, Busch H (eds): *Methods in Cancer Research*, Vol. 16, *Cancer Drug Development.* New York, Academic Press, 1979, pp 165-245.

released by the body to meet a demand for new cells. This process of commitment to cell division is tightly regulated for nondividing tissues in order to maintain normal body functions.

Similar to normal cells, many cancer cells are dormant and exist in $G_0$. However, the processes that regulate their commitment to division are abnormal and less stringent, leading to an increased growth fraction of the cancer cell population relative to normal cells. Recent studies have helped to clarify the biologic events that determine this commitment to begin cell division. These experiments have provided new insights into the biologic differences between cancer and normal cells and have thus helped explain the basis of neoplastic growth.

Cells are lost from the proliferating population in mainly two ways. Normal *terminal differentiation* creates a cell that never divides again; terminal differentiation of normal cells is closely balanced by cell proliferation. Neoplastic cells can be defective in terminal differentiation. As a consequence, the cell population increases. Conversely, cells can be lost through *death*. An example would be necrosis at the center of a tumor. Although inadequate nutrition is probably responsible, other studies suggest that genetic properties exist to regulate cell death in certain tissues, independent of nutrition. Some tumors undergo major cell death that nearly balances proliferation, and as a result, the tumor mass increases very slowly (Steel, 1967). Interventions to increase the rate of tumor cell loss, even slightly, could possibly shift this balance so as to make the tumor regress.

**Mitogens and Extracellular Factors** Circulating mitogens, including some *physiologic hormones*, stimulate cell division in normal tissues, which respond through the expression of specific receptors. Human cancers that arise in hormone-sensitive tissues can also respond to physiologic hormones through specific receptors. Hormonal manipulations are of therapeutic benefit in prostate, breast, uterine, and some ovarian cancers (Kodama and Kodama, 1983). In addition to their common occurrence in breast cancer cells, estrogen and/or progesterone receptors have been demonstrated in ovarian and endometrial cancers and in some cervical adenocarcinomas (Sledge and McGuire, 1983), suggesting that circulating hormones could play a role in the growth of these gynecologic neoplasms.

Monoclonal antibodies to estrogen receptors have been developed. Fluorescent tagging of these antibodies has identified marked heterogeneity in the expression of estrogen receptors among breast cancer cells from individual biopsy specimens (McCarty et al, 1985). This heterogeneity may be due to the evolution of receptor-negative clones within the tumor mass. However, an alternative explanation is suggested by studies of mouse teratocarcinoma cells, in which receptors for epidermal growth factor (EGF) increase after the induction of differentiation into a nonmalignant phenotype (Rees et al, 1979). Similarly, human cancer cells may retain some capacity for differentiation that includes the development of hormone receptors in later states. In this case,

stem cells of the neoplasm would be mostly receptor-negative and would produce receptors (becoming hormone-sensitive) only later—i.e., a subpopulation may begin commitment to a more differentiated phenotype. In support of this hypothesis may be the observation that histologic differentiation tends to correlate with the presence of hormone receptors in uterine, cervical, and breast cancer (Ford et al, 1983). In terms of therapy, this hypothesis may explain the poor correlation between the presence of hormone receptors and the clinical response to hormonal therapy observed in some tumors: the receptor-positive cells, which are already committed to differentiation, would be part of the cell loss population, so that hormonal therapy would have little effect on receptor-negative stem cells.

In addition to altered internal properties related to energy metabolism or cell division, which provide overall growth advantages for cancer cells, several properties that operate external to the cell appear to be critical for growth, invasion, or metastatic spread. *Angiogenesis* is such a property, defined as the ability of tumors to recruit new blood vessels providing essential nutrients for tumor growth. The importance of angiogenesis for growth of solid tumors has been demonstrated in animal tumor explants, which grow to only 2 to 3 mm in diameter when angiogenesis is blocked (Folkman et al, 1989).

Growth parameters can vary dramatically within a single tumor, depending on its proximity to blood vessels. Autoradiographic studies of animal tumors have revealed that cancer cells near blood vessels had an average LI of 74% and a growth fraction of nearly 100%, whereas cells distant from blood vessels had growth parameters that were about half these values (Tannock, 1968). Some types of animal tumors can be reliably induced by local implantation of carcinogens: these and other pre-neoplastic tissues show angiogenesis preceding the growth of visible cancers, further supporting the importance of this property in neoplasia (Folkman et al, 1989).

Recent studies have shown that angiogenesis results from diffusible factors that appear near growing neoplasms, so-called "tumor angiogenesis factors." These proteins stimulate the migration of normal endothelial cells from nearby blood vessels, forming afferent and efferent loops that become new blood vessels supplying the tumor mass (Folkman et al, 1989). Angiogenesis factors are also produced by some normal cells, possibly induced as a secondary process by growing neoplasms. For example, heparin or heparin subunits, which can have angiogenic properties, are released from mast cells surrounding solid tumors. Some benign tumors and normal tissues also produce potent angiogenesis factors under special conditions, such as the developing follicle of the normal ovary, which exhibits rapid growth of new blood vessels in the capillary sheath surrounding the follicle at the time of ovulation (Nicolson, 1982). Angiogenesis factors have also been detected in other physiologic processes, such as wound healing or inflammatory conditions. These observations indicate that angiogenesis factors are not unique to neoplasms but are normal cell components that may be abnormally expressed by neoplasms or induced from normal host cells during the initial growth of the tumor.

***Tumor Spread in Vivo*** *Metastasis* is a complex process that depends on specific properties of cancer cells related to the normal microenvironment of the host. Regional metastases can be explained by anatomic or mechanical spread of tumor emboli through efferent veins or lymphatics; however, distant organ metastases frequently establish unique patterns of colonization, indicating that unique tumor-host interactions play a role.

In reviewing the patterns of metastases in human solid tumors, numerous examples can be found of malignant tumors that tend to metastasize to particular secondary locations (Nicolson, 1982). The Krukenberg adenocarcinoma is one example in which metastatic spread from the primary site (gastrointestinal tract) to the secondary site (ovary) cannot be fully explained by passive mechanical processes. Another example is clear cell carcinoma of the kidney, one of the most frequent types of metastases found in the thyroid gland. Specific patterns of metastatic colonization have also been discovered in several transplantable animal tumors, and these models have been used extensively to analyze the biologic properties involved in the metastatic process. One of the most widely used tumor models for these studies is the murine B16 melanoma, in which subclones have been selected that preferentially metastasize to ovary, brain, or lung (Nicolson, 1982).

*Cell-surface properties* of metastatic tumors in animals have been the subject of numerous investigations related to the pathophysiology of metastatic and invasive properties. Specific alterations in cell-surface properties have also been described as an early event in the malignant transformation of animal cells in vitro, a topic that will be reviewed later. Treating the surface of some animal tumor cells with enzymes such as trypsin or neuraminidase significantly lowers their metastatic potential without affecting total viability. Similarly, nontoxic doses of tunicamycin, which inhibits the glycosylation of proteins, can prevent metastasis of B16 melanoma in mice. These experiments suggest that sialogalactoproteins on cell surfaces are necessary for the metastatic process. However, other studies with human tumor cells and different animal tumors do not support these observations.

*Enzymatic properties* of neoplasms are presumed to be one of the most important features of cancer cells that lead to metastases or invasion. Models of neoplastic transformation in animal cells also demonstrate a dramatic increase in cell-released or cell surface-bound degradative enzymes. In terms of the pathogenesis of metastases and invasion, such enzymes may be essential for degrading the extracellular matrix of normal tissue, promoting infiltration by malignant cells, preventing cell-cell contacts that inhibit cell division, or activating host products that could aid in the metastatic process.

Several types of degradative enzymes have been identified as surface-associated or secreted products of animal tumors or human biopsy specimens, and their possible functions have been reviewed (Nicolson, 1982). Some of the most commonly detected enzymes include collagenases, glycosidases, and proteases, particularly cathepsins. Cathepsins are thiol proteases that are increased and exhibit abnormal intracellular distribution in clinical biopsy specimens of cervical, gastric, colon, and breast cancers (Pietras and Roberts, 1981). In patients with breast cancer, cathepsin D content of tumor tissues may be an independent predictor of relapse and survival (Tandon et al, 1990; Thorpe et al, 1989). Results were somewhat different in biopsy samples of colon cancers, in that the level of cathepsin B activity was higher in limited cancers (Dukes' A) than in more advanced cancers (Dukes' B, C, and D), suggesting an important role for these proteases in the early progression of colorectal cancers (Murnane et al, 1991). Experiments in animal models indicate that metastases can be prevented by inhibitors of these or related enzymes, and the observation that hyaline cartilage is almost never affected by metastases has been related to the inhibitory effects of this type of tissue on degradative enzymes.

*Fibrin deposition* has been detected in the early stages of tumor spread in animal systems, suggesting that fibrin deposition around tumor cells in the microcirculation aids in the metastatic process. Plasminogen activator, a serine protease that rapidly converts plasminogen to plasmin, has been found in many animal tumors and biopsy specimens of human cancers. Plasmin has numerous actions, including feedback stimulation of plasminogen activator, degradation of some basement membrane components, activation of tissue collagenases, and enzymatic cleavage of fibrin clots. A functional role proposed for tumor-derived plasminogen activator is to allow tumor emboli to escape this fibrin meshwork, leading to tissue invasion. Some subclones of metastatic animal tumors produce plasminogen activator at levels that correlate with their relative metastatic potential. In some experiments, blocking plasminogen activator pathways reduces metastatic potential of human tumor cell lines (Need and Messmore, 1990). Clinical studies have suggested that levels of fibrinolytic activity in biopsy samples correspond to the degree of invasion and metastasis (Spremulli and Dexter, 1983). However, the role of plasminogen activator in the metastatic process is not universal, since many experiments conducted on animal tumors show no difference in the production of this enzyme between high and low metastatic subclones. Furthermore, large amounts of plasminogen activator are released in nonmalignant conditions.

In contrast to these studies relating metastases to fibrinolysis, several tumors release *procoagulant substances*, which promote the formation of fibrin and other clotting factors. While fibrinolytic activity may play a role in tissue infiltration, activation of clotting factors may be important in the initial steps of vascular implantation by tumor cells. In many experimental systems, dramatic reduction in metastatic spread can be seen after treatment with anticoagulants such as coumarin. However, altered clotting is not a consistent finding, and several studies have shown no change in clotting factors during metastatic spread or even negative correlations between metastatic potential and the release of procoagulants (Nand and Messmore, 1990).

Clinical studies of anticoagulants in human cancer also suggest that the clotting system plays a major role in some human malignancies. One study of patients with carcinoma of the uterine cervix reported increased survival and an almost 50% reduction in the recurrence rate among women who received anticoagulants to prevent thromboembolic complications (Nicolson, 1982). Similarly, clinical outcome was improved by the addition of warfarin to a chemotherapy program for patients with small cell lung cancer, but no major benefit was observed in patients with non–small cell lung cancer or with colorectal, head and neck, or prostate cancer (Zacharski et al, 1984). However, it is difficult to reach definitive conclusions about the role of clotting or procoagulants in human cancer, since most clinical studies are small, retrospective, or poorly controlled (Zacharski et al, 1979).

In addition to the possible role of plasma clotting or fibrinolysis in metastasis, *platelet-tumor interactions* have been linked to this process. The metabolism of arachidonic acid in tumor cells, platelets, and the vessel wall is one biochemical pathway that has been proposed to promote attachment to and penetration of vessel walls by tumor cells (Nicolson, 1982). Drug manipulations of arachidonic acid, or other steps of platelet activation are currently under investigation as possible strategies for preventing metastases. In retrospective studies, aspirin ingestion correlated with a reduced risk of death from colon cancer (Thun et al, 1991), but it is not clear if this was due to reduced invasion potential, change in detection rates for early lesions, or other mechanisms. Clinical trials are in progress to evaluate aspirin ingestion for preventing cancer.

Normal tissues as well can produce factors that promote the growth of neoplasms. Several investigators have reported that human *macrophages* or macrophage subpopulations promote the growth of human tumor cells in culture. Many of these studies have utilized a bilayer agar system developed by Hamburger, Salmon, and others (Hamburger and Salmon, 1977; Salmon et al, 1978) in which the in vitro growth of clonogenic cells obtained from clinical tumor samples is measured (see next paragraph). Studies with human ovarian tumor cells show that selective depletion of macrophages from the tumor samples can decrease tumor cell growth by more than 90%, while the readdition of macrophages can restore tumor cell growth in a dose-dependent manner (Hamburger and White, 1981). In addition, some animal tumor models suggest that macrophages exhibit growth-promoting activity in vivo (Hewlett et al, 1977), although other models suggest that macrophages can inhibit tumor cell growth.

Several laboratories are attempting to define the biologic properties of human cancer and to assess new forms of treatment using the *bilayer agar system* (Pratt and Ruddon, 1979). This technique has been termed the "human tumor stem cell assay" by Salmon and coworkers, who presume that the system selects for the most important stem cells of human cancers by detecting cells that form anchorage-independent colonies in soft agar (Salmon et al, 1978). Although correlations between clinical response to chemotherapy and drug sensitivity or resistance in vitro appear promising in early studies of ovarian cancer, improvements in methodology will be needed for studies of other types of human cancers (Selby et al, 1983). A major drawback of this method is the low plating efficiency, which is well under 1% for most human tumor samples. Other methods for growing human tumor cells in vitro report plating efficiencies greater than 10%, suggesting that the bilayer agar system selects for small subpopulations of neoplastic cells that grow well in the agar substrate. This system also uses anchorage independence—i.e., the ability of cells to grow without attachment to the culture plate—as a means of selecting neoplastic cells. Although anchorage independence is a feature of many neoplastic cells in culture, other studies indicate that this property correlates poorly with tumorigenicity (Stiles et al, 1976).

New methodologies have been developed to test the response of clinical tumor samples in vitro to various drugs or biologic therapies (Rotman et al, 1988; Weisenthal et al, 1988). Such methods do not require growth of tumor cell colonies, and they do not select for cells that survive in the agar media. Because these features permit a higher frequency of testing with clinical tumor samples, they may provide a more reliable tool for use in clinical practice. Early studies have demonstrated correlations between assay results and clinical responses in ovarian cancer, small cell lung cancer, and other tumors (Leone et al, 1991; Gazdar et al, 1990).

Human tumors that grow in culture systems demonstrate that most growth factors are not species-specific. Successful growth of human cancer cells generally depends on careful selection and screening of the bovine and/or horse serum used in the culture medium. Many human tumors also grow in athymic nude mice, which are immunologically deficient in their ability to reject foreign tissue grafts (Stiles et al, 1976). Short-term growth of clinical biopsy specimens and passaged human tumor cells has also been demonstrated in the subrenal capsule of mice, especially after immunosuppression with irradiation, cyclosporine, or cyclophosphamide (Fingert et al, 1987). These models also demonstrate that external factors which promote the growth of human cancer are not specific to humans. In addition, they provide experimental systems for investigating those biologic mechanisms which determine the abnormal growth of human cancer, both in culture and in the living host.

## Normal and Transformed Cells in Culture

***Properties of Cells in Culture*** Mammalian cells, both normal and tumor derived, can be grown and compared in culture (Baserga, 1985; Pardee, 1989). Neoplastic properties reside within single cells, and these properties—important in vivo—can be more readily investigated using cell culture techniques. Cultured cells are generally maintained in a medium containing salts, amino acids, glucose, vitamins, and serum. In recent years, it has been possible to substitute purified hormones and growth factors for serum (Bettger et al, 1981).

Most normal and tumor cells introduced into culture

directly from tissues do not grow, possibly because culture techniques have been designed and optimized for fibroblasts. Therefore, much of our knowledge about the properties of normal versus transformed cells derives from studies using cultured fibroblasts. Since this cell type is easily cultured, it is the most apt to grow out of a tissue explant. Fibroblastic cells were among the first to be developed into established cell lines. In addition, much has been learned from hematopoietic cells (Crabtree, 1989).

After 30 to 50 population doublings, the proliferative activity of human fibroblasts gradually slows down and eventually ceases (Hayflick and Moorhead, 1961). Such cells are said to senesce, and they are referred to as a "cell strain." Cells of very young or embryonic rodents behave quite differently as the population ages. Proliferation declines, and a small subpopulation begins to overgrow the culture. These predominant cells are immortal, i.e., they can be propagated indefinitely in culture (Rafferty, 1975; Todaro and Green, 1963). Such populations are called "cell lines." Human and chick cells generally cannot be established into cell lines; rodent cells, on the other hand, can be rather easily established (Ponten, 1976).

Cell lines can be cloned, and the clones can be expanded to produce a large population of genetically uniform cells, the properties of which change only gradually with age. However, cell lines often undergo chromosomal changes in the course of their establishment and hence are not normal (see "Genetic Information" later in this chapter). Nonetheless, cell lines that are nontumorigenic in animals have been established, so that one can still inquire into the mechanism by which such cells become tumorigenic.

Among the most commonly used cell lines for studying transformation are embryonic mouse (3T3) fibroblasts. These cells flatten out on a solid plastic substratum and grow until they have formed a monolayer (Todaro and Green, 1963). Growth (proliferation) ceases when they begin to come into close contact with one another (a feedback mechanism called density dependence or contact inhibition). Proliferation also ceases when they are forced to assume a rounded form in a semisolid substratum such as agar or methycellulose (anchorage dependence), or when serum factors or nutrients are removed from the medium. Thus, their growth state can be manipulated in culture. Despite their chromosomal abnormalities, 3T3 cells usually will not form tumors in animals. However, they can readily be transformed to exhibit tumorigenicity after treatment with carcinogens, oncogenes, or tumor viruses (Ponten, 1976).

Although many principles regarding the control of proliferation by normal (nontumorigenic) cells have been discovered using fibroblasts, most naturally occurring cancers are epithelial in origin. Some culture systems have been developed for the study of epithelial, hematopoietic (Crabtree, 1989), or very early embryonic cells (Sager and Kovac, 1978). In general, the broad aspects of growth control that characterize fibroblasts apply to these other cell types as well. For example, nutrient or hormonal insufficiency will generally arrest

the growth of these other cell types, as will a semisolid substratum if they are anchorage-dependent (as are epithelial cells); these cells will generally arrest growth in the same part of the cell cycle ($G_1$) as do fibroblasts.

***Assay Systems for Normal versus Transformed Cells in Culture*** Tumorigenic cells in culture are less sensitive to the presence of other cells in their immediate vicinity than are normal cells. One common characteristic of tumorigenic cells in culture is their ability to reach cell densities that are severalfold higher than those of nontumorigenic cells. This property of transformed cells is the basis for the "focus formation assay," discussed later.

Another feature of cancer cells' interactions in culture is that their growth tends to be physically disorganized. Nontumorigenic cultured cells often cease growth as a well-ordered monolayer. In contrast, transformed cells often randomly crisscross each other, forming local piles of viable and necrotic cells. This behavior of tumor cells in culture reflects their behavior in vivo.

Anchorage-dependent cells in vivo usually lie on an extracellular matrix (ECM), composed largely of glycoprotein, that stimulates growth (Hay, 1985). In culture, the cells require specially treated plastic for attachment and on which they can secrete ECM material. Secreted molecules include collagen, fibronectin, laminin, and proteoglycan, and they vary with the cell type. In general, the ECM promotes the growth of cells in culture. Transformed cells are often partially or completely independent of the ECM for optimal growth, and they may secrete much less matrix material (Hawkes and Wang, 1982; Liotta, 1986). Moreover, they often secrete substances that destroy the organizing structures of the basement membrane (e.g., plasminogen activator).

Various changes are seen on or near the cell membrane (Alitalo and Vaheri, 1982). Intracellular proteases are activated (Reich et al, 1975; Murnane et al, 1991). Specialized proteins (e.g., vinculin) connect the intracellular cytoskeleton to the ECM through the plasma membrane (Geiger, 1983; Hynes, 1987). Cytoskeletal filaments are responsible for maintaining cell shape, and it has been proposed that the ECM participates in this shape control by means of these adhesion proteins (Gospodarowicz et al, 1979; Liotta, 1986). The cytoskeleton of tumor cells tends to be less well organized, and the actin filaments are less highly polymerized (Pollack et al, 1975). Agents that disrupt microtubules affect density-dependent growth. Because protein synthesis can be sensitive to the organization of the cytoskeleton filaments (Wittelsberger et al, 1981), any disruption in this structure might lead to altered regulation of the cell cycle. Cytoskeletal abnormalities would not inhibit the growth of tumor cells, since these cells have less stringent protein and RNA synthesis requirements for passage through the $G_1$ phase.

To grow in culture, nontumorigenic cells generally require high serum (10%) and nutrient concentrations, a solid substratum (for anchorage-dependent cells), and a relatively uncrowded environment. Cells that have been transformed to become tumorigenic (e.g., by carcinogens or viruses) or cells derived from a tumor often have lower serum and nutrient requirements for growth. Moreover, they continue to proliferate on a semisolid substratum or when the culture dish becomes crowded (Macpherson and Montagnier, 1964; Dulbecco, 1970). These differences in the behavior of transformed cells in culture are not strict correlates of tumorigenicity but are nonetheless indicators of faulty growth control. Consequently, these differences have been exploited in order to develop an assay to detect the transformed phenotype in culture.

Two types of assays are most commonly used to identify transformed cells. In the first, the cells to be tested are suspended at low density within a semisolid medium. For a population of mostly anchorage-dependent cells, only a transformed or tumorigenic cell will grow into a macroscopic colony suspended in the medium. In the second assay, the focus formation assay, a subconfluent monolayer of normal cells (generally 3T3 fibroblasts) is mixed with putative transformed cells. The cells are then allowed to grow to confluence. At this point, the normal cells will cease proliferating, whereas the transformed cells will continue to grow, forming a local pile or focus of dense cells (Fig. 1-2). This method has been used extensively to discover and characterize carcinogens and oncogenes (see "Genetic Information" later in this chapter).

Other differences between normal and transformed cells (e.g., their dissimilar serum and nutrient requirements), as well as variations in the assay systems described above, have been used to distinguish these cells from each other in culture. Each assay allows the observation of one end point in the transformation process (i.e., release from anchorage dependence or contact inhibition). However, in order to understand transfor-mation, we must first examine in finer detail the mechanisms by which normal cells control their growth.

### Growth Regulation by Normal and Transformed Cells in Culture

Cells in culture provide a simple, controllable system for studying growth regulation by extracellular conditions. With a single cell type in culture, one can ask, what regulates proliferation and how? For most normal fetal and adult cells, the decision of whether to proliferate or arrest growth is governed by conditions outside the cell. Certain factors can induce proliferation or differentiation in the appropriate cell type. Similarly, a particular ECM or another cell type may stimulate or inhibit proliferation or differentiation depending upon the target cell.

The growth cycle of higher eukaryotes can be divided into four discrete periods: mitosis (M), when the nuclear and cytoplasmic contents are actually divided into two daughter cells; $G_1$, the period following M and preceding the start of DNA synthesis; S, the DNA synthetic phase; and $G_2$, which follows S and precedes M (Fig. 1-1). The distribution of cells among the four phases of the cell cycle varies enormously, depending upon the cell type and the culture conditions. For the commonly used 3T3 cells, the durations of M, $G_1$, S, and $G_2$ are approximately 30 minutes, 6 hours, 8 hours, and 2 hours, respectively.

For untransformed cells, the cycle is not free-running; rather, it is highly regulated (Pardee, 1989). The $G_1$ period appears to be very important in this regard. The major growth controls are in effect during this phase, prior to the initiation of DNA synthesis (Fig. 1-1). Thus, during $G_1$, the cell must assess whether conditions are permissive and sufficient for replicating its genome and partitioning into daughter cells. If conditions are not

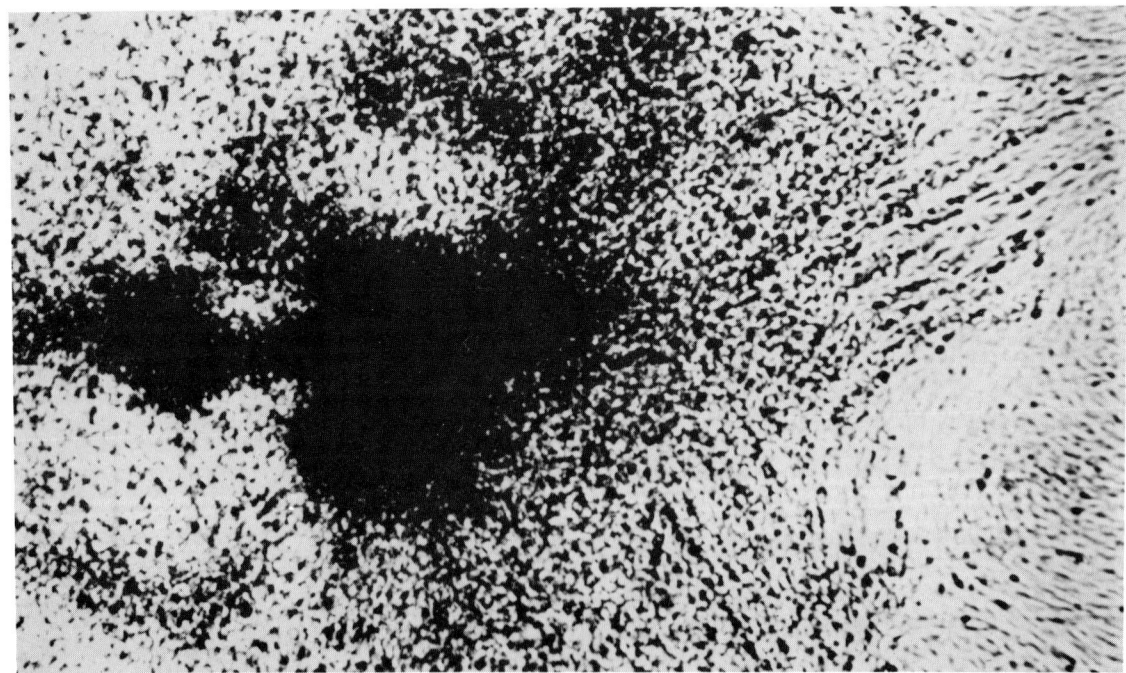

FIGURE 1-2 A focus of hamster fibroblasts transfected with an activated *ras* oncogene (pEJ).

favorable, the $G_1$ period may lengthen considerably or the cells may enter a viable, nonproliferating state ($G_0$) with an unduplicated DNA content. Both in vivo and in culture, cells may spend relatively long periods of time—even their entire lifetime—in this state, depending on the cell type.

Most adult cells in vivo are in a nonproliferating, quiescent state, termed $G_0$. Such cells have an unduplicated DNA content, as do cells in $G_1$. $G_0$ cells can be very active functionally and metabolically; they may produce enzymes, structural proteins, hormones, and other substances characteristic of the particular cell type. However, they do not proliferate unless stimulated to do so. These stimuli may be specific growth factors or loss of other cells in the population through death or differentiation (Baserga, 1985).

Once a cell has entered the S phase, it is generally committed to complete the cycle through the M phase and to divide, although control points may possibly exist in the $G_2$ period as well. Integrity of the newly replicated DNA seems to be an important control factor in the initiation of M. Cells that have incurred damage to their DNA can spend abnormally long periods of time in $G_2$, and so delay M (Lau and Pardee, 1982). Thus, during $G_2$, the cells appear to assess whether the DNA is sufficiently intact to be passed on to daughter cells.

3T3 cells rapidly cease to proliferate when they have grown to a confluent monolayer or when they are placed into a medium containing a suboptimal serum concentration (0.5%). They will remain with an unduplicated DNA content in a viable state ($G_0$) for many weeks, provided that essential nutrients are continually supplied. There is some disagreement as to whether $G_0$ (in culture) is a distinct metabolic state or simply a protracted $G_1$. However, many biochemical differences exist between quiescent cells in $G_0$ and cycling cells in $G_1$ (Baserga, 1985).

Some tumor-forming cells, such as 3T3 cells transformed by a DNA virus, may be incapable of entering a quiescent state. Such cells continue to proliferate very slowly under conditions that would cause normal cells to become quiescent. Eventually they die, ending with a random cell-cycle distribution. Despite high culture densities or inadequate serum, some fraction of cells transformed by chemicals or RNA viruses continues to proliferate—behavior attributable to escape of the tumor cells from the requirement for specific growth factors.

Cultured normal fibroblasts in a quiescent state can be stimulated to resume proliferation. Therefore, these cells have provided a valuable experimental system for studying control of the initiation of growth, DNA synthesis, and subsequent completion of the cell cycle. The steps involved in the switch from quiescence to proliferation and vice versa appear to be central for neoplasia and have been investigated to the greatest extent in 3T3 cells. Although the details may vary, growth control in other cell types will probably be similar in broad outline. Fresh 10% serum added to a quiescent 3T3 culture, produced by confluence or serum insufficiency,

will stimulate DNA synthesis to start after about 12 hours.

At least three *growth factors* present in serum have been found to be necessary for this resumption of proliferation: platelet- or fibroblast-derived growth factor (PDGF or FGF), epidermal growth factor (EGF), and insulin-like growth factor (IGF-1 or somatomedin C). These are small polypeptides that act by binding to specific receptors on the cell surface (Goustin et al, 1986). PDGF is a protein contained within alpha granules of circulating platelets, and it appears to have important physiologic functions for the maintenance of vascular endothelium and wound healing by inducing the growth of fibroblasts and other connective tissue cells at the site of trauma (Scher et al, 1979). EGF is a small protein that stimulates growth of many epithelial cells (Carpenter and Cohen, 1979). These two factors, together with IGF-1 (or insulin at a very high concentration), can induce DNA synthesis in 3T3 and other untransformed cells (Rothstein, 1982).

While these polypeptide growth factors are clearly necessary for growth of certain normal cells, most animal and human cancer cells do not require all of them. Two main mechanisms have been proposed to explain the loss of this growth-factor requirement in cancer cells. First, alterations in growth-related biochemical pathways could arise within cancer cells so as to allow continued growth in the absence of these external signals. Second, tumor cells can produce abnormal growth factors, such as TGF-alpha, that activate their own receptors, leading to continuous autostimulation. Several animal and human tumors have been shown to produce potent autostimulatory or *autocrine* growth factors, some of which can induce normal cells to behave like malignant cells in terms of their growth properties in culture. Abnormal production of these autocrine growth factors may be an early step in the pathophysiology of cancer. Some secreted factors negatively influence cell proliferation; of these, TGF-beta has been most extensively studied (Sporn and Roberts, 1989).

Specific genes, called *proto-oncogenes*, are abnormally expressed, overproduced, or mutated in several human neoplasms (see "Genetic Information" later in this chapter). Proto-oncogenes are the normal cellular forms of certain genes, the *oncogenes*, that are found in mutant form in some human tumor cells and in animal retroviruses that induce neoplastic transformation. Different oncogenes probably intervene in different ways. They may directly cause a cell to produce its own growth factor, as in the case of the sis oncogene, which codes for a PDGF-like molecule. This discovery provides a direct link between a genetic event in neoplasia and the abnormal growth properties of cancer due to production of an autocrine (autostimulatory) growth factor (Deuel et al, 1983).

Oncogenes also intervene at other points in the chain between the growth factor and its ultimate function, e.g., by producing aberrant growth-factor receptors or altering the cell's internal metabolism. For example, oncogenes could cause the continuous production of some second messenger protein, inducing cell division that is otherwise triggered in nonmalignant cells by growth factor-receptor interactions.

The fms gene, which is found in some leukemias and produces a protein similar to the colony-stimulating factor (CSF) receptor, has been implicated in the growth of leukemia cells (Ashmun et al, 1989). Another example is the erbB-2 gene, also called HER-2/neu, which is similar to the gene for the epidermal growth factor receptor (EGFR). Expression of HER-2/neu has been found to be increased in breast, ovarian, gastric, and other neoplasms; in some patients with breast and ovarian cancer, this increased expression may be linked to prognosis (Tandon et al, 1989a; Thor et al, 1989; Slamon et al, 1989).

The proteins encoded by oncogenes display diverse characteristics. Some are located on the plasma membrane, others in the nucleus, and still others on intramembranous or cytoskeletal structures. Some are protein kinases, others glycoproteins, and some bind to chromatin. This subject has previously been reviewed (Bishop, 1987), and more information should be forthcoming from ongoing intensive investigations. Results of these studies are already providing a much clearer picture not only of the genetics but also of the controlling events that are altered in cancer cells. Here, we will discuss a few examples of aberrant regulation by some oncogenes.

The emergence of 3T3 cells from confluent quiescence ($G_0$) into the cell cycle requires the sequential action of growth factors. First, the cells enter a state of competence, after which they actually progress in time through $G_1$ toward S. PDGF (or FGF) will render a quiescent cell competent to respond to the progression factors in plasma (i.e., plasma that is free of platelets and thus designated platelet-poor plasma [PPP]). During exponential growth, competence to initiate another round of replication is acquired prior to M in the previous cycle (Scher et al, 1979). The ability to enter a quiescent state is an important aspect of normal growth control.

Competent 3T3 cells require at least EGF and IGF-1 in order to initiate DNA synthesis. Cells must also be able to synthesize protein at a rapid rate in order to reach a control point, called the *restriction (or R) point* (Pardee, 1989), located about 2 hours prior to the start of S. Even modest inhibition of protein synthesis by drugs like cycloheximide or by amino acid insufficiency will greatly increase the interval from M to R without significantly affecting the durations of the other phases of the cell cycle. This $G_1$-specific need for rapid protein synthesis suggests that an unstable R protein must be synthesized up to a critical amount before cells can pass the R point (Rossow et al, 1979; Croy and Pardee, 1983). Many tumor cells do not require this rapid protein synthesis. In some tumorigenic cells, R-protein function, synthesis, or degradation may be specifically altered.

Results of recent studies suggest that at least three control points exist in the emergence from quiescence of 3T3 cells: competence, V, and R, located approximately 12, 6, and 2 hours, respectively, prior to the start of S. Successful passage through these points requires a

linked sequence: in turn, PDGF (competence), some protein synthesis and EGF (V), and rapid protein synthesis and IGF-1 (R). Once the cells enter the S phase, they are committed to complete the cycle through M. Tumor cells may be abnormally regulated at several of these control points.

A relaxation at one or more of these control points could give a growth advantage in such a way that a cell's chance of undergoing the additional changes seen in mature tumors is increased (Baserga, 1985; Denhardt, 1986). A class of compounds known as *tumor promoters*, commonly phorbol esters, enhance tumorigenesis in vivo after treatment with an *initiator compound*, usually a mutagen (Weinstein, 1988). According to a two-step model of carcinogenesis, the initiator may be responsible for the primary insult or mutation, and the promoter may allow its expression by stimulating cell growth. Phorbol esters activate a membrane-bound protein kinase (Housey et al, 1988). Tumor promoters may cooperate synergistically with growth factors like EGF in stimulating the proliferation of cultured cells. The fact that tumor promoters are growth-stimulatory (but are not themselves carcinogenic) emphasizes the importance of cell proliferation as a primary requisite for establishing cancer.

## Neoplasia at the Subcellular Level: Signal Transmission from Membrane to Nucleus

At the molecular level, cell proliferation requires that all cellular components be duplicated so that a new cell can be produced (Baserga, 1985). In contrast, quiescent cells approximately maintain their molecular composition and change only gradually with time. Some molecules, such as DNA, are simply not made in these cells. Other molecules, of which proteins are a major example, are constantly being synthesized and degraded, being maintained at a steady-state level. The average half-life of a protein in quiescent cells is on the order of a few days. Protein synthesis goes on in quiescent cells at about one-third the rate of that in rapidly growing cells. Turnover of many cell components takes place, and a quiescent cell is still metabolically very active.

When quiescent cells in culture are stimulated by the addition of serum, they activate a chain of events (Rozengurt, 1986; Bourne, 1988). These changes occur during various time periods. Within a few minutes, the transport of nutrients into the cell is increased, a process that does not require new protein synthesis. Within one hour, a set of "immediate early" messenger RNAs is produced, including those encoding the fos and myc proto-oncogenes. Then, over a few hours, the rates of RNA and protein synthesis increase severalfold. The protein-synthesizing machinery is activated; ribosomes are assembled into polysomes; and ribosomal and other proteins are phosphorylated, thus presumably becoming activated (Chambard et al, 1983; Rubin et al, 1983). Much later (after about 12 hours in 3T3 cells), DNA synthesis starts. The cells then pass through the S, $G_2$, and M phases in sequence and finally divide and commence the next cycle.

Cell fusion studies show that cell proliferation—particularly progress through $G_1$—depends on positive intracellular inducers (Yanishevsky and Stein, 1981). Cultured cells at different stages in the cell cycle can be fused in order to determine whether positive inducers of DNA synthesis accumulate during $G_1$. The cellular cytoplasm contains a substance capable of inducing DNA synthesis in early $G_1$ nuclei, and this inducer seems to be present in higher quantities toward the end of $G_1$ and in early S (Rao and Sunkara, 1978). It could possibly be the labile R protein, the accumulation of which is required for passage through the R point (Pardee, 1989).

In asking questions about important events of growth control inside the cell, it is important to separate regulatory events from processes necessary for survival—the so-called housekeeping functions. Normal and transformed cells have in common many requirements for survival; the difference between the two types of cells tends to be in their regulatory functions. Nevertheless, a derangement in regulatory function can result in an altered set of housekeeping functions. For example, some normal fibroblasts terminally differentiate into adipocytes, which have lost their capacity for proliferation and have a unique set of enzymes directed toward fat storage and mobilization (see the next section of this chapter, "Differentiation and Cancer"). When these fibroblasts are transformed to exhibit tumorigenicity, they lose their ability to differentiate terminally. The seminal change in this transformation is not the inability to express fat-metabolizing enzymes but rather the inability to cease proliferating.

Qualitatively, the biochemistry of growth appears to be very similar in tumor and normal cells (Weber, 1983). During the past several decades, enormous efforts have been directed toward detecting differences in metabolism between these types of cells; however, universal,

fundamental differences have not yet been discovered. There is no obvious biochemical marker that distinguishes tumor cells in general from nontumor cells. The classic example of this approach to understanding cancer was the hypothesis proposed by Otto Warburg in the 1920s that tumor cells are better able to use carbohydrates (for energy) under anaerobic conditions than are normal cells. This observation is true of a number of tumors but was shown not to be a general characteristic. Nonetheless, it is still an interesting aspect of cancer cell biology. More likely, it is a property gained later, one that permits tumor cells to utilize energy supplies for rapid growth more effectively than can normal cells.

The fundamental difference probably lies in a relaxation of the regulatory requirements for cell growth (Pardee, 1987). Whereas normal cells require physiologic levels of growth factors, a related tumor cell must be able to proliferate at hypophysiologic levels. The question then becomes, how does transformation at the biochemical level make the supply of growth factors from outside the cells less important? And what metabolic reactions are turned on by these growth factors?

The first event in cell activation is the binding of growth factors to specific receptors on the cell membrane (Fig. 1-3). There may be 100,000 or so specific receptors per cell with which growth factors combine tightly and specifically (Goustin et al, 1986; Sporn and Roberts, 1989). In several cases, the first change observed after binding is activation of protein kinases. They phosphorylate proteins, sometimes at tyrosine residues, which are unusual sites for this reaction. Phosphorylation is known to change the functions of proteins, such as the catalytic activities of enzymes and the binding of proteins to DNA. In fact, many growth-factor receptors are themselves protein kinases; when

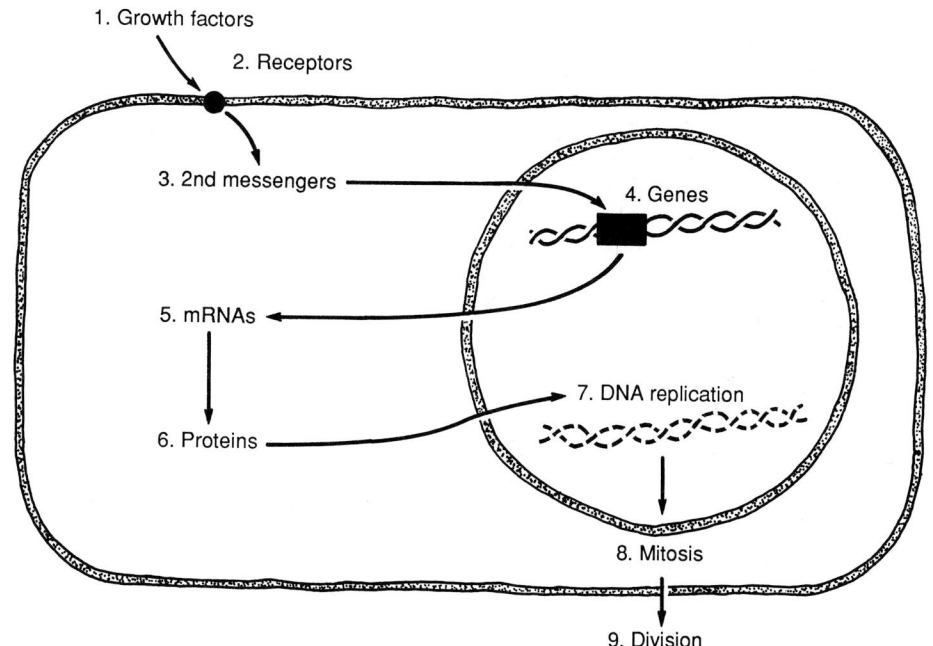

FIGURE 1-3 Steps in the process of cell activation. (See text for detailed description of events.)

the factor binds to a receptor's extracellular site, it activates the intracellular kinase of the same transmembrane molecule (Riedel et al, 1989).

Shortly thereafter, a variety of molecules change concentrations. These are collectively called "second messengers" and include calcium and hydrogen ions (Perona and Serrano, 1988) and organic compounds, of which phosphatidylinositol and diacylglycerol are important in activating intracellular kinases (Berridge, 1987). One set of proto-oncogene proteins named *ras* is involved in signal transduction during mid-$G_1$, although their exact actions are not yet clear (McCormick, 1989). In essence, the cells are switched on to synthesize major macromolecules and other cell components and can be conceived of as reassembling their machinery for active metabolism.

PDGF activates some of the initial events brought about by serum. During the first few hours, it causes novel mRNAs to appear in small numbers, and specific new proteins are produced. Thus, PDGF appears to be a key factor in turning on the growth of quiescent cells (Denhardt et al, 1986).

Along with this general increase in metabolic activity are changes in cell morphology. The structure of the cytoskeleton, composed of various filaments and microtubules, is modified, as seen on microscopy (Cold Spring Harbor Symposium, 1982). Actin, the major structural component of microfilaments, is produced more rapidly. Some enzyme activities also change dramatically; ornithine decarboxylase, a catalyst for polyamine production, is a striking example (Scalabrino and Feriola, 1981). Other changes include increased transmembrane ion fluxes, alterations in the concentration of cyclic AMP (cAMP), and increased accumulation of cyclin proteins. Within a few hours after the addition of serum or a mixture of selected growth factors, cells rapidly increase their rates of mRNA and protein synthesis. During this time, more than a dozen novel proteins appear (Croy and Pardee, 1983).

A gene is activated to produce RNAs by the binding of proteins to specific DNA sequences that lie upstream of the coding sequences (Mitchell and Tjian, 1989; Johnson and McKnight, 1989). Some of these binding proteins have been identified as products of proto-oncogenes such as fos and jun (Distel and Spiegelman, 1988), which combine to form a tightly bound complex. How stimuli generated by growth factors alter the binding of these transcriptional regulators to DNA is not yet clear, although protein phosphorylations, catalyzed by kinases, have been implicated.

The growth factor IGF-1 appears to be necessary toward the end of the $G_1$ period (Leof et al, 1982). In order to proceed to DNA synthesis, these cells require rapid protein synthesis until about 2 hours before the S phase. A variety of experiments has led to the idea that the cell must make a sufficient amount of a special protein in order to begin DNA synthesis and that this protein is unstable, having a half-life of only about 2.5 hours in 3T3 cells. Therefore, unless the general synthesis of proteins is rapid, degradation of this special protein will prevent its accumulation (Croy and Pardee, 1983). It is of great interest that in a variety of tumor-

forming cells, this protein is not rapidly degraded and therefore is much more easily accumulated than in their normal counterparts. This difference seems to be one of the few distinctive molecular changes in tumor versus normal cells (Pardee, 1989).

Just prior to the onset of DNA synthesis (S phase), a variety of other events occur. During the 2-hour period immediately preceding the S phase, biochemical changes associated with DNA synthesis occur. A number of mRNAs and enzymes required for the production of DNA building blocks and for the synthesis of DNA itself increase dramatically. Furthermore, prior to the onset of DNA synthesis, these enzyme molecules are located outside the nucleus in the cytoplasm, where they are synthesized on ribosomes. By the time DNA synthesis starts, they have migrated to the nucleus. Furthermore, they cosediment upon centrifugation as a multienzyme complex of high molecular weight. This complex, termed *replitase*, appears to be the machinery underlying efficient DNA synthesis; it contains many enyzmes known to be involved in this process (Reddy and Pardee, 1980; Tubo and Berezney, 1987). Recently, the onset of DNA replication at the start of the S phase has been investigated with in vitro systems (Challberg and Kelly, 1989; Stillman, 1988). These experiments reveal that enzymes with DNA unwinding activity may constitute the final factor.

When DNA synthesis has commenced, a cell becomes relatively independent of external growth-controlling factors. Of course, it needs essential nutrients such as amino acids, required for making new proteins. However, such a cell is not subject to external growth control and will complete its synthesis of DNA unless it is poisoned by drugs or other toxins. It will go through the events of $G_2$ and mitosis and will finally divide to form two daughter cells. Whether or not it then passes through another cycle depends once more upon external conditions during $G_1$; if these are not appropriate, it will become arrested before it reinitiates DNA synthesis.

At present, only the general sequence of control events, passing from the medium to the nucleus, and extending in time from the activation of a $G_0$ cell to its division some 24 hours later, has been determined. A great deal needs to be fitted into this framework before we will have a clear understanding of cell growth and its control. Growth controls are relaxed at several points in tumor-forming cells. Important novel components are being discovered, such as the p53 protein (Finlay et al, 1989) and the product of the retinoblastoma gene (Ludlow et al, 1989).

## DIFFERENTIATION AND CANCER

### Anaplasia in Vivo

***Loss of Differentiation Markers*** A major morphologic criterion for the diagnosis of cancer is *anaplasia*, which can be defined as the reversion of cells to a more primitive or less differentiated state. While invasion, metastasis, and neoplasia are properties that help define malignancy at the level of gross pathology, anaplasia—the abnormal appearance of cells in terms of positional or cytologic differentiation—is characteristic of cancer at the level of microscopic histopathology. Experimental tumors demonstrate that defective differentiation (anaplasia) and abnormal growth (neoplasia) are not independent properties of cancer cells; rather, they appear to be clearly associated, both in the initial stages of malignant transformation and in the later stages of tumor progression (Yuspa and Morgan, 1981). Not only does the organization of the tissue generally appear disrupted, but histochemical staining often reveals unusual or inappropriate cell types. The abnormal cells frequently appear less well differentiated than in normal tissue and are reminiscent of more primitive or embryonic cells.

Since morphologic markers for differentiation have been relatively easy to quantify in human hematologic malignancies, these neoplasms have been most commonly used for experimental analysis of the properties of differentiation related to the malignant phenotype. HL60, a continuous cell line derived from a patient with promyelocytic leukemia, can be treated with several agents that induce differentiation to mature macrophages or granulocytes. This differentiation process corresponds directly to loss of growth and other neoplastic properties.

While these experimental systems suggest that numerous external factors may be important in the differentiation process of malignant or premalignant conditions, other studies point to host-derived factors as possible mediators of differentiation. Normal myeloblasts require protein(s) called *colony-stimulating factors* (CSF) or *macrophage and granulocyte inducer* (MGI), derived from various malignant or normal tissues (Sachs, 1980*a*), for viability, normal proliferation, and differentiation. In mice, some types of myeloid leukemia cells also differentiate in response to CSF or MGI. This differentiation also results in the loss of malignant properties. While viability, proliferation, and differentiation are tightly coupled in normal myeloid cells, these properties appear to be uncoupled in leukemia cells, leading to uncontrolled proliferation.

A few differentiation markers have been described in solid tumors derived from various histologic cell types. Histochemical analyses of mammalian ovaries reveal an increased accumulation of intracellular lipid bodies during normal development. Oil Red O, a fast-acting stain for lipid droplets in cells, has been utilized as a differentiation marker for ovarian serous cystadenocarcinomas. Using clinical samples of ovarian cancer, investigators compared the proliferative capacity (labeling index [LI] and clonogenicity in soft agar) of tumor cells with the presence of Oil Red O–positive cells and found a close association between increased proliferative capacity and loss of this differentiation marker (Mackillop and Buick, 1982).

A similar relationship between proliferative capacity and loss of differentiation was reported in a patient with malignant ascites from serous adenocarcinoma of the ovary (Mackillop et al, 1983). Seven consecutive ascites tumor samples were obtained from the same patient over a 9-month period, and the cancer cells were analyzed in vitro for LI, agar clonogenicity, and lipid staining. Cell-surface expression of *carcinoembryonic antigen* (CEA) was also analyzed as a potential marker for an undifferentiated or oncofetal phenotype. Table 1-4 presents some of the data from this clinical study, illustrating the general correlation between proliferative capacity and loss of differentiation.

***Expression of Oncofetal Markers in Cancer*** Many tumors abnormally express increased levels of cell surface–associated or secreted products that are usually produced only by fetal or trophoblastic cells. Fetal gut cells normally produce CEA; this oncofetal product in colon cancers was first attributed to abnormal expression of fetal antigens specific to the histologic origin of the neoplasm. Later studies showed this antigen to be produced by prostate, lung, breast, and other cancers not clearly related to fetal gut. Elevated CEA has also been reported in over 80% of recurrent cervical cancers and 35% of ovarian cancers. *Alpha-fetoprotein* (AFP) is elevated in 50 to 70% of patients with primary liver carcinoma, but this protein is also found in teratocarcinomas and in nearly 100% of endodermal sinus tumors. In a recent study of children with resected immature teratomas of the ovary and other sites, elevated serum AFP at initial diagnosis was found to be a significant predictor of later recurrence of malignancy (Malogolowkin et al, 1989). CEA and AFP levels are elevated in several nonmalignant conditions as well (Bast and Knapp, 1983).

*CA125* is a high molecular weight glycoprotein ex-

---

TABLE 1-4  Tumor Proliferation and Differentiation in Serial Samples from a Patient with Ovarian Cancer

| Sample | Labeling Index (Average % Tumor) | Clonogenicity in Agar (Average Colonies per $10^5$ Cells) | CEA-Positive Cells (%) | Oil Red O–Negative Cells (%) |
|---|---|---|---|---|
| 1 | 1.7 | 98 | N.D. | N.D. |
| 2 | 2.5 | N.D. | 0.9 | 52 |
| 3 | 1.6 | 68 | 1.7 | 60 |
| 5 | 3.5 | 554 | 3.6 | 90 |
| 7 | 6.8 | 650 | 5.7 | 95 |

CEA = Carcinoembryonic antigen; N.D. = not done.
*Source:* Mackillop WJ, et al: Tumor progression studied by analysis of cellular features of serial ascitic ovarian carcinoma tumors. *Cancer Res* 43:874-878, 1983.

pressed in coelomic epithelium during embryonic development as well as in most nonmucinous epithelial ovarian cancers. Using monoclonal antibodies, researchers have developed sensitive techniques to monitor levels of this antigen in patients with ovarian cancer. Several studies have shown that rising or falling levels of CA125 reflect clinical disease progression or regression, respectively (Schwartz et al, 1987). However, this assay is not always predictive of residual tumor, since one study showed that 6 of 14 patients with normal CA125 values after initial chemotherapy still had residual cancer as documented by surgical exploration (Atack et al, 1986). This antigen is found in over 50% of patients with endometrial cancer and is also elevated in patients with lung, pancreatic, hepatic, and other malignancies (Schwartz et al, 1987). Numerous other antigens, including LASA, NB70-K, TA-4, and SCC, have been detected in the serum of patients with gynecologic malignancies, and early studies suggest that serum analysis for one or more of these antigens can be useful in predicting the therapeutic response and/or tumor recurrence.

Sensitive immunoassays for subunits of human chorionic gonadotropin (hCG) demonstrate this glycoprotein in many nontrophoblastic gynecologic cancers. A urinary gonadotropin fragment (UGF) is cleared rapidly from the circulation, so detection is greatly increased in urine compared to serum. In recent clinical studies, elevated UGF levels have been found in about two-thirds of women with gynecologic cancers, and current trials are evaluating UGF levels to predict tumor response, recurrence, or as a screening tool for early diagnosis (Nam et al, 1990).

***Abnormal Differentiation in Cancer Pathogenesis*** There is a close association between malignant behavior and abnormal differentiation in both human cancers and experimental tumors. This observation suggests that for some cancers neoplastic properties are a direct result of the abnormal expression of normal, differentiation-related genes rather than the normal expression of abnormal genes (Pitot, 1981). If aberrant differentiation is a condition for the pathogenesis of cancer, it follows that some of the biologic properties of the differentiated state should confer an advantage for tumor cells. Differentiation involves many products, the one being used as a marker (e.g., CA125 or UGF) not necessarily being the product that leads to abnormal growth.

Although most studies of oncofetal products do not suggest a clear functional property for markers, these products do provide important diagnostic tools in the evaluation of treatment response, occult tumor masses, and so on. For example, *involucrin*, the cell envelope precursor protein, is greatly reduced in squamous carcinoma cells. This has been proposed as a potential aid in diagnosing cervical and vaginal disease (Warhol et al, 1982). However, some studies do support a functional role for aberrant differentiation in the origin or progression of malignancies. CEA can function as an adhesion protein and promotes cell-cell contact within a growing neoplasm, possibly leading to alterations in cell structure or in the microenvironment. Depressed

immune function in patients with elevated serum levels of human chorionic gonadotropin (hCG) may contribute to the progression of cancer by suppressing physiologic immune reactions to the growing tumor. AFP could have a similar effect on the immune system, since the growth of experimental tumors in mice can be accelerated by cotreatment with this antigen (Gershwin et al, 1980).

Another proposed relationship between oncofetal products and tumor progression is based on the observed similarity between maternal tolerance to the growing fetus and immunologic tolerance to a growing cancer (Salmon, 1980). Oncofetal products could act to increase tolerance directly (such as suppressive effects of hCG on lymphocyte function), or they could act indirectly by signaling macrophages or other host cells to produce inhibitors of the immune response and/or tumor-specific growth factors. Macrophages can also respond to the presence of fetal antigens (or hormones produced by the placenta or trophoblasts) by secreting prostaglandins and other growth-promoting factors that may assist normal fetal development.

As discussed earlier (under "Neoplasia"), the expression of genetic programs for fetal metabolism could provide selective growth advantages to cancer cells. Numerous *fetal or placental isoenzymes* have been reported in hepatomas, sarcomas, mammary cancers, and other experimental tumors, and related studies indicate increased activity of these enzymes under conditions that offer an obvious growth advantage to neoplastic cells (Weinhouse, 1982). One such protein is termed the *Regan isoenzyme of alkaline phosphatase*, an enzyme commonly found in ovarian, testicular, and pancreatic cancers and abundant in the normal-term placenta.

Cancer cells produce many secreted or cell surface–associated products that probably play a role in growth, invasion, or metastases (discussed earlier). Several of these products can also be identified in normal fetal, embryonic, or placental tissues. *Plasminogen activator* may promote metastases by leading to the degradation of fibrin clots. In addition to its presence at high levels in many human and experimental cancers, this enzyme is a constituent of normal early embryos. Angiogenesis factors appear to be important for the growth of solid tumors; they are also produced by developing embryos, which require an ingrowth of capillaries from nearby blood vessels (Nicolson, 1982).

Another property of cancer that may affect growth by abnormal differentiation is the production of *hormone receptors*. A general correlation between histologic differentiation and the presence of steroid hormone receptors has been recognized in breast cancer, and a similar correlation was observed in a study of endometrial cancer (Allegra et al, 1983). Improved survival has also been correlated with the presence of estrogen receptors in carcinoma of the cervix; further studies are needed to determine whether this is an independent prognostic factor, as reported for breast cancer (Martin et al, 1982). In some cancers, production of hormone receptors could be viewed as the expression of a normal, differentiated function that promotes tumor growth by permitting stimulation from physiologic hormones (seen in the rapid growth of some breast cancers during pregnancy). However, many cancers demonstrate stronger correlations between decreased histologic differentiation, receptor negativity, and poor prognosis. This suggests that loss of hormone receptors is a more important phenomenon correlated with tumor progression.

***Therapeutic Implications of Abnormal Differentiation in Cancer*** Close associations between abnormal differentiation and the malignant phenotype present a therapeutic challenge to manipulate the key differentiation properties that influence cancer growth. Alterations in the physiologic hormonal milieu have clear therapeutic benefits in prostate, breast, and uterine cancers, and new methods for detecting hormone receptors in subgroups of patients with ovarian and cervical cancer may lead to similar benefits for those patients with receptor-positive gynecologic neoplasms. *Müllerian inhibitory factor*, a hormone that evokes natural regression of müllerian ducts in the developing male embryo, could provide a treatment modality for those specific gynecologic cancers that retain the differentiated function to regress in the presence of this physiologic regulator (Donahoe et al, 1982).

The development of assays for *retinoid-binding proteins* (RBP) may lead to similar therapeutic strategies using retinoids to promote the differentiation of cancers (Chytil and Ong, 1982). Numerous experimental tumors can be induced to differentiate by retinoids, carotene, or other analogues of vitamin A. While this differentiation leads to cessation of growth and tumor regression in most experimental systems, some tumors become more aggressive with retinoid treatment, so that the ultimate action of these drugs may be related to tumor type, the host's environment, or other unknown factors. RBP have been detected in human cancers of the cervix, ovary, endometrium and other solid tumors; some studies suggest that the presence of RBP in cancer cell lines can predict a patient's responsiveness to retinoid treatment, similar to the case with estrogen or progesterone receptors and hormonal therapy.

Clinical trials are under way to test the effectiveness of retinoids in preventing breast cancer. Other trials are ongoing in patients with premalignant lesions of the cervix, lung, and oral cavity, and early results suggest a beneficial effect in producing regression of some high-risk lesions, especially oral leukoplakia (Cheson et al, 1986). Retinoids have also induced rapid differentiation of a human promyelocytic cell line (HL60) in culture, and retinoid therapy of clinical promyelocytic leukemia has produced objective remissions (Warrell et al, 1991).

Some current *cancer chemotherapeutic agents* may produce regression or cures by inducing a more differentiated phenotype. Dramatic differentiation of HL60 cells can be induced in culture by sublethal concentrations of cytosine arabinoside or thioguanine; both these drugs have been valuable in the clinical therapy of leukemia, although very few patients obtain long-term remissions with these treatments used as single agents. Similarly, azacytidine has produced some documented remissions in patients with preleukemic syndromes, and

hexamethyl-bisacetamide (HMBA) is being evaluated in clinical trials to study its potential as a differentiating agent for both hematologic and solid tumors (Cheson et al, 1986). Experiments with a choriocarcinoma cell line indicate that differentiation can be induced by methotrexate under proper conditions (Friedman and Skehan, 1979), suggesting that the dramatic responses produced in this disease may be due in part to drug-induced differentiation. Benign teratomas are frequently discovered during surgical resection of residual masses, found after aggressive chemotherapy of malignant embryonal carcinomas. Although some of these teratomas are likely to predate the malignancies, it is also possible that chemotherapy produces regression of some cancers by promoting differentiation.

*Mithramycin* has been used to treat hypercalcemia in patients with chronic myeloid leukemia (CML), and unexpected clinical responses have been observed in patients with blast-phase CML. Laboratory studies suggest that a differentiating effect of mithramycin is responsible for these results (Koller and Miller, 1986).

The molecular mechanism(s) for this proposed differentiating action of chemotherapy remain(s) unclear, as do the exact molecular events produced by retinoids and other agents (see "Molecular Studies of Defective Differentiation" later in this chapter). Some studies suggest an alteration in the expression of certain oncogenes—e.g., the down-regulation of c-myb, c-myc, c-abl, or other proto-oncogenes—while others suggest that increased expression of certain genes may be important. For example, azacytidine is useful in some children with thalassemia and in adults with preleukemic syndromes. Azacytidine induces the expression of fetal hemoglobin genes in children with thalassemia, and both clinical and laboratory studies suggest that drug-induced alterations in DNA methylation are key events controlling genetic expression of this hemoglobin (Ley et al, 1982).

## Differentiation and Tumorigenesis: Cells in Culture

***Differentiation Patterns Seen in Tumor Cells*** The abnormal differentiation seen in most tumors in vivo can, in many cases, be observed and studied in culture. By studying the differentiated properties of normal and tumor cells in culture, we can begin to understand the mechanisms underlying the abnormal differentiation shown by tumor cells and its relationship to the loss of growth control.

The abnormal differentiation of most tumor cells often takes the form of "dedifferentiation" or a reversion to a more primitive or embryonic cell type. Cells at a more primitive stage of differentiation are often multipotential and thus readily give rise to other cell types (Hall, 1983; Blau et al, 1985). Most important, embryonic cells often display traits that endow them with a selective growth advantage over adult cells. Typically, embryonic cells have a high proliferative capacity and are capable of extensive migration; they also produce factors that increase the supply of blood (and therefore nutrients) and that degrade basement membranes and other support structures, thereby facilitating invasiveness (Hall, 1983). These are, of course, the very traits commonly found in adult tumor cells.

Aberrant differentiation can cause excessive cell growth. In healthy tissue, a balance between cell growth and loss is achieved. In many tissues, cell growth is restricted to a select subpopulation; these stem cells often have the ability to terminally differentiate into nonproliferating cell types and to do so in a controlled manner. Cell loss commonly occurs through terminal differentiation followed by cell death. Mutations that partially or completely inhibit terminal differentiation will result in unbalanced cell proliferation and therefore uncontrolled growth of the tissue.

Several types of cells can be grown in culture and induced to terminally differentiate by manipulation of the culture conditions. Generally, such cells are differentiated stem cells, i.e., cells that already express some specialized functions. In culture, as in vivo, differentiated stem cells have the ability to proliferate and to further differentiate into a restricted number of new cell types. These cells express new differentiated functions and irreversibly lose the ability to proliferate. One exception is embryonal carcinoma cells, some of which retain the ability to differentiate into many different cell types (Mintz and Fleischman, 1981). Some examples of such culture systems and the conditions for differentiation are given in Table 1-5.

An important lesson that has been learned from cell-culture studies is that transformation by chemical carcinogens or by oncogenes generally blocks terminal differentiation (Graf and Beug, 1983; Ke et al, 1988; Pecoraro et al, 1989; Coppola et al, 1989). Indeed, failure to terminally differentiate under the appropriate culture conditions is a common, although not universal, feature of naturally occurring tumor cells. This has been well studied in a number of epithelial cell cancers, particularly squamous cell cancers of the head and neck region (Rheinwald and Beckett, 1980) and in leukemia cells (Lotem and Sachs, 1982). In many cases of natural and experimentally induced tumors, the cells have not entirely lost all differentiated functions. Rather, the terminal pattern of differentiated functions is incompletely expressed, so that the cells do not stop dividing. The introduction of defined oncogenes into differentiating cells clearly shows that aberrant differentiation and continued proliferation can be brought about by the same transforming event.

Even after tumorigenic transformation, some cells can be induced to terminally differentiate in culture. Table 1-5 also lists some transformed cell lines and the culture conditions that cause terminal differentiation. After such cells have been induced to differentiate, their ability to form tumors in immunosuppressed or syngeneic animals is often stably suppressed. As discussed earlier, the ability of certain tumor cells to undergo terminal differentiation in response to natural or xenobiotic agents has provided the rationale for using differentiating agents to augment chemotherapy.

***General Mechanisms of Differentiation and Anaplasia*** Normal stem cells are multipotential, having the capacity for self-renewal as well as for differentiation. Some stem cells have already undergone differentiation, so that only a single cell type or lineage emerges; others are totipotential and capable of differentiating to cell types of many lineages. Often, stem cells have the characteristics of established cell lines; for example, they may proliferate well in culture and may not undergo cellular senescence. One mechanism by which aberrant differentiation in tumor cells might arise is through one or more mutations that render a primitive stem cell unable—either partly or completely—to respond to the normal signals for differentiation. A second possibility is that an already differentiated cell might sustain a mutation in a gene responsible for initiating or maintaining the differentiated state. Were either of these cells later to proliferate, they would produce clones of undifferentiated or incompletely differentiated cells. A third possibility is that a cell responsible for maintaining the

TABLE 1-5 Induction of Terminal Differentiation in Culture

| Stem Cell | Differentiated Cell(s) | Inducers of Differentiation |
| --- | --- | --- |
| Preadipocyte | Adipocyte | High cell density, insulin, glucocorticoids |
| Basal keratinocyte | Cornified envelope keratinocyte | High cell density, calcium, retinoid-deficient |
| Myoblast | Myotube | High cell density, growth factor–deficient medium |
| Embryonal carcinoma | Endoderm (some cell lines) | Retinoic acid |
| | Multiple cell types | Retinoids, serum deprivation, spontaneous |
| Erythroleukemia | Terminal erythroid cell | Dimethylsulfoxide, hexamethylene-bisacetamide |
| Promyelocytic leukemia | Granulocyte | Dimethylsulfoxide |
| | Monocyte/macrophage | Phorbol esters, 1,25-dihydroxy-vitamin $D_3$ |

differentiated state of other cells might suffer a genetic change that disrupts its function. For example, some cells produce hormones or an extracellular matrix (ECM) that acts as a signal for the differentiation of distal or adjacent cells. A mutation could cause a cell of this type to produce an abnormal hormone or ECM or to fail to produce the proper signal at all. Such cells would then induce an abnormal state of differentiation or growth in the target cells. As the mutated cells proliferate, the number of aberrantly regulated target cells would increase.

Clearly, then, conditions that reactivate select portions of an embryonic program of gene expression (or that inactivate portions of an adult program of gene expression) could generate cells having many of the properties of malignant tumor cells. Many of the embryonic gene products found in tumor cells—molecules such as CA125—may not themselves confer a growth advantage or malignant phenotype. Rather, the appearance of these embryonic markers most likely reflects a change in one or more regulatory molecules that, in turn, controls the expression of an entire battery of embryonic genes, including those that confer a growth advantage. In addition, mutations that alter the local cellular environment can also have profound effects on growth and differentiation. The importance of the immediate cellular environment in controlling cellular behavior is most clearly illustrated by embryonal carcinoma cells, which will be discussed further below.

***Cell Biology*** Studies of differentiation in cell culture suggest that cell-cycle regulation, particularly of the $G_1$ period, is important for differentiation. For example, preadipocyte cell lines proliferate indefinitely as growth-controlled, fibroblastic cultures; when the cells reach confluence and arrest growth, they differentiate into nonproliferating, mature adipocytes. Several aspects of the relationships among growth, differentiation, and tumorigenesis are interesting. First, full expression of the differentiated program occurs after the cells have ceased dividing. Like most terminally differentiated cells, they irreversibly arrest growth with a $G_1$ DNA content. However, prior to the initiation of morphologic and biochemical differentiation, the cells arrest in a reversible differentiation-specific $G_1$ state that has been termed $G_{1D}$. Transformed preadipocytes are unable to differentiate into terminally nonproliferating adipocytes and they consistently fail to arrest growth in $G_{1D}$ (Wille et al, 1982).

The commitment to terminal differentiation often occurs in the $G_1$ phase of the cell cycle. Murine myoblasts become committed to differentiate into nonproliferating myotubes after mitogens, notably fibroblast-derived growth factor, have been withdrawn from cells in $G_1$ (Nadal-Ginard, 1978; Linkhart et al, 1980; Lathrop et al, 1985). In the earlier section on "Neoplasia," we discussed the importance of the $G_1$ period in modulating the response to growth factors. The finding that myoblast differentiation is controlled by growth factors active in $G_1$ lends support to the idea that differentiation and hormonal control of $G_1$ are somehow linked. Thus,

it is not surprising that tumor cells show both an abnormal response to growth factors (Goustin et al, 1986) and aberrant differentiation. On the other hand, once a muscle cell has differentiated, it expresses factors in its cytoplasm that can induce the expression of muscle-specific genes in fetal fibroblasts (Chiu and Blau, 1984). Taken together, these observations suggest that differentiation involves the induction, possibly in the $G_1$ phase of the cell cycle, of dominant, trans-acting factors produced by one gene that in turn induce and maintain the expression of other differentiation-specific genes. Only recently have candidates for such developmentally regulated, trans-acting factors been identified through molecular cloning. As discussed below, these factors tend to be nuclear, DNA-binding proteins.

There is also evidence in some cells that one or more rounds of DNA synthesis are needed for differentiation (Edgar and McGhee, 1988). In these cases, DNA synthesis may be needed to alter the pattern of DNA methylation. The methylation of DNA on cytosine residues is believed to affect the structures of chromatin (Keshet et al, 1986) and to contribute to the selectivity of gene expression during development, presumably by affecting the accessibility of critical trans-acting differentiation factors (Felsenfeld and McGhee, 1982; Kolata, 1985). During development, changes in DNA methylation are commonly introduced following DNA replication. However, certain pharmacologic agents, notably 5-azacytidine, can inhibit DNA methylation in any replicating cell. Indeed, 5-azacytidine promotes differentiation of a number of cells in culture (Jones and Taylor, 1980; Sager and Kovac, 1982). Since undermethylated DNA is usually transcriptionally active (Felsenfeld and McGhee, 1982), 5-azacytidine may induce differentiation by causing demethylation, thereby derepressing the genes coding for the switch to differentiated phenotypes.

Cancer is ultimately the result of stable genetic alterations. However, the effects of oncogenic mutations can be indirect. As noted earlier, cells can grow and differentiate abnormally as a result of mutations in other cells that affect the local cellular environment. A good example of this type of indirect or epigenetic control is the behavior of *embryonal carcinoma (EC) cells*. EC cells are the undifferentiated stem cells from teratocarcinomas, malignant tumors that contain disorganized, differentiated tissue from all three germ layers. EC cells have much in common with the normal, totipotential embryonic stem cells that first appear as a discrete cluster called the *inner cell mass* (ICM) in the blastocyst (Martin, 1980). Both EC cells and ICM cells can be grown as continually proliferating cell lines in culture. The striking feature about the behavior of these cell types—one from a malignant tumor (the EC cell) and the other from a normal embryo (the ICM cell)—is that both can give rise to malignant tumors or to normal embryos, depending upon the environment in which the cell is placed. Either cell type can be manually injected into a normal blastocyst, and the injected blastocyst will develop normally in utero. In some cases, live young are born, and these animals have normal differentiated tissues of all three germ layers that were derived from the injected cell. Alternatively, either cell type can be injected into an animal at an ectopic (nonuterine) site, and teratocarcinomas will form (Mintz and Fleischman, 1981; Martin, 1981). This ability to behave as a normal embryonic stem cell or as a malignant stem cell, depending upon the local cellular environment, is depicted in Figure 1-4.

In culture, EC and ICM cells behave like transformed cells. They grow in low serum concentrations on a semisolid support and do not show contact inhibition. Upon differentiation, cell proliferation slows down or ceases, and the cells acquire many of the characteristics of untransformed cells and lose their tumorigenicity (Speers, 1982). The signals that induce the differentiation of these cells in culture include retinoids and some chemicals. In addition, the extraembryonic cells of the blastocyst, in particular the trophectoderm, also exert an antiproliferative effect on the cells (Pierce et al, 1982). This supports the idea that some tumor cells arising as a result of abnormal differentiation can be controlled by providing them with a suitable embryonic environment.

**Molecular Biology** In recent years, a small number of genes have been identified that are potential master regulators of developmental-specific or differentiation-specific gene expression. Although the concept of genes that serve as master switches for differentiation programs has been considered for some time, only recently have candidate genes been cloned and their functions studied by transfection into cultured cells or early embryos.

*Homeotic genes* were classically and most thoroughly described as genetic loci that determined the developmental fates of primitive, spatially distinct cell popula-

tions in the embryo of the fruit fly *Drosophila* (Harding et al, 1985). Similar genes have since been identified in the genomes of higher organisms (Colberg-Poley et al, 1985). Different homeotic genes are expressed at different times during embryonic development and to varying extents in differentiated cells of adult organisms; moreover, such genes are expressed in EC cells and their expression changes during differentiation (Colberg-Poley et al, 1985; Jackson et al, 1985; LaRosa and Gudas, 1988). Some homeotic gene products appear to be growth factors (Bender, 1985), whereas others have strong structural similarities to DNA binding proteins (Hogan, 1985).

Other differentiation master-switch genes have been identified that appear to function only in cells of a restricted lineage. For example, two genes, MyoD and myd, have recently been shown to control the determination of a multipotential mesenchymal stem cell into a monopotent myoblast (Davis et al, 1987; Pinney et al, 1988). Another gene, myogenin, has been shown to control differentiation into mature skeletal muscle (Wright et al, 1989). Since the myogenic lineage involves highly proliferative stem cells that terminally differentiate into muscle cells, disruption of the function of MyoD, myd, or myogenin could select for cells that cannot terminally differentiate and thus have the potential to form a tumor.

**Molecular Studies of Defective Differentiation** Differentiation is expressed at the subcellular level as well as at the levels of tissue and cell. Each differentiated cell type exhibits its own pattern of enzymes, proteins, and other molecules. Furthermore, the spatial arrangements of these molecules differ in variously differentiated cells. At the molecular level, these differentiated properties become scrambled in tumor cells, as does differentiation at the higher levels. Tumors tend to lose differentiated properties as they progress, and novel properties not usually exhibited by the cell of origin can also arise. In a set of Morris hepatoma cells showing different degrees of malignancy, aberrant enzyme patterns approached those of neonatal liver (Potter, 1968). The derangement of differentiation appears to be related to tumor progression—i.e., the more a tumor progresses, the greater the modifications of normal differentiation patterns.

What differentiated molecular properties are changed in tumors? These changes are numerous indeed, affecting virtually all cell components. On the exterior of tumor cells, decreases in fibronectin, an ECM protein, have been extensively studied. As with most such changes, loss of fibronectin is not universal, but alterations in the distribution of this protein are often seen (Chen et al, 1979). Increases in plasminogen activator (a protease) have been frequently reported for cultured tumor cells, as discussed earlier. This protease may strip various proteins from the cell surface in addition to converting plasminogen to plasmin (Reich et al, 1975). Various tumorigenic cells are better agglutinated than are normal cells by plant proteins known as lectins. The membranes of neoplastic cells show a variety of changes in molecular composition, including protein, glycolipid,

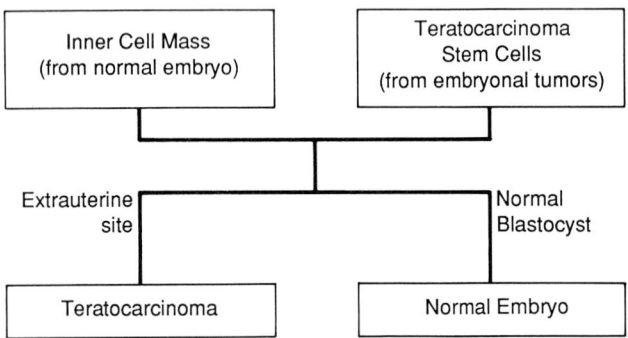

FIGURE 1-4 Tumorigenicity and differentiation of malignant teratocarcinoma stem cells and cells of inner cell mass (ICM) are controlled by the cellular environment. The ICM of a normal mouse embryo can be implanted into a blastocyst of a genetically different mouse strain. There it will participate in normal development and contribute cells to a viable, chimeric mouse. However, if placed at an extrauterine site (such as a testis or kidney), it will form a malignant teratocarcinoma. Stem cells from malignant teratocarcinomas, on the other hand, will participate in normal development if they are implanted into a blastocyst, although they form teratocarcinomas if implanted elsewhere. Thus, both differentiation and tumorigenicity in the teratocarcinoma stem cell and the normal ICM cells are controlled by the immediate cellular environment.

and antigens (Hynes and Fox, 1980). There are also changes in hormone receptors and transport systems. Gap junctions, which connect adjacent cells, are generally decreased between tumor cells, and the flow of small molecules between these cells is correspondingly reduced—a property modified by protein kinases (Wiener and Loewenstein, 1983).

Within the cell, numerous changes in structure and enzymology occur. Microfilaments in normal cells are aligned in parallel arrays, which tend to be disrupted in tumor cells (McClain and Edelman, 1980). The nuclear morphology is often changed, and this has been proposed as one of the most characteristic markers of malignancy (Smith et al, 1979). Numerous enzyme changes between normal and transformed cells have been described, mostly in studies of hepatomas. Many of these are related to biosynthesis and energy metabolism rather than to differentiated properties (Weber, 1983). In normal liver certain enzyme activities vary widely depending upon nutrition. In hepatoma cells, these enzymes tend to be fixed, each tumor cell having an enzyme level that is within the normal range but that does not vary with external conditions (Pitot, 1981). Among the differentiation products of interest are keratins; carcinoma cell lines produce different types of keratins and involucrins that differ from those of their cell of origin (Warhol et al, 1982).

These observations show that the normal patterns of enzyme and metabolite production are altered when differentiated cells become tumorigenic. However, little is known regarding the molecular mechanism underlying these changes. More knowledge about the molecular basis of normal differentiation should help to elucidate the basis for its modifications in cancer.

The fundamental event that leads to differentiation is *alteration of gene expression*. Under conditions of differentiation, the sensitivity to DNAse cleavage of genes involved in making specific products is changed, indicating conformational DNA alterations (Cold Spring Harbor Symposium, 1982). As discussed earlier, DNA is sometimes modified by decreased or increased methylation of cytosine residues, and it is of interest that 5-azacytidine both decreases methylation and greatly affects gene expression and differentiation. One change related to differentiation is altered attachment of poly-ADP-ribose to proteins such as histones (Althaus et al, 1982). All these results suggest that important changes in chromatin structure are triggered by various differentiating agents. These changes must not be readily reversed, since normal differentiation is, in general, irreversible. Furthermore, cell fusion experiments between a differentiated cell and its precursor show that the differentiated property is usually dominant and controls gene expression in the hybrid (Weiss, 1982).

Aberrant differentiation is often correlated with chromosome rearrangement in cancer cells. Moving a gene to another location can change its level of expression or prevent it from being expressed. Changes in chromosomal structure and activity lead to the production of numerous new products, as demonstrated by

discoveries of new messenger RNA and proteins in differentiated cells. Most of these are probably terminal expressions of the altered genes rather than causes of differentiation modification.

In summary, the best current hypothesis is that selected sets of genes are switched off or on by the action of external factors during normal differentiation. These events are perturbed in tumor cells, perhaps by rearrangements or mutations in chromosomal structure. Incorrect sets of genes are thereby switched on, or products of genes necessary for differentiation are decreased in other sets of genes. At present, the basic mechanism that allows or prevents gene expression is unknown but may well involve DNA methylation, poly-ADP-ribosylation, and changes in chromosomal proteins such as histones and high mobility group (hMG) proteins.

## GENETIC INFORMATION

### In Vivo Studies

***Chromosome Changes*** Cancer genetics has been among the most rapidly developing areas of medical research in the last decade. With discoveries of chromosomal and genetic abnormalities in human neoplasia (Rowley and Testa, 1982), exciting new insights into the possible etiologies of cancer have been gained and new strategies for diagnosis, prevention, or treatment may result. In this section, we shall review two areas of genetic research that have been closely linked to cancer in humans: (1) chromosomal aberrations related to the etiology and/or prognosis of neoplasms, and (2) specific cancer-related gene sequences—oncogenes—that have been discovered in numerous human cancers.

Several lines of evidence point to the importance of chromosomal abnormalities in the etiology and progression of cancer. In order to review recent findings in this field, it is helpful to define terms used in studies of chromosomal abnormalities. *Random changes* are chromosomal deletions, additions, rearrangements, or other aberrations that have no consistent pattern among neoplasms of the same histologic type. In contrast, *nonrandom changes* are chromosomal defects that occur with relative consistency in cancers of one histologic type. In certain malignancies, nonrandom changes occur frequently, such as altered chromosome 1 in cervical cancer, chromosome 6 in ovarian cancer, chromosome 3 in small cell lung cancer, and chromosome 12 in testicular cancer. Other neoplasms exhibit nonrandom aberrations in a minority of patients, and statistical methods can be used to evaluate their significance in a given series of patients (Brodeur et al, 1982).

*Specific chromosomal abnormalities* are nonrandom changes associated with only one type of neoplasm or with a group of neoplasms that are histologically similar. *Nonspecific abnormalities* are nonrandom changes that can be found in several unrelated cancers. Chromosome 1 abnormalities are found as nonrandom changes in ovarian cancer, melanoma, and other tumors; therefore, this particular change in cervical cancers is nonrandom and nonspecific. Alternatively, the changes in chromosome 3 of small cell lung cancers have not been well described in other human cancers, so these changes are nonrandom and specific. Similarly, alterations in chromosome 12 are frequent in both testicular and extragonadal germ cell neoplasms, and these changes have not been well described in other malignancies.

*Chromosome banding* is one of several histochemical methods that permit sensitive identification of individual chromosomes. Developed in the 1970s, these methods tremendously improved the sensitivity of chromosome analysis—comparable to the development of two-dimensional computed axial tomographic (CAT) scanning in radiology. It was once thought that chromosome aberrations occurred in only about 50% of patients with acute leukemia, but recent banding techniques have demonstrated about 10 times as many small chromosomal defects (Yunis et al, 1981). Improved methods for in vitro cultivation of human cancers (described in the earlier section on "Neoplasia") and these new banding techniques have greatly improved studies of specific chromosomal abnormalities.

Compelling evidence for the role of chromosomal abnormalities in the pathogenesis of cancer is the high frequency of specific nonrandom changes that occur in certain neoplasms. These changes often consist of chromosomal translocations, deletions, or numerical alterations. The first human neoplasms shown to have frequent nonrandom changes were leukemias and lymphomas, such as the 9,22 translocation that has been found in over 90% of patients with chronic myelogenous leukemia (Yunis, 1983). Consistent nonrandom defects have now been reported in most types of leukemia and lymphoma. One reason that most early studies were done with leukemias and lymphomas is the relative technical advantage of obtaining viable mitotic tumor cells in these diseases.

Before the 1970s, a major difference was observed in the number of solid tumors versus leukemias and/or lymphomas having specific nonrandom chromosomal abnormalities. This difference led some investigators to suggest that nonrandom aberrations were the exception and not the rule, i.e., that cytogenetic changes in cancer either were epiphenomenal or were primary events in only limited types of hematologic or lymphatic malignancies. However, recent developments in cell culture and banding techniques have provided increasing evidence for nonrandom chromosomal changes that also occur in solid tumors.

Nonrandom and possibly specific cytogenetic changes have been reported in patients with papillary serous adenocarcinoma of the ovary (Wake et al, 1980). A serial study of 12 patients revealed that all tumors exhibited a deletion from chromosome 6, an addition to chromosome 14, or a reciprocal translocation between these two chromosomes. This study also revealed chromosome 1 abnormalities in 9 of 12 cases. Chromosome 1 abnormalities have been found in other studies of ovarian cancers. Unlike the changes in chromosomes 6 and 14, alterations in chromosome 1 appear

to be nonspecific. Nonrandom chromosomal abnormalities in various gynecologic neoplasms have been reviewed, and an altered chromosome 1 also appears to be the most common finding in this group of neoplasms, including squamous cell carcinoma of the cervix (Atkin, 1981).

Common chromosomal abnormalities include translocations and deletions. Specific translocations are the hallmark of many leukemias and lymphomas. It has been possible to show that, in some cases, particular oncogenes have been moved to transcriptionally active regions as a result of the translocation. Increased (unbalanced) gene expression may be a common outcome of translocations. For instance, trisomy of chromosome 15 is a characteristic of a murine leukemia (Klein, 1981). Moreover, specific chromosomal regions may be amplified in some tumors, giving rise to a homogeneous staining region (HSR), a nonbanding, amplified stretch of chromosome that interrupts the normal banding pattern, or to double minutes (DM), small acentric chromosomal fragments. HSRs and DM are seen in tumor cells. They are also generated by cultured cells exposed to increasingly high concentrations of certain drugs (e.g., methotrexate). These HSRs and DM can code for overproduction of enzymes that confer drug resistance, such as dihydrofolate reductase, which leads to methotrexate resistance (Schimke, 1982).

Deletions of specific chromosomal regions are also common findings in human cancers. In contrast to HSRs and DM, which appear to confer a growth advantage in some cancers by directly coding for protein products that are advantageous for cell survival, allelic deletions may increase malignant properties through the loss of "tumor suppressor genes." Such allelic deletions appear to be important in the pathogenesis of retinoblastomas and acoustic neuromas. Sequences on chromosome 11 are lost in a high proportion of patients with Wilms' tumor of the kidney, and one study found that about 40% of patients with bladder cancer had a similar loss of sequences from the 11p chromosome arm (Fearon et al, 1985).

Recent evidence also points to specific deletions involved in breast, lung, and colon cancers. For example, in a study of 56 human colon cancers (Vogelstein et al, 1989), 75% of the tumors showed a loss of alleles from the same two chromosome arms (17p and 18q). Prognosis was also linked to the number of chromosomal deletions, expressed as the fraction of chromosomal arms with deletions divided by the number of chromosomal arms evaluable in the patient's normal cells. In fact, this computation of allelic deletions predicted both tumor recurrence and prognosis independent of other clinical variables (such as Dukes' classification), suggesting a new approach to prognostic assesment that could be used in clinical practice.

A technique used to assay allelic deletions, or other subchromosomal changes, is termed *restriction fragment length polymorphisms* (RFLPs). DNA polymorphisms are normal variations of specific DNA sequences that occur in the human population. Since they are inherited, they can be used to distinguish the maternal and paternal copies of a gene. Sensitive detection can be achieved by first cutting the DNA with restriction enzymes, the cutting locations of which are sensitive to the presence of a polymorphism, and then treating the DNA fragments with radioactive, cloned copies of the target gene. These cloned copies will hybridize to gene fragments from tumor or normal cells. By comparing DNA from normal and tumor tissue, this technique can detect whether one or the other allele of a gene was lost during tumorigenesis (Fearon et al, 1985; Vogelstein et al, 1989).

It is not clear what role chromosomal changes play in tumorigenesis. Chromosomal changes accompany the immortalization of cultured cell lines. The ease with which nontumorigenic cell lines are transformed suggests that they may be preneoplastic. Tumorigenesis is usually accompanied by general chromosomal instability. It has been suggested that the cellular environment within a tumor is abnormal and may apply strong selective pressure for unusual phenotypes, including those disposed to large, rapid changes in the chromosomes. Alternatively, a mechanism for chromosome rearrangement could be activated. The genome of eukaryotes and prokaryotes can undergo a variety of changes by the process of transposition. Transpositions (specific genetic rearrangements) normally occur during lymphocyte differentiation for antibody production. Aberrant transpositions could create and sustain much of the genetic instability seen in tumors (Cairns, 1981; Cairns and Logan, 1983).

**Inherited Chromosomal Abnormalities** Another line of evidence pointing to chromosomal aberrations in the etiology of cancer is the close association between certain premalignant or high-risk conditions and nonrandom chromosomal abnormalities. These conditions can be grouped into three types: (1) inherited abnormalities that predispose to specific neoplasms; (2) acquired changes due to drugs, viruses, radiation, or other agents that are known carcinogens; and (3) abnormalities present in tissues that are histologically premalignant.

A small group of neoplasms are clearly linked to inherited or congenital syndromes characterized by chromosomal abnormalities. Pediatric malignancies that have been attributed to specific nonrandom chromosomal abnormalities include (1) Wilms' tumor and chromosome 11 deletion (associated with congenital aniridia), (2) retinoblastoma and chromosome 13 deletion, and (3) acute leukemia and trisomy of chromosome 21 (Down's syndrome). A review of patients with Klinefelter's syndrome (XXY) has suggested that this condition is also associated with an increased risk for extragonadal germ cell tumors (Schimke et al, 1983). Familial adenomatous polyposis (FAP) is closely linked to inherited abnormalities on chromosome 5q21, and losses from this chromosome region are one of the earliest genetic changes found in sporadic colorectal cancers and preneoplastic adenomas (Winawer et al, 1991). These chromosomal abnormalities are not sufficient for the development of cancer in any of the cases mentioned, since tumors develop in only a fraction of the affected population. For example, only 40% of patients with aniridia and deletion of chromosome 11 develop Wilms'

tumor. It is more likely that these inherited or congenital chromosomal defects provide conditions that either allow other oncogenic events to occur or confer susceptibility to transformation by other events.

**Acquired Chromosomal Abnormalities** Chromosomal abnormalities can be a consistent early finding after exposure to environmental agents known to cause cancer. In rodents, nonrandom chromosomal aberrations are among the first changes produced by certain carcinogens, and these chromosomal defects are consistently found in the tumors that later arise in these animals. Clinical studies support a connection between chromosomal defects and carcinogen-induced malignancies. Specific abnormalities of chromosome 5, 7, or 8 have been detected in subgroups of patients with acute nonlymphocytic leukemia, and this same subgroup had a history of increased exposure to suspected environmental carcinogens (Yunis, 1983). Alterations of chromosomes 3, 5, 7, or 17 have also been frequently observed in patients with acute leukemia that occurs after previous treatment with chemotherapy and/or radiation (Sandberg et al, 1982).

Patients receiving curative therapy for Hodgkin's disease are at higher risk for the later development of leukemia or lymphoma. One study of patients who received curative treatment with chemotherapy and/or radiation revealed a high incidence of random chromosomal abnormalities in bone marrow stem cells and lymphocytes (Lawler et al, 1982). These chromosomal abnormalities were evident more than 3 years after treatment was completed, and the degree of chromosomal rearrangement was highly correlated with the types of treatment that are probably the most carcinogenic. Since treatment with alkylating agents in ovarian cancer is also associated with an increased risk for leukemia, these results suggest that random or nonrandom chromosomal aberrations could be a marker for patients at highest risk for the development of leukemia after cytotoxic chemotherapy. Prospective studies are in progress to analyze chromosomal changes in adult or pediatric patients who have received such therapy.

The acquisition of chromosomal abnormalities in human cells is a complex event that depends on several interrelated processes. Total organ functions related to metabolism, activation, or excretion of potential carcinogens are critical properties, and the individual biologic response of target tissues is also important. For example, increased spontaneous chromosomal rearrangements are observed in colon cells and fibroblasts from patients with familial polyposis, a syndrome associated with a high risk for colon cancer (Delhanty et al, 1983; Winawer et al, 1991). Bloom's syndrome, ataxia telangiectasia, and xeroderma pigmentosum are also inherited syndromes in which the risk for malignancy may be related to increased spontaneous or induced chromosomal aberrations, possibly resulting from abnormal DNA repair of genetic damage, either spontaneous or induced by environmental agents (Setlow, 1978).

In the general population, carcinogens appear preferentially to alter discrete areas of certain chromosomes, termed *fragile sites*. Spontaneous chromosomal defects at fragile sites can be produced in vitro under special conditions, such as low folic acid and thymidine levels in the culture medium. Some of the chromosome areas suspected to be fragile sites are also associated with malignancies that may be induced by environmental carcinogens, such as chromosome 3 in small cell carcinoma of the lung, which has been associated with heavy smoking (Yunis, 1983). These findings suggest that fragile sites may serve as predisposing factors for chromosomal abnormalities that are induced by carcinogens and lead to cancer.

### Chromosomal Abnormalities in Premalignant Conditions

Chromosomal defects in premalignant or precursor lesions also support the concept that chromosomal abnormalities are early events in the pathogenesis of malignancy. Compared with the published reports of studies using cancer cells, relatively few studies have analyzed chromosomal abnormalities in premalignant tissues owing to several problems: (1) methods for cell culture of benign human tissue are not well developed; (2) less biopsy material is usually available; and (3) histologic sources of premalignant tissues are not well defined for many neoplasms.

In one study of early ovarian tumors analyzed with banding techniques, no cytogenetic abnormalities were found in seven cases of benign cystadenomas of the ovary (Knoerr-Gaertner et al, 1977). However, chromosomal defects were detected in all seven cystadenomas with borderline malignant histologies, and five of these early lesions revealed nonrandom changes in chromosome 10. This finding contrasts with reports of altered chromosomes 1, 6, and/or 14 in advanced ovarian cancer. Such differences between chromosomal abnormalities in early versus advanced neoplasms can be explained in several ways. One hypothesis is that the defects noted in early tumors are permissive events that lead to early malignant properties, whereas the changes noted in advanced tumors are related to later disease progression, possibly through increased expression of critical growth-related properties. Alternatively, these later stages of tumor progression could be related to the loss of normal genes that regulate cell growth, often called "tumor suppressor genes" or "anti-oncogenes" (Sager, 1989).

Abnormal chromosome patterns have also been reported in small series of patients with endometrial hyperplasia, fibroadenomas of the breast, and premalignant intraepithelial lesions of the cervix. By means of banding techniques, two patients with endometrial hyperplasia were found to have chromosomal defects similar to those in other patients with histologically confirmed endometrial carcinoma (Trent and Davis, 1979). In a retrospective analysis of patients with premalignant cervical lesions, the degree of cytogenetic abnormalities correlated with subsequent progression to invasive carcinoma (Fu et al, 1981). The method used in this study was flow cytometry, an automated technique that can rapidly detect alterations in total chromosomal content (abnormal ploidy) but not specific chromosomal changes as seen with banding. Although cytogenetic abnormalities generally correlated with more serious

prognostic lesions of the cervix, 15% of the group with an abnormal chromosomal content were later found to have normal biopsies without specific therapy. This observation supports the concept that cytogenetic changes alone are not sufficient for malignant progression (see "Inherited Chromosomal Abnormalities" discussed earlier).

### Chromosomal Abnormalities and Tumor Progression

In addition to cytogenetic defects in premalignant lesions, several cancers exhibit additional specific or nonspecific chromosomal abnormalities during progression to more aggressive disease. Trisomy of chromosome 8, 19, 21, or 22 can be found in many patients with aggressive forms of chronic myelogenous leukemia, and the appearance of these chromosomal abnormalities during the stable phase often predicts the rapid development of aggressive disease and a poor prognosis. A few studies have used banding techniques to analyze specific chromosomal changes in early versus advanced solid tumors, but most investigators have used flow cytometry or related techniques to determine the relationship between ploidy and stage of disease or prognosis. In most reports, patients with near-diploid tumors had an earlier stage of disease and/or a better prognosis than did those with aneuploid tumors. This relation between tumor aggressiveness and ploidy has been observed in cancers of the bladder, colon, lung, and breast (Clark et al, 1989).

The relation between prognosis and ploidy has also been studied in several gynecologic cancers. Near-diploid tumors are associated with a more favorable prognosis in uterine and ovarian cancer. In a study of 157 patients with ovarian cancer, risk of death from malignancy was twofold higher in patients with aneuploid tumors; this risk increased to sixfold in patients with greater aneuploidy (Kallioniemi et al, 1988). However, a relatively large study of patients with squamous cell carcinomas of the cervix indicated a different trend, since patients with near-diploid tumors had a worse overall prognosis (Atkin and Kay, 1979). The reason for this reported difference between cervical cancer and other gynecologic malignancies remains unclear.

Few studies have reported serial cytogenetic changes during progression of solid tumors to a more aggressive state. Over a 9-month period, seven chromosome analyses were reported from one patient with malignant ascites from ovarian cancer (Mackillop et al, 1983). Investigations of the biologic behavior of the tumor cells in vitro revealed a progressive proliferative capacity and decreasing markers for differentiation (see earlier section on "Differentiation and Cancer"). Karyotyping revealed no gross chromosomal changes over the same period of time, although increased DM chromatin bodies and loss of the X chromosome were observed. Since the patient was taking methotrexate for psoriasis at the time of this study, the increase in DM bodies could have been due to the selection of clones with amplified genetic material for dihydrofolate reductase—a phenomenon also observed in patients treated with methotrexate for small cell carcinoma of the lung.

Progression of cytogenetic changes has been studied

in transplantable animal tumors during serial passage, and these reveal a striking association between new chromosomal alterations and progression to more malignant properties (Isaacs et al, 1982). These experiments suggest that such alterations are linked to genetic instability, resulting in new clones of cells with a distinct growth advantage.

Since many drugs used for cancer treatment are mutagenic, it has been proposed that cancer therapy may promote genetic instability in the cancer cells that survive the therapy, leading to cells that are resistant to the same therapy by means of selection. However, few clinical studies have verified this hypothesis, and some experiments using L1210 (mouse) leukemia cells show that the emergence of drug-resistant clones is not due to treatment but rather represents the outgrowth of preexisting resistant cells from the original tumor (Kim et al, 1981).

***Chromosomal Abnormalities and Oncogenes*** The molecular mechanism by which chromosomal defects lead to cancer was an area of intense investigation throughout the last decade. The discovery of specific gene sequences in tumor-producing viruses (viral oncogenes) that have similar expression in animal and human neoplasms (cellular oncogenes) has led to new insights into the connections among chromosomal abnormalities, specific gene expression, and the origins of cancer. Oncogenes were first discovered in viruses that produce tumors in animals, and several closely related gene sequences have been found in human neoplasms. Although some oncogenes show increased expression in some human cancers, normal cells also express oncogene-related sequences. Thus, it is not merely the presence of oncogenes that leads to neoplasia; their abnormal structure, activation, or altered expression also appears to be critical in the pathogenesis of some malignancies.

A direct connection between chromosomal abnormalities and oncogene expression is illustrated by Burkitt's lymphoma. C-myc expression in Burkitt's lymphoma has been reported to be increased up to 20 times normal. These tumors frequently contain a nonrandom translocation between chromosomes 8 and 14. The donor site of chromosome 8 normally contains the c-myc oncogene, and the receptor site on chromosome 14 codes for immunoglobulin synthesis by B lymphocytes. This specific translocation in Burkitt's lymphoma most likely leads to activation of the c-myc oncogene (in addition to a slight alteration in sequence) by relocating the c-myc sequence from chromosome 8 to reside next to promoter sequences on chromosome 14 that normally activate immunoglobulin synthesis (Sager, 1983). B-cell malignancies in mice have also been found to have similar chromosome translocations that move the c-myc oncogene next to the immunoglobulin region.

In the last decade, new techniques for analyzing oncogene alterations in small, clinical tumor samples have been developed, providing a feasible approach to study biopsy samples from individual patients (Bishop, 1987; Tandon et al, 1989a). Alterations in oncogene amplification and/or expression are found in several tumor types, and the list is growing at a rapid pace (Table 1-

**TABLE 1-6** Proto-Oncogenes in Human Tumors

| Neoplasm | Proto-Oncogene(s) |
|---|---|
| Cystadenocarcinoma of ovary | HER-2/neu, c-myc, N-myc, Ha-ras, Ki-ras |
| Squamous cell carcinoma of uterine cervix | c-myc, Ha-ras, EGFR |
| Adenocarcinoma of endometrium | fms, Ha-ras, Ki-ras, c-myc, EGFR |
| Adenocarcinoma of breast | HER-2/neu, c-myc, Ha-ras, Ki-ras, EGFR, c-myb, int-2, hst |
| Adenocarcinoma of stomach | HER-2/neu, EGFR, c-myc |
| Adenocarcinoma of lung | Ki-ras |
| Small cell carcinoma of lung | L-myc, N-myc, c-myc, fos, jun, myb |
| Neuroblastoma | N-myc |
| Glioblastoma | EGFR, N-myc, c-myc, gli |
| Burkitt's lymphoma | c-myc, c-abl |
| Chronic myelogenous leukemia | c-abl, Ha-ras |
| Acute myelogenous leukemia | c-myc, c-sis, c-fms, Ha-ras, c-abl |
| Multiple myeloma | c-myc |
| Colorectal, bladder, prostate, others | Ki-ras, Ha-ras |

6). In addition to improving our understanding of the mechanism(s) of tumor growth, these studies may provide assistance in diagnosis as well as practical information about individual patient prognosis. N-myc amplification in neuroblastoma correlates closely with poor prognosis following conventional treatment, and measurement of this oncogene is a useful means of determining which patients should receive more aggressive treatments (Brodeur et al, 1988).

HER-2/neu amplification was reported to predict poor clinical outcome in patients with node-positive breast cancer. Early studies have suggested that amplification of this gene and/or its protein product is independent of other prognostic variables. In this way, it could be used in clinical programs, i.e., to assign more aggressive adjuvant chemotherapy to those patients with a worse prognosis (Tandon et al, 1989a). In contrast, other studies have used monoclonal antibodies to the HER-2/neu protein product, and initial results suggest that HER-2/neu protein expression correlates with poor prognosis, but only in subgroups of patients with large (T3 to T4) primary breast cancers (Thor et al, 1989).

Amplification of an oncogene and/or increased expression of its protein product does not always correlate with poor prognosis or other measures of more aggressive malignant behavior. For example, prognosis was improved in some patients with breast cancers that expressed higher levels of the c-myb gene (Guerin et al, 1989), and a slight improvement in survival was reported for patients with malignant glioma that expressed higher levels of epidermal growth factor receptor and other proto-oncogenes (Bigner et al, 1988). In other studies, high levels of an oncogene or its protein have not been related to prognosis or tumor progression (Bishop, 1987). In such cases oncogene expression may be a *result* of neoplastic growth and not its cause. Variations in the techniques used to measure oncogenes or their products may also lead to different conclusions about relationships to prognosis (Bigner et al, 1988; Tandon et al, 1989*a*). In other situations, an analysis of multiple clinical variables in larger patient groups may be required to determine which subgroups exhibit a correlation between prognosis and oncogene expression (Thor et al, 1989).

In some tumors, elevated oncogene expression could come about through a higher gene dosage, possibly caused by chromosomal duplication through nondisjunction, resulting in trisomy or tetraploidy. For example, if oncogene expression on chromosome 8 is also related to malignant progression of chronic myelogenous leukemia, trisomy of chromosome 8 seen in patients with aggressive disease could play a critical role.

Another proposed mechanism linking chromosomal changes to oncogene expression is the loss of normal suppressor genes (Sager, 1989). This hypothesis is based on the concept that oncogene expression in normal cells is tightly controlled by specific DNA suppressor genes, the loss of which can lead to cancer. Such a mechanism has been well described in patients with inherited forms of retinoblastoma, in which loss of the retinoblastoma (Rb) gene function leads to malignancy. Some researchers have also noted a loss of Rb gene function in small cell lung cancer. Sequential loss of the DCC and p53 genes has been observed in the transition from preneoplastic adenoma to invasive carcinoma of the colon, and this observation may have a role in future strategies for screening, follow-up, or identification of high-risk patients (Winawer et al, 1991). It has been generally observed that deletions of other specific bands or segments are common abnormalities in human solid tumors; some of these may be similar to the Rb gene, where loss leads to uncontrolled expression of one or more malignant properties. This general hypothesis is also supported by experiments in culture that demonstrate complete suppression of the malignant phenotype when cell hybrids are produced by fusing human cancer and normal cells (Sager, 1989).

## Proto-Oncogenes in Gynecologic Malignancies

Gynecologic neoplasms demonstrate a variety of changes in the expression of proto-oncogenes. These changes include amplifications, mutations, and increased production of protein products. To date, no single change has been 100% consistent in any one type of malignancy, and the results of several studies have been conflicting, possibly owing to differences in analytic techniques.

Gene amplification and/or an increased expression of HER-2/neu has been observed in 20 to 26 percent of ovarian cystadenocarcinomas (Zhang et al, 1989; Slamon et al, 1989). In a retrospective clinical study of 87 patients, HER-2/neu gene amplification correlated closely with patient survival (Table 1-7), and an analysis of the HER-2/neu protein content of tumor cells dem-

### TABLE 1-7 HER-2/neu Gene Amplification and Expression in Ovarian Cancer

| Gene Copy Number | Median Survival Time (days) | Log Rank Test (P value) |
|---|---|---|
| 1 | 1,879 | < 0.0001 |
| 2 to 5 | 959 | |
| Over 5 | 243 | |
| *Protein level by histochemistry:* | | |
| 0 to 1+ | 1,960 | 0.0126 |
| 2+ | 1,093 | |
| Over 2+ | 417 | |

*Source:* Slamon DJ, Godolphin W, Jones LA, Holt JA, Wong SG, Keith DE, Levin WJ, Stuart SG, Udove J, Ullrich A, Press MF: Studies of the HER-2/neu proto-oncogene in human breast and ovarian cancer. *Science* 244:707-712, 1989.

onstrated a similar relation to prognosis (Slamon et al, 1989).

Amplification or increased expression of the Ki-ras or Ha-ras oncogenes has been found in 10 to 20% of ovarian cancers (Zhou et al, 1988; Van de Veer et al, 1988). Deletion or rearrangement of one Ha-ras allele was also observed in six of 17 patients with ovarian cancer (Lee et al, 1989). Increased expression of the myc protein product, termed p62c-myc, has been observed in 22 out of 22 mucinous cystadenocarcinomas of the ovary (100%) (Polacarz et al, 1989). Although no clear relationship with prognosis has been observed in these studies of altered ras or myc expression, further studies are in progress. Some investigators have observed consistent differences in immunohistochemical staining for myc protein in normal ovary compared with that in tumors of "borderline" malignancy, suggesting that such staining could be useful in diagnosis (Watson et al, 1987).

Increased expression of ras or myc proteins has also been observed in squamous cell carcinomas of the uterine cervix (Riou, 1988). In one study of 31 patients, 16 with elevated c-myc protein had worse disease-free and total survival rates and a greater tendency to develop extrapelvic metastatic disease (Sowani et al, 1989). Similarly, amplification of the c-myc and/or c-Ha-ras genes has been correlated with clinical stage and prognosis (Riou et al, 1984). In contrast, other studies demonstrated high levels of c-myc protein in nonmalignant tissues, and no correlation between protein expression and prognosis (Hendy et al, 1987). A correlation between prognosis and expression of the ras protein, called p21, was studied in 170 squamous cell carcinomas of the cervix; p21-positive tumors correlated with a worse prognosis in most histologic subtypes (Sagae et al, 1989); however, this correlation was not seen in patients with the small cell subtype. Other studies have noted a high frequency (36 to 40%) of deletions for one of the Ha-ras alleles (Riou et al, 1988).

Increased expression of the ras p21 protein has also been noted in up to 95% of grade 2 and 3 adenocarcinomas of the endometrium (Long et al, 1988). In this same study, p21 was observed in only two of 11 grade 1 tumors. Endometrial adenocarcinomas also demonstrate increased expression of Ki-ras, c-myc, erbB, and fms (Kacinski et al, 1988). In a recent study of 21 endometrial neoplasms, fms expression correlated with aggressive clinical behavior and poor outcome. These results suggested that analysis of fms expression in initial endometrial biopsies may be of help in preoperative management (Kacinski et al, 1988).

## Genetic Aspects of Cells in Culture

***Clonal Nature of Cancer*** There is much evidence to indicate that cancer is due to genetic changes originating in a single cell. First, the billions of cells in a naturally occurring or experimentally induced tumor display a common genetic background—a strong indication of a unicellular origin. The cells may have in common a chromosomal abnormality (Yunis, 1983), or they may express an isoenzyme characteristic of one X chromosome but not the other (Fialkow, 1979). RFLP analysis has also confirmed the clonal origin of human tumors (Vogelstein et al, 1985). Second, a single tumorigenic cell can produce a mature tumor in the appropriate animal, as discussed earlier (Skipper, 1982). Third, susceptibility to several specific cancers appears to be inherited, sometimes as a Mendelian dominant trait with a high degree of penetrance (Mulvihill, 1977). Fourth, many known carcinogens are mutagenic; thus, compounds known to produce hereditary damage to DNA in a single cell are also likely to produce tumors.

These four types of evidence show the importance of genetic changes in the initiation and progression of cancer. For at least one tumor (embryonal carcinoma), however, progression in experimental animals is governed entirely by the cells' immediate environment.

***Transformation in Culture*** Many tumors are clonal (unicellular) in origin. Therefore, it is both appropriate and feasible to study transformation at the cellular level using cells in culture. Cultured cells can be treated with a variety of oncogenic agents, and their conversion to a transformed phenotype can be studied in a relatively controlled environment. As described below, there are several ways in which cultured cells can be transformed, and these are relevant to the transformations seen in naturally occurring tumors.

Transformation can be spontaneous. In the discussion of growth control, it was pointed out that most cells in the adult organism are in a nonproliferating state. By contrast, cultured cells are generally kept in a dividing state. Cell cultures are usually maintained so as to minimize selection for any rare cell having a growth advantage over its neighbors. Nonetheless, spontaneous transformants occasionally do arise and will dominate the population in time. The basis for spontaneous transformation is unknown; such cells may arise because of a rare mutation. Established rodent cell lines are particularly susceptible to spontaneous transformation, while human cell strains are not (Ponten, 1976). One reason for this difference might be that cell lines are karyotypically abnormal and not necessarily stable (Rothfels and Parker, 1959; Todaro and Green, 1963). This instability could greatly increase the chances of a mutational rearrangement to more relaxed growth control. Spontaneously transformed mouse 3T3 cells can be deliberately generated by long-term passaging at high population densities, which selects for contact inhibition–independent cells; such cells are tumorigenic.

Does the generation of spontaneous transformants in culture tell us anything about the development of cancers in vivo? Certain agents (e.g., phorbol esters) or physical stimuli (e.g., foreign bodies known to increase tumorigenesis) may do so by simply stimulating local cell proliferation (Upton, 1982). Any "spontaneous" mutation that results in diminished growth control would give a cell the opportunity for clonal expansion under the influence of the stimulus and thus further selection. This scenario is related to the two-step model of carcinogenesis (initiation as the mutagenic event and promotion as the growth stimulus) (Berenblum, 1975).

Cultured cells of both human (rarely) and rodent origin can be transformed by chemical carcinogens or radiation to exhibit tumorigenicity (Ishii et al, 1977; Kakunaga, 1973, 1978; Kennedy et al, 1980). After a brief period of proliferation, they will form foci on a cell monolayer or colonies in a semisolid medium. Subsequently, the derived transformants can be tested for tumor-forming ability in experimental animals. A few agents that block transformation have been reported (Boothman and Pardee, 1989).

The mutagenic potential of radiation and chemical carcinogens is well known. Most of these agents cause well-defined defects in DNA: strand breaks, crosslinks, and chemical additions. In some cases, the fixed mutation has also been well characterized: base substitutions, deletions, additions, or frame shift mutations (Auerbach, 1976; Rinkus and Legator, 1979). Moreover, the somatic mutation frequencies of compounds such as benzo($a$)pyrene or *N*-methyl-*N*-nitrosoguanidine correlate well with the frequency of transformations induced by these agents (Barrett and Ts'o, 1978). Thus, there is strong circumstantial evidence for a mutational origin in carcinogenesis by chemicals and radiation. The difficulty in demonstrating a clear cause-and-effect relationship between a single mutation and tumor formation probably stems from the fact that a mutation may be an important but insufficient step in tumorigenesis.

***Oncogenes*** In recent years, it has been possible to introduce, or *transfect*, specific DNA into cultured cells. The recipient cells are generally monolayer fibroblasts, the most common of which are 3T3 cells derived from an NIH strain of mouse (NIH 3T3 cells). The exogenous DNA may be a single purified gene (usually cloned into a bacterial plasmid), or it may be total cellular DNA. In the simplest experiments, mutant cells deficient in thymidine kinase (TK) were transfected with DNA fragments coding for herpes simplex virus TK or with naked total DNA from a cell line expressing normal TK activity (Wigler et al, 1978). The mutant cells acquired and expressed functional TK activity after transfection. The efficiency of stable transfection varies depending upon the recipient cells and is generally low (Cooper et al, 1982). However, the uptake of transfecting DNA is reproducible and can result in the stable integration of an exogenously added gene into the recipient chromosome (Robbins et al, 1981).

Transfection has been used with success to demonstrate the existence of discrete cellular genes that are responsible for the transformed phenotype (oncogenes). The cellular DNA from several human tumors or chemically transformed rodent cells causes foci to appear on a monolayer of untransformed NIH 3T3 cells (Fig. 1-2). Cells isolated from a focus and grown in culture are tumorigenic (Shih et al, 1979; Krontiris and Cooper, 1981). Thus, DNA from the tumor cells contains specific sequences that transfer the transformed phenotype to an untransformed cell. The functions of some oncogenes have already been mentioned, at least some of which are involved in growth regulation. In a later section ("Viral Transforming Genes"), we will discuss the identity of some of these genes and the changes that might be responsible for their transforming ability. Despite the fact that a single altered oncogene can transform NIH 3T3 cells, at least two different oncogenes are found in a human promyelocytic leukemia line, and primary fibroblasts require at least two oncogenic alterations for transformation (Murray et al, 1983; Land et al, 1983).

The DNA from untransformed cells will generally not induce foci in NIH 3T3 cells or will do so only at frequencies much below those of DNA isolated from transformed cells. However, if the untransformed DNA is sheared to small fragments (30.0 to 0.5 kb) before transfection, its ability to induce foci is greatly increased. This result suggests that normal cells contain genes that are potentially transforming but are generally regulated by adjacent sequences. After shearing, these genes could be separated from their regulatory sequences (Cooper et al, 1982) and may then be either overexpressed or expressed inappropriately, depending on where they integrate in the chromosome.

**Suppression of Transformed Cells** Suppression is a most intriguing phenomenon of transformed cells. When normal and transformed cells in culture are fused, the initially resulting hybrid cells are not tumorigenic (Stanbridge et al, 1982; Sager, 1989). Normal cells apparently contain genetic information that suppresses the transformed phenotype. Hybrid cells, resulting from either inter- or intraspecies fusions, gradually lose chromosomes as they proliferate in culture. The emergence of tumorigenicity in hybrid cells has been traced to the loss of specific chromosomes, suggesting that these chromosomes bear the putative suppressor genes. (Suppressor genes could also be inactivated by mutation or by disruption due to chromosome translocation.) The phenomenon of suppression lends credence to the idea that tumorigenesis is a multistep process involving both activation of positive growth regulators and inactivation of negative regulators or of genes required to maintain genetic stability.

## Molecular Genetics

**DNA Changes Caused by Carcinogens** Some carcinogens are themselves reactive, but others must first be activated by metabolism (Hanawalt et al, 1979). A set of oxidative enzymes commonly known as the P-450 system, which are found in the microsomal cell fraction, can activate carcinogens. Although activated carcinogens can also modify RNA and protein, their carcinogenic action is generally attributed to reactions with DNA. The changes in DNA are varied and correspond to the variety of carcinogens. For example, monofunctional alkylating agents (such as methyl methanesulfonate) alkylate DNA bases at several sites—e.g., converting adenine to 3-methyladenine or guanine to 6-0-methylguanine. Bi- or trifunctional alkylating agents (such as nitrogen mustard [HN2] or thiotepa) crosslink DNA chains. Agents such as aflatoxin or benzo-(*a*)pyrene, after being activated, add to DNA as bulky organic groups. Ultraviolet light creates thymine dimers and other changes in DNA, whereas x-rays produce chemical radicals within the cell that create DNA strand breaks.

These changes in DNA structure are only a first step in carcinogenesis. Most changes are eliminated by repair mechanisms that remove damaged DNA structures and replace them with normal components (Hanawalt et al, 1979). If a damaged base is replaced by the original one, there is no permanent harm to the cell. But when a different base is substituted as a result of repair, the point mutation can be lethal or mutagenic. Correlations between mutagenicity and carcinogenicity suggest that point mutations in DNA may be carcinogenic. However, this correlation may reflect only the ability of carcinogens to cause both changes (mutations and cancers) in more or less equal proportion; for example, chromosome rearrangements, observed in carcinogen-treated cells, are common in cancer cells and may be more important than point mutations (Sager, 1989).

As discussed previously, methylation of cytosine residues is another change in DNA structure (Ehrlich and Wang, 1981; Doerfler, 1983). Most studies have shown that a decrease in methylation is associated with gene activation. When compared with DNA from normal colon tissue, DNA from benign polyps and malignant colorectal cancers is substantially hypomethylated (Goelz et al, 1985).

**Viral Transforming Genes** An oncogenic virus converts a normal cell into a transformed or tumor cell by introducing a new piece of genetic information. Such a viral transforming gene (oncogene) can be either *DNA or RNA*, the latter being transcribed into DNA within the recipient cell. The DNA tumor virus studied most intensively at the molecular level is *simian virus 40* (SV40) (Tooze, 1980a; Ludlow et al, 1989). It contains a single, circular, double-stranded DNA molecule of 5,226 base pairs that have been completely sequenced. The A gene, containing about 2,630 base pairs, is responsible for transformation. Its naked DNA can convert normal cells into tumor cells. Mutations within this DNA can destroy or alter their tumorigenic ability. The A gene codes for two viral proteins, the T and t antigens, both of which appear to be involved in the transformation process; T has been studied more than t. Microinjection of the T protein into recipient cells can activate their growth. This protein binds to the replication origin of the SV40 genome and also has ATPase activity.

Several viruses are known to cause tumors at high frequencies in animals. In humans, it has been difficult to demonstrate viral oncogenesis unambiguously, but there is evidence that DNA viruses such as herpes viruses (Epstein-Barr virus and herpes simplex types 1 and 2), human papillomavirus, hepatitis B, and a newly isolated RNA virus (human T-cell leukemia virus) are potentially oncogenic in humans.

*Retroviruses* are small RNA viruses that cause tumors in animals. They fall into two classes: (1) those that cause tumors with low efficiency and long latency periods; and (2) rarer, highly oncogenic and acutely transforming retroviruses. At some point in their evolution, the acutely transforming viruses acquired certain cellular gene sequences, and these have profound effects when introduced into infected mammalian cells. These acquired sequences are responsible for the vigorous transforming ability of some retroviruses. Conditional and nonconditional mutations affecting oncogenic properties have been mapped to these segments (Bishop, 1987). The transforming viral genes have been termed *v-oncogenes*, while the homologous cellular sequences from which they are derived are termed proto-oncogenes. Mutated or unregulated forms of proto-oncogenes are termed *c-oncogenes*. Proto-oncogenes have been highly conserved throughout eukaryotic evolution; v-oncogenes are modified (Duesberg, 1983).

The retroviruses are oncogenic by virtue of their ability to introduce aberrantly regulated genes into the cell, demonstrating that these genes play an important role in cancer. Several dozen different oncogenes have been found in retroviruses (Bishop, 1987). Not all oncogenes identified by transfection of tumor cell DNA are carried by retroviruses. In certain tumors, including some of human origin, c-oncogenes appear to be either overexpressed or specifically mutated. It is not known whether activation or misregulation of these genes is an initiating or later event in nonviral tumorigenesis.

Because these genes are carried by viruses, they can be purified and used to probe the expression (transcription) of proto-oncogenes and c-oncogenes in a variety of normal, transformed, or tumor-derived cells. One of the best studied oncogenes is *src*, present in the genome of the Rous sarcoma virus (RSV). Transformation by RSV results in marked overproduction of the src protein kinase. This is a tyrosine-specific protein kinase (pp60src) located on the cytoplasmic side of the plasma membrane. Transformation by a temperature-sensitive RSV results in the temperature sensitivity of the transformed phenotype and also of catalytic activity of the pp60src. Thus, this virus is oncogenic by virtue of its ability to produce a modified cellular protein kinase that presumably is growth regulatory.

Cells transformed by the v-sis oncogene produce their own PDGF-like molecule. The v-sis gene codes for an aberrant PDGF molecule that might be a more potent or more complete mitogen. This state of readiness to respond to progression factors may be sufficient to give the transformed cells a growth advantage.

Viral transformation appears to convert a normal cell into the tumor cell in a single step, as opposed to the multistep carcinogenesis observed with other agents. However, viruses effect this conversion in only a very limited number of recipient cells. It is not yet clear, however, that viral oncogenes immediately cause cancer. They may accomplish one of the several steps required for tumorigenicity; the usual recipient NIH 3T3 cell is special and has already undergone other required steps. It is likely that further changes occur in the cell after infection with oncogene DNA. Recently, it has become evident that more than one oncogene transfection is required for tumorigenic transformation (Cairns and Logan, 1983), and these may destabilize other genes in the chromosomes. Viral oncogenes have flanking sequences called long terminal repeats (LTR). These repeats are inserted by the virus adjacent to host material, and it is thought that they can act to promote the activities of host genes. The detailed mechanism of action of these viral genes remains to be clarified.

Both alleles of a cell's retinoblastoma gene must be inactivated for the disease to appear; therefore, one normal allele suppresses. Rapid progress is being made at the molecular level in elucidating the function of this gene. Its protein product blocks progression through the cell cycle until it is phosphorylated near the start of S phase (Ludlow et al, 1989). This protein also is inactivated by products of DNA viruses, such as the T antigen of SV40. These results provide an explanation for how these viruses bypass cell proliferation controls. Transfection of the retinoblastoma gene has been reported to suppress tumor cells (Huang et al, 1989). Another suppressing protein is p53, originally thought to be an oncogene because a mutated p53 transforms NIH 3T3 cells (Finlay et al, 1989). It, too, is bound by T antigen. How these several proteins interact is still not clear. Isolation of suppressing genes is difficult, using the negative assay of inhibition of proliferation, but a few such genes have been obtained, including one that suppresses growth of cells transformed by the ras oncogene (Noda et al, 1989).

## SUMMARY

Cancer is characterized by three fundamental properties that distinguish it from normal tissue. These can be defined as follows: (1) neoplasia, or the abnormal growth of cancer cells compared with normal cells; (2) anaplasia, or the loss of differentiation according to specific histologic criteria; and (3) genetic alterations in chromosomal structure and/or in the expression of particular DNA sequences. Recently, investigations of these biologic properties in normal compared with neoplastic cells have led to dramatic advances in our understanding of how cancers develop and grow. Such breakthroughs offer the hope for new, more effective treatment and prevention strategies.

# REFERENCES

Alitalo L, Vaheri A: Pericellular matrix in malignant transformation. *Adv Cancer Res* 37:111-158, 1982.

Allegra J, Day T, Carlson J, Wittliff J: Combination hormonal therapy in the treatment of advanced endometrial cancer. *Proc Am Soc Clin Oncol* 2:14, 1983.

Althaus FR, Lawrence SD, Sattler GL, Pitot HC: ADP-ribosyltransferase activity in cultured hepatocytes. *J Biol Chem* 257:5528-5535, 1982.

Ashmun RA, Look AT, Roberts WM, Roussel MF, Seremetis S, Ohtsuka M, Sherr CJ: Monoclonal antibodies to the human CSF-1 receptor detect epitopes on normal mononuclear phagocytes and on human myeloid leukemia blast cells. *Blood* 73:827-837, 1989.

Atack DB, Nisker JA, Allen HH, Tustanoff ER, Levin L: CA125 surveillance and second-look laparotomy in ovarian carcinoma. *Am J Obstet Gynecol* 154:287-289, 1986.

Atkin BB, Kay R: Prognostic significance of modal DNA value and other factors in malignant tumours, based on 1465 cases. *Br J Cancer* 40:210-221, 1979.

Atkin NB: Chromosome changes in cancer. In Coppelson M (ed): *Gynecologic Oncology*. New York, Churchill Livingstone, 1981, pp 66-78.

Auerbach C: *Mutation Research: Problems, Results and Perspectives*. London, Chapman and Hall, 1976.

Barrett JC, Ts'o POP: Relationship between somatic mutation and neoplastic transformation. *Proc Natl Acad Sci [USA]*, 75:3297-3301, 1978.

Baserga R: *Multiplication and Division in Mammalian Cells*. New York, Marcel Dekker, 1976.

Baserga R: Resting cells and the G1 phase of the cell cycle. *J Cell Physiol* 95:377-386, 1978.

Baserga R: *The Biology of Cell Reproduction*. Cambridge, MA, Harvard University Press, 1985.

Bast RC, Knapp RC: The immunobiology of ovarian cancer. In Griffiths CT, Fuller AF Jr (eds): *Gynecologic Oncology*. The Hague, Martinus Nijhoff, 1983, pp 187-226.

Bender W: Homeotic gene products as growth factors. *Cell* 43:559-560, 1985.

Bennington JL: Cellular kinetics of invasive squamous carcinoma of the human cervix. *Cancer Res* 29:1082-1088, 1969.

Berenblum I: Sequential aspects of chemical carcinogenesis: Skin. In Becker FF (ed): *Cancer*, Vol 1. New York, Plenum Publishing Co, 1975, pp. 323-344.

Berridge MJ: Inositol triphosphate and diacylglycerol, two interacting second messengers. *Ann Rev Biochem* 56:159-193, 1987.

Bettger WJ, Boyce ST, Walthall BJ, Ham RG: Rapid clonal growth and serial passage of human diploid fibroblasts in a lipid-enriched synthetic medium supplemented with epidermal growth factor, insulin, and dexamethasone. *Proc Natl Acad Sci [USA]* 78:5588-5592, 1981.

Bigner SH, Burger PC, Wong AJ, Werner MH, Hamilton SR, Muhlbaier LH, Vogelstein B, Bigner DD: Gene amplification in malignant human gliomas: Clinical and histopathologic aspects. *J Neuropathol Exp Neurol* 47:191-205, 1988.

Bishop JM: The molecular genetics of cancer. *Science* 235:305-311, 1987.

Bishop JM: The molecular genetics of cancer: *Leukemia* 2:199-208, 1988.

Blau HM, Pavlath GK, Hardeman EC, Chiu CP, Silberstein L, Webster SG, Miller SC, Webster C: Plasticity of the differentiated state. *Science* 230:758-766, 1985.

Boothman DA, Pardee AB: Inhibition of radiation-induced neoplastic transformation by beta-lapachone. *Proc Natl Acad Sci [USA]* 86:4963-4967, 1989.

Bourne HR: Signals past, present, and future. In Cold Spring Harbor Symposia on Quantitative Biology, Vol 53, New York, Cold Spring Harbor Laboratory, 1988, pp 1019-1031.

Breitman TR, Collins SJ, Keene BR: Terminal differentiation of human promyelocytic leukemic cells in primary culture in response to retinoic acid. *Blood* 57:1000-1004, 1981.

Bresciani F, Paoluzi R, Benassi M, Nervi C, Casale C, Ziparo E: Cell kinetics and growth of squamous cell carcinomas in man. *Cancer Res* 34:2405-2415, 1974.

Brodeur GM, Seeger RC, Barrett A, Berthold F, Castleberry RP, D'Angio G, De Bernardi B, Evans AE, Favrot M, Freeman AI: International criteria for diagnosis, staging, and response to treatment in patients with neuroblastoma. *J Clin Oncol* 6:1874-1881, 1988.

Brodeur GM, Tsiatis AA, Williams DL, Luthardt FW, Green AA: Statistical analysis of cytogenetic abnormalities in human cancer cells. *Cancer Genet Cytogenet* 7:137-152, 1982.

Cairns J: The origin of human cancers. *Nature* 289:353-357, 1981.

Cairns J, Logan J: Step by step into carcinogenesis. *Nature* 304:582-583, 1983.

Carpenter G, Cohen S: Epidermal growth factor. *Ann Rev Biochem* 48:193-216, 1979.

Challberg MD, Kelly TJ: Animal virus DNA replication. *Ann Rev Biochem* 58:671-717, 1989.

Chambard JC, Franchi A, LeCam A, Pouyssegur J: Growth factor–stimulated protein phosphorylation in G0/G1-arrested fibroblasts. *J Biol Chem* 258:1706-1713, 1983.

Chen LB, Summerhayes I, Hsieh P, Gallimore PH: Possible role of fibronectin in malignancy. *J Supramolec Struct* 12:139-150, 1979.

Cherington PV, Pardee AB: On the basis of loss of the EGF growth requirement by transformed cells. In Cold Spring Harbor Conferences on Cell Proliferation, Vol 9, *Growth of Cells in Hormonally Defined Media*. New York, Cold Spring Harbor Laboratory, 1982.

Cheson BD, Jasperse DM, Chun HG, Friedman MA: Differentiating agents in the treatment of human malignancies. *Cancer Treat Rev* 13:129-145, 1986.

Chiu CP, Blau HM: Reprogramming of cell differentiation in the absence of DNA synthesis. *Cell* 37:359-365, 1984.

Chytil F, Ong DE: Retinoid-binding proteins and human cancer. In Arnott MS, van Eys J, Wang YM (eds): *Molecular Interrelations of Nutrition and Cancer*. New York, Raven Press, 1982, pp 409-416.

Clark GM, Dressler LG, Owens MA, Pounds G, Oldaker T, McGuire WL: Prediction of relapse or survival in patients with node-negative breast cancer by DNA flow cytometry. *N Engl J Med* 320:627-633, 1989.

Clarkson B, Ota K, Ohkita T, O'Connor A: Kinetics of proliferation of cancer cells in neoplastic effusions in man. *Cancer* 1118:1189-1213, 1965.

Cold Spring Harbor Symposium on Quantitative Biology, Vol 46: *Organization of the Cytoplasm*. New York, Cold Spring Harbor Laboratory, 1982.

Colberg-Poley AM, Voss SD, Chowdhury K, Gruss P: Structural analysis of murine genes containing homeobox sequences and their expression in embryonal carcinoma cells. *Nature* 314:713-718, 1985.

Cooper GM, Lan MA, Krontiris TG, Gougin G: Analysis of cellular transforming genes by transfection. *Adv Virol Oncol* 1:243-257, 1982.

Coppola JA, Parker JM, Schuler, GD, Cole MD: Continued withdrawal from the cell cycle and regulation of cellular genes in mouse erythroleukemia cells blocked in differentiation by the c-myc oncogene. *Molec Cell Biol* 9:1714-1720, 1989.

Crabtree GR: Contingent genetic regulatory events in T lymphocyte activation. *Science* 243:355-361, 1989.

Croy RG, Pardee AB: Enhanced synthesis and stabilization of Mr 68,000 protein in transformed BALB/c-3T3 cells: Candidate for restriction point control of cell growth. *Proc Natl Acad Sci [USA]* 80:4699-4703, 1983.

Darmon M, Stallcup WB, Pittman QJ: Induction of neural differentiation by serum deprivation in cultures of the embryonal carcinoma cell line 1003. *Exp Cell Res* 138:73-78, 1982.

Davis RL, Weintraub H, Lassar AB: Expression of a single transfected cDNA converts fibroblasts to myoblasts. *Cell* 51:987-1000, 1987.

Delhanty JJA, Davis MB, Wood J: Chromosome instability in lymphocytes, fibroblasts, and colon epithelial-like cells from patients with familial polyposis coli. *Cancer Genet Cytogenet* 8:27-50, 1983.

Denhardt DT, Edwards DR, Parfett CLJ: Gene expression during the mammalian cell cycle. *Biochim Biophys Acta* 865:83-125, 1986.

Deuel TF, Huang JS, Huang SS, Stroobant P, Waterfield MD: Expression of a platelet-derived growth factor–like protein in simian sarcoma virus transformed cells. *Science* 221:1348-1350, 1983.

Distel RJ, Spiegelman BM: Involvement of fos as a trans-acting factor in adipogenic gene expression. *Progr Clin Biol Res* 284:187-209, 1988.

Doerfler W: DNA methylation and gene activation. *Ann Rev Biochem* 52:93-124, 1983.

Donahoe PK, Budzik GP, Telstad R, Mudgett-Hunter M, Fuller AF Jr, Hutson JJ, Ikawa H, Hayashi A, MacLaughlin D: Müllerian inhibitory substance—An update. *Rec Progr Hormone Res* 38:279-330, 1982.

Duesberg PH: Retroviral transforming genes in normal cells? *Nature* 304:219-226, 1983.

Dulbecco R: Topoinhibition and serum requirement for transformed and untransformed cells. *Nature* 227:802-806, 1970.

Edgar LG, McGhee JD: DNA synthesis and the control of embryonic gene expression in *C. elegans*. *Cell* 53:589-599, 1988.

Ehrlich M, Wang RY-H: 5-Methylcytosine in eukaryotic DNA. *Science* 212:1350-1357, 1981.

Elias PM, Williams MC: Retinoids, cancer and the skin. *Arch Dermatol* 117:160-181, 1981.

Fabrikant JI, Cherry J: The kinetics of cellular proliferation in normal and malignant tissues. *J Surg Oncol* 1:23-47, 1969.

Fakuda K, Iwasaka T, Hachisuga TD, Sugimon HK, Taugitomi H, Mutch F: Immunocytochemical detection of S-phase cells in normal and neoplastic cervical epithelium by anti-BrDu monoclonal antibody. *Anal Quant Cytol Histol* 12:135-138, 1990.

Fearon ER, Feinberg AP, Hamilton SR, Vogelstein B: Loss of genes on the short arm of chromosome 11 in bladder cancer. *Nature* 318:377-380, 1985.

Feinberg AP, Vogelstein B: Hypomethylation distinguishes genes of some human cancers from their normal counterparts. *Nature* 301:89-92, 1983.

Felsenfeld G, McGhee J: Methylation and gene control. *Nature* 296:602-603, 1982.

Fettig O, Sievers R: 3H-index und mittlere Generationszeit des menschlichen Portiokarzinoms und seiner Vorstufen. *Beitr Pathol* 133:83-100, 1966.

Fialkow PJ: Clonal origin of human tumors. *Ann Rev Med* 20:135-143, 1979.

Fingert HJ, Chen Z, Mizrahi N, Gajewski WH, Bamberg MP, Kradin RL: Rapid growth of human cancer cells in a mouse model with fibrin clot subrenal capsule assay. *Cancer Res* 47:3824-3829, 1987.

Finlay CA, Hinds PW, Levine AJ: The p53 proto-oncogene can act as a suppressor of transformation. *Cell* 57:1083-1093, 1989.

Folkman J: Tumor invasion and metastasis. In Liotta LA, Hart IR (eds): *Pathogenesis of Cancer*. The Hague, Martinus Nijhoff, 1982, pp 167-176.

Folkman J, Watson K, Ingber D, Hanahan D: Induction of angiogenesis during the transition from hyperplasia to neoplasia. *Nature* 339:58-61, 1989.

Ford LC, Berek JS, Lagasse LD, Hacker NF, Heins YL, DeLange RJ: Estrogen and progesterone receptor sites in malignancies of the uterine cervix, vagina, and vulva. *Gynecol Oncol* 15:27-31, 1983.

Foulds L: *Neoplastic Development*, Vols I and II. New York, Academic Press, 1975.

Friedman SJ, Skehan P: Morphological differentiation of human choriocarcinoma cells induced by methotrexate. *Cancer Res* 39: 1960-1967, 1979.

Fu Y-S, Regan JW, Richart RM: Definition of precursors. *Gynecol Oncol* 12:5220-5231, 1981.

Gazdar AF, Steinberg SM, Russell EK, Oie H, Ghosh B, Cotelingham J, Minna J, Ihde D: Correlation of in vitro drug-sensitivity testing results with response to chemotherapy and survival in extensive-stage small cell lung cancer: A prospective clinical trial. *J Natl Cancer Inst* 82:117-124, 1990.

Geiger B: Membrane-cytoskeletal interaction. *Biochim Biophys Acta* 737:305-341, 1983.

Gershwin ME, Castles JJ, Makishima R: Accelerated plasmacytoma formation in mice treated with alpha-fetoprotein. *J Natl Cancer Instit* 64:145-150, 1980.

Goelz SE, Vogelstein B, Hamilton SR, Feinberg AP: Hypomethylation of DNA from benign and malignant human colon neoplasms. *Science* 228:187-190, 1985.

Goldin A, Shepartz SA, Venditti JM, DeVita VT Jr: Historical development and current strategy of the National Cancer Institute Drug Development Program (Chap 5). In Devita VT Jr, Busch H (eds): *Methods in Cancer Research*, Vol l6: *Cancer Drug Development*. New York, Academic Press, 1979, pp 165-245.

Gospodarowicz D, Moran JS: Review on growth factors. *Ann Rev Biochem* 45:531-558, 1976.

Gospodarowicz D, Vlodavsky I, Greenburg G, Johnson LK: Cellular shape is determined by the extracellular matrix and is responsible for the control of cellular growth and function. In Sato GH, Ross R (eds): *Hormones and Cell Culture*. New York, Cold Spring Harbor Laboratory, 1979, pp 561-592.

Goustin AS, Leof EB, Shipley GD, Moses HL: Growth factors and cancer. *Cancer Res* 46:1015-1025, 1986.

Graf T, Beug H: Role of the v-erbA and v-erbB oncogenes of avian erythroblastosis virus in erythroid cell transformation. *Cell* 34:7-9, 1983.

Green H, Meuth M: An established pre-adiposite cell line and its differentiation in culture. *Cell* 3:127-133, 1974.

Green MR: Where the products of oncogenes and anti-oncogenes meet. *Cell* 56:1-3, 1989.

Guerin M, Le MG, Travagli JP, Riou GF: Expression of c-myb and pS2 genes in inflammatory breast cancer: Association with a longer relapse-free survival. *Proc Am Soc Clin Oncol* 8:30, 1989.

Hall AK: Stem cell is a stem cell is a stem cell. *Cell* 33:11-12, 1983.

Hamburger AW, Salmon SE: Primary bioassay of human tumor stem cells. *Science* 197:461-463, 1977.

Hamburger AW, White CP: Interaction between macrophages and human tumor clonogenic cells. *Stem Cells* 1:209-223, 1981.

Hanawalt PC, Cooper PK, Ganesan AK, Smith CA: DNA repair in bacteria and mammalian cells. *Ann Rev Biochem* 48:783-836, 1979.

Harding K, Wedeen C, McGinnis W, Levine M: Spatially regulated expression of homeotic genes in *Drosophila*. *Science* 229:1236-1242, 1985.

Hawkes S, Wang JL: *Extracellular Matrix*. New York, Academic Press, 1982.

Hay ED (ed): *Cell Biology of Extracellular Matrix*. New York, Plenum Press, 1981.

Hayflick L, Moorhead PS: The serial cultivation of human diploid cell strains. *Exp Cell Res* 25:585-621, 1961.

Heath J, Bell S, Rees AR: Appearance of functional insulin receptors during the differentiation of embryonal carcinoma cells. *J Cell Biol* 91:293-297, 1981.

Hellman S, DeVita VT Jr: Principles of cancer biology: Kinetics of cellular proliferation. In DeVita VT Jr, Hellman S, Rosenberg SA (eds): *Cancer—Principles and Practice of Oncology*, 2nd ed. Philadelphia, JB Lippincott Co, 1982, pp 73-78.

Hendy IP, Cox H, Evan GI, Watson JV: Flow cytometric quantitation of DNA and c-myc oncoprotein in archival biopsies of uterine cervix neoplasia. *Br J Cancer* 55:275-282, 1987.

Heppner GH, Miller BE: Therapeutic implications of tumor heterogeneity. *Semin Oncol* 16:91-105, 1989.

Hewlett G, Opitz HG, Schlumberger HD, Lemke H: Growth regulation of a murine lymphoma cell line by a 2-mercaptoethanol or macrophage-activated serum factor. *Eur J Immunol* 7:781-785, 1977.

Hochhauser SJ, Stein JL, Stein GS: Gene expression and cell cycle regulation. *Int Rev Cytol* 71:96-243, 1981.

Hogan B: Homeo boxes and strings for the packaging of genes? *Nature* 314:670-671, 1985.

Housey GM, Johnson MD, Hsiao WL, O'Brian CA, Murphy JP, Kirschmeier P, Weinstein IB: Overproduction of protein kinase C causes disordered growth control in rat fibroblasts. *Cell* 52:343-354, 1988.

Huang HJS, Yee JK, Shew JY, Chen PL, Bookstein R, Friedmann T, Lee EY, Lee WH: Suppression of the neoplastic phenotype by replacement of the RB gene in human cancer cells. *Science* 242:1563-1566, 1989.

Hynes RO: Integrins: A family of cell surface receptors. *Cell* 48:549-554, 1987.

Hynes RO, Fox CF (eds): *Tumor Cell Surfaces and Malignancy*. New York, Alan R Liss, 1980.

Igo-Kemenes T, Horz W, Zachau HG: Chromatin. *Ann Rev Biochem* 51:89-121, 1982.

Isaacs JT, Wake N, Coffey DS, Sandberg AA: Genetic stability coupled to clonal selection as a mechanism for tumor progression in the

Dunning R-3327 rat prostatic adenocarcinoma system. *Cancer Res* 42:2353-2361, 1982.

Ishii Y, Elliot JA, Mishra NK, Lieberman MW: Quantitative studies of transformation by chemical carcinogen and ultraviolet radiation using a subclone of BHK2l clone l3 Syrian hamster cells. *Cancer Res* 37:2023-2029, 1977.

Jackson IJ, Schofield P, Hogan B: A mouse homeobox gene is expressed during embryogenesis and in adult kidney. *Nature* 317:745-747, 1985.

Johnson PF, McKnight SL: Eukaryotic transcriptional regulatory proteins. *Ann Rev Biochem* 58:799-840, 1989.

Jones PA, Taylor SM: Cellular differentiation, cytidine analogues and DNA methylation. *Cell* 28:85-93, 1980.

Kacinski BM, Carter D, Mittal K, Kohorn EI, Bloodgood RS, Donahue J, Donofrio L, Edwards R, Schwartz PE, Chambers JT: High level expression of fms proto-oncogene mRNA is observed in clinically aggressive human endometrial adenocarcinomas. *Int J Radiat Oncol Biol Phys* 15:823-829, 1988.

Kakunaga T: A quantitative system for assay of malignant transformation by chemical carcinogens using a clone derived from Balb/3T3. *Int J Cancer* 12:463-473, 1973.

Kakunaga T: Neoplastic transformation of human diploid fibroblast cells by chemical carcinogens. *Proc Natl Acad Sci [USA]* 75:1334-1338, 1978.

Kallioniemi O, Punnonen R, Mattila J, Lehtinen M, Koivula T: Prognostic significance of DNA index, multiploidy, and S-phase fraction in ovarian cancer. *Cancer* 61:334-339, 1988.

Ke Y, Reddel R, Gerwin BI, Miyashita M, McMenamin M, Lechner JF, Harris CC: Human bronchial epithelial cells with integrated SV40 virus T antigens retain the ability to undergo squamous differentiation. *Differentiation* 38:60-66, 1988.

Kennedy AR, Fox M, Murphy G, Little JB: Relationship between x-ray exposure and malignant transformation in C3Hl0T l/2 cells. *Proc Natl Acad Sci [USA]* 77:7262-7266, 1980.

Keshet I, Lieman-Hurwitz J, Cedar H: DNA methylation affects the formation of active chromatin. *Cell* 44:535-543, 1986.

Kim K, Blechman WJ, Riddle VGH, Pardee AB: Basis of observed resistance of Ll2l0 leukemia in mice to methotrexate, 6-thioguanine, 6-methylmercaptopurine riboside, 6-mercaptopurine, 5-fluorouracil and l-B-D arabinofuranosylcytosine administered in different combinations. *Cancer Res* 41:4529-4534, 1981.

Klein G: The role of gene dosage and genetic transpositions in carcinogenesis. *Nature* 294:313-318, 1981.

Knoerr-Gaertner H, Schuhmann R, Kraus H, Uebele-Kallhardt B: Comparative cytogenetic and histologic studies on early malignant transformation in mesothelial tumors of the ovary. *Hum Genet* 35:281-297, 1977.

Kodama M, Kodama T: Relation between steroid metabolism of the host and genesis of cancers of the breast, uterine cervix and endometrium. *Adv Cancer Res* 38:77-120, 1983.

Kolata G: Fitting methylation into development. *Science* 228:1183-1184, 1985.

Koller CA, Miller DM: Preliminary observations on the therapy of the myeloid blast phase of chronic granulocytic leukemia with plicamycin and hydroxyurea. *N Engl J Med* 315:1433-1438, 1986.

Koller CA, Campbell VW, Polansky DA, Mulhern A, Miller DM: In vivo differentiation of blast-phase chronic granulocytic leukemia. *J Clin Invest* 76:365-369, 1985.

Krontiris TG, Cooper GM: Transforming activity of human tumor DNAs. *Proc Natl Acad Sci [USA]* 78:1181-1184, 1981.

Land H, Parada LF, Weinberg RA: Tumorigenic conversion of primary embryo fibroblasts requires at least two cooperating oncogenes. *Nature* 304:596-601, 1983.

LaRosa GJ, Gudas LJ: Early retinoic acid—induced F9 teratocarcinoma stem cell gene REA-l: Alternate splicing creates transcripts for a homeobox-containing protein and one lacking the homeobox. *Molec Cell Biol* 8:3906-3917, 1988.

Lathrop B, Thomas K, Glaser L: Control of myogenic differentiation by fibroblast growth factor is mediated by position in the G1 phase of the cell cycle. *J Cell Biol* 101:2194-2198, 1985.

Lau CC, Pardee AB: Mechanism by which caffeine potentiates lethality of nitrogen mustard. *Proc Natl Acad Sci [USA]* 79:2942-2946, 1982.

Lawler SD, Summersgill BM, McElvain TJ: Cytogenetic studies in patients previously treated for Hodgkin's disease. *Cancer Genet Cytogenet* 5:25-35, 1982.

Lee JH, Kavanagh JJ, Wharton JT, Wildrick DM, Blick M: Allele loss at the c-Ha-ras1 locus in human ovarian cancer. *Cancer Res* 49:1220-1222, 1989.

Lehman JM, Speers WC, Swartzendruber DE, Pierce GB: Neoplastic differentiation: Characteristics of cell lines derived from a murine teratocarcinoma. *J Cell Physiol* 84:13-28, 1974.

Leof EB, Wharton W, Van Wyk JJ, Pledger WJ: Epidermal growth factor and somatomedin C regulate Gl progression in competent Balb/c3T3 cells. *Exp Cell Res* 141:107-115, 1982.

Leone LA, Meitner PA, Myers TJ, Grace WR, Gajewski WH, Fingert HJ, Rotman B: Predictive value of the Fluorescent Cytoprint Assay (FCA): A retrospective correlation study of *in vitro* chemosensitivity and individual responses to chemotherapy. *Cancer Invest* 9:491-503, 1991.

Ley TJ, DeSimone J, Anagnou NP, Keller GH, Humphries RR, Turner PH, Young NS, Heller P, Nienhuis AW: 5-Azacytidine selectively increases gamma globulin synthesis in a patient with beta$^+$ thalassemia. *N Engl J Med* 307:1469-1475, 1982.

Liau G, Ong DE, Chytil F: Interaction of retinol/cellular retinol-binding protein complex with isolated nuclei and nuclear components. *J Cell Biol* 91:63-68, 1981.

Linkhart TA, Clegg CH, Hauschka SD: Control of mouse myoblast commitment to terminal differentiation by mitogens. *J Supramol Struct* 14:483-498, 1980.

Liotta LA: Tumor invasion and metastases—Role of the extracellular matrix. *Cancer Res* 46:1-7, 1986.

Long CA, O'Brien TJ, Sanders MM, Bard DS, Quirk JG: Ras oncogene is expressed in adenocarcinoma of the endometrium. *Am J Obstet Gynecol* 159:1512-1516, 1988.

Lotem J, Sachs L: Mechanisms that uncouple growth and differentiation in myeloid leukemia cells: Restoration of requirement for normal growth-inducing protein without restoring induction of differentiation-inducing protein. *Proc Natl Acad Sci [USA]* 79:4347-4351, 1982.

Ludlow JW, De Caprio JA, Huang CM, Lee WH, Paucha E, Livingston DM: SV40 large T antigen binds preferentially to an under-phosphorylated member of the retinoblastoma susceptibility gene product family. *Cell* 56:57-65, 1989.

Mackillop WJ, Buick RN: Cellular heterogeneity in human ovarian carcinoma studied by density gradient fractionation. *Stem Cells* 1:355-366, 1982.

Mackillop WJ, Trent JM, Stewart SS, Buick RN: Tumor progression studied by analysis of cellular features of serial ascitic ovarian carcinoma tumors. *Cancer Res* 43:874-878, 1983.

Macpherson I, Montagnier L: Agar suspension culture for the selective assay of cells transformed by polyoma virus. *Virology* 23:291-294, 1964.

Malogolowkin MH, Ortega JA, Krailo M, Gonzalez O, Mahour GH, Landing BH, Siegel SE: Immature teratomas: Identification of patients at risk for malignant recurrence. *J Natl Cancer Instit* 81:870-874, 1989.

Martin GR: Teratocarcinomas and mammalian embryogenesis. *Science* 209:768-776, 1980.

Martin, GR: Isolation of a pluripotent cell line from early mouse embryos cultured in medium conditioned by teratocarcinoma stem cells. *Proc Natl Acad Sci [USA]* 78:7634-7638, 1981.

Martin GR, Evans MG: Differentiation of clonal lines of teratocarcinoma cells: Formation of embryoid bodies in vitro. *Proc Natl Acad Sci [USA]* 72:1441-1445, 1975.

Martin JD, Hahnel R, McCartney AJ, Woodings T: Prognostic value of estrogen receptors in cancer of the uterine cervix. *N Engl J Med* 306:485, 1982.

Mathis D, Oudet P, Chambon P: Structure of transcribing chromatin. *Progr NA Res Mol Biol* 24:2-55, 1980.

McCarty KS, Miller LS, Cox EB, Konrath J: Estrogen receptor analyses. Correlation of biochemical and immunohistochemical methods using monoclonal antireceptor antibodies. *Arch Pathol Lab Med* 109:716-721, 1985.

McClain DA, Edelman GM: Density dependent inhibition of cell growth by agents that disrupt microtubules. *Proc Natl Acad Sci [USA]* 77:2748-2752, 1980.

McCormick F: Ras GTPase activating protein: Signal transmitter and signal terminator. *Cell* 56:5-8, 1989.

McGuire WL, Clark GM: Prognostic factors in breast cancer. *Semin Surg Oncol* 5:102-110, 1989.

Medrano EE, Pardee AB: Prevalent deficiency in tumor cells of cycloheximide-induced cycle arrest. *Proc Natl Acad Sci [USA]* 77:4123-4126, 1980.

Metcalf D: *Hematopoietic Colonies*. New York, Springer-Verlag, 1977.

Meyer JS: Growth and cell kinetic measurements in human tumors. *Pathol Ann* 16(2):53-81, 1981.

Mintz B, Fleischman RA: Teratocarcinoma and other neoplasms as developmental defects in gene expression. *Adv Cancer Res* 34:211-278, 1981.

Mitchell PJ, Tjian R: Transcriptional regulation in mammalian cells by sequence-specific DNA binding proteins. *Science* 245:371-378, 1989.

Mulvihill JJ: Genetic repertory of human cancer. *Progr Cancer Res Ther* 3:137-143, 1977.

Murnane MJ, Sheahan K, Ozdemirli M, Shuja S: Stage-specific increases in cathepsin B messenger RNA content in human colorectal carcinoma. *Cancer Res* 51:1137-1142, 1991.

Murray MJ, Cunningham JM, Parada LF, Dautry F, Lebowitz P, Weinberg RA: The HL-60 transforming sequence: A ras oncogene coexisting with altered myc genes in hematopoietic tumors. *Cell* 33:749-757, 1983.

Nadal-Ginard B: Commitment, fusion and biochemical differentiation of a myogenic cell line in the absence of DNA synthesis. *Cell* 15:855-864, 1978.

Nam JH, Cole LA, Chambers JT, Schwartz PE: Urinary gonadotropin fragment, a new tumor marker. *Gynecol Oncol* 36:383-390, 1990.

Nand S, Messmore H: Hemostasis in Malignancy. *Am J Hematol* 35:45-55, 1990.

Nicolson GL: Cancer metastasis: Organ colonization and the cell-surface properties of malignant cells. *Biochim Biophys Acta* 695:113-176, 1982.

Noda M, Kitayama H, Matsuzaki T, Sugimoto Y, Okayama H, Bassin RH, Ikawa Y: Detection of genes with a potential for suppressing the transformed phenotype associated with activated ras genes. *Proc Natl Acad Sci [USA]* 86:162-166, 1989.

Oren M, Maltzman W, Levine A: Post-translational regulation of the 54K cellular tumor antigen in normal and transformed cells. *Molec Cell Biol* 1:101-110, 1981.

Pai SB, Steele VE, Nettesheim P: Identification of early carcinogen-induced changes in nutritional and substrate requirements in cultured tracheal epithelial cells. *Carcinogenesis* 3:1201-1206, 1982.

Pardee AB: A restriction point for control of normal animal cell proliferation. *Proc Natl Acad Sci [USA]* 71:1286-1290, 1974.

Pardee AB: Principles of cancer biology. In DeVita VT Jr, Hellman S, Rosenberg SA (eds): *Cancer—Principles and Practice of Oncology*, 2nd ed. Philadelphia, JB Lippincott Co, 1982, pp 59-72.

Pardee AB: Molecules involved in proliferation of normal and cancer cells. *Cancer Res* 47:1488-1491, 1987.

Pardee AB: G1 events and regulation of cell proliferation. *Science* 246:603-608, 1989.

Pardee AB, Medrano EE, Rossow PW: A labile protein model for growth control of mammalian cells. In Ritzen M, et al (eds): *The Biology of Normal Human Growth*. New York, Raven Press, 1981, pp 59-69.

Parshad RR, Sanford KK, Jones GM: Chromatid damage after G2 phase X-irradiation of cells from cancer-prone individuals implicates deficiency in DNA repair. *Proc Natl Acad Sci [USA]* 80:5612-5616, 1983.

Pecoraro G, Morgan D, Defendi V: Differential effects of human papillomavirus type 6, 16, and 18 DNAs on immortalization and transformation of human cervical epithelial cells. *Proc Natl Acad Sci [USA]* 86:563-567, 1989.

Perona R, Serrano R: Increased pH and tumorigenicity of fibroblasts expressing a yeast proton pump. *Nature* 334:438-440, 1988.

Pierce BG, Pantazis GG, Caldwell JE, Wells RS: Specificity of the control of tumor formation by the blastocyst. *Cancer Res* 42:1082-1087, 1982.

Pietras RJ, Roberts JA: Cathepsin B–like enzymes. *J Biol Chem* 256:8536-8544, 1981.

Pinney DF, Pearson-White SH, Konieczny SF, Latham KE, Emerson CP: Myogenic lineage determination and differentiation: Evidence for a regulatory gene pathway. *Cell* 53:781-793, 1988.

Pitot HC: *Fundamentals of Oncology*. New York, Marcel Dekker, 1981, p 19.

Polacarz SV, Hey NA, Stephenson TJ, Hill AS: C-myc oncogene product p62c-myc in ovarian mucinous neoplasms: Immunohistochemical study correlated with malignancy. *J Clin Pathol* 42:148-152, 1989.

Pollack R, Osborn M, Weber K: Patterns of organization of actin and myosin in normal and transformed cultured cells. *Proc Natl Acad Sci [USA]* 72:994-998, 1975.

Ponten J: The relationship between in vitro transformation and tumor formation in vivo. *Biochim Biophys Acta* 458:397-422, 1976.

Potter VR: Mechanisms of carcinogenesis in relation to studies on minimal deviation hepatomas. In *Exploitable Molecular Mechanisms and Neoplasia*. Austin, University of Texas Press, 1968, pp 587-610.

Pratt WB, Ruddon RW: *The Anticancer Drugs*. New York, Oxford University Press, 1979.

Rafferty KA Jr: Epithelial cells: Growth in culture of normal and neoplastic forms. *Adv Cancer Res* 21:249-272, 1975.

Rao PN, Sunkara PS: *Cell Cycle Regulation*. New York, Academic Press, 1978, pp 133-147.

Rao PN, Johnson RT, Sperling K (eds): *Premature Chromosome Condensation*. New York, Academic Press, 1982.

Reddy GPV, Pardee AB: Multienzyme complex for metabolic channeling in mammalian DNA replication. *Proc Natl Acad Sci [USA]* 77:3312-3316, 1980.

Rees AR, Adamson ED, Grahm CF: Epidermal growth factor receptors increase during differentiation of embryonal carcinoma cells. *Nature* 281:309-311, 1979.

Reich E, Rifkin D, Shaw T (eds): *Proteases and Biological Control*. New York, Cold Spring Harbor Laboratory, 1975, pp 1-1021.

Rheinwald JG, Beckett MA: Defective terminal differentiation in culture as a consistent and selectable character of malignant human keratinocytes. *Cell* 22:629-632, 1980.

Riddle VGH, Rossow PW, Boorstein RJ, Adonizio ML, Pardee AB: Can a fibroblast teach a lymphocyte anything useful? In Kaplan JG (ed): *The Molecular Basis of Immune Cell Function*. Amsterdam, Elsevier/North-Holland Biomedical Press, 1979, pp 29-37.

Riedel H, Dull TJ, Honegger AM, Schlessinger J, Ullrich A: Cytoplasmic domains determine signal specificity, cellular routine characteristics and influence ligand binding of epidermal growth factor and insulin receptors. *EMBO J* 8:2943-2954, 1989.

Rinkus SJ, Legator MS: Chemical characterization of 465 known or suspected carcinogens and their correlation with mutagenic activity in the *Salmonella typhimurium* system. *Cancer Res* 39:3289-3318, 1979.

Riou GF: Proto-oncogenes and prognosis in early carcinoma of the uterine cervix. *Cancer Surv* 7:441-456, 1988.

Riou GF, Barrois M, Sheng ZM, Duvillard P, Lhomme C: Somatic deletions and mutations of c-Ha-ras gene in human cervical cancers. *Oncogene* 3:329-333, 1988.

Riou GF, Barrois M, Tordjam I, Dutronquay V, Orth G: Presence de génomes de papillomavirus et amplification des oncogénes c-myc et c-Ha-ras dans des cancers envahissants du col de l'uterus. *CR Acad Sci* 299:575-580, 1984.

Rissino A: Two multipotent embryonal carcinoma cell lines irreversibly differentiate in defined media. *Dev Biol* 95:126-136, 1983.

Robbins DM, Ripley S, Henderson AS, Axel R: Transforming DNA integrates into the host chromosome. *Cell* 23:29-39, 1981.

Rosenstraus MJ, Sundell CL, Liskay RM: Cell cycle characteristics of undifferentiated and differentiating embryonal carcinoma cells. *Dev Biol* 89:516-520, 1982.

Rossow PW, Riddle VGH, Pardee AB: Synthesis of labile, serum-dependent protein in early GI controls animal cell growth. *Proc Natl Acad Sci [USA]* 76:4446-4450, 1979.

Rothfels K, Parker RC: The karyotypes of cell lines recently established from normal mouse tissue. *J Exp Zool* 142:507-519, 1959.

Rothstein H: Regulation of the cell cycle by somatomedins. *Int Rev Cytol* 78:127-232, 1982.

Rotman B, Teplitz C, Dickinson K, Cozzolino JP: Individual human tumors in short-term micro-organ cultures: Chemosensitivity testing by fluorescent cytoprinting. *In Vitro Cell Dev Biol* 24:1137-1146, 1988.

Rowley JF, Testa JR: Chromosome abnormalities in malignant hematologic disease. *Adv Cancer Res* 36:103-148, 1982.

Rozengurt E: Early signals in the mitogenic response. *Science* 234:161-166, 1986.

Rubin JB, Shia MA, Pilch PF: Stimulation of tyrosine specific phosphorylation in vitro by insulin-like growth factor 1. *Nature* 305:438-440, 1983.

Sachs L: Constitutive uncoupling of pathways of gene expression that control growth and differentiation in myeloid leukemia: A model for the origin and progression of malignancy. *Proc Natl Acad Sci [USA]* 77:6152-6156, 1980a.

Sachs L: Constitutive uncoupling of the controls in growth and differentiation in myeloid leukemia and the development of cancer. *J Natl Cancer Instit* 65:675-679, 1980b.

Sagae S, Kuzumaki N, Hisada T, Mugikura Y, Kudo R, Hashimoto M: Ras oncogene expression and prognosis of invasive squamous cell carcinomas of the uterine cervix. *Cancer* 63:1577-1582, 1989.

Sager R: Genomic rearrangements and the origin of cancer. In German J (ed): *Chromosome Mutation and Neoplasia.* New York, Alan R Liss, 1983, pp 333-346.

Sager R: Tumor suppressor genes: The puzzle and the promise. *Science* 246:1406-1412, 1989.

Sager R, Kovac PE: Genetic analysis of tumorigenesis. Expression of tumor-forming ability in hamster hybrid cell lines. *J Somatic Cell Genet* 4:375-392, 1978.

Sager R, Kovac PE: Pre-adipocyte determination either by insulin or by 5-azacytidine. *Proc Natl Acad Sci [USA]* 79:480-484, 1982.

Salmon SE: Perspectives on future directions. In Salmon SE (ed): *Cloning of Human Tumor Stem Cells.* New York, Alan R Liss, 1980, pp 315-327.

Salmon SE, Hamburger AW, Soehnlen B, Durie BGM, Alberts DS, Moon TE: Quantitation of differential sensitivity of human tumor stem cells to anticancer drugs. *N Engl J Med* 298:1321-1327, 1978.

Sandberg AA, Abe S, Kowalczyk JR, Zedgenidze A, Teuchi J, Kakati S: Chromosomes and causation of human cancer and leukemia. 1. Cytogenetics of leukemias complicating other disease. *Cancer Genet Cytogenet* 7:95-136, 1982.

Scalabrino G, Feriola ME: Polyamines in mammalian tumors, Part 1. *Adv Cancer Res* 35:152-268, 1981.

Scalabrino G, Feriola ME: Polyamines in mammalian tumors, Part 2. *Adv Cancer Res* 36:12-102, 1982.

Scher CD, Shepard RC, Antoniades HN, Stiles CD: Platelet-derived growth factor and the regulation of the mammalian fibroblast cell cycle. *Biochim Biophys Acta* 560:217-241, 1979.

Scher W, Scher BM, Waxman S: Nuclear events during differentiation of erythroleukemia cells. In Dunn DCR (ed): *Current Concepts in Erythropoiesis.* Chichester, John Wiley and Sons, Ltd, 1983.

Schimke RN, Madigan CM, Silver BJ, Fabian CJ, Stephens RL: Choriocarcinoma, thyrotoxicosis, and the Klinefelter syndrome. *Cancer Genet Cytogenet* 9:108, 1983.

Schimke RT (ed): *Gene Amplification.* New York, Cold Spring Harbor Laboratory, 1982.

Schwartz PE, Setsuko KC, Chambers JT, Gutmann J, Katopodis N, Foemmel R: Circulating tumor markers in the monitoring of gynecologic malignancies. *Cancer* 60:353-361, 1987.

Scott RE, Hoerl BJ, Willie JJ, Florine DL, Krawisz BR, Kankatsu Y: Coupling of preadipocyte growth arrest and differentiation. II. A cell cycle model for the physiological control of cell proliferation. *J Cell Biol* 94:400-405, 1982.

Selby P, Buick RN, Tannock I: A critical appraisal of the "human tumor stem-cell assay." *N Engl J Med* 308:129-134, 1983.

Shih S, Shilo BZ, Goldfarb MP, Dannenberg A, Weinberg RA: Passage of phenotypes of chemically transformed cells via transfection of DNA and chromatin. *Proc Natl Acad Sci [USA]* 76:5714-5718, 1979.

Skipper HE, Schabel FM Jr: Quantitative and cytokinetic studies in experimental tumor systems. In Holland JF, Frei E III (eds): *Cancer Medicine.* Philadelphia, Lea and Febiger, 1982, pp 663-684.

Slamon DJ, Godolphin W, Jones LA, Holt JA, Wong SG, Keith DE, Levin WJ, Stuart SG, Udove J, Ullrich A, Press MF: Studies of the HER-2/neu proto-oncogene in human breast and ovarian cancer. *Science* 244:707-712, 1989.

Sledge GW Jr, McGuire WL: Steroid receptors in human breast cancer. *Adv Cancer Res* 38:61-76, 1983.

Smith HS, Springer EL, Hackett AJ: Nuclear ultrastructure of epithelial cell lines derived from human carcinomas and nonmalignant tissues. *Cancer Res* 39:332-344, 1979.

Sowani A, Ong G, Dische S, Quinn C, White J, Soutter P, Waxman J, Sikora K: C-myc oncogene expression and clinical outcome in carcinoma of the cervix. *Molec Cell Probes* 3:117-123, 1989.

Speers WC: Conversion of malignant murine embryonal carcinomas to benign teratocarcinomas by chemical induction of differentiation in vivo. *Cancer Res* 42:1843-1849, 1982.

Sporn MB, Roberts, AB: Role of retinoids in differentiation and carcinogenesis. *Cancer Res* 43:3034-3040, 1983.

Sporn MB, Roberts AB (eds): *Peptide Growth Factors and Their Receptors.* Heidelberg, Springer-Verlag, 1989.

Spremulli EN, Dexter DL: Human tumor cell heterogeneity and metastasis. *J Clin Oncol* 1:496-509, 1983.

Stanbridge EJ, Der CJ, Doersen CJ, Hishimi RY, Peehl DM, Weissman BE, Wilkinson JE: Human cell hybrids: Analysis of transformation and tumorigenicity. *Science* 215:252-259, 1982.

Steel GG: Cell loss as a factor in the growth rate of human tumors. *Eur J Cancer* 3:381-387, 1967.

Stevens LC: The development of transplantable teratocarcinomas from intratesticular grafts of pre- and post-implantation mouse embryos. *Dev Biol* 21:364-382, 1970.

Stiles CD: The molecular biology of platelet-derived growth factors. *Cell* 33:653-655, 1983.

Stiles CD, Desmond W, Chuman LM, Sato G, Saier MH Jr: Relationship of cell growth behavior in vitro to tumorigenicity in athymic nude mice. *Cancer Res* 36:3300-3305, 1976.

Stillman B : Initiation of eukaryotic DNA replication in vitro. *Bioassays* 9:56-60, 1988.

Strickland S, Mahdavi V: The induction of differentiation in teratocarcinoma stem cells by retinoic acid. *Cell* 15:393-403, 1978.

Tandon AK, Clark GM, Chamness GC, Ullrich A, McGuire WL: HER-2/neu oncogene protein and prognosis in breast cancer. *J Clin Oncol* 7:1120-1128, 1989a.

Tandon AK, Clark GM, Chamness GC, Chirgwin J, McGuire W: Cathepsin D and prognosis in breast cancer. *N Engl J Med* 322:297-302, 1990.

Tannock IF: The relation between cell proliferation and the vascular system in a transplanted mouse mammary tumour. *Br J Cancer* 22:258-273, 1968.

Tannock I: Cell kinetics and chemotherapy: A critical review. *Cancer Treat Rep* 62:1117-1133, 1978.

Thor AD, Schwartz LH, Koerner FC, Edgerton SM, Skates SJ, Yin S, McKenzie SJ, Panicali DL, Marks PJ, Fingert HJ, Wood WC: Analysis of c-erbB-2 expression in breast carcinomas with clinical follow-up. *Cancer Res* 49:7147-7152, 1989.

Thorpe SM, Rochefort H, Garcia M, Freiss G, Christiensen IJ, Khalaf S, Paolucci F, Pau B, Rasmussen BB, Rose C: Association between high concentrations of Mr 52,000 cathepsin D and poor prognosis in primary human breast cancer. *Cancer Res* 49:6008-6014, 1989.

Thun MJ, Namboodiri MM, Heath CW: Aspirin use and reduced risk of colon cancer. *N Engl J Med* 325:1593-1596, 1991.

Todaro GJ, Green H: Quantitative studies of the growth of mouse embryo cells in culture and their development into established lines. *J Cell Biol* 17:299-313, 1963.

Tooze J (ed): *DNA Tumor Viruses.* New York, Cold Spring Harbor Laboratory, 1980a.

Tooze J (ed): *RNA Tumor Viruses.* New York, Cold Spring Harbor Laboratory, 1980b.

Trent J, Davis JR: D-group chromosome abnormalities in endometrial cancer and hyperplasia. *Lancet* 2:361, 1979.

Tubo RA, Berezney R: Pre-replicative association of multiple replicative enzyme activities with the nuclear matrix during rat liver regeneration. *J Biol Chem* 262:1148-1154, 1987.

Upton A: Principles of cancer biology: Etiology and prevention of cancer. In DeVita VT Jr, Hellman S, Rosenberg SA (eds): *Cancer—Principles and Practice of Oncology,* 2nd ed. Philadelphia, JB Lippincott Co, 1982, pp 33-58.

Van't Veer LJ, Hermens R, Van den Berg-Bakker LA, Cheng NC, Fleuren GJ, Bos JL, Cleton FJ, Schrier PI: Ras oncogene activation in human ovarian carcinoma. *Oncogene* 2:157-165, 1988.

Vogelstein B, Fearon ER, Hamilton SR, Feinberg AP: Use of restriction fragment length polymorphisms to determine the clonal origin of human tumors. *Science* 227:642-645, 1985.

Vogelstein B, Fearon ER, Kern SE, Hamilton SR, Preisinger AC, Nakamura Y, White R: Allelotype of colorectal carcinomas. *Science* 242:207-211, 1989.

Wake N, Hreshchyshyn MM, Piver SM, Matsui S, Sandberg AA: Specific cytogenetic changes in ovarian cancer involving chromosomes 6 and 14. *Cancer Res* 40:4512-4518, 1980.

Warhol MJ, Antonioli DA, Pinkus GS, Burke L, Rice R: Immunoperoxidase staining for involucrin: A potential diagnostic aid in cervicovaginal pathology. *Human Pathol* 13:1095-1100, 1982.

Warrell RP, Frankel SR, Miller WH, Scheinberg DA, Itri LM, Hittelman WN, Vyas R, Andreef M, Tafuri A, Jakubowski A, Gabrilove J, Gordon M, Dmitrovsky E: Differentiation therapy of acute promyelocytic leukemia with tretinoin (all-trans-retinoic acid). *N Engl J Med* 324:1385-1393, 1991.

Watson JV, Curling OM, Munn CF, Hudson CN: Oncogene expression in ovarian cancer: A pilot study of c-myc oncoprotein in serous papillary ovarian cancer. *Gynecol Oncol* 28:137-150, 1987.

Weber G: Differential carbohydrate metabolism in tumor and host. In Arnott MS, van Eys J, Wan YM (eds): *Molecular Interrelations of Nutrition and Cancer.* New York, Raven Press, 1982, pp 191-208.

Weber G: Biochemical strategy of cancer cells and the design of chemotherapy: G.H.A. Clowes Memorial Lecture. *Cancer Res* 43:3466-3492, 1983.

Weinhouse G: Changing perceptions of carbohydrate metabolism of tumors. In Arnott MS, van Eys J, Wang YM (eds): *Molecular Interrelations of Nutrition and Cancer.* New York, Raven Press, 1982, pp 167-181.

Weinstein IB: The origins of human cancer: Molecular mechanisms of carcinogenesis and their implications for cancer prevention and treatment. *Cancer Res* 48:4135-4143, 1988.

Weisenthal LM, Lippman ME: Clonogenic and nonclonogenic in vitro chemosensitivity assays. *Cancer Treat Rep* 69:615-632, 1985.

Weisenthal LM, Dill PL, Kurnick NB, Lippman ME: Comparison of dye exclusion assays with a clonogenic assay in the determination of drug-induced cytotoxicity. *Cancer Res* 43:258-264, 1983.

Weisenthal LM, Su YZ, Duarte TE, Nagourney RA: Non-clonogenic, in vitro assays for predicting sensitivity to cancer chemotherapy. *Progr Clin Biol Res* 276:75-92, 1988.

Weiss MC: Cell hybridization: A tool for the study of cell differentiation. In Caskey CT, Robbins DC (eds): *Somatic Cell Genetics.* New York, Plenum Publishing Co, 1982, pp 169-175.

Wheelock EF, Weishold KJ, Levich J: The tumor dormant state. *Adv Cancer Res* 34:107-140, 1981.

Wiener EC, Loewenstein WR: Correction of cell-cell communication defect by introduction of a protein kinase into mutant cells. *Nature* 305:433-435, 1983.

Wigler M, Pellicer A, Silverstein S, Axel R: Biochemical transfer of single-copy eucaryotic genes using total cellular DNA as donor. *Cell* 14:725-731, 1978.

Wille JJ, Maercklein PB, Scott RE: Neoplastic transformation and defective control of cell proliferation and differentiation. *Cancer Res* 42:5139-5146, 1982.

Winawer SJ, Zauber AG, Stewart E, O'Brien MJ: The natural history of colorectal cancer. *Cancer* 67:1143-1149, 1991.

Wittelsberger SC, Kleene K, Penman S: Progressive loss of shape-responsive metabolic controls in cells with increasingly transformed phenotype. *Cell* 24:859-866, 1981.

Wright WE, Sasoon D, Lin VK: Myogenin, a factor regulating myogenesis, has a homologous domain to Myo D. *Cell* 56:607-617, 1989.

Yanishevsky RM, Stein GH: Regulation of the cell cycle in eucaryotic cells. *Int Rev Cytol* 69:223-259, 1981.

Yunis JJ: The chromosomal basis of human neoplasia. *Science* 221:227-235, 1983.

Yunis JJ, Bloomfield CD, Ensrud K: All patients with acute nonlymphocytic leukemia may have a chromosomal defect. *N Engl J Med* 305:135-139, 1981.

Yuspa SH, Morgan DL: Mouse skin cells resistant to terminal differentiation associated with initiation of carcinogenic transformation. *Nature* 293:72-74, 1981.

Yuspa SH, Vass W, Scolnick E: Altered growth and differentiation of cultured mouse epidermal cells infected with oncogenic retroviruses: Contrasting effects of viruses and chemicals. *Cancer Res* 43:6021-6030, 1983.

Zacharski LR, Henderson WG, Rickles FR, Forman WB, Cornell CJ, Forcier RJ, Edwards RL, Headley E, Kim SH, O'Donnell JF: Effect of warfarin anticoagulation on survival in carcinoma of the lung, colon, head and neck, and prostate. *Cancer* 53:2046-2052, 1984.

Zacharski LR, Henderson WG, Rickles FR, Forman WB, Cornell CJ Jr, Forcier FJ, Harpower HW, Johnson RO: Rationale and experimental design for the VA Cooperative Study of Anticoagulation (warfarin) in the treatment of cancer. *Cancer* 44:732-741, 1979.

Zhang X, Silva E, Gershenson D, Hung MC: Amplification and rearrangement of c-erb B in carcinomas of the human female genital tract. *Oncogene* 4:985-989, 1989.

Zhou DJ, Gonzalez-Cadavid N, Ahuja H, Battifora H, Moore GE, Cline MJ: A unique pattern of proto-oncogene abnormalities in ovarian adenocarcinomas. *Cancer* 62:1573-1576, 1988.

# Chapter 2

# Tumor Invasion and Metastasis: Pathogenesis and Therapeutic Implications

*William P. Peters*     *Emil Frei III*

Malignant neoplasms are characterized by two fundamental properties: the capacity to expand locally by invasion and distantly by metastasis. These two phenomena are interrelated and constitute the major cause of morbidity and mortality from cancer. Information about the biology of tumor invasion and metastasis, provided by pathologists and clinicians, has been largely descriptive. Only during the past 15 years has this subject come under scientific scrutiny. With the advent of tumor biology, and particularly the sciences of cell biology, genetics, tissue culture, biochemistry, and cytokinetics, additional fundamental and quantitative information has been recently acquired. Although major advances in prevention and therapy are still awaited, the outlines of such interventions are emerging and should become clear in the reasonably near future.

Here we will review the process of neoplastic transformation, the evolution of preoplasia to primary neoplasia, the monoclonal origin of neoplastic transformation, and clonal evolution; the characteristics of primary neoplasms in terms of mechanisms of invasion; the process of tumor cell release from the primary lesion; circulation of tumor cells in the blood; tumor cell embolization and selection of the site of metastasis; early invasion; protection from the host; and finally, the kinetics of growth of the metastatic lesion. Throughout, the emphasis will be put on the pathogenic mechanisms involved. Although major advances in prevention and therapy are still awaited, initial therapeutic trials are already under way to assess ways to alter the formation of metastases.

## THE PROCESS OF TRANSFORMATION

The development of preoplasia and its transition to neoplastic disease are outlined in Figure 2-1A. For most major tumors (for example, those of the skin, lung, breast, stomach, prostate, or bladder), preoplastic events have been linked to environmental factors. These environmental factors interact with host target tissue either to mutagenize or otherwise to activate latent oncogenes, resulting in oncogenic products, several of which have been identified. The multistep nature of preoplasia and neoplasia has long been appreciated by clinicians and pathologists who have observed, for example, the gradual transition of aging skin that has been subjected to ultraviolet irradiation through a series of changes from preneoplstic actinic keratoses to carcinoma in situ and neoplasia.

Preoplasia may be a progressive, stable, or reversible process (Fig. 2-1B); it may be reversed through withdrawal of the offending environmental factors. Recently, therapeutic interventions (chemoprevention) have been directed toward this preoplastic process. For example, vitamin A is known to be essential to the maintenance and differentiation of normal epithelial tissues (Sporn et al, 1976). Experimentally, vitamin A deprivation leads to dysplastic and metaplastic changes in normal tissues, which may progress to neoplasia. In a controlled study, the British have demonstrated that vitamin A analogue 13-cis-retinoic acid significantly reduced preoplastic changes in the bronchial mucosa of heavy smokers (Gouveia et al, 1982). More recently, similar observations have been made by American investigators who showed that the risk for cancer was reduced in such patients (Hong et al, 1990). Whether ongoing trials will confirm that this is a successful and practical approach to diminishing the risk of cancer in such patients remains to be determined.

At some point in this multistep process, the line of transformation to neoplasia is crossed, and neoplastic disease occurs. The distinctions between late preoplasia and early neoplasia—particularly between some forms of benign and malignant disease—may present problems. Local invasion and distant metastasis, the subjects of this chapter, have been and remain the only requisite and unequivocal characteristics of neoplastic disease.

By means of genetic techniques, the initial neoplastic transformation has been shown to be monoclonal in origin in most cases (Fialkow, 1976; Fialkow et al, 1977, 1978). The experimental technique most appropriate for exploring this question involves analysis of glucose-6-phosphate dehydrogenase (G6PD) isozymes. This enzyme is carried on the X chromosome and as such is, in women, subject to lyonization. Approximately 35% of black women are heterozygous for this enzyme, i.e., isozyme A will be present on one X chromosome of the zygote and isozyme B on the other. Early in embryonic life, a random X chromosome in the individual cell becomes inactive (lyonization) and produces the Barr body (Lyon, 1972). Thus, in such individuals, genetic mosaicism occurs in normal tissues; about half of the cells contain G6PD isozyme A (GdA) and the remainder contain G6PD isozyme B (GdB). If the neoplastic event were polyclonal in origin, one

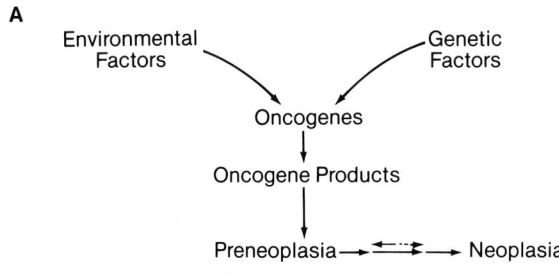

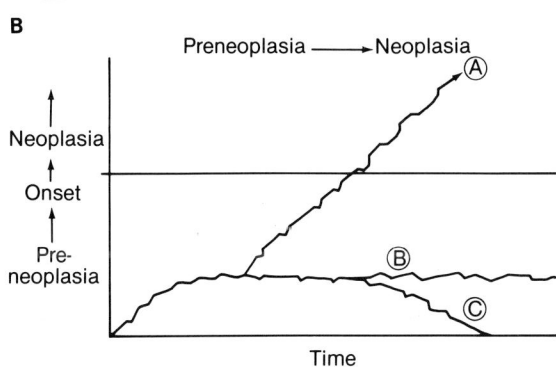

FIGURE 2-1 *Top:* In the progression from the normal state to neoplasia, environmental and genetic factors appear to interact, leading to activation of oncogenes and subsequent production of oncogene products. The latter appears to be a first step in the development of neoplasia, leading to preneoplastic states and, if other conditions are appropriate, eventually to a full neoplastic state.
*Bottom:* The dividing line between preneoplasia and neoplasia is not always clear, and the progression to neoplasia is not necessarily always completed. (A) After the preneoplastic state has been induced, additional environmental or genetic influences may lead to the development of a frankly neoplastic state. (B) The preneoplastic change that had been induced remains in a stable state. (C) Withdrawal of outside offending agents that maintain the preneoplastic state or treatment with differentiating agents can reverse the preneoplastic phenotype.

would expect tumors to contain mixtures of cells with both A and B isozymes, and analysis should reveal the presence of both enzymes in mixtures derived from cell homogenates. In fact, the vast majority of tumors are either all GdA or all GdB, indicating that they are of monoclonal origin. The isoenzymes are determined from lysates of tissues that are prepared and analyzed by starch gel electrophoresis. In view of the nature of preneoplasia, it is possible that neoplastic change arises in several cells in the lung, for example, but that a single transformed cell, for temporal or cytokinetic reasons, becomes dominant. Thus, monoclonality may in part be the result of a selection process.

## PRIMARY GROWTH

While growth is the most obvious property of neoplasms, it is their invasive properties that result in the morbidity related to the disease. *Invasion* refers to the capacity of primary tumors to encroach upon and erode adjacent tissues (Fig. 2-2). While pressure was initially

## TUMOR INVASION

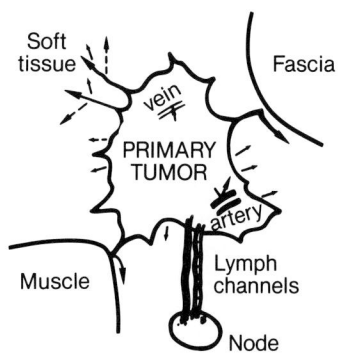

--→ = TUMOR PRODUCTS PROMOTING INVASION
PROTEOLYTIC ENZYMES
HYALURONIDASE
COLLAGENASE

HOST FACTORS RESTRAINING GROWTH
RIGID OR DENSE TISSUES
TUMOR IMMUNITY, ENDOCRINE FACTORS, ETC.

FIGURE 2-2 Growth and expansion of primary tumors depend upon mechanical and enzymatic factors as well as intrinsic genetic heterogeneity. Primary tumors tend to expand along lines of least resistance, invading soft tissue and tending to be inhibited from crossing fascial planes. Invasion of primary tumor into vessels will preferentially be into venous channels, given the more rigid structure of arteries. Spread will occur locally but also via lymphatic channels. The tumors will produce proteolytic enzymes, hyaluronidase, and collagenase (see text), which will help to promote invasion of underlying tissues. Other factors such as host immunity and endocrine factors will influence the growth and spread of primary neoplasms.

thought to be important to tumor growth, it probably plays a relatively minor role in the invasion process. As will be discussed below, tumor angiogenesis factor must be produced for vascularization and rapid growth of the tumor to occur. The most rapidly growing cells (as noted by indices of tritiated thymidine DNA labeling) tend to be immediately adjacent to blood vessels and at the periphery, particularly in the advancing columns of the tumor (Tannock, 1968). Not surprisingly, tumors tend to invade along lines of least resistance, including particularly invasion of veins in preference to arteries and invasion of the soft tissue matrix rather than fascia, muscle, or bone. Certain mediators that also influence tumor invasion will be discussed below. Finally, certain tumors have a tropism for and tend to invade along fascial planes, nerve fibers, and peritoneal surfaces.

Tumors may grow in size from a single cell to approximately a million cells, supported by nutrients such as metabolites and oxygen supplied by diffusion; however, simple diffusion is inadequate to allow growth beyond this point. Using a variety of techniques, particularly involving the rabbit cornea, Gimbrone and colleagues have demonstrated that tumors produce a diffusible, nondialyzable substance, not yet completely characterized, which he has called *tumor angiogenesis factor* (TAF) (Gimbrone et al, 1974). TAF stimulates normal adjacent endothelium, causing proliferation of vessels and thus neovascularization of the tumor, permitting continued, rapid tumor growth.

## NEOPLASTIC PROGRESSION IN TUMOR CELL HETEROGENEITY

Beginning in the 1950s, Foulds, while studying the mouse mammary tumor, described a phenomenon of tumor evolution leading to tumor heterogeneity, which he termed *neoplastic progression* (1969). He described this tumor progression as the acquisition of permanent, irreversible qualitative changes of one or more characteristics in a neoplasm and postulated that this derived from *clonal evolution due to genetic instability*. Heterogeneity allows for variation and selection, and this concept and subsequent related experiments have contributed enormously to our understanding of the nature and manifestations of invasion and metastases as well as the biologic behavior of tumors and problems of treatment. Nowell confirmed and extended these studies through cytogenetic analyses of human leukemia (1976). The monoclonal origin of tumors suggests that one cell from the enormous number (greater than $10^{13}$) in the human body is rendered malignant and is subsequently able to proliferate, invade, and metastasize (Fig. 2-3).

In the early preclinical stages of tumor development, one would expect substantial homogeneity. However, experimental evidence suggests that phenotypic and cytogenetic heterogeneity can develop early in the natural history of tumors (Foulds, 1969), and that by the time of clinical detection a tumor may exhibit substantial clinical heterogeneity (Fidler and Hart, 1982; Fidler et al, 1981; Kripke et al, 1978). This is particularly evident with certain tumors such as melanomas, which are manifested clinically by variations in pigment production in cutaneous metastases. Heterogeneity may be evident in multiple phenotypes such as histology, pigment production, hormone receptors, and immunologic characteristics, including antigen expression, drug sensitivity, metastatic capacity, mutation frequency, and mediator production (Baylan et al, 1978; Biorklund et al, 1980; Colcher et al, 1981; Fidler and Hart, 1981; Siracky, 1979; Sluyser and Van Nie, 1974; Trope, 1982; Trope et al, 1975, 1980).

Under the microscope, one sees substantial heterogeneity, in terms of the morphology of individual tumor cells within a given tumor, as well as in the degree of cellular differentiation. As the tumor progressively increases in size, genetic instability, as manifested by clonal evolution, results in increasing aneuploidy and therefore phenotypic variation (Fig. 2-3). This progression, along with the crowding of the tumor as it grows, causes an increased proportion of daughter cells to die or drop out of the cycle, i.e., to enter a resting phase ($G_0$). As will be described later, this leads to greater cell loss and a decreasing growth fraction, which are characteristics of larger tumors and represent a phenomenon well described by Gompertzian growth kinetics (Steel, 1977). Human breast cancer has been shown to display heterogeneity with respect to surface antigen representation in studies using a monoclonal antibody (Colcher et al, 1981) and in studies in estrogen receptors that indicate similar phenotypic heterogeneity (Sluyser and Van Nie, 1974). Almost 20 years ago, it was recognized

## Clonal Evolution of Human Neoplasia

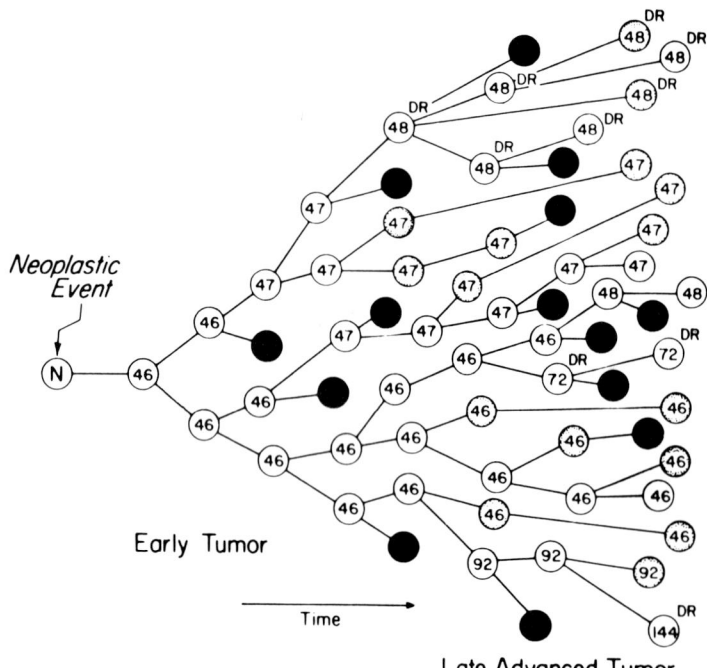

**● = Death. Terminal Differentiation, Lethal Mutant, Cell Loss**

**DR = Drug Resistant Mutant**

**㊻ = Resting Cell, i.e., $G_1$ or $G_2$ Block**

FIGURE 2-3 Most human tumors are monoclonal in origin, i.e., the neoplastic event occurs in a single normal cell that undergoes clonal expansion. During clonal expansion, there is genetic instability (a high mutation rate [see text], resulting in clonal evolution to progressive heterogeneity. Thus, as the tumor increases in size and age, the growth fraction is lower and there is increasing cell death, aneuploidy, and heterogeneity in terms of the metastatic potential of individual clones, antigenicity, hormone receptors, and response to chemotherapy.

that different clones isolated in vitro from a single human metastasis could exhibit substantial variation in response to the antitumor agent BCNU, a nitrosourea (Barranco et al, 1973). Numerous subsequent studies have confirmed this variation in response to cytotoxic agents (Biorklund et al, 1980; Siracky, 1979; Trope, 1983; Trope et al, 1975, 1980).

Fidler and Kripke (1977), employing the fluctuation analysis orginally applied in microbial systems by Luria and Delbruck (1943), have shown that cells within primary tumors are heterogeneous with respect to metastatic potential. Experiments were performed on the murine model of melanoma, B16. In this study, a single cell suspension of the parental tumor was divided into aliquots and injected intravenously into mice. As expected, the number of pulmonary metastases in the individual mice receiving such injections was relatively constant. In a parallel experiment, individual cells of the parent B16 melanoma were cloned in vitro. The individual cell clones were expanded, and the expanded lines were then used to inoculate a series of animals. If each cell had possessed the equivalent capacity for metastasis, the cell lines derived from cloned cells should have had equal potential in terms of the development of metastases. However, there was considerable variation (fluctuation) among the clones in terms of the number of pulmonary metastases that were formed, suggesting that the cells present in the initial population varied considerably in their ability to form pulmonary metastases. Clones vary in their capacity to form pulmonary metastases, indicating that at the time of the cloning process, the individual cells differed from each other in this capacity. Therefore, metastases represent a selection process.

The preceding experiment was performed in a long-established B16 cell line that would be expected to have undergone substantial clonal evolution. To exclude the possibility that the metastatic heterogeneity found in the B16 melanoma might have been introduced as a result of lengthy in vivo and in vitro cultivation, Kripke et al (1978) performed similar experiments involving newly induced primary and ultraviolet radiation–induced fibrosarcoma (UV-2231) and the K1735 melanoma syngeneic to C3H/HeN. Mice were evaluated as above but with tumor after only five in vitro passages. Results were similar to those obtained with the B16 melanoma. In fact, the cloned cell lines from these tumors varied greatly in their ability to grow in subcutaneous sites as well as to produce spontaneous metastasis in distant organs. These experiments demonstrate that metastatic potential is a property for which heterogeneity develops early in the natural history of the tumor.

It appears that heterogeneity for a single phenotype does not appear to be unlimited; as they grow, tumors possess areas of apparent homogeneity for a given phenotype, or "zones." Claus Trope, using a primary mouse melanoma, found that certain regions of the melanoma were pigmented and others were not (Trope, 1982). If one transplanted fragments taken from the melanotic area, one had (at least initially) relatively homogeneous melanotic tumors, whereas the opposite was true when fragments were obtained from amelanotic areas. On the other hand, cell suspensions prepared from the original tumor maintained their diversity. In terms of therapeutic response, these results imply that different areas of even an individual tumor may not respond in a similar manner (Fidler and Hart, 1981) and that different metastatic or even primary lesions might be expected to show considerable variation in their response to individual antitumor agents (Talmadge, 1985)—a phenomenon often observed clinically.

The cause of heterogeneity appears to be clonal evolution due to genetic instability. Clonal evolution was first observed in chronic myelogenous leukemia. As patients entered the advanced stage of their disease, a series of progressive cytogenetic abnormalities developed, indicating the evolution of additional clones (Nowell, 1976). Such genetic instability might be expected to be a positive and correlative feature in the selection of cells for more neoplastic behavior, such as survival, invasion, metastases, drug resistance, and so on.

An increase in mutation rates may be intrinsic to the tumor, since these rates may increase in the absence of host factors (e.g., mutation rates to drug resistance in vitro) or their increase may be promoted by the neoplastic environment. This issue was addressed by Cifone and Fidler (1981), who studied the relative mutation rates of cell lines selected for high and low metastatic potential. If clonal evolution is a positive attribute for neoplastic behavior and survival, one would expect mutation rates to be higher in cells with greater metastatic potential. In several systems, mutation rates to ouabain and 6-thioguanine resistance were found to be four to seven times higher in the cell lines having high metastatic potential compared with those having low metastatic potential (Table 2-1), suggesting that cells possessing metastatic potential are intrinsically more unstable genetically.

Furthermore, microenvironmental factors may promote mutations in tumors, particularly solid tumors. Macrophages and other phagocytizing cells that commonly surround or infiltrate tumors may, during the phagocytosis and killing process, produce and release potential mutagens, such as superoxides and peroxides (Weitzman and Stossel, 1981). In addition, in the past few years, highly specific reciprocal chromosomal translocations and deletions have been found to characterize certain cancers, with specific deletions present in many solid tumors (Jackey et al, 1983; Sutherland, 1979; Sutherland and Hinton, 1981; Yunis, 1983). It has been found that these rearrangements tend to occur at "fragile sites" on the chromosomes. Some form of compromise within the tumor microenvironment, such as a decrease in metabolites or oxygen supply, may lead to more frequent cytogenetic changes, particularly at these fragile sites (Jackey et al, 1983). Anticancer therapies such as radiation or alkylating agent chemotherapy may also cause cytogenetic, chromosomal, or genetic changes. Thus, presumably, both intrinsic genetic instability and environmental factors may contribute to the clonal evolution of tumors.

TABLE 2-1 Metastasis and Mutation Rates

| Line | Metastatic Potential | Selecting Agent | Rate of Mutation* | Fold Increase |
|---|---|---|---|---|
| UV2237 | Low | Ouabain | 0.16 | — |
| Fibrosarcoma | High | Ouabain | 0.73 | 4.6 |
| K1735 | Low | Thioguanine | 0.08 | — |
| Melanoma | High | Thioguanine | 0.61 | 7.0 |

* Mutation rate ($\times 10^6$ per cell generation).
Note: Cell lines with high and low metastatic potential were selected in vivo from UV2237 and K1735 parental lines. In vitro, they were tested for their rate of spontaneous mutation and resistance to the selecting agents ouabain and 6-thioguanine. In the cell lines derived from tumors with high metastatic potential, there was an increased mutation rate.
*Source:* Modified from Cifone MA, and Fidler IJ: Increasing metastatic potential is associated with increasing genetic instability of clones isolated from murine neoplasms. *Proc Natl Acad Sci, USA*, 78:6949, 1981.

## RELEASE OF TUMOR CELLS INTO THE BLOOD

Factors that cause the release of cells from the primary tumor into the circulation are incompletely understood. In transplanted tumors in animals, it has been shown that the primary lesion must reach a certain size before tumor cells appear in the blood and metastases occur (Skipper, personal communication). For a given tumor type, this critical size tends to be relatively constant, although there may be considerable variation among different types of tumors. In a quantitative sense, the more tumor cells present in the primary lesion, presumably the greater the risk that an individual cell will invade the bloodstream. Clearly, however, other factors operate as well.

Tumor neovasculature is known to be abnormal in several respects. For example, these vessels are characterized by loose endothelial junctions, which explains the high protein content in the interstitium of tumors and the high concentration of radionuclide colloids within tumors, presumably due to a "leaky" blood-tumor barrier. These junctions are particularly loose at the advancing edge of the columns of proliferating tumor cells (Goldacrer and Sylven, 1962). Loose endothelial junctions allow tumor cells to enter the vascular system. Fibronectin is a large, sticky protein that promotes coherence of normal tissues as well as some tumor tissues. There is evidence that the capacity of experimental tumors to metastasize is inversely related to their fibronectin production, supporting the earlier suggestion that tumors are less coherent than normal tissues and thus capable of metastasizing (Yamada and Olden, 1978). The motility and deformability of tumor cells presumably relates to their capacity to invade and metastasize and to produce mediators that may promote invasiveness and ultimately the possible invasion of blood vessels. External trauma of the tumor (as a result of surgery, for example) may play a role in increasing the number of circulating tumor cells in certain settings.

Tumors can vary substantially in their capacity to be tumorigenic and metastatic. When the K1735 melanoma was evaluated in seven different subpopulations of cells, there was substantial variation between clones and their tumorigenic and metastatic behavior (Auker-

man et al, 1986; Fidler et al, 1981; Kripke et al, 1978). Three of the cloned cells were tumorigenic but not metastatic, whereas the other four cloned lines consisted of cells that were tumorigenic and highly metastatic. Hence, the biologic behavior of these lines differed in a clear and qualitative manner.

## CIRCULATING TUMOR CELLS

Traditionally, tumors have been characterized as initially metastasizing via vascular channels or via regional lymph nodes and then to the vascular system. The distinction between these two mechanistic descriptions is not always clear and frequently overlaps. In any event, in earlier studies involving Millipore filtration, it was observed that tumor cells were commonly found in the peripheral blood of patients with "localized" cancer and that the correlation between the presence of these cells and the prognosis was not particularly good (Butler and Gullino, 1975; Fisher and Turnbull, 1955). Tumor cells in the blood may circulate as single cells (Liotta et al, 1974) or as clumps (Fidler, 1970) and may have adherent lymphoid cells or platelets, factors which influence their capacity to produce metastases (Fidler, 1970; Karpatkin and Pearlstein, 1981; Liotta et al, 1976; Zeidman, 1975).

Experimental studies have shed considerable light on the quantitative importance of tumor cells in the peripheral blood. If tumor cells are labeled with [131]I-uridine (a thymidine analogue incorporated into cells making DNA) and are injected intravenously, the body burden of tumor cells can be determined precisely, since dying cells rapidly release [131]I, which appears in the urine and can be quantitated, and viable cells can be localized. After injection, 99% of such cells are rapidly destroyed and less than 1% appear in the lungs, where they remain temporarily (Fidler, 1970). Less than 0.1% of the cells will persist in the lung or move on to other sites to establish metastases. Thus, even in syngeneic systems, the environment in which metastases may be established is hostile, and the capacity to produce metastases is very limited. Cells that succeed in this difficult task truly represent the fittest.

In these experiments, cell lines that varied in their

capacity to form metastases were eliminated from the circulation at different rates. Three days after intravenous injection, only highly metastatic lines were still viable in the lungs and lymph nodes. Cells from nonmetastatic lines were not found (Price et al, 1986). Thus, for these cell lines that are arrested in the pulmonary bed, definitive selection for cells that form pulmonary colonies occurred between 1 and 24 hours after inoculation, so that most of the cells of the high metastatic lines were eliminated (more than 80%) as were essentially all the cells in the low metastatic lines (more than 99%).

## THE CLONAL ORIGIN OF METASTASES

Metastases might develop as a result of the establishment of individual cells or clumps of cells. Observations by Talmadge et al (1982) demonstrate the clonal origin of experimental metastatic lesions. In this study, mouse melanoma cells in culture were sublethally irradiated, a process that often produces aneuploidy and nonspecific changes but in some cells will produce marker chromosomes that characterize the progeny of such cells and differ from cell to cell in the original population. The sublethally irradiated population of cells was injected intravenously into syngeneic mice, and the resultant metastatic tumors were analyzed cytogenetically. Chromosomal markers differed among the different metastases, but within a given metastasis, the same marker chromosomes characterized all of the scorable metaphases, indicating that experimental metastases are clonal in origin.

Such observations have important implications for therapy. If the phenotype of drug resistance varies substantially among the individual cells present in the primary tumor, and metastases are formed from individual cells, one might expect considerable heterogeneity in drug sensitivity among metastatic lesions. Indeed, subsequent studies by Talmadge have shown this (Talmadge, 1985).

Drug sensitivity of individual metastases was scored in cell lines derived from individual pulmonary metastases. The ability of a given agent to kill various metastatic lesions differed by more than 10-fold, demonstrating considerable heterogeneity for drug sensitivity among metastatic lesions. Other investigators have noted substantial heterogeneity in other tumor models, such as the C3H mammary tumor treated with chemo-immunotherapy (Fischer and Saffer, 1982).

## INITIATION OF THE METASTATIC PROCESS

Events surrounding the initial development of metastases are incompletely understood, although one pathogenic model has been suggested (Fig. 2-4). The process of cancer metastasis involves a long series of sequential and interrelated steps, any of which can be rate-limiting, since the failure at any one of the steps aborts the

metastatic process (Poste and Fidler, 1980). Tumor cells may circulate individually or as clumps, and there is evidence that clumps of cells may be more readily arrested in capillaries and produce metastases. In experimental studies, it has been found that clumps comprising four to five tumor cells are optimal for producing pulmonary metastases, presumably due to mechanical factors. Lymphocytes and/or platelets may be attached to circulating tumor cells and appear to influence metastatic potential. Morphologic studies by Kramer indicate that as tumor cells come in contact with the endothelial surface, endothelial junctions retract and the tumor attaches to the basement membrane.

For a specific tumor host organ, metastasis receptors may be involved (see The Distribution of Metastases below). Production of mediators from the tumor, or from the associated platelet release phenomenon, may contribute to the trapping and entry of the tumor cell. For example, some tumors exhibit collagenase IV lytic activity. Collagenase IV is a 60,000-dalton metallopro-

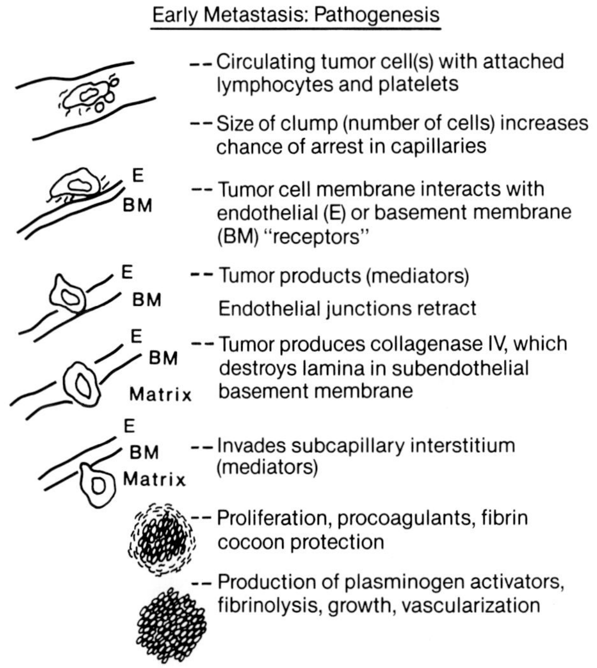

Early Metastasis: Pathogenesis

-- Circulating tumor cell(s) with attached lymphocytes and platelets

-- Size of clump (number of cells) increases chance of arrest in capillaries

-- Tumor cell membrane interacts with endothelial (E) or basement membrane (BM) "receptors"

-- Tumor products (mediators) Endothelial junctions retract

-- Tumor produces collagenase IV, which destroys lamina in subendothelial basement membrane

-- Invades subcapillary interstitium (mediators)

-- Proliferation, procoagulants, fibrin cocoon protection

-- Production of plasminogen activators, fibrinolysis, growth, vascularization

FIGURE 2-4 Tumor cells may circulate individually or as clumps. Evidence suggests that clumps of tumor cells may be more efficient than single cells in promoting metastases. Often the circulating tumor cells have attached lymphocytes and platelets that appear to influence metastatic potential. The tumor cell membrane interacts with endothelial (E) or basement membrane (BM) receptors. After attachment to the vessel wall, tumor products cause the endothelial junctions to retract, and the tumor cell becomes attached to the subendothelial basement membrane. The invasive cell then releases enzymes that can degrade elements of the basement membrane, allowing the tumor cell to invade the subcapillary interstitium. Cells that cannot degrade components of the extracellular matrix in any given organ will be unable to invade that organ and will eventually pass on to another organ or die in the bloodstream. After escape from the vessel, there is proliferation, often with the tumor being protected by a fibrin cocoon. Finally, with continued growth, plasminogen activators are produced. Fibrinolysis of the protective cocoon, growth, and neovascularization through the production of tumor angiogenesis factors (TAF) occur.

tein that produces "specific cleavage" of type IV collagen, a major component of the basement membrane, and results in destruction of the lamina on the subendothelial basement membrane (Fig. 2-4) (Liotta and Stetler-Stevenson, 1989). This may allow migration of the tumor cell into the interstitial connective tissue matrix. In Table 2-2, this type IV collagenolytic metalloproteinase activity and the metastatic potential are listed for several cell lines, including cell populations with low and high metastatic potential as well as normal cells. There appears to be a good correlation between metastatic potential and the ability to degrade collagenase IV. Other intrinsic properties of the tumor cell, such as motility and deformability, as well as the production of mediators, may affect such invasion in the subendothelial region (Hay, 1981; Yusa et al, 1989; Kao and Stern, 1986; Zimmerman and Keller, 1987; Liotta and Schiffmann, 1988). The tumor cell may then undergo limited proliferation and produce procoagulants, thus becoming enmeshed in a fibrin cocoon. Dvorak has presented evidence that this cocoon may protect the early microscopic metastasis from host attack. The subsequent production of plasminogen activators may, at the appropriate time, permit the tumor to dissolve the cocoon and continue to grow (Liotta et al, 1977, 1979, 1980; Dvorak et al, 1979).

## TUMOR CELL MEDIATORS

There is evidence that mediators may play a major role in tumor invasion and metastasis. The connective tissue matrix is composed of glycoproteins, proteoglycans, collagen, and elastin. The distribution of these four substances varies for different connective tissues, and with the exception of elastin, the materials are often qualitatively different for the various tissues. Thus, destruction of the matrix requires a complex of proteases with optimal variability so as to be effective in different tissues. Procoagulants, plasminogen activators, and plasmin have already been discussed. Collagenase type IV is specific for collagen in the basement membrane

and is therefore important to the early metastatic process, whereas collagenases I, II, and III appear to have other substrate specificities. Cathepsin B has been demonstrated to be markedly increased in breast cancer cells and in metastatic subpopulations of the B16 melanoma. Other proteolytic enzymes under increasing study include hyaluronidase, proteoglycan-degrading activity, chondroitinases, keratinases, and elastases. The importance of TAF and fibronectin were noted earlier. Although emphasis is placed on the production of these mediators by tumors, it should be appreciated that lysosomal enzymes released by normal phagocytes that surround the tumors may also play a major role in modifying the matrix. Experiments designed to evaluate the importance of specific enzymes and site-specific metastases are just beginning to be done and may be expected to yield important clinical implications.

## THE DISTRIBUTION OF METASTASES

It was long thought that simple factors, such as blood supply, determined the distribution of metastases. This mechanical explanation implied that all tumor cells were equally capable of establishing metastases and that the soil was the critical factor in determining where tumors developed. One would predict from this explanation that metastasis would follow a random distribution. Yet, extensive clinical observation has indicated that metastases are nonrandom: breast cancer cells frequently metastasize to bone, liver, and lung; soft tissue sarcoma will metastasize to the lung; lung cancer will metastasize to the brain, liver, kidneys, and adrenals, whereas ovarian cancers tend to metastasize locally within the peritoneum. For the individual patient—and for the disease in general—patterns of metastases may be characteristic and represent a nonrandom distribution.

One of the seminal experiments in the science of metastasis was conducted by Fidler, who addressed the issue of whether individual cells in a primary tumor had variable metastatic potential (Fidler, 1973). In these experiments, parental B16 melanoma cells were injected into the tail vein of a syngeneic mouse, and a small number of pulmonary metastases occurred. Fidler cultured these metastases and injected expanded clones into the tail veins of syngeneic recipient mice, repeating the process for 10 transfer generations. If the cells responsible for pulmonary metastases were from a random sample of tumor cells within the primary, and all cells possessed an equal capacity for pulmonary metastases, the number of pulmonary metastases that occurred after multiple lung selection and transfer experiments should remain the same. In fact, there was a marked selection process, such that in B16 F10 (the tenth transfer generation), the number of pulmonary metastases produced by a given inoculation was 100-fold greater than that of the parental line. Similarly, by the same process, a B16 line was developed that produced metastases in the brain, specifically between the cerebral cortex and the olfactory bulb (Brunson et al, 1978). In subsequent experiments by several investiga-

| TABLE 2-2 Metastasis and Type IV Collagenolytic Metalloproteinase Activity | | |
| --- | --- | --- |
| Tissue | Collagenase IV Activity (CPM/$10^5$ Cells) | Incidence of Metastasis (%) |
| Normal fibroblasts | Not done | 0 |
| Transformed mouse fibroblasts, | | |
| B77 (Rous) | 140 | 5 |
| B16 (F1) | 180 | 0 |
| B16 (F10) | 355 | 30 |
| B16 (high metastatic) | 1,150 | 80 |
| AA6 (from B77) | 3,800 | 100 |
| PMT (T241) | 4,200 | 100 |

*Source:* Modified from Liotta LA, et al: Role of collagenases in tumor cell invasion. *Cancer Metastasis Rev* 1:277, 1982.

tors, cell lines from the original parental population have been developed that have a high capacity to produce metastases to several different anatomic sites.

Intercarotid injection of K1735 melanoma produced lesions only in the brain parenchyma, whereas B16 melanoma produced only meningeal growths (Schackert and Fidler, 1988). These results demonstrate specificity for metastatic growth in different regions of a single organ that is not dependent on initial patterns of cell arrest in the microvasculature, and they raise the possibility of specific binding sites for endothelial cells and tumor proliferative responses to local growth factors. This would imply an important interaction between the metastasizing cells and their new environment that is critical for their development.

What is the pathogenesis of this nonrandom distribution of metastases? The cell membrane of the tumor appears to be critical to the selective organ tropism, since there seems to be a specific interaction between this membrane and the endothelium or basement membrane of a particular organ. The murine melanoma B16 in culture sheds vesicles into the medium. Nicolson (1977) took membrane vesicles derived from a high lung metastatic cell line (B16 F10), mixed them with cells from a low lung metastatic line (B16 F1), and fused the membranes with polyethylene glycol. The resultant cells showed a substantially increased capacity to produce pulmonary metastases in mice (Nicolson, 1977; Poste

and Fidler, 1980). This increased potential for metastases is short-lived, consistent with the expected turnover of membrane proteins.

In an elegant experiment, shown in Figure 2-5, Nicolson (1977) found that a hepatic oncofetal antigen may play a role in the organ specificity of metastasis of a liver-metastasizing lymphoma. Using the RAW117 murine lymphoma, a subpopulation that exhibited preferential metastasis to the liver was selected by serial transfer. Aggregation of fetal liver cells occurred in the tumor subpopulation, suggesting that the tumor cells had a specific oncofetal antigen on their surface. Antibodies against the oncofetal hepatic aggregating antigen were prepared. Such antibodies inhibited the aggregation of fetal liver cells with the tumor cells and also decreased the "homing" capacity of the tumors to the liver (Nicolson, 1982a,b).

These experiments clearly demonstrate that in this model, selection of a metastatic population with homing potential for the liver was associated with appearance of an oncofetal hepatic antigen on the surface of the metastatic tumor. It is also worthwhile to note that this murine lymphoma, which is associated with a C-type RNA tumor virus, had in the parental cell significant amounts of GP70, the envelope glycoprotein of the murine tumor virus, but with the selection of the population metastatic for the liver, the antigen expression of this GP70 on the tumor cell was greatly reduced. Bio-

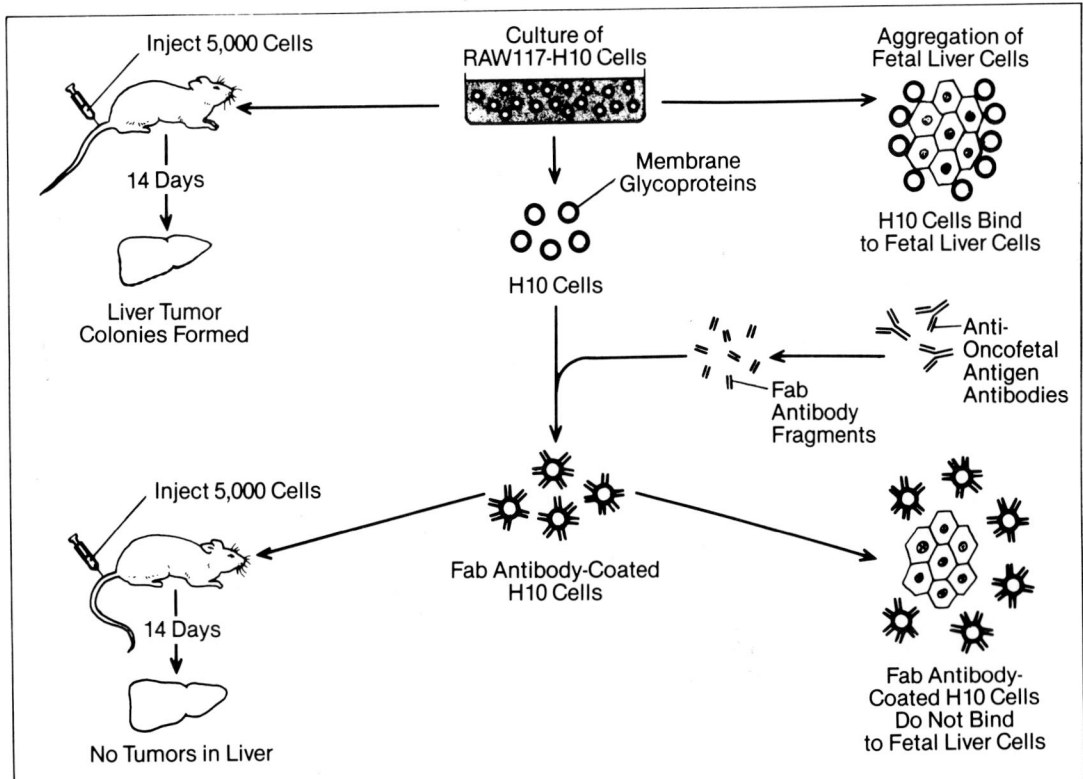

**FIGURE 2-5** Nicolson showed that an oncofetal hepatic antigen plays a major role in the metastatic "homing" of RAW117-H10 cells. If these cells are injected intravenously into a mouse (*top left*), a large number of hepatic metastases are formed. If, however, these cells are coated with antibody directed against the oncofetal hepatic antigen, a similar inoculation of tumor cells does not produce hepatic metastases (*bottom left*). H10 cells sufficiently bind aggregates of fetal liver cells owing to the presence of surface oncofetal antigen. However, when they are treated with antibodies directed against the fetal antigen, aggregation of fetal liver cells with tumor cells is blocked. (From Nicolson GL: Cell surfaces and cancer metastasis. *Hosp Pract* 17(8):75, 1982. Drawing by Nancy Lou Makris.)

chemical cell membrane proteins clearly indicate differences among cell lines with differing anatomic metastatic potential (Nicolson, 1977, 1982a).

The importance of this provocative observation remains to be determined. Loss of an antigen associated with an increased metastatic potential suggests that an immunologic relationship may be involved in allowing the metastatic cell to escape host control. Nevertheless, this is another clear demonstration of the heterogeneity of antigenic phenotypes present in parental populations. Thus, the seed as well as the soil is important to the development of metastases.

Finally, the nonrandomness of metastases is almost certainly—at least experimentally and probably clinically—the result of mediators. Activated B cells, including myeloma cells, produce a polypeptide known as *osteoclastic activating factor (OAF)*, a material that will activate proximate osteoclasts with resultant bone resorption (Mundy et al, 1974). Cells capable of producing OAF, such as myeloma and breast cancer cells, are presumably capable of transforming otherwise hostile environments of the bony cortex into compatible ones. In experimental animals and in human breast cancers with bone tropism, increased $PGE_2$ production has been demonstrated (Powles et al, 1973). This material will also activate osteoclasts and thus may help promote bone metastases. In the V2 rabbit breast carcinoma, this phenomenon has been conclusively demonstrated. Further, in this model, inhibition of cyclooxygenase by aspirin and related agents reduced the number of osseous metastatic lesions in one study (Powles et al, 1973).

## IMMUNITY AND METASTASES

The soil hypothesis for metastases, first presented by Paget in 1900, was extended by Fidler in 1973 to include the importance of the seed. Some have suggested that a third critical component of metastases is immunity. However, the relationship between immunity and the development of metastases is unclear. For example, immunosuppression does not generally increase metastasis; indeed, for appropriate tumors, the nude mouse is not particularly susceptible to metastasis. Natural killer (NK) cells have been postulated to play a major role in immunosurveillance. However, by serial exposure in vitro and selection, B16 melanoma cells resistant to killing by NK cells have been produced. Surprisingly, such B16 melanoma cells produce fewer, not more, metastases when injected intravenously compared with the parental cells. On the other hand, immune adherence of lymphocytes to circulating tumor cells appears to enhance metastatic potential in experimental systems. At this time, the conclusion must be that there is no simple relation between immunosuppression and metastatic potential.

Other factors may be important in determining the distribution of metastases in experimental models. For example, when colorectal carcinomas were injected intravenously in nude mice, there was no correlation between the experimental lung metastases and the clinical stage of the original neoplasm. However, intrasplenic injection, in which the primary metastatic site would be the liver, correlated closely with clinical extent of disease (Morikawa et al, 1988a and 1988b).

## GROWTH OF TUMORS

Once the primary tumor, particularly the metastasis is established and vascularized, growth (potentially exponential) may occur. Growth rates as measured by volume doubling time may vary substantially for different tumors (Steel, 1977; Shackney et al, 1978). A distribution of doubling times for testicular cancer and colon cancer follows a reasonable, logarithmically normal pattern, but the median doubling time for rapidly growing testicular carcinoma is 21 days, whereas for the slow-growing colon carcinoma it is 100 days. The clinical implications of this finding are suggested in Figure 2-6, in which the median volume doubling times of various tumors, ranging from the very rapidly growing choriocarcinoma to the slow-growing tumors such as colon cancer and prostate carcinoma, are presented in descending order. A strong correlation exists between rapidity of growth and response to chemotherapy. Indeed, this correlation leads to the conclusion that one of the most important discriminants for response to chemotherapy, including curative chemotherapy, is the tumor growth rate or—more precisely—the tumor volume doubling time (Steel, 1977; Shackney et al, 1978; Malaise et al, 1973).

Accordingly, more fundamental cytokinetic studies addressing this issue have been conducted. The technique of tritiated thymidine autoradiography with measurements of the percentage of labeled mitoses has been used to study this problem (Steel, 1977) (Fig. 2-7). In an asynchronous population of cells in culture, tritiated thymidine will label only the S phase (the DNA-synthesizing) cohort of cells. Following flash labeling, the percentage of labeled mitoses is plotted as a function of time. As the S-phase, flash-labeled cohort of cells moves through the cell cycle, it will describe a curve that provides much cytokinetic information. Thus, the S period and the $G_2$ period can be easily obtained, and if a second wave of mitosis occurs—or even if it does not—the generation time ($T_c$) of cells can usually be calculated.

In Table 2-3, characteristics of the various solid tumors that have been studied cytokinetically, in particular the percentage of labeled mitoses, are presented. The tumor types are arranged in descending order from volume doubling times of 21 to 100 days. Note that the $T_c$ is 1.5 to 4.0 days and is independent of the doubling time. Thus, the previous facile explanation that volume doubling time is a function of the cycling time of proliferating cells is not tenable. Mendelson speculated that this discrepancy resulted from the fact that many cells within a primary tumor were nonproliferating and introduced the term *growth fraction*, which was an expression of the proportion of tumor cells in the proliferative cycle relative to the total number of tumor cells (Steel, 1977).

## Metastatic Human Cancer: Correlation of Doubling Time with Response to Chemotherapy

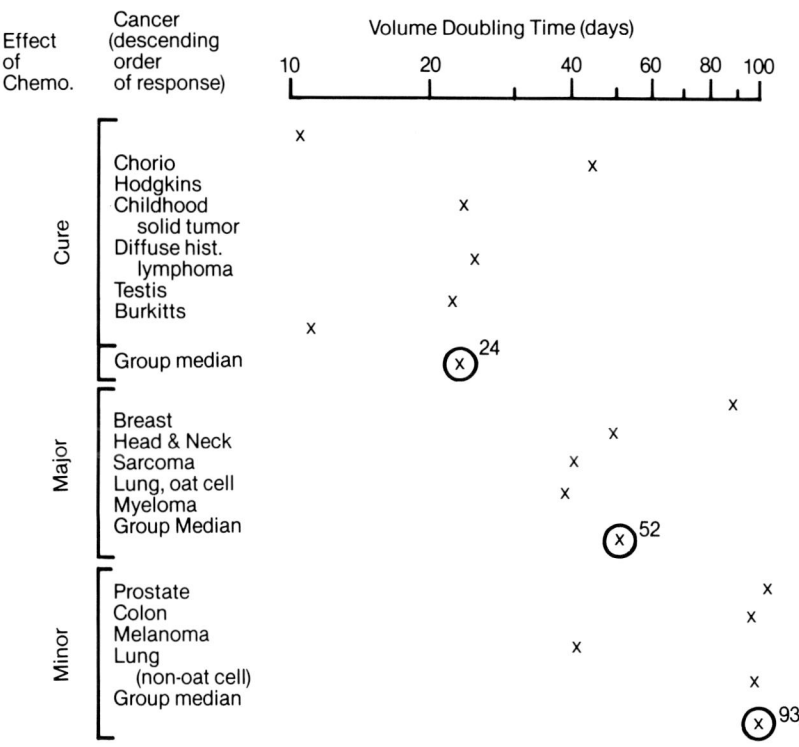

FIGURE 2-6   Volume doubling time of the tumor has a strong effect on the curative potential of chemotherapy. The strong correlation between the rapidity of growth and the response to chemotherapy suggests that the volume doubling time is one of the most important discriminants of response to chemotherapy.

There are several ways of determining growth fraction, the most common of which involves the labeling index with tritiated thymidine cells within a tumor divided by the labeling index, assuming that 100% of the cells are proliferating. The latter can be determined from the percent label mitosis (PLM) curve by the ratio of the S period ($T_s$) to the intermitotic or cycle time ($T_c$). This was done for a series of tumors, and the results are summarized in Table 2-3. It is evident that the major determinant of volume doubling time is the growth fraction. Thus, for tumors with rapid proliferative thrusts, as evidenced by short volume doubling times of 24 to 40 days, the growth fraction is high. In contrast, for indolent, slow-growing tumors such as breast and colon carcinomas, less than 5% of the cells may be in a proliferative cycle.

The relationship of such cytokinetic studies to the dynamics of growth of experimental solid tumors has long been noted. When the tumor is small and grows rapidly, its growth may indeed be almost exponential; however, as it increases in size, the growth rate decreases, as indicated by an increase in the doubling time. This change correlates only slightly with the cell cycle time ($T_c$) of the proliferating cells within the tumor. The resulting Gompertzian curve—i.e., a decreased growth rate with increasing size—is largely a function of the decrease in growth fraction. Thus, the small early tumors have a growth fraction of 80% or better, but as the tumor increases in size, an increasing proportion of cells drop out of the cycle, so that only 10% of the cells of a large tumor are in the cycle. There are several explanations for the decreasing growth fraction and increasing cell death as tumors increase in size. Tumors have, in fact, a greater proliferative capacity than the endothelium and may outgrow their blood supplies. Thus, it has been demonstrated that the growth fraction decreases for tumor cells that are more distant from capillaries. The metabolite and oxygen gradients are at least partially responsible (Steel, 1977; Malaise et al, 1973; Frindel et al, 1968).

A more recent relevant and powerful technique for the cytokinetic study of solid tumors relates to tumor stem cells (Hamburger and Salmon, 1977). Thus, certain cells within tumors are capable of producing a large family of descendent cells, for example, a colony. In vivo assay techniques allow meaningful quantitative assessment of tumor stem cells. For the clinic, in vitro clonogenic assays have been developed and are undergoing steady refinement and improvement, although their clinical relevance has not yet been established. If such an assay were to demonstrate good correlation with clinical tumor growth, it would have major importance in the development of therapeutic stategies for human neoplastic disease.

## IMPLICATIONS FOR THERAPY

As the study of the biology of tumor invasion and metastasis has proceeded, it has become clear that there are many sites at which the neoplastic process might possibly be halted. The first and most prominent inter-

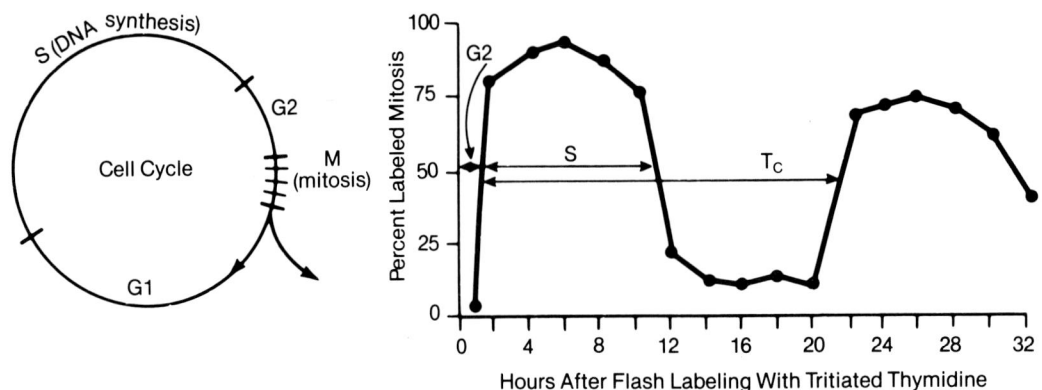

KINETICS OF ESTABLISHED NEOPLASTIC CELL LINES in vitro
Schematic

$T(time)_{G2} = 2$ hrs.
$T_S = 8$ hrs.
$T_C^{(a)} = 20$ hrs.
$T_{G1} = T_C - (T_S + T_{G2}) = 10$ hrs.

(a)$T_C$ = Time of cycle = generation time.

Labeling index = percent labeled cells.
If 100% of cells are in proliferating pool (PP),

labeling index should equal $\frac{T_S}{T_C}$.

$\frac{\text{Labeling index}}{T_S/T_C}$ = Proportion of cells in proliferating pool.

**FIGURE 2-7** The time of cycle ($T_c$) (or the generation time) can be determined by flash labeling tumor cell populations with tritiated thymidine. In an asynchronous population of cells in culture, tritiated thymidine will label only cells in the DNA-synthesizing (S) phase of the cell cycle. Hence, after flash labeling, the percentage of labeled mitoses will increase after a delay (which is equivalent to $G_2$), and the duration of the S phase will be described by the width of the percent labeled mitoses curve. If sufficient time is allowed to pass, a second wave of mitosis occurs from which one can calculate $T_c$ (see text).

vention is to control the environmental factors responsible for the majority of preneoplastic events. Placebo-controlled randomized comparative trials have demonstrated that 13-cis-retinoic acid can prevent the development of second malignant tumors in patients with head and neck cancer (Hong et al, 1990). Applied appropriately to high-risk populations, this approach has the potential for markedly reducing the development of neoplastic disease in patients who are clearly at high risk. Firm cancer control efforts to avoid exposure to carcinogens (e.g., cigarettes) would also have major therapeutic effects. Second, it may be possible to modify

invasion by the use of substances that affect the cyto-skeleton of cells, and therefore their mobility and deformability. Efforts to do this would thereby lead to a greater localization of the primary tumor and a decrease in the frequency of metastasis. Third, the initial establishment of a metastatic lesion may be perturbed by attacking coagulation mechanisms. Considerable preclinical evidence as well as ongoing clinical experience supports this approach, particularly with the use of warfarin to reduce the number and extent of metastatic lesions in small cell carcinoma of the lung (Azcharaski et al, 1981).

**TABLE 2-3**  Human Solid Tumors: Doubling Time (DT), Generation Time ($T_c$), and Growth Fraction (GF)

| Tumor | Number of Patients Studied | Technique* | DT (Days) | $T_c$ (Days) | $T_s$ (Hours) | GF† (%) |
|---|---|---|---|---|---|---|
| Diffuse histiocytic lymphoma | 1 | PLM, DL | 21 | 2 | 14 | 24-86 |
| Lung (oat cell) | 1 | PLM | 40 | 2-3 | 18 | 67 |
| Melanoma | 7 | PLM, DL | 42 | 2-3 | 14-21 | 14 |
| Head and neck | 5 | PLM | 55 | 1-3 | 11-28 | |
| Breast | 5 | PLM | 90 | 1.5-4.0 | 13-24 | 3 |
| Colon | 10 | DL‡ | 100 | 2.5-3.0 | 17 | 1.5 |

* PLM = percentage of labeled mitosis curve; DL = double labeling technique for determining $T_s$.
† GF = $\frac{\text{tumor cells in cycle}}{\text{total number tumor cells}} = \frac{\text{LI (all cells)}}{\text{LI (proliferating cells)}} = \frac{\text{LI}}{T_s/T_c}$ where LI = the percentage of tumor cells in DNA synthesis at one point in time, i.e., the percentage of cells that label with tritiated thymidine.
‡ Estimated mean value of $T_c$ from the growth fraction determined by the DNA polymerase technique.

Through the science of metastasis and tumor heterogeneity, multiple phenotypes for drug resistance as well as for hormonal and immunologic characteristics of the tumor cells have been demonstrated in the parental population. This has profound implications for the development of therapeutic strategies, and approaches that attempt to be curative will have to take into account the marked heterogeneity in drug sensitivity and other phenotypes that are present. Clearly, the use of single-agent chemotherapy is unlikely to be curative in this setting; at the minimum, the use of combinations of agents—whether chemical, hormonal, or immunologic—will be needed for a successful therapeutic strategy to be devised. Finally, other mediators of the metastatic process (such as TAF) may be inhibited by certain products (such as protamine) and that metastasis to certain sites may be decreased by the use of $PGE_2$, which is capable of activating osteoclasts. There is experimental evidence to support these approaches, although to date clinical success has been limited (Powles et al, 1976). Overall, the biology of tumor invasion and metastasis holds promise for providing guidance in developing successful therapeutic strategies.

## REFERENCES

Aukerman SL, Price JE, Fidler IJ: Different deficiencies in the prevention of tumorigenic, low-metastatic murine K1735b melanoma cells from producing metastases. *J Natl Cancer Inst* 77:915, 1986.

Azcharaski LR, Henderson WG, Nickles FR, Forman WB, Cornell CJ, Forcier RJ, Edwards R, Headly E, Kim SH, O'Donald JR, O'Dell R, Tornyos K, Kivaan HC: Effect of warfarin on survival in small cell carcinoma of the lungs. *JAMA* 245:831-835, 1981.

Barranco S, Drewinko B, Humphrey RM: Differential response by human melanoma cells to 1,3-bis-(2-chloroethyl)-1 nitrosourea and bleomycin. *Mutation Res* 19:277-280, 1973.

Baylan SD, Weissberger WR, Eggleston JC, et al: Variable content of histaminase, L-dopa decarboxylase and calcitonin in small cell carcinoma of the lung: Biological and clinical implications. *N Engl J Med* 290:105-110, 1978.

Biorklund A, Hakansson L, Stemstan B, Trope C, Akerman M: Heterogeneity of non-Hodgkin's lymphomas as regards sensitivity to cytotoxic drug: An *in vitro* study. *Eur J Cancer* 16:647-654, 1980.

Brunson KW, Beattie G, Nicholson GL: Selection and altered properties of brain-colonizing metastatic melanoma. *Nature* 272:543-545, 1978.

Butler TP, Gullino PM: Quantitation of cells setting into efferent blood of mammary adenocarcinoma. *Cancer Res* 35:512-516, 1975.

Cifone MA, Fidler IJ: Increasing metastatic potential is associated with increasing genetic instability of clones isolated from murine neoplasms. *Proc Natl Acad Sci USA* 78:6949-6952, 1981.

Colcher D, Hand PH, Nati M, Schlom J: A spectrum of monoclonal antibodies reactive with human mammary tumor cells. *Proc Natl Acad Sci USA* 78:3199-3203, 1981.

Dvorak HF, Orenstein NS, Caravelle AC, Churchill WA, Giovinco P: Induction of a fibrin gel investment. *J Immunol* 122:166-174, 1979.

Fialkow PJ: Clonal origin of human tumors. *Biochem Biophys Acta* 458:283-291, 1976.

Fialkow PJ, Denman AM, Jakobson RJ, Lowenthal MN: Chronic myelocytic leukemia: Origin of some lymphocytes from leukemic stem cells. *J Clin Invest* 62:815-823, 1978.

Failkow PJ, Jakobson RJ, Papyannopoulou T: Chronic myelocytic leukemia: Clonal origin in a stem cell common to the granulocyte, erythrocyte, platelet and monocyte/macrophage. *Am J Med* 63:125-130, 1977.

Fidler IJ: Metastasis: Quantitative analysis of distribution and fate of tumor emboli labelled with $^{125}$-1-5-iodo-2$^1$ deoxyuridine. *J Natl Cancer Inst* 45:773-782, 1970.

Fidler IJ: Selection of successive tumor lines for metastases. *Nature (New Biol)* 242:148-149, 1973.

Fidler IJ, Hart IR: Biological and experimental consequences of the zonal composition of solid tumors. *Cancer Res* 41:3266-3267, 1981.

Fidler IJ, Hart IR: Biological diversity in metastatic neoplasms: Origins and implications. *Science* 217:998-1003, 1982.

Fidler IJ, Kripke ML: Metastasis results from pre-existent variant cells within a malignant tumor. *Science* 197:893-895, 1977.

Fidler IJ, Gruys E, Cifone MA, Barnes ZB, Bucana C: Demonstration of multiple phenotypic diversity in the murine melanoma of recent origin. *J Natl Cancer Inst* 67:947-956, 1981.

Fischer B, Saffer EA: Heterogeneity of tumor growth during chemoimmunotherapy. Observations in a murine model. In Fidler IJ, White RJ (eds): *Designs of Models for Testing Cancer Therapeutic Agents.* New York, Van Nostrand-Reinhold Co. 1982, pp 114-125.

Fisher ER, Turnbull RB Jr: Cytologic demonstration and significance of tumor cells in the mesenteric venous blood of patients with colorectal cancer. *Surg Gynecol Obstet* 100:102-108, 1955.

Foulds L: *Neoplastic Development.* London, Academic Press, 1969.

Frindel E, Malaise E, Tubiana M: Cell proliferation kinetics in five solid tumors. *Cancer* 22:611-620, 1968.

Gimbrone MA, Cotran RS, Folkman J: Tumor growth and neovascularization: An experimental model using rabbit cornea. *J Natl Cancer Inst* 52:413-427, 1974.

Goldacrer J, Sylven B: Access of blood borne dyes to various tumor regions. *Br J Cancer* 16:306-322, 1962.

Gouveia J, Mathe G, Herrend T, et al: Degree of bronchial metaplasia in heavy smokers and its regression after treatment with a retinoid. *Lancet* 1:710-712, 1982.

Hamburger AW, Salmon SE: Primary assay of human tumor stem cells. *Science* 197:461-473, 1977.

Hay ED (ed): *Cell Biology of the Extracellular Matrix.* New York, Plenum Press, 1981.

Hong WK, Lippman SM, Itri L, Karp DB, Lee JS, Byers R, Kramer A, et al: Prevention of second malignant tumors in head and neck cancer with 13-cis-retinoic acid (13cRA): Placebo controlled, double blind randomized trial. *Proc Am Soc Clin Oncol* 9:171(661), 1990a.

Hong WK, Lippman S, Itri LM, et al: Prevention of second primary tumors with isotretinoin in squamous cell carcinoma of the head and neck. *N Engl J Med* 323:795-801, 1990b.

Jackey PB, Beak B, Sutherland GR: Fragile sites in chromosomes: Possible model for the study of spontaneous chromosomal breakage. *Science* 220:69-70, 1983.

Kadish JL, Butterfield CE, Folkman J: The effect of fibrin on cultured vascular endothelial cells. *Tissue and Cell* 11:99-106, 1979.

Kao PT, Stern R: Elastases in human breast carcinoma cell lines. *Cancer Res* 46:1355, 1986.

Karpatkin S, Pearlstein E: Role of platelets in tumor cell metastases. *Ann Intern Med* 95:636-641, 1981.

Kramer S: Cancer of the head and neck: A challenge and a dilemma. *Semin Oncol* 4:353-355, 1977.

Kripke ML, Gruys E, Fidler IJ: Metastatic heterogeneity of cells from an ultraviolet light induced murine fibrosarcoma of recent origin. *Cancer Res* 38:2962-2967, 1978.

Liotta LA, Schiffermann E: Tumor motility factors. *Cancer Surv* 7:631, 1988.

Liotta LA, Stetler-Stevenson W: Metalloproteinases and malignant conversion: Does correlation imply causality? *J Natl Cancer Inst* 81:556, 1989.

Liotta LA, Abe S, Gehron-Robey P, Martin GR: Preferential digestion of basement membrane collagen by an enzyme derived from a metastatic murine tumor. *Proc Natl Acad Sci USA* 76:2268-2272, 1979.

Liotta LA, Kleinerman JN, Catanzaro P, Rymbrant D: Degradation of the basement membrane by tumor cells. *J Natl Cancer Inst* 58:1427-1431, 1977.

Liotta LA, Kleinerman JN, Saidel GM: Quantitative relationships of intravascular tumor cells, tumor vessels and pulmonary metastasis following tumor implantation. *Cancer Res* 34:997-1004, 1974.

Liotta LA, Saidel GM, Kleinerman JN: Stochastic model of metastasis formation. *Biometrics* 32:535-550, 1976.

Liotta LA, Thorgeirsson AP, Garbina S: Role of collagenases in tumor cell invasion. *Cancer Metastasis Rev* 1:277-288, 1982.

Liotta LA, Tryggvason K, Garbisa S, Hart I, Foltz CM, Shafie S:

Metastatic potential correlates with enzymatic degradation of basement membrane collagen. *Nature* 284:67-68, 1980.

Luria SE, Delbruck M: Mutations of bacteria from virus sensitivity to virus resistance. *Genetics* 28:491-511, 1943.

Lyon MF: X chromosome inactivation and developmental patterns in mammals. *Biol Rev* 47:1-35, 1972.

Malaise E, Shavaudra N, Tubiana M: The relationship between growth labelling index and histologic type of tumors. *Eur J Cancer* 9:305-312, 1973.

Morikawa K, Walker SM, Jessup JM, Fidler IJ: *In vivo* selection of highly metastatic cells from surgical specimens of different human colon carcinomas implanted into nude mice. *Cancer Res* 48:1943, 1988a.

Morikawa K, Walker SM, Makajima M, Pathak S, Jessup JM, Fidler IJ: Influence of organ environment on the growth, selection and metastasis of human cloned carcinoma cells in nude mice. *Cancer Res* 48:6863, 1988b.

Mundy GR, Luben RA, Raisz LG, et al: Bone resorbing ability in supernatants from lymphoid cell lines. *N Engl J Med* 290:867-871, 1974.

Nicholson GL: Cell surface antigen heterogeneity in blood borne tumor metastasis. In Owens AH Jr, Coffey DS, Baylin SB (eds): *Tumor Cell Heterogeneity.* New York, Academic Press, 1982a, pp 83-97.

Nicholson GL: Cell surfaces and cancer metastasis. *Hosp Pract* 17:75-86, 1982b.

Nicholson GL: Cellular interactions in blood borne metastasis: Metastatic spread to specific secondary sites. In Day SB, et al, (eds): *Cancer Invasion and Metastasis: Biological Mechanisms in Therapy.* New York, Raven Press, 1977.

Nowell P: The clonal evolution of tumor cell populations. *Science* 194:23-28, 1976.

Poste G, Fidler IJ: The pathogenesis of cancer metastasis. *Nature* 283:139-146, 1980.

Powles TJ, Clark SA, Easty DM, Easty GC, Neville AM: The inhibition by aspirin and indomethacin of osteolytic tumor deposits and hypercalcemia in rats with Walker tumor and if possible application to human breast cancer elements. *Br J Cancer* 28:316-321, 1973.

Powles TJ, Dow M, Easty GC, Easty DM, Neville AM: Breast cancer, bone metastasis and histio-osteolytic effect of aspirin. *Lancet* 1:608-610, 1976.

Price JE, Aukerman SL, Fidler IJ: Evidence of the process of murine melanoma and metastasis is sequential and selective and contains stochastic elements. *Cancer Res* 46:5172, 1986.

Schackert G, Fidler IJ: Site-specific metastasis of mouse melanomas and a fibrosarcoma in the brain or the meninges of syngeneic animals. *Cancer Res* 48:3478, 1988.

Shackney SE, McCormack GW, Cuchural GV: Growth rate patterns of solid tumors and their relationship to responsiveness to therapy. *Ann Intern Med* 89:107-121, 1978.

Siracky J: An approach to the problem of heterogeneity of human tumor cell populations. *Br J Cancer* 39:570-577, 1979.

Sluyser N, Van Nie R: Estrogen receptor content and hormone responsive growth of mouse mammary tumors. *Cancer Res* 34:3253-3257, 1974.

Sporn MB, Dunlop NM, Newton DL, Smith JM: Prevention of chemical carcinogenesis by vitamin A and the synthetic analogs (retinoids). *Fed Proc* 35:1332-1338, 1976.

Steel GG: *Growth Kinetics of Tumors.* New York, Oxford University Press, 1977.

Sutherland GR: Heritable fragile sites on human chromosomes. II. Distribution, phenotypic effects and cytogenetics. *Am J Hum Genet* 31:136-148, 1979.

Sutherland GR, Hinton L: Heritable fragile sites on human chromosomes. VI. Characterization of the fragile site at 12q13. *Am J Hum Genet* 57:217-219, 1981.

Talmadge JE: The evolution of diversity within tumors and metastases. In Kaiser HE (ed): *Progressive Stages of Neoplastic Growth.* Oxford, Pergamon Press, 1984, pp 276-285.

Talmadge JE, Wolman SR, Fidler IJ: Evidence for the clonal origin of spontaneous metastases. *Science* 217:361-363, 1982.

Tannock IF: The relationships between cell proliferation and the vascular system in transplanted mouse mammary tumour. *Br J Cancer* 22:258-273, 1968.

Trope C: Different susceptibilities of tumor cell subpopulations to cytotoxic agents. In Fidler IJ, White RJ (eds): *Design of Models for Testing Cancer Therapeutic Agents.* New York, D. Van Nostrand, 1982, pp 64-79.

Trope C, Apergrin K, Kullander S, et al: Heterogeneous response of disseminated human ovarian cancer to cytostatics *in vitro. Acta Obstet Gynecol Scand* 32:29-36, 1980.

Trope C, Hakansson L, Dencker H: Heterogeneity of human adenocarcinomas of the colon and the stomach as regards sensitivity to cytostatic agents. *Neoplasma* 22:423-430, 1975.

Weitzman SA, Stossel TP: Mutagenicity caused by human phagocytes. *Science* 212:546-547, 1981.

Yamada KM, Olden K: Fibronectins: Adhesive glycoproteins of cell surface and blood. *Nature* 275:179-184, 1978.

Yunis JJ: The chromosomal basis of human neoplasia. *Science* 212:227-236, 1983.

Yusa T, Blood CH, Zetter BR: Tumor cell interactions with elastin: Implications for pulmonary metastasis. *Am Rev Resp Dis* 140:1458, 1989.

Zeidman I: Critical comments. In Ruben P (ed): *Current Concepts in Cancer,* Vol. I. New York, Pergamon Press, 1975, pp 107-108.

Zimmerman A, Keller HU: Locomotion of tumor cells as an element of invasion in metastasis. *Biomed Pharmacother* 41:337, 1987.

# Chapter 3 | Viral Oncogenesis

*Ellen E. Sheets*

## VIRUSES AND CANCER

The concept that viruses may cause cancer is by no means novel or recent. With regard to cervical cancer, medical textbooks in the 1840s cited as its cause "animalcules," which, based on the description, were actually viruses (Walshe, 1844). The possibility that viruses were responsible for cervical cancer arose from epidemiologic studies in which cancer appeared to be sexually transmitted. Probably the earliest of these was a study by Rigoni-Stern in 1842, in which he found that uterine cancer was relatively rare among sexually inactive women (i.e., those who were unmarried or cloistered). In the 1950s, his findings gained support from more extensive epidemiologic data that refined the concept of sexual transmission by distinguishing two statistically significant risk factors: age of first intercourse and number of sexual partners (Gagnon, 1950; Jones et al, 1958).

Modern techniques in molecular biology, developed in the 1970s and 1980s, have enabled us to seek a scientific basis for the role of viruses in oncogenesis. The most notable evidence is the ever-increasing body of data implicating *human papillomavirus* (HPV) as the cause of cervical cancer. Although this association is strong, it is still not clear whether HPV acts alone or in concert with other carcinogens. Other viruses suspected of being carcinogenic are hepatitis B virus in primary liver cell carcinoma, Epstein-Barr virus in Burkitt's lymphoma, and cytomegalovirus in cancer of the prostate.

Definitive proof of a viral etiology for any cancer requires that the following criteria, known as *Koch's postulates* (Aurelian, 1983; Koch, 1890) be met:

1. The microorganism must be regularly isolated from patients with the illness.
2. It must be grown in (pure) culture.
3. When this (pure) culture is inoculated into a susceptible animal species, it should induce symptoms typical of the disease.
4. It should be possible to re-isolate the microorganism from the infected animals.

Absolute proof that a virus was the cause of a human cancer would require that an antiviral vaccine successfully prevent its development. In the absence of definitive etiologic proof, potential human tumor viruses should be followed through the lines of evidence that support their role in cancer induction.

Here we will focus on data for DNA viruses, as exemplified by HPV and its association with cervical cancer. Similar information regarding other viruses can be found in appropriate reviews (Epstein and Achong, 1986; Shaftner and Popper, 1987).

## Mechanisms of Viral Infection

Before we discuss how viruses might cause cell transformation and subsequent tumors, it is helpful to review the way in which viruses can interact with their host cell (i.e., establish an infection). There are three major types of virus-cell interactions—permissive, nonpermissive transformable, and nonpermissive nontransferable—and the type of interaction depends on the specific virus and cell being evaluated.

Not all cells are hosts for all viruses. Specific patterns of tropism, or preference, can occur for viral families and, to certain degree, within families. When a host cell is *permissive*, the virus enters and sets up its DNA in a separate, circular, or episomal form to allow for synthesis of viral DNA, RNA, and viral proteins. Mature viral particles are formed and then released, usually through cell lysis.

When nonpermissive cells allow the virus to enter, the viral DNA will still be episomal; however, complete synthesis of viral DNA, RNA, and proteins does not occur and mature viral particles are not formed. This may occur when those host-cell functions necessary for viral replication are lacking. As yet, these functions are not well defined. It is in these nonpermissive transferable cells that viruses can be associated with cell transformation, a process that requires viral DNA to become integrated into the host-cell DNA. Subsequently, viral and host-cell functions are lost, the host-cell phenotype is altered, and transformation can occur. Integration of viral DNA appears to be a rare event and may require prior viral protein synthesis.

The most common type of virus-cell interaction is *nonpermissive nontransformable*, in which the virus either is unable to enter the cell or cannot remain viable within the cell. This may be due to a whole range of factors, the more prominent of which are lack of cell functions that allow for viral entry, lack of functions to support the virus (called an abortive infection), or lack of factors necessary for transformation.

## Cell Transformation

The concept of cell transformation is important to an understanding of viral oncogenesis. A common misconception is that changes affecting a cell in vitro reflect identical changes in vivo that lead to tumor formation. Although numerous cell characteristics have been associated with an altered or transformed state, no specific characteristic defines a cell as being transformed. Transformation is best defined as one cell being transformed relative to another, usually the parent cell. Table 3-1 lists the major categories of transformed cell character-

TABLE 3-1   Characteristics of Transformed Cells

- Loss of contact inhibition of movement and growth.
- Alteration in morphology.
- Alteration in cell growth properties.
- Increased ability to survive prolonged culture in vitro.
- Reduced serum requirement for growth.
- Ability to grow in soft agar.
- Altered cell-surface properties.
- Karyotypic abnormalities.
- Ability to form tumors in susceptible animals.
- Presence of virus-specific cellular functions.
- Increased resistance to superinfection by the transforming virus.

Modified from Mackowiak PA: Microbial oncogenesis. *Am J Med* 82:79-97, 1987.

istics (Abercrombie, 1979; Rapp and Westmoreland, 1976).

# PROPERTIES OF PAPILLOMAVIRUSES

The papillomaviruses are strictly epitheliotropic (Table 3-2), including benign epithelial or fibroepithelial proliferations of the skin and mucosa in humans and a variety of animal species. Usually these tumors are self-limiting and regress; however, carcinomas have been reported to develop in association with longstanding papillomas. References to HPV-related infections can be found as early as the Roman-Hellenistic era in descriptions of the classic condylomas (exophytic warts) found on the external genitalia of both men and women. It was not until the late 1970s when Meisels et al, (1976, 1977) identified flat and endophytic "inverted" condylomatous lesions of the cervix that a possible role for HPV in cervical neoplasia was recognized.

Papillomaviruses are members of *Papovaviridae*, a DNA-containing family of animal viruses. Papillomavirus virions are nonenveloped iscosahedrons containing circular, double-stranded genomes of approximately $5 \times 10^6$ daltons. This translates into about 8,000 base pairs.

Initially, studies focused on shope (rabbit) and bovine (cow) papillomaviruses, since there was no suitable tissue culture system for propagating the virus in vitro. Now, with isolation and cloning of HPV DNA from virions obtained from clinical specimens, essentially all known HPVs have been completely sequenced (Lorinez

et al, 1986; Gissmann et al, 1982; Dartmann et al, 1986). These studies have shown that the HPV genomes sequenced to date are of similar size, have a low guanine and cytosine content, and exhibit similar overall genetic organization. The eight, long open reading frames (ORF) from which proteins are formed are located at similar positions on a single strand of viral DNA and are highly conserved. This means that these regions of DNA sequences are very similar, if not identical, between the different HPV types.

## Viral Genetic Function

Although most of what is known about the genetic function of various portions of the HPV genome comes from studies of animal papillomaviruses interacting with mouse fibroblasts, it is still valuable to examine these data relative to human disease. Essentially, three functional portions of the papillomavirus genome have been defined: the upstream regulatory region (URR), the early (E) region, and the late (L) region (Fig. 3-1).

The URR represents about 15% of the viral genome and is a noncoding region, i.e., it does not give rise to any protein formation. This region contains the origin of DNA replication for the virus, several promoters (sequences that initiate viral mRNA transcription), and several enhancers (sequences that speed up RNA transcription). Enhancers can bind to the viral genome, thus

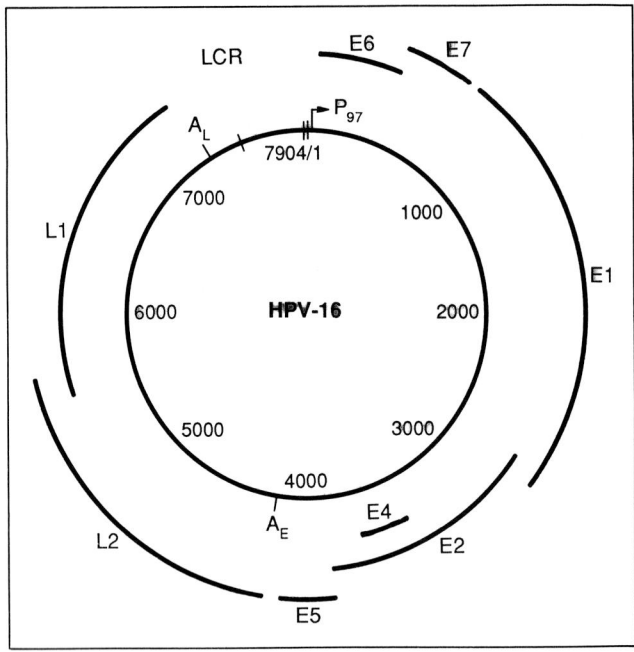

**Figure 3-1** Genomic map of HPV-16 deduced from DNA sequencing. Nucleotide numbers are noted within the circular map, with transcription occurring clockwise. The major open reading frames (designated E1 to E7, L1 and L2) are shown. The only promoter yet in HPV-16 is designated $P_{97}$. $A_E$ and $A_L$ represent the putative polyadenylation signals for early and late transcripts, respectively. The viral long control region (LCR), which contains the putative viral transcriptional and replication regulatory elements, is noted. (From Howley PM, Schlegel R: The human papillomaviruses. An overview. *Am J Med* 85[Suppl 2A]:155, 1988.)

TABLE 3-2   Clinical Association of Human Papillomaviruses (HPV)

| Types of Lesions | HPV Type(s) |
| --- | --- |
| Epidermodysplasia | 5, 8, 9, 12, 14, 15 |
| Verruciformis | 17, 19-25 |
| Genital tract lesions | 6, 11, 16, 18, 30, 31, 33, 35, 39, possibly 50s |

regulating the production of other viral proteins, or can bind to host receptors, thus inducing a conducive host environment (Lusky and Botchan, 1984; Yang et al, 1985; Baker and Howley, 1987).

Most genetic divergence among viral types occurs in the URR and these differences may be correlated with changes in virulence and oncogenic potential (Broker, 1987). Recently, these differences provided the basis for type-specific diagnostic probes by polymerase chain reaction (Chow et al, 1987).

The E region represents about 45% of the viral genome and contains at least seven ORFs, all of which code for proteins that either control viral DNA replication or maintain cell transformation. The ORFs were named according to relative size and not their actual location within the E region. The functions of individual ORFs are as follows:

- [ ] E1 ORF controls the episomal replication of viral DNA. When E1 is preserved, the viral genome cannot integrate (or become part of) the host-cell chromosome (Broker, 1987; Lusky and Botchan, 1985).
- [ ] E7 ORF helps regulate episomal DNA replication and may also play a role in malignant transformation (Lusky and Botchan, 1986).
- [ ] E2 ORF may be important for initiating or maintaining "benign" cellular transformations.
- [ ] E5 ORF produces a 7,000-dalton protein that binds to cytoplasmic membranes, leading to cell transformation. Loss of E5 favors integration of viral DNA into the cellular chromosome (Broker, 1987).
- [ ] E6 ORF produces a 18,000-dalton protein that leads to a change of growth properties in cell culture and appears to be involved in "malignant" cell transformation. Conservation and transcription of E6 have been observed in biopsy specimens of all HPV-containing human tumors and cervical-derived cell lines (Broker, 1987).
- [ ] E4 ORF produces proteins thought to contain messages that initiate the onset of koilocytotic changes, and this frame is usually deleted from carcinomas.

The L region contains about 40% of the viral genome, and its two ORFs code for capsid proteins (Kurman et al, 1983).

Some intriguing outcomes of molecular comparisons of HPV clinical isolates have been the demonstration of numerous subtypes of the virus (Coggin and zur Hausen, 1979), the preferential association of individual HPV subtypes with distinct clinical papillomas, and the observation that specific types of papillomatous lesions appear to be associated with multiple types of HPV (Table 3-2) (Krzyzck et al, 1980; Orth, et al, 1978; Green et al, 1982; Gissmann et al, 1983). At the molecular level, each subtype exhibits distinct DNA restriction enzyme cleavage patterns and antigenic heterogeneity of their capsid proteins (Gissmann et al, 1980; Orth et al, 1977). Such molecular heterogeneity has served to complicate the search for both HPV DNA and antigens in human tissue.

# CRITERIA FOR VIRAL ONCOGENESIS

Since it is not possible to utilize Koch's postulates exactly to prove a viral etiology for cancer, the following minimal criteria should ideally be met in order to support the concept of a tumor virus:

1. Infection with the agent should be sufficiently frequent in the population to account for the frequency of the tumor in question.
2. A 1:1 correlation must be demonstrated between occurrence of the tumor and evidence of infection with the virus.
3. The agent should exhibit oncogenic potential either after direct inoculation into laboratory animals or by demonstrating the tumorigenicity of cells transformed in vitro by the virus.
4. The agent, its nucleic acid, and/or its proteins must be present in tumor cells at some stage of tumor development.

## Incidence of Viral Infection in Cervical Cancer

Cancer epidemiology is difficult to interpret since genetic variation and social environmental factors often influence the development and subsequent progression of the disease. Although a detailed discussion of these factors is beyond the scope of this chapter, they do interfere with attempts to define the relationship between a possible etiologic agent and its rate of occurrence (Larsen et al, 1988). In the case of cervical cancer, this problem is compounded, since simple, prospective, large-volume studies of HPV are virtually impossible. There is no culture system to allow its detection, and investigators must rely on hybridization techniques to look for specific viral types.

Such data further suffer from differences in DNA hybdrization techniques, with some methods yielding better sensitivity and specificity than others. In general, between 10 and 23% of the asymptomatic female population between age 15 and 50 carries some type of HPV. Obviously, high-risk populations such as those seen at sexually transmitted disease clinics, have an overall higher rate of infection; however, they are not generally asymptomatic nor do they represent a large segment of the population (Kiviat et al, 1989; Wickenden et al, 1987; de Villiers et al, 1987). It is also possible that all types of HPV DNA have not been identified, so that DNA hybridization data should be considered the lowest estimate of the infection rate.

Serologic data for HPV are sparse but significant. Before the studies by Baird (1983), most serologic investigations of HPV infection had been limited to the study of skin warts and had utilized relatively insensitive techniques. Using a group-specific bovine papillomavirus antigen common to all papillomaviruses in conjunction with the sensitive solid-phase enzyme linked immunosorbent assay (ELISA) to test serum from patients with anogenital warts, cervical intraepithelial neoplasia (CIN), or cervical squamous carcinoma, Baird showed that antibody titers were higher in patients in all three groups compared with controls. The three groups were 95%, 60%, and 93% seropositive, respectively, whereas controls were essentially seronegative. Data for herpes simplex virus type 2 (HSV-2) have varied depending on how the study was controlled. The general consensus is that antibodies against HSV-2 are not more common in cancer patients than in appropriately matched control subjects (Vonka et al, 1984).

## HPV DNA, RNA, and Proteins in Cervical Cancer Cell Lines and Tumors

Several techniques can be used to detect viral DNA in any given sample of cells. Hybridization with a nick-translated, cloned viral DNA probe labeled with radioactive phosphorus ($^{32}$P) or selenium ($^{35}$S) to extracted sample DNA can be achieved with a sensitivity in the range of one copy/cell (Southern blot). This probe or the use of an immunoenhancement technique (e.g., biotin streptavidin) can be applied to cells or tissue sections in situ (Ostrow et al, 1987). One most be aware, however, that the total viral genome may not be present.

Data substantiating the presence of HPV DNA in cervical cancer cell lines and human tumor samples abound (Woodworth et al, 1988; Pecoraro et al, 1989; McCance et al, 1988; Wilczynski et al, 1988; Durst et al, 1983). Early hybridization studies were conducted before the plurality of HPV subtypes was known. More recently, this has been taken into account, and essentially all immortal cell lines and 80 to 90% of cervical cancers contain HPV DNA. The type of HPV DNA varies with the clinical lesion, whereas cell lines such as HeLa and Ca-Ski appear to harbor HPV 16 or 18. Which HPV is found seems to depend on the histologic grade of the preinvasive lesions, with type 6 or 11 found in cervical condylomas or cervical intraepithelial neoplasia grade I (CIN I) and types 16, 18, 31, 33, 35, 43, and 44 found in CIN II or III. Invasive squamous cell cervical cancers, regardless of grade, are associated with HPV types 16, 18, 33, 35, and 39 (Howley and Schlegel, 1988). Only now are we beginning to investigate possible differences in clinical course associated with different viral types. In women with Stage IB cervical cancer, Walker et al (1989) demonstrated retrospectively that the presence of HPV 18 was associated with a statistically greater chance of recurrence, irrespective of tumor histology or grade.

When viral RNA is detected in either cell lines or clinical samples, it indicates that the virus is not dormant. In addition, post-transcriptional splicing of RNA may be a mechanism by which the transformational ability of the same or different viral types can be controlled. RNA for HPV has been found in cervical cancers, and HPV types 16, 18, and 31 do have splicing sites (Gissmann and Schwarz, 1986). Specifically, HPV 16 and 18 have splicing sites within the E6 ORF. These sites lead to a smaller version of the E6 protein, termed E6* (Smotkin and Wettstein, 1986). The properties of this transcript may be important in transformation and carcinogenesis. In other recently isolated RNAs part of the viral message is deleted and replaced with RNA of

host-cell origin. The importance of these RNAs is not yet clear.

The presence of viral proteins also indicates viral activity. As noted previously, HPV proteins are divided into E and L regions. E region proteins play a role in viral replication and transformation, which the L region proteins are thought to be structural units of the viral particle. L region proteins are important in that antibodies can be made to the antigens and used to detect the presence of the virus in either tissue samples or sera. The importance of the E region proteins is much more complex and appears to vary greatly with the specific region. A large body of data has begun to accumulate implicating E6 and E7 proteins as important in host-cell transformation (Sato et al, 1989; Bedell et al, 1987).

## Oncogenic Potential of HPV

Although the causal association between the presence of a virus and cancer can be strong, such as between HPV and cervical cancer, it does not provide enough evidence to prove the oncogenicity of the virus. Transformation of normal cells to a malignant phenotype is a multistage process accomplished by different viruses using different mechanisms.

Four distinct mechanisms of transformation by viruses have been identified to date: (1) the stable introduction and expression of essential viral replicative genes that also have transforming functions into cellular DNA, (2) transduction of cellular genes with oncogenic potential by their incorporation into viral genomes accompanied by their release from normal control mechanisms, (3) insertion of strong promoter sequences adjacent to cellular oncogenes, and (4) genetic alternation in the cellular DNA sequences that activate cellular oncogenes.

While all four mechanisms have been associated with transformation by retroviruses, the oncogenic DNA viruses (adenoviruses, polyomavirus, and SV40) appear to transform cells in culture by the stable insertion of protein-coding sequences into cellular DNA (mechanism 1 above) (Tooze, 1980). The transforming proteins of these viruses play essential roles early in the viral replicative cycle; in transformed cells, their expression is required continuously in order to maintain the transformed phenotype. Moreover, for polyomaviruses and adenoviruses, the cooperative interaction of multiple viral proteins is apparently essential to establish the fully transformed phenotype.

In *polyomavirus*, the interactions of specific viral proteins have been implicated in the induction of individual transformed cell phenotypes—e.g., growth of dense foci in high serum, growth of continuous cell lines in low serum, and loss of anchorage-dependence. Cooperating viral proteins are encoded in overlapping genes (Rassoulzadegan et al, 1982). With *adenoviruses*, the genes for cooperating proteins lie adjacent to one another (Graham et al, 1974). In both cases, however, the genes for cooperating proteins lie within a single defined segment of the genome. Importantly, the fact that different cell lines transformed by the same virus may exhibit different phenotypic properties depending upon which proteins are expressed indicates that different transformation assays (focus formation, immortalization, colony formation in soft agar, and so on) can yield different results with respect to the viral genes (proteins) involved in transformation.

As the DNA from HPV-related infections has been isolated and sequenced, investigators have been able to determine that HPV 16 and 18 can be found integrated into the cellular DNA. Obviously this follows the pattern of transformation outlined in the first mechanism above. Although HPV 16 has been found in episomal form in some CIN lesions, it is found only in an integrated form in immortal cervical cancer cell lines and invasive cancers. At present, it is not possible to create cervical cancers by injecting HPV into laboratory animals; however, mouse cell lines that have been transformed by bovine papillomavirus can cause tumors in nude mice (Dvoretzky et al, 1980). HPV 16 can transform immortalized mouse cells and convert them into a tumorigenic state and can immortalize primary human cells in vitro (Yasumoto et al, 1986; Pirisi et al, 1987). The immortalized cells do not create tumors in nude mice. It is not yet clear what is missing in this transformation, so that a tumor cannot form. Many researchers are now interested in how transformation occurs and is controlled in HPV-infected cells. Using techniques that allow either the entire genome or fragments of DNA to be introduced into cells, the viral genome can be investigated in more detail. Separation of DNA fragments created by digestion of viral DNA with subsequent transection of different fragments into receptive cells allows the transformation potential of that genomic region to be evaluated (Howley et al, 1986). Even more revealing has been the characterization of sites of integration in cell lines and tumors.

Iwasaka et al (1988) inserted the full genome of either HPV 16 or 18 into Syrian hamster embryo cells immortalized by HSV-2. Morphologic transformation occurred in these cells and caused tumors when injected into nude mice. Tumors did not occur when cells without HSV-2 were utilized. Pecoraro et al (1989) evaluated the differential transforming ability of HPV 16, 18, and 6 on the same cell line. HPV 6 did not integrate into the cellular DNA but remained in a stable, episomal form. No transformation of the cells occurred. The changes in growth properties and morphology differed when HPV 16 or 18 was used to transform the same cell lines, and integration did occur. Intriguingly, this differential growth may reflect similar progressive oncogenic processes that result in cervical cancer in vivo.

Evaluations of integration sites have yielded information about the cellular DNA surrounding the site and have supported the apparent importance of the E6 or E7 ORFs. Durst et al (1987) looked at cellular sequences surrounding integrated DNA in four cell lines and two primary tumors. In the two tumors, HPV 16 was integrated in a region that also contains the *c-src-1* and *c-raf-1* oncogenes. In cell lines, integration also occurred near known cellular oncogenes. Specifically, the HPV 18 integration site in HeLa cells is near *c-myc*,

and *c-myc* RNA levels are elevated in HeLa relative to other cervical carcinoma cell lines. These preliminary support the concept of *cis*-activation of cellular oncogenes by HPV, which may play a role in a malignant transformation. Data reviewed by Cannizzaro et al (1988) further support the concept that HPV is integrated in cell lines and primary tumors near fragile sites, oncogenes, and chromosome breakpoints characteristic of hematologic malignancies and solid tumors. Choo et al (1987) evaluated seven separate cervical cancer specimens and noted that although the E2 reading frame was invariably lost, E6/E7 was highly retained.

## HPV in Tumor Cells During Tumor Development

Because cancer takes years to progress, as is certainly the case for cervical cancer, it is exceedingly difficult—if not impossible—to prove that a lesion progresses from simple infection to cancer. In cervical cancer, the histologic progression from early grades of intraepithelial neoplasia to carcinoma in situ and finally to invasive cancer is widely accepted. The logical approach would be to look for those invasive tumors that have associated preinvasive lesions in proximity and probe for HPV DNA. Several investigators have done this, with the interesting result that more than one type of HPV is often present in these areas (Crissman et al, 1985; Boon and Kok, 1985; Kadish et al, 1986). In addition, latency of HPV infection has been established—an important point, since the number of patients who are reexposed or are carriers is much higher than the number who actually develop preinvasive or invasive disease (Ferenczy et al, 1985).

## SUMMARY

Definitive proof of an etiologic role for HPV in cervical cancer has not yet been established. However, a review of the data has revealed certain points essential to indirect support of a viral cause of cancer, based on the criteria cited earlier:

1. HPV infection appears to be sufficiently frequent in the population to account for the frequency of cervical cancer.
2. The fact that a 1:1 correlation between the occurrence of any HPV type and cervical cancer has not been definitively demonstrated may have several explanations:
   a. Not all viral types have been isolated.
   b. The technique of DNA hybridization for small fragments of the genome is not sensitive enough.
   c. Cervical cancer may be caused by more than one viral agent, acting either alone or synergistically.
3. Either direct or indirect evidence for the oncogenic potential of HPV has been reported. Although HPV has not induced tumors after direct inoculation of laboratory animals, cells transformed under certain conditions in vitro have been found to be tumorigenic.

4.  HPV DNA, RNA, and proteins have been detected in the vast majority of cervical cancer cell lines and tumor specimens. These findings provide strong support for HPV's etiologic role in the development of this disease. Whatever the mechanism of transformation by HPV, zur Hausen (1977, 1982) has postulated a synergistic effect involving HSV-2 and HPV in the genesis of human genital cancer on the basis of (a) the frequent occurrence of genital infection with HPV and the less frequent conversion of papillomatous lesions to cancer, (b) possible simultaneous infection with HSV-2, and (c) the apparent inability to detect HSV-2 DNA readily in cervical carcinoma biopsy specimens. The hypothesis proposes that HSV-2 provides an "initiating" function and HPV a "promoting" function. The model can actually be changed to use any known carcinogens (such as those found in cigarette smoke) as the initiator, not just HSV-2. This model provides a mechanism whereby cervical tumors, like other tumors, may develop through several stages involving initiation and promotion.

The model described above is clearly only conjectural and will require further epidemiologic and experimental substantiation. Despite these uncertainties, the body of evidence implicating HPV in the development of gynecologic tumors is very impressive. Should HPV (and/or HSV-2) be shown to play an essential role in one or more stages of malignant conversion, the prospect for intervention and control of genital tumors will be at hand.

## REFERENCES

Abercrombie M: Contact inhibition and malignancy. *Nature* 281:259-262, 1979.

Aurelian L: Herpes viruses and cervical cancer. In Phillips LA (ed): *Viruses Associated With Human Cancer.* New York, Marcel Dekker, 1983, pp 79-135.

Baird PJ: Serological evidence for the association of papillomavirus and cervical neoplasia. *Lancet* 2:17, 1983.

Baker CC, Howley PM: Differential promoter utilization by bovine papillomavirus in transformed cells and productively infected wart tissues. *EMBO J* 6:1027-1035, 1987.

Bedell MA, Jones KH, Laimins LA: The E6-E7 region of human papilloma virus type 18 is sufficient for transformation of NIH 3T3 and rat-1 cells. *J Virol* 61:3635-3640, 1987.

Boon ME, Kok LP: Koilocytotic lesions of the cervix: The interrelation of morphometric features the presence of papilloma-virus antigens and the degree of koilocytosis. *Histopathology* 9:751-763, 1985.

Broker TR: Structure and genetic expression of papillomaviruses. *Obstet Gynecol Clin NA* 14:329-348, 1987.

Cannizzaro LA, Durst M, Mendez MJ, Hecht BK: Regional chromosomal localization of human papillomavirus integration sites near fragile sites, oncogenes, and cancer chromosome breakpoints. *Cancer Genet Cytogenet* 33:93-98, 1988.

Choo KIB, Pan, Han SH: Integration of human papilloma type 16 into cellular DNA of cervical carcinoma; preferential deletion of the long control region and the E6/E7 open reading frames. *Virology* 16:259-261, 1987.

Chow LT, Hirochilea H, Nasser M, et al: Human papillomavirus gene expression. In Steinberg BM, Brandsma JL, Taichman LB (eds): *Papillomaviruses. Cancer Cells 5.* New York, Cold Spring Harbor Laboratory, 1987.

Coggin JR, zur Hausen H: Workshop on papilloma viruses and cancer. *Cancer Res* 39:545-546, 1979.

Crissman JD, Makuch R, Budhraja M: Histopathologic grading of squamous cell carcinoma of the uterine cervix. An evaluation of 70 stage IB patients. *Cancer* 55:1590-1596, 1985.

Danos O, Katinka M, Yanio M: Papillomavirus genomes: Sequences and consequences. *J Invest Dermatol* 83:7s-11s, 1984.

Dartmann K, Schwarz E, Gissman L, et al: The nucleotide sequence and genome organization of human papilloma virus type. *Virology* 151:124-130, 1986.

de Villiers EM, Wagner D, Schneider A, Wesch H, et al: Human papillomavirus infections in women with and without abnormal cervical cytology. *Lancet* 2: 703-706, 1987.

Durst M, Croce CM, Gissmann L, et al: Papillomavirus sequences integrate near cellular oncogenes in some cervical carcinomas. *Proc Natl Acad Sci [USA]* 84:1070-1074, 1987.

Durst M, Gissmann L, Ikenberg H, zur Hausen H: A papillomavirus DNA from a cervical carcinoma and its prevalence in cancer biopsy samples from different geographic regions. *Proc Natl Acad Sci [USA]* 80:3812-3815, 1983.

Dvoretsky I, Shober R, Chattopdhyay SK, Lowy DR: A quantitative in vitro focus assay for bovine papillomavirus. *Virology* 103:369-375, 1980.

Epstein MA, Achong BG (eds): *The Epstein-Barr Virus: Recent Advances.* London, William Heinemann, 1986.

Ferenczy A, Mitai M, Nagai N, et al: Latent papillomavirus and recurring genital warts. *N Engl J Med* 313:748-754, 1985.

Gagnon F: Contribution to the study of the etiology and prevention of cancer of the cervix of the uterus. *Am J Obstet Gynecol* 60:516-522, 1950.

Gissmann L, Schwarz E: Persistence and expression of human papillomavirus DNA in genital cancer. CIBA Foundation Symposium: *Papillomaviruses, Vol 120.* New York, John Wiley & Sons, 1986, pp 190-207.

Gissmann L, Dichl V, Schulz-Conlon HJ, et al: Molecular cloning and characteristics of human papillomavirus DNA derived from a laryngeal papilloma. *J Virol* 44:393-396, 1982.

Gissmann L, Pfister H, zur Hausen H: Human papillomavirus (HPV): Characterization of four different isolates. *Virology* 76:569-580, 1980.

Gissmann L, Wolnik L, Ikenberg H, Kolodovsky U, Schnurch HG, zur Hausen H: Human papillomavirus types 6 and 11 DNA sequences in genital and laryngeal papillomas and in some cervical cancers. *Proc Natl Acad Sci [USA]* 80:560-563, 1983.

Graham FL, Abrahams PJ, Mulder C, Hiejneker HL, Warnaar SO, DeVires FAJ, Fiers W, van der EB AJ: Studies on in vitro transformation by DNA and DNA fragments of human adenoviruses and simian virus 40. Cold Spring Harbor Symposium on Quantitative Biology 39:637-650, 1974.

Green M, Brackmann KH, Sanders PR, Lowenstein PM, Freel JH, Eisinger M, Switlyk SA: Isolation of a human papillomavirus from a patient with epidermodysplasia verruciformis: Presence of related viral DNA genomes in human urogenital tumors. *Proc Natl Acad Sci [USA]* 79:4437-4441, 1982.

Howley PM, Schlegel R: The human papillomaviruses. An overview. *Am J Med* 85(supp 2A):155-158, 1988.

Howley PM, Young YC, Spalholz BA, Rabson MS: Papillomavirus transforming functions. CIBA Foundation Symposium: *Papillomaviruses, Vol 120.* New York, John Wiley & Sons, 1986, pp 39-52.

Iwasaka T, Yokoyama M, Hayashi Y, Sugimori H: Combined herpes simplex virus type 2 and human papillomavirus type 16 or 18 deoxyribonucleic acid leads to oncogenic transformation. *Am J Obstet Gynecol* 159:1251-1255, 1988.

Jones EG, MacDonald I, Breslow L: A study of epidemiologic factors in carcinoma of the uterine cervix. *Am J Obstet Gynecol* 76:726-735, 1958.

Kadish AS, Burk RD, Kress Y, et al: Human papillomaviruses of different types in precancerous lesions of the uterine cervix: Histologic, immunocytochemical and ultrastructural studies. *Human Pathol* 17:384-392, 1986.

Kiviat NB, Koutsky LA, Paavonen JA, et al: Prevalence of genital papillomavirus infection among women attending a college student health clinic or a sexually transmitted disease clinic. *J Infect Dis* 159:1424-1477, 1989.

Krzyzek RA, Watts SL, Anderson DL, Faras AJ, Pass F: Anogenital warts contain several distinct species of human papillomaviruses. *J Virol* 36:236-244, 1980.

Kurman RJ, Jensen AB, Lancaster WD: Papillomavirus infection of the cervix. 2. Relationship to intraepithelial neoplasia based on the presence of specific viral structural proteins. *Am J Surg Pathol* 7:39-52, 1983.

Larsen PM, Vetner M, Hansen K, Fey SJ: Future trends in cervical cancer. *Cancer Lett* 41:123-137, 1988.

Lorinez AT, Lancaster WD, Temple GF: Cloning and characterization of the DNA of a new human papillomavirus from a woman with dysplasia of the uterine cervix. *J Virol* 58:225-229, 1986.

Lusky M, Botchan MR: Characterization of the bovine papillomavirus plasmid maintenance sequences. *Cell* 36:391-401, 1984.

Lusky M, Botchan MR: Genetic analysis of bovine papillomavirus type I transacting replication factors. *J Virol* 53:935-965, 1985.

Lusky M, Botchan MR: Transient replication of bovine papillomavirus type I plasmids. *Cis* and *trans* requirements. *Proc Natl Acad Sci [USA]* 83:3609-3613. 1986.

McCance DJ, Kopan R, Fuchs E, Laimins LA: Human papillomavirus type 16 alters human epithelial cell differentiation in vitro. *Proc Natl Acad Sci [USA]* 85:7169-7173, 1988.

Meisels A, Fortin R: Condylomatous lesions of the cervix and vagina. I. Cytologic patterns. *Acta Cytol* 20:505-509, 1973.

Meisels A, Fortin R, Roy M: Condylomatous lesions of the cervix and vagina. II. Cytologic, colposcopic and histopathologic study. *Acta Cytol* 21:379-389, 1977.

Orth G, Favre M, Croissant O: Characterization of a new type of human papillomavirus that causes skin warts. *J Virol* 24:108-120, 1977.

Orth G, Jablonska S, Favre M, Croissant O, Jarzabek-Chrzelska M, Rzesa G: Characterization of two types of human papillomaviruses in lesions of epidermodysplasia verruciformis. *Proc Natl Acad Sci [USA]* 75:1537-1541, 1978.

Ostrow RS, Krzyzek R, Pass F, Faras AJ: Identification of a novel human papillomavirus in cutaneous warts of meat-handlers. *Virology* 108:21-27, 1981.

Ostrow RS, Manias DA, Clark BA, et al: Detection of human papillomavirus DNA in invasive carcinomas of the cervix by in situ hybridization. *Cancer Res* 47:649-653, 1987.

Pecoraro G, Morgan D, Defendi V: Differential effects of human papillomavirus type 6, 16, 18, DNAs on immortalization and transformation of human cervical epithelial cells. *Proc Nat Acad Sci [USA]* 86:563-567, 1989.

Phelps WC, Yee CL, Munger K, Howley PM: The human papillomavirus type 16 E7 gene encodes transactivation and transformation function similar to those of adenovirus EIA. *Cell* 53:539-547, 1988.

Pirisi L, Yasumoto S, Feller M, et al: Transformation of human fibroblasts and keratinocytes with human papillomavirus type 16 DNA. *J Virol* 61:1061-1066, 1987.

Rapp F, Westmoreland D: Cell transformation by DNA containing viruses. *Biochim Biophys Acta* 458:167-211, 1976.

Rassoulzadegan M, Cowie A, Carr A, et al: The roles of individual polyomaviruses early proteins in oncogenic transformation. *Nature* 300:713-718, 1982.

Rigoni-Stern D: Fatti statistici relativi alle malattie cancerose. *Gior Servire Progr Pathol Terap* 2:507-517, 1842.

Sato H, Furuno A, Yoshiike K: Expression of human papillomaviruses type 16 E7 gene induces DNA synthesis of rat 3Y1 cells. *Virology* 168:195-199, 1989.

Shaftner F, Popper H (eds): *Progress in Liver Disease*. Orlando, Florida, Grune and Stratton, 1987.

Smotkin D, Wettstein OF: Transcription of human papillomavirus type 16 early genes in a cervical cancer and a cancer derived cell line and identification of the E7 protein. *Proc Natl Acad Sci [USA]* 83:4680-4684, 1986.

Storey A, Pim D, Murray A, Osborn K, Banks L, Crawford C: Comparison of the in vitro transforming activities of human papillomavirus types. *EMBO J* 7:1815-1820, 1988.

Tooze J: DNA tumor viruses. In Tooze J (ed): *Molecular Biology of Tumor Viruses (Part 2)*, 2nd ed. New York, Cold Spring Harbor Laboratory, 1980.

Vonka V, Kanka J, Hirsh I, et al: Prospective study on the relationship between cervical neoplasia and herpes simplex type-2 virus. II. Herpes simplex type-2 antibody presence in sera taken at enrollment. *Int J Cancer* 33:61-66, 1984.

von Knebel Doeberitz M, Oltersdorf T, Schwarz E, Gissmann L: Correlation of modified human papilloma virus early gene expression with altered growth properties in C4-1 cervical carcinoma cells. *Cancer Res* 48:3780-3786, 1988.

Walker J, Bloss JO, Liao S, et al: Human papillomavirus genotype as a prognostic indicator in carcinoma of the uterine cervix. *OB/GYN* 74:781-785, 1989.

Walshe WH: *The Anatomy, Physiology, Pathology and Treatment of Cancer* Boston, W.D. Ticknor, 1844, pp 349-350.

Wickenden C, Malcolm AD, Byrne M, et al: Prevalence of HPV DNA and viral copy numbers in cervical scrapes from women with normal and abnormal cervices. *J Pathol* 153:127-135, 1987.

Wilczynski SP, Walker J, Liao SY, Bergen S, Berman M: Adenocarcinoma of the cervix associated with human papillomavirus. *Cancer* 62:1331-1336, 1988.

Woodworth CD, Bowden PE, Doniger J, et al: Characterization of normal human exocervical epithelial cells immortalized in vitro by papillomavirus types 16 and 18 DNA. *Cancer Res* 48:4620-4628, 1988.

Yang YC, Okayama H, Howley PM: Bovine papillomavirus contains multiple transforming genes. *Proc Natl Acad Sci [USA]* 82:1030-1064, 1985.

Yasumoto S, Burkhardt AL, Doniger J, DiPaolo JA: Human papillomavirus type 16 DNA induced malignant transformation of NIH 3T3 cells. *J Virol* 57:572-577, 1986.

zur Hausen H: Human papillomaviruses and their possible role in squamous cell carcinomas. *Curr Top Microbiol Immunol* 78:1-30, 1977.

zur Hausen H: Human genital cancer: Synergism between two virus infections or synergism between a virus infection and initiating events? *Lancet* 2:1370-1372, 1982.

# Chapter 4 | Gynecologic Tumor Immunology

*Robert C. Bast, Jr.*     *Michael A. Bookman*

*Robert C. Knapp*

## TUMOR-ASSOCIATED ANTIGENS

Cellular and humoral immune responses have evolved to recognize and eliminate pathogens that bear antigenic molecules not found in normal host tissues. According to a central concept of contemporary tumor immunology, tumor cells also bear antigens not found on normal tissues that permit the host to identify and destroy a tumor as foreign (Klein, 1966; Herberman, 1977; Old, 1981). Specific tumor-associated antigens that mediate the rejection of tumor transplants have been defined in animal systems. How frequently comparable antigens are associated with human cancers remains to be resolved. Yet many antigens are expressed by both human tumor cells and normal cells in the adult or fetus, including histocompatibility, oncofetal, differentiation, and lineage-associated antigens.

### Tumor-Specific Transplantation Antigens

At the turn of the century, investigators began to ask whether tumors could be transplanted from one animal to another. Such tumor transplants were usually rejected within a few days. Repeated tumor transplants in the same animal were rejected even more promptly. Eventually, it became apparent that exactly the same phenomenon could be observed when normal tissues or organs were transplanted between genetically nonidentical individuals. Rejection of tumor transplants was mediated by the immunologic recognition of foreign histocompatibility antigens rather than by recognition of specific antigens associated only with tumor cells.

With the development of inbred strains of mice in the early 1940s, it was possible to reexamine whether tumor cells bore specific antigens capable of mediating resistance to tumor transplantation (Gross, 1943; Foley, 1953; Prehn and Main, 1957). Some of the first critical studies were performed with sarcomas that developed in inbred mice following the injection of polycyclic hydrocarbon carcinogens. Progressive tumor growth was observed following the injection of sarcoma cells into healthy recipients from the same inbred strain. If a tumor transplant was excised or its blood supply ligated prior to the formation of metastases, the "cured" mouse resisted rechallenge with the same number of tumor cells that would grow progressively in a nonimmune recipient. The cured mouse would, however, accept a graft of normal skin from the tumor donor, confirming that the donor and recipient shared the same histocompatibility antigens.

Transplantation resistance was relative rather than absolute. Although an immune mouse would reject up to 10,000 times as many tumor cells as a nonimmune recipient, a dose of tumor could usually be found that would overcome the transplantation resistance of the host. Specific resistance to tumor growth depended primarily upon T lymphocytes rather than upon antibodies. Each antigen detected in a new chemically induced tumor appeared to be distinct (Old and Boyse, 1964; Baldwin and Price, 1975). If tumors A, B, and C were induced with the same chemical in different mice, a mouse immunized with tumor A could reject only tumor A but not tumor B or tumor C. Conversely, when tumors were induced by an oncogenic virus, all tumors induced by a single virus exhibited a common antigen (Habel, 1961). Over the last three decades, these distinctions have been modified. Tumors induced by some viruses exhibit unique or "private" antigens (Morton et al, 1969; Vaage, 1968). Alternatively, some chemically induced tumors share common oncofetal antigens that may mediate transplantation resistance. Many "spontaneous" tumors that have not been induced intentionally with chemical or viral carcinogens appear to lack tumor-specific transplantation antigens. Among 44 spontaneous rat tumors, only seven were found to be immunogenic on transplantation (Baldwin, 1983). In many, but not all, animal tumor models, rejection is mediated by T lymphocytes that recognize not only the specific transplantation resistance antigens of the tumor but also the histocompatibility antigens of the host (Wagner et al, 1980).

Thus, even under optimal circumstances in which healthy animals are actively immunized with tumor tissue, the resistance to tumor growth is not absolute and may not be expressed against all cancers. Moreover, the ability of T lymphocytes to recognize tumor cells generally requires co-recognition of the host's own histocompatibility antigens together with tumor-associated transplantation resistance antigens.

Recent advances in molecular biology have permitted chemical characterization of antigens that mediate tumor-specific transplantation resistance in animal models (Thurin, 1990). One of the antigens associated with a chemically induced murine fibrosarcoma is a 96-kD cell-surface glycoprotein (Srivastava et al, 1987) with a primary amino acid sequence, resembling that of certain human tumor associated glycoproteins (Srivastava and Old, 1989). In another murine tumor system, a single point mutation alters a 60-kD protein, permitting recognition by murine T cells (Lurquin et al, 1989).

Evidence for the existence of tumor-specific transplantation resistance in humans has been assembled from several sources. Spontaneous regressions occur in a very small fraction of renal cell cancers and melanomas, although it is not certain that these relate to an immune response of the host to tumor. Autologous tumor cell extracts have produced delayed cutaneous reactivity after injection into cancer patients, but it is not clear whether this reactivity would induce rejection of a vascularized tumor. In cell culture, proliferation of lymphocytes has been observed in the presence of autologous tumor cells from a majority of patients with solid tumors (Vose and Howell, 1983). Lymphocytes from cancer patients can lyse autologous tumor cells in as many as 35% of cases (Vose and Howell, 1983; Vanky et al, 1984). Cytotoxic T-cell clones have been isolated from the blood, lymph nodes, or tumor tissue of patients with different cancers. Availability of recombinant interleukin-2 (IL-2) has permitted prolonged growth of human T cells in cell culture and the isolation of antigen-specific T-cell clones. Cytotoxic T lymphocytes grown in the presence of IL-2 have recognized unique antigens associated with breast cancer, pancreatic cancer, and melanoma. In general, MHC restriction is important for human tumor immunity mediated by antigen-specific T lymphocytes (Okubo et al, 1989).

Thus, the patient's own tumor cells are the most relevant target for studying T-cell-mediated antitumor activity and provide the most relevant components for potential vaccines. Perhaps the most compelling evidence for human tumor-specific transplantation resistance has been provided by studies of cloned cytotoxic lymphocytes from melanoma patients, which lyse only autologous tumor cells and home to tumor sites after adoptive transfer (Fisher et al, 1989). Although the majority of antigens are recognized in the context of host major histocompatibility complex (MHC) determinants, T cells from patients with breast and pancreatic cancer can recognize exposed areas in the protein core of tumor-associated mucin molecules that have undergone abnormal glycosylation (Jerome et al, 1990). The core protein has been cloned and found to contain numerous repeating subunits of 20 amino acids that create multiple identical epitopes on the same mucin molecule and that may circumvent the requirement for recognition in the context of MHC antigens (Burchell et al, 1989).

Only a few studies of specific cellular immunity have been performed in gynecologic cancer patients. Tumor growth was inhibited in vitro with allogeneic lymphocytes from patients with cervical and ovarian cancer (DiSaia, 1975). In some studies, "blocking factors" were found in the patient's serum that inhibited the cytotoxic activity of lymphocytes. Patients with progressively growing tumors had such factors, whereas patients who were in complete remission did not (Dini and Faiferman, 1980; Pattillo et al, 1979*a,b,* and *c*). Lymphocytes from ovarian cancer patients proliferated in the presence of autologous tumor cells (Hudson et al, 1976) and T-cell clones have demonstrated relative specificity for autologous tumor cells in a small number of cases (Ferrini et al, 1985). Recently, additional cytotoxic T-cell clones have been grown from tumor-associated lymphocyte infiltrates in the presence of IL-2 and autologous ovarian cancer cells (Ioannides et al, 1990). At least three different antigenic epitopes have been defined that are recognized in the context of MHC determinants.

The potential role of the humoral immune response in tumor rejection is less well defined than that of cellular immunity, but patients with melanoma, renal cell carcinoma, and glioblastoma can produce immunoglobulins that bind to these neoplasms. In the case of melanoma, three types of antibodies have been identified: (1) antibodies reactive only with autologous tumor; (2) antibodies reactive only with autologous and allogeneic tumor cells; and (3) antibodies broadly reactive with multiple malignant and benign tissues. Some 75% of patients with melanoma can produce antibodies that bind to autologous tumor cells, but only 5% are of type 1 and 7% of type 2 (Old, 1981). An antibody that reacted only with autologous melanoma was used to identify a unique FD antigenic determinant or epitope on a 90-kd cell-surface molecule associated with a single cell line (Real et al, 1984). Murine monoclonal antibodies bind to different epitopes on this molecule and can also bind to similar molecules on tumor cells from most melanoma patients (Furukawa et al, 1989), suggesting that unique epitopes may be expressed on molecules that are widely distributed among tumor cells from different individuals.

## Histocompatibility Antigens

Both class I and class II MHC antigens are associated with gynecologic tumors. Class I human leukocyte antigens A, B, and C (HLA-A, HLA-B, and HLA-C) each contain two polypeptide chains (Kindt and Robinson, 1984). A polymorphic 42-kD chain is noncovalently linked to an invariant 12-kD chain known as beta$_2$ microglobulin. Class II MHC antigens consist of two covalently linked polymorphic polypeptide chains of up to 33 and 29 kD. The T-cell receptor generally recognizes antigenic peptides only after they have bound to class I or class II MHC molecules on the surface of antigen-presenting cells such as macrophages and B cells. Exogenous protein antigens are taken up through endosomes and are bound to class II MHC products, whereas endogenous viral and cell-surface antigens are associated with class I products during synthesis and cell-membrane expression.

CD8$^+$ T cells interact primarily with class I MHC antigens and CD4$^+$ T cells interact primarily with class II determinants. In general, cytotoxic and suppressor T-cell phenotypes have been more often associated with CD8$^+$ cells, whereas helper-inducer phenotypes have been associated with CD4$^+$ cells. However, the opposite associations have been described in a minority of T cells. Class I MHC antigens are widely expressed on most human tissues, with the exception of germ cells, placenta, and erythrocytes. Thus, many tumor cells can directly activate CD8$^+$ T lymphocytes without additional antigen processing. Class II MHC determinants are not commonly expressed on tumor cells and are restricted to lymphocytes, macrophages, and endothelial cells. Epithelial cells can, however, express Class II antigens, particularly after treatment with gamma-interferon.

In the normal ovary, class I MHC determinants are found on the surface epithelium, stroma, and follicles. Class II determinants are generally not detected in the normal ovary, with the exception of weak expression on vascular endothelium. Approximately 80% of epithelial ovarian carcinomas express class I determinants, judged by binding of monoclonal antibodies directed against the nonpolymorphic region of the HLA molecule (Kabawat et al, 1983b). Interestingly, some 40% of epithelial ovarian carcinomas express class II antigens. Similar ectopic expression of class II antigen has been observed in melanomas and in a small fraction of other epithelial tumors (Daar et al, 1982). Whether or not this reflects endogenous interferon production and whether Class II antigen expression permits the host to recognize tumors more readily remain to be determined. When ovarian cancers that stimulated proliferation of autologous lymphocytes were compared with those which did not, a similar fraction of HLA-DR$^+$ tumors (50 to 54%) was observed in each group (Di Bello et al, 1988). Expression of Class II MHC antigens has not correlated with survival among patients with advanced disease (Festenstein et al, 1990).

In patients treated for trophoblastic disease, immune complexes containing antibody and HLA fragments appeared in the serum after chemotherapy-induced tumor regression (Rayner et al, 1981; Lahey et al, 1984). The HLA determinants were of paternal origin, consistent with the presence of tumor-associated HLA in the immune complexes. MHC antigens have been difficult to demonstrate on nonmalignant human trophoblast cells (Faulk and Temple, 1976). Using in situ hybridization, low or undetectable levels of class I HLA mRNA were detected in syncytial trophoblast, whereas mRNA was readily demonstrable in cytotrophoblast (Hunt et al, 1988). Cytotrophoblast bound one of three murine monoclonal antibodies against monomorphic HLA determinants, whereas synctial trophoblast failed to bind any of the reagents and adjacent fetal mesenchymal cells bound all three. Human antibodies against paternal histocompatibility antigens have been detected in serum from 40% of primiparas during 16- to 24-week molar gestations (Bagshawe and Lawler, 1974).

Immunologic recognition of paternal antigens has long been considered one mechanism by which gestational trophoblastic neoplasms are controlled. This may account, in part, for the remarkable response of these tumors to single-agent chemotherapy. Several reports have addressed the question of whether sharing of histocompatibility antigens between patients with choriocarcinoma and their husbands might favor progressive tumor growth. In early studies, histocompatibility for certain HLA sites was more common than expected in patients with disseminated trophoblastic disease (Morgensen et al, 1969), and histocompatibility was more frequent with choriocarcinomas than with invasive moles (Tomoda et al, 1976). On the other hand, when the histocompatibility type of the child antecedent to a choriocarcinoma was determined, HLA-compatible children were infrequent (Lawler et al, 1971; Lewis and Terasaki, 1971). In long-term survivors of choriocarcinoma, there has been neither an unusual frequency of any particular HLA type nor an unusual degree of HLA compatibility between patients with choriocarcinoma and their husbands (Berkowitz et al, 1981).

From these data, it appears that histocompatibility between patients and their husbands is not a prerequisite for the development of choriocarcinoma. However, this does not preclude a contribution from the immune response against histocompatibility antigens to the elimination of established tumor. Indeed, patients may differ in their immune response to histocompatibility antigens in general and to certain alloantigens in particular. Both lymphocyte-mediated cytotoxicity (Currie, 1967) and complement-dependent cytotoxicity (Loke and Ballard, 1973) have been observed against trophoblastic cells in culture. Of interest, an improved prognosis for patients with gestational trophoblastic neoplasms has been correlated with the presence of a peritumoral mononuclear infiltrate (reviewed in Berkowitz et al, 1984).

## Viral Antigens

Over the last decade certain strains of human papilloma-virus (HPV) have been implicated in the pathogenesis of cervical cancer (see Chapter 3). Relevant viral DNA sequences can be detected in cervical tissue using Southern transfers or in situ hybridization. Antibodies against the E4 and E7 proteins of type 16 HPV have been detected in human sera. Antibodies against E7 were observed 14 times more frequently in cervical cancer patients than in controls (Yajima et al, 1988). Earlier immunoepidemiologic data had also linked human cervical carcinoma with herpesvirus type 2 (HSV-2) in addition to papillomavirus (Rapp, 1981; Dürst et al, 1983). HSV-2 antigens were detected in cervical carcinoma cells but not in normal squamous epithelium. Antibodies against HSV-2 have been found in a majority of patients with cervical carcinoma but not in all individuals with the disease (Rawls et al, 1968). Although herpesvirus DNA and RNA can be found in tumor cells from many individuals with the disease (Frenkel et al, 1972), it has not been determined whether herpesvirus contributes to the pathogenesis of cervical cancer.

Expression of viral antigens by human tumors has also been observed in nongynecologic neoplasms. Burkitt's lymphoma and nasopharyngeal carcinoma have been associated with Epstein-Barr virus antigens. The most convincing evidence for the viral induction of a human neoplasm has been obtained with the human T-cell lymphotropic virus type 1 (HTLV-1) associated with sporadic cases of lymphoblastic leukemia in Japan, Africa, and the Caribbean (Gallo et al, 1982). Patients with the disease generally develop antibodies reactive with virus-transformed tumor cells. A small fraction of apparently healthy individuals exhibit antibodies against HTLV-1 consistent with the successful resolution of a previous infection. Whether or not an immune response prevents or inhibits development of the neoplasm is not known.

## Oncofetal Antigens

Certain antigens can be detected during embryonic development but not in normal adult tissues. Some of these antigens are reexpressed when adult tissues undergo neoplastic change.

***Carcinoembryonic Antigen (CEA)*** CEA is a glycoprotein of approximately 200 kD that contains a substantial amount of carbohydrate. Recent studies suggest that the amino-acid sequence of the protein portion of CEA is related to that of the immunoglobulins. The antigen is expressed in the fetal gut and is found in a variety of gastrointestinal neoplasms, including carcinomas of the colon and rectum, stomach, and pancreas. The molecule may be important for the adhesion of tumor cells to vascular endothelium, since injection of CEA along with human colorectal cancer cells increases the number of lung metastases observed in nude mice (Jessup et al, 1990). Circulating CEA can be detected in sera from patients with nongastrointestinal malignancies, including carcinomas of the breast, lung, bladder, prostate, and female reproductive organs (Zamcheck and Kupchik, 1980). Approximately half the patients with cervical cancer or epithelial ovarian carcinoma exhibit a modest elevation of serum CEA (Stall and Martin, 1981). In most cases of ovarian cancer, the antigen is not sufficiently elevated to provide a useful marker for monitoring disease progression or regression during treatment. The most significant elevations have been observed in advanced disease, in tumors of mucinous histology, and in poorly differentiated neoplasms.

***Alpha-fetoprotein (AFP)*** AFP, a glycoprotein of 69 kD, is associated with hepatomas and testicular germ cell tumors (McIntire and Waldmann, 1980). Although it is not often of value in following patients with epithelial ovarian cancer, it is useful as a marker for certain germ cell neoplasms of the ovary. AFP is usually elevated in embryonal tumors and in endodermal sinus tumors but not in choriocarcinomas. In contrast, human chorionic gonadotropin (hCG) is elevated in choriocarcinomas and in some embryonal tumors. Given the current success in treating germ cell neoplasms with conservative surgical resection and combination chemotherapy, AFP has become an important marker.

## Differentiation and Lineage-Associated Antigens

Heteroantisera have been developed against both cervical and ovarian tumor-associated differentiation antigens. In an early report, TA-4, a glycoprotein of 48 kD, was detected in sera from 52% of 25 patients with cervical carcinoma but in only 2% of 58 controls (Kato et al, 1979). Antigen levels correlated with the disease course in patients followed sequentially. Several ovarian carcinoma-associated antigens have been recognized by antibodies raised in rabbits, including the ovarian cystadenocarcinoma-associated antigen (OCAA), ovarian tumor-associated antigen (OCA) (Bhattacharya and Barlow, 1979; Knauf and Urbach, 1980) and a 70-kd component of OCA, designated NB/70K.

With the development of murine monoclonal antibodies, new markers have been defined for human ovarian and cervical carcinomas. The technique originally described by Kohler and Milstein (1975) has permitted the production of an essentially unlimited amount of chemically pure immunoglobulin of defined specificity. Mice have been immunized with foreign antigens, and antibody-forming cells from spleens of the immune mice have been fused with a murine myeloma cell line. The "hybridomas" formed can be grown on a selective medium that permits survival of only the somatic cell hybrids. Since there are at least 100,000 different antibody specificities, as many different hybridomas can potentially be obtained. Finding the small number of hybridomas that produce immunoglobulins that bind to tumor-associated antigens poses a formidable technical problem. Once identified, however, hybridomas will continue to proliferate in vitro or in the abdominal cavity of mice, producing an essentially unlimited amount of pure immunoglobulin with defined reactivity.

***Squamous Cell Carcinoma (SCC) Antigen*** Isoelectric focusing can distinguish at least 14 components of the TA-4 antigen ranging in molecular weight from 42 to 48 kD. One of these components has been designated the SCC antigen. Multiple murine monoclonal or goat polyclonal antibodies have been prepared against different determinants or epitopes shared by the SCC antigen and other members of the family of TA-4 molecules. A double determinant assay has been developed in which antigen is trapped specifically using one of the anti-SCC antibodies that has been bound to a solid-phase immunoabsorbent. A second anti-SCC antibody against a distinct epitope is radiolabeled and used as a probe to detect bound antigen. The SCC antigen is caught as a "sandwich" in the double-determinant assay, and the bound radioactivity is proportional to the amount of antigen present in serum or body fluids.

Among sera from 381 healthy subjects, SCC antigen levels ranged from 0.5 to 6.7 ng/ml (Kato and de Bruijn, 1987). Approximately 95% of healthy donors had SCC antigen levels below 2.5 ng/ml. Elevated values have been observed in some 8% of patients with benign gynecologic disorders (de Bruijn et al, 1987), whereas more than 80% of patients with the benign skin diseases pemphigus and eczema had elevated SCC levels (Duk et al, 1989). In eight studies that included 547 patients with clinically active carcinoma of the cervix, 54% of the subjects had SCC antigen levels above 2.0 to 2.5 ng/ml. Antigen levels correlated with stage of disease. High levels of antigen have been detected in normal squamous epithelium, and serum levels in patients with cervical cancer are elevated by infiltrative growth, by increasing tumor mass, and possibly by maintenance of differentiation (Crombach et al, 1989). Abnormal values were sometimes encountered in patients with cervical intraepithelial neoplasia (CIN), but cervical cytology and colposcopy were substantially more sensitive techniques for early detection. Adenocarcinomas of the cervix were less frequently associated with abnormal SCC antigen levels than were squamous carcinomas. Elevation of SCC (above 4 ng/ml) during 1 to 14 months of followup after primary therapy was a poor prognostic factor, with a specificity of 90% and a sensitivity of 63% for predicting recurrence of cervical cancer in 40 patients (Maiman et al, 1989*b*). Persistent elevations may be a more useful indicator of recurrent disease than the occurrence of a single abnormal value (Duk et al, 1990). These elevations correlated with the clinical

TABLE 4-1  Monoclonal Antibodies That React With Epithelial Ovarian Carcinomas

| Source of Immunogen | Antibody(ies) | Investigator(s) |
|---|---|---|
| Ovarian carcinoma cells or cyst fluid | OC 125 | Bast et al, 1981 |
| | 1D3 | Bhattacharya et al, 1982, |
| | | Gangopadhyay et al, 1985 |
| | MOV-1,MOV-2 | Tagliabue et al, 1985 |
| | | Miotti et al, 1985 |
| | | Mariani-Costantini et al, 1985 |
| | OC 133 | Berkowitz et al, 1983 |
| | MD144,MF61,MF116 | Mattes et al, 1984 |
| | OV632 | Fleuren et al, 1984, 1987 |
| | $4F_4,7A_{10}$ | Bhattacharya et al, 1984 |
| | $2C_8,2F_7$ | Bhattacharya et al, 1985a |
| | 8C3,10D6 | Bharracharya et al, 1985b |
| | 3C2,4C7 | Tsuji et al, 1985 |
| | MU78,MT334,MQ49 | Mattes et al, 1985 |
| | OM-1 | de Kretser et al, 1985 |
| | UMNWR-2 | Wahl and Piko, 1985 |
| | WB12123 | Knauf et al, 1986, Knauf, 1988 |
| | OV-TL 3 | Poels et al, 1986a and b |
| | MOV-18,MOV-19 | Miotti et al, 1986 |
| | 8C,10B | Baumal et al, 1986 |
| | MS2B6* | Smith et al, 1987 |
| | 3G8C2* | Carsetti et al, 1987 |
| | MT179,MW162, | Mattes et al, 1987, 1989 |
| | MW207,MX35 | |
| | 5G6.4 | Rodriguez-Rodriguez et al, 1987 |
| | OM-A,OM-B,OM-C | Sakakibara et al, 1988 |
| | COC166-9 | He-nian, 1988 |
| | 1B3* | Werner et al, 1989 |
| | OVB1 | Kurrasch et al, 1989 |
| | CF511 | Ohkawa et al, 1989 |
| | OV-TL 16,OV-TL 23 | Boerman et al, 1989 |
| | MH99 | Mattes et al, 1989 |
| | OV-TL 15,OV-TL 30 | Boerman et al, 1990 |
| | OV-TL 31 | |
| | HMD4* | Cui et al, 1990 |
| | Ki-OC I-6-2 | Mettler et al, 1990 |
| | AC6C3* | Freedman et al, 1991 |
| Endometrial carcinoma | MH55,MH94 | Mattes et al, 1984 |
| | MSN-1 | Poropatich et al, 1990 |
| Colorectal carcinoma | 19-9 | Koprowski et al, 1979 |
| Pancreatic carcinoma | DUPAN-2 | Metzgar et al, 1982 |
| | | Lan et al, 1985 |
| Lung carcinoma | 130-22 | Matsuoka et al, 1987 |
| Laryngeal carcinoma | Ca-1 | Woods et al, 1982 |
| Epidermoid carcinoma | AR-3 | Prat et al, 1985 |
| Osteogenic sarcoma | 791-T36 | Embleton et al, 1981 |
| Breast carcinoma | F36/22 | Croghan et al, 1983, 1984 |
| | DF3 | Sekine et al, 1985a and b |
| | B72.3 | Colcher et al, 1983, |
| | | Kuroki et al, 1990 |
| | 260F9,454C11, | Frankel et al, 1985 |
| | 280D11,245E7 | |
| | BTMA8 | Boyer et al, 1989 |
| | | Liao et al, 1987 |
| Immune complex antigens | FEN-1 | Giancotti et al, 1986 |
| | 5E3 | Murray et al, 1988 |
| Benign cust fluid | — | Bara et al, 1984 |
| | 121SLE | Herrero-Zabeleta et al, 1985 |
| Defined antigens: | | |
| Milk fat globule protein(s) | HMFG2,AUA1 | Epenetos et al, 1982 |
| | MAM-6 | Hilkens et al, 1984 |
| | IIID5 | Krohn et al, 1985 |
| | ICO-21, ICO-22 | Iakubovskaia et al, 1990 |
| | ICO-26, ICO-29 | |

*(continued)*

TABLE 4-1    Monoclonal Antibodies That React With Epithelial Ovarian Carcinomas *(continued)*

| Source of Immunogen | Antibody(ies) | Investigator(s) |
|---|---|---|
| Placental alkaline phosphatase | NDOG2 | Sunderland et al, 1984, Davies et al, 1985 |
| | E6 | DcGrootc ct al, 1983 |
| Galactosyl transferase | | Chatterjee et al, 1984 |
| Lacto-N-fucopentaose | GA 29-1 | Cox et al, 1986 |
| Immunosuppressive acidic protein | MI1,MI2 | |
| Manganese superoxide dismutase | — | Ishikawa et al, 1990 |
| P-glycoprotein (MDR1) | C219,JSB-1 | Rubin et al, 1990 |
| | C219 | Rutledge et al, 1990 |

course in 87% of 15 patients monitored during chemotherapy for advanced disease (Ngan et al, 1989). Elevated SCC antigen levels have been encountered in sera from patients with squamous cell carcinomas that arise at other sites, including the vulva, head and neck, esophagus, and lung.

**CA 125**    The first murine monoclonal antibody reported to react with human ovarian carcinoma was designated OC 125 (Bast et al, 1981). OC 125 binds to an antigenic determinant (CA 125) associated with a high-molecular-weight glycoprotein, which contains subunits of approximately 220 kD. Chemical analysis indicates that CA 125 is likely to be a conformational peptide determinant (Davis et al, 1986). Multiple CA 125 determinants are present on each antigen molecule. CA 125 is associated with more than 80% of nonmucinous epithelial ovarian carcinomas studied in tissue sections. During embryonic development, CA 125 determinants can be found in the coelomic epithelium and in the müllerian duct (Kabawat et al, 1983a). Trace amounts of the antigen can be detected in adult tissue derived from these anlage, including the pleura, pericardium, and peritoneum, as well as epithelial cells lining the fallopian tube, endometrium, and endocervix. CA 125 is also expressed in the amnion, accounting for the presence of large amounts of antigen in amniotic fluid (Niloff et al, 1984b).

A double-determinant immunoradiometric assay has been developed that uses the OC 125 antibody to both trap and detect molecules with multiple identical CA 125 determinants (Bast et al, 1983b; Klug et al, 1984). CA 125 activities are arbitrarily defined on a scale of 1 to more than 20,000 units. Using this assay, sera from less than 1% of apparently healthy individuals have greater than 35 U/ml of CA 125, whereas more than 80% of patients with clinically apparent epithelial ovarian cancer have levels exceeding this value. A number of benign gynecologic conditions can increase CA 125, including severe endometriosis, adenomyosis, pelvic inflammatory disease, first-trimester of normal pregnancy, and rarely menstruation. Conditions that inflame the pleura, pericardium, and peritoneum can elevate CA 125, as can renal failure and severe liver disease, particularly when associated with ascites.

CA 125 is not a specific marker for ovarian cancer among patients with malignancy for which the primary site is unknown. Antigen levels can be elevated in a majority of patients with endometrial, fallopian tube, endocervical, and pancreatic cancers as well as in a minority of patients with cancers of the breast, lung, and colon (Niloff et al, 1984a).

In patients with ovarian cancer, increases or decreases in CA 125 have paralleled disease activity in 80 to 93% of the cases monitored. Elevation of CA 125 has been observed from 1 to 14 (median = 3) months prior to the clinical detection of recurrent disease (Knapp et al, 1985). Persistently rising levels of CA 125 that double outside the normal range have generally indicated progressive disease. If CA 125 is persistently elevated during therapy, prognosis is very poor. One woman in five who undergoes a second-look surveillance procedure will have an elevated CA 125 (above 35 U/ml). When elevated in this setting, CA 125 has a positive predictive value of 96% for indicating persistence of disease (Jacobs and Bast, 1989). CA 125 can, however, return to levels below 35 U/ml and small amounts of disease can be found at second-look laparotomy in up to 60% of cases. The rate of decline in CA 125 levels during treatment also has prognostic significance when an apparent half-life of over 20 days is associated with persistence of disease at second look and a shortened survival (van der Burg et al, 1988; Hunter et al, 1990). Since the physiologic half-life of circulating CA 125 antigen is approximately 4.8 days, a longer apparent half-life is thought to reflect persistence of tumor following cytoreductive surgery and during combination chemotherapy.

CA 125 may aid preoperatively in distinguishing benign from malignant adnexal masses, particularly in postmenopausal patients (Einhorn et al, 1986; Malkasian et al, 1988; Soper et al, 1990). When diagnostic laparotomy reveals ovarian carcinoma, the surgeon may not feel comfortable carrying out an aggressive cytoreductive procedure. In this setting, a biopsy specimen is obtained, the abdomen closed, and the patient referred for a second definitive procedure. A serum marker with a high positive predictive value for malignancy might prompt preoperative referral of patients to a surgeon skilled in the staging and cytoreductive removal of ovarian cancer, sparing the patient both the discomfort and cost of a second procedure. In a study of 343 postmenopausal women with adnexal masses, a preoperative CA 125 above 95 U/ml had a positive predictive value of 96% for indicating the presence of gynecologic malignancy (Zurawski et al, personal communication). A negative predictive value of CA 125 in this setting is not sufficiently high, however, to recommend delaying exploration of a patient with a pelvic mass and a normal antigen value who is otherwise an appropriate surgical candidate.

Preliminary data suggest that antigens defined by monoclonal antibodies might facilitate early detection of ovarian cancer. In one fortuitous case, CA 125 levels were elevated 12 months prior to the clinical diagnosis of a primary Stage III epithelial ovarian carcinoma (Bast et al, 1985). From a study of serum samples stored in the JANUS bank of Oslo, Norway, 50% of women destined to develop ovarian cancer within 18 months had levels of CA 125 exceeding 30 U/ml (Zurawski et al, 1988). At the time of diagnosis, approximately 60% of patients with Stage I or II ovarian cancer have had CA 125 levels above 35 U/ml (Jacobs and Bast, 1989). Elevated antigen levels (above 65 U/ml) were found in 0.6% of 915 apparently healthy nuns over 40 years of age (Zurawski et al, 1987).

Given the prevalence of ovarian cancer in the U.S. and the U.K., a specificity slightly greater than 99.6% would be required to assure that no more than 10 laparotomies were performed for each case of ovarian cancer diagnosed. In a study of 4,000 healthy women in London, a specificity in excess of 99.6% was attained with a combination of CA 125 and transabdominal ultrasound or CA 125 and vaginal examination, but not with any single method (Jacobs et al, 1988). In a larger trial of 22,000 women in the U.K., modest elevations of CA 125 (30 U/ml) triggered vaginal examination and ultrasound (Jacobs, personal communication). Some 11 cases of ovarian cancer were detected and eight were missed using this approach. Four laparotomies were performed for each case of ovarian cancer detected.

Another approach to early detection has involved CA 125 monitoring over time. In an initial phase I investigation of 1,082 apparently healthy women in the Stockholm area, an elevated CA 125 (>35 U/ml) prompted repeat CA 125 determinations every 3 months, with pelvic examination and ultrasound done every 6 months. The only patient to have a progressively rising CA 125 was found to have a mixed mesodermal ovarian malignancy 20 months after the initial elevation of antigen (Zurawski et al, 1990). In a subsequent phase II study 5,550 apparently healthy women were followed with annual CA 125 determinations (Einhorn et al, 1990). Serum CA 125 values exceeding 30 to 35 U/ml triggered more intensive surveillance using pelvic examination and ultrasound. Among postmenopausal women, abnormal antigen values (above 30 U/ml) were found in less than 2%, suggesting that the test would have adequate specificity to conduct a larger trial. Six cases of ovarian cancer were detected and three were missed by this approach. Although the numbers are small, four of the six cases detected were in Stage I or II. Larger randomized trials with up to 70,000 women in each arm will be required to test whether CA 125 used in combination with transabdominal or transvaginal ultrasound will detect a sufficient number of patients with early-stage ovarian cancer to prolong survival. During the course of such a trial a serum bank could be established that would facilitate the prompt evaluation of new serum markers.

### Other Serum Markers Defined by Monoclonal Antibodies

By means of the monoclonal technology, a number of other antibodies have been developed that react with human ovarian carcinomas (Table 4-1). These antibodies bind to a wide variety of antigens ranging from high molecular weight mucins to cell-surface glycolipids (Table 4-2). In contrast to CA 125, the ID3 antibody reacts with mucinous tumors preferentially (Bhattacharya et al, 1982). The MOV-1 and MOV-2 antibodies react with both mucinous and nonmucinous neoplasms (Colnaghi et al, 1982; Tagliabue et al, 1985).

In some cases, monoclonal antibodies have been prepared against tumors that arise from other organs but that cross-react with ovarian carcinomas (Table 4-1). The DUPAN-2 antibody was raised against a pancreatic carcinoma (Metzgar et al, 1982), the NS 19-9 antibody against a poorly differentiated colorectal carcinoma (Koprowski et al, 1979), and B72.3 against a breast carcinoma (Schlom et al, 1985).

Some of the antigens recognized by monoclonal antibodies remain associated with the cell surface, whereas others are shed. Several antigens that can be detected in serum have been evaluated as markers that would improve the sensitivity or specificity of CA 125. Promising complementarity has been found between CA 125 and HMFG2 (Ward et al, 1987), placental alkaline phosphatase (Ward et al, 1987), lipid associated sialic acid (LASA) (Schwartz et al, 1987), urinary gonadotropin fragment (Nam et al, 1989), and macrophage colony stimulating factor (Kacinski et al, 1989; Xu et al, submitted for publication). Use of a panel of markers in combination might detect a larger fraction of patients with early-stage disease. Conversely, use of TAG 72 and CA 15-3 in combination with CA 125 has improved the specificity of CA 125 for distinguishing authentic elevations of the antigen in ovarian cancers from false-positive elevations in benign disease (Bast et al, 1991) as well as for discriminating malignant from benign pelvic masses (Einhorn et al, 1989; Soper et al, 1990).

### Immunoscintigraphy

Both conventional polyclonal and novel monoclonal reagents have been used to localize occult ovarian carcinomas by radionuclide imaging. Iodine-131, iodine-123, and indium-111 have been conjugated with immunoglobulins. Conjugates have been prepared with antibodies against CEA (Van Nagell et al, 1980), human milk-fat globule protein (Epenetos et al, 1982; Epenetos et al, 1985a; Granowska et al, 1986a and b), placental alkaline phosphatase (Epenetos, 1985b; Davies et al, 1985), CA 125 (Haisma et al, 1988), an osteogenic sarcoma–associated antigen (Embleton et al, 1981), and TAG 72 (Brown et al, 1990). Small intraperitoneal implants have sometimes been imaged more effectively by intraperitoneal rather than intravenous administration of radionuclide conjugates. Large retroperitoneal and intraperitoneal tumor depos-

TABLE 4-2   Antigens Associated With Human Epithelial Ovarian Carcinomas Defined by Monoclonal Antibodies

| Antigen | Monoclonal Antibody(ies) | Investigator(s) |
|---|---|---|
| High molecular weight glycoproteins (>200 kd) | OC125 | Bast et al, 1981 |
| | | Masuho et al, 1984 |
| | | Davis et al, 1986*a* and *b* |
| | 130-22 | Matsuoka et al, 1987 |
| | CF511 | Ohkawa et al, 1989 |
| | 41B4 | Boyer et al, 1989 |
| Mucin-like glycoproteins | NS 19-9* | Koprowski et al, 1979 |
| | | Charpin et al, 1982 |
| | 1D3 | Bhattacharya et al, 1982 |
| | MOV1,MOV2* | Tagliabue et al, 1985 |
| | | Miotti et al, 1985 |
| | DUPAN-2* | Metzgar et al, 1982 |
| | | Lan et al, 1985 |
| | F36/22* | Papsidero et al, 1983 |
| | | Croghan et al, 1983, 1984 |
| | DF3 | Kufe et al, 1984 |
| | | Sekine et al, 1985a and *b* |
| | B72.3 | Colcher et al, 1983 |
| | | Meltzer and Macy, 1989 |
| | Ca2,Ca3 | Bramwell et al, 1985 |
| | HMFG1,HMFG2, AUA1 | Epenetos et al, 1982 |
| | MW162,MT334,MQ49* | Mattes et al, 1985, 1987 |
| | MAM-6 | Hilkens et al, 1984 |
| | 2G3,369F10, 200F9,493D1 | Boyer et al, 1989 |
| p200/100/60/40 | 113F1 | Boyer et al, 1989 |
| p185 (HER/2-*neu*) | 454C11,520C9,741F8 | Xu et al (in press) |
| | RC1,RC3,PB3,TA1 | |
| | ID5,BD5,OD3,RC6 | |
| p170 (EGFR) | 225,528 | Berchuck et al, 1990 |
| gp170 (MDR1) | C219,JSB-1 | Rubin et al, 1990 |
| | C219 | Rutledge et al, 1990 |
| gp105 | MF116 | Mattes et al, 1984 |
| p95 (transferrin receptor) | 454E4,454A12 | Boyer et al, 1989 |
| p90 | 8C,10B | Baumal et al, 1986 |
| | SP-2 | Scambia et al, 1987 |
| p80 | OC 133 | Berkowitz et al, 1983 |
| | Ki-OC I-6-2 | Mettler et al, 1990 |
| p72 | 791-T36 | Embleton et al, 1981 |
| | 9C6 | Boyer et al, 1989 |
| p70 | NB12123 | Knauf et al, 1986 |
| p67 | MH99 | Mattes et al, 1987 |
| p66 | 33F8 | Boyer et al, 1989 |
| p61/65 | 677B8 | Boyer et al, 1989 |
| p60 | $2C_8, 2F_7$ | Bhattacharya et al, 1985a and b |
| p55 | 260F9 | Frankel et al, 1985 |
| | | Boyer et al, 1989 |
| | HMD4* | Cui et al, 1990 |
| p48 | $4F_4, 7A_{10}$ | Bhattacharya et al, 1984 |
| p47 (galactosyl transferase) | | Chatterjee et al, 1984 |
| p40-42 | 317G5 | Frankel et al, 1985 |
| | | Boyer et al, 1989 |
| | KS-1/4 | Apelgren et al, 1990 |
| p38 | MOV18,MOV19 | Miotti et al, 1986 |
| p37 | MW207 | Mattes et al, 1987 |
| p32 | AC6C3** | Freedman et al, 1991 |
| p2-5 | MU78 | Mattes et al, 1985 |
| Glycolipids | NS 19-9** | Koprowski et al, 1979 |
| | MOV-1,MOV-2* | Tagliabue et al, 1985 |
| | MD144,MF61 | Mattes et al, 1984 |
| lacto-N-fucopentaose | GA29-1 | Cox et al, 1986 |

its have generally been detected most effectively after intravenous injection.

Imaging depends upon differences in activity between the tumor and blood pool. Circulating antigen can pre-vent antibody from reaching tumor sites and can pro-long clearance of radionuclide conjugates complexed with antigen in blood. Circulating CA 125 appears to affect the use of OC 125 to image tumors (Zalutsky et al, 1988), whereas circulating CEA does not affect imaging using antibodies against epitopes on this antigen (Goldenberg et al, 1978). With different conjugates, label has appeared in liver, gastrointestinal tract, ascites fluid, and in urine, producing artifacts or preventing the detection of small nodules.

Despite these limitations, recurrent tumor has been detected in a majority of cases (Epenetos et al, 1982; Shepherd et al, 1983). Sensitivity for detecting the persistence of intraperitoneal tumor may range as high as 90%, with reported specificities in the 80 to 90% range. Nodules as small as 0.8 cm have been identified, although immunoscintigraphy has failed to detect lesions as large as 7 cm. Consequently, the technique should be regarded as a complement to more conventional methods of imaging such as computed tomographic (CT) scanning, magnetic resonance imaging (MRI), and ultrasound. However, the diagnostic accuracy of these other modalities is limited. CT, for example, exhibits a sensitivity of 32% and a specificity of 77% in predicting persistence of disease prior to second-look surveillance procedures (Clarke-Pearson et al, 1986). In a review of 116 patients with a variety of different tumor types imaged by different techniques, 10% of patients had recurrent tumor that was visualized only by immunoscintigraphy (Baum et al, 1988).

In primary ovarian carcinoma, sensitivity has been promising but specificity limited. Primary malignant disease could be localized in 19 of 20 patients imaged with $^{123}$I-labeled HMFG2, but scans were also positive in five of 10 patients with benign pelvic lesions (Granowska et al, 1986a and b). When immunoscintigraphy with $^{111}$In-labeled B72.3 was used prior to laparotomy in 108 patients with ovarian cancer, antibody imaging exhibited higher sensitivity (69% vs. 44%) but lower specificity (57% vs. 79%) than CT imaging and correctly detected tumor in 19 patients with negative CT scans (Mann et al, 1990). Surgeons found the information valuable for locating disease intraoperatively in 28% of cases.

Repeated injection of murine immunoglobulin has evoked a human antimouse immunoglobulin response. Although severe allergic reactions have generally not occurred following repeated injection of murine monoclonal antibodies, human antimurine antibodies may hasten the clearance of radionuclide conjugates in vivo and interfere with in vitro monitoring assays such as CA 125 that utilize murine monoclonal antibodies.

# IMMUNOLOGIC INTERACTIONS BETWEEN TUMOR AND HOST

## Cellular and Humoral Immunity

For more than two decades, immunologists have appreciated that small lymphocytes could be divided into two major categories: T cells and B cells (Table 4-3). B cells are responsible for antibody production and bear small amounts of immunoglobulin as an integral part of their cell-surface membrane (Cooper et al, 1984). Binding of antigen to antibody on the B-cell surface triggers proliferation and differentiation to antibody-producing plasma cells. Antibodies formed by B cells fall into five different classes: IgM, IgG, IgA, IgD, and IgE. Some of these classes are further divided into subclasses, such as IgG1 to IgG4 (Table 4-4).

Antibodies are made up of heavy and light polypeptide chains. The class and function of each antibody molecule are specified by the carboxy-terminal portion of each heavy chain (Table 4-4). Binding to antigen is mediated through structures defined by the unique amino-acid sequences of the N-terminal portion of both heavy and light chains. Hypervariable complementarity-determining regions (CDRs) make particularly important contributions to the antibody binding site. Antibody diversity is generated by (1) somatic recombination of genes specifying portions of the heavy and light chains, (2) association of different heavy and light chains, and (3) somatic mutation of recombined genes. Humoral immunity mediated by specific antibodies eliminates a number of gram-positive organisms and limits the spread of certain viral infections. IgE binds strongly to mast cells and basophils mediating immediate hypersensitivity reactions such as anaphylaxis.

In early studies, T lymphocytes were recognized by their ability to bind sheep erythrocytes, forming "E rosettes." More recently, heteroantisera and monoclonal reagents have been used to define "clusters of differentiation," or "CD groups." Some CD groups are characteristic of T cells. In addition, each T cell bears a distinctive antigen-receptor complex that contains a 90 kD transmembrane heterodimer (Ti) linked noncovalently to a 5-peptide CD3 protein complex (Hedrick et al, 1989). The Ti can contain either alpha/beta (more than 95%) or gamma/delta (2 to 5%) chains. Diversity in the Ti is generated by somatic recombination of gene segments resembling that observed in B cells, but somatic mutation apparently does not occur. When specific antigen binds to the receptor complex, signals are transduced through the phosphoinositol or tyrosine kinase pathways, activating T cells which then proliferate, form mediators, and regulate the activities of B lymphocytes, monocytes, and other T cells. T cells are ultimately responsible for delayed hypersensitivity, rejection of organ transplants, and resistance to certain pathogens that are destroyed by macrophages (including fungi, mycobacteria, *Listeria monocytogenes*, and *Salmonella*).

Subsets of T cells serve different functions. *T-inducer cells* ($T_{ind}$) facilitate the proliferation and differentiation of B cells, macrophages, and other T cells. A subset of $T_{ind}$ cells prompts the formation of *T-suppressor cells* ($T_s$). $T_s$ cells inhibit $T_{ind}$ cells, ultimately inhibiting the proliferation and differentiation of cytotoxic T cells ($T_s$), B cells, and macrophages. Induction and suppression can be produced by either direct cell-cell interaction or the release of mediators. T-inducer cells release a number of cytokines, including at least six interleukins and granulocyte-macrophage colony stimulating (GM-CSF) (Tables 4-5 and 4-6). Inducer cells also produce factors that attract, arrest, and activate macrophages. Interaction of $T_{ind}$ cells and macrophages is essential for delayed cutaneous reactivity.

**TABLE 4-3** Phenotype and Functions of Human Lymphoreticular Cells

| | Cell Type | | | |
|---|---|---|---|---|
| | T | B | Null | Monocyte/ Macrophage |
| **Phenotype** | | | | |
| Surface membrane immunoglobulin | − | + | − | − |
| Fc Receptors | +/− | + | +/− | + |
| C3 Receptors | − | + | − | + |
| Ia | +/−* | + | +/− | + |
| CD-3 | + | − | − | − |
| **Function** | | | | |
| Antibody formation | − | + | − | − |
| Tumor cell killing | + | − | + | + |
| Induction | + | − | − | − |
| Suppression | + | − | − | + |
| Proliferation to | | | | |
| Phytohemagglutinin | + | +/− | − | − |
| Concanavalin A | + | +/− | − | − |
| Pokeweed mitogen | + | + | − | − |
| Alloantigens | + | − | − | − |
| Soluble proteins | + | − | − | − |
| Mediator production | | | | |
| Macrophage-inhibiting factor | + | +/− | − | − |
| Lymphocyte-inhibiting factor | + | +/− | − | − |
| Interleukin 1 | − | +/− | − | + |
| Interleukin 2 | + | − | − | − |
| Antibody-dependent toxicity | +/−* | − | + | + |
| Natural killing | − | − | + | − |

*Present when activated.
*Source:* Adapted from Bast RC Jr: Effects of cancers and their treatment on host immunity. In Holland JF, Frei E III (eds): *Cancer Medicine*, 2nd ed. Philadelphia, Lea & Febiger, 1982, p 1137.

One of the most potent macrophage-activating factors described to date is gamma interferon, but interleukin-4 (IL-4) and GM-CSF can also stimulate macrophage function (reviewed in Meltzer and Macy, 1989). Interferons are glycoproteins that confer resistance to viral infection on otherwise susceptible cells. In addition to gamma interferon, which is produced primarily by activated T lymphocytes, alpha interferon is synthesized by a variety of cell types, including other leukocytes, and beta interferon is released by fibroblasts. Each interferon has distinctive molecular and pharmacologic properties (Borden, 1983). Treatment of ovarian cancer cell lines with gamma interferon increases the expression of Class I and Class II MHC antigens (Boyer et al, 1989) as well as TAG 72 and CEA (Greiner et al, 1986).

**TABLE 4-4** Properties of Different Human Immunoglobulins

| Anti-body | Heavy Chain | Serum Concentration (mg/ml) | Molecular Weight (daltons) ($\times 10^3$) | Binding to Complement, Activation | | Mediation of ADCC | Receptors on Mast Cells and Basophils |
|---|---|---|---|---|---|---|---|
| | | | | Classic Pathway | Alternate Pathway | | |
| IgG1 | α1 | 9 | 160 | + + | + | − | − |
| IgG2 | α2 | 3 | 160 | +/− | + | − | − |
| IgG3 | α3 | 1 | 160 | + + + | + | + | − |
| IgG4 | α4 | 0.5 | 160 | − | ? | +/− | + |
| IgA1 | α1 | 3 | 170 | − | + | − | − |
| IgA2 | α2 | 0.5 | 170 | − | + | − | − |
| IgM | μ | 1.5 | 900 | + + + | + | − | − |
| IgD | δ | 0.03 | 184 | − | − | − | − |
| IgE | ε | 0.00005 | 188 | − | + | ? | + + |

ADCC = Antibody-dependent cell-mediated cytotoxicity.
*Source:* Adapted from Turner MW: The immunoglobulins. In Holborow EJ, Reeves WG (eds): *Immunology in Medicine*, 2nd ed. London, Academic Press, 1977, by permission of Grune and Stratton.

TABLE 4-5  Sources, Characteristics, and Effects of Human Interleukins and Cytokines

| Factor | Sources | Characteristics | Effects on B Cells | Effects on Other Cells | Other Names |
|---|---|---|---|---|---|
| IL-1 | Monocyte and macrophage lines; dendritic cells Natural killer cells; B cell lines; T cell lines; endothelial cells; fibroblasts; astrocytes; keratinocytes | IL-1α 15-17 kD, pI 5.0 IL-1B 15-17 kD pI 7.0 | —Differentiation of activated B cells with IL-6 —Proliferation of activated B cells with IL-5 | —Lymphokine release from activated T cells and fibroblasts —Growth of fibroblasts, synovial cells, endothelial cells —Tissue catabolism —Release of PGE$_2$, collagenase, and acute phase reactants —Fever —Chemotaxins for neutrophils, macrophages, and lymphocytes —Increased NK activity | Endogenous pyrogen (EP); lymphocyte-activating factor (LAF); B-cell-activating factor (BAF); leukocyte endogenous mediator (LEM) |
| IL-2 | Activated T cells | 15 kD, pI 6.8, 7.1 | —Proliferation of B cells with IL-4 or after stimulation with *Staphylococcus aureus* Cowan (SAC) —Proliferation of CLL B cells —Differentiation of B cell lines or SAC-stimulated B cells | —Growth of activated T cells —Lymphokine production by T cells —Increased NK activity —Increased LAK cell activity —Increased monocyte cytotoxicity | T-cell-derived growth factor (TCGF); T-cell-maturation stimulating factor (TMF/TSF); Killer helper factor (KHF); T-cell-replacing factor (TRF) |
| IL-3 | Activated T cell clones Myelomonocytic cell lines (mouse) | 14-28 kD | —Supports growth of pre-B cell lines (mouse) | —Stimulates growth of multipotential stem cells | Multiple colony stimulating factor (multi-CSF) |
| IL-4 | Activated T cells | 15-20 kD (mouse) pI 6.4-6.7, 7.4-7.6, 8.5-8.7 | —Increased B cell proliferation —Increased Fc receptor and Class II MHC antigen expression on B cells —Increased IgE secretion —Release of CD23 | —Growth factor for T cells | B-cell growth factor (BCGF); B-cell-stimulating factor-1 (BSF-1); B-cell-stimulating factor p1 (BSFp1); Macrophage fusion factor (MFF); Macrophage-activating factor (MAF) |
| IL-5 | T cells | 45-60 kD pI 5.5 (mouse) | —Increased IgM and IgA secretion by stimulated B cells | —Induced eosinophil differentiation | T-cell replacing factor (TRF); eosinophil differentiation factor (EDF); B cell growth factor II (BCG-2); Killer helper factor (KHF); IgA-enhancing factor (IgAEF); Eosinophil colony-stimulating factor (EO-CSF) |
| IL-6 | Monocytes; HTLV-transformed T cells; fibroblasts; carcinoma cells; sarcoma cells | 34 kD, pI 4.9 (19-21 kD by SDS) | —Increased growth of plasmacytoma cell hybridomas —Increased Ig secretion by EBV stimulated cells | —Production of acute phase reactants | Hybridoma growth factor (HGF); Interferon B2 (IFNB2); B-cell-stimulating factor (BSF-2); B-cell-differentiation factor |
| IFN-α | Leukocytes Macrophages | 20 kD (15 genes) | | —Antiviral activity —Increased MHC Class I expression —Antiproliferative activity | Alpha-interferon, type I interferon |
| IFN-β | Fibroblasts Epithelial cells | 20 kD | | —Antiviral activity —Increased MHC Class I expression —Antproliferative activity | Beta interferon; type I interferon |

*(continued)*

TABLE 4-5   Sources, Characteristics, and Effects of Human Interleukins and Cytokines *(continued)*

| Factor | Sources | Characteristics | Effects on B Cells | Effects on Other Cells | Other Names |
|---|---|---|---|---|---|
| IFN-γ | T cells LGL | 20-25 kD by SDS-Page 40-60 kD | —Increased proliferation of anti-Ig and SAC-stimulated B cells<br>—Increased proliferation and differentiation of CLL cells with IL-2<br>—Increased IL-4 induced proliferation of anti-Ig-stimulated tonsillar B cells<br>—Decreased IL-4 induced activity of B cell lines. | —Increased MHC Class II expression by endothelial cells; fibroblasts; myelomonocytic cells<br>—Increased antimicrobial and antitumor activity by macrophage<br>—Increased NK cell activity | Gamma-interferon; type II interferon; macrophage-activating factor (MAF) |
| TNF-α | Macrophages; T cells; thymocytes; endothelial cells | 40 kD | | —Cytotoxic or cytostatic effects for certain cell lines; fever; cachexia; neutrophil; chemotaxis<br>↑ endothelial cell coagulant activity; endothelial cell adhesion molecules; bone resorption; tumor; necrosis | —Tumor necrosis factor-alpha; cachectin |
| TNF-β | T cells | | | —Cytotoxic or cytostatic for selected cell lines | —Tumor necrosis factor-beta; lymphotoxin |

Adapted from O'Garra et al (1988) and Rosenberg et al (1988).
NK = Natural killer cells; CLL = chronic lymphocytic leukemia; LAK = lymphocyte-activated killer cells; MHC = major histocompatibility complex; HTLV = human T-cell lymphotropic virus; EBV = Epstein-Barr virus.

Macrophages can also participate in immunoregulation, facilitating or inhibiting immunologic reactions. The immune response to many antigens is initiated when $T_{ind}$ cells interact with a specific antigen associated with Class II histocompatibility determinants on the surface of macrophages. In addition to presenting antigens, macrophages release a mediator, interleukin 1 (IL-1), a 14-kD glycoprotein that induces the expression of receptors for IL-2 on the surface of T cells (Lachman, 1983). Thus, macrophages stimulate the proliferation of T cells through antigen presentation and the release of IL-1. Conversely, activated macrophages inhibit the proliferation and differentiation of T cells and B cells. Given these complex interactions of lymphocytes and macrophages, failure to produce an antibody may relate to a defect in B cells, inadequate T-inducer cell function,

TABLE 4-6   Human Hematopoietic Colony-Stimulating Factors

| Factor | Molecular Weight (kd) | Cellular Source | Hematopoietic Precursors Found in Colonies |
|---|---|---|---|
| G-CSF | 18-22 | Monocytes<br>Fibroblasts | Neutrophils |
| GM-CSF | 14-35 | T cell<br>Endothelial cells<br>Fibroblasts | Neutrophils, monocytes, eosinophils, erythroid, megakaryocytes |
| IL-3 | 14-18 | T cells | Neutrophils, monocytes, eosinophils, basophils, erythroid, megakaryocytes |
| M-CSF | 34-45 (×2)<br>18-26 (×2) | Fibroblasts<br>Endothelial cells<br>Carcinoma cells | Monocytes |

Adapted from Clarke and Kamen (1987).

an excess of T-suppressor cells, inappropriate antigen presentation, or an excess of activated macrophages.

## Mechanisms of Tumor Cell Killing

Components of the immune response, such as T lymphocytes, natural killer (NK) cells, activated macrophages, granulocytes, and antibodies, can destroy tumor cells in vitro through a number of different mechanisms.

**T-Cell Cytotoxicity** Tumor-specific transplantation resistance in murine models is mediated by T lymphocytes. In cell culture, murine CD8$^+$ T cells are required to lyse tumors. In vivo CD4$^+$ T-inducer cells are required for tumor-specific transplantation resistance in some systems, whereas both CD4$^+$ and CD8$^+$ T cells are required in other systems. The mechanism of human T cell cytotoxicity has been studied most extensively using histoincompatible targets. CD8$^+$ T cells are cytotoxic for targets that bear different Class I MHC antigens, whereas CD4$^+$ T cells kill targets that express different Class II determinants. Direct contact between viable T cells and target cells is required. Binding of the T cell to the target through a specific receptor results in irreversible membrane damage and loss of osmotic integrity. This process requires glucose and divalent cations. Although the exact mechanism by which membrane damage occurs has not been defined, it may involve release of a "lymphotoxin," direct membrane-membrane interaction, transmembrane signaling that triggers autodestruction, release of a perforin or the activity of phospholipase (reviewed in Berke, 1989). When gynecologic tumors have been studied, T lymphocytes have been found to be the predominant mononuclear cells within ovarian carcinomas (Kabawat et al, 1983b). T cells with inducer and cytotoxic/suppressor phenotypes are present. Infiltrates of T$_{ind}$ cells have also been identified at the implantation site of complete moles (Berkowitz et al, 1984).

**Natural Killer (NK) Cells** Lymphocytes from apparently normal individuals can inhibit the growth of certain tumors in cell culture. Morphologically, this NK activity is associated with large granular lymphocytes (LGL) (Herberman and Oldham, 1983). Most of these cells bear FcRIII receptors for the carboxy-terminal portion of the IgG heavy chain, and many NK cells express T-cell–associated antigens. Destruction of tumor targets by NK cells does not require previous exposure to tumor cell antigens. Tumor cells are usually killed more readily by NK cells than are normal targets, but not all tumors are equally susceptible to NK activity. K562, a human erythroleukemia cell line, has most frequently been the target for measuring NK activity in vitro. Killing of autologous tumors has been difficult to demonstrate, and many human tumors contain relatively few NK cells. Ovarian carcinoma cells can sometimes be destroyed in vitro by autologous NK cells, but cells with NK phenotype or function are infrequently associated with tumor tissue or peritoneal fluid in vivo. For tumor cell killing, contact between NK cells and tumor targets

is generally required. The exact mechanism of cytotoxicity is unknown but may relate to perforins within LGL granules, superoxide production or serine protease activity. NK activity is augmented by incubation with interferon or IL-2, and NK cells may contribute to the clinical antitumor activity of interferon, interferon inducers, or bacterial immunostimulants (Herberman and Santoni, 1984). NK activity is inhibited by prostaglandins, glucocorticoids, cyclophosphamide, and antigen-antibody complexes.

**Macrophage-Mediated Cytotoxicity** Tumoricidal and tumoristatic effects have been documented with macrophages obtained from the peritoneal cavities of mice treated with bacillus Calmette-Guerin (BCG) or *Corynebacterium parvum* (Nathan et al, 1980; Adams et al, 1983). Activation of macrophages for tumor cell killing occurs in different stages (Johnson et al, 1984). Resident peritoneal cells must be incubated in vitro to respond to different lymphokines. After in vitro incubation, macrophages can be partially activated by treatment with gamma-interferon (Nathan et al, 1983), IL-4 or GM-CSF. Full activation, however, requires additional incubation with endotoxin, maleylated proteins, or certain products of lymphocytes or tumor cells. Activated macrophages kill tumor cells preferentially and bind more avidly to neoplastic cells than to normal cells (Hibbs, 1973). The actual mechanism by which macrophages inflict membrane damage is not completely defined but may relate to the generation of reactive oxygen species, release of tumor necrosis factor, or intercellular transfer of lysosomal enzymes. Different tumor cells may be destroyed by different mechanisms. Activated macrophages synthesize prostaglandin, which may limit additional macrophage activation and which can suppress the activities of T cells and NK cells. Prostaglandins have also been implicated in the stimulation of ovarian tumor growth in clonogenic assays (Salmon and Hamburger, 1978). Substantial variation has been observed in the macrophage content of different human tumors. In animal systems, tumor-derived chemotactic and inhibitory factors have been described. In addition, lymphocytes that infiltrate tumors may release factors that attract and activate macrophages. The functional state of macrophages within the tumor may be as important as the number of macrophages that infiltrate the neoplasm.

**Antibody-Mediated Tumor Cell Killing** With few exceptions, simple binding of an antibody to a tumor cell has not been sufficient to inhibit tumor growth. Antibodies that bind to growth factors or their receptors can sometimes downregulate tumor growth. Binding of antibody to certain cell-surface determinants can trigger programmed cell death or apoptosis. Two more general mechanisms have been described by which antibody can mediate cytotoxicity. In one, the antibody activates a series of serum complement components (C1 to C9) (Sandberg, 1981); in the other, antibody serves as a bridge assuring close contact between tumor cells and leukocyte effectors (Henney and Gillis, 1984).

The latter mechanism is known as antibody-dependent cell-mediated cytotoxicity (ADCC). Potential effector cells for ADCC include granulocytes, activated macrophages, and non-T, non-B (null) lymphocytes. Two forms of ADCC have been described. In conventional ADCC (Henney and Gillis, 1984) antibody binds initially to tumor cells, whereas in a novel form of ADCC antibody binds to effectors, subsequently triggering tumoricidal activity after linking the effector to a tumor target (Adams et al, 1983). IgG antibodies can mediate either complement-dependent or antibody-dependent cell-mediated cytotoxicity (see Table 4-4). IgM antibodies are generally not effective for ADCC but are more efficient than IgG in mediating complement-dependent lysis. Circulating immune complexes (CIC) can potentially inhibit both forms of antibody-dependent lysis. The number of functionally active cellular effectors that accumulate within the tumor bed may also limit ADCC.

***Neutrophil-Mediated Lysis*** After stimulation with phorbol myristate acetate, human granulocytes can lyse human ovarian cancer cells taken directly from patients (Lichtenstein et al, 1989). In contrast to T-cell-mediated cytotoxicity, more than 8 hours of contact between neutrophils and tumor cells are required to observe significant lysis.

## Immunocompetence of Patients With Gynecologic Cancer

Several factors affect immunocompetence in gynecologic cancer, including the underlying neoplasm, nutritional status, and previous therapy (Bast, 1982). If several immunologic functions are monitored, different tumors can be associated with different immunologic profiles (see Table 4-3). In general, however, immunocompetence varies inversely with tumor burden and directly with nutritional status. Distinctive patterns of immunosuppression are associated with surgery, radiotherapy, and chemotherapy. Interestingly, administration of some cytotoxic drugs in conventional dosages may not depress all immunologic parameters (Kohorn and Klein-Angerer, 1984).

Many clinical studies have monitored nonspecific indices of immunocompetence. T and B cells have been enumerated, and the response to mitogens or non-tumor-associated antigens has been measured in vitro. These studies have been influenced by the techniques used to isolate peripheral blood mononuclear cells (Check et al, 1980). In only a few instances have specific responses to tumor-associated antigens been studied. Despite these limitations, correlations have been found between decreased immunocompetence and a poor prognosis. Whether or not immunologic tests will improve on more conventional staging in gauging prognosis remains to be demonstrated.

***Nonspecific Assays of Immunocompetence*** Among the solid tumors, ovarian cancer is unusual in that B-cell function is decreased prior to treatment (Mandell et al, 1979). In this regard, it is similar to chronic lymphocytic leukemia or multiple myeloma and unlike most other epithelial carcinomas or sarcomas (Table 4-7). The mitogenic response to pokeweed mitogen is diminished and the formation of antibody is impaired after primary immunization with keyhole-limpet hemocyanin. When T cells are enumerated, taking advantage of their ability to form E rosettes, T-cell levels are reduced prior to treatment (Crowther et al, 1981a), but T-cell function remains relatively intact, as evidenced by the proliferation of lymphocytes in the presence of mitogens in vitro or by delayed cutaneous reactivity (DCR) in vivo. In contrast to patients with ovarian cancer, women with untreated cervical cancer exhibit T-cell deficiency (Ishiguro et al, 1980; Sawanobori et al, 1977; Pillai et al, 1987), as do one-third of patients with advanced endometrial carcinoma. B cells and IgG levels can actually be increased in cervical cancer patients, despite a relative deficiency of CD4$^+$ inducer cells (Pillai et al, 1987).

DCR to contact allergens depends upon both T cells and monocytes and is impaired in the majority of patients with advanced ovarian, cervical, and endometrial carcinoma (Sharma et al, 1979; Khoo and MacKay, 1974; Khoo et al, 1979; Nalick et al, 1974). A complete lack of reactivity is, however, unusual. Impaired reactivity to contact allergens such as dinitrochlorobenzene (DNCB) correlates inversely with tumor stage and is associated with a poor prognosis.

Normal peripheral blood NK activity has been observed in patients with cervical dysplasia or carcinoma-in-situ (Neill and Norval, 1984). Although the number of large granular lymphocytes is similar in patients with localized or disseminated cervical carcinomas, both NK and ADCC are decreased in advanced disease (Satam et al, 1986).

NK activity and macrophage-mediated cytotoxicity are decreased in the peripheral blood and ascites fluid from ovarian cancer patients (Mantovani et al, 1980a and 1980b). The number of T and NK cells is lower in ascites than in peripheral blood. NK activity can be boosted in vitro by treatment with interferon. In some

---

**TABLE 4-7** Immunocompetence in Different Malignancies

B-cell defects
  Chronic lymphocytic leukemia
  Multiple myeloma
  Ovarian carcinoma
T-cell defects
  Hodgkin's disease
  Disseminated carcinomas*
  Kaposi's sarcoma/AIDS
Monocyte defects
  Carcinomas and sarcomas
  Hodgkin's disease
Granulocyte defects
  Acute lymphoblastic leukemia
  Acute myelogenous leukemia
  Chronic myelogenous leukemia
  Multiple myeloma

*Including endometrial and cervical carcinoma.
*Source:* Bast RC Jr: Principles of cancer biology: Tumor immunology. In DeVita V Jr, Hellman S, Rosenberg S (eds): *Cancer: Principles and Practice of Oncology,* 2nd ed. Philadelphia, JB Lippincott Co, 1985, p 141.

cases, killing of autologous as well as allogeneic tumor cells can be demonstrated (Mantovani et al, 1980*a*; Shau et al, 1983). Both cellular and humoral inhibitors of natural killing have been described. Adherent macrophages have inhibited NK function in some studies (Uchida et al, 1984) but not in others (Mantovani et al, 1980*a*). A poorly adherent, nonphagocytic lymphocyte population can also inhibit NK activity (Allavena et al, 1981). Peritoneal cells from patients with minimal residual ovarian cancer release a low molecular weight (<2 kd) inhibitor of NK function (Lichtenstein et al, 1985). In some cases, humoral inhibitory factors can be isolated from benign as well as tumor-bearing ascites, suggesting that their production is related to the host's response rather than a result of the tumor. Suppressors of T, B, and NK cells have been described. Immunosuppressive acidic protein is elevated in serum from a majority of gynecologic cancer patients (Sawada et al, 1984).

A majority of patients have mononuclear inflammatory cells in ascites capable of mediating ADCC (Mantovani et al, 1979; Haskill et al, 1982), but mononuclear cells derived from solid tumors may lack ADCC effector activity against certain targets (Haskill et al, 1982). Within solid tumors or ascites fluid, macrophages might either inhibit or stimulate tumor growth depending upon the relative number of cells, their stage of activation, and the relative susceptibility of the tumor to macrophage-mediated damage. Macrophages can potentiate the growth of ovarian tumor colonies in clonogenic assays (Salmon and Hamburger, 1978). Stimulation can sometimes be abolished by indomethacin, implicating prostaglandins in this reaction. T-inducer cells may also be important for maintaining the stimulatory activity of macrophages (Hamburger et al, 1984). Seven of 11 ovarian tumors have proved susceptible to macrophage mediated killing, but cells from the remaining tumors were actually stimulated by the presence of macrophages.

Recent studies have documented that ovarian cancer cells produce macrophage colony stimulating factor (M-CSF) (Kacinski et al, 1988; Ramakrishnan et al, 1989). More than half of ovarian cancers express the proto-oncogene c-*fms* that encodes the M-CSF (CSF-1) receptor, raising the possibility that ovarian tumor growth could be stimulated by autocrine production of M-CSF (Kacinski et al, 1988; Baiocchi et al, 1991; Tyson et al, 1991). In addition, M-CSF is a potent chemoattractant for monocytes and can stimulate the proliferation of tumor associated macrophages which also express high levels of c-*fms* (Bottazzi et al, 1990). Tumor associated macrophages can, in turn, produce IL-6 (Erroi et al 1989) and tumor necrosis factor-alpha that can stimulate the growth of some ovarian cancers (Wu et al, *in press*). IL-6 can also be expressed by ovarian tumor cells (Watson et al, 1990). Consequently, both autocrine and paracrine growth regulation might stimulate growth of ovarian cancer.

***Specific Assays of Immunocompetence*** Patients with ovarian and cervical carcinomas can sometimes develop DCR to extracts of their own tumors (Wells et al, 1973; Levin et al, 1976; Cerni et al, 1979), and DCR is also observed with tumor extracts from other patients. Lymphocytes from patients with ovarian cancer in remission can proliferate in the presence of extracts of ovarian tumor or fetal ovary (Levin et al, 1975); those from parous women will also proliferate in the presence of tumor-associated antigens, suggesting that oncofetal antigens might be expressed by tumor cells (Crowther et al, 1981*b*). A more recent study documented lymphocyte proliferation in the presence of autologous tumor cells from 49% of 43 patients (Allavena et al, 1988).

Lymphokine-activated killer (LAK) cells can be generated by incubating the peripheral blood lymphocytes of ovarian cancer patients with IL-2 (Allavena et al, 1986). Tumor-infiltrating lymphocytes (TIL) from a majority of patients can also be induced to lyse autologous tumor cells after incubation of the effectors with IL-2. TIL cultured in the presence of IL-2 plus tumor necrosis factor-alpha showed significantly higher cytotoxicity against autologous targets than did TIL cultured in IL-2 alone (Wang et al, 1989).

Leukocyte migration has been inhibited by autologous or allogeneic tumor extracts in patients with cervical and ovarian carcinoma (Chen et al, 1973; Melnick and Barber, 1975; Faiferman et al, 1977; Rivera et al, 1979). Reactivity appeared to be organ site-specific. Plasma from the majority of ovarian cancer patients enhanced the migration of autologous leukocytes. In early studies, lymphocytes from a majority of patients with ovarian carcinoma proved cytotoxic for an allogeneic ovarian carcinoma cell line in tissue culture. Lymphocytes from more than two-thirds of patients with cervical cancer lysed an allogeneic cervical carcinoma. Factors have been identified that blocked the cytotoxicity of lymphocytes for cervical and ovarian carcinoma cells (Kohorn et al, 1978; Pattillo et al, 1979*a*), and persistent blocking activity has been associated with a poor prognosis. In other systems, blocking factors have been better characterized. Free antigen, free antibody, or antigen-antibody complexes can all contribute to blocking activity.

Antibodies capable of binding to ovarian or cervical carcinomas have been detected with complement-mediated cytotoxicity and indirect immunofluorescence (DiSaia et al, 1973; Matsunago et al, 1979; van de Linde et al, 1981; Dawson et al, 1983). In most cases, the specificity of these antibodies has not been well characterized. Circulating immune complexes (CIC) have been observed in patients with ovarian (Poulton et al, 1978; Clayton et al, 1982), cervical (Seth et al, 1979), and endometrial carcinoma (Cauchi et al, 1980), as well as in individuals with trophoblastic disease (Lahey et al, 1984). In the case of ovarian carcinoma, some investigators have identified complexes readily (Silburn et al, 1983), whereas others have had more difficulty. Immune complex levels have risen prior to the recurrence of epithelial ovarian cancer in some studies (Clayton et al, 1982), but not in others (Runowicz et al, 1989). Tumor-associated antigens have been isolated from ovarian complexes in ascites fluid (Stolbach et al, 1979). In patients with gestational trophoblastic neoplasms, CIC increased transiently following complete regression of the tumor, and paternal histocompatibility antigens have been identified in these complexes (Lahey et al, 1984).

# IMMUNOTHERAPY OF GYNECOLOGIC MALIGNANCY

Immunotherapy has traditionally been divided into active and passive forms. In active immunotherapy, immunostimulants or tumor-cell vaccines are given directly to the patient to stimulate endogenous immunity. In passive immunotherapy, antibodies or mononuclear cells from putatively immune donors have been transferred to the tumor-bearing host to provide exogenous immunity. Both active and passive immunotherapy have been attempted in patients with gynecologic cancers. Trials of active immunotherapy were initiated at the turn of the century when William B. Coley induced regression of ovarian and cervical carcinomas in small numbers of patients by injecting toxins produced by *Streptococcus pyogenes* and *Serratia marcescens* (Nauts, 1977). Passive immunotherapy using lymphocytes, heteroantisera, and monoclonal antibodies has been attempted clinically only within the last decade.

## Active Immunotherapy

***Immunostimulants*** Direct contact between immunostimulants and tumor cells has favored active immunotherapy. Perhaps the most striking example of active immunotherapy is direct intralesional injection with the tuberculosis vaccine bacillus Calmette-Guerin (BCG) in patients with multiple small cutaneous metastases from malignant melanoma (Bast et al, 1974). In this setting, the intratumoral injection of BCG produces regression in more than 60% of lesions. If patients are selected for immunocompetence, more than 90% of directly injected lesions will regress. In approximately 15% of cases, noninjected lesions will also regress. Regression of noninjected nodules is, however, largely limited to other cutaneous metastases. Regression of lymph node metastases is much less common, and there are only a few reports in which visceral metastases have responded to the injection of cutaneous lesions. Antitumor activity of BCG has also been demonstrated after intravesical instillation of the organism in patients with recurrent bladder cancers, suggesting that regional therapy can be effective against tumors growing from mucosal surfaces (Pinsky et al, 1982; Lamm et al, 1982). The mechanism of BCG's local antitumor activity is not completely understood, but activated macrophages, cytotoxic lymphokines, NK cells, and augmentation of tumor-specific immunity have all been implicated. A similar approach has been used to treat serosal implants of ovarian carcinoma using heat-killed *Corynebacterium parvum*. Intraperitoneal administration of *C. parvum* has led to regression of ascites and pleural effusions (Webb et al, 1978; Miller et al, 1980; Mantovani et al, 1981; Bast et al, 1983*a*; Currie et al, 1983). Objective regression

of small tumor nodules has been observed in 6 of 21 cases (Bast et al, 1983*a*; Berek et al, 1984*b*). Although effector function was difficult to demonstrate in peritoneal cells prior to treatment (Berek et al, 1984*a*), both NK and AD were augmented by treatment with this organism (Bast et al, 1983*a*; Lichtenstein et al, 1984*a*). In a study of cervical carcinoma, *C. parvum* was injected into the cervix 10 days prior to surgery in 22 patients; as a control, an additional 21 patients received no preoperative immunotherapy (Mignot et al, 1981). After the injection, there was an increase in the number of peripheral blood T cells, the degree of phytohemagglutinin (PHA) reactivity in vitro, and immunoreactivity to DNCB in vivo (Mignot, 1982). After 2 years, 29% of the control group had relapsed compared with only 5% who had received *C. parvum*.

In most forms of malignancy, systemic treatment with bacterial immunostimulants has not affected tumor growth in carefully controlled trials. Complete Freund's adjuvant or BCG has been administered to gynecologic cancer patients in several series (Graham and Graham, 1962; Hudson et al, 1976; Rao et al, 1977; Wanebo et al, 1977; Olkowski et al, 1978; Alberts and Moon, 1980; Gall et al, 1980). Although most of these studies also failed to produce convincing results, a randomized concurrently controlled trial was conducted by the Southwest Oncology Group in which the application of BCG by scarification increased response rates and prolonged the survival of ovarian cancer patients treated with cyclophosphamide and doxorubicin (Alberts and Moon, 1980). However, two subsequent randomized studies failed to confirm that BCG augmented the effects of cytotoxic chemotherapy (Alberts et al, 1989*a* and 1989*b*). Historically controlled studies suggested that *C. parvum* enhanced the antitumor activity of melphalan (Creasman et al, 1979) and 5-fluorouracil [5-FU]-doxorubicin-cyclophosphamide (Rao et al, 1977), but significant benefit has not been observed in concurrently randomized studies (Wanebo et al, 1977; Barlow et al, 1980). OK-432 is prepared from a strain of *Streptococcus pyogenes* that exhibits low virulence by treatment with heat and penicillin. Administration of OK-432 after primary therapy of cervical cancer improved 3-year recurrence-free survival from 59% to 72% in a randomized concurrently controlled trial (Cervical Cancer Immunotherapy Study Group, 1987).

***Contact Allergens*** Topical immunotherapy has been attempted in vulvar, vaginal, and cervical carcinoma using 5-FU and DNCB (Mansell et al, 1975; Krupp and Bohm, 1978; Guthrie and Way, 1979). DNCB induces DCR, whereas 5-FU induces both a local hypersensitivity response and exerts a direct cytotoxic effect on tumor cells. Regression of vulvar carcinoma in situ was observed in approximately 60% of patients treated with DNCB in early reports, but more recent studies have produced less promising results. Vaginal intraepithelial neoplasia was successfully treated with local DNCB application in seven women with three or more dysplastic vaginal smears after hysterectomy (Guthrie and Way, 1975). Cytology returned to normal in these patients within 2 to 35 months of followup. Among 180 women with positive cervical cytologic findings and no clinical evidence of invasive cancer, topical DNCB produced long-term control in 26% (Guthrie and Way, 1979). Therapy with DNCB was associated with marked vulvar discomfort, while 5-FU produced somewhat less discomfort (Hull et al, 1976) and in one report eradicated vaginal carcinoma in situ in six of eight patients treated and followed for 1.1 to 6.9 years (Piver et al, 1979). In another series, topical 5-FU controlled cervical intraepithelial neoplasia or upper vaginal cancer in six of 11 patients (Pride and Chuprevich, 1982). Consequently, topical immunotherapy can sometimes be effective but may not be sufficiently reliable to replace standard methods for outpatient management of these conditions. In principle, however, human tumor cells can be destroyed by an inflammatory response at sites of DCR evoked by DNCB.

**Immunorestorative Agents** In contrast to immunostimulants such as BCG and C. *parvum*, which boost normal immunologic reactivity to supranormal levels, levamisole is an immunorestorative agent that raises a suboptimal response to within a normal range. In patients with Dukes' C-stage colon cancer, adjuvant treatment with 5-FU and levamisole has decreased the rate of recurrence in two randomized studies (Hamilton et al, 1990). In women with ovarian cancer, however, the addition of levamisole to chemoradiotherapy had no beneficial effect upon survival and may have actually shortened survival in patients with Stage II disease (Khoo et al, 1984). Systemic immunotherapy with both BCG and levamisole has been used in patients with cervical carcinoma without definite benefit (Olkowski et al, 1978). Most studies of immunostimulants and immunorestorative agents have failed to monitor response to tumor-associated antigens and have not taken into account the complex immunoregulatory interactions of T cells and macrophages.

**Vaccines** A few studies have utilized tumor-cell vaccines in an attempt to augment specific antitumor immunity. In some cases, tumor cells have been superinfected with virus to increase their immunogenicity (Freedman et al, 1980). Regional intraperitoneal or intracavitary therapy using viral oncolysates produced objective partial remissions in 2 of 40 patients with refractory ovarian cancer and stabilized ascites in seven (Freedman et al 1988). Responses may relate to activation of NK cells (Lotzova et al, 1986), development of T-cell-mediated delayed hypersensitivity, or an augmented hormonal response to virus- or tumor-associated antigens. Regression of metastatic gestational choriocarcinoma has been reported after systemic immunization with paternal cells (Cinander et al, 1961), although active systemic immunotherapy has not been consistently effective in trophoblastic disease.

**Interferons** Recent trials have centered on the use of purified mediators. In some cases, recombinant DNA technology has permitted biologically active substances such as interferon to be produced in large quantities and with a high degree of purity. Interferon was admin-

istered topically to patients with early-stage cervical carcinoma for 3 weeks prior to surgical removal of the tumor (Mignot, 1982). In nine of the 15 patients studied, interferon was also administered intramuscularly. Tumors may have decreased in size during treatment, but precise measurements were not provided. Subsequent trials with recombinant alpha-interferon have documented only one possible response among 18 patients treated (Einhorn et al, 1983).

In clonogenic assays, alpha-interferon inhibited the growth of up to 70% of ovarian tumor specimens from ascites fluid. Cells isolated from solid tumors appeared less susceptible to interferon than did cells from ascites (Epstein et al, 1980). Systemic administration of alpha- or beta-interferon has had only a modest effect in patients with ovarian carcinoma (Einhorn et al, 1982; Freedman et al, 1983; Kanazawa et al, 1984; Niloff et al, 1985). Overall, no more than 10% of patients have responded to systemic therapy. Administration of interferon by the intraperitoneal route is more promising. In one pilot study, five of 11 (45%) surgically restaged patients with lesions smaller than 5 mm before treatment showed either a complete or a partial response (Berek et al, 1985). Intraperitoneal administration of alpha-interferon has been associated with increased NK effector function (Lichtenstein et al, 1988). Systemic administration of gamma-interferon produced four responses among 14 patients with ovarian cancer in relapse. Alpha-interferon has been given in combination with doxorubicin or cisplatin. The most promising results were achieved when alpha-interferon and cisplatin were both given by the intraperitoneal route to patients with minimal residual disease, producing pathologically complete responses in seven of 14 cases (Nardi et al, 1990). In animal models, additive effects have been observed between tumor necrosis factor (TNF)-alpha and interferon gamma that can upregulate TNF receptors (Balkwill et al, 1987).

## Passive Immunotherapy

**Adoptive Immunotherapy With Lymphoreticular Cells** Human ovarian cancers have been reported to regress after being infused with mesenteric lymph node cells from pigs immunized with human tumor tissue (Turner and Symes, 1979). Activity of xenogeneic lymphocytes may be limited by the body's rapid rejection of foreign cells. Given the availability of recombinant IL-2, human lymphocytes can now be grown ex vivo to produce activation of large granular lymphocytes, NK cells and lymphocyte-activated killer (LAK) cells with antitumor activity that is not major histocompatability complex (MHC)-restricted. Administration of IL-2 and IL-2-activated autologous lymphocytes has produced objective remissions in approximately 20% of patients with metastatic melanoma and renal cell carcinoma. Similar response rates have been produced with IL-2 alone. An anecdotal partial response has been observed after intravenous injection of LAK cells and IL-2 in a patient with ovarian carcinoma (West et al, 1987). Intraperitoneal injection of IL-2 and LAK cells produced partial remissions in two of 10 patients. Systemic side effects were reduced, although peritoneal irritation, fibrosis and fluid loculation were observed (Steis et al, 1990).

Tumor infiltrating lymphocytes (TIL) can be activated with IL-2 ex vivo and are more potent than LAK cells in murine models. TIL specifically reactive with tumor have been successfully derived from patients with melanoma and evaluated in clinical trials (Rosenberg et al, 1988). [111]In-labeled TIL have localized to tumor sites, consistent with the possibility that TIL are more specific than LAK cells (Fisher et al, 1989). Immunohistochemical studies indicate that T cells are the most prevalent leukocytes that infiltrate ovarian cancers, and T cells have been cloned from ovarian cancer ascites in the presence of phytohemagglutinin and irradiated spleen cells (Ferrini et al, 1985). A portion of CD3[+] T-cell clones lysed autologous ovarian cancer cells preferentially and lysis could be blocked with anti-CD8[+] antibody, characteristic of conventional class I MHC-restricted cytotoxic T lymphocytes. Incubation with high concentrations of IL-2 favored the production of non-MHC-restricted LAK cells from TIL of solid tumors (Heo et al, 1988), whereas incubation with low concentrations of IL-2 and TNF-alpha generated CD8[+] T cells that lysed autologous tumor cells preferentially (Li et al, 1989). Clinical trials of TIL-mediated therapy in ovarian cancer have not yet been reported.

***Serotherapy With Polyclonal Antibodies*** Serotherapy has been evaluated most extensively in ovarian cancer. In animal models, intraperitoneal injection of specific heteroantiserum raised in rabbits against a murine ovarian carcinoma suppressed the growth of intraperitoneal tumor transplants (Order et al, 1973 and 1974). Increased antitumor activity was observed with a combination of *C. parvum* and specific heteroantiserum (Knapp and Berkowitz, 1977; Bast et al, 1979). Doses and schedules of *C. parvum* that potentiated the efficacy of heteroantiserum in vivo attracted and activated peritoneal cells for more effective ADCC in vitro. Among the peritoneal cells, activated macrophages appeared to be particularly important effectors for ADCC, although polymorphonuclear leukocytes and lymphocytes could also contribute to the killing of tumor. In the absence of antibody, polymorphonuclear leukocytes may be important as early effectors of tumor killing. In addition, neutrophils can recruit macrophages that exert additional tumor activity (Lichtenstein et al, 1984*b*). A clinical trial was performed in Stage III ovarian cancer in which chemotherapy and radiotherapy were administered with or without serotherapy using polyclonal antibodies raised in different species. Patients received chemotherapy, intraperitoneal [32]P, and total abdominal radiation with or without ovarian antitumor serum. Initial studies suggested that patients who had received antiserum did at least as well as those who had not (Hernandez et al, 1982).

***Serotherapy With Monoclonal Antibodies*** A number of antibodies have been produced that react with ovarian tumor-associated antigens (See Tables 4-1 and 4-2). Most of these reagents are of murine origin, although several human monoclonal antibodies have now been described. The monoclonal technology has permitted the production of essentially unlimited amounts of immunoglobulin of defined specificity. Despite the administration of antibody in extraordinarily high dosage, serotherapy with murine monoclonal antibodies may be limited by a number of factors, including circulating antigen, antigenic modulation, heterogeneity of antigen expression, and the development of immunity to foreign immunoglobulin. A number of potential antigenic targets, such as CA 125, are shed into the circulation in large quantities (Bast et al, 1983*b*). Circulating antigen can affect the localization of some antibodies (Zalutsky et al, 1988). Binding of anti-CD10 antibodies to the common acute lymphoblastic leukemia antigen on leukemic cells results in the modulation of all CD10 antigen from the cell surface within hours (Ritz et al, 1980). Fortunately, most of the ovarian tumor-associated antigens that have been studied in detail do not modulate in the presence of antibody. Substantial heterogeneity in antigen expression has been observed within and between different breast and ovarian carcinomas (Boyer et al, 1989). When 16 different antigens were measured, each of 14 ovarian cancers exhibited a distinctive combination of determinants. However, the use of four or five antibodies in combination can overcome this degree of heterogeneity. In some studies changes in antigenic phenotype have been observed over time (Welch et al, 1990), whereas in others similar expression of antigens has been observed at different points in time (Rubin et al, 1989; Berchuck et al, 1990). Human anti-murine antibodies (HAMA) have developed in a majority of patients treated with monoclonal serotherapy. Attempts to circumvent the HAMA response to foreign protein have utilized immunosuppressive agents and genetic restructuring of antibodies to substitute human for murine sequences in the constant regions of the immunoglobulin genes.

The major limitation of serotherapy with unconjugated antibodies may, however, be the availability of host effector mechanisms. With the exception of antibodies directed against the extracellular domains of the epidermal growth factor receptor or the *c-erb*B-2 (HER-2/*neu*) oncogene product (Vollmar et al, 1987; Drebin et al, 1988), simply binding monoclonal antibodies to antigens on the surface of tumor cells generally fails to inhibit their growth. Moreover, many murine monoclonal antibodies cooperate inefficiently with human complement components. Few functional effectors of ADCC may be present within ovarian tumors. Conjugation of antibodies with cytotoxic drugs, toxins, or isotopes may avoid the limitations of human effector mechanisms.

Radioconjugates of murine monoclonal antibodies with [131]I have been most extensively evaluated. Both beta and gamma rays are emitted by this isotope. Emissions from radioconjugates that bind to tumor cells could destroy adjacent tumor cells that failed to bind immunoconjugate; however, normal tissues could also be damaged by radiation. In a study by Epenetos et al (1987), [131]I-conjugates with HMFG1, HMFG2, AUA1, and H17E2 were administered intraperitoneally to 36 patients with ovarian cancer. Myelotoxicity limited treatment at doses above 100 mCi. Antitumor activity correlated inversely with tumor volume in that no responses were observed in eight patients with nodules larger than 2 cm, two of 15 partial responses occurred with nodules smaller than 2 cm, and three of six complete responses were documented against microscopic disease. In a separate trial of intraperitoneal therapy with [131]I-HMFG2 and [131]I-AUA1, progressive tumor growth was encountered in each of six evaluable patients with small-volume disease, whereas transient improvement was observed in three of four patients with ascites alone. Failure to control ascites formation in one patient was associated with a subpopulation of antigen-negative cells (Ward et al, 1988). A phase I study has also been completed in 29 patients who were given [131]I-labeled OC 125 F(ab')$_2$ intraperitoneally (Muto et al, 1990). Both myelosuppression and gastrointestinal toxicity were observed in a majority of patients who received doses in excess of 100 mCi. [90]Y emits only beta rays with a range of 3 to 6 mm. To the extent that longer-range gamma irradiation affects the bone marrow, myelotoxicity might be reduced with [90]Y chelates, provided that the conjugate was cleared promptly from the circulation and that the isotope remained firmly associated with the immunoglobulin. When 19 patients with ovarian cancer were treated intraperitoneal with [90]Y-labeled monoclonal antibodies, myelotoxicity was once again dose-limiting (Stewart et al, 1988). [90]Y released from chelates accumulated in bone, irradiating the marrow.

Toxins derived from plants or bacteria have been conjugated to murine monoclonal antibodies that mediate the selective binding of the immunotoxin to tumor cells in preference to normal tissues. After binding, the immunotoxin is taken up into endosomes. Within the endosome, the toxin moiety dissociates from immunoglobulin and is translocated into the cytoplasmic compartment where ribosomal protein synthesis is inhibited catalytically. Only those antigens that traffic through endosomes after interacting with antibody make appropriate targets for immunotoxins. Consequently, not all monoclonal antibodies have provided suitable carriers for toxins.

The most intensively studied conjugates have contained the A chain of ricin (RTA) or *Pseudomonas* exotoxin (PE). Whole ricin has been isolated from castor beans and contains RTA covalently linked to a B chain. The B chain binds to galactose residues on the surface of a variety of normal cells, facilitating the internalization and translocation of RTA that contains N-glycosidase activity capable of inactivating the 60S ribosomal subunit. In immunotoxins, the broad reactivity of the B chain is replaced by the more restricted specificity of the monoclonal antibody. PE consists of a single peptide chain with distinct domains that mediate binding, internalization, and catalysis. Once internalized, PE ribosylates and inactivates elongation factor 2.

In theory, immunotoxins should bind exclusively to tumor, inhibiting protein synthesis, and bystander damage of normal tissues should not be observed. In order to control tumor growth, however, immunotoxins must bind to every clonogenic tumor cell. Consequently, immunotoxins prepared with several different antibodies may be required to compensate for antigenic heterogeneity. Use of immunotoxins in combination can exert additive or synergistic antitumor activity (Yu et al, 1990; Crews et al, submitted). Should subadditive effects be observed with normal tissues, a substantial therapeutic advantage could be achieved. Very low levels of antigen in normal tissue may, however, facilitate internalization of toxin. Given qualitative and quantitative differences in antigen expression between species, studies of antitumor activity in nude-mouse heterograft models may not predict clinical toxicity. Phase I clinical trials have been conducted with 454A12(anti-transferrin receptor)-RTA, OVB3-PE and 260F9(anti-p55)-RTA. In each case, distinctive neurotoxicities have proved to be dose-limiting. Immunohistochemical studies have indicated that transferrin receptor is preferentially expressed by capillary endothelial cells of the basal ganglia; OVB3 binds to cerebellar cells and p55 can be found in the myelin sheaths of peripheral nerves. Thus, toxicities observed to date appear related to the specificity of the monoclonal antibody rather than to toxicity of the dissociated toxins. Choice of more specific antibodies and molecular engineering of conjugates should produce more clinically useful reagents.

Bispecific antibodies have been created by chemical conjugation or molecular engineering of two separate monoclonal reagents. By combining antibodies reactive with tumor-associated antigens and antibodies that bind to different immune effectors, close association can be achieved between tumor cells and T cells, NK cells, LAK cells, or activated macrophages. Bispecific antibodies and activated human effectors have proven cytotoxic for ovarian cancer cells ex vivo (Mezzanzanica et al, 1988). Such an approach might combine the potency of both serotherapy and adoptive immunotherapy of cellular effectors.

***Future Directions*** Ultimately, immunotherapy will need to be evaluated in patients with minimal residual disease. Given the high rate of relapse in patients who have received platinum-based therapy despite negative surgical surveillance procedures, immunologic reagents might be evaluated in complete responders. Whether administering biologic agents intraperitoneally, intravenously, or by a combination of routes will prove optimal remains to be determined. Considering the heterogeneity in antigen expression as well as differences in susceptibility to immunologic effectors within and between different gynecologic cancers, multiple reagents or approaches will be required to eliminate all clonogenic tumor cells. Given the distinctive biology of gynecologic cancers, immunologic approaches continue to hold promise for more effective management of patients with these neoplasms.

## REFERENCES

Adams DO, Lewis JG, Johnson WJ: Multiple modes of cellular injury by macrophages: Requirement for different forms of effector activation. *Progr Immunol* 13:1009-1018, 1983.

Alberts DS, Mason-Liddil N, O'Toole RV, et al: Randomized phase III trial of chemoimmunotherapy in patients with previously untreated stages III and IV suboptimal disease ovarian cancer: A Southwest Oncology Group study. *Gynecol Oncol* 32:8-15, 1989*a*.

Alberts DS, Mason-Liddil N, O'Toole RV, et al: Randomized phase III trial of chemoimmunotherapy in patients with previously untreated stage III, optimal disease ovarian cancer. A Southwest Oncology Group Study. *Gynecol Oncol* 32:16-21, 1989*b*.

Alberts DS, Moon TE: Randomized trial of chemotherapy versus chemoimmunotherapy for advanced ovarian carcinoma: A preliminary report of a Southwest Oncology Group Study. NCI Second International Conference on Immunotherapy of Cancer: *Present Status of Trials in Man*, 1980, p 13.

Allavena P, Introna M, Mangioni C, Mantovani A: Inhibition of natural killer activity by tumor-associated lymphoid cells from ascites ovarian carcinomas. *J Natl Cancer Inst* 67:319-325, 1981.

Allavena P, Lo Presti P, Di Bello M, et al: Proliferative response of lymphocytes from ovarian cancer patients to autologous tumor cells. *Cancer Immunol Immunother* 27:69-76, 1988.

Allavena P, Zanaboni F, Rossini S, et al: Lymphokine-activated killer activity of tumor-associated and peripheral blood lymphocytes isolated from patients with ascites ovarian tumors. *J Natl Cancer Inst* 77:863-868, 1986.

Apelgren LD, Zimmerman DL, Briggs SL, Bumol TF: Antitumor activity of the monoclonal antibody-vinca alkaloid immunoconjugate LY203725 (KS1/4-4-desacetylvinblastine-3-carboxhydrazide) in a nude mouse model of human ovarian cancer. *Cancer Res* 50:3540-3544, 1990.

Aurelian L, Strand BC, Smith MF: Immunodiagnostic potential of a virus-coded, tumor-associated antigen (AG-4) in cervical cancer. *Cancer* 39:1834-1849, 1977.

Bagshawe K, Lawler S: The immunogenicity of the placenta and trophoblast. In Edwards RG, Howe CW, Johnson MH (eds): *Immunobiology of Trophoblast*. London, Cambridge University Press, 1974, pp 171-191.

Baiocchi G, Kavanagh JJ, Talpaz M, et al: Expression of the macrophage colony-stimulating factor and its receptor in gynecologic malignancies. *Cancer* 67:990-996, 1991.

Baldwin RW: Specific antitumor immunity and its role in host resistance to tumors. In Herberman RB (ed): *Basic and Clinical Tumor Immunology*. Boston, Martinus Nijhoff, 1983, pp 107-128.

Baldwin RW, Price MR: Neoantigen expression in chemical carcinogenesis. In Becker FF (ed): *Cancer: A Comprehensive Treatise*. New York, Plenum Press, 1975, pp 353-383.

Balkwill FR, Ward BG, Moodie E, Fiers W: Therapeutic potential of tumor necrosis factor-alpha and gamma-interferon in experimental human ovarian cancer. *Cancer Res* 47:4755-4758, 1987.

Bara J, Lependu J, Cartron JP, et al: Monoclonal antibodies against mucin of an ovarian mucinous cyst fluid. International Meeting on Monoclonal Antibody in Oncology, 1984.

Bara J, Zabaleta EH, Mollicone R, et al: Distribution of GICA in normal gastrointestinal and endocervical mucosae and in mucinous ovarian cysts using antibody NS 19-9. *Am J Clin Pathol* 85:152-159, 1986.

Barlow JJ, Piver MS, Lele SB: High-dose methotrexate with "rescue" plus cyclophosphamide as initial chemotherapy in ovarian adenocarcinoma. A randomized trial with observations on the influence of *C. parvum* immunotherapy. *Cancer* 46:1333-1338, 1980.

Bast RC Jr: Effects of cancers and their treatment on host immunity. In Holland JF, Frei E III (eds): *Cancer Medicine*, 2nd ed. Philadelphia, Lea & Febiger, 1982, pp 1134-1173.

Bast RC Jr: Principles of cancer biology: Tumor immunology. In DeVita V Jr, Hellman S, Rosenberg S (eds): *Cancer: Principles and Practice of Oncology*, 2nd ed. Philadelphia, JB Lippincott Co, 1985, pp 125-150.

Bast RC Jr, Berek JS, Obrist R, et al: Intraperitoneal immunotherapy of human ovarian carcinoma with *Corynebacterium parvum*. *Cancer Res* 43:1395-1401, 1983*a*.

Bast RC Jr, Feeney M, Lazarus H, et al: Reactivity of a monoclonal antibody with human ovarian carcinoma. *J Clin Invest* 68:1331-1337, 1981.

Bast RC Jr, Klug TL, Schaetzl E, et al: Monitoring human ovarian carcinoma with a combination of CA 125, CA 19-9 and carcinoembryonic antigen. *Am J Obstet Gynecol* 149:553-559, 1984.

Bast RC Jr, Klug TL, St John E, et al: A radio-immunoassay using a monoclonal antibody to monitor the course of epithelial ovarian cancer. *N Engl J Med* 309:883-887, 1983*b*.

Bast RC Jr, Knapp RC, Mitchell A, et al: Immunotherapy of a murine ovarian carcinoma with *Corynebacterium parvum* and specific heteroantiserum. I. Activation of peritoneal cells to mediate antibody-dependent cytotoxicity. *J Immunol* 123:1945-1951, 1979.

Bast RC Jr, Knauf S, Epenetos A, et al: Coordinate elevation of serum markers in ovarian cancer but not in benign disease. *Cancer* 68:1758-1763, 1991.

Bast RC Jr, Siegal FP, Runowicz C, et al: Elevation of serum CA 125 prior to diagnosis of an epithelial ovarian carcinoma. *Gynecol Oncol* 22:115-120, 1985.

Bast RC Jr, Zbar B, Borsos T, Rapp HJ: BCG and cancer. *N Engl J Med* 290:1413-1420 and 1458-1469, 1974.

Baum RP, Lorenz M, Hottenrott C, et al: Radioimmunoscintigraphy using monoclonal antibodies to CEA, CA 19-9, and CA 125. *Int J Biol Markers* 3:177-184, 1988.

Baumal R, Law J, Buick RN, et al: Monoclonal antibodies to an epithelial ovarian adenocarcinoma: Distinctive reactivity with xenografts of the original tumor and a cultured cell line. *Cancer Res* 46:3994-4000, 1986.

Berchuck A, Bast RC Jr: New directions in diagnosing, monitoring and detecting epithelial ovarian cancer. *Adv Oncol* 6:18-22, 1990.

Berchuck A, Olt GJ, Soisson AP, et al: Heterogeneity of antigen expression in advanced epithelial ovarian cancer. *Obstet Gynecol* 162:883-888, 1990.

Berek JS, Bast RC Jr, Lichtenstein A, et al: Lymphocyte cytotoxicity in the peritoneal cavity and blood of patients with ovarian cancer. *Obstet Gynecol* 64:708-714, 1984*a*.

Berek JS, Hacker NF, Lichtenstein A, et al: Intraperitoneal recombinant alpha interferon for "salvage" immunotherapy in stage III epithelial ovarian cancer. A Gynecologic Oncology Group Study. *Cancer Res* 45:4447-4453, 1985.

Berek J, Knapp R, Hacker N, et al: Intraperitoneal immunotherapy of human ovarian carcinoma with *Corynebacterium parvum*. *Proc Am Soc Clin Oncol* 3:173, 1984*b*.

Berke G: Functions and mechanisms of lysis induced by cytotoxic T lymphocytes and natural killer cells. In Paul WE (ed): *Fundamental Immunology*, 2nd ed. New York, Raven Press, 1989, pp 735-764.

Berkowitz RS, Goldstein DP, Hoch EJ, Anderson DJ: Immunobiology of molar pregnancy and gestational trophobastic tumors. *J Reprod Med* 29:796-801, 1984.

Berkowitz RS, Hornig-Rohan J, Martin-Alosco S, et al: HL-A antigen frequency distribution in patients with gestational choriocarcinoma and their husbands. *Placenta* 3(Suppl):263-267, 1981.

Berkowitz RS, Kabawat S, Lazarus H, et al: Comparison of a rabbit heteroantiserum and a murine monoclonal antibody raised against a human epithelial ovarian carcinoma cell line. *Am J Obstet Gynecol* 146:607-612, 1983.

Bhattacharya M, Barlow JJ: Ovarian cystadenocarcinoma-associated antigen (OCAA). In Herberman RB (ed): *Compendium of Assays for Immunodiagnosis of Human Cancer*. New York, Elsevier–North Holland, 1979, pp 527-531.

Bhattacharya M, Chatterjee SK, Barlow JJ: Identification of a human cancer-associated antigen defined with monoclonal antibody. *Cancer Res* 44:4528-4534, 1984.

Bhattacharya M, Chatterjee SK, Barlow JJ, Fuji H: Monoclonal antibodies recognizing tumor-associated antigen of human ovarian mucinous cystadenocarcinomas. *Cancer Res* 42:1650-1654, 1982.

Bhattacharya M, Chatterjee SK, Gangopadhyay A, Barlow JJ: Production and characterization of monoclonal antibody to 60-kD glycoprotein in ovarian carcinoma. *Hybridoma* 4:153-162, 1985*a*.

Bhattacharya M, Chatterjee SK, Gangopadhyay A, Barlow JJ: Production of murine monoclonal antibodies against cell-surface antigens of human ovarian carcinoma. *J Surg Oncol* 30:209-214, 1985*b*.

Boerman O, Makkink K, Massuger L, et al: Monoclonal antibodies against ovarian carcinoma-associated antigens, raised by immunization with cyst fluids. *Anticancer Res* 9:551-558, 1989.

Boerman OC, Makkink WK, Thomas CM, et al: Monoclonal antibodies that discriminate between human ovarian carcinomas and benign ovarian tumours. *Eur J Cancer* 26:117-127, 1990.

Borden EC: Interferons and cancer: How the promise is being kept. *Interferon* 5:43-83, 1983.

Bottazzi B, Erba E, Nobili N, et al: A paracrine circuit in the regulation of the proliferation of macrophages infiltrating murine sarcomas. *J Immunol* 15:2409-2412, 1990.

Boyer CM, Borowitz MJ, McCarty KS Jr, et al: Heterogeneity of antigen expression in benign and malignant breast and ovarian epithelial cells. *Int J Cancer* 43:55-60, 1989.

Bramwell ME, Ghosh AK, Smith WD, et al: Ca2 and Ca3. New monoclonal antibodies evaluated as tumor markers in serous effusions. *Cancer* 56:105-110, 1985.

Branconi F, Amunni G, Bonazza M, et al: Monoclonal antibodies in serological, immunoscintigraphic and immuno-cytochemical diagnosis of epithelial ovarian cancer. *Eur J Gynaecol Oncol* 10:262-267, 1989.

Brown BA, Dearborn CB, Drozynski CA, Sands H: Pharmacokinetics of $^{99m}$Tc-methallothionein-B72.3 and its F(ab') Z fragment. *Cancer Res* 50(Suppl):835S-839S, 1990.

Burchell J, Taylor-Papadimitriou M, Boshell S, et al: A short sequence, within the amino acid tandem repeat of a cancer-associated mucin, contains immunodominant epitopes. *Int J Cancer* 44:691, 1989.

Carsetti R, Freedman RS, Edwards CL, et al: Human monoclonal antibodies derived from peripheral blood lymphocytes of patients with ovarian carcinoma. *Eur J Gynaecol Oncol* 8:480, 1987.

Cauchi MN, Goriup D, Riglar C, et al: Cancer of the endometrium—A multiparametric study. *Gynecol Obstet Invest* 11:65-74, 1980.

Cerni C, Tatra G, Berger R, Micksche M: Cell-mediated immunity in patients with cervical cancer. *Oncology* 36:164-170, 1979.

Cervical Cancer Immunotherapy Study Group: Immunotherapy using the streptococcal preparation OK-432 for the treatment of uterine cervical cancer. *Cancer* 60:2394-2402, 1987.

Charpin C, Bhan AK, Zurawski VR Jr, Scully RE: Carcinoembryonic antigen (CEA) and carbohydrate determinant 19-9 (CA 19-9) localization in 121 primary and metastatic ovarian tumors: An immunohistochemical study with the use of monoclonal antibodies. *Int J Gynecol Pathol* 1:231-245, 1982.

Chatterjee SK, Bhattacharya M, Barlow JJ: Murine monoclonal antibodies against galactosyltransferase from the ascites of ovarian cancer patients. *Cancer Res* 44:5725-5732, 1984.

Check IJ, Hunter RL, Rosenberg KD, Herbst AL: Prediction of survival in gynecological cancer based on imunological tests. *Cancer Res* 40:4612-4616, 1980.

Chen SY, Koffler D, Cohen CJ: Cell-mediated immunity in patients with ovarian carcinoma. *Am J Obstet Gynecol* 115:467-470, 1973.

Cinander B, Hayley MA, Rider WD, Warwick OH: Immunotherapy of a patient with choriocarcinoma. *Can Med Assoc J* 84:306-309, 1961.

Clarke SC, Kamen R: The human hematopoietic colony stimulating factors. *Science* 236:1229-1236, 1987.

Clarke-Pearson DL, Bandy LC, Dudzinski M, et al: Computed tomography in evaluaton of patients with ovarian carcinoma in complete clinical remission. Correlation with surgical-pathologic findings. *JAMA* 255:627-630, 1986.

Clayton LA, Gall SA, Dawson JR, Creasman WT: Immune complexes in ovarian cancer. *Gynecol Oncol* 13:203-212, 1982.

Colcher D, Hand PH, Nuti M, Schlom J: Differential binding to human mammary and non-mammary tumors of monoclonal antibodies reactive with carcinoembryonic antigen. *Cancer Invest* 1:127-138, 1983.

Colnaghi MI, Canaveri S, Dellatorre G, et al: Monoclonal antibodies directed against human tumors. Proceedings of the 13th Cancer Congress, 1982, p 55.

Cooper MD, Kearney J, Scher I: B lymphocytes. In Paul WE (ed): *Fundamental Immunology*. New York, Raven Press, 1984, pp 43-55.

Cox CJ, Freedman RG, Fritsche HA: Lacto-N-fucopentaose III activity in the serum of patients with ovarian cancer. *Gynecol Obstet Invest* 21:164-168, 1986.

Creasman WT, Gall SA, Blessing JA, et al: Chemoimmunotherapy in the management of primary stage III ovarian cancer: A Gynecologic Oncology Group study. *Cancer Treat Rep* 63:319-323, 1979.

Crews JR, Maier LA, Yu YH, et al: A combination of two immunotoxins exerts synergistic antitumor activity gainst a human breast cancer cell line (*Submitted for publication*).

Croghan GA, Papsidero LD, Valenzuela LA, et al: Tissue distribution of an epithelial and tumor-associated antigen recognized by monoclonal antibody F36/22. *Cancer Res* 43:4980-4988, 1983.

Croghan GA, Wingate MB, Gamarra M, et al: Reactivity of monoclonal antibody F36/22 with human ovarian adenocarcinomas. *Cancer Res* 44:1954-1962, 1984.

Crombach G, Scharl A, Vierbuchen M, et al: Detection of squamous cell carcinoma antigen in normal squamous epithelial and in squamous cell carcinomas of the uterine cervix. *Cancer* 63:1337-1342, 1989.

Crowther ME, Poulton TA, Hudson CN: E-rosette-forming cells and cell-mediated immunity in ovarian cancer. *Eur J Gynaecol Oncol* 2:1-8, 1981a.

Crowther ME, Poulton TA, Hudson CN: The relationship between cellular responses of parous women and ovarian cancer patients to tumour extracts. *J Obstet Gynaecol* 1:263-267, 1981b.

Cui H, Qian HN, Feng J, et al: A human monoclonal antibody HMD4 against ovarian carcinoma associated antigen. *Chin Med J* 103:478-484, 1990.

Currie GA: Immunological studies of trophoblast in vitro. *J Obstet Gynaecol Br Commonw* 74:841-848, 1967.

Currie JL, Gall S, Weed JC Jr, and Creasman WT: Intracavitary *Corynebacterium parvum* for treatment of malignant effusions. *Gynecol Oncol* 16:6-14, 1983.

Daar AS, Fuggle SV, Ting A, Fabre JW: Anomalous expression of HLA-DR antigens on human colorectal cancer cells. *J Immunol* 129:447-449, 1982.

Davies JO, Davies ER, Howe K, et al: Practical applications of a monoclonal antibody (NDOG2) against placental alkaline phosphatase in ovarian cancer. *J R Soc Med* 78:899-905, 1985.

Davis HM, Zurawski VR Jr, Bast RC Jr, Klug TC: Characterization of the CA 125 antigen associated with human epithelial ovarian carcinomas. *Cancer Res* 46:6143-6148, 1986.

Dawson JR, Lutz PM, Shau H: The humoral response to gynecologic malignancies and its role in the regulation of tumor growth. A review. *Am J Reprod Immunol* 3:12-17, 1983.

de Bruijn HW, Bouma J, Boonstra H, Aalders JG: Serum levels of SCC in squamous cell carcinoma of the cervix. In Klapdor R (ed): *New Tumour Markers and Their Monoclonal Antibodies*. 4th Symposium on Tumour Markers. Hamburg, Stuttgart, Georg Thieme Verlag, 1987, pp 204-210.

De Groote G, De Waele P, Van de Voorde A, et al: Use of monoclonal antibodies to detect human placental alkaline phosphatase. *Clin Chem* 29:115-119, 1983.

de Kretser TA, Thorne HJ, Jacobs DJ, Jose DG: The sebaceous gland antigen defined by the OM-1 monoclonal antibody is expressed at high density on the surface of ovarian carcinoma cells. *Eur J Cancer Clin Oncol* 21:1019-1035, 1985.

Di Bello M, Lucchini V, Chiari S, et al: DR antigen expression on ovarian carcinoma cells does not correlate with their capacity to elicit an autologous proliferative response. *Cancer Immunol Immunother* 27:63-68, 1988.

Dini MM, Faiferman I: Cytotoxic blocking activity in invasive squamous cell carcinoma of the human uterine cervix. *Cancer* 46:2573-2576, 1980.

DiSaia PJ: Immunological aspects of gynecological malignancies. *J Reprod Med* 14:17-20, 1975.

DiSaia PJ, Nalick RH, Townsend DE: Antibody cytotoxity studies in ovarian and cervical malignancies. *Obstet Gynecol* 42:664-650, 1973.

Drebin JA, Link VC, Greene MI: Monoclonal antibodies reactive with distinct domains of the neu oncogene-encoded P185 molecule exert synergistic anti-tumor effects in vivo. *Oncogene* 2:273-277, 1988.

Duk JM, de Bruijn HW, Groenier KH, et al: Cancer of the uterine cervix: Sensitivity and specificity of serum squamous cell carcinoma antigen determinations. *Gynecol Oncol* 39:186-194, 1990.

Duk JM, van Voorst Vader PC, ten Hoor KA, et al: Elevated levels of squamous cell carcinoma antigen in patients with a benign disease of the skin. *Cancer* 64:1652-1656, 1989.

Dürst M, Gissmann L, Ikenberg H, zur Hausen H: A papillomavirus DNA from a cervical carcinoma and its prevalence in cancer biopsy samples from different geographic regions. *Proc Natl Acad Sci USA* 80:3812-3815, 1983.

Einhorn N, Bast RC Jr, Knapp RC, et al: Preoperative evaluation of serum CA 125 levels in patients with primary epithelial ovarian cancer. *Obstet Gynecol* 67:414-416, 1986.

Einhorn N, Bertelsen K, Björkholm E, et al: Recombinant leukocyte interferon in metastatic or recurrent cervical cancer. Proceedings of the 13th International Congress of Chemotherapy. Vienna, 8E 12.5.4, 1983.

Einhorn N, Cantrell K, Einhorn S, Strander H: Human leukocyte interferon therapy for advanced ovarian carcinoma. *Am J Clin Oncol* 5:167-172, 1982.

Einhorn N, Knapp RC, Bast RC Jr, Zurawski VR Jr: The CA 125 assay used in conjunction with CA 15-3 and TAG-72 assays for discrimination between malignant and nonmalignant diseases of the ovary. *Acta Oncol* 28:655-657, 1989.

Einhorn N, Sjovall K, Schoenfeld DA, et al: Early detection of ovarian cancer using the CA 125 radioimmunoassay (RIA). *Proc Am Soc Clin Oncol* 9:157, 1990.

Einhorn N, Zurawski VR, Knapp RC, Bast RC: Preoperative elevation of CA 125, CA 72 and CA 15-3 in patients with nonmucinous epithelial ovarian cancer. *Proc Am Assoc Cancer Res* 28:357, 1987.

Embleton MJ, Gunn B, Byers VS, Baldwin RW: Antitumor reactions of monoclonal antibody against a human osteogenic-sarcoma cell line. *Br J Cancer* 43:582-587, 1981.

Epenetos AA, Britton KE, Mather S, et al: Targeting of iodine-123-labelled tumour-associated monoclonal antibodies to ovarian, breast, and gastrointestinal tumours. *Lancet* 2:999-1005, 1982.

Epenetos AA, Munro AJ, Stewart S, et al: Antibody-guided irradiation of advanced ovarian cancer with intraperitoneally administered radiolabeled monoclonal antibodies. *J Clin Oncol* 5:1890-1899, 1987.

Epenetos AA, Shepherd J, Britton KE, et al: [123]I radioiodinated antibody imaging of occult ovarian cancer. *Cancer* 55:984-987, 1985a.

Epenetos AA, Snook D, Hooker G, et al: Indium-111 labelled monoclonal antibody to placental alkaline phosphatase in detection of neoplasms of testis, ovary, and cervix. *Lancet* 2:350-353, 1985b.

Epstein LB, Shen JT, Abele JS, Reese CC: Further experience in testing the sensitivity of human ovarian carcinoma cells to interferon in an in vitro semisolid agar culture system: Comparison of solid and ascitic forms of the tumor. In Salmon S, Hamburger A (eds): *Cloning of Human Tumor Stem Cells*. New York, Alan R. Liss, 1980, pp 277-290.

Erroi A, Sironi M, Chiaffarino F, et al: IL-1 and IL-6 release by tumor-associated macrophages from human ovarian carcinoma. *Int J Cancer* 44:795-801, 1989.

Faiferman I, Gleicher N, Cohen CJ, Koffler D: Leukocyte migration in ovarian carcinoma: Comparison of inhibitory activity of tumor extracts. *J Natl Cancer Inst* 59:1593-1597, 1977.

Faulk WP, Temple A: Distribution of beta2 microglobulin and HLA in chorionic villi of human placentae. *Nature* 262:799-802, 1976.

Ferrini S, Biassoni R, Moretta A, et al: Clonal analysis of T lymphocytes isolated from ovarian carcinoma ascitic fluid. Phenotypic and functional characterizaton of T-cell clones capable of lysing autologous carcinoma cells. *Int J Cancer* 36:337-343, 1985.

Festenstein H, Bridges J, Navarrete C: MHC expression on tumours including ovarian cancer. In Sharp F, Mason WP, Leake RE (eds): *Ovarian Cancer: Biological and Therapeutic Challenges*. London, Chapman and Hall Medical, 1990, pp 97-112.

Fisher B, Packard BS, Read EJ, et al: Tumor localization of adoptively transferred indium-111 labeled tumor infiltrating lymphocytes in patients with metastatic melanoma. *J Clin Oncol* 7:250-261, 1989.

Fleuren GJ, Coerkamp EG, Nap M: Immunohistological characterization of a monoclonal antibody directed against non-mucinous ovarian carcinomas. International Meeting on Monoclonal Antibodies in Ocology. *Clin Applica* 1984, p A5.

Fleuren GJ, Coerkamp EG, Nap M, et al: Immunohistological characterization of a monoclonal antibody (OV632) against epithelial ovarian carcinomas. *Virchows Arch [A]* 410:481-486, 1987.

Foley EJ: Antigenic properties of methylcholanthrene-induced tumors in mice of the strain of origin. *Cancer Res* 13:835-837, 1953.

Frankel AE, Ring DB, Tringale F, Hsieh-Ma ST: Tissue distribution of breast cancer-associated antigens defined by monoclonal antibodies. *J Biol Response Mod* 4:273-286, 1985.

Freedman RS, Bowen JM, Herson J, et al: Virus-modified homologous tumor-cell extract in the treatment of vulvar carcinoma. *Cancer Immunol Immunother* 8:33-38, 1980.

Freedman RS, Ioannides CG, Tommasovic B, et al: Development of a cell surface reacting human monoclonal antibody recognizing ovarian and certain other malignancies. *Hybridoma* 10:21-33, 1991.

Freedman RS, Edwards CL, Bowen JM, et al: Viral oncolysates in patients with advanced ovarian cancer. *Gynecol Oncol* 29:337-347, 1988.

Freedman RS, Gutterman JU, Wharton JT, Rutledge FN: Leukocyte interferon (IFNa) in patients with epithelial ovarian carcinoma. *J Biol Resp Mod* 2:133-138, 1983.

Frenkel N, Roizman B, Cassai E, Nahmias A: A DNA fragment of herpes simplex 2 and its transcription in human cervical cancer tissue. *Proc Natl Acad Sci USA* 69:3784-3789, 1972.

Furukawa K, Furukawa K, Real FX, et al: A unique antigenic epitope of human melanoma is carried on the common melanoma glycoprotein gp95/p97. *J Exp Med* 169:585-590, 1989.

Gall SA, Blessing JA, DiSaia PJ, Creasman WT: The effect of chemoimmunotherapy in the treatment of primary stage III epithelial ovarian cancer: A Gynecologic Oncology Group study. In NCI Second International Conference on Immunotherapy of Cancer: *Present Status of Trials in Man*, 1980, p 13.

Gallo RC, Wong-Staal F: Retroviruses as etiologic agents of some animal and human leukemias and lymphomas and as tools for elucidating the molecular mechanism of leukemogenesis. *Blood* 60:545-557, 1982.

Gangopadhyay A, Bhattacharya M, Chatterjee SK, et al: Immunoperoxidase localization of a high-molecular-weight mucin recognized by monoclonal antibody 1D3. *Cancer Res* 45:1744-1752, 1985.

Ghazizadeh M, Oguro T, Sasaaki Y, et al: Immunohistochemical and ultrastructural localization of T antigen in ovarian tumors. *Am J Clin Pathol* 93:315-321, 1990.

Giancotti FR, Dorsett BH, Cronin WJ, et al: Ovarian cancer associated antibodies recovered from ascites: Reagents for preparing the monoclonal antibody FEN-1. *Clin Res* 34:494A, 1986.

Giancotti FR, Dorsett BH, Kim KT, et al: Immunohistochemical characterization of a monoclonal antibody detecting an endometrioid ovarian cancer-associated antigen. *Int J Gynecol Pathol* 9:253-262, 1990.

Goldenberg DM, DeLand F, Kin E, et al: Use of radiolabeled antibodies to carcinoembryonic antigen for the detection and localization of diverse cancers by external photoscanning. *N Engl J Med* 298:1384-1388, 1978.

Graham JB, Graham RM: The effect of vaccine on cancer patients. *Surg Gynecol Obstet* 109:131-138, 1962.

Granowska M, Britton KE, Shepherd JH, et al: A prospective study of [123]I-labeled monoclonal antibody imaging in ovarian cancer. *J Clin Oncol* 4:730-736, 1986a.

Granowska M, Nimmon CC, Britton KE: Immunoscintigraphy of ovarian cancer by means of HMFG2 monoclonal antibody. In Winkler C (ed): *Nuclear Medicine in Clinical Oncology. Current Status and Future Aspects*. New York, Springer-Verlag, 1986b, pp 171-176.

Greiner JS, Fisher PB, Pestka S, Schlom J: Differential effects of recombinant human leukocyte interferons on cell surface antigen expression. *Cancer Res* 46:4984-4990, 1986.

Gross L: Intradermal immunization of C3H mice against a sarcoma that originated in an animal of the same line. *Cancer Res* 3:326-333, 1943.

Guthrie D, Way S: Immunotherapy of non-clinical vaginal cancer. *Lancet* 2:1242-1243, 1975.

Guthrie D, Way S: Failure of topical DNCB immunotherapy in most patients with non-clinical carcinoma of the cervix. *Br J Cancer* 39:445-448, 1979.

Habel K: Resistance of polyoma virus immune animals to transplanted polyoma tumors. *Proc Soc Exp Biol Med* 106:722-725, 1961.

Haisma HJ, Moseley KR, Battaile A, et al: Distribution and pharmacokinetics of radiolabeled monoclonal antibody OC 125 after intravenous and intraperitoneal administration in gynecologic tumors. *Am J Obstet Gynecol* 159:843-848, 1988.

Hamburger AW, White CP, Dunn FE: Modulation of tumor colony growth by irradiated accessory cells. Fourth Conference on Tumor Cloning, Tucson, Arizona, 1984.

Hamilton JM, Sznol M, Friedman MA: 5-Fluorouracil plus levamisole: Effective adjuvant treatment for colon cancer. In DeVita VT, Hellman S, Rosenberg SA (eds): *Important Advances in Oncology*. Philadelphia, J.B. Lippincott Co, 1990, pp 115-130.

Haskill S, Koren H, Becker S, et al: Mononuclear-cell infiltration in ovarian cancer. III. Suppressor-cell and ADCC activity of macrophages from ascitic and solid ovarian tumours. *Br J Cancer* 45:747-753, 1982.

Hedrick SM: T lymphocyte receptors. In Paul WE (ed): *Fundamental Immunology*. 2nd ed. New York, Raven Press, 1989, pp 291-313.

He-nian Q: Immunohistological analysis of monoclonal antibody COC166-9 against primary ovarian epithelial cancer. *Chung-hua Ping Li Hsueh Tsa Chih* 17:207-209, 1988.

Henney CS, Gillis S: Cell-mediated cytotoxicity. In Paul WE (ed): *Fundamental Immunology.* New York, Raven Press, 1984, pp 669-684.

Heo DS, Whiteside TL, Kanbour A, Herberman RB: Lymphocytes infiltrating human ovarian tumors. I. Role of Leu-19 (NKH1)-positive recombinant IL-2-activated cultures of lymphocytes infiltrating human ovarian tumors. *J Immunol* 140:4042-4049, 1988.

Herberman RB: Immunogenicity of tumor antigens. *Biochim Biophys Acta* 473:93-119, 1977.

Herberman RB, Oldham RK: Cell-mediated cytotoxicity against human tumors: Lessons learned and future prospects. *J Biol Response Mod* 2:111-120, 1983.

Herberman RB, Santoni A: Regulation of natural killer cell activity. In Mihich E (ed): *Biological Responses in Cancer: Progress Toward Potential Applications II.* New York, Plenum Press, 1984, pp 121-144.

Hernandez E, Rosenshein NB, Pino y Torres J, et al: Ip immunotherapy and chemotherapy in advanced epithelial ovarian cancer. *Cancer Treat Rep* 66:1981-1982, 1982.

Herrero-Zabaleta ME, Gautier R, Burtin P, Bara J: Monoclonal antibody against a sialylated Lewis antigen isolated from an ovarian mucinous cyst. *Tumour Biol* 6:391-400, 1985.

Hibbs JB Jr: Macrophage nonimmunologic recognition: Target cell factors related to contact inhibition. *Science* 180:868-870, 1973.

Hilkens J, Buijs F, Hilgers J, et al: Monoclonal antibodies against human milk-fat globule membranes detecting differentiation antigens of the mammary gland and its tumors. *Int J Cancer* 34:197-206, 1984.

Hudson CN, Levin L, McHardy JE, et al: Active specific immunotherapy for ovarian cancer. *Lancet* 2:877-879, 1976.

Hull MG, Bowen-Simpkins P, Paintin DB: 5-Fluorouracil versus immunotherapy for non-clinical vaginal cancer. *Lancet* 1:588, 1976.

Hunt JS, Fishback JL, Andrews GK, Wood GW: Expression of class I HLA genes by trophoblast cells. Analysis by in situ hybridization. *J Immunol* 140:1293-1299, 1988.

Hunter VJ, Daly L, Helms M, et al: The prognostic significance of CA 125 half-life in ovarian cancer patients who have received primary chemotherapy after surgical cytoreduction. *Am J Obstet Gynecol* 163:1164-1167, 1990.

Iakubovskaia RI, Kazachkina NI, Karmakova TA, et al: Study of the integral antigen of the membranes of fatty globules of human milk. *Eksp Onkol* 12:61-65, 1990.

Ioannides CG, Freedman RS, Platsoucas CD, et al: Cytotoxic T cell clones isolated from ovarian tumor-infiltrating lymphocytes recognize multiple antigenic epitopes on autologous tumor cells. *J Immunol* 146:1700-1707, 1991.

Ioannides CG, Platsoucas CD, Patenia R: T-cell functions in ovarian cancer patients treated with viral oncolysates: I. Increased helper activity to immunoglobulin production. *Anticancer Res* 10:645-653, 1990.

Ishiguro T, Sugitachi I, Katoh K: T and B lymphocytes in patients with squamous cell carcinoma of the uterine cervix. *Gynecol Oncol* 9:80-85, 1980.

Ishikawa M, Yaginuma Y, Hayashi H, et al: Reactivity of a monoclonal antibody to manganese superoxide dismutase with human ovarian carcinoma. *Cancer Res* 50:2538-2542, 1990.

Jacobs I, Bast RC Jr: The CA 125 tumour-associated antigen: A review of the literature. *Human Reproduction* 4:1-12, 1989.

Jacobs I, Stabile I, Bridges J, et al: Multimodal approach to screening for ovarian cancer. *Lancet* 1:268-271, 1988.

Jerome KR, Barnd DL, Boyer CM, et al: Adenocarcinoma reactive cytotoxic T lymphocytes recognize an epitope present on the protein core of mucin molecules. In Lotze MT, Finn OJ (eds): *Cellular Immunity and The Immunotherapy of Cancer.* New York, Wiley-Liss Inc, 1990, pp 321-328.

Jessup JM, Wagner H, Toth CA, et al: Carcinoembryonic antigen may promote metastasis by cell adhesion. *Proc Am Assoc Cancer Res* 31:65, 1990.

Johnson WJ, Somers SD, Adams DO: Expression and development of macrophage activation for tumor cytotoxicity. *Contemp Top Immunobiol* 13:127-146, 1984.

Kabawat SE, Bast RC Jr, Bhan AK, et al: Tissue distribution of a coelomic-epithelium-related antigen recognized by the monoclonal antibody OC125. *Int J Gynecol Pathol* 2:275-285, 1983a.

Kabawat SE, Bast RC Jr, Welch WR, et al: Expression of major histocompatibility antigens and nature of inflammatory cellular infiltrate in ovarian neoplasms. *Int J Cancer* 32:547-554, 1983b.

Kacinski BM, Bloodgood RS, Carter D, et al: M-CSF (CSF-1), its receptor the FMS protein, and other lymphohematopoietic factors and receptors involved in macrophage activation (IL-3, G-IFN, GM-CSF) play important roles in producing the proliferative and invasive characteristics of human ovarian, endometrial, and other adenocarcinomas in vivo and in vitro. Cold Spring Harbor Symposium, 1988, p 117.

Kacinski BM, Carter D, Korhorn EI, et al: Markedly elevated plasma levels of a tumor-produced cytokine CSF-1 (M-CSF), the macrophage colony-stimulating factor are seen in ovarian carcinoma patients with active gynecological neoplasms. *Soc Gynecol Invest*, p 182, 1989.

Kanazawa K, Honma S, Yuzawa H, Takeuchi S: Clinical effects of human fibroblast interferon in advanced gynecological cancers. *Gan To Kagaku Ryoho* 11:1276-1283, 1984.

Kato H, de Bruijn HW (eds): *Tumor Markers in the Management of Squamous Cell Carcinoma of the Cervix and Vagina.* Excerpta Medica, 1987.

Kato H, Miyauchi F, Morioka H, et al: Tumor antigen of human cervical squamous cell carcinoma. Correlation of circulating levels with disease progress. *Cancer* 43:585-590, 1979.

Khoo SK, MacKay EV: Immunologic reactivity of female patients with genital cancer: Status in preinvasive, locally invasive, and disseminated disease. *Am J Obstet Gynecol* 119:1018-1025, 1974.

Khoo SK, MacKay EV, Daunter B: Dinitrochlorobenzene reactivity of women with cancer of the ovary, cervix and corpus uteri. *Int J Gynaecol Obstet* 17:58-62, 1979.

Khoo SK, Whitaker SV, Jones IS, Thomas DA: Levamisole as adjuvant to chemotherapy of ovarian cancer. Results of a randomized trial and 4-year follow-up *Cancer* 54:986-990, 1984.

Kindt TJ, Robinson MA: Major histocompatibility complex antigens. In Paul WE (ed): *Fundamental Immunology.* New York, Raven Press, 1984, pp 347-377.

Klein G: Tumor antigens. *Annu Rev Microbiol* 20:223-252, 1966.

Klug TL, Bast RC Jr, Niloff JM, et al: Monoclonal antibody immunoradiometric assay for an antigenic determinant (CA 125) associated with human epithelial ovarian carcinomas. *Cancer Res* 44:1048-1053, 1984.

Knapp RC, Berkowitz RS: *Corynebacterium parvum* as an immunotherapeutic agent in an ovarian cancer model. *Am J Obstet Gynecol* 128:782-786, 1977.

Knapp RC, Lavin PT, Schaetzl E, et al: Elevation of CA 125 prior to recurrence of ovarian cancer. *Gynecol Oncol* 20:263-264, 1985.

Knauf S: Clinical evaluation of ovarian tumor antigen NB/70K: Monoclonal antibody assays for distinguishing ovarian cancer from other gynecologic disease. *Am J Obstet Gynecol* 158:1067-1072, 1988.

Knauf S, Urbach GI: A study of ovarian cancer patients using a radioimmunoassay for human ovarian tumor-associated antigen OCA. *Am J Obstet Gynecol* 138:1222-1223, 1980.

Knauf S, Kalwas J, Helmkamp BF, et al: Monoclonal antibodies against human ovarian tumor associated antigen NB/70K: Preparation and use in a radioimmunoassay for measuring NB/70K in serum. *Cancer Immunol Immunother* 21:217-225, 1986.

Kohler G, Milstein C: Continuous cultures of fused cells secreting antibody of predefined specificity. *Nature* 256:495-497, 1975.

Kohorn EI, Klein-Angerer S: The effect of chemotherapy on lymphocyte subpopulations and cell-mediated cytotoxicity in patients with ovarian carcinoma. *Gynecol Oncol* 19:60-66, 1984.

Kohorn EI, Mitchell MS, Dwyer JM, et al: Effect of radiation on cell-mediated cytotoxicity and lymphocyte subpopulations in patients with ovarian carcinoma. *Cancer* 41:1040-1048, 1978.

Koprowski H, Steplewski Z, Mitchell K, et al: Colorectal carcinoma antigens detected by hybridoma antibodies. *Somatic Cell Genet* 5:957-971, 1979.

Krohn K, Ashorn R, Helle M: Generation of monoclonal antibodies to human milk-fat globule membrane antigens, with special reference to a precipitable secretory product of breast and ovarian carcinomas. *Tumour Biol* 6:13-23, 1985.

Krupp PJ, Bohm JW: 5-Fluorouracil topical treatment of in situ vulvar cancer. A preliminary report. *Obstet Gynecol* 51:702-706, 1978.

Kufe D, Inghirami G, Abe M, et al: Differential reactivity of a novel monoclonal antibody (DF3) with human malignant versus benign breast tumors. *Hybridoma* 3:223-232, 1984.

Kuroki M, Fernsten PD, Wunderlich D, et al: Serological mapping of the TAG-72 tumor-associated antigen using 19 distinct monoclonal antibodies. *Cancer Res* 50:4872-4879, 1990.

Kurrasch RH, Rutherford AV, Rick ME, et al: Characterization of a monoclonal antibody, OVB1, which binds to a unique determinant in human ovarian carcinomas and myeloid cells. *J Histochem Cytochem* 37:57-67, 1989.

Lachman LB: Human interleukin 1: Purification and properties. *Fed Proc* 42:2639-2645, 1983.

Lahey SJ, Steele G Jr, Berkowitz R, et al: Identification of material with paternal HLA antigen immunoreactivity from purported circulating immune complexes in patients with gestational trophoblastic neoplasia. *J Natl Cancer Inst* 72:983-990, 1984.

Lamm DL, Thor DE, Harris SC, et al: Intravesical and percutaneous BCG immunotherapy of recurrent superficial bladder cancer. In Terry WD, Rosenberg SA (eds): *Immunotherapy of Human Cancer.* New York, Elsevier-North Holland, 1982, pp 315-322.

Lan MS, Finn OJ, Fernsten PD, Metzgar RS: Isolation and properties of a human pancreatic adenocarcinoma-associated antigen DU-PAN-2. *Cancer Res* 45:305-310, 1985.

Lawler SD, Klouda PT, Bagshawe KD: The HL-A system in trophoblastic neoplasia. *Lancet* 2:834-837, 1971.

Levin L, McHardy JE, Curling OM, Hudson CN: Tumor antigenicity in ovarian cancer. *Br J Cancer* 32:152-159, 1975.

Levin L, McHardy JE, Poulton TA, et al: Tumor associated immunity and immunocompetence in ovarian cancer. *Br J Obstet Gynaecol* 83:393-399, 1976.

Lewis JL Jr, Terasaki PI: HL-A leukocyte antigen studies in women with gestational trophoblastic neoplasms. *Am J Obstet Gynecol* 111:547-554, 1971.

Li D, Wang Y, Yao X, et al: Treatment of patients with malignant pleural effusions due to advanced lung cancer by transfer of autologous LAK cells combined with RIL-2 or RIL-2 alone. *Proc Chin Acad Med Sci Peking Union Med Coll* 5:51-55, 1990a.

Li SG, Elferink DG, de Vries RR: Phenotypic and functional characterization of human suppressor T-cell clones: II. Activation by *Mycobacterium leprae* presented by HLA-DR molecules to alpha beta T-cell receptors. *Hum Immunol* 28:11-26, 1990b.

Li WY, Lusheng S, Kanbour A, et al: Lymphocytes infiltrating human ovarian tumors: Synergy between tumor necrosis factor α and interleukin 2 in the generation of CD8⁺ effectors from tumor-infiltrating lymphocytes. *Cancer Res* 49:5979-5985, 1989.

Liao SK, Avner BP, Meranda C, Kanamaru T: Monoclonal antibody BTMA8 with apparent selective specificity for adenocarcinomas of breast, colorectum, ovary and pancreas. *Proc Annu Meet Am Assoc Cancer Res* 28:362-363, 1987.

Lichtenstein AK, Berek J, Bast R Jr, et al: Activation of peritoneal lymphocyte cytotoxicity in patients with ovarian cancer by intraperitoneal treatment with *Corynebacterium parvum*. *J Biol Response Mod* 3:371-378, 1984a.

Lichtenstein AK, Berek J, Kahle J, Zighelboim J: Role of inflammatory neutrophils in antitumor effects induced by intraperitoneal administration of *Corynebacterium parvum* in mice. *Cancer Res* 44:5118-5123, 1984b.

Lichtenstein AK, Berek J, Zighelboim J: Natural killer inhibitory substance produced by the peritoneal cells of patients with ovarian cancer. *J Natl Cancer Inst* 74:349-355, 1985.

Lichtenstein AK, Seelig M, Berek J, Zighelboim J: Human neutrophil-mediated lysis of ovarian cancer cells. *Blood* 74:805-809, 1989.

Lichtenstein AK, Spina C, Berek JS, et al: Intraperitoneal administration of human recombinant interferon-alpha in patients with ovarian cancer: Effects on lymphocyte phenotype and cytotoxicity. *Cancer Res* 48:5853-5859, 1988.

Loke YW, Ballard AC: Blood group A antigens on human trophoblast cells. *Nature* 245:329-330, 1973.

Lotzova E: Therapeutic possibilities of virus-modified tumor cell extracts and interleukin-2 in human ovarian cancer. *Nat Immun Cell Growth Regul* 5:277-282, 1986.

Lurquin C, Van Pel A, Mariame B, et al: Structure of the gene of Tumor-transplantation antigen P91A: The mutated exon encodes a peptide recognized with Ld by cytolytic T cells. *Cell* 58:293-303, 1989.

Maiman M, Feuer G, Fruchter RG, et al: Identification of the gas-trointestinal and pancreatic cancer-associated antigen levels in invasive cervical carcinoma. *Gynecol Oncol* 34:312-316, 1989a.

Maiman M, Feuer G, Fruchter RG, et al: Value of squamous cell carcinoma antigen levels in invasive cervical carcinoma. *Gynecol Oncol* 34:312-316, 1989b.

Malkasian GD Jr, Knapp RC, Lavin PT, et al: Preoperative evaluation of serum CA 125 in premenopausal and postmenopausal patients with pelvic masses: Discrimination of benign from malignant disease. *Am J Obstet Gynecol* 159:341-346, 1988.

Mandell GL, Fisher RI, Bostick F, Young RC: Ovarian cancer: A solid tumor with evidence of normal cellular immune function but abnormal B cell function. *Am J Med* 66:621-624, 1979.

Mann W, Surwit E, Krag D, et al: Immunoscintigraphy of ovarian cancer with indium IN-111-CYT-103. Symposium on the Biology and Therapy of Ovarian Cancer, Marble Island, Vermont, 1990.

Mansell PW, Litwin MS, Ichinose H, Krementz ET: Delayed hypersensitivity to 5-fluorouracil following topical chemotherapy of cutaneous cancers. *Cancer Res* 35:1288-1294, 1975.

Mantovani A, Allavena P, Sessa C, et al: Natural killer activity of lymphoid cells isolated from human ascitic ovarian tumors. *Int J Cancer* 25:573-582, 1980a.

Mantovani A, Peri G, Polentarutti N, et al: Effects on in vitro tumor growth of macrophages isolated from human ascitic ovarian tumors. *Int J Cancer* 23:157-164, 1979.

Mantovani A, Polentarutti N, Peri G, et al: Cytotoxicity on tumor cells of peripheral blood monocytes and tumor associated macrophages in patients with ascites ovarian tumors. *J Natl Cancer Inst* 64:1307-1315, 1980b.

Mantovani A, Sessa C, Peri G, et al: Intraperitoneal administration of *Corynebacterium parvum* in patients with ascitic ovarian tumors resistant to chemotherapy: Effects on cytotoxicity of tumor-associated macrophages and NK cells. *Int J Cancer* 27:437-446, 1981.

Mariani-Costantini R, Agresti R, Colnaghi MI, et al: Characterization of the specificity by immunohistology of a monoclonal antibody to a novel epithelial antigen of ovarian carcinomas. *Pathol Res Pract* 180:169-180, 1985.

Masuho Y, Zalutsky M, Knapp RC, Bast RC Jr: Interaction of monoclonal antibodies with cell surface antigens of human ovarian carcinoma. *Cancer Res* 44:2813-2819, 1984.

Matsunago K, Mashiba H, Gojobori M, Jimi S: Antibody-dependent cell-mediated cytotoxicity of sera from cancer patients against cultured cervical cancer cell lines. *Gann* 70:1-7, 1979.

Matsuoka Y, Nakashima T, Endo K, et al: Recognition of ovarian cancer antigen CA125 by murine monoclonal antibody produced by immunization of lung cancer cells. *Cancer Res* 47:6335-6340, 1987.

Mattes MJ, Cordon-Cardo C, Lewis JL Jr, et al: Cell surface antigens of human ovarian and endometrial carcinoma defined by mouse monoclonal antibodies. *Proc Natl Acad Sci USA* 81:568-572, 1984.

Mattes MJ, Lloyd KO, Lewis JL Jr: Binding parameters of monoclonal antibodies reacting with ovarian carcinoma ascites cells. *Cancer Immunol Immunother* 28:199-207, 1989.

Mattes MJ, Look K, Furukawa K, et al: Mouse monoclonal antibodies to human epithelial differentiation antigens expressed on the surface of ovarian carcinoma ascites cells. *Cancer Res* 47:6741-6750, 1987.

Mattes MJ, Look K, Lewis JL Jr, et al: Three mouse monoclonal antibodies to human differentiation antigens: Reactivity with two mucin-like antigens and with connective tissue fibers. *J Histochem Cytochem* 33:1095-1102, 1985.

McIntire KR, Waldmann TA: Measurement of alpha-fetoprotein. In Rose NR, Friedman H (eds): *Manual of Clinical Immunology.* 2nd ed. Washington, DC, American Society for Microbiology, 1980, p 936-943.

Melnick H, Barber HRK: Cellular immunologic responsiveness to extracts of ovarian epithelial tumors. *Gynecol Oncol* 3:77-86, 1975.

Meltzer MS, Macy CA: Delayed-type hypersensitivity and the induction of activated cytotoxic macrophages. In Paul WE (ed): *Fundamental Immunology*, 2nd ed. New York, Raven Press, 1989, pp 765-777.

Mettler L, Radzun HJ, Salmassi A, et al: Six new monoclonal antibodies to serous, mucinous, and poorly differentiated ovarian adenocarcinomas. *Cancer* 65:1525-1532, 1990.

Metzgar RS, Gaillard MT, Levine SJ, et al: Antigens of human pancreatic adenocarcinoma cells defined by murine monoclonal antibodies. *Cancer Res* 42:601-608, 1982.

Mezzanzanica D, Canevari S, Menard S, et al: Human ovarian carcinoma lysis by cytotoxic T cells targeted by bispecific monoclonal antibodies: Analysis of the antibody components. *Int J Cancer* 41:609-615, 1988.

Mignot MH: Preoperative immune stimulation by local *C. parvum* treatment in carcinoma of the cervix. (Thesis at the Free University of Amsterdam). Amsterdam, Mondeel, 1982, p 45.

Mignot MH, Lens JW, Drexhage HA, et al: Lower relapse rates after neighborhood injection of *Corynebacterium parvum* in operable cervix carcinoma. *Br J Cancer* 44:856-862, 1981.

Miller JW, Hunter AM, Horne NW: Intrapleural immunotherapy with *Corynebacterium parvum* in recurrent malignant pleural effusions. *Thorax* 35:856-858, 1980.

Miotti S, Aguanno S, Canevari S, et al: Biochemical analysis of human ovarian cancer-associated antigens defined by murine monoclonal antibodies. *Cancer Res* 45:826-832, 1985.

Miotti S, Tagliabue E, Menard S, Colnaghi MI: Two new monoclonal antibodies identify an ovarian carcinoma: A molecule with a more restricted tumor specificity. *Tumor Biol* 7:289-300, 1986.

Mitsuyasu RT, Li SN, Champlin RE, Gale RP: Abnormal T-lymphocyte colonies (CFU-TL) following bone marrow transplantation. *Exp Hematol* 14:1049-1055, 1986.

Morgensen B, Kissmeyer-Nielsen F, Hauge M: Histocompatibility antigens on the HL-A locus in gestational choriocarcinoma. *Transplant Proc* 1:76-79, 1969.

Morton DL, Miller GF, Wood DA: Demonstration of tumor-specific immunity against antigens unrelated to the mammary tumor virus in spontaneous mammary adenocarcinomas. *J Natl Cancer Inst* 42:289-301, 1969.

Murray T, Elliott AT, Wheldon TE, et al: Immunoscintigraphy of human ovarian cancer xenografts using a radiolabelled monoclonal antibody to human pregnancy serum-derived immune complexes. *Nucl Med Commun* 9:505-511, 1988.

Muto MG, Finkler NJ, Howes AE, et al: The intraperitoneal radioimmunotherapy of refractory ovarian carcinoma utilizing I-131 labeled OC 125. Symposium on the Biology and Therapy of Ovarian Cancer, Marble Island, Vermont, 1990.

Nalick RH, DiSaia PJ, Rea TH, Morrow CP: Immunocompetence and prognosis in patients with gynecologic cancer. *Gynecol Oncol* 2:8192, 1974.

Nam JH, Chambers JT, Schwartz PE, Cole L: UGF—A marker for pelvic malignancies. II. In the management of patients with ovarian and cervical cancer. Second Meeting International Gynecologic Oncology Society, 1989, pp 305.

Nardi M, Cognetti F, Pollera CF, et al: Intraperitoneal recombinant alpha-2-interferon alternating with cisplatin as salvage therapy for minimal residual-disease ovarian cancer: A phase II study. *J Clin Oncol* 8:1036-1041, 1990.

Nathan CF, Murray HW, Cohn ZA: The macrophage as an effector cell. *N Engl J Med* 303:622-626, 1980.

Nathan CF, Murray HW, Wiebe ME, Rubin BY: Identification of interferon-gamma as the lymphokine that activates human macrophage oxidative metabolism and antimicrobial activity. *J Exp Med* 158:670-689, 1983.

Nauts HC: Beneficial effects of acute concurrent infection, inflammation, fever, or immunotherapy (bacterial toxins) on ovarian and uterine cancer. *Cancer Res Inst Monog* 17:1-122, 1977.

Neill W, Norval M: Natural killer cell activity in patients with abnormalities of the uterine cervix. *Gynecol Obstet Invest* 18:122-128, 1984.

Ngan HY, Wong LC, Chan SY, Ma HK: Use of serum squamous cell carcinoma antigen assays in chemotherapy treatment of cervical cancer. *Gynecol Oncol* 35:259-262, 1989.

Niloff JM, Klug TL, Schaetzl E, et al: Elevation of serum CA 125 in carcinomas of the fallopian tube, endometrium, and endocervix. *Am J Obstet Gynecol* 148:1057-1058, 1984a.

Niloff JM, Knapp RC, Jones G, et al: Recombinant leukocyte alpha interferon in advanced ovarian carcinoma. *Cancer Treat Rep* 69:895-896, 1985.

Niloff JM, Knapp RC, Schaetzl E, et al: CA 125 antigen levels in obstetric and gynecologic patients. *Obstet Gynecol* 64:703-707, 1984b.

Noda K, Teshima K, Tekeuti K, et al: Immunotherapy using the streptoccocal preparation OK-432 for the treatment of uterine cervical cancer. Cervical cancer immunotherapy study group *Gynecol Oncol* 35:367-372, 1989.

O'Garra A, Vonland S, De France T, Christiansen J: "B cell factors" are pleiotropic. *Immunol Today* 9:45-54, 1988.

Ohkawa K, Tsukada Y, Murae M, et al: Serum levels and biochemical characteristics of human ovarian carcinoma-associated antigen defined by murine monoclonal antibody CF511. *Br J Cancer* 60:953-960, 1989.

Okubo M, Sato N, Wada Y, et al: Identification by monoclonal antibody of the tumor antigen of an autologous breast cancer cell that is involved in cytotoxicity by a cytotoxic T-cell clone. *Cancer Res* 49:3950-3954, 1989.

Old LJ: Cancer immunology: The search for specificity. *Cancer Res* 41:361-375, 1981.

Old LJ, Boyse EA: Immunology of experimental tumors. *Annu Rev Med* 15:167-186, 1964.

Olkowski ZL, McLaren JR, Skeen MJ: Effects of combined immunotherapy with levamisole and bacillus Calmette-Guerin on immunocompetence of patients with squamous cell carcinoma of the cervix, head and neck, and lung undergoing radiation therapy. *Cancer Treat Rep* 62:1651-1661, 1978.

Order SE, Donahue V, Knapp R: Immunotherapy of ovarian carcinoma: An experimental model. *Cancer* 32:573-579, 1973.

Order SE, Kirkman R, Knapp R: Serologic immunotherapy: Results and probable mechanism of action. *Cancer* 34:175-183, 1974.

Papsidero LD, Croghan GA, O'Connell M, et al: Monoclonal antibodies (F36/22 and M7/105) to human breast carcinoma. *Cancer Res* 43:1741-1747, 1983.

Pattillo RA, Ruckert AC, Story MR, et al: Immunodiagnosis in ovarian cancer: Blocking factor activity. *Am J Obstet Gynecol* 133:791, 1979a.

Pattillo RA, Ruckert AC, Story MT, Mattingly RF: Immunodiagnosis in ovarian cancer cells in vitro. *Cancer Res* 39:1185, 1979b.

Pattillo RA, Story MT, Uckert CF: Expression of cell-mediated immunity and blocking factor using a new line of ovarian cancer cells in vitro. *Cancer Res* 39:1185, 1979c.

Pillai MR, Balaram P, Padmanabhan TK, Nair MD: Monoclonal antibody defined phenotypes of peripheral blood lymphocytes in cancer of the uterine cervix. *Am J Reprod Immunol Microbiol* 14:141-143, 1987.

Pinsky CM, Camacho FJ, Kerr D, et al: Treatment of superficial bladder cancer with intravesical BCG. In Terry WD, Rosenberg SA (eds): *Immunotherapy of Human Cancer.* New York, Elsevier–North Holland, 1982, pp 309-313.

Piver MS, Barlow JJ, Tsukada Y, et al: Postirradiation squamous cell carcinoma in situ of the vagina: Treatment by topical 20 percent 5-fluorouracil cream. *Am J Obstet Gynecol* 135:377-380, 1979.

Poels LG, Kenemans P: A new monoclonal antibody (OV-TL3) against human ovarian carcinoma that does not react with circulating tumour antigens. *Br J Cancer,* 54:529-530, 1986a.

Poels LG, Peters D, van Megen Y, et al: Monoclonal antibody against human ovarian tumor-associated antigens. *J Natl Cancer Inst* 76:781-791, 1986b.

Poropatich C, Nozawa S, Rojas M, et al: MSN-1 antibody in the evaluation of female genital tract adenocarcinomas. *Int J Gynecol Pathol* 9:73-79, 1990.

Poulton TA, Crowther ME, Hay FC, Nineham LJ: Immune complexes in ovarian cancer. *Lancet* 2:72-73, 1978.

Prat M, Morra I, Bussolati G, Comoglio PM: CAR-3: A monoclonal antibody-defined antigen expressed on human carcinomas. *Cancer Res* 45:5799-5807, 1985.

Prehn RT, Main JM: Immunity to methylcholanthrene-induced sarcomas. *J Natl Cancer Inst* 18:769-778, 1957.

Pride GL, Chuprevich TW: Topical 5-fluorouracil treatment of transformation zone intraepithelial neoplasia of cervix and vagina. *Obstet Gynecol* 60:467-472, 1982.

Ramakrishnan S, Xu FJ, Brandt SJ, et al: Constitutive production of macrophage colony-stimulating factor by human ovarian and breast cancer cell lines. *J Clin Invest* 83:921-926, 1989.

Rao BB, Wanebo HJ, Ochoa M, et al: Intravenous *Corynebacterium parvum:* An adjuvant to chemotherapy for resistant advanced ovarian cancer. *Cancer* 39:514-526, 1977.

Rapp F: Herpes simplex virus type 2 and cervical cancer. In Hickey RC (ed): *Current Problems in Cancer,* Vol. 6, No 4. Chicago, Year Book Medical Publishers, 1981, pp 1-18.

Rawls WE, Laurel D, Melnick JL, et al: A search for viruses in smegma, premalignant and early malignant cervical tissues: The isolation of herpes viruses with distinct antigenic properties. *Am J Epidemiol* 87:647-655, 1968.

Rayner AA, Berkowitz R, Steele GD Jr, et al: Serial circulating immune complex concentrations in patients with gestational trophoblastic neoplasia. *Surg Forum* 32:462-465, 1981.

Real FX, Mattes MJ, Houghton AN, et al: Class 1 (unique) tumor antigens of human melanoma. Identification of a 90,000 dalton cell surface glycoprotein by autologous antibody. *J Exp Med* 160:1219-1233, 1984.

Ritz J, Pesanedo JM, Notis-McConarty J, Schlossman SF: Modulation of human acute lymphoblastic leukemia antigen induced by monoclonal antibody in vitro. *J Immunol* 125:1506-1514, 1980.

Rivera ES, Hersh EM, Bowen JM, et al: Leukocyte migration inhibition assay of tumor immunity in patients with cervical squamous cell carcinoma. *Cancer* 43:2297-2305, 1979.

Rodriguez-Rodriguez L, Liebert M, Natale R, Wahl R: Monoclonal antibody (5G6.4) against ovarian carcinoma shows inhibition of in vitro colony formation. *Gynecol Oncol* 27:382-388, 1987.

Rosenberg SA, Packard BS, Aebersold PM, et al: Use of tumor-infiltrating lymphocytes and interleukin-2 in the immunotherapy of patients with metastatic melanoma. A preliminary report. *N Engl J Med* 319:1676-1680, 1988.

Rubin SC, Finstad CL, Hoskins WJ, et al: A longitudinal study of antigen expression in epithelial ovarian cancer. *Gynecol Oncol* 34:389-394, 1989.

Rubin SC, Finstad CL, Hoskins WJ, et al: Expression of P-glycoprotein in epithelial ovarian cancer: Evaluation as a marker of multidrug resistance. *Am J Obstet Gynecol* 163:69-73, 1990.

Runowicz CD, Cohen CJ, Adelsberg BR: Immune complexes in ovarian carcinoma. *Gynecol Oncol* 32:350-353, 1989.

Rutledge ML, Robey-Cafferty SS, Silva EG, Bruner JM: Monoclonal antibody C219 detection of the multidrug-resistant protein P-glycoprotein in routinely processed tissues: A study of 36 cases of ovarian carcinoma. *Mod Pathol* 3:298-301, 1990.

Sakakibara K, Ueda R, Ohta M, et al: Three novel mouse monoclonal antibodies, OM-A, OM-B, and OM-C, reactive with mucinous type ovarian tumors. *Cancer Res* 48:4639-4645, 1988.

Salmon SE, Hamburger AW: Immunoproliferation and cancer: A common macrophage-derived promoter substance. *Lancet* 1:1289-1290, 1978.

Sandberg AL: Complement. In Oppenheim JJ, Rosenstreich DL, Potter M (eds): *Cellular Functions in Immunity and Inflammation.* New York, Elsevier–North Holland, 1981, pp 373-395.

Satam MN, Suraiya JN, Nadkarni JJ: Natural killer and antibody-dependent cellular cytotoxicity in cervical carcinoma patients. *Cancer Immunol Immunother* 23:56-59, 1986.

Sawada M, Okudaira Y, Matsui Y, Shimizu Y: Immunosuppressive acidic protein in patients with gynecologic cancer. *Cancer* 54:652-656, 1984.

Sawanobori S, Ashman RB, Nahmias AJ, et al: Rosette formation and inhibition in cervical dysplasia and carcinoma in situ. *Cancer Res* 37:4332-4335, 1977.

Scambia G, Iacobelli S, Arno E, et al: Tumor associated antigen 90K in gynecological neoplasms. *Eur J Gynaecol Oncol* 8:481-482, 1987.

Schlom J, Greiner P, Hand P, et al: Human breast cancer markers defined by monoclonal antibodies. In Sell S, Reisfeld R (eds): *Monoclonal Antibodies in Cancer.* Clifton, New Jersey, Humana Press, 1985, pp 247-277.

Schwartz PE, Chambers SK, Chambers JT, et al: Circulating tumor markers in monitoring of gynecological malignancies. *Cancer* 60:353-361, 1987.

Sekine H, Hayes DF, Ohno T, et al: Circulating DF3 and CA125 antigen levels in serum from patients with epithelial ovarian carcinoma. *J Clin Oncol* 3:1355-1363, 1985a.

Sekine H, Ohno T, Kufe DW: Purification and characterization of a high molecular weight glycoprotein detectable in human milk and breast carcinomas. *J Immunol* 135:3610-3615, 1985b.

Seth P, Balachandran N, Malaviya AN, Kumar R: Circulating immune complexes in carcinoma of uterine cervix. *Clin Exp Immunol* 38:77-82, 1979.

Sharma D, Gupta RM, Kadian V: Clinical and immunological study of patients with cancer of the cervix. *Indian J Med Res* 70:793-800, 1979.

Shau H, Koren HS, Dawson JR: Human natural killing against ovarian carcinoma. *Br J Cancer* 47:687-695, 1983.

Shepherd JH, Epenetos AA, Britton KE, et al: Radioimmune diagnosis of ovarian carcinoma using tumor associated monoclonal antibodies. *Proc Soc Gynecol Oncol* 14:12, 1983.

Silburn PA, Khoo SK, Daunter B, et al: Types of immune complexes in the ascitic fluid of women with carcinoma of the ovary. *Int Arch Allergy Appl Immunol* 71:219-223, 1983.

Smith LH, Yin A, Bieber M, Teng NN: Generation of human monoclonal antibodies to cancer-associated antigens using limited numbers of patient lymphocytes. *J Immunol Methods* 105:263-273, 1987.

Soper JT, Hunter VJ, Daly L, et al: Preoperative serum tumor associated antigen levels in women with pelvic masses. *Obstet Gynecol* 75:249-254, 1990.

Srivastava PK, Old LJ: Identification of a human homologue of the murine tumor rejection antigen GP96. *Cancer Res* 49:1341-1343, 1989.

Srivastava PK, Chen YT, Old LJ: 5'-Structural analysis of genes encoding polymorphic antigens of chemically induced tumors. *Proc Natl Acad Sci USA* 84:3807-3811, 1987.

Stall KE, Martin EW Jr: Plasma carcinoembryonic antigen levels in ovarian cancer patients: A chart review and survey of published data. *J Reprod Med* 26:73-79, 1981.

Steis R, Urba W, Van der Molen L, et al: Intraperitoneal lymphokine-activated killer cell and interleukin-2 therapy for malignancies limited to the peritoneal cavity. *J Clin Oncol* 6:1618-1629, 1990.

Stewart JS, Hird V, Snook D: Intraperitoneal ¹³¹I- and ⁹⁰Y-labelled monoclonal antibodies for ovarian cancer: Pharmacokinetics and normal tissue dosimetry. *Int J Cancer* 3:71-76, 1988.

Stolbach L, Pitt A, Gandbhir L, et al: Ovarian cancer patient antibodies and their relationship to ovarian cancer associated markers. In Herberman RB (ed): *Compendium of Assays for Immunodiagnosis of Human Cancer.* New York, Elsevier–North Holland 1979, pp 553-557.

Sunderland CA, Davies JO, Stirrat GM: Immunohistology of normal and ovarian cancer tissue with a monoclonal antibody to placental alkaline phosphatase. *Cancer Res* 44:4496-4502, 1984.

Tagliabue E, Menard S, Della Torre G, et al: Generation of monoclonal antibodies reacting with human epithelial ovarian cancer. *Cancer Res* 45:379-385, 1985.

Thurin J: Characterization and molecular biology of tumor-associated antigens. *Cur Opin Immunol* 2:702-707, 1990.

Tomoda Y, Fuma M, Saiki N, et al: Immunologic studies in patients with trophoblastic neoplasia. *Am J Obstet Gynecol* 126:661-667, 1976.

Tsuji Y, Suzuki T, Nishiura H, et al: Identification of two different surface epitopes of human ovarian epithelial carcinomas by monoclonal antibodies. *Cancer Res* 45:2358-2362, 1985.

Turner GM, Symes MO: The use of sensitized pig lymph-node cells in the treatment of carcinoma of the ovary. *Br J Cancer* 40:823, 1979.

Turner MW: The immunoglobulins. In Holborow EJ, Reeves WG (eds): *Immunology in Medicine,* 2nd ed. London, Academic Press, 1977.

Tyson FL, Boyer CM, Kaufman R, et al: Overexpression and amplification of the HER-2/*neu* (c-*erb*B-2) proto-oncogene in epithelial ovarian tumors and cell lines. *Am J Obstet Gynecol* 165:640-646, 1991.

Uchida A, Colot M, Micksche M: Suppression of natural killer cell activity by adherent effusion cells of cancer patients. Suppression of motility, binding capacity and lethal hit of NK cells. *Br J Cancer* 49:17-23, 1984.

Vaage J: Nonvirus-associated antigens in virus-induced mouse mammary tumors. *Cancer Res* 28:2477-2483, 1968.

van de Linde AW, Streefkerk M, te Velde ER, et al: Tumor specific antibodies in sera from patients with squamous cell carcinoma of the uterine cervix. Detection by a membrane immunoflorescence assay on cultured cervical carcinoma cells. *Cancer Immunol Immunother* 11:201-206, 1981.

van der Burg ME, Lammes FB, van Putten WL, Stoter G: Ovarian cancer: The prognostic value of serum half-life of CA125 during induction chemotherapy. *Gynecol Oncol* 30:307-312, 1988.

van Nagell JR Jr, Kim E, Casper S, et al: Radioimmunodetection of primary and metastatic ovarian cancer using radiolabelled antibodies to carcinoembryonic antigen. *Cancer Res* 40:502-506, 1980.

Vanky F, Masucci MG, Bejarano MT, Klein E: Lysis of tumor biopsy cells by blood lymphocyte subsets of various densities. Autologous and allogeneic studies. *Int J Cancer* 33:185-192, 1984.

Vollmar AM, Banker DE, Mendelsohn J, Herschman HR: Toxicity of ligand and antibody-directed ricin A-chain conjugates recognizing the epidermal growth factor receptor. *J Cell Physiol* 131:418-425, 1987.

Vose BM, Howell A: Cultured human antitumour T cells and their potential for therapy. In Herberman RB (ed): *Basic and Clinical Tumor Immunology*. Boston, Martinus Nijhoff, 1983, pp 129-157.

Wagner H, Pfizenmaier K, Rollinghoff M: The role of the major histocompatibility gene complex in murine cytotoxic T cell responses. *Adv Cancer Res* 31:77-124, 1980.

Wahl R, Piko C: Intraperitoneal (IP) delivery of radiolabeled monoclonal antibody to IP-induced xenografts of human ovarian cancers. *Proc Am Assoc Cancer Res* 26:298, 1985.

Wanebo HJ, Ochoa M Jr, Gunther U, et al: Randomized chemoimmunotherapy trial of CAF and intravenous *C. parvum* for resistant ovarian carcinoma. Preliminary results. *Proc Am Assoc Cancer Res* 18:225, 1977.

Wang YL, Si LS, Kanbour A, et al: Lymphocytes infiltrating human ovarian tumors: Synergy between tumor necrosis factor alpha and interleukin 2 in the generation of CD8[+] effectors from tumor-infiltrating lymphocytes. *Cancer Res* 49:5979-5985, 1989.

Ward BG, Cruickshank DJ, Tucker DF, Love S: Independent expression in serum of three tumor-associated antigens: CA125, placental alkaline phosphatase and HMFG-2 in ovarian cancer. *Br J Obstet Gynaecol* 94:696-698, 1987.

Ward B, Mather S, Shepherd J, et al: The treatment of intraperitoneal malignant disease with monoclonal antibody guided [131]I radiotherapy. *Br J Cancer* 58:658-662, 1988.

Watson J, Sensintaffar JL, Berek JS, Martinez-Maza O: Constitutive production of interleukin 6 by ovarian cancer cell lines and by primary ovarian tumor cultures. *Cancer Res* 50:6959-6965, 1990.

Webb HE, Oaten SW, Pike CP: Treatment of malignant ascitic and pleural effusion with *Corynebacterium parvum*. *Br Med J* 1:338-340, 1978.

Welch WR, Niloff JM, Anderson D, et al: Heterogeneity of antigen expression in advanced epithelial ovarian cancer. *Obstet Gynecol* 162:883-888, 1990.

Wells SA Jr, Melewicz FC, Christiansen C, Ketcham AS: Delayed cutaneous hypersensitivity reactions to membrane extracts of carcinomatous cells of the cervix uteri. *Surg Gynecol Obstet* 136:717-720, 1973.

Werner M, Ahlert T, Bastert G: Human monoclonal antibodies directed against ovarian carcinoma. *Gynecol Oncol* 34:148-154, 1989.

West WH, Tauer KW, Yannelli JR, et al: Constant-infusion recombinant interleukin-2 in adoptive immunotherapy of advanced cancer. *N Engl J Med* 316:898-905, 1987.

Woods JC, Harris H, Spriggs AI, McGee JO: A new marker for human cancer cells. 3. Immunocytochemical detection of malignant cells in serous fluids with the Ca-1 antibody. *Lancet* 2:512-515, 1982.

Wu S, Rodabaugh K, Martinez-Maza O, et al: Stimulation of ovarian tumor cell proliferation with monocyte products including interleukin-1-alpha, interleukin-6 and tumor necrosis factor-alpha. *Am J Obstet Gynecol* (in press).

Xu CX, Lin L, Huang YY, et al: Purge of malignant cells from bone marrow by hematoporphyrin derivatives and light exposure in vitro. *Chung Kuo Yao Li Hsueh Pao* 11:72-75, 1990.

Xu FJ, Ramakrishnan S, Daly L, et al: Increased serum levels of macrophage colony-stimulating factor in ovarian cancer. *Am J Obstet Gynecol* (in press).

Xu FJ, Rodriguez GC, Whitaker R, Boente M, Berchuck A, McKenzie S, Houston L, Boyer CM, Bast RC Jr: Antibodies against immunochemically distinct epitopes on the extracellular domain of HER-2/*neu* (c-*erb* B-2) inhibit growth of breast and ovarian cancer cell lines. *Proc Amer Assoc Cancer Res* 32:260, 1991.

Yajima H, Noda T, de Villiers EM, et al: Isolation of a new type of human papillomavirus (HPV52b) with a transforming activity from cervical cancer tissue. *Cancer Res* 48:7164-7172, 1988.

Yu SC, Bao YH, Li X: Effect of autologous bone marrow transfusion on cancer patients with impaired hemopoietic function. *Chung Hua Fang She I Hsueh Yu Fang Hu Tsa Chih* 4:5-9, 1984.

Yu YH, Crews S, Ramakrishnan S, et al: Use of immunotoxins in combination to inhibit clonogenic growth of human breast carcinoma cells. *Cancer Res* 50:3231-3238, 1990.

Zalutsky MR, Knapp RC, Bast RC Jr: Influence of circulating antigen on blood pool activity of a radioiodinated monoclonal antibody. *Nucl Med Biol* 15:431-437, 1988.

Zamcheck N, Kupchik HZ: Summary of clinical use and limitations of the carcinoembryonic antigen assay and some methodological considerations. In Rose NR, Friedman H (eds): *Manual of Clinical Immunology*. 2nd ed. Washington, DC, American Society for Microbiology, 1980, pp 919-935.

Zurawski VR Jr, Broderick SF, Pickens P, et al: Serum CA 125 levels in a group of nonhospitalized women: Relevance for the early detection of ovarian cancer. *Obstet Gynecol* 69:606-611, 1987.

Zurawski VR Jr, Orjaseter H, Andersen A, Jellum E: Elevated serum CA 125 levels prior to diagnosis of ovarian neoplasia: Relevance for early detection of ovarian cancer. *Int J Cancer* 42:677-680, 1988.

Zurawski VR Jr, Sjovall K, Schoenfeld DA, et al: Prospective evaluation of serum CA 125 levels in a normal population, Phase I: The specificities of single and serial determinations in testing for ovarian cancer. *Gynecol Oncol* 36:299-305, 1990.

# Chapter 5 | Chemotherapy in Gynecologic Oncology

*Robert C. Young*

## ANTINEOPLASTIC DRUGS: CLINICAL PHARMACOLOGY AND MECHANISMS OF ACTION

### General Principles

With the large number of antineoplastic drugs now available to physicians, selecting the appropriate drug(s) for a particular tumor is becoming increasingly complex. Obviously, the more we know about the clinical pharmacology and mechanisms of action of an antineoplastic agent, the more rational can be its use. Fortunately, certain general principles may help guide the physician in choosing the proper drugs or classes of drugs. In addition, differences among these agents with respect to their mechanism of action, absorption, distribution, metabolism, and excretion will influence their effectiveness in vivo. Since all chemotherapeutic agents are toxic to normal tissues, specific toxicities must also be considered. Thus, the choice of any particular agent depends upon a mosaic of information patched together from knowledge of cellular kinetics, clinical pharmacology, toxicity, and mechanisms of action.

When compared with other classes of drugs, antineoplastic agents are unique in that they have a relatively narrow therapeutic index. Therefore, the decision to use these agents at all must be made with great care, taking into account several important issues (Table 5-1). Of major importance is the natural history of the disease. Use of antineoplastic agents should be restricted to patients whose malignancy has been established histologically; any tendency to employ these agents as part of a diagnostic trial should be resisted. Furthermore, the decision to employ chemotherapy is clearly influenced by the physician's knowledge of the extent of the disease and its rate of progression.

A second major consideration involves the patient's unique circumstances and probable tolerance of the antineoplastic drug therapy. The patient's age and general health as well as any complicating illnesses, the extent of previous treatment, and any residual functional compromise also affect this decision. In addition, emotional, social, and even financial concerns must be respected and taken into account. Antineoplastic drug therapy should not be instituted if the physician is not prepared and equipped to monitor the patient's response carefully and to treat inherent toxicities. Instead, the patient should be referred to a physician or facility that can provide such care. Because all these agents cause significant toxicity, some means of measuring their effect on the tumor must be available. It is inappropriate to ad-

minister chemotherapeutic drugs unless their benefit can be objectively determined.

Finally, the decision to proceed with antineoplastic drug treatment depends upon the likelihood of achieving a beneficial response. All cancers do not respond to chemotherapy in quantitatively and qualitatively similar ways. In general, human tumors can be grouped according to the likelihood of a successful outcome from such treatment. For example, there are some tumors for which chemotherapy has been curative for *most* patients (e.g., choriocarcinoma, ovarian germ cell tumors). Obviously, a decision *not* to treat patients with diseases known to be curable with chemotherapy would have to be weighed very carefully. Even substantial toxicities would be acceptable if the probability of long-term survival was high. There is another group of cancers for which chemotherapy has improved patient survival but has not restored a normal life expectancy (e.g., epithelial ovarian cancer). Patients with tumors of these types usually benefit from chemotherapy. Obviously, such patients should receive therapy, when appropriate, unless there is a clear reason why they should not. A third group of cancers respond to chemotherapy, but survival has not been improved for a significant number of patients (e.g., cervical carcinoma, endometrial carcinoma). Finally, in certain cancers, only marginal or no responses to chemotherapy have been achieved. In this last group, the use of chemotherapy should be restricted and particular emphasis given to including such patients in well-structured prospective clinical trials.

Obviously, decision to embark on antineoplastic drug therapy is a complex one. Optimal patient care demands a careful review of the many factors discussed above in order to maximize the possibilities for improving the patient's survival and quality of life. Once the decision to utilize chemotherapy has been made, the appropriate drug or drug regimen must be selected. The physician is aided in this task by the fact that chemotherapeutic agents can be conveniently grouped into several classes having similar pharmacologic properties, mechanisms of action, and toxicities. The most important classes are the alkylating agents, antimetabolites, antitumor antibiotics, vinca alkaloids, and hormones; the rest have been grouped here under the heading "Miscellaneous Compounds."

### Alkylating Agents

Although several hundred alkylating compounds exist, only a few are commonly used. These include nitrogen mustard (Mustargen), cyclophosphamide (Endoxan,

**TABLE 5-1  Guidelines to Be Considered Before Using Antineoplastic Drugs**

1. Natural history of the malignancy
   a. Diagnosis made by biopsy
   b. Rapidity of progression
   c. Extent of disease spread
2. Patient circumstances and tolerance
   a. Age, general health, underlying diseases
   b. Extent of previous treatment
   c. Adequate facilities to evaluate, monitor, and treat potential drug toxicities
   d. The patient's emotional, social, and financial factors
   e. Determination of the objective response to treatment
3. Probability of achieving a useful response
   a. Cancers in which chemotherapy is curative in some patients
   b. Cancers in which chemotherapy has improved survival
   c. Cancers that respond to treatment but for which improved survival has not been clearly demonstrated
   d. Cancers showing marginal or no response to chemotherapy

Cytoxan), chlorambucil (Leukeran), melphalan (Alkeeran), triethylenethiophosphoramide (Thiotepa), busulfan (Myleran) and Ifosfamide. Their primary mechanism of action involves the production of extremely unstable alkyl groups that react with many organic compounds. The antineoplastic properties of these drugs are primarily based upon the alkylation of nucleic acids, particularly DNA. Such reactions produce breaks and cross-linking in double-stranded DNA and interfere with with DNA replication as well as with transcription of RNA. Because the alkylating agents share some of the characteristic effects of irradiation, they are often called *radiomimetic*. Most of the effective alkylating agents are polyfunctional and possess two or more potentially unstable alkyl groups per molecule. Alkylating agents tend to be cross-resistant to other agents in the same class, presumably because of the common production of similar alkyl groups. Differences in their activity for specific diseases apparently relate not so much to different mechanisms of action as to differences in absorption, tissue specificity, plasma clearance, and rates of degradation. Some of the basic characteristics of the commonly used alkylating agents are shown in Table 5-2.

In addition to the more common alkylating agents, several antineoplastic agents of different types are generally classed with the alkylating agents, although their mechanism of action is less well defined and may not be exclusively alkylation. These are the nitrosoureas (BCNU [carmustine], CCNU [lomustine], methyl CCNU [semustine]), DTIC (dacarbazine), cis-dichlorodiammine platinum (cisplatin), and carboplatin.

## Antimetabolites

Antimetabolites work by interacting with vital intracellular enzymes, leading either to inactivation of the enzyme or to synthesis of a fraudulent product incapable of normal function. Structurally they resemble analogues of the normal purines and pyrimidines required

for cell replication or the normal metabolites required for cell function. Whether or not they need to undergo biotransformation to active drugs, antimetabolites usually act in one of several ways to disrupt cell growth or proliferation:

1. They may substitute for a normal metabolite that is crucial to a vital metabolic pathway; an example of such a drug is the antimetabolite 6-thioguanine.
2. They may work by binding tightly to inhibitors of a vital enzyme; such inhibition is seen with methotrexate and the inactivation of dihydrofolate reductase.
3. They may temporarily occupy a catalytic site of a key enzyme; cytosine arabinoside is believed to work primarily by this mechanism.
4. Finally, an antimetabolite may compete with a normal metabolite acting at an enzyme-regulatory site to alter the catalytic rate of a vital enzyme; there is some evidence that 6-mercaptopurine works, at least in part, by this mechanism.

In spite of these different basic mechanisms, the final common pathway of each of these drugs is the disruption of vital functions crucial to the cell's viability. Since such effects are generally more disruptive to proliferating cells, the antimetabolites are generally classed as cell cycle–specific agents. Although hundreds of antimetabolites have been synthesized and tested, only a handful are in widespread clinical use. They are methotrexate, a folate antagonist; 6-mercaptopurine (6-MP, Purinethol) and 6-thioguanine, both purine antagonists; 5-fluorouracil (5-FU, fluorouracil) and 5-azacytidine, both pyrimidine antagonists; cytosine arabinoside (Ara-C, Cytosar), a pyrimidine nucleoside analogue; and hydroxyurea (Hydrea), an antimetabolite that acts by inhibiting ribonucleotide reductase. The important characteristics of these agents are shown in Table 5-3. In most instances, the antimetabolites are utilized not as single drugs but in combinations.

## Antitumor Antibiotics

The antitumor antibiotics have generally been isolated as natural products from soil fungi. Although most of these agents have extremely complex and widely divergent chemical structures, they generally function by forming complexes with DNA, thus inhibiting DNA, RNA, and protein synthesis. This class of agents is generally felt to be cell cycle–nonspecific. Since the antitumor antibiotics inhibit cellular functions common to both neoplastic and normal cells, their therapeutic index is rather narrow. Actinomycin D (dactinomycin, Cosmegen), bleomycin (Blenoxane), mitomycin-C (Mutamycin), doxorubicin (Adriamycin), daunorubicin (rubidomycin, daunomycin), and mithramycin (Mithracin) belong to this class of agents. Some of the important characteristics of the antitumor antibiotics are listed in Table 5-4.

## Vinca Alkaloids

The vinca alkaloids are derived from a species of the periwinkle plant. Their chemical structures are complex,

**TABLE 5-2** Alkylating Agents

| Compound | Route of Administration | Dosage Form | Typical Treatment Schedule | Usual Toxicities | Diseases Treated |
|---|---|---|---|---|---|
| Nitrogen mustard | IV, intracavitary | Powder, 10 mg (unstable after mixing) | IV: 0.4 mg/kg (Mustargen, HN$_2$) as a single dose or 0.1 mg/kg qd × 4 | Nausea and vomiting myelosuppression, local vesicant | Ovarian carcinoma; malignant pleural or pericardial effusions |
| Cyclophosphamide (Cytoxan) | Oral, IV | 25-mg and 50-mg tablets; 100-, 200-, and 500-mg vials | Oral: 1.5 to 3.0 mg/kg/day IV: 10 to 50 mg/kg q 1-4 wk | Myelosuppression, cystitis ± bladder fibrosis, alopecia, hepatitis, amenorrhea, and azoospermia | Breast, ovary, soft tissue sarcomas |
| Chlorambucil (Leukeran) | Oral | 2-mg tablets | 0.03-0.10 mg/kg/day | Myelosuppression, gastrointestinal distress, dermatitis, hepatotoxicity | Ovarian carcinoma |
| Melphalan (Alkeran, L-PAM) | Oral | 2-mg tablets | 0.2 mg/kg/day × 5 days q 4-6 wk | Myelosuppression, nausea and vomiting (rare), mucosal ulceration (rare) | Ovarian, breast carcinoma |
| Triethylenethiophosphoramide (TSPA, Thiotepa) | IV, intracavitary, intravesical | 15-mg vials | IV: 0.8 mg/kg q 4-6 wk; Intracavitary: 45-60 mg in 10 ml sterile water; Intravesical: 60 mg in 30-60 mg sterile water | Myelosuppression, nausea and vomiting, headaches and fever (rare) | Ovarian carcinoma, intracavitary for malignant effusions, breast cancer, bladder cancer (intravesical) |
| Busulfan (Myleran) | Oral | 2-mg tablets | 4-6 mg/m$^2$ as an oral loading dose | Myelosuppression (may be prolonged), pulmonary fibrosis, alopecia, amenorrhea, and sterility | Chronic myelogenous leukemia |
| Nitrosoureas (BCNU, CCNU) | IV, oral | 100-mg vial; 10-, 40-, and 100-mg capsules | IV: 150-200 mg/m$^2$ g 6 wk; Oral: 130 mg/m$^2$ q 6 wk | Delayed myelosuppression, nausea and vomiting, local pain and pigmentation | Gastrointestinal neoplasms, gliomas |
| Cis-dichlorodiammine platinum (cisplatin) | IV | 10-mg vial | IV: 15-20 mg/m$^2$ × 5 q 3 wk or 50-75 mg/m$^2$ × 1 q 3 wk | Nephrotoxicity, tinnitus and hearing loss, nausea and vomiting, myelosuppression | Ovarian carcinoma, germ cell tumors of the ovary; cervical carcinoma |
| Dacarbazine (DTIC) | IV | 100- and 200-mg vials | 2.0-4.5 mg/kg/day × 5-10 q 4 wk | Myelosuppression, nausea and vomiting, flu-like syndrome, hepatotoxicity | Uterine sarcomas, soft tissue sarcomas |
| Ifosfamide | IV | | 1.2 gm/m$^2$/day × 5 | Myelosuppression, nemonhagic cystitis | Cervix, ovary |

with the two most active compounds differing only in a small side chain on the parent compound. Nevertheless, this small alteration significantly changes the compound's antitumor spectrum as well as its toxicity. These two agents act primarily by binding to vital microtubular proteins within the cell. These proteins are present in high concentrations in neural tissue and are a vital part of the contractile protein in the mitotic spindle formed at the time of cell division. By inhibiting mitotic spindle formation, they block cell division by causing mitotic arrest. At higher concentrations, the drugs affect nucleic acid and protein synthesis as well. The two important members of this group are vincristine (Oncovin) and vinblastine (Velban), the pharmacologic and clinical features of which are listed in Table 5-5.

## Hormones

Another class of agents used in the treatment of cancer are hormones. While not strictly antineoplastic in action, these agents play an important role in cancer management. All classes of steroid hormones seem to share similar mechanisms of action. Whether secreted by endocrine tissues or given as drugs, steroids freely permeate cell membranes. Inside cells, they bind to proteins in the cytoplasm. These steroid-receptor complexes then penetrate the nucleus and bind to chromatin—an interaction that alters the patterns of gene transcription and thereby the newly synthesized messenger RNA. Eventually these messenger RNAs are translated into new proteins responsible for hormonally induced antitumor effects. Steroid-induced effects therefore depend on the

**TABLE 5-3** Antimetabolites

| Compound | Route of Administration | Dosage Form | Typical Treatment Schedule | Usual Toxicities | Diseases Treated |
|---|---|---|---|---|---|
| 6-Mercaptopurine (Purinethol, 6-MP) | IV or PO | 50-mg tablets | Oral: 2.5 mg/kg/day | Myelosuppression, hepatotoxicity, nausea and vomiting, anorexia, mucosal ulcerations | Leukemias |
| 6-Thioguanine (thioguanine, 6-TG) | IV or PO | 75-mg vials, 40-mg tablets | IV: 100-300 mg infusions<br>Oral: 2-3 mg/kg bid | Myelosuppression, nausea and vomiting, anorexia, nephrotoxicity, hepatotoxicity | Acute leukemia |
| 5-Fluorouracil (fluorouracil, 5-FU) | IV | 500-mg ampules | 10-15 mg/kg/wk | Myelosuppression, nausea and vomiting, anorexia, alopecia | Gastrointestinal carcinoma, breast cancer, ovarian carcinoma |
| Cytosine arabinoside (Ar-C, Cytosar, cytarabine) | IV intrathecal | 100- and 500-mg vials | Pulse therapy: 2-3 mg/kg bid × 7 days<br>Continuous infusion: 2-3 mg/kg qd × 7 days<br>Intrathecal: 10-30 mg/m² 1-3 × /wk | Myelosuppression, mucosal ulceration, nausea and vomiting, hepatotoxicity | Leukemias, carcinomatous meningitis |
| 5-Azacytidine | IV | 100-mg vial | Weekly: 500 mg/m² IV<br>Daily: 150-200 mg/m²/day × 5 days | Nausea and vomiting, diarrhea, myelosuppression, hepatotoxicity, fever | Acute myelogenous leukemia |
| Methotrexate (MTX, amethopterin) | PO, IV, intrathecal | 2.5-mg tablets; 5-, 20-, and 50-mg vials | Oral: 15-30 mg/day × 5 days<br>IV: 240 mg/m² with leukovorin rescue<br>Intrathecal: 12-15 mg/m² 1-3 × wk | Mucosal ulceration, myelosuppression, hepatotoxicity, allergic pneumonitis, With intrathecal: meningeal irritation | Choriocarcinoma, breast cancer, ovarian cancer, osteogenic sarcoma (adjuvant) |
| Hydroxurea (Hydrea) | PO, IV | 50-mg capsules, 2-gm vial for injection | Oral: 1-2 gm/m²/day<br>IV: 1-2 gm/m²/day | Myelosuppression, nausea and vomiting, anorexia | Cervical carcinoma |

presence of steroid receptors within the cell, and any defect in the chain of transport into the nucleus could render the cell unresponsive to these hormones. By means of hormone-receptor assays, physicians have been able to determine the probability of a response to hormone therapy in patients with breast cancer and endometrial cancer. The various hormones commonly in use are listed in Table 5-6.

## Miscellaneous Compounds and New Drugs

In addition to those antineoplastic drugs which fit into the general classes listed above, there are a group of agents that are in common use although their mechanisms of action are unique or poorly understood. The characteristics of the more commonly used of these drugs are shown in Table 5-7.

Because of the wide range of agents available and their narrow margin of safety, the clinician must pay careful attention to the details of drug administration, drug interaction, and both common and uncommon toxicities. This brief discussion serves only to highlight some of the general aspects of drug treatment. More

detailed reviews should be consulted before such therapy is undertaken (Haskell, 1985; Chabner, 1982).

Finally, research in the use of antineoplastic drug therapy has established that combination chemotherapy is, in many diseases, more effective than single-drug treatment. The rationale for such treatment and its results will now be discussed.

## PRINCIPLES OF COMBINATION CHEMOTHERAPY

Combinations of antineoplastic agents are now commonly used in the management of cancer patients. Such treatment is based on a firm theoretical rationale that grew out of studies of cellular kinetics, biochemical drug action, drug interactions, drug resistance, and tumor heterogeneity. At present, combination chemotherapy is the accepted approach to the treatment of choriocarcinoma and ovarian germ cell tumors as well as many pediatric solid tumors, such as Wilms' tumor and rhabdomyosarcoma among others.

TABLE 5-4  Antitumor Antibiotics

| Compound | Route of Administration | Dosage Form | Typical Treatment Schedule | Usual Toxicities | Diseases Treated |
|---|---|---|---|---|---|
| Actinomycin D (dactinomycin, Cosmegen) | IV | 0.5-mg vials | 0.3-0.5 mg/m² IV × 5 days or 0.5 mg/m² IV weekly q 2-4 wk | Nausea and vomiting, skin necrosis, mucosal ulceration, myelosuppression | Germ cell ovarian tumors; Wilms' tumor; Ewings tumor; choriocarcinoma, soft tissue sarcoma |
| Bleomycin (Blenoxane) | IV or IM | 15 units of the base/ampule | 10-20 units/m² IV or IM 1-2 × wk for a dose of 400 units For effusions: 60-120 units | Fever, dermatologic reactions, pulmonary toxicity, anaphylactic reactions, myelosuppression | Cervical carcinoma, germ cell ovarian tumors; malignant effusions |
| Mitomycin C (Mutamycin) | IV | 5-mg vial | 10-20 mg/m² IV q 6-8 wk | Myelosuppression, local vesicant, nausea and vomiting, mucosal ulcerations, nephrotoxicity | Breast cancer |
| Doxorubicin (Adriamycin, hydroxydaunomycin) | IV | 10- and 50-mg vial | IV: 60-90 mg/m² q 3 wk or 20-35 mg/m² qd × 3 q 3 wk | Myelosuppression, alopecia, cardiotoxicity, local vesicant, nausea and vomiting, mucosal ulcerations | Breast cancer, endometrial cancer, ovarian cancer |
| Daunorubicin (rubidomycin, daunomycin) | IV | 20-mg vial | 30-60 mg/m² daily for 2-3 days | Myelosuppression, alopecia, cardiotoxicity, local vesicant, nausea and vomiting, mucosal ulcerations | Acute leukemias, solid tumors of childhood |
| Mithramycin (Mithracin) | IV | 2.5-mg vial | 20-50 μg/kg/day q 4-6 wk Hypercalcemia: 25 μg/kg IV × 1 q 3-4 days | Nausea and vomiting, hemorrhagic diathesis hepatotoxicity, fever, myelosuppression, facial flushing | Testicular carcinoma, hypercalcemia of malignancy |

Interest in combination chemotherapy developed because of the following limitations inherent in single-agent chemotherapy:

1. The toxicity of single agents limits the duration of therapy and the dose that can be tolerated, thus restricting the amount of tumor-cell kill possible.
2. Adaptive mechanisms allow a fraction of the resistant neoplastic cells to survive and eventually regrow in spite of lethal effects produced in the bulk of the tumor.
3. Spontaneous drug resistance.
4. Pleiotropic drug resistance.

Some of the mechanisms of resistance to particular antineoplastic drugs are listed in Table 5-8. Since most of the major limitations of single-drug therapy cannot be corrected by simple alterations in the amount or

TABLE 5-5  The Vinca Alkaloids

| Compound | Route of Administration | Dosage Form | Typical Treatment Schedule | Usual Toxicities | Diseases Treated |
|---|---|---|---|---|---|
| Vincristine (Oncovin) | IV | 1- and 5-mg vials | 0.01-0.03 mg/kg/wk | Neurotoxicity, alopecia, myelosuppression, cranial nerve palsies, gastrointestinal distress | Ovarian germ cell tumors; sarcomas; childhood solid tumors |
| Vinblastine (Velban) | IV | 10-mg vials | 5-6 mg/m² q 1-2 wk | Myelosuppression, alopecia, nausea and vomiting, neurotoxicity | Germ cell ovarian cancers; choriocarcinoma |

TABLE 5-6  Hormones

| Compound | Route of Administration | Dosage Form | Typical Treatment Schedule | Usual Toxicities | Diseases Treated |
|---|---|---|---|---|---|
| Estrogens<br>Diethylstilbestrol | Oral | 0.1- to 25-mg tablets | Brest cancer: 15 mg qd | Gynecomastia, nausea and vomiting, fluid retention, change in libido, hypercalcemia | Breast cancer |
| Progestins<br>Hydroxyprogcstcronc caproate (Delalutin) | IM | In oil 125 and 250 mg/ml | 1 gm biw | Fluid retention, epithelial changes in genital tract, nausea, sterile abscesses from injections | Endometrial carcinoma; ovarian carcinoma |
| Medroxyprogesterone acetate (Depo-Provera) | IM, oral | IM: susension 50 mg/ml<br>Oral: 2.5 and 10 mg | 300 mg IM q wk | | |
| Megestrol acetate (Megace) | Oral | 20-mg tablets | 20 mg PO bid | | |
| Androgens<br>Testosterone propionate (Oreton propionate) | IM | In oil, 100 mg/ml | 50-200 mg 2-3 times/wk | Virilization in females, change in libido, fluid retention, cholestatic jaundice, hypercalcemia | Breast cancer |
| Fluoxymesterone (Halotestin) | Oral | 2-, 5-, and 10-mg tablets | 10-40 mg daily | | |
| Corticosteroids<br>Prednisone | Oral | 1-, 2.5-, 5-, and 20-mg tablets | 40-120 mg qd | Fluid retention, hypertension, diabetes mellitus, gastric irritation, potassium loss, psychosis | Breast cancer, neurologic symptoms from metastatic disease |
| Dexamethasone (Decadron) | Oral<br>IV or IM | 0.25, 0.5-, 0.75- and 1.5-mg tablets | 0.5-4 mg qd | | |
| Tamoxifen | Oral | 2-, 5-, and 10-mg tablets | 2-12 mg/m$^2$ bid | Myelosuppression, retinitis | Breast cancer, ovarian carcinoma |

schedule of dosing, drugs are now more frequently used in combination.

## Cellular Kinetics

Drug combinations have several definite theoretical advantages (DeVita et al, 1975). Evidence from studies of cellular kinetics provides a rationale for combining antineoplastic agents. Various classes of agents have different cell-killing characteristics depending on the proliferative state of the tumor. (This topic was discussed in considerable detail in Chapter 2.) The use of several drugs having different kinetic characteristics allows more extensive reduction of a huge tumor load than can be achieved with single agents.

Consider the use of combinations of drugs with different characteristic sites of activity or mechanisms of action to induce a marked regression of tumor. If one were to administer a cell cycle–nonspecific agent that produces a 2-log kill in a host bearing a tumor mass with $10^9$ cells, and no further therapy were given, the tumor would simply regrow. Cell death would be delayed only temporarily. If a cell cycle–nonspecific agent produces this amount of cell kill, theoretically a cell cycle–sensitive agent would be effective against the new cells entering the cell cycle. Simply by alternating, or

using in sequence, cell cycle–specific and cell cycle–nonspecific agents, one can theoretically produce consistent, repetitive log kill in tumors; finally, after using such agents in combination and in the proper sequence, one may produce the magnitude of log kill required to induce a cure.

## Biochemical Drug Action

The different biochemical effects of antineoplastic drugs also provide a rationale for combination chemotherapy. Although there are few potentially exploitable and unique biochemical differences between cancer and normal cells, there is evidence for differential sensitivity between normal and tumorous tissues. In addition, the various biochemical mechanisms of action can be useful in developing new combinations or explaining the success of empirically derived regimens. Combinations can be designed to incorporate agents that produce different biochemical lesions and work by attacking multiple sites in biosynthetic pathways. Alternatively, they may be designed to inhibit several processes involved in the maintenance and function of vital macromolecules.

Two such biochemical concepts, known as *sequential* and *concurrent blockade*, illustrate the rational design of drug combinations. *Sequential blockade* is the si-

TABLE 5-7   Miscellaneous Agents

| Compound | Route of Administration | Dosage Form | Typical Treatment Schedule | Usual Toxicities | Diseases Treated |
|---|---|---|---|---|---|
| Procarbazine (Matulane, methyl-hydrazine) | Oral | 50-mg capsules | 100-200 mg/m² daily | Myelosuppression, CNS toxicity, peripheral neuropathy, nausea and vomiting, dermatitis | Hodgkin's disease, lymphomas |
| Mitotane (Lysodren, *o,p*¹-DDD) | Oral | 500-mg tablets | 8-10 g daily | Nausea and vomiting, CNS reactions, dermatitis, adrenal insufficiency | Adrenocortical carcinoma |
| Streptozotocin | IV | 1-gm vial | 1-1.5 g/m² q wk × 4 | Nausea and vomiting, myelosuppression, nephrotoxicity, hepatotoxicity, hypoglycemia | Malignant insulinoma, Hodgkin's disease, carcinoid tumors |
| L-Asparaginase (Crasnitin, Colaspase, Elspar, L-ASP) | IV | 10,000 units/vial | 1,000 units IV/kg/day for 10 days | Hypersensitivity reactions, neurotoxicity, hepatotoxicity, pancreatitis, hyperglycemia | Acute lymphoblastic leukemia, lymphomas |
| Hexamethylmelamine | Oral | 50- and 10-mg capsules | 4-8 mg/kg/day | Nausea and vomiting, myelosuppression, neurotoxicity, skin rashes | Ovarian carcinoma, breast cancer, oat cell carcinoma of lung |
| Taxol | IV | 135-250 mg/m² 24 hour infusion | 3 weeks | Hypersensitivity reactions, myelosuppression, neurotoxicity | Ovarian carcinoma breast cancer |

multaneous inhibition of sequential enzymes in a single biochemical pathway. An example of this approach might be the inhibition of de novo purine synthesis by the combination of azaserine and 6-mercaptopurine. *Concurrent blockade* involves the simultaneous inhibition of parallel enzymatic pathways that lead to the same end product. An example of this kind of inhibition is the interaction of azaserine, a glutamine antagonist that inhibits de novo purine biosynthesis, and 6-thioguanine, which inhibits the reutilization of preformed purines.

TABLE 5-8   Mechanisms of Resistance to Anticancer Drugs

| Mechanism | Examples |
|---|---|
| Insufficient activation of drug | 6-Mercaptopurine, 5-fluorouracil |
| Insufficient drug uptake or defective drug transport | Methotrexate, daunomycin |
| Increased inactivation | Arabinosyl cytosine |
| Increased utilization of an alternative biochemical pathway (salvage) | Antimetabolites |
| Increased concentration of the target enzyme | Methotrexate |
| Decreased requirement for a specific metabolic product | L-Asparaginase |
| Rapid DNA repair of a drug-related lesion | Alkylating agents |
| Gene amplification | Methotrexate |

A third major biochemical rationale for combination chemotherapy is termed *complementary inhibition*. According to this concept, drugs are combined that produce biochemical lesions at different sites in the synthesis of polymeric molecules such as DNA, RNA, and protein. Drugs are categorized as inhibitors of the synthesis of polymer precursors (e.g., the antimetabolites) or as agents that directly attack a preformed molecule (e.g., the alkylating agents or antibiotics). One would predict success from a combination that interferes with both the synthesis and function of a vital molecule such as DNA, RNA, or protein at multiple sites. Thus, the combination of an antimetabolite and an alkylating agent prevents the syntheses of a given polymeric molecule, while the antimetabolite also impedes the repair of DNA, which has been cross-linked by the alkylating agent. Clinical and experimental studies have defined many examples of effective combinations of alkylating agents and antimetabolites such as cyclophosphamide and methotrexate in ovarian carcinoma (MECY) and cyclophosphamide (Cytoxan), methotrexate, and 5-fluorouracil (CMF) in adjuvant therapy for breast cancer.

## Drug Interactions

Drug interactions, which have been studied more completely in animals than in humans, may be described as synergistic, additive, or antagonistic. Combinations that improve therapy because of either increased antitumor activity or decreased toxicity are felt to be synergistic. With additive therapies, antitumor activity is enhanced but in amounts roughly equal to the sum of both agents acting singly. Unfortunately, antitumor agents may sometimes antagonize each other's actions, producing less of a therapeutic effect than when they are used singly.

Drugs used in combination also interact with other drugs administered during therapy, or they may be influenced by certain metabolic factors in the individual patient. These drug interactions may have important consequences, and some of the more important ones are listed in Table 5-9. A detailed review of the subject of antitumor drug interactions has been published by Warren and Bender (1977). Some common in vivo interactions include (1) the increased toxicity of doxorubicin in patients with impaired biliary excretion; (2) the displacement of methotrexate from its transport protein by the concomitant administration of either aspirin or sulfonamides; (3) the possible disruption of the metabolism of 6-mercaptopurine, a purine analogue, by allopurinol, a xanthine oxidase inhibitor used to reduce excessive uric acid formation during cancer treatment (believed to result in increased toxicity when the two drugs are used in combination); and (4) the increased toxicity of methotrexate in patients with impaired renal function due to compromised drug excretion.

## Spontaneous Drug Resistance

Among the most important factors providing a rationale for combination chemotherapy is the problem of spontaneous drug resistance. Although early principles of cancer chemotherapy were based on insights gained through the use of antibiotics, one important observation received little attention—i.e., the apparently inherent capacity of bacteria to mutate toward resistance to antibiotics they had never encountered. Because the absolute number of resistant organisms depended on when the mutation occurred, the size of the resistant population in bacteria would vary. Studies subsequently proved conclusively that resistance occurred not as a result of selection but spontaneously.

The implications of this important work for cancer chemotherapy have been reviewed by Goldie and Coldman (1979). In mammalian systems there is evidence that spontaneous and permanent mutation to phenotypic drug resistance could occur in genetically unstable, rapidly growing malignant cell lines (Baker and Ling, 1978) but that such mutations were not seen in normal hematopoietic cell populations. This observation suggested that most mammalian cells start with intrinsic sensitivity to anticancer drugs but simply develop spontaneous resistance at variable rates. The clinical implications of such a concept are manifold. First, it explains why a tumor that is initially sensitive to chemotherapy subsequently becomes resistant and ultimately proves lethal. It also explains why marrow toxicity always occurs after retreatment with drugs even when they are ineffective against the tumor.

***The Goldie-Coldman Model*** Goldie and Coldman developed a mathematical model relating curability to the time of appearance of a singly or doubly resistant cell line. Assuming a mutation rate approximating the natural mutation frequency, their model predicted that the resistant fraction in tumors of the same size and type will vary depending on the rate of mutation and the point at which a mutation develops. Given such assumptions, the proportion of resistant cells in any given mass is likely to be small, and the initial response to a treatment should not be influenced by the number of resistant cells. In clinical practice, this means that complete remission can be attained even if a resistant cell line is present. However, failure to cure (i.e., relapse from a complete remission) would depend directly on the presence of resistant cell lines.

This model of spontaneous drug resistance also explains some of the unusual clinical observations of tumor heterogeneity. It suggests that fluctuation in phenotypic resistance may also be associated with preferential sites of metastases, since drug sensitivity fluctuates in different lines isolated from different metastatic sites. According to these latter data and the Goldie-Coldman model, metastases in different organs in the same patient may respond differently to the same drugs. Some experimental data using the Goldie-Coldman assumptions have been studied for cyclophosphamide and arabinosyl cytosine (Skipper, 1978). Using the same dose and schedule for each drug, the curability of mouse tumor lessens as the size of the tumor increases from $10^5$ to $10^8$ cells, fitting the pattern of cells with a mutation rate of approximately $10^{-7}$. These studies suggest an inherent rationale for the idea of spontaneous drug resistance in human tumors.

***Implication for Chemotherapy*** Computer-assisted programs to develop strategies for managing treatable cancers with chemotherapy have been developed (Goldie et al, 1982) and have the following clinical implications:

1. Tumors are curable with chemotherapy if no permanently resistant cell lines are present and if chemotherapy is begun before such cells develop.

TABLE 5-9 Drug Interactions Important in Cancer Treatment

| Interaction | Examples |
|---|---|
| Alterations in renal function that influence rates of renal excretion | Methotrexate, cis-dichloro-diammine platinum |
| Alterations in hepatic metabolism or biliary excretion of drugs | Doxorubicin, vincristine |
| Interaction at plasma or blood transport sites | Methotrexate with sulfonamides |
| Drug interaction during intestinal absorption | Methotrexate with neomycin |
| Interaction at a cellular receptor site | Procarbazine and tricyclic antidepressants |
| Direct chemical interaction | Cis-dichlorodiammine platinum and mannitol |
| Drug interaction by accelerated or impeded metabolism | 6-Mercaptopurine with allopurinol; cyclophosphamide with phenobarbital |

2. If only one drug (or therapy) is used, curability diminishes rapidly with the occurrence of a single resistant cell line.
3. Minimizing the emergence of drug-resistant clones requires the early application of multiple effective drugs or therapies.
4. Spontaneous mutation to resistance occurs at about the natural frequency of $10^{-5}$ or $10^{-6}$ and is a stepwise function from sensitivity to resistance to each of the applied therapies.
5. The Goldie-Coldman model predicts that alternating cycles of treatment would be superior to the sequential use of single drugs, since the latter approach would allow for a doubly resistant line to develop and regrow.
6. Using this model, two equally effective combinations of drug would have to be available. At present, this is obviously possible for only a few human tumors. Nevertheless, success in treating Hodgkin's disease using alternating sequences of MOPP (nitrogen mustard, Oncovin, procarbazine, and prednisone) and ABVD (Adriamycin, bleomycin, vinblastine, DTIC) (Santoro et al, 1982) and in treating diffuse large-cell lymphoma using ProMACE and MOPP (Fisher et al, 1983) have improved rates of disease-free and overall survival, even though these alternating sequences were not given in a way that would optimally exploit the implied benefits of the spontaneous resistance model.

Spontaneous drug resistance may explain why adjuvant chemotherapy after surgical resection of tumor may be more effective than the same treatment in patients with clinically evident disease. In addition, it suggests that the time to first drug treatment may be critical. If a resistant line can develop spontaneously in weeks, adjuvant therapy should be started as soon as possible. Of interest in this regard is the adjuvant breast cancer study (Nissen-Meyer, 1979) in which the 10-year survival benefit reported by four of the participating hospitals was not seen in the hospital that delayed adjuvant chemotherapy for 2 to 4 weeks after surgery.

Spontaneous mutation to drug resistance is likely to be influenced by the cause of initial tumor development. In lung cancer, for example, the association with multiple carcinogenic chemicals in cigarette smoke may cause the spontaneous mutation rate to be higher than the natural frequency. If so, numerous drug-resistant cells may be present even before tumors become clinically evident, accounting for the failure of drugs to predictably cure lung cancer. Although initial response rates and even complete remission rates might be high, the emergence of these drug-resistant clones would preclude curability.

The concept of spontaneous drug resistance in tumors has important implications for the design of future chemotherapy trials. First, combination chemotherapy rather than single-agent therapy is likely to be more effective as an adjuvant, as it is for most of the successful treatment programs for patients with clinically evident disease. Second, adjuvant chemotherapy is not likely to be effective unless micrometastases are treated as intensively as is clinically evident disease involving the same tumor type. Third, drugs that produce partial responses in patients with clinically evident disease should not always be expected to produce better results (cures) in the adjuvant setting. Fourth, treatment may not need to last as long as was previously thought if the number of drugs and the intensity of their administration are sufficient to eradicate relatively small numbers of resistant tumor cells. In fact, a lengthy period of adjuvant therapy might actually accelerate the growth of a resistant population by enhancing its mutation rate.

## Pleiotropic Drug Resistance

If success or failure of drug treatment depends upon the spontaneous appearance of resistant cells in a tumor, what is the nature of this resistance and can it be manipulated and overcome? A wide variety of mechanisms (described earlier in this chapter) can confer resistance to a particular drug or family of drugs; however, under certain circumstances, resistance to one specific drug can confer cross-resistance to structurally dissimilar drugs having different mechanisms of action. This phenomenon, which has profound implications for cancer treatment, is known as *pleiotropic drug resistance*. Initially described in murine tumors, this phenomenon is commonly seen among patients who are unresponsive to salvage chemotherapy, which includes single drugs or even combinations of drugs to which the tumor had not been exposed previously. Epithelial ovarian carcinoma is a good example of this phenomenon.

Initial studies indicated that acquired drug resistance developed through the selection of cells with generally less penetrable membranes. Among the drugs demonstrating pleiotropic drug resistance were the anthracyclines, vinca alkaloids, actinomycin-D and Taxol. Studies suggested that pleiotropic drug resistance might be due to an impaired ability to accumulate and retain these drugs (Juliano and Ling, 1976). Furthermore, in such pleiotropically resistant cells, Ling and coworkers have demonstrated a "P-glycoprotein" having a molecular weight of 170,000 that appears to be a marker for this type of drug resistance. Chinese hamster ovary cells selected in colchicine are highly resistant to anthracyclines, vincristine, and actinomycin D. This P-glycoprotein is directly related to the expression of resistance, and cells that revert from resistant to sensitive lose this membrane glycoprotein. In addition, one can use DNA from resistant cells to transfer pleiotropic resistance to unexposed cells (Debenham et al, 1982).

## Clinical Implications

Where does all this new information leave the clinician interested in the optimal use of cancer drugs? Several observations suggest some promising therapeutic avenues not yet sufficiently explored. First, cells that appear to develop pleiotropic drug resistance often develop *collateral sensitivity* to other chemotherapeutic agents, including cyclophosphamide, glucocorticoids, and local anesthetics (Bech-Hanson et al, 1976). By further characterizing the patterns of this collateral sensitivity and defining the mechanisms and magnitude of its effect, one may be able to exploit it clinically.

The second major area of potential attack on drug resistance involves drugs for which the mechanism of resistance is at least partially known. In ovarian cancer, melphalan remains one of the most active chemotherapeutic agents. Nevertheless, resistance develops in most patients, and retreatment with other alkylating agents or other drugs is generally not successful. It has been demonstrated that melphalan-resistant murine leukemia cells have increased intracellular levels of glutathione critical for the metabolism of the drug to its inactive metabolite (Suzukake et al, 1982 and 1983). By reducing intracellular glutathione by the nutritional restriction of L-cysteine, the sensitivity to melphalan can be restored (Suzukake et al, 1982).

We have carried out similar studies in human ovarian cancer cells in which melphalan resistance either had been induced by serial exposure to the drug or had existed in cell lines derived from patients clinically resistant to the agent (Hamilton et al, 1985). In contrast to melphalan-resistant murine tumor cells, these resistant human ovarian cancer cell lines had the same transport characteristics as melphalan-sensitive cell lines (Green et al, 1984). In the human cell lines, resistance is associated with increased levels of glutathione, and sensitivity can be restored by the presence of a specific inhibitor of glutathione synthesis such as buthionine sulfoximine (Green et al, 1984). Studies involving a unique intraperitoneal nude mouse model have demonstrated that melphalan cytotoxicity can be restored in human ovarian cancer cells in vivo (Hamilton et al, 1985). Clinical trials in patients with ovarian cancer resistant to alkylating agents are now under way using buthionine sulfoximine (Ozols, personal communication).

An interesting characteristic of vinca alkaloid and anthracycline resistance is that it can apparently be reversed by certain calcium-channel blockers and calmodulin inhibitors. The calcium-channel blocker verapamil, used to treat supraventricular arrhythmias, hypertension, and angina, has been shown to reverse resistance in several tumors (Tsuruo et al, 1981). It has been suggested that verapamil increases the uptake or decreases the efflux of these drugs in resistant cells and, in so doing, reverses permeability-dependent resistance.

Using established human ovarian cancer cell lines, we have been able to confirm this in vitro effect. However, it appears that potentiation may occur with only certain drugs; verapamil did not potentiate the effects of melphalan in a melphalan-resistant ovarian cancer cell line, nor did it potentiate the cytotoxicity of doxorubicin in a human fibroblast cell line established from the same patient from which the ovarian cancer cell line was established (Rogan et al, 1984). Verapamil inhibits the efflux of doxorubicin from resistant ovarian cancer lines. These laboratory studies prompted a clinical trial of doxorubicin (Adriamycin) and verapamil in patients with ovarian cancer refractory to initial combination chemotherapy (Ozols et al, 1987). Unfortunately, it was not possible to reverse Adriamycin drug resistance clin-

ically at doses of verapamil associated with toxicity. Further studies are under way using other calcium-channel blockers.

Whether any of these approaches to reversing drug resistance will be clinically successful remains to be demonstrated. Nevertheless, it is clear that clinical trials can be designed to address the problem of drug resistance. All current evidence suggests that the probability of success will be enhanced if combinations of drugs are used.

If the pleiotropic phenotype is a common cause of resistance to anticancer drugs in human cancers, the availability of monoclonal antibodies to detect this phenotype at the time of diagnosis may allow (a) drug combinations to be designed so as to circumvent the resistance or (b) resistant lines to be attacked directly using monoclonals linked to toxins or radioisotopes. Such treatments might be used either as initial therapy or to eradicate resistant cells that remain after induction treatment has resulted in complete or good partial remission. If one can identify and predict a general pathway to the development of collateral sensitivity in human tumors, collaterally effective drugs that may have been overlooked as potentially useful anticancer agents for initial treatment may be effectively interspersed with other active drugs. Indeed, one can envision alternating cycles of combination chemotherapy that include combinations made up of some drugs predicted or known to be made collaterally effective in the face of the development of a pleiotropic resistant phenotype.

With this theoretical and experimental background in mind, it is important to outline the general principles that have guided the development of successful combinations in clinical use (Table 5-10). These guidelines cannot always be applied in every instance, and some toxicities will overlap. Nevertheless, these general concepts are a central feature in most of the currently successful regimens.

## Dose Intensity

While it has long been known that the selection of a particular drug or regimen has a critical effect on therapeutic outcome, it is now becoming clear that the intensity of drug administration may be as important as drug selection. The concept of dose intensity is based on the amount of drug administered over time and has been developed through a series of retrospective studies

---

**TABLE 5-10 Principles Used in Design of Combination Chemotherapy**

Drugs must be active as single agents against the particular tumor.

Drugs should have different mechanisms of action to minimize the emergence of drug resistance.

Drugs should have a biochemical basis for either additive or synergistic effects.

Drugs should have different spectra of toxicity so that they can be used in full therapeutic doses.

Drugs should be administered intermittently so that cell killing is enhanced and immunosuppression is not continuous.

(Hryniuk, 1988). The first analysis utilized data from a large number of trials in patients with advanced breast cancer (Hryniuk and Bush, 1987). Subsequent studies by this group have focused on advanced ovarian cancer, adjuvant therapy of breast cancer, and adjuvant colon cancer (Hryniuk et al, 1987).

Any analysis of dose intensity requires that each drug in a regimen be converted to a certain standard dose rate (most commonly $mg/m^2/wk$) independent of the schedule of drug administration. Once a particular regimen has been expressed in this uniform terminology, the regimen can be compared with the dose intensity of any standard regimen, and the relative dose intensity of each drug in the regimen can then be summated to determine the relative dose intensity of the particular regimen vis-à-vis the standard. One can then compare dose intensity with outcome as measured by overall response rates or by median survival.

If one applies a dose intensity analysis to multiple regimens employed to treat advanced breast cancer and compares these with a standard cyclophosphamide, methotrexate, and 5-FU (CMF) regimen, a correlation between the dose intensity and overall response rate emerges. This correlation becomes even clearer when outcome is compared with the actual doses of drug received rather than projected doses. Similar analysis of cyclophosphamide, Adriamycin, and 5-FU (CAF) regimens in adjuvant breast cancer yields similar results. Levin and Hryniuk (1987) have now performed dose-intensity analyses in advanced ovarian cancer. In each instance, the dose intensity of the compared regimens correlated well with outcome. Studies in ovarian cancer suggest that cisplatin is the drug for which proper dose intensity is most important.

Although most of the data on the importance of dose intensity has been retrospective, several subsequent studies prospectively performed have fit the retrospectively generated data. In a recent study, Tannock et al (1988) tested two different dose-intensity schedules of CMF in advanced breast cancer. These regimens were relatively low-dose, and relative dose intensities were 19% and 34% of the standard, respectively; they produced overall response rates of 11% and 30%. These data fit well with the previously established dose-intensity relationships from a retrospective analysis (Hryniuk and Bush, 1987). More recently a prospective test of the hypothesis has been completed in advanced breast cancer (Hryniuk et al, 1988). Thirty-one patients were treated with an intensive CAF regimen. On the basis of the retrospectively derived dose-intensity data, they predicted that patients who received a dose intensity of 0.8 of their CAF should have a response rate of 80%. The patients actually received 0.78 of the planned dose, and the overall response rate was 74%, correlating closely with the regression curve from the retrospective study. This prospective test of the hypothesis lends credence to the importance of dose intensity in advanced breast cancer. However, preliminary results from a dose intensity study by the GOG advanced ovarian cancer do not show a benefit for a dose intense cyclophosphamide/cisplatimis regimen.

Although these studies are still preliminary, they do suggest a number of important concepts for future clin-

ical trials. First, dose intensity should be considered prospectively in the design of new drug regimens for clinical trials. Second, in subsequent adjuvant trials adequate drug dose intensity should be utilized before assuming that adjuvant therapy is inactive. Third, careful analysis of new regimens should enable the independent contributions of each agent to the overall success of the combination to be properly evaluated. These studies emphasize that a regimen is not intense just because it is so described. Furthermore, it is not dose-intensive just because it produces more toxicity. Finally, it is not yet clear what relationship exists between dose intensity and total dose of drug.

## Novel Approaches to Administering Chemotherapy

Although chemotherapy is for the most part administered by the systemic route, using either oral, intramuscular, or intravenous approaches, there are unique situations in which the regional use of chemotherapy has been studied. For example, when primary tumors or their metastases are confined to certain organs or particular regions of the body or when a unique pharmacokinetic circumstance favors rapid and localized regional clearance (i.e., liver and 5-FU, brain and BCNU), a theoretical rationale for regional chemotherapy exists.

Intraarterial drug administration has been widely studied in a variety of areas including pelvic infusion for cervical cancer, localized rectal carcinoma recurrences, intracarotid therapy for head and neck cancer, and intracarotid administration of nitrosoureas for brain tumors. In general, these approaches have sometimes produced higher response rates but rarely have demonstrated improved survival and are associated with significant serious local toxicities. Currently, these approaches remain experimental.

Intracavitary chemotherapy has been utilized for cancers confined to body cavities and to control effusions in the peritoneum, pleura, or pericardium. The rationale for such an approach is based on the fact that for many chemotherapeutic agents the clearance from a body cavity is slower than systemic clearance, which results in a substantial differential concentration between the cavity and the systemic circulation. The technique has been most extensively studied in ovarian cancer, in which disease usually remains confined within the intraperitoneal space. Many chemotherapeutic agents have now been studied, including 5-FU, Adriamycin, cisplatin, cytarabarine, L-PAM, and others (Brenner, 1986). In general, phase I studies of these agents have all demonstrated a clear pharmacologic advantage for intraperitoneal chemotherapy (Myers, 1985). Because of the limited penetration (1 to 3 mm) of most drugs, the major role for this approach would appear to be in patients with minimal residual disease.

Two recent trials have established cisplatin as the current intraperitoneal drug of choice in ovarian cancer. In the first, in which 19 patients were treated with intraperitoneal cisplatin at $50 \ mg/m^2$ in 2 liters (Cohen, 1985), 32% had no evidence of disease at repeat surgical reevaluation. Similar results were achieved using doses of 60 to $150 \ mg/m^2$ in 2 liters every 2 to 3 weeks × 6, with sodium thiosulfate used as a rescue agent (ten Bokkel Huinink et al, 1985). In this trial, 33% of patients had negative results on laparotomy after therapy. It is not clear what the survival advantage of such an approach will be, nor is it clear whether this approach is superior to other salvage approaches. One long-term followup study has reported an actuarial 2-year survival rate of 74% for patients with minimal residual disease treated with a variety of intraperitoneal therapies (Markman et al, 1986).

The development of reliable pumps and safe long-term venous access catheters to administer infusion chemotherapy has allowed an extensive investigation of anticancer drug infusion. The rationale for the approach is based upon (1) cell kinetic principles that suggest significant activity only in actively cycling cells, (2) the relatively short half-lives of certain chemotherapeutic agents, and (3) the concentration time concepts of drug transport across tumor cell membranes. In general, these studies have not been done in a randomized manner, or when randomized, have failed to demonstrate substantial benefit over bolus chemotherapy. However, several drugs with short half-lives or unique toxicities appear to have an improved therapeutic index when given by intravenous continuous infusion; these include bleomycin, Ara-C, and Adriamycin (Vogelzang, 1984)

### Evaluation of Therapeutic Response

Once a combination regimen has been selected, it is necessary to have some standardized way to evaluate the patient's response to drug treatment The terms *complete and partial remission* are frequently used and are a convenient way to describe responses and compare various regimens. *Complete remission* refers to the complete disappearance of all objective evidence of tumor as well as a resolution of all signs and symptoms referable to the tumor. Complete remission is generally associated with a prolongation of survival. *Partial remission* refers to a 50% or greater reduction in the size of all measurable lesions, along with some degree of subjective improvement and the absence of any new lesions during treatment. Partial remissions generally translate into improved well-being for the patient but only occasionally improve overall survival. Finally, a variety of terms have been used to designate lesser responses, but these are rarely associated with any significant improvement in survival.

As with any form of treatment, patients vary in their tolerance and response to combination chemotherapy. Because of the toxicity and narrow margin of safety inherent in combination chemotherapy regimens, it is necessary to adjust the treatment to the particular patient. One convenient method of doing this is through the application of a *sliding scale*. A typical scheme is shown in Table 5-11. The principle behind a sliding scale is that doses are modified during the subsequent course of therapy according to the degree of toxicity experienced during the preceding course. Doses of myelosuppressive agents can be reduced if the patient proves to be very sensitive to the regimen, but these can be returned to full levels if tolerance improves because of the response to treatment and improvement in overall

**TABLE 5-11  Sliding Scale for Adjustment of Therapy Based Upon Myelosuppression**

| If the white blood count before starting the new course is | Then the dosage is adjusted to |
|---|---|
| > 4,000/mm$^3$ | 100% of all drugs |
| 3,999 to 3,000/mm$^3$ | 100% of nonmyelotoxic agents, 50% of each myelotoxic agent |
| 2,999 to 2,000/mm$^3$ | 100% of nonmyelotoxic agents, 25% of each myelotoxic agent |
| 1,999 to 1,000/mm$^3$ | 50% of nonmyelotoxic agents, 25% of myelotoxic agents |
| 999 to 0/mm$^3$ | No drug until recovery |
| If the platelet count before starting the new course is | Then the dosage is adjusted to |
| > 100,000/mm$^3$ | 100% of all drugs |
| 50,000 to 100,000/mm$^3$ | 50% of myelotoxic drugs |
| < 50,000/mm$^3$ | No drug until recovery |

well-being. This system offers the physician the best opportunity to administer the maximum amount of therapy possible. Obviously, the sliding scale depicted is based only upon hematotoxicity. If the drugs used cause substantial degrees of other toxicities, one must employ sliding scales based on these other toxicities in order to minimize toxicity but maximize the therapeutic effect.

A large number of combination regimens are now being used in gynecologic malignancies, and it would be impossible to discuss them all in detail here. Many have become established as treatments of choice for particular tumors, while others are experimental. When evaluating any particular combination, one should consider its importance on the basis of several different criteria: (1) Is the combination chemotherapy now the treatment of choice in a particular stage of that disease? (2) Has the regimen been utilized for a number of years and has it been demonstrated to be effective by more than one investigator? (3) Has the regimen been reported with adequate discussion of the toxicities inherent in the program? (4) Does the regimen contain unusual forms of treatment that require unique facilities? (5) Does the combination comprise drugs that are available commercially? Using this kind of evaluation scheme, the clinician can put most of the combination chemotherapy regimens being used in gynecologic oncology into some sort of rank order in terms of importance, effectiveness, and safety.

## CLINICAL TRIALS AND FUTURE APPLICATIONS OF CHEMOTHERAPY IN GYNECOLOGIC CANCER

The gynecologic malignancies are a challenging group of diseases that vary widely in their biologic characteristics and natural histories. Despite this heterogeneity, management of these diseases has historically been highly standardized. Therapy has almost always involved initial surgery followed by radiotherapy. Nevertheless, there is reason to conclude that for each type of gynecologic cancer, some patients might benefit from systemic chemotherapy administered in concert with, or instead of, conventional surgical or radiotherapeutic management. Important prognostic factors crucial to the identification of these patients must be clarified; in addition, the current status of conventional therapies for each of the prognostic groups must be better defined. In this section, the existing as well as the potential roles of systemic chemotherapy will be discussed along with recommendations for future research.

## Ovarian Carcinoma

Although not the most common of the gynecologic malignancies, epithelian ovarian cancer is the most commonly fatal. Of the 21,000 new patients identified yearly, approximately 12,500 will die. During the past decade, a better understanding of the natural history of ovarian cancer has resulted in carefully designed therapeutic trials, which in turn have significantly improved the prognosis for many patients. These earlier studies provide the foundation for future clinical research in the treatment of epithelial ovarian cancer.

The overall response rates and survival appear to be influenced by a variety of prognostic factors, including stage of disease, extent of residual tumor, and histologic grade in addition to the nature of the response to initial therapy (Young et al, 1982). These important prognostic factors are listed in Table 5-12, and their influence on the results of therapy in advanced ovarian cancer is substantial. When studies are published without a clear statement about these factors, it becomes extremely difficult to interpret the results, and comparisons between studies are virtually impossible. Several studies have suggested that in addition to the factors listed above, age, Karnofsky index, and prior treatment are also important.

***Value of Surgical Staging Prior to Therapy*** Careful initial staging in apparent early disease has led to a better understanding of the sites at high risk for undetected disease. This, in turn, has explained the high failure rate associated with local therapeutic modalities in early ovarian cancer. In one such study (Young et al, 1983), systematic restaging was performed prospectively in 100 patients referred with a diagnosis of early (Stage IA to IIB) ovarian cancer. Prior to referral, only 25% of these patients had had an initial surgical incision that was adequate to allow complete evaluation of the pelvis and the abdominal cavity. As a result of careful restaging, including laparatomy if necessary, 31 (77%) actually had Stage III disease. Sites of unsuspected disease were most frequently the pelvic peritoneum, ascites fluid, other pelvic tissue, paraaortic nodes, and diaphragms.

Thus, it is clear that a major reason why local treatment fails in many patients with apparently localized disease is that they have unsuspected extrapelvic metas-

**TABLE 5-12** Ovarian Cancer: Factors Influencing Survival

| Stage | 5-Year Survival (%) |
|---|---|
| Ia and Ib | 61-65 |
| Ic | 52 |
| II | 40 |
| III | 5 |
| IV | 3 |

*Histologic Type*
Within each stage, the histologic type of epithelial tumor may have an effect on survival.

*Histologic Grade*
An independent prognostic factor within each stage.

| | *Volume of Tumor* | |
|---|---|---|
| Stage | Residual Tumor (cm) | 5-Year Survival (%) |
| II | 0-1 | 53 |
| | 3-6 | 22 |
| III | None | 63 |
| | 0-1 | 41 |
| | 1-2 | 15 |
| | 3-6 | 8 |
| IV | 0-1 | 20 |
| | >1 | 0 |

*Source:* Smith JP, Day TG: Review of ovarian cancer at the University of Texas Medical Center, M.D. Anderson Hospital and Tumor Institute. *Am J Obstet Gynecol* 135:984-993, 1979.

tases that are not being treated by surgery or pelvic irradiation. Understanding the patterns of spread in early ovarian cancer has allowed us to interpret more accurately the results of earlier published studies on the treatment of patients with Stage I and Stage II disease (Hreshchyshyn et al, 1980; Delclos, 1983; Dembo et al, 1978).

Of significance, none of these early studies required comprehensive surgical staging prior to therapy. Based on data from the aforementioned staging studies, it is probable that some of these patients had undetected extrapelvic spread of disease that would make some relapses inevitable. However, the recently published Gynecologic Oncology Group (GOG) study (Young et al, 1990) required comprehensive pretreatment staging. In the first trial, 81 patients with well-differentiated or moderately well-differentiated cancers confined to the ovaries (Stages IA and IB) were assigned to receive either no chemotherapy or melphalan (0.2 mg/kg body weight/day for 5 days, repeated every 4 to 6 weeks for up to 12 cycles). After a median followup of more than 6 years there were no significant differences between the patients given no chemotherapy and those treated with melphalan with respect to either 5-year disease-free survival (91 vs. 98% [p = 0.41]) or overall survival (94 vs. 98% [p = 0.43]).

In the second trial, 141 patients with poorly differentiated Stage I tumors or with cancer outside the ovaries but limited to the pelvis (Stage II) were randomly assigned to treatment with either melphalan (in the same regimen as above) or a single intraperitoneal dose of

$^{32}$P (15 mCi) at the time of surgery. In this trial (median followup > 6 years) the outcomes for the two treatment groups were similar with respect to 5-year disease-free survival (80% in both groups) and overall survival (81% with melphalan vs. 78% with $^{32}$P [p = 0.48]).

This study makes it clear that comprehensive staging at the time of surgical resection in patients with localized ovarian cancer can serve to identify those patients (as defined by the first trial) who can be followed without adjuvant chemotherapy; the remaining patients with localized ovarian cancer should receive adjuvant therapy and, with adjuvant melphalan or intraperitoneal $^{32}$P, should have a 5-year disease-free survival of about 80%.

**Approach to Therapy** Unfortunately, only 25 to 30% of women present with early disease, and the vast majority of patients with epithelial ovarian cancer have Stage III or IV disease at the time of initial diagnosis. The standard approach to treating for Stage III to IV disease has been initial surgery (including a bilateral salpingo-oophorectomy, hysterectomy, and omentectomy) to remove as much tumor as possible followed by combination chemotherapy.

A major role for chemotherapy in advanced epithelial ovarian cancer was established when it was demonstrated that patients who responded to melphalan showed improved survival compared with patients who did not respond (Smith et al, 1972). This observation has been confirmed in other studies, and chemotherapy trials have been aimed at improving upon the 40% response rate achieved with single agents.

One of the first studies to demonstrate significantly improved survival with any combination in a prospective comparison with a standard alkylating agent was published over 10 years ago (Young et al, 1978). Eighty previously untreated patients were randomized to receive either melphalan in conventional doses or HexaCAF (hexamethylmelamine, cyclophosphamide, methotrexate, and 5-fluorouracil). Treatment with the four-drug combination achieved a significantly higher overall response rate (75% vs. 54%, [p <0.05]), more complete remissions (33% vs. 16%, [p = 0.06]), and significantly longer median survival (29 vs. 17 months, [p <0.02]). However, HexaCAF was most effective in patients with minimal residual disease. The toxicity of the combination was greater than that of the single agent, primarily because of greater hematologic toxicity, along with nausea, vomiting, and alopecia.

Dutch investigators confirmed the activity of the HexaCAF combination in previously untreated patients (overall response rate 57%, with 30% complete remission) but also demonstrated that, in previously treated patients, HexaCAF has a much lower overall response rate (3 of 13, [25%]), no complete remissions, and increased toxicity (Neijt et al, 1979). That study emphasizes the marked reduction of activity of any regimen used as second-line therapy in advanced ovarian cancer.

Subsequently, a series of trials randomly comparing single-agent chemotherapy (generally alkylating agents) with combination chemotherapy has been published. Generally, these trials show improved rates of response, disease-free survival, overall survival, or all three. A summary of trials demonstrating improved survival are shown in Table 5-13. In addition to the HexaCAF study, two other prospective randomized trials have demonstrated better survival. The first was a multiinstitutional Swedish study comparing melphalan plus Adriamycin with melphalan alone in 142 patients with bulky Stage III and Stage IV disease (Trope, 1981). The combination was found to be superior to the single agent in overall response (63% vs. 40%, [p < 0.01]), duration of response (23 + vs. 8.1 months, [p < 0.001]), and overall median survival (16.8 + vs. 10.7 months, [p < 0.03]).

The second was a trial at the Mayo Clinic involving 41 patients; 2-year survival was 52% with cyclophosphamide/cisplatin compared with 19% with cyclophosphamide alone (Decker et al, 1982). The projected median survivals were 40 months and 16 months, respectively.

Several clinical trials in the treatment of advanced ovarian cancer have utilized maintenance alkylating agent therapy for several years. These trials have failed to show a benefit for such maintenance and have reported leukemias in long-term survivors. In light of the dangers of prolonged alkylating agent therapy and the absence of demonstrated benefit, this approach should be abandoned.

A number of general conclusions emerge from this series of prospective randomized trials. Combination chemotherapy continues to result in higher overall response rates and higher complete response rates than those achieved with single agents, although in some studies survival is not altered significantly. Nevertheless, long-term disease-free survival, although uncommon, is more often seen with combinations, particularly when the dose intensity is adequate. Several newer combinations may be more effective than those originally used in the prospective comparisons using single alkylating agents.

At present, it would appear that the chances of achieving a complete remission in advanced ovarian carcinoma are best when initial therapy is begun with an effective combination regimen administered in full therapeutic doses. Many studies now use combination chemotherapy as initial treatment in advanced disease. The published studies have either been single-arm studies or randomized trials in which two or more combinations have been compared. A summary of a representative group of these trials is given in Table 5-14. Most of these studies now contain sufficient information about prognostic factors, response duration, and survival to allow realistic comparisons with currently established combination chemotherapy regimens or single agents.

Several groups have reported results of two-, three-, and four-drug combinations in nonrandomized studies in previously untreated Stage III and Stage IV disease. Most of these trials have used combinations of cisplatin, Adriamycin, cyclophosphamide, hexamethylmelamine, methotrexate, or 5-FU. Overall response rates have ranged from 60 to 80%, with clinical complete remissions seen in approximately 40 to 50% of patients. Careful restaging demonstrates that approximately half of those found clinically to be free of disease actually have residual disease at second-look laparotomy. As a

**TABLE 5-13** Combination Chemotherapy vs. Single Agents in Previously Untreated Advanced Carcinoma: Results of Clinical Trials

| Regimen | Results | Reference |
|---|---|---|
| *Trials Demonstrating Increased Complete Response Rates and/or Disease-Free Survival* | | |
| CHAD vs. LPAM | 38% CR vs. 21% CR: progression-free survival increased for CHAD | Vogl et al, 1983 |
| CHF vs. LPAM | 85% RR vs. 57% RR; 50% CR vs.17% CR | Delgado et al, 1985 |
| AC vs. C | Improved progression-free survival with AC in patients with minimal residual disease | Edmonson et al, 1979 |
| PAC vs. CLB | RR: 68% vs. 26%, p = 0.0004 PCR: 26% vs. 15% | Williams et al, 1985 |
| *Trials Demonstrating Improved Survival* | | |
| HexaCAF vs. LPAM | 75% RR vs. 43%; 33% CR vs. 16%; median survival 29 vs. 17 months | Young et al, 1978 |
| A + LPAM vs. LPAM | 67% RR vs. 40%; 23+ vs. 8.1 months for duration of response; median survival 17 vs. 11 months | Trope et al, 1981 |
| CP vs. C | 2-year disease-free interval: 52% vs. 10%; 2-year survival: 62% vs. 19% | Decker et al, 1982 |

CHAD = cyclophosphamide, hexamethylmelamine, Adriamycin, cisplatin; LPAM = melphalan; CHF = cyclophosphamide, hexamethylmelamine, fluorouracil; AC = Adriamycin, cyclophosphamide; C = cyclophosphamide; PAC = cisplatin, Adriamycin, cyclophosphamide; CLB = chlorambucil; HexaCAF = hexamethylmelamine, cyclophosphamide, methotrexate, 5-fluorouracil; CP = cyclophosphamide, cisplatin. CR = complete response; RR = response rate (complete and partial); PCR = pathologic complete response.

result, approximately 25 to 30% of all patients treated with combination chemotherapy will be free of disease at restaging, and it is this subset of patients for whom disease-free survival is prolonged. At present, there does not seem to be a striking difference between combinations, although the addition of cisplatin appears beneficial. Randomized trials comparing platinum-containing combinations have generally demonstrated equivalent results in terms of survival.

Recently, several well-designed trials have been performed testing various combination regimens in an attempt to define the relative contributions of each individual drug as well as the combinations themselves. Some of the more significant studies are summarized in Table 5-15.

Neijt et al (1984) compared CHAP-5 (cyclophosphamide, hexamethylmelamine, Adriamycin, and cisplatin) with HexaCAF and demonstrated a statistically greater response rate (79% vs. 50%) and complete remission rate (30% vs. 17%) as well as an improved disease-free survival (19.5 vs. 6.8 months) and improved overall survival (30.7 vs. 19.6 months) for the CHAP-5 combination. Ten year follow up on this study has confirmed the superiority of the platinium-containing CHAP-5 combination.

The Gynecologic Oncology Group (GOG) compared AC (Adriamycin and cyclophosphamide) with PAC (cisplatin, Adriamycin and cyclophosphamide) in 227 patients with measurable disease (Omura et al, 1986). The complete response rate was 51% for CAP and 26% for AC (p = <0.0001). The progression-free interval (13 vs. 7.7 months) and overall survival (19.7 vs. 15.7 months) were statistically better with the platinum-con-

taining combination. These trials provide substantial evidence for the importance of platinum in any ovarian cancer regimen. Indeed, it is not clear whether the addition of other agents to regimens that include full dose intensities of cyclophosphamide and cisplatin is necessary or beneficial. In a large trial comparing CHAP-5 with CP (cyclophosphamide and cisplatin), the overall response rate (78% vs. 76%) and the pathologically documented complete response rate (34% vs. 37%) were similar for the two regimens (Neijt et al, 1987). Another study compared CP with HCAP (hexamethylmelamine, cyclophosphamide, doxorubicin, and cisplatin) in 181 patients (Edmonson et al, 1985). At a median followup of 30 months the two regimens led to identical rates of survivals (24.6 months). A similar experience was demonstrated in the analysis of the GOG trial comparing CAP with CP. In this trial, the percentage of negative second-look laparotomies was similar (39% vs. 38%) as were the times to disease progression and survival for the two arms. Based on the available data, there is very little evidence that any combination regimen produces better results than the two-drug CP regimen used in full therapeutic doses.

***Intraperitoneal Chemotherapy*** The technique of intraperitoneal (IP) chemotherapy is based on several observations unique to both the disease itself and the pharmacologic behavior of chemotherapeutic agents. Several unique aspects of ovarian cancer make intraperitoneal treatment potentially appropriate: (1) the disease remains confined to the IP space throughout most of its natural history; (2) currently available combination chemotherapy produces clinically complete responses in

TABLE 5-14    Results of Combination Chemotherapy in Advanced Ovarian Carcinoma

| Regimen | Schedule | Total Evaluable Patients | Complete and Partial Remissions (%) | No. of Clinical CR (%) | No. of Pathologic CR (%) |
|---|---|---|---|---|---|
| PAC (Ehrlich et al, 1979) | | 56 | 44/56 (79) | 23/56 (41) | 10/56 (18) |
| Cisplatin | 20 mg/m$^2$ IV day x 5 q 4 wk | | | | |
| Adriamycin | 50 mg/m$^2$ IV day 1 q 4 wk | | | | |
| Cyclophosphamide | 750 mg/m$^2$ IV day 1 q 4 wk | | | | |
| A-C (Dana Farber) (Parker et al, 1980) | | 41 | 35/41 (83) | 20/41 (48) | 12/41 (29) |
| Cyclophosphamide | 500 mg/m$^2$ IV | | | | |
| Adriamycin | 40 mg/m$^2$ | | | | |
| HexaCAF (NCI) (Young et al, 1978) | | 40 | 30/40 (75) | Not stated | 13/40 (33) |
| Hexamethylmelamine | 150 mg/m$^2$ PO qd x 14 | | | | |
| Cyclophosphamide | 150 mg/m$^2$ PO qd x 14 | | | | |
| Methotrexate | 40 mg/m$^2$ IV days 1 and 8 | | | | |
| 5-Fluorouracil | 600 mg/m$^2$ IV days 1 and 8 | | | | |
| CHAD (Greco et al, 1981) | | 46 | 45/46 (98) | 35/46 (76) | 14/46 (30) |
| Cyclophosphamide | 600 mg/m$^2$ IV day 1 | | | | |
| Hexamethylmelamine | 200 mg/m$^2$ PO days 8 to 22 | | | | |
| Adriamycin | 25 mg/m$^2$ IV day 1 | | | | |
| Cisplatin | 50 mg/m$^2$ IV day 1 | | | | |
| CHEX-UP (Louie et al, 1986) | | 62 | 43/62 (69) | 29/62 (47) | 12/62 (19) |
| Cyclophosphamide | 150 mg/m$^2$ PO days 2-8 and 2-16 | | | | |
| Hexamethylmelamine | 150 mg/m$^2$ PO days 2-8 and 9-16 | | | | |
| 5-Fluorouracil | 600 mg/m$^2$ IV days 1 and 8 | | | | |
| Cisplatin | 30 mg/m$^2$ IV days 1 and 8 | | | | |
| CHAP-5 (Neijt et al, 1987) | | 84 | 66/84 (79) | Not stated | 25/84 (30) |
| Cyclophosphamide | 100 mg/m$^2$ PO days 15 to 29 | | | | |
| Hexamethylmelamine | 150 mg/m$^2$ PO days 15 to 29 | | | | |
| Adriamycin | 35 mg/m$^2$ IV day 1 | | | | |
| Cisplatin | 20 mg/m$^2$ IV days 1 to 5 | | | | |
| PC (Neijt et al, 1987) | | 52 | Not stated | Not stated | 12/52 (23) |
| Cisplatin | 20 mg/m$^2$ IV days 1 to 5 | | | | |
| Cyclophosphamide | 600 mg/m$^2$ IV day 4 | | | | |

CR = complete response

TABLE 5-15    Randomized Comparisons of Combination Chemotherapy in Advanced Ovarian Adenocarcinoma

| Study | Results | Reference |
|---|---|---|
| CHAP-5 vs. HexaCAF | 79% RR vs. 50%; 30% CR vs. 17%; median survival 31 vs. 20 months | Neijt et al, 1984 |
| PAC vs. AC | 51% CR vs. 26% in patients with measurable disease. Response duration (15 vs. 9 months), progression-free interval (13 vs. 7 months), and overall survival (20 vs. 16 months), all statistically significant. | Omura et al, 1986 |
| CHAP-5 vs. CP | 78% RR vs. 76%; PCR 34% vs. 37% and no differences in survival. | Neijt et al, 1987 |
| HCAP vs. CP | Survival at 30 months equivalent for the two regimens (24.6 months). | Edmonson, 1985 |

CR = complete response; RR = response rate (complete and partial); PCR = pathologic complete response.

about 40% of patients, but at least half these patients have minimal residual disease; and (3) a dose-response effect is seen for some drugs, such that cytotoxic drug concentrations may be achieved by IP but not by IV administration.

The pharmacologic principles on which IP therapy is based center on the difference between peritoneal clearance and clearance from the systemic circulation. The slower the peritoneal clearance of a drug, the greater the potential pharmacologic advantage. Peritoneal clearance is a function of the drug's molecular weight and hydrophilic properties. High molecular weight compounds with a low lipid solubility are cleared slowly, leading to an increased pharmacologic advantage. Two other properties are necessary for a drug to be useful in the IP treatment of ovarian cancer: (1) the concentrations achievable in the peritoneal cavity must be cytotoxic to ovarian cancer cells and (2) the cytotoxic drug concentration should produce no more than an acceptable degree of peritoneal irritation.

IP chemotherapy is not a new technique in the management of patients with ovarian cancer. In the past antineoplastic agents have been injected directly into the peritoneal cavity to aid in the control of malignant ascites. The major differences between previous methods of IP chemotherapy and current techniques are (1) use of a semipermanent Tenckhoff dialysis catheter or the Port-a-Cath system and (2) delivery of the antineoplastic agents in a large volume (2 liters of dialysate) instead of in 50 to 100 ml of saline. A maximum pharmacologic advantage for IP chemotherapy will be achieved by the repetitive administration of a drug in a large volume to allow for its uniform distribution throughout the peritoneal cavity.

Although the most significant threat to prolonged catheter usage is infection, the overall incidence of this complication is still relatively low (3 of 78, [3.8%]). In a few cases outflow or inflow obstruction develops, but in most instances this condition responds to repositioning of the catheter. Gradually, only drug inflow becomes possible and no significant drainage occurs. A large number of phase I and II trials have now demonstrated a pharmacologic advantage for intermittent administration of a large volume (2 liters) of drug-containing dialysate via a Tenckhoff dialysis catheter. The ratio of

peak peritoneal level to peak plasma level varies from 30 to as much as 2,000, depending upon the drug used.

Similar investigations using cisplatinum suggest that peak IP concentrations exceed the peak plasma concentrations six- to eightfold (Howell et al, 1982). Free platinum concentrations in ascites were 30 times greater than those achieved with a similar IV dose (Casper et al, 1982).

Although the pharmacologic success of IP chemotherapy has been established, its therapeutic benefit is still unclear. Early trials established that patients with minimal residual disease are most likely to respond and that responses in bulky disease are uncommon. Two studies using IP cisplatin have established this drug as the current IP drug of choice (Cohen, 1985; ten Bokkel Huinink et al, 1985). A summary of the study design and results are listed in Table 5-16.

In one study, the survival of patients treated with IP cisplatin depended upon the extent of residual disease (Markman et al, 1986). For patients with bulky residual disease, the median survival was 6.5 months. In contrast, for those with minimal residual disease before therapy, the 2-year actuarial survival was 74%. Nevertheless, the survival of patients with microscopic residual, positive washings, or minimal residual disease is variable, and the true survival benefit of this approach will be established only with prospective trials.

At present, the use of IP therapy remains experimental. Cisplatin appears to be the current drug of choice, and IP therapy does not appear to be useful in patients with bulky residual disease. Studies with combination chemotherapy administered intraperitoneally are now in progress, as are studies using IP therapy as part of initial induction. Perhaps the greatest potential for IP therapy is among those patients who have had a good but only partial response to induction chemotherapy and have residual microscopic disease.

Another potential role for IP chemotherapy is in patients who have responded completely to chemotherapy, since this group remains at risk for relapse. IP therapy needs to be evaluated further in other clinical situations, for example, as adjuvant therapy in high-risk patients with early-stage disease and combined with systemic treatment as part of the induction therapy for patients with Stage III disease.

| TABLE 5-16    Results of Intraperitoneal Cisplatin in Minimal Residual Ovarian Cancer | | |
|---|---|---|
| | Mt Sinai (Cohen, 1985) | Netherlands Cancer Institute (ten Bokkel Huinink, 1985) |
| Patient eligibility: | Small-volume disease after induction chemotherapy | |
| No. of patients | 23 | 21 |
| Cisplatin dose | 50 mg/m$^2$ in 2 L every 3 weeks | 60 to 150 mg/m$^2$ in 2 L every 2 to 3 weeks |
| No. of cycles | 6 | 6 to 10 |
| Sodium thiosulfate | Not used | If toxicity developed in previous cycle |
| Catheter | Temporary catheter in 75% of patients | Tenckhoff |
| Results | 6/19 (32%) negative laparotomy | 7/21 (33%) negative laparotomy |

The optimal drug for IP therapy also remains to be determined. As previously discussed, it should be a cytotoxic drug that offers a marked pharmacologic advantage but does not cause prohibitive local toxicity. The development of sterile peritonitis has been a major problem in several studies of IP therapy in ovarian cancer.

***Future Trials in Ovarian Cancer*** In Stage I disease with a favorable prognosis, the previously discussed GOG-Ovarian Cancer Study Group study has established that no adjuvant therapy is necessary. For Stage II and unfavorable Stage I disease (ascites, poorly differentiated tumors), the optimal therapy needs to be determined. Since combination chemotherapy is generally more effective than melphalan alone in advanced ovarian cancer, and since patients with a small volume of tumor have a high probability of achieving complete remission with combination chemotherapy, it is appropriate for adjuvant trials in Stage II ovarian cancer to compare $^{32}$P with a more active drug combination. A randomized GOG trial comparing $^{32}$P with three cycles of cyclophosphamide-cisplatin is now under way in this group of carefully staged patients. Experimental approaches such as IP immunotherapy and chemotherapy are potentially useful modalities in patients with small volume disease. In any case, it is mandatory that patients be accurately staged prior to entry into early-stage protocols.

In patients with advanced disease, the role of surgery needs to be critically evaluated in terms of its impact upon subsequent therapy and survival. In patients with nonbulky disease, total abdominal radiotherapy of the type advocated by the Princess Margaret group should be compared with combination chemotherapy (Dembo et al, 1978). It is in this group of patients that IP chemotherapy should also be explored. In patients with bulky disease, approaches involving combined modalities require further evaluation. The timing of cytoreduction and the integration of radiation and chemotherapy (both IV and IP) will likely affect the results of therapy. In addition, the optimal induction chemotherapy regimen and the dose and schedule of administration remain to be defined for patients with advanced disease. Furthermore, since there appears to be a poorly defined but significant relapse rate among patients with pathologically documented complete remission, the role of IP therapy after negative second-look laparotomy needs to be assessed.

## Malignant Germ Cell Tumors of the Ovary

The malignant germ cell tumors of the ovary are an uncommon and heterogeneous group of tumors that constitute less than 5% of ovarian neoplasms. They predominate in childhood and early adolescence. The histologic types vary greatly in their natural histories and prognoses. For many years these tumors were categorized into cell types with a good prognosis (i.e., dysgerminomas) and aggressive cell types with a worse prognosis, (i.e., endodermal sinus tumor, malignant teratoma, and embryonal and mixed germ cell tumors). The dysgerminomas were radiosensitive but cureable in over 86% of the cases with local resection and post-operative radiotherapy. At the other extreme were the aggressive germ cell tumors, which historically have had a poor prognosis even when treated at an early stage. Several early series report an overall 10% survival rate with surgical and/or radiation management for this group of tumors (Kurman and Norris, 1976; Norris et al, 1976).

Review of a large group of patients with aggressive germ cell tumors indicates that clinical stage is of limited prognostic significance (Cangir et al, 1978). Most patients have occult or demonstrable dissemination of tumor at the time of diagnosis and as a consequence are not curable with a local therapeutic modality. Proper management must take into account the prognosis of the histologic types as well as the importance of early dissemination.

Pure dysgerminomas are highly radiosensitive, and modern radiotherapy techniques following surgical resection have contributed significantly to the successful management of these tumors. A cure rate of better than 90% is expected for the Stage I and II tumors following such therapy, and in some treatment centers a long-term survival rate of 70% has been reported for patients with advanced or recurrent dysgerminomas (Krepart et al, 1978). However, extensive radiation therapy is sterilizing in these women, and in light of the activity of cisplatin, vinblastine, bleomycin (PVB) in testicular seminoma, this tumor has recently been treated with combination chemotherapy. Seven patients with Stage III or IV dysgerminomas (four of whom had not responded to previous radiation) were treated with PVB (Smales and Peckham, 1987). All seven showed a complete response, and six have been free of disease for more than one year. A recent study from the GOG using PVB or PEB (Etoposide substitute for Vinblastine) achieved a 94% complete remission rate in patients with advanced (Stage III & IV) dysgerminomas. This suggests that combination chemotherapy should replace irradiation as the therapy of choice for these tumors.

In contrast, the other germ cell tumors have not been managed successfully with aggressive surgery with or without radiation despite apparently adequate control of the disease with surgery (Kurman and Norris, 1976; Norris et al, 1976; Cangir et al, 1978). Even in patients with early-stage disease, survival rates have been poor. More advanced stages of these aggressive germ cell tumors were once uniformly fatal with surgical resection alone. Irradiation alone has added little to improving the outlook in these patients (D'Angio and Tefft, 1967).

Experience with combination drug therapy using vincristine, actinomycin D, and cyclophosphamide (VAC) indicates that chemotherapy dramatically alters the prognosis of these aggressive tumors (Slayton et al, 1978). Initial programs began drug therapy within 2 weeks of surgery and continued treatment for 2 years. At 2 years, 40 to 50% of patients with advanced endodermal sinus tumors, malignant teratomas, and embryonal tumors were still alive without evidence of disease. It is important to note that this survival benefit is limited to those patients who have minimal residual disease at the time chemotherapy is initiated.

The successful experience with combination chemotherapy including PVB in the primary management of advanced testicular germ cell cancers and etoposide (VP-16) in refractory testicular cancers led to the use of these drug regimens in the management of ovarian germ cell tumors, and evidence indicates that PVB is very active.

Collected experience from published series indicates that 53 out of 61 patients treated with PVB are alive without evidence of disease. Recently, platinum/VP-16/bleomycin has been used by the Royal Marsden group in nine patients (six with Stage III or IV disease) (Smales and Peckham, 1987). Eight of the nine are disease-free at 6 to 62 + months. Although no randomized trials have compared VAC with PVB or PVP-16B, the latter two regimens have become the therapy of choice for the aggressive germ cell ovarian tumors. The development of effective chemotherapy regimens for germ cell tumors has resulted in a dramatic survival benefit in all stages of this disease.

Now the optimal duration of chemotherapy in advanced disease as well as in adjuvant therapy will need to be defined. In addition, the need for second-look laparotomy in these patients must be questioned, since the results in the vast majority of those laparotomies in patients with no clinical evidence of disease and with normal markers have been negative.

## Carcinoma of the Cervix

Although the incidence of cervical carcinoma is decreasing in the United States and management approaches for in situ or microinvasive cervical carcinoma have been highly successful, improvement in the management of invasive cervical carcinoma has failed to match this achievement. Approximately 5,600 of the 13,000 patients seen each year with invasive cervical carcinoma die of either recurrent or disseminated disease.

The current staging classification for carcinoma of the cervix is based on the extent of local disease. Although the clinical stage correlates with the success of current treatment, it does not reflect the presence of nodal metastases and thus fails to define those patients with occult dissemination. Involvement of pelvic nodes is not infrequent when invasion is greater than 3 mm. In Stage IB the incidence of nodal metastases is reported to range from 10 to 29%, including a 6% incidence of paraaortic nodal metastases (Boronow, 1977; Hoskins et al, 1976). Metastasis to paraaortic nodes occurs in 20 to 29% of patients with invasive disease. In addition to nodal metastases, the size of the primary lesion has also been correlated with the response to therapy and survival.

The 5-year survival of patients with Stage I cervical cancer is 70 to 80% after radical hysterectomy or local radiation therapy (Marcial, 1976). Although local disease is adequately controlled with either modality, treatment failures occur primarily because neither of these modalities adequately controls disease that has spread to regional nodes (Delgado, 1978; Lagasse et al, 1974). Radiation has been the primary form of treatment for patients with advanced cervical cancer. Although the primary disease is often controlled in these patients, many will have paraaortic node metastases that are inadequately treated with current modalities, including

lymphadenectomy or extended-field irradiation. One explanation for the failure of these current therapeutic modalities in paraaortic node metastases is that in many of these patients disease has spread beyond even the most extensive radiation therapy field.

About 35% of all patients with invasive carcinoma of the cervix will experience local recurrence (Van Nagell et al, 1978). A small number of highly selective patients with recurrent small central lesions may benefit from radical surgery; in the remaining patients, irradiation is often limited by previous surgery (Evans et al, 1975). Overall survival among patients with local recurrent disease has been 3 to 19%.

This information defines various subsets of patients with cervical carcinoma who might benefit from some form of effective systemic therapy, if such therapy can be identified. These include many patients with early disease and most of those with advanced disease who have paraaortic node metastases and are therefore at high risk for recurrence despite apparent local control with currently available techniques. The great majority of patients with locally recurrent disease and patients with distant metastatic disease would also benefit from effective systemic therapy. Although this means that many patients would potentially benefit from such treatment, drug therapy has been inadequately studied.

Much of the experience with systemic therapy in cervical cancer has involved patients with advanced recurrent disease who have not responded to radiation and surgery. In this group, drug therapy is difficult both to administer and to evaluate in terms of response owing to several major factors: (1) decreased pelvic vascular perfusion, (2) limited bone marrow reserve, and (3) pelvic fibrosis and adhesions as a result of previous surgery and radiotherapy. Many of the drugs that showed limited activity in these patients may be found to have a greater effect if administered earlier in the course of the disease (for example, as adjuvant therapy in a patient with clinical Stage I disease with metastases to the paraaortic nodes).

Although a wide variety of chemotherapeutic agents have demonstrated some activity in cervical carcinoma (Table 5-17), the magnitude of this activity is limited. Only 5-FU, Dibromodulcitol cisplatin, and Ifosfamide have demonstrated significant activity in well-designed studies with adequate patient numbers (Thigpen et al, 1987; Thigpen et al, 1981). Cisplatin is the single chemotherapeutic agent with the best documented activity. The GOG treated 497 patients using three separate dose schedules and demonstrated responses in approximately 25%, with complete responses in 10%. Response rates did not vary with dose schedule. The median duration of response was 4 months, and median survival was 6.5 months. Significant renal toxicity and myelosuppression were seen with all cisplatin dose schedules.

***Combination Chemotherapy in Cervical Carcinoma*** There have been many published studies of combination chemotherapy for advanced cervical carcinoma. Several studies show complete response rates of 10 to 29%, suggesting some enhancement of overall effect compared with single agents. Table 5-18 lists combination

TABLE 5-17   Results of Single-Agent Chemotherapy in Cervical Carcinoma

| Drugs | No. of Responders/Total Treated | % Overall Response |
|---|---|---|
| *Alkylating Agents* | | |
| Cyclophosphamide | 31/228 | 14 |
| Chlorambucil | 11/44 | 25 |
| Dibromodulcitol | 4/15 | 27 |
| Dianhydrogalactitol | 7/36 | 17 |
| Ifosfamide | 10/30 | 30 |
| *Antimetabolites* | | |
| 5-Fluorouracil | 68/348 | 20 |
| Methotrexate | 12/77 | 16 |
| *Mitotic Inhibitors* | | |
| Vincristine | 10/44 | 23 |
| *Antitumor Antibiotics* | | |
| Doxorubicin (Adriamycin) | 8/78 | 10 |
| Bleomycin | 17/172 | 10 |
| *Other Agents* | | |
| Cisplatin | 21/52 | 40 |
| Iproplatin | 7/36 | 21 |
| Carboplatin | 11/39 | 28 |
| Piperazinedione | 5/38 | 13 |

chemotherapy regimens in which reasonable numbers of evaluable patients have been studied, and response rates appear to exceed those achieved with single agents. However, most of these studies have not prospectively compared combination therapy to standard single agents, and the combinations are invariably associated with increased toxicity. Although some of these combinations produce higher response rates, none has been convincingly shown to be more effective than single-agent cisplatin.

*Intraarterial infusion* of drugs in advanced cervical carcinoma has theoretical appeal in light of the decrease in pelvic vascular perfusion resulting from surgical and radiation therapy. An arterial infusion would be expected to increase the concentration of the drugs in tissue. Unfortunately, efforts to exploit this potential advantage have been unsuccessful and toxicity has been significant. Morrow et al (977) evaluated continuous pelvic arterial infusion of bleomycin in 20 patients with locally recurrent cervical carcinoma. Substantial toxicity was observed with little evidence of tumor response. Similar negative results were reported by Swenerton and associates (1979), who administered a bleomycin–mitomycin C–vincristine combination as an arterial infusion. A study from Japan reported encouraging results with an intraarterial infusion of bleomycin immediately prior to the delivery of 4,000 to 5,000 rads to the pelvis. Unfortunately, the authors' assertion that bleomycin was beneficial because it acted as a radiation sensitizer is impossible to evaluate given the study design (Ohta, 1978). In summary, despite the theoretical rationale, there is no evidence to support the hypothesis that intraarterial chemotherapy is advantageous in cervical cancer. Because of the morbidity associated with such therapy, it cannot be recommended at this time.

**Chemotherapy as a Radiosensitizer**   Chemotherapy has been used as a radiation sensitizer in several studies of cervical carcinoma. Two prospective trials compared hydroxyurea or placebo combined with irradiation in patients with Stages IIB and IV cervical cancer (Hreshchyshyn et al, 1979; Piver et al, 1983). In the 104 evaluable patients randomized to treatment, the response rate for the hydroxyurea-treated group was 68% compared with 48% for the group given placebo. The duration of progression-free intervals and survival were also significantly better for patients treated with hydroxyurea, but hematologic toxicity was more common and more severe in this group. Unfortunately, both trials had significant design defects, not all patients were surgically staged, and substantial numbers of randomized patients were inevaluable. Other studies with effective radiotherapy alone in similar stages of cervical cancer have produced rates of survival and tumor control similar to those observed with the addition of hydroxyurea in the two series published. In spite of defects in trial design and drug selection, these two randomized trials do suggest a potential role for radiation sensitizers in

TABLE 5-18   Results of Combination Chemotherapy in Cervical Carcinoma

| Regimen | Evaluable Patients | No. of Responses (%) | Complete Responses (%) |
|---|---|---|---|
| Doxorubicin (Adriamycin) and methotrexate | 59 | 39 (66%) | 13 (22%) |
| | 24 | 7 (28%) | 0 (0%) |
| Doxorubicin and methyl CCNU | 31 | 14 (45%) | 9 (29%) |
| Doxorubicin and cisplatin | 19 | 6 (31%) | 2 (10%) |
| Mitomycin C and bleomycin | 33 | 12 (36%) | 5 (15%) |
| Mitomycin C, vincristine, and bleomycin | 91 | 46 (51%) | 14 (15%) |
| Mitomycin C, vincristine, bleomycin, and cisplatin | 14 | 6 (43%) | 4 (29%) |
| Cisplatin, bleomycin, and vinblastine | 33 | 22 (66%) | 6 (18%) |
| Cisplatin, bleomycin, vincristine, and methotrexate | 15 | 10 (66%) | 3 (20%) |

cervical carcinoma. More recent studies have utilized cisplatin as a radiation sensitizer in cervical carcinoma (Choo al, 1986; Twiggs et al, 1986). Significantly higher complete response rates in Stage I and II patients were seen in the group receiving cisplatin radiosensitization (55%) compared with those treated with radiation alone (20%), but no differences in local recurrence rates or survival were reported. The role of this or any other radiation sensitizer in cervical carcinoma therefore remains unproved.

Based on the information to date, a variety of important studies should be considered in an effort to improve therapy for cervical carcinoma and to define properly the role (if any) of chemotherapy in primary management. Patients with paraaortic node metastases should be entered in prospective trials to test the role of adjuvant systemic therapy. The initial experience with cisplatin in advanced disease is encouraging and indicates a potential role for this drug as adjuvant therapy. Further evaluation of new radiotherapeutic techniques, particularly those incorporating radiation sensitizers, should be carried out and compared with the proposed adjuvant drug therapy.

Effective systemic chemotherapy could assume a prominent role in the treatment of patients in whom local disease is not controlled with irradiation, in those with localized recurrences not amenable to surgical resection, and in those with extrapelvic disease. Newly designed drug combinations that include cisplatin or novel approaches will be required to improve this condition.

## Endometrial Carcinoma

In spite of the fact that endometrial carcinoma is believed to have a much better prognosis than many of the other gynecologic malignancies, stage for stage its prognosis is similar to that of epithelial ovarian carcinoma. Its improved prognosis is the result not of available therapy but rather of the high frequency with which the disease is diagnosed in its early stage with well-differentiated histology and with limited myometrial invasion. Since the incidence of endometrial carcinoma is on the increase in the United States, more effective approaches to this disease must still be sought.

Three prognostic factors have been identified that help to discriminate between the subset of patients with poor prognoses and those expected to be cured with local therapy: poorly differentiated (high-grade) histology, deep myometrial invasion and regional node metastasis. Although patients with Grade 3 tumors, deep myometrial invasion, and/or regional node metastases require a more aggressive management approach, it is not clear what approach is best. Radical surgery, including extensive lymphadenectomy, has not been shown to improve survival in these patients (Rutledge, 1974). The role of *radiotherapy* in patients with Stage I disease is controversial. No prospective study has ever demonstrated increased survival among patients treated with adjuvant irradiation. Nevertheless, an argument can be made for adjuvant therapy in high-risk Stage I

disease. This conclusion is supported by the results of a prospectively randomized trial in Stage I endometrial cancer in which patients received either postoperative pelvic irradiation or surgery alone (Candiani et al, 1978). Patients treated with pelvic irradiation showed a significant decrease in pelvic recurrence. A similar reduction in pelvic recurrence and the virtual elimination of vaginal recurrence have been shown in a number of retrospective reviews (Salazar et al, 1978c). However, it should be reiterated, that patients at high risk continue to have a poor prognosis despite this apparent local control of disease.

The failure of surgery or irradiation to control disease in some Stage I patients is almost certainly a result of early dissemination of disease outside the pelvis. Evidence for such early dissemination in these patients with Grade 3 tumors or deep myometrial invasion has been reported in a multicenter staging study of endometrial cancer (Lewis et al, 1970). Pelvic and paraaortic node metastases in patients with Grade 3 tumors were documented in 36% and 28%, respectively, and in 43% and 21% of those with deep myometrial invasion. The survival rate of patients with nodal metastases is poor. In a review of 32 cases collected from the literature, Morrow et al (1973) found a 60% recurrence rate among patients with pelvic node metastases who underwent surgical resection of tumor followed by pelvic irradiation. One explanation for this poor response to pelvic irradiation is the high incidence (60%) of concomitant paraaortic node metastases in patients with pelvic node metastases. Patients with paraaortic metastases are not curable with current treatments. Considering the experience with paraaortic node irradiation in cervical cancer, it is not likely that extending the irradiation field to include these nodes will improve the survival of these patients.

Stage II endometrial cancer is currently managed with a combination of *preoperative irradiation and surgery*. However, there is a 33% relapse rate among patients with Grade 3 tumors (Bruckman et al, 1978), and pelvic node metastases occur in 36% and paraaortic node metastases in 22% of all patients with Stage II endometrial cancer (Kottmeier, 1977; Cox et al, 1980). These subsets of patients with a poor prognosis should be candidates for study of additional systemic treatment.

The survival rate of patients with Stage III or IV endometrial cancer managed with surgery and pelvic irradiation is low. In addition, patients with recurrent endometrial cancer have a 10% salvage rate with surgical and radiotherapeutic management. Isolated vaginal recurrences are associated with long-term survival rate of 20%. The outlook in these patients is particularly dismal when pelvic radiation therapy has been previously administered.

The most commonly used systemic treatment in advanced endometrial cancer has been *progestational drug therapy*. Synthetic progestational agents have been the most commonly used systemic treatment of recurrent endometrial carcinoma. Collected publications indicate overall response rates of 30% to 37%. Responses to systemic progestogen therapy are associated with prolonged survival (Kneale, 1986). Median survival of responders ranges from 23 to 29 months compared with 6 months for patients who do not respond. In general, well-differentiated tumors respond more often than those with poorly differentiated histology. Additional factors influencing response include disease-free interval, age, and presence of areas of squamous metaplasia within the tumor. Metastases in the lung, vagina, lymph nodes, or soft tissues are more likely to respond to hormone therapy. Extensive pelvic recurrences rarely respond.

Multiple studies now document the correlation between the progesterone-receptor content of endometrial tumors and their response to progesterone therapy. Although well-differentiated tumors tend to have higher progesterone-receptor activity, receptor positivity is a better prognostic factor than grade (Ehrlich et al, 1981). One large study documented that the mean progesterone-binding capacity in endometrial carcinoma was inversely related to tumor grade. In that study, 88% of progesterone-responsive tumors were progesterone receptor–positive and 94% of patients who did not respond to progestogen therapy were progesterone receptor–negative. Although progestogens are widely used, there is no evidence that a particular hormone preparation is more effective. Those most commonly used include hydroxyprogesterone (Delalutin) or medroxyprogesterone (Depo-Provera). Oral megesterol acetate (Megace) appears to produce similar results. Patients are treated continuously until there is evidence of recurrence or the development of distant metastases.

Alternative endocrine therapy has been investigated, including tamoxifen (Swenerton et al, 1980) and danazol; both appear to have some activity. Several studies have documented a response rate of 30 to 39% for tamoxifen, and well-differentiated tumors respond more commonly. Attempts have been made to induce progesterone receptor and thereby increase the response to hormone therapy. In one study, an increase in the number of progesterone receptors was documented, but the overall response rate was 33%—not significantly different from that achieved with progesterone alone. Other studies on the modulation of progesterone receptors in endometrial cancer are needed.

Single-agent chemotherapy for endometrial carcinoma has not been studied extensively. Published information can be used only to suggest activity because small numbers of patients with an admixture of prognostic factors have generally been included in these studies. A list of the single agents that appear to have some activity in advanced endometrial cancer are listed in Table 5-19. Of the drugs listed, only doxorubicin, hexamethylmelamine, and cisplatin appear to have well-established activity (Deppe et al, 1984; Cohen, 1986). These drugs produce overall response rates in 30 to 40% of patients. Doxorubicin (Adriamycin) has been the single drug most extensively studied and appears to be the current drug of choice. Forty-three patients with advanced or recurrent endometrial carcinoma were treated, and 37% responded with 26% clinical complete regressions of disease (Thigpen et al, 1979). The median survival was 14 months for complete responders, 6.8

| TABLE 5-19 | Results of Chemotherapy in Endometrial Carcinoma | |
| --- | --- | --- |
| Drugs | No. of Responders/Total Treated | Response Rate |
| *Alkylating Agents* | | |
| Cyclophosphamide | 7/33 | 21% |
| Nitrogen mustard | 3/11 | 27% |
| *Antimetabolites* | | |
| 5-Fluorouracil | 10/43 | 23% |
| *Antitumor Antibiotics* | | |
| Doxorubicin (Adriamycin) | 33/92 | 36% |
| Bleomycin | 3/8 | 37% |
| *Miscellaneous* | | |
| Hexamethylmelamine | 6/20 | 30% |
| Cisplatin | 11/26 | 42% |
| Cisplatin | 4/13 | 31% |

months for partial responders, and 3.5 months for patients without significant response.

Cisplatin produces responses in 46% of patients when used at full doses (100 mg/m²) and in patients not previously treated (Seski et al, 1982). In contrast, the same drug has achieved a 4% response rate when used as second-line treatment. Studies of combination chemotherapy for advanced endometrial carcinoma has been limited. Those employing the two most active single agents, doxorubicin and cisplatin, report higher response rates (30 to 90%) but have been used only in small numbers of patients. One randomized study comparing this two-drug regimen with doxorubicin alone produced a 45% response rate for the two-drug combination and 20% for single-agent Adriamycin (Chauvergne et al, 1986). A three-drug combination—cisplatin, Adriamycin, and cyclophosphamide (PAC)—produced a 45% response rate in 209 patients but was associated with significant hematopoietic toxicity (Turbow et al, 1982). Another study with the same three drugs in slightly different doses and schedules produced a 58% response rate, including 28% complete remissions. Although the two-drug combination (Adriamycin, cisplatin) and the three-drug combination (PAC) appear to have some increased activity in single-arm studies, any definite benefit must be confirmed by prospective comparisons to Adriamycin alone. Other trials have used combination chemotherapy with hormones, but the independent contribution of each modality cannot be assessed in these small single-arm studies. These few pilot studies indicate a potential role for systemic chemotherapy in advanced endometrial carcinoma. If significant activity is documented in advanced disease, active regimens should be evaluated as adjuvant therapy in patients at high risk for recurrence after standard management.

Systemic chemotherapy is a therapeutic modality with a potential role both as adjuvant therapy in patients at high risk with early disease and as primary therapy in patients with advanced disease. Careful evaluation of systemic chemotherapy is warranted (1) in patients with Stage III or IV endometrial cancer; (2) in those with recurrent disease, including vaginal recurrence; and (3) as postoperative adjuvant therapy in clinical Stage I and II disease when there is evidence of paraaortic metastases. If adjuvant therapy improves the disease-free survival rate in patients with positive paraaortic nodes, studies of adjuvant therapy in patients with pelvic node metastases or deep myometrial invasion would be indicated.

Hormonal therapy will continue to play a role in the management of many patients. The progesterone-receptor assay will allow the selection of patients likely to benefit from therapy with a progestational agent. However, because of the low incidence of progesterone receptors in the more aggressive tumors, cytotoxic therapy should have a more prominent role in patients who require systemic therapy.

## Uterine Sarcoma

Uterine sarcomas account for 1 to 5% of all uterine malignancies. In contrast to the more common uterine adenocarcinomas, 50% of patients with Stage I uterine sarcomas die despite surgery plus irradiation. In 96% of those patients, extrapelvic metastases develop. The tendency of these tumors to disseminate makes these patients appropriate candidates for study using adjuvant systemic therapy.

The extent of the tumor at the time of diagnosis is an important prognostic factor for survival in the patient with uterine sarcoma (Salazar et al, 1978a). Even in Stage I disease after complete surgical resection and local irradiation, the survival rate is only 50%. Patients with Stage II to IV disease have a 20% survival rate. Mean survival of those in whom primary therapy fails is 9 months (Salazar et al, 1978b).

Stage for stage, there is no significant difference in survival among patients whose tumors are histologic variants of uterine sarcoma, i.e., leiomyosarcoma, mixed mesodermal sarcoma, and endometrial stromal sarcoma. Leiomyosarcomas, however, occur in younger patients and tend to be localized to the uterine corpus in 80% of cases (Gallup and Cordray, 1979).

Current management of uterine sarcomas is directed toward controlling local disease. Surgical resection alone results in a 5-year survival rate of 56% in patients with Stage I disease; the addition of adjuvant pelvic irradiation has no impact on their survival (Salazar et al, 1978b and 1978c). When disease recurs after initial treatment, it is usually at extrapelvic sites: 70% in the upper abdomen, 60% in lung, 20% in bone, and 5% in brain. Fifty percent of the patients who do not respond to primary therapy have recurrent disease at both pelvic and extrapelvic sites. Isolated pelvic recurrences are rare.

Because a large number of patients with uterine sarcomas show systemic spread of the disease—even in the earliest clinical stage—interest in systemic chemotherapy has grown. Chemotherapy has generally been unsuccessful in prolonging survival in patients with metastatic leiomyosarcomas, and single-agent therapy produces a clinical response only rarely. Twelve patients treated with a combination of dacarbazine (DTIC) and doxorubicin had higher response rates and more prolonged survival compared with historical controls (Gottlieb et al, 1976). However, the patients were younger and had less prior treatment with radiation and chemotherapy. Postoperative pelvic irradiation and chemotherapy with vincristine, actinomycin D, and cyclophosphamide (VAC) was used by Smith (1975), who reported survival times of 10 to 40 months in seven of eight patients with advanced disease. However, this 87% partial response rate has not been reported by others, and toxicity was considerable. In another study, six patients with metastatic disease were treated with vincristine, doxorubicin, and DTIC, and three complete responses and one partial response were observed (Azizi et al, 1979).

The GOG has conducted two separate prospective clinical trials for metastatic uterine sarcomas. In one study comparing doxorubicin alone with the doxorubicin/DTIC combination, the response rates were not statistically different (15.1% versus 10.8%) (Omura et al, 1983). The toxicity of the combination, however, was significantly greater, and doxorubicin alone had a better therapeutic index. Only 12 of 226 patients (5.3%) showed complete clinical responses, and median survival was 15 months, compared with 8 months for the 17 patients with a partial response (7.5%), 9 months for the 39 patients with stable disease (17.3%), and 3.5 months for the 78 patients with progressive disease on therapy (34.5%). A second study by the GOG compared doxorubicin with doxorubicin plus cyclophosphamide. The response rate and survival was the same for each group (Muss et al, 1985). The total response rate has been only 9.3%, with 70% of the patients dead at 2 years.

The addition of cisplatin to doxorubicin has resulted in several impressive complete responses in a small series; however, this regimen needs to be more extensively studied.

***Adjuvant Chemotherapy*** On the basis of uncontrolled studies, it has been suggested that doxorubicin might be useful as adjuvant treatment in completely resected Stage I and II disease. Unfortunately, a prospective study of adjuvant doxorubicin in early-stage disease conducted by the GOG did not demonstrate any significant benefit in disease-free or overall survival for patients who received doxorubicin (Omura et al, 1985).

In a 9-year retrospective experience from the M. D. Anderson Hospital, 34 patients with Stage I and II disease were treated with adjuvant chemotherapy using the VAC regimen, VA, or AC for 3 to 4 months; results were compared with those for 37 patients who received no adjuvant chemotherapy (Hannigan et al, 1983). The researchers concluded that neither the probability of survival nor the disease-free interval was improved by the addition of these particular adjuvant chemotherapies.

VAC combination chemotherapy was given after surgery to 17 patients with Stages I and II uterine sarcoma. Five of 10 patients evaluable at 3 years were free of disease, but this result is similar to the results for those treated with either surgery alone or with surgery plus postoperative pelvic radiation treatment (Buchsbaum et al, 1979).

Currently, there is no evidence that either adjunctive radiation or chemotherapy improves the survival of patients with uterine sarcoma. This is true for all the histologic subtypes. Pelvic radiation may be useful for the control of pelvic disease, but results are mixed.

Nevertheless, the natural history of the uterine sarcomas indicates that occult dissemination occurs early in the course of the disease. At this time, patients with evidence of extrapelvic extension, high-grade histology, or metastatic disease should be considered for protocols that include aggressive postsurgical systemic therapy. Although there is some evidence that systemic chemotherapy will improve survival in patients with advanced disease, further evaluation of the benefit of such chemotherapy in the adjuvant setting is required. Because of the small number of patients with uterine sarcoma, large randomized studies will be difficult to complete.

## Gestational Trophoblastic Disease

Gestational trophoblastic disease (GTD) continues to be the most sensitive of all neoplastic growths, with an expected long-term disease-free survival of 90% or more among patients receiving appropriate management. Recent attention has therefore focused on poor prognostic features that allow investigators to study patients who are still inadequately treated with methotrexate or actinomycin D given alone or together. The principal poor-risk factors appear to be cerebral or hepatic metastases, high serum beta-human chorionic gonadotropin (β-hCG) levels (range, 40,000 to 100,000 IU/liter), previous treatment, symptoms lasting longer than 4 months, and the development of disease after a term pregnancy. The prognosis for these patients at high risk treated with a single-drug regimen is poor. Although intensive therapy with aggressive combination chemotherapy improves the prognosis in this high-risk group, the cure rate is not as high as that achieved for the good-prognosis group, and toxicity is substantial. Such patients should receive an aggressive combination regimen along with whole-brain irradiation if central nervous system metastases are detected.

Patients with poor-risk factors should receive initial combination chemotherapy. The most common regimen used is methotrexate, actinomycin D, and chlorambucil (triple therapy), with courses repeated as required until 3 successive weeks of normal β-hCG levels are achieved. Other effective regimens include EMA-CO or CHAM-OCA regimens (Bagshawe, 1976, Newland, 1986), MAC (methotrexate, actinomycin D, cyclophosphamide), or PVB (cisplatin, vinblastine, bleomycin). Using these regimens, complete responses are generally achieved in approximately 80% of patients, although generally lower responses (60 to 70%) are seen in patients with hepatic or cerebral metastases.

Salvage chemotherapy for patients who do not respond to initial induction therapy for high-risk disease has generally employed six or seven drug combinations.

Although many of these early trials achieved some salvage, small numbers of patients were included. One salvage regimen using high-dose cisplatin, vincristine, and methotrexate with leucovorin achieved durable, complete remissions in 35% of previous failures. With the identification of VP-16 and cisplatin as active agents in a salvage setting, several investigators have used these drugs in new regimens.

After the failure of conventional triple therapy, PVB led to complete remission in 50% of patients, although only 20% (2 of 11) had a sustained complete remission. More recently, high-dose methotrexate with leucovorin rescue, VP-16, and bleomycin were used in nine patients unresponsive to initial therapy with the modified Bagshawe regimen. Eight (89%) achieved a sustained remission for more than 2 years; however, bone marrow toxicity was universal and substantial.

Although the successful use of systemic chemotherapy in the management of gestational trophoblastic disease is well established, two areas still require investigation. First, the sensitive assay for hCG titer now allows more precise tailoring of established drug therapy. This can be used to reduce the toxicity of current treatments by allowing fewer courses of therapy. Second, a group of patients at high risk for failure with conventional treatment is now well defined. New treatment approaches with combination chemotherapy regimens have proved beneficial even in previously refractory cases. The development of even more successful combination regimens with newly identified drugs appears reasonable. Unfortunately, the various regimens have usually been developed and used primarily at single institutions, and the relative merits of one regimen versus another in patients with a poor prognosis remain to be established.

## REFERENCES

Azizi F, Bitran J, Javehari G, et al: Remission of uterine leiomyosarcomas treated with vincristine, Adriamycin and dimethyltriazeno-imidazole carboximide. *Am J Obstet Gynecol* 133:379, 1979.

Bagshawe KD: Treatment of trophoblastic tumors. *Ann Acad Med* 5:273, 1976.

Baker RM, Ling V: Membrane mutants of mammalian cells in culture. In Korn ED (ed): *Methods in Membrane Biology*, Vol 19. New York, Plenum Press, 1978, p 337.

Bech-Hanson NT, Till JE, Ling V: Pleiotropic phenotype of colchicine-resistant CHO cells: Cross-resistance and collateral sensitivity. *J Cell Physiol* 88:23, 1976.

Boronow RC: Stage I cervix cancer and pelvic node metastases. *Am J Obstet Gynecol* 127:135, 1977.

Brenner DE: Intraperitoneal chemotherapy. A review. *J Clin Oncol* 4:1135-1147, 1986.

Bruckman JE, Goodman BL, Murthy A, Marck A: Combined irradiation and surgery in the treatment of stage II carcinoma of the endometrium. *Cancer* 42:1146, 1978.

Buchsbaum HJ, Lifshitz S, Blyth JG: Prophylactic chemotherapy in stages I and II uterine sarcoma. *Gynecol Oncol* 8:346, 1979.

Candiani GB, Mangioni C, Murz MM: Surgery in endometrial cancer: Age, route and operability in 854 stage I and II fresh consecutive cases: 1955-1976. *Gynecol Oncol* 6:363, 1978.

Cangir A, Smith JP, van Eys J: Improved prognosis in children with ovarian cancers following modified VAC (vincristine, sulfate, dactinomycin, and cyclophosphamide) chemotherapy. *Cancer* 42:1234, 1978.

Casper ES, Kelsen DP, Alcock NW, Lewis JL Jr: Pharmacokinetic study of intraperitoneal cisplatin in patients with malignant ascites. *Proc Am Soc Clin Oncol* 1:22, 1982.

Chabner BA: *Pharmacologic Principles of Cancer Treatment.* Philadelphia, WB Saunders Co, 1982.

Chauvergne J, Granger C, Mage PH, et al: Chimiotherapie palliative des cancers de l'endometre. *Rev Fr Gynecol Obstet* 81:547, 1986.

Choo YC, Choy TK, Wong C, et al: Potentiation of radiotherapy by cis-dichlorodiammine platinum (II) in advanced cervical carcinoma. *Gynecol Oncol* 23:94, 1986.

Cohen CJ: Cytotoxic chemotherapy for patients with endometrial carcinoma. *Clin Obstet Gynecol* 13:811, 1986.

Cohen CJ: Surgical considerations in ovarian cancer. *Semin Oncol* 12:53-56, 1985.

Cox JD, Komaki R, Wilson JF, Greenberg M: Locally advanced adenocarcinoma of the endometrium: Results of irradiation with and without subsequent hysterectomy. *Cancer* 45:715, 1980.

D'Angio GJ, Tefft M: Radiation therapy in the management of children with gynecologic cancers. *Ann NY Acad Sci* 142:675, 1967.

Debenham PG, Kartner N, Simonovitch L, Riordan JR, Ling V: DNA-mediated transfer of multiple drug resistance and plasma membrane glycoprotein expression. *Mol Cell Biol* 2:881, 1982.

Decker DG, Fleming TR, Malkasian GD, Webb MJ, Jeffries JA, Edmonson JH: Cyclophosphamide and cis-platinum in combination: Treatment program for Stage III and IV ovarian carcinoma. *Obstet Gynecol* 60:481, 1982.

Delclos L: *International Symposium on Combined Modalities Approach to Gynecologic Cancer.* Mexico City, Mexico, May 19-20, 1983, p 61.

Delgado G: Stage IB squamous cancer of the cervix: The choice of treatment. *Obstet Gynecol Surv* 33:174, 1978.

Delgado G, Smith FP, McLaughlin EF, et al: Single agent vs combination chemotherapy for ovarian cancer. *Am J Clin Oncol* 8:33-37, 1985.

Dembo AJ, Bush RS, Beale FA, et al: Ovarian carcinoma: Improved survival following abdomino-pelvic irradiation in patients with a completed pelvic operation. *Am J Obstet Gynecol* 134:793, 1978.

Deppe G, Malviya VK, Zbella E: Non-hormonal chemotherapy in endometrial cancer: A review. *Wien Klin Wochenschr* 96:747, 1984.

DeVita VT, Young RC, Canellos GP: Combination versus single agent chemotherapy: A review of the basis for selection of drug treatment in cancer. *Cancer* 35:98, 1975.

Edmonson JH, Fleming TR, Decker DG, et al: Different chemotherapeutic sensitivities and host factors affecting prognosis in advanced ovarian carcinoma versus minimal residual disease. *Cancer Treat Rep* 63:241-247, 1979.

Edmonson JH, McCormack GW, Fleming TR, et al: Comparison of cyclophosphamide plus cisplatinum versus hexamethylmelamine, cyclophosphamide, doxorubicin, and cisplatinum in combination as initial chemotherapy for Stage III and IV ovarian carcinomas. *Cancer Treat Rep* 69:1243, 1985.

Ehrlich CE, Einhorn L, Williams SD, et al: Chemotherapy for stage III-IV epithelial ovarian cancer with cis-dichlorodiammineplatinum (II), Adriamycin, and cyclophosphamide: A preliminary report. *Cancer Treat Rep* 63:281-288, 1979.

Ehrlich CE, Young PCM, Cleary RE: Cytoplasmic progesterone and estradiol receptors in normal, hyperplastic, and carcinomatous endometrial: Therapeutic implications. *Am J Obstet Gynecol* 141:539-546, 1981.

Evans SR, Hilaris BS, Barber HRK: External vs. interstitial irradiation in unresectable recurrent cancer of the cervix. *Cancer* 28:1284, 1975.

Fisher RI, DeVita VT, Hubbard SM, Longo DL, Wesley R, Chabner BA, Young RC: Diffuse aggressive lymphomas: Increased survival after alternating flexible sequences of ProMACE and MOPP chemotherapy. *Ann Intern Med* 98:304, 1983.

Gallup DG, Cordray DR: Leiomyosarcoma of the uterus: Case reports and a review. *Obstet Gynecol Surv* 34:300, 1979.

Goldie JH, Coldman AJ: A mathematic model for relating the drug sensitivity of tumors to their spontaneous mutation rate. *Cancer Treat Rep* 63:1727, 1979.

Goldie JH, Coldman AJ, Gudauskas GA: Rationale for the use of non-cross-resistant chemotherapy. *Cancer Treat Rep* 66:439, 1982.

Gottlieb JA, Benjamin RS, Baker LH, et al: Role of DTIC in the chemotherapy of sarcomas. *Cancer Chemother Rep* 60:199, 1976.

Greco FA, Julian CG, Richardson RL, et al: Advanced ovarian cancer: Brief intensive combination chemotherapy and second-look operation. *Obstet Gynecol* 58:199-206, 1981.

Green JA, Vistica DT, Young RC, et al: Potentiation of melphalan cytotoxicity in human ovarian cancer cell lines by glutathione depletion. *Cancer Res* 44:5427-5431, 1984.

Hamilton TC, Young RC, McKoy WM, et al: Characterization of a human ovarian carcinoma cell line (NIH:OVCAR-3) with androgen and estrogen receptors. *Cancer Res* 43:5379-5389, 1983.

Hamilton TC, Winker MA, Louie KG, et al: Augmentation of Adriamycin, melphalan, and cisplatin cytotoxicity in drug-resistant and sensitive human ovarian carcinoma cell lines by butethamine sulfoximine–mediated glutathione depletion. *Biochem Pharmacol* 34:2583-2586, 1985.

Hannigan EV, Freedman RS, Rutledge FN: Adjuvant chemotherapy in early uterine sarcoma. *Gynecol Oncol* 15:56, 1983.

Haskell CM: Principles of cancer chemotherapy. In Haskell CM (ed): *Cancer Treatment,* 2nd ed. Philadelphia, WB Saunders Co, 1985.

Hoskins WJ, Ford JH, Lutz MH, Averette HE: Radical hysterectomy and pelvic lymphadenectomy for the management of early invasive cancer of the cervix. *Gynecol Oncol* 4:278, 1976.

Howell SB, Pfeifle L, Wung WE, Olshen RA, Lucas WE, Yon JL, Green M: Intraperitoneal cis-platin with systemic thiosulfate protection. *Ann Intern Med* 97:845, 1982.

Hreshchyshyn MM, Aron BS, Boronow RC, Franklin EN, Shingleton HM, Blessing JA: Hydroxyurea or placebo combined with radiation to treat stages IIIB and IV cervical cancer confined to the pelvis. *Int J Radiat Oncol Biol Phys* 5:317-322, 1979.

Hreshchyshyn MM, Park RC, Blessing JA, et al: The role of adjuvant therapy in stage I ovarian cancer. *Am J Obstet Gynecol* 138:139, 1980.

Hryniuk WM: The importance of dose intensity in the outcome of chemotherapy. In Hellman S, DeVita V, Rosenberg S (eds): *Important Advances in Oncology.* Philadelphia, JB Lippincott Co, 1988, pp 121-141.

Hryniuk WM, Bush H: The importance of dose intensity in chemotherapy metastatic breast cancer. *J Clin Oncol* 5:756-767, 1987.

Hryniuk WM, Figueredo A, Goodyear M: Application of dose intensity to problems in chemotherapy of breast and colorectal cancer. *Semin Oncol* 14:3-11, 1987.

Juliano RL, Ling V: A surface glycoprotein modulating drug permeability in Chinese hamster ovary cell mutants. *Biochem Biophys Acta* 455:152, 1976.

Kneale BLG: Adjunctive and therapeutic progestins in endometrial cancer. *Clin Obstet Gynecol* 13:789, 1986.

Kottmeier HL (ed): *Annual Report on Results of Treatment,* Vol 16. Radiumhemmet, Stockholm, 1977.

Krepart G, Smith JP, Rutledge F, Delclos L: The treatment for dysgerminoma of the ovary. *Cancer* 41:986, 1978.

Kurman RJ, Norris HJ: Endodermal sinus tumor of the ovary: A clinical and pathologic analysis of 71 cases. *Cancer* 38:2404, 1976.

Lagasse LD, Smith ML, Moore JG, et al: The effect of radiation therapy on pelvic lymph node involvement in stage I carcinoma of the cervix. *Am J Obstet Gynecol* 119:328, 1974.

Levin L, Hryniuk W: Dose intensity analysis of chemotherapy regimens in ovarian cancer. *J Clin Oncol* 5:756-767, 1987.

Lewis BV, Stallworthy JA, Condell R: Adenocarcinoma of the body of the uterus. *J Obstet Gynaecol Br Commonw* 77:343, 1970.

Louie KG, Hamilton TC, Winker MA, et al: Adriamycin accumulation and metabolism in Adriamycin-sensitive and resistant human ovarian cancer cell lines. *Biochem Pharmacol* 35:467-472, 1986.

Marcial VA: Carcinoma of the cervix: Present status and future. *Cancer* 39:945, 1976.

Markman M, Howell S, Cleary S, et al: Survival following cisplatin based intraperitoneal chemotherapy for refractory ovarian carcinoma. *Proc Am Soc Clin Oncol* 5:113, 1986.

Morrow CP, DiSaia PJ, Mangan CF, Lagasse LD: Continuous pelvic arterial infusion with bleomycin for squamous carcinoma of the cervix recurrent after irradiation therapy. *Cancer Treat Rep* 61:1403, 1977.

Morrow CP, DiSaia PJ, Townsend DE: Current management of endometrial carcinoma. *Obstet Gynecol* 42:399, 1973.

Muss HB, Bundy B, DiSaia PJ, et al: Treatment of recurrent or advanced uterine sarcoma: A randomized trial of doxorubicin versus doxorubicin and cyclophosphamide (a phase III trial of the Gynecologic Oncology Group). *Cancer* 55:1648, 1985.

Myers C: The clinical setting and pharmacology of intraperitoneal chemotherapy: An overview. *Semin Oncol* 12:12-16, 1985.

Neijt JP, ten Bokkel Huinink WW, van der Burg MEL: Randomized trial comparing two combination chemotherapy regimens (CHAP-5 vs. CP) in advanced ovarian carcinoma. *J Clin Oncol* 5:1157-1168, 1987.

Neijt JP, van der Burg MEL, Vriesendorp R, et al: Randomized trial comparing two combination chemotherapy regimens (Hexa-CAF vs. CHAP-5) in advanced ovarian carcinoma. *Lancet* 2:594-598, 1984

Newlands, ES, Bagshawe, KD, Begent, RHJ, et al: Development in chemotherapy for medium- and high-risk patients with geotation trophoblastic tumors (1979-1984). *BR J Obstet Gynecol* 93:63, 1986.

Neijt JP, Vanlindert ACM, Vendrijk CPJ, et al: Hexa-CAF combination chemotherapy and other multiple drug regimens in advanced ovarian carcinoma: Present and future. *Neth J Med* 22:38, 1979.

Nissen-Meyer R: Breast cancer. In Jones, Salmon SE (eds): *Adjuvant Therapy of Cancer*, Vol II. New York, Grune and Stratton, 1979, p 207.

Norris HJ, Zirkin HJ, Benson WL: Immature (malignant) teratoma of the ovary: A clinical and pathologic study of 58 cases. *Cancer* 37:2359, 1976.

Ohta A: Basic and clinical studies on the simultaneous combination treatment of cervical cancer with a carcinostatic agent and radiation. *J Tokyo Med Coll* 36:529, 1978.

Omura GA, Blessing JA, Major F, et al: A randomized trial of Adriamycin versus no adjuvant chemotherapy in stage I and II uterine sarcomas. *J Clin Oncol* 9:1240, 1985.

Omura G, Blessing JA, Ehrlich CE, et al: A randomized trial of cyclophosphamide and doxorubicin with or without cisplatin in advanced ovarian carcinoma. *Cancer* 57:1725-1730, 1986.

Omura G, Major F: Phase III trial of Adriamycin versus Adriamycin and DTIC in the treatment of stage III, IV, or recurrent uterine sarcomas. *Cancer* 52:40, 1983.

Ozols RF, Cunnion RE, Klecher RW Jr, et al: Verapamil and Adriamycin in the treatment of drug resistant ovarian cancer patients. *J Clin Oncol* 5:641-647, 1987.

Parker LM, Griffiths CT, Yankee RA, et al: Combination chemotherapy with Adriamycin-cyclophosphamide for advanced ovarian carcinoma. *Cancer* 46:669-674, 1980.

Piver MS, Barlow JJ, Vongtama V, et al: Hydroxyurea: A radiation potentiator in carcinoma of the uterine cervix. *Am J Obstet Gynecol* 174:803, 1983.

Rogan AM, Hamilton TC, Young RC, Ozols RF: In Salmon S (ed): *Proceedings of the 4th Human Tumor Cloning Conference*. Orlando, Florida, Grune and Stratton, 1984, pp 383-388.

Rutledge F: The role of radical hysterectomy in adenocarcinoma of endometrium. *Gynecol Oncol* 2:331, 1974.

Salazar OM, Bonfiglio TA, Patten SF, Keller BE, Feldstein ML, Dunne ME, Rudolph JH: Uterine sarcomas: Analysis of failures with special emphasis on the use of adjuvant radiation therapy. *Cancer* 42:1161, 1978a.

Salazar OM, Bonfiglio TA, Patten SF, Keller BE, Feldstein ML, Dunne ME, Rudolph JH: Uterine sarcomas: Natural history, treatment and prognosis. *Cancer* 42:1152, 1978b.

Salazar OM, Feldstein ML, DePapp EW, Bonfiglio TA, Keller BE, Rubin P, Rudolph JH: The management of clinical stage I endometrial carcinoma. *Cancer* 41:1-16, 1978c.

Santoro A, Bonadonna G, Bonfante V, Valagussa P: Alternating drug combinations in the treatment of advanced Hodgkin's disease. *N Engl J Med* 306:770, 1982.

Seski JC, Edwards CL, Herson J, et al: Cisplatin chemotherapy for disseminated endometrial cancer. *Obstet Gynecol* 59:225, 1982.

Skipper HE: Reasons for success and failure in treatment of murine leukemias with drugs now employed in treating human leukemias. *Cancer Chemother Rep* 1:1, 1978.

Slayton RE, Hreshchyshyn MM, Silverberg SG, Shingleton HM, Park RC, DiSaia PJ, Blessing JA: Treatment of malignant ovarian germ cell tumors: Response to vincristine, dactinomycin, and cyclophosphamide. *Cancer* 42:390, 1978.

Smales E, Peckham MJ: Chemotherapy of germ cell ovarian tumors. *Eur J Cancer Clin Oncol* 23:469-473, 1987.

Smith JP: Chemotherapy in gynecologic cancer. *Clin Obstet Gynecol* 18:109, 1975.

Smith JP, Rutledge F, Wharton JT: Chemotherapy of ovarian cancer. *Cancer* 30:1565, 1972.

Suzukake K, Petro BJ, Vistica DT: Reduction in glutathione content of L-PAM resistant L1210 cells confers drug sensitivity. *Biochem Pharmacol* 31:121, 1982.

Suzukake K, Vistica BP, Vistica DT: Dechlorination of L-phenylalanine mustard sensitive and resistant cells and its relationship to intracellular glutathione content. *Biochem Pharmacol* 32:165, 1983.

Swenerton KD: Treatment of advanced endometrial adenocarcinoma with tamoxifen. *Cancer Treat Rep* 64:805-811, 1980.

Swenerton KS, Evers JA, White GW, Boyes DA: Intermittent pelvic infusion with vincristine, bleomycin, and mitomycin C for advanced recurrent carcinoma of the cervix. *Cancer Treat Rep* 63:1379, 1979.

Tannock IF, Boyd NF, DeBoer G, et al: A randomized trial of two dose levels of cyclophosphamide, methotrexate, and fluorouracil chemotherapy for patients with metastatic breast cancer. *J Clin Oncol* 6:1377-1387, 1988.

ten Bokkel Huinink WW, Dubbelman R, Aartsen E, et al: Experimental and clinical results with intraperitoneal cisplatin. *Semin Oncol* 12:43-46, 1985.

Thigpen JT: Single agent chemotherapy in carcinoma of the cervix. In Surwit EA, Alberts DS (eds): *Cervix Cancer*. Boston, Martinus Nijhoff, 1987, pp 119-136.

Thigpen JT, Buchsbaum HJ, Mangan C, Blessing JA: Phase II of Adriamycin in the treatment of advanced or recurrent endometrial carcinoma: A Gynecologic Oncology Group study. *Cancer Treat Rep* 63:21, 1979.

Thigpen JT, Shingleton H, Homesley H, et al: Cisplatinum in treatment of advanced or recurrent squamous cell carcinoma of the cervix: A phase II study of the Gynecologic Oncology Group. *Cancer* 48:899-903, 1981.

Trope C: A prospective randomized trial comparison of melphalan vs. melphalan-Adriamycin in advanced ovarian carcinoma. *Proc Am Soc Clin Oncol* 22:469, 1981.

Tsuruo T, Lida H, Tsukagoshi S, Sakurai Y: Overcoming of vincristine resistance in P388 leukemia *in vivo* and *in vitro* through enhanced cytotoxicity of vincristine and vinblastine by verapamil. *Cancer Res* 41:1967, 1981.

Turbow MD, Thornton J, Ballon S, et al: Chemotherapy of advanced endometrial carcinoma with platinum, Adriamycin and cyclophosphamide. *Proc Am Soc Clin Oncol* 1:108, 1982.

Twiggs LB, Potash RA, McIntyre S, et al: Concurrent weekly cisplatinum and radiotherapy in advanced cervical cancer: A preliminary dose escalating toxicity study. *Gynecol Oncol* 24:143, 1986.

Van Nagell JR, Donaldson ES, Gay EC: Evaluation and treatment of patients with invasive cervical cancer. *Surg Clin N Am* 58:67, 1978.

Vogelzang N: Continuous infusion chemotherapy: A critical review. *J Clin Oncol* 2:1289-1304, 1984.

Vogl SE, Pagano M, Davis T, et al: Platinum based combination chemotherapy versus melphalan for advanced ovarian carcinoma. *Proc Int Congr Chemother* 207:9-13, 1983.

Warren RD, Bender RA: Drug interactions with antineoplastic agents. *Cancer Treat Rep* 61:1231, 1977.

Williams CJ, Mead GM, Macbeth FR, et al: Cisplatin combination chemotherapy versus chlorambucil in advanced ovarian carcinoma: Mature results of a randomized trial. *J Clin Oncol* 3:1455-1462, 1985.

Young RC, Chabner BA, Hubbard SM, Fisher RI, Bender RA, Anderson T, Simon RM, DeVita VT: Advanced ovarian adenocarcinoma: A prospective clinical trial of melphalan (L-PAM) vs. combination chemotherapy (Hexa-CAF). *N Engl J Med* 299:1261, 1978.

Young RC, Decker DG, Wharton JT, et al: Staging laparotomy in early ovarian cancer. *JAMA* 250:3072-3076, 1983.

Young RC, Myers CE, Ozols RF, Hogan WM: Cancer of the ovary: Chemotherapy in advanced disease. *Int J Radiol Oncol Biol Phys* 8:889, 1982.

Young RC, Walton LA, Ellenberg SS, et al: Adjuvant therapy in stage I and stage II epithelial ovarian cancer. *N Engl J Med* 322:1017, 1990.

# Chapter 6 | The Radiobiologic Basis for Radiation Therapy

*James A. Belli*

The utility and efficacy of radiation in the treatment of human neoplastic disease are based upon extensive empiric experience and observation. Improvements in radiotherapy will be made only if we can gain a thorough understanding of the biologic effects of this modality. This chapter will describe briefly the physical principles underlying the interaction of electromagnetic and particulate radiation with matter; examine the details of the response of mammalian cells to radiation; identify factors that are important in modifying cell and tissue responses to radiation; and identify potential approaches in experimental radiation therapy, particularly as these apply to the treatment of gynecologic cancer.

There is, however, a caveat. The perceptive reader will recognize that the major contribution of cellular radiation biology to radiation therapy has been to establish the information base used to explain the success of an empiric radiotherapeutic approach. The vast increase in our understanding of the response of mammalian cells to radiation has not generally led to changes in radiation therapy techniques based upon biologic information. Nonetheless, radiobiologic insights provide the basis for the appreciation and understanding of radiation as a major modality in the treatment of human neoplastic diseases.

It is not my purpose here to present an exhaustive review of the substantial literature on mammalian cell radiation biology. For the reader who wishes to review in detail some of the principles considered in this chapter, a number of monographs are available (Elkind and Whitmore, 1967; Hall, 1978; Alper, 1979).

## PHYSICAL AND CHEMICAL INTERACTIONS

### Physical Considerations

Radiation can be conveniently divided into two types: electromagnetic and particulate. *Electromagnetic radiation* consists of "packets" of energy (quanta) characterized by energy and wavelength (photons). Visible light, ultraviolet light, infrared light, and x-rays are well-known examples of this type of radiation. *Particulate radiation* consists of particles with mass and, except in the case of neutrons, charge. Examples are electrons, protons, alpha particles, neutrons, negative pi ($\pi$) mesons, and certain stripped atomic nuclei (e.g., neon, argon, and silicon).

The absorption events of radiation, whether particulate or electromagnetic (photons), result in changes at the atomic and subatomic levels that are precisely known. For example, absorption of a photon by an atom of the irradiated material can result in excitation or ionization. *Excitation* results when an orbital electron changes to a higher energy level; the electron remains within the influence of the nucleus. *Ionization* occurs when the absorption event causes ejection of an electron from its orbit. These events are accompanied by release of substantial amounts of energy, particularly in the ionization process, which is sufficient to break most chemical bonds.

Electromagnetic radiation is of two types: x-rays (roentgen rays) and gamma rays. Their biologic effects are comparable; the difference resides in their production or source. *X-rays* are produced in a machine capable of accelerating electrons across a large potential difference and against a suitable target material. The resulting interactions between the electrons and the target material produce x-rays that are used therapeutically. A modern linear accelerator is an example of such a facility. *Gamma rays* are also photons but are produced as a consequence of the decay of certain radioactive isotopes. The most common example is radioactive cobalt ($^{60}$Co), the decay properties and characteristics of which result in the emission of photons of electromagnetic radiation. These photons (gamma rays) can also be used radiotherapeutically. The biologic and therapeutic effects of these beams are the same.

### Chemical Considerations

The biologic effects of radiation absorption begin with the initial, instantaneous physical interactions described briefly above. These are followed by rapid chemical reactions that can be described as either indirect or direct. Direct effects result when a photon or particle is absorbed in a molecule of biologic importance, and the expression of the resultant molecular change is eventually identified as a biologic effect. However, living systems consist predominantly of water, and indirect effects are based upon the ionization events produced by energy absorption in this important molecule.

Important chemical species produced by the irradiation of water are the hydrated electron, the hydroxyl (OH) radical, hydrogen peroxide ($H_2O_2$), the perhydroxyl radical ($O_2H$), and free electrons. Because of their state of ionization, these chemical species, except for hydrogen peroxide, are highly reactive, and the majority of them react with each other to re-form water. However, if the diffusion distances and proximity of important biologic macromolecules are appropriate, interaction with these molecules will occur within $10^{-10}$ second. The resultant chemical reactions lead to altered macromolecular conformations that are eventually expressed as biologic damage. Obviously, because of the abundance of water within living systems, registration of damage by ionizing radiation is generally mediated through initial interactions in water molecules, hence the term *indirect effect*.

The radiation dose is specified in terms of units related to the ionization reduced in a standard volume of air at standard temperature and pressure (roentgen). A more appropriate measure of radiation dose is the *rad*, which is defined as the absorption of 100 erg per gram of absorbing material. More recently, the rad has been replaced by the Gray; 1 Gray equals 100 rads and 1 rad equals 1 centigray (cGy).

## MAMMALIAN CELL RADIATION BIOLOGY

### Biologic End Points of Radiation Effects

The biologic expression of radiation damage may be one of a range of effects, from death of the organism to mutation of a single gene. The expression of damage registered at the time of energy absorption may occur within seconds or may take hundreds of years, spanning several generations.

The common designation for quantitation of animal death is the lethal dose-50 ($LD_{50}$), usually specified for a particulr length of time after irradiation. $LD_{50}$ refers to that radiation dose which will kill 50% of a population exposed to total-body irradiation within a specified length of time. $LD_{50(30)}$ for humans (i.e., that dose which will kill 50% of individuals given total-body irradiation within 30 days) is approximately 450 cGy. Animal death is the result of the interaction of a variety of responses in cells and tissues as modified by host defense mechanisms and can be related to cellular events occurring at the time of irradiation.

At the other end of the spectrum, one can measure mutation rates, production of benign and malignant neoplasms, and chromosomal aberrations. Mutations and carcinogenic effects are particularly important because these end points have been used to establish permissible levels of exposure for radiation workers and populations exposed to radiation. The study of chromosomal aberrations has fundamental biologic importance to our understanding of cell biology in general and radiation effects in particular. The important chromosomal aberrations consequent to radiation exposure are ring chromosomes, dicentrics, anaphase bridges (chromatids), and chromosome fragments.

However important these biologic effects are to our fundamental understanding of radiation effects in biologic systems, they are not directly relevant to the end point of interest to the oncologist. The success or failure of a particular therapeutic strategy in human neoplastic disease depends upon the presence or absence of tumor cells that retain the capacity to divide in an unlimited fashion. If one or more cells retain this capacity, tumor will recur in the region toward which the initial strategy was directed. On the other hand, if the capacity for unlimited division of tumor cells in the treated region has been completely suppressed, tumor will not recur.

Thus, with regard to radiation, the mammalian cell end point that determines the success or failure of a therapeutic strategy is the capacity for cells to divide without limit in the treated volume.

Analysis of irradiated cells to determine whether they expressed unlimited division as an end point began with the work of Puck and his associates (Puck and Marcus, 1956; Puck et al, 1957) and continued with the in vivo work of Hewitt (1958) and Hewitt and Wilson (1959). Subsequently, radiation survival responses were described for bone marrow stem cells in vivo (Till and McCulloch, 1961), intestinal crypt cells (Withers and Elkind, 1970), and stem cells of the skin (Withers, 1967).

It is common to express cell death after irradiation as interphase or mitotic. *Interphase death* was originally used to describe the radiation effects on mature, peripheral lymphocytes. These cells are exquisitely sensitive to irradiation, disappearing from the circulation very rapidly in response to small doses of total-body irradiation in experimental animals and humans. Thus, the term *interphase* refers to the effects of radiation on cell populations that have reached the end of their reproductive history. *Mitotic death* is used to describe inactivation of cells that are actively dividing. Unfortunately, it has been used to indicate that cell death following irradiation occurs *during* mitosis. Cell death can occur at any point in the cell cycle of dividing cells; in fact, if the cell enters mitosis following irradiation, it is likely to complete that event. More precisely, therefore, the term *interphase death* should be used to refer to the inactivation of cells in *nondividing* populations and *mitotic death* to the sterilization of cells within a *dividing* population.

### Properties of Mammalian Cell Survival Curves

An important characteristic of continuous lines of mammalian cells grown in culture is their capacity to attach to a suitable surface. After attachment, viable cells begin dividing and, when an appropriate time has elapsed, the progeny of the original plated cell form a colony that is visible macroscopically. When stained, the number of colonies can be scored and related to the original number of cells plated. This ratio indicates the fraction of cells in the original population capable of unlimited division and can also be used to determine the surviving fraction of cells after a particular radiation dose.

When a known number of cells is exposed to different doses of radiation and colony formation is scored (as described above), the survival fraction, which decreases with increasing dose, can be determined. The resulting data can be plotted on semilogarithmic coordinates because the probability of absorption of an initial photon can be described by Poisson statistics. This approach predicts that absorption of a particular quantum of energy is determined by predictable probabilities and that subsequent absorption events are independent of those which have already occurred.

When mammalian cells in culture are irradiated with graded doses of radiation, survival fractions are produced which, when plotted on semilogarithmic coordi-

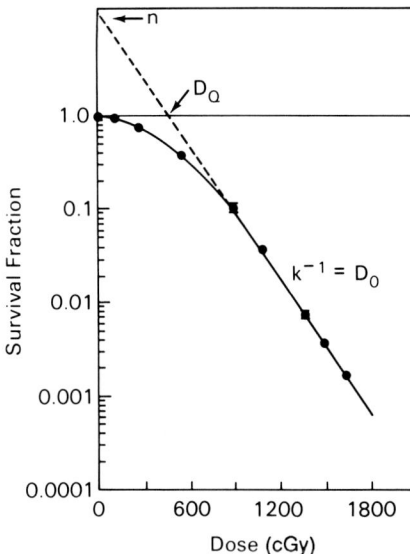

FIGURE 6-1 Single-dose survival curve for mammalian cells in culture. The curve starts with an initial threshold, followed by an exponential decrement in survival. The reciprocal of the slope ($k$) is $D_0$, the dose required to reduce survival fraction by $e^{-1}$ on the straight-line portion of the curve. The extrapolation number ($n$) is the number to which the straight-line portion of the curve extrapolates back to dose = 0. $D_Q$ is the intersection of this back-extrapolate with the dose axis at survival fraction = 1. (See text for discussion.)

nates, result in the survival curve shown in Figure 6-1. This survival curve has the following characteristics:

1. The curve starts with an initial threshold region. This means that at low radiation doses, little if any cell killing is observed. In addition, the slope of the survival curve in the region of a low radiation dose is constantly changing.

2. The threshold region of the survival curve is followed by an exponential decrement in survival as the radiation dose increases. The incremental decrease in survival per incremental increase in radiation dose is a constant, i.e., the straight-line portion of the survival curve can be described by a constant slope ($-k$). It is convenient to describe this slope by the dose which reduces survival by a factor of $e^{-1} = 0.368$. This value is defined as $D_0$. Because $D_0$ is related to the slope of the exponential portion of the survival curve, it is a direct measure of the radiosensitivity of the cells being studied. The radiosensitivity of any cell population is defined as the rate of survival decrement relative to the radiation dose. Thus, as $D_0$ increases, radiation sensitivity decreases; as $D_0$ decreases, radiation sensitivity increases. The concept of radiation sensitivity as defined in this way has important implications for the response of tumors in human populations.

3. Graphic extrapolation of the straightline (exponential) portion of the survival curve to its intersection with the zero-dose axis yields a number, greater than 1, which has been defined as the *extrapolation number* ($n$). The value of the extrapolation number is directly related to the extent of the threshold of the single-dose radiation survival curve. The definition of the extrapolation number leads to a closer

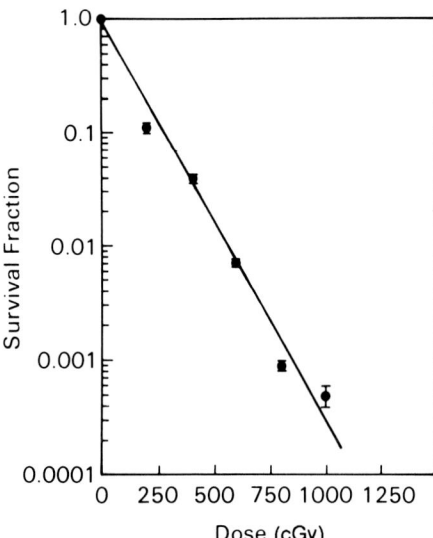

FIGURE 6-2 Example of exponential survival curve showing no threshold, as compared with the curve in Figure 6-1.

examination of the biologic implications of the threshold region of the radiation survival curve. In Figure 6-2, a survival curve is shown which does not have a threshold, i.e., the decrement of survival with increasing doses of radiation begins exponentially at the zero dose. The implication of such a survival curve is that cells being irradiated express radiation injury in an all-or-none fashion; that is, if damaged, the cell will not survive (divide indefinitely). In other words, all radiation doses—no matter how small—will kill cells.

Returning to Figure 6-1, we see that the initial portion of the survival curve has a threshold, implying that the cells being irradiated are capable of sustaining a given level of radiation damage without being killed relative to their capacity for unlimited division. Damage registered at the time of irradiation that does *not* result in cell death has been termed *sublethal injury* (see later). Most mammalian cells are capable of accumulating sublethal radiation damage and do not express exponential survival until the registration of sublethal injury has been saturated.

4. Another measure of the amount of sublethal damage tolerated by mammalian cells is the quasi-threshold dose ($D_Q$). This dose is given by the intersection of the back-extrapolate of the exponential portion of the survival curve with the dose axis when the survival fraction equals 1 (Fig. 6-1). It is convenient to look upon $D_Q$ as the radiation dose necessary to reach saturation of sublethal injury. The $D_Q$, extrapolation number, and $D_0$ are related by the following equation:

$$D_Q = D_0 \ln(n)$$

In summary, the single-dose radiation survival curve for mammalian cells in culture can be described by $D_0$, which is the dose necessary to reduce survival by $e^{-1}$ on the exponential portion of the survival curve and defines the radiosensitivity of the population being studied. The extrapolation number, usually greater than 1, is a measure of the amount of sublethal injury a cell population is capable of accumulating before an exponential response is observed. $D_Q$ is the radiation dose required to reach saturation of sublethal damage. Once this point is reached, cells require only one additional inactivating event (exponential survival) before being inactivated.

## The Oxygen Effect

The influence of molecular oxygen on the radiation response of normal and neoplastic tissues is important to the radiation therapist. On purely biologic grounds, the oxygen effect is one of the most important in radiation biology and has been studied extensively in bacterial systems (Alper, 1961 and 1967; Alper and Howard-Flanders, 1956), in mammalian cells in vitro (Dewey, 1960; Elkind et al, 1965; Revesz and Littbrand, 1964), and in vivo (Belli and Andrews, 1963; Deschner and Gray, 1959; Berry and Andrews, 1961). Figure 6-3 shows the differences in single-dose radiation survival properties of mammalian cells in the presence or absence of oxygen. The following features are important:

1.  The ratio of the slope of the oxic curve relative to that of the hypoxic curve is 2.5 to 3.5. This means that, in the exponential portion of the survival curves, a radiation dose 2.5 to 3.5 times higher is needed to produce the same survival fraction in the absence of oxygen compared with the dose required when oxygen is present.
2.  The extrapolation number for both curves is equal, suggesting that the presence or absence of oxygen does not influence the level of sublethal injury tolerated by cells. When survival curves of mammalian cells vary only with respect to the final slope, the curves can be described by a dose-modifying factor (DMF), which, in the case of the oxygen effect, is

termed the *oxygen enhancement ratio (OER)*. For a large variety of mammalian cells, both normal and abnormal, the OER falls within the range of 2.5 to 3.5.

3.  The oxygen effect is a classic example of a means of producing a change in radiation sensitivity, since the effect is expressed almost exclusively by a change in the slope of the single-dose radiation survival curve.

One of the important features of tumor growth is that foci of hypoxic cells may appear when cells are displaced more than 150 μm away from a capillary (Thomlinson, 1977; Thomlinson and Gray, 1955). This distance is the effective diffusion distance for oxygen, and cells so displaced will, in all likelihood, be deficient with regard to oxygen tension (pO2). The significance of the presence of hypoxic cells in human tumors with regard to the probability of local control with radiation has not been firmly established. It can be argued that hypoxic cells within a tumor mass have, geographically, entered a physiologic state that will eventually lead to cell death.

The issue of hypoxic cells in human neoplastic disease may be important in the radiation therapy of at least two types of tumors of the female reproductive tract. In advanced carcinoma of the cervix, the probability of local control of pelvic disease with external-beam radiation is, unfortunately, low. This experience may reflect the presence of large numbers of hypoxic tumor cells. In another instance, women with carcinoma of the ovary who present with ascites are more effectively treated with chemotherapeutic agents and/or whole-abdomen irradiation following paracentesis and/or surgical debulking. Whether or not the improved efficacy of these modalities is due to reduction of tumor burden or removal of populations of hypoxic cells cannot be determined from current clinical information. Suffice it to say, however, that both radiation and, to a lesser extent, chemotherapeutic agents are more effective when tumor cells are well oxygenated and the tumor cell burden is low.

Figure 6-4 demonstrates the relationship between pO2 and relative radiation sensitivity. Note that the OER increases rapidly with small increases in pO2 and reaches a maximum value between 20 and 30 mm Hg at 37°C. This level of pO2 is well within the range of the pO2 of venous blood, and significant changes in radiation sensitivity are observed only at very low pO2 values.

In summary, oxygen is an important modifier of radiation sensitivity, and mammalian cells are 2.5 to 3.5 times more resistant when irradiated in the absence of oxygen. Whether or not this effect influences the probability of local control of human tumors is not known. Nevertheless, the role of oxygen in determining radiotherapeutic results is being actively investigated in the clinic and laboratory.

## Reoxygenation

Consider the case of a solid tumor large enough to contain a certain proportion of hypoxic cells. Further,

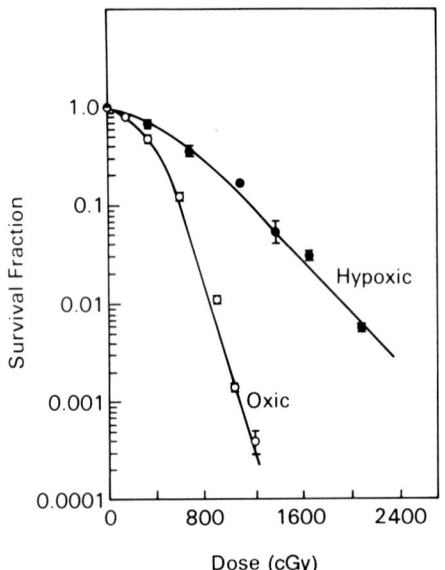

**FIGURE 6-3** Survival properties of mammalian cells in culture under oxic or hypoxic conditions. The ratio of the final slopes is the oxygen enhancement ratio (OER), usually 2.5 to 3.5.

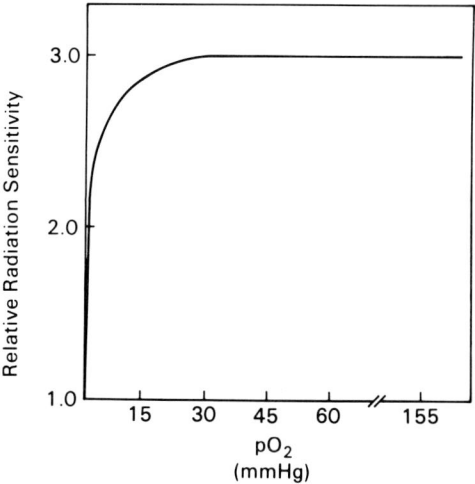

FIGURE 6-4 Relationship between relative radiation sensitivity and $pO_2$. Relative radiation sensitivity increases rapidly with small increases in oxygen tension and reaches a maximum below the $pO_2$ of venous blood.

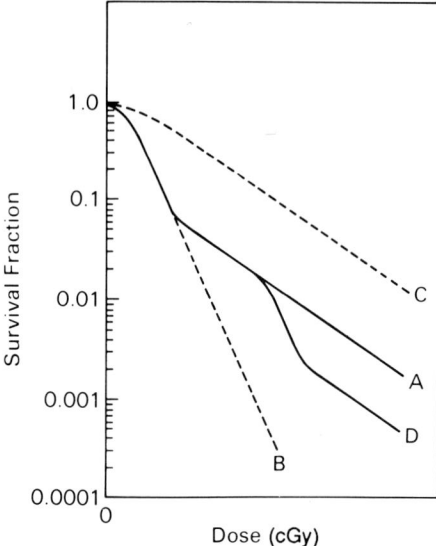

FIGURE 6-5 Curve A represents the single-dose survival fraction of a population of cells in which 10% of the population is hypoxic. Note the inflection point when the survival fraction equals 0.07. The dashed curves (B and C) represent the single-dose survival curves for fully oxic and fully hypoxic populations, respectively. After a radiation dose to reduce survival to about 0.02, followed by a time interval, curve D results when survivors are irradiated to variable second doses. Note that the initial portion of curve D has the same slope as that of curve B and that the eventual slope of curve D is parallel to that of curve C. This indicates that the survivors that were hypoxic at the time of the initial irradiation have reestablished complex survival curve properties, indicating reoxygenation.

assume that this proportion of hypoxic cells is approximately 10%. If one were to determine the single-dose survival curve for *all* the cells in this tumor, curve A shown in Figure 6-5 would result. The dashed curves represent the single-dose survival curves for the fully oxygenated (curve B) and fully hypoxic (curve C) populations. At low radiation doses, the predominant population (i.e., the oxygenated cells, 90%) dominates in the net survival fraction. As the radiation dose increases and cell killing of oxygenated cells becomes more prominent, the hypoxic population contributes to most of the net survivors, even though this population represents only 10% of the total. The final slope of curve A is therefore similar to the final slope of a completely hypoxic population.

If the radiation dose is sufficiently large—i.e., if the survival fraction is on the terminal slope of curve A—it can be assumed that relatively few of the survivors represent initially oxygenated cells. If time is allowed to elapse, the initial single-dose survival curve is recapitulated (curve D). This finding can be interpreted to mean that in the time elapsed after the initial radiation dose, previously hypoxic cells were reoxygenated and the hypoxic fraction was reduced to 10%.

This phenomenon has been described in experimental mouse tumors (van Putten and Kallman, 1968), and the time for reoxygenation has been estimated to be less than 24 hours. Upon close examination, this time course would be considered short to account for the physiologic changes needed for reoxygenation of previously hypoxic cells. First, even though well-oxygenated cells may have been reproductively sterilized by radiation, a substantial proportion may continue to metabolize and require oxygen for extended periods of time. This would result in a persistent nutritional disadvantage, including the lack of oxygen, for hypoxic cells. Second, reorganization of vascular structures consequent to the loss of cells from tumor cell populations would probably require longer periods of time than those required for the

"radiobiologic" reoxygenation observed in experimental animal tumor systems. For these reasons, it is not possible to state whether or not reoxygenation plays an important role in the response of human tumors to fractionated radiation.

## CELL-CYCLE EFFECTS

Mammalian cells growing exponentially are distributed randomly throughout the four compartments of the cell cycle (Fig. 6-6). These compartments have been designated $G_1$, S, $G_2$, and M to represent the presynthetic phase, DNA synthesis, the postsynthetic phase, and mitosis, respectively. Compartmental analysis of the cell cycle depends upon the observation of certain morphologic events. First among these is *mitosis*. In an appropriately stained population of exponentially growing mammalian cells, the proportion of cells in mitosis can be scored and the mitotic index—i.e., the ratio of cells undergoing mitosis to the total cell population observed—can be estimated. In most mammalian cell populations, the mitotic index is in the range of 2 to 7%.

The second directly observable event is the period of *DNA synthesis*. To estimate the proportion of cells in DNA synthesis, exponentially growing cells are exposed to a precursor of DNA that has been labeled with an appropriate isotope (usually tritium). During a brief

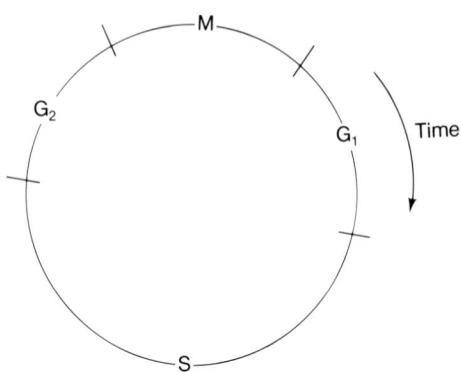

FIGURE 6-6 The cell cycle. M = mitosis; $G_1$ = presynthetic phase; S = DNA synthetic phase; $G_2$ = postsynthetic phase. The time required to traverse the entire cycle is the generation time, and each compartment contains proportions of cells equal to the total time occupied by that compartment within the cycle.

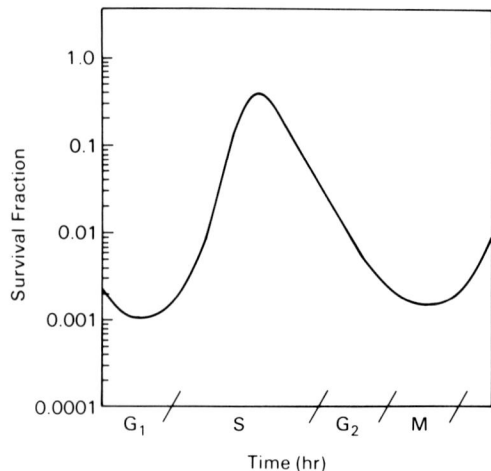

FIGURE 6-7 Variation in survival relative to radiation can be considered a function of the cell-cycle phase. Middle and late S constitute a resistant phase, and $G_2$ and M are sensitive phases. $G_1$ may be sensitive and/or resistant, depending upon its length.

exposure to the labeled precursor, only cells replicating DNA will be labeled, and these cells can be identified by appropriate autoradiographic techniques. The labeling index gives the proportion of cells in DNA synthesis (usually 50 to 65%).

The estimation of $G_1$ and $G_2$ utilizing autoradiographic techniques is time-consuming and laborious. However, more recently, flow cytometric techniques have become available in which cells appropriately stained with a DNA-specific fluorescent compound can be analyzed directly to determine their distribution throughout the cell cycle.

Important considerations in understanding the cell cycle are that (1) in exponentially growing populations, the proportion of cells in each of the four compartments remains constant; (2) the proportion of cells in each compartment is roughly proportional to the time required for completion of that particular cellular activity; (3) important macromolecular events occur between each division; and (4) accurate estimates of cell-cycle distributions can be obtained rapidly with modern technology.

Experimentally, it is possible to obtain cell populations in which the majority of cells are in a single compartment of the cell cycle and progress synchronously through subsequent compartments. Terasima and Tolmach (1963) synchronized cells in mitosis and determined the radiation survival properties as cells progressed through subsequent compartments. Similar determinations have been made for a variety of cell lines in cultures, and while the details of response may vary, the following general conclusions have been found: (1) when cells are in the process of DNA synthesis, they are most resistant to radiation; (2) when cells are in $G_2$ or mitosis, they are most radiation-sensitive; and (3) cells in $G_1$ may be sensitive if the time in the compartment is short, or they may exhibit a period of increased resistance when $G_1$ occupies a more significant portion of the total cell-cycle time. These generalizations are shown schematically in Figure 6-7.

It follows from these considerations that when an *asynchronous* population is irradiated with a sufficiently

large dose of radiation, the majority of the survivors represent cells that were in resistant response states at the time of exposure. Because these cells represent cells in DNA synthesis and because DNA synthesis occupies the majority of the cell-cycle time, a complex survival curve such as that depicted in Figure 6-5 (curve A) will not be observed with most cell types. Clearly, radiation can be considered a classic cell-cycle–specific agent. By implication, therefore, the radiation response of human tumors may be related to cell-cycle distributions of tumor cells. In addition, normal tissue responses may be dependent upon similar kinetic considerations.

## REPAIR OF RADIATION DAMAGE

### Levels of Damage

Operationally, damage registered in mammalian cells at the time of exposure to ionizing radiation can be of three types: (1) *lethal damage*, in which (when registered) suppression of unlimited division occurs under any circumstance; (2) *sublethal damage*, in which (when registered) cells with this level of damage eventually express unlimited division, and accumulation of this class of damage is the important implication of the presence of a threshold in a mammalian cell radiation survival curve; and (3) *potentially lethal damage*, which may be reparable to a nonlethal state if suitable postirradiation conditions are provided; if repair does not take place, conversion to a lethal state may occur and unlimited division will be suppressed. Note that characterization of these classes of radiation damage, particularly at the molecular level, is not possible; therefore, these are only operational definitions.

The concept of sublethal injury prompted Elkind and his associates to initiate a series of important studies in the repair of sublethal injury (Elkind and Sutton, 1960; Elkind et al, 1961; Elkind, 1965). The essential features of their observations are shown schematically in Figures

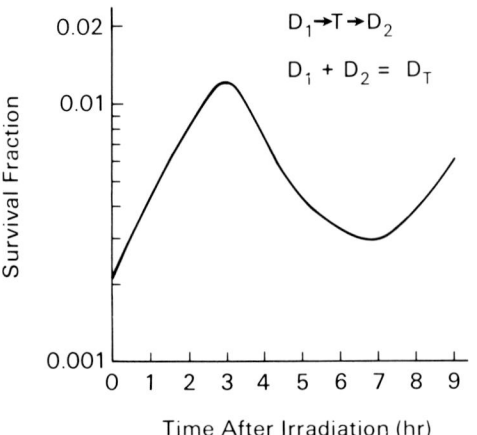

**FIGURE 6-8** Survival fluctuation as a function of the time between two equal radiation doses. The survival fraction at time zero is that observed when the total dose is delivered in one fraction. Survival increases to a maximum, followed by a decrease and a second increase. (See text for discussion.)

6-8 and 6-9. The survival fluctuations shown in Figure 6-8 represent those that result when a total radiation dose is divided into two fractions separated by variable lengths of time. Survival rapidly increases to a maximum, followed by a survival decrement and a second survival increase. Thus, the proportion of cells capable of unlimited division is greater when a total dose is divided into two fractions compared with survival when the total dose is delivered without interruption.

The survival decrease and second increase can be explained on the basis of the cell-cycle effects described

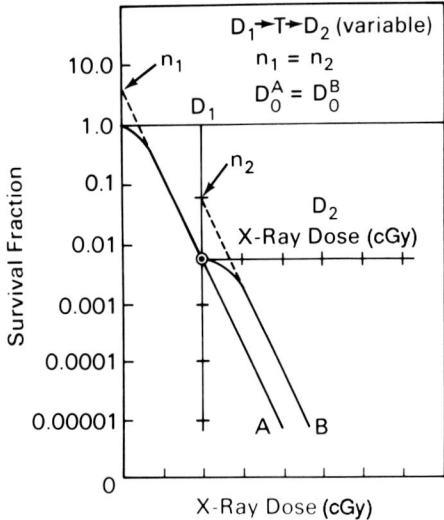

**FIGURE 6-9** Schematic curves showing survival-curve properties of cells surviving a conditioning radiation dose ($D_1$). Curve A represents the single-dose survival curve. Curve B is the survival curve of survivors to $D_1$ after a sufficient time has elapsed for complete repair of sublethal radiation injury (See text for discussion.) (From Belli JA, Piro AJ: *Principles of Radiation Biology.* Brookhaven National Laboratory Symposium on Interactions of Radiation and Host Immune Defense Mechanisms in Malignancy, Brookhaven National Laboratory Publication No. 50418, 1974, pp 99–118.)

above. The first radiation dose inactivates those cells which are in sensitive cell-cycle compartments at the time of exposure. As time is allowed to elapse before the second exposure, these surviving cells progress into cell-cycle compartments that are radiation-sensitive. If cells are irradiated during these cell-cycle shifts, net survival will decrease because of the change in the radiation response state. The second increase can be ascribed to both cell division and progression into radiation-resistant cell-cycle compartments. Thus, the survival fluctuations shown in Figure 6-8 can be ascribed to the repair of sublethal radiation injury and progression, after the initial radiation dose, into cell-cycle–dependent radiation response states.

The single-dose survival curve (A) shown in Figure 6-9 was obtained by irradiating mammalian cells with graded radiation doses. Consider the survivors irradiated with a level of radiation sufficiently high to reduce survival to the exponential portion of the survival curve ($D_1$). The single-dose survival curve had an initial extrapolation number of $n_1$. If the survivors to $D_1$ are given sufficient time and are then irradiated with variable second doses, survival curve B results. This survival curve has an extrapolation number of $n_2$. Note that the extrapolation number and $D_0$ of the fractionated survival curve are equal to those for cells not previously irradiated ($D_0^A = D_0^B$; $n_1^A = n_2^B$).

The important implication of these findings is that cells that have experienced saturation of sublethal injury will eventually regain their capacity to accumulate additional sublethal damage. This interpretation satisfies an important criterion for repair. Thus, surviving irradiated mammalian cells, if allowed sufficient time, will respond to subsequent exposure to x-rays as if the previous radiation dose had not been delivered.

These observations have important implications in terms of the consequences of fractionated and protracted radiation therapy. For example, a patient with carcinoma of the cervix treated with external-beam radiation is treated over a period of weeks, during which small amounts of radiation are delivered each day. The schematic survival curves in Figure 6-10 show that the net biologic effect of a total dose of radiation is less if the dose is delivered in multiple fractions rather than as a single exposure. Curve A is a schematic single-dose radiation survival curve. Curves B, C, D, and E represent the single-dose survival curves for cells exposed to fractions $D_1$, $D_2$, $D_3$, and $D_4$, (with $D_5$, and $D_1$ representing additional fractions). The dashed survival curve (F) is the net survival response of cells exposed to multiple fractions. It is clear that a single dose of radiation is more effective in producing cell kill than the same total dose delivered in multiple fractions. Clearly, other factors are important in the use of fractionated radiation to treat neoplastic disease, but the repair of sublethal injury between fractions probably plays an important role.

## Potentially Lethal Damage

This class of damage was defined above as that which, under ordinary circumstances, would be expressed as

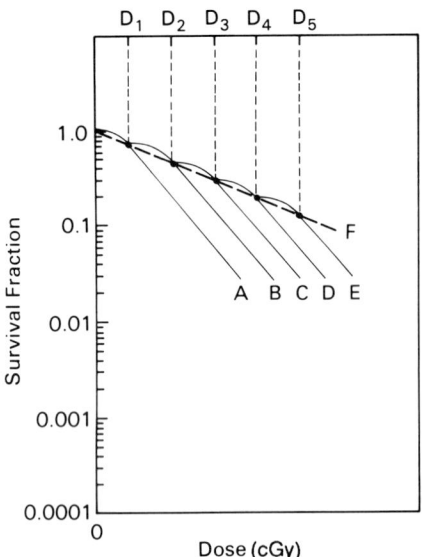

FIGURE 6-10 Schematic representation of the effect of fractionated-dose versus single-dose on survival. Curve A is the single-dose survival curve. Curve B is the survival curve following a single fractional dose. Curves C, D, and E represent survival curves following two, three, and four fractions, respectively. Curve F is the survival curve following $D_1$, $D_2$, $D_3$, $D_4$, and $D_5$.

lethal injury. However, if appropriate postirradiation conditions are provided, part of the registered damage may exist in a labile injury state that may be fixed to a lethal event or repaired, permitting unlimited division. There is now substantial evidence that survival of irradiated mammalian cells depends upon postirradiation conditions (Phillips and Tolmach, 1966; Belli and Shelton, 1969; Whitmore and Gulyas, 1967; Little, 1969; Belli et al, 1970). The general conclusion appears to be that when irradiated mammalian cells are provided with postirradiation conditions that are deficient with regard to cell growth, fluctuations in survival are observed that strongly suggest the repair of potentially lethal radiation injury. Figure 6-11A schematically depicts cell survival

after a *single* radiation exposure when cells are placed in a deficient postirradiation condition.

Conditions that promote an increase in survival after a single exposure to radiation include protein synthesis inhibitors (Phillips and Tolmach, 1966), a balanced salt solution (Belli and Shelton, 1969), low temperature (Whitmore and Gulyas, 1967), cells in the plateau phase of growth (Little, 1969; Belli et al, 1970), and hypoxia (Belli et al, 1970). The increase in survival as a consequence of the repair of potentially lethal damage, unlike that following the repair of sublethal injury, is due to a change in $D_0$ (Fig. 6-11B).

Recently, attempts have been made to establish the relationship between radiocurability and repair of potentially lethal injury using primary explants of human tumors (Weichselbaum et al, 1977). Although no clear correlation was found, such a relationship appeared to exist in cells isolated from human osteosarcoma (non-radiation-responsive) that were found to have a large capacity for repair of potentially lethal injury compared with tumors considered to be radiation responsive.

In summary, potentially lethal injury is that class of radiation damage the presence and repair of which are determined by an increase in survival following a *single* dose of radiation under environmental conditions that are deficient with regard to cell division. Whether or not this repair property plays a role in the response of tumors to fractionated radiation has not been clarified.

## DRUG–RADIATION DAMAGE INTERACTIONS

The advent of multiagent chemotherapeutic regimens in the treatment of cancer requires a detailed understanding of the interaction between these agents and radiation. Patients are likely to experience increased complications, both acute and late, as the consequence of interactions between drugs and radiation. In general, modification of the response to radiation by single or multiple cytotoxic drugs may be defined as additive, synergistic, or antagonistic. When two agents produce

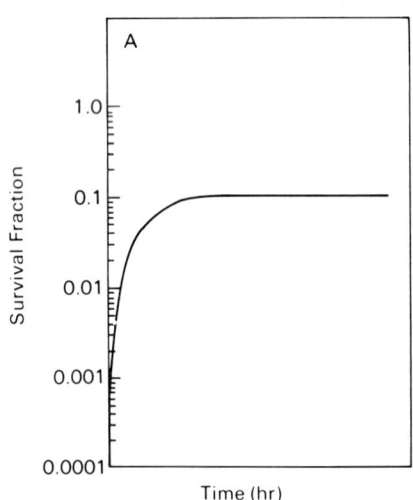

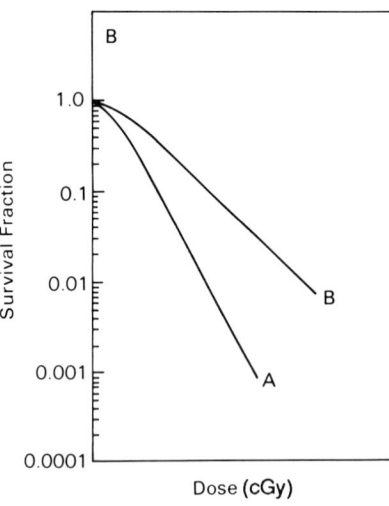

FIGURE 6-11 (A) Survival following a single radiation dose in terms of time after exposure. The survival increase is taken to indicate the repair of potentially lethal radiation injury.

(B) Repair of potentially lethal injury following variable single doses. Curve A represents the single-dose survival curve with no repair interval following irradiation. Curve B is the survival curve that results when cells are allowed time for complete repair of potentially lethal injury following variable single doses. Note that the survival increase is predominantly due to a change in the final slope.

*additive* effects, the total effect of the combination is equal to that produced by each agent independently. *Synergistic* effects result when the total effect of two agents is greater than the predicted effect of each agent by itself. *Antagonistic* interactions occur when the effect is less than that produced by each agent alone (protection).

Important interactions occur between chemotherapeutic agents and radiation. Some of these interactions have been studied extensively under well-controlled conditions, including the interactions between radiation and actinomycin D, doxorubicin (Adriamycin), halogenated pyrimidines, methotrexate, 5-fluorouracil, and cis-platinum. These chemotherapeutic agents interfere with repair of sublethal injury (actinomycin D, halogenated pyrimidines) and the capacity to accumulate sublethal injury (doxorubicin, methotrexate).

Another aspect of such damage interaction is that delayed effects can be observed when chemotherapeutic agents are delivered much later than irradiation. This is particularly true of actinomycin D and doxorubicin; acute reactions can be produced by these drugs when they are delivered some time after irradiation. These reactions can occur in the skin, mucous membranes, esophagus, heart, bladder, and gastrointestinal tract. Actinomycin D and doxorubicin are classic examples of drugs that produce so-called "recall reactions."

## EXPERIMENTAL RADIOTHERAPEUTIC APPROACHES

### General Considerations

Recently, a number of experimental approaches to radiation therapy have been examined in an effort to increase the efficacy of radiation for controlling local human neoplastic disease. These include (1) particulate radiation (including neutrons), (2) hyperthermia, and (3) agents that differentially sensitize hypoxic cells to radiation (hypoxic-cell sensitizers).

### Particulate Radiation

Neutrons, alpha particles, certain stripped atomic nuclei, electrons, and protons share the physical characteristics of mass and charge (except for neutrons, which are neutral). As a consequence, deposition of energy along the absorption track of the particle is greater than that observed with photons. Particles have high linear energy transfer (LET) characteristics. Except for neutrons and electrons, the dose distribution of charged particles in tissue is characterized by the absorption curve shown in Figure 6-12. As a particle enters tissue, it loses very little of its energy until it nears the end of its track, when energy deposition becomes rapid and high in a very small tissue volume. In contrast, the absorption of photons in tissue exhibits an exponential relationship (i.e., the dose is higher at or near the surface than at depth). The absorption of neutrons follows a curve similar to that of photons and does not show the peak of high-density energy distribution shown in Figure 6-12.

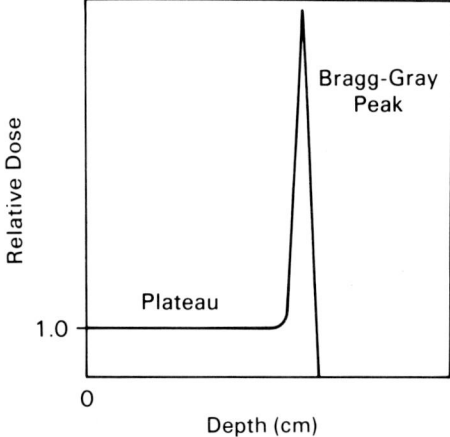

**FIGURE 6-12** Bragg-Gray curve depicting the dose distribution in absorbing material for charged particles. Note that the relative dose is low at and below the surface until the particle nears the end of its track and releases its energy in a very small volume.

Apart from these differences in physical characteristics, particles exhibit radiotherapeutic attraction for at least two biologic reasons. First, the survival curve for mammalian cells exposed to particulate radiation generally has no threshold. This implies that damage registered by particulate radiation is either lethal or nonlethal; the accumulation of sublethal injury is not possible. In addition, cells exposed to particles are less capable of showing increases in survival after fractionated particulate irradiation (i.e., sublethal damage is not repaired). Second, cells exposed to particles under hypoxic conditions do not demonstrate increased resistance. In fact, for most mammalian cells studied, the OER following exposure to particles approaches 1. Therefore, in those human tumors suspected of having a large proportion of hypoxic cells, treatment with particles such as neutrons may increase the probability of local control.

### Hyperthermia

Preheating mammalian cells 41 to 43°C prior to irradiation changes the single-dose survival properties, characterized by (1) a decrease in $D_0$ and increased radiation sensitivity, and (2) loss of the threshold of the survival curve. High temperature by itself is toxic to mammalian cells. There is good evidence that hypoxic cells are more sensitive to heat than are well-oxygenated cells. In addition, it has been found that thermotolerance can develop after a single heat exposure. Thus, hyperthermia, either alone or in combination with radiation, produces effects that are similar to those produced by particulate radiation, as discussed above.

Methods of local heating include ultrasound, shortwave diathermy, radiofrequency currents, and microwaves. All are currently being studied clinically. Unsettled issues include (1) the sequence of heat and radiation, (2) the interval between each modality, (3) specification of heat distributions in normal and neoplastic tissues at depth, and (4) determination of whether or not fractionated heat will result in thermo-tolerance of neoplastic cells.

### Sensitizers of Hypoxic Cells to Radiation

Nitroimidazoles are electron-affinic compounds (of which metronidazole [Flagyl] is an example) that differentially sensitize hypoxic cells to radiation. These compounds mimic oxygen in their modification of single-dose radiation responses. Clinically useful hypoxic-cell sensitizers must have the following characteristics (Hall, 1978):

1. The compound should selectively sensitize hypoxic cells at concentrations that result in acceptable toxicity to normal tissues.
2. The compound should be metabolically stable and not subject to rapid breakdown.
3. The compound must be soluble in water or lipid and must have the capacity to diffuse over large distances in order to exert its effect on hypoxic cells within tumor tissues.
4. The compound must be capable of sensitizing hypoxic cells to radiation throughout all phases of the cell cycle.
5. The compound should be effective at the relatively low daily radiation doses used in conventional fractionated radiation therapy.

The attraction of hypoxic-cell radiation sensitizers is based upon the assumption that hypoxic tumor cells influence the probability of local control after radiation therapy. As stated above, the question of whether or not hypoxic tumor cells are important in this regard has not been answered. Thus far, metronidazole and mizonidazole have been studied in clinical trials; far more experience has been obtained with the latter compound. However, its use in the clinic has been compromised by its substantial peripheral neurotoxicity. Attempts to modify molecular conformation and composition to avoid this toxicity are important aspects of current research regarding hypoxic-cell radiation sensitizers.

As the foregoing discussion demonstrates, the major directions in experimental radiation therapy—use of particles, hyperthermia, and hypoxic-cell radiation sensitizers—are toward the reproductive inactivation of hypoxic cells during fractionated radiation therapy. This is particularly important in late-stage carcinoma of the cervix, in which large tumor masses may include a substantial proportion of hypoxic cells. It is anticipated that continued progress in these areas of research will improve cancer control rates locally, in gynecologic cancer, and in tumors at other anatomic sites.

## SUMMARY

This brief review of the response of mammalian cells to radiation under a variety of environmental and experimental conditions has highlighted the following points:

1. The single-dose radiation survival curve of mammalian cells under well-controlled conditions, in which reproductive survival is measured as an end point, is characterized by an initial threshold, implying that mammalian cells are capable of accumulating sublethal injury followed by an exponential survival response.
2. The reciprocal of the final slope of the survival curve ($D_0$) is a direct measure of the radiation sensitivity of the cells being studied.
3. Mammalian cells are capable of repairing sublethal radiation injury if sufficient time is allowed between multiple radiation exposures.
4. Potentially lethal injury is reparable if mammalian cells are provided with environments deficient in the nutrients required for cell division after a *single* exposure.
5. As cells progress through the phases of their cycle, important changes in radiation response occur. In general, cells in mitosis and in $G_2$ are most sensitive and cells in S are most resistant. $G_1$ is a special compartment in which a resistant response state may occur if the phase is long enough.
6. Hypoxic cells are 2.5 to 3.5 times more resistant to single doses of radiation than are well-oxygenated cells. Whether or not hypoxic tumor cells are important in determining the probability of local tumor control is not yet clear.
7. Important interactions occur between chemotherapeutic agents and radiation. These interactions are characterized by changes in the single-dose radiation survival curve with regard to the threshold and final slope.
8. Important directions in experimental radiation therapy include the use of particulate radiation, hyperthermia, and hypoxic-cell radiation sensitizers. This research is directed specifically toward suppression of damage repair and differential sensitization of hypoxic tumor cells.

Understanding the biologic basis for radiation therapy can only increase the cooperation and collaboration between radiation, medical, and surgical oncologists. Successful collaboration demands an appreciation by all concerned of the important issues in each specialty. Like the surgical and medical oncologists, the radiation oncologist has a substantial body of experimental and clinical experience on which to base the effective and intelligent use of radiation. Local tumor control is the goal of both the surgeon and the radiation oncologist. The use of adjuvant chemotherapeutic agents for distant micrometastatic disease requires a detailed knowledge of the interaction between drugs and radiation and the influence of these interactions on surgically stressed tissues. As we begin to understand better the cellular processes that occur after irradiation and how these processes are influenced by surgical procedures and the use of chemotherapeutic agents, a more rational approach to combined management of human cancer will result.

## REFERENCES

Alper T: Variability in the oxygen effect observed with microorganisms. Part II. *Escherichia coli* B. *Int J Radiat Biol* 3:369-377, 1961.

Alper T: A characteristic of the lethal effect of ionizing radiation on "Her" bacterial strains. *Mutation Res* 4:15-20, 1967.

Alper T: *Cellular Radiobiology.* Cambridge, Cambridge University Press, 1979.

Alper T, Howard-Flanders P: The role of oxygen in modifying the radiosensitivity of *E. coli* B. *Nature (Lond)* 178:978-979, 1956.

Belli JA, Andrews JR: Relationship between tumor growth and radiosensitivity. *J Natl Cancer Instit* 31:689-703, 1963.

Belli JA, Dicus GJ, Nagle W: Repair of radiation damage as a factor in preoperative radiation therapy. *Front Radiat Ther Oncol* 5:40-57, 1970.

Belli JA, Shelton M: Potentially lethal radiation damage. Repair by mammalian cells in culture. *Science* 165:490-492, 1969.

Berry RJ, Andrews JR: Quantitative relationships between radiation dose and the reproductive capacity in a mammalian system *in vivo*. *Radiology* 77:824-830, 1961.

Deschner EE, Gray LH: Influence of oxygen tension on x-ray–induced chromosomal damage in Ehrlich ascites tumor cells irradiated *in vitro* and *in vivo*. *Radiat Res* 11:115-146, 1959.

Dewey DL: Effect of oxygen and nitric oxide on the radiosensitivity of human cells in tissue culture. *Nature (Lond)* 186:780-782, 1960.

Elkind MM: Repair of x-ray damage in mammalian cells. *Japan J Genet* 40:176-193, 1965.

Elkind MM, Sutton-Gilbert H: Radiation response of mammalian cells grown in culture. I. Repair of x-ray damage in surviving Chinese hamster cells. *Radiat Res* 13:556-593, 1960.

Elkind MM, Sutton-Gilbert H, Moses WB, Alescio T, Swain RW: Radiation response of mammalian cells grown in culture. V. Temperature dependence of the repair of x-ray damage in surviving cells (aerobic and hypoxic). *Radiat Res* 25:359-376, 1965.

Elkind MM, Whitmore E: *The Radiobiology of Cultured Mammalian Cells.* New York, Gordon and Breach, 1967.

Elkind MM, Sutton-Gilbert H, Moses WB: Postirradiation survival kinetics of mammalian cells grown in culture. *J Cell Comp Physiol* 58 (Suppl 1):113-134, 1961.

Hall EJ: *Radiobiology for the Radiologist*, 2nd ed. New York, Harper & Row, 1978.

Hewitt HB: Studies of the dissemination and quantitative transplantation of a lymphocytic leukemia of CBA mice. *Br J Cancer* 12:378-401, 1958.

Hewitt HB, Wilson CWA: Survival curves for tumor cells irradiated *in vivo*. *Br. J Cancer* 13:69-75, 1959.

Little JB: Repair of sub-lethal and potentially lethal radiation damage in plateau phase cultures of human cells. *Nature (Lond)* 224:804-806, 1969.

Phillips RA, Tolmach LJ: Repair of potentially lethal damage in x-irradiated HeLa cells. *Radiat Res* 29:413-432, 1966.

Puck TT, Marcus PI: Action of x-rays on mammalian cells. *J Exp Med* 103:653-666, 1956.

Puck TT, Morkovin D, Marcus PI, Cieciura SJ: Action of x-rays on mammalian cells. II. Survival curves of cells from normal human tissues. *J Exp Med* 106:483-500, 1957.

Revesz L, Littbrand B: Variation in the relative sensitivity of closely related neoplastic cell lines irradiated in culture in the presence or absence of oxygen. *Nature (Lond)* 203:742-744, 1964.

Terasima R, Tolmach LJ: X-ray sensitivity and DNA synthesis in synchronous populations of HeLa cells. *Science* 140:490-492, 1963.

Thomlinson RH: Hypoxia and tumors. *J Clin Pathol* Suppl 30(*R Coll Pathol*) 11:105-113(263), 1977.

Thomlinson RH, Gray LH: The histological structure of some human lung cancers and the possible implications for radiotherapy. *Br J Cancer* 9:539-549, 1955.

Till JWE, McCulloch EA: A direct measurement of the radiation sensitivity of normal mouse bone marrow stem cells. *Ratiat Res* 14:213-222, 1961.

van Putten LM, Kallman RF: Oxygen status of a transplantable tumor during fractionated radiotherapy. *J Natl Cancer Instit* 40:441-451, 1968.

Weichselbaum RR, Little JB, Nove J: Response of human osteosarcoma *in vitro* to irradiation: Evidence for unusual cellular repair activity. *Int J Radiat Biol* 31:295-299, 1977.

Whitmore GF, Gulyas S: Studies on recovery processes in mouse L cells. *Natl Cancer Inst Monogr* 24:141-156, 1967.

Withers HR: The dose-survival relationship for irradiation of epithelial cells of mouse skin. *Br J Radiol* 40:187-194, 1967.

Withers HR, Elkind MM: Microcolony survival assay for cells of mouse intestinal mucosa exposed to radiations. *Int J Radiat Biol* 17:261-267, 1970.

# *Chapter 7* | **The Practice of Radiotherapy**

**Lee M. Chin    Anthony E. Howes**

Soon after artificial x-rays and natural radioactivity were discovered at the turn of the century, ionizing radiation began to be applied to the diagnosis and treatment of diseases. In the wake of Roentgen's discovery of x-rays in 1895, reports of radiation effects appeared, with skin erythema and epilation among the first clinically observed phenomena. Indeed, in those early days there were no established units for measuring radiation, so that doses were frequently described in terms of their effects—e.g., "erythema doses." Today, however, ionizing radiation is one of the most carefully monitored and thoroughly studied therapeutic agents.

The biologic effects of ionizing radiation result from the absorption of radiation energy by living tissue. Although the effects differ for different types of radiation, they can ultimately be related to the absorption of energy and its distribution as a result of tissue interactions. The fundamental objective of radiotherapy is to deliver a dose of ionizing radiation sufficient to destroy all malignant cells within a given target volume without inflicting intolerable injury on associated normal cells and tissues. To optimize the therapeutic result, we must understand how radiation interacts with matter; how these interactions produce biochemical changes and subsequent biologic effects; and how these effects can be quantified, modified, and controlled in a given clinical situation.

The preceding chapter dealt with the biologic processes that occur when cells are exposed to radiation. In this chapter, we will address issues of physical dosimetry and treatment planning for tumors and normal tissues of importance in gynecologic oncology.

## FUNDAMENTAL CONCEPTS OF MATTER AND RADIATION

The fundamental building block of matter is the atom, which consists of a nuclear core and a peripheral "cloud" of orbiting electrons. The nuclear core has a radius of about $10^{-12}$ cm (nuclear radius) and contains neutrons and protons. Surrounding the nucleus are electrons that move in various orbits or shells with orbital radii of about $10^{-8}$ cm (atomic radius). Electrons are held in their orbits by the attractive force of the nucleus, and the energy required to keep each electron in the atomic configuration is called its *binding energy*. Atoms differ from one another in the composition of their nuclei and in the number and configuration of the orbiting electrons. In a neutral atom, the number of electrons constitutes the atomic number Z. Atoms range from the simple (hydrogen, $Z = 1$) to the complex (hahnium, $Z = 105$), and each atom has its own characteristic chemical and physical properties.

An electron has a very small mass ($9.1 \times 10^{-31}$ kg) and carries a negative charge ($1.6 \times 10^{-19}$ C). Protons have a mass about 1,860 times larger than that of electrons and carry a positive charge. Neutrons, on the other hand, have a mass comparable to that of protons but carry no charge. Therefore, the mass of an atom is concentrated in a core of $10^{-12}$ cm; however, the size of the atom is really defined by the radii of the orbiting electrons and increases with increasing Z.

Since the atom normally exists in an electrically neutral state, the number of electrons and protons must be equal; therefore, the atomic number Z conventionally denotes the number of protons or electrons in a neutral atom. For this reason, Z is used to identify the individual elements.

The atomic mass, conventionally denoted by the symbol A, is the total number of protons and neutrons in the nucleus. Atoms consisting of nuclei with the same number of protons (the same Z) but a different number of neutrons are called *isotopes*. Isotopes may be stable or unstable. In general, unstable isotopes have an unbalanced number of protons and neutrons and seek to reach an equilibrium by ejecting one or more particles from the nucleus until a stable isotope results. During this process, energy is released, often in the form of ionizing radiation. The classic designations for the emitted radiations are alpha, beta, and gamma radiations. *Alpha particles* are, in essence, positively charged helium nuclei. *Beta particles* are electrons. *Gamma rays* are electromagnetic waves that oscillate at various frequencies. The product of the frequency and the wavelength is the speed of the wave; for electromagnetic waves traveling in a vacuum, this is the speed of light. According to the quantum description of nature, the energy of the electromagnetic wave travels in discrete bundles. These discrete energy bundles are called *quanta* or *photons*. The energy of the photon is directly proportional to the frequency of the wave. Figure 7-1 shows the relationship of frequency, wavelength, and the energy of the electromagnetic radiation.

Radioactive nuclides may emit one or more types of radiation. They exist in nature, and some may be artificially produced. Artificial radioactive isotopes can be produced by bombarding neutral atoms with high-energy particles, often neutrons, to disrupt the balance of the nuclear core. An example is radioactive cobalt-60, produced by bombarding stable cobalt-59 with neutrons in a nuclear reactor. The resulting unstable cobalt-60 emits two beta particles and two gamma rays before reaching nickel-60, a stable atom. The physical half-life of cobalt-60 is 5.26 years, which is the time required for the activity of the radioactive nuclide to be halved. The gamma rays emitted from cobalt-60 as the result of nuclear transitions are electromagnetic radiations oscillating at frequencies of about $10^{20}$ hertz (Hz).

X-rays are also electromagnetic radiations with frequencies of about $10^{17}$ Hz. X-rays and gamma rays differ only in that x-rays result from electron interactions *outside* the atomic nucleus, whereas gamma rays result from energy balance processes *inside* the nucleus. In radiation therapy, the electromagnetic radiations used are x-rays and gamma rays (with frequencies above $10^{18}$ Hz) because of their penetration characteristics. However, other particulate radiations, such as energetic electrons, $\pi$-mesons, protons, neutrons, and helium and carbon atoms, are also used or are under investigation. This discussion will be limited to treatments with photons, since most medical centers use these sources.

Elements with atomic numbers between 1 (hydrogen) and 92 (uranium) exist naturally, while those with atomic numbers between 93 and 105 are produced artificially. Most lighter atoms have at least one stable nuclear configuration; most heavier atoms are radioactive. There are three radioactive decay series, each of which begins with a long-lived radioactive parent and ends with a stable nuclide. Many natural radioactive

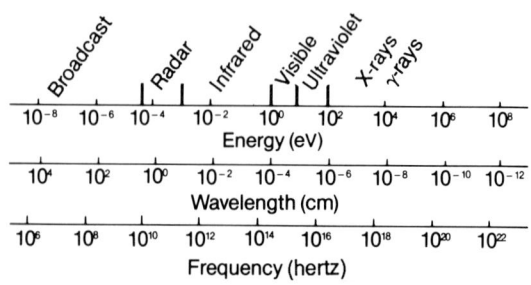

FIGURE 7-1 The electromagnetic spectrum. Wavelengths and frequencies corresponding to the photon energies are indicated. The energy is proportional to the frequency, and the frequency of the electromagnetic wave in a vacuum is equal to the speed of light divided by the wavelength.

nuclides belong to one of the three series. Of particular importance in radiation therapy is the uranium-238 series, which decays to lead-206.

*Radium*, one of the most commonly used radioactive sources for interstitial treatment of cancer, is the sixth decay product of the uranium-238 series. It disintegrates with a half-life of 1,622 years to form the gaseous element radon-222. In 94.5% of the cases of radium decay, one alpha particle is emitted with energy equaling 4.78 MeV. (One MeV is $10^6$ electron volts; an electron volt is the energy required to move an electron through an electric potential of 1 volt.) The rest of the disintegrations produce an alpha particle of energy 4.60 MeV followed by a gamma ray of energy 0.18 MeV. The daughter atom then decays through another eight steps to reach lead-206. During this involved sequence of events, alpha particles, beta particles, and various gamma photons are emitted. It is primarily the gamma photons that are used therapeutically.

When either radium or radon is used for therapeutic purposes, the radioactive substance is encapsulated in a platinum-iridium or gold container—usually a tube or needle—that will absorb all the alpha and practically all the beta particles. Generally, only gamma rays penetrate the walls of the container. Radium and its daughters emit many gamma rays, and the average photon energy is about 0.8 MeV. If a sample of radium is sealed in a tube, the decay products of radon gas accumulate until a state of radioactive equilibrium is established. When this occurs, any element in this series of disintegration products decays at the same rate as it is being produced—i.e., all the daughters decay with the half-life of the parent (1,622 years). For this reason, a sealed radium source with its various radon daughters emitting penetrating gamma rays can be considered to have a constant radioactive strength for many years.

Other radioactive sources frequently used in radiotherapy are cesium-137, iridium-192, gold-198, iodine-125, and cobalt-60. Cesium-137 is a fission product, and the latter four are artificially produced through nuclear reactions. Like radium, they are encapsulated or sealed. These radioactive sources pose serious problems in terms of radiation protection, since they emit high-energy gamma radiation continuously and must be stored in lead containers when not in use.

*Cobalt-60* is the most common teletherapy source for external-beam radiation therapy and is sometimes used in interstitial treatment as well. As mentioned before, cobalt-60 is produced by bombarding stable cobalt-59 with neutrons. It decays with a half-life of 5.26 years, emitting two gamma photons per disintegration with energies of 1.17 and 1.33 MeV (average = 1.25 MeV). These photons can penetrate tissue to a depth sufficient to treat deep-seated tumors. When cobalt-60 is the source of the external beam, it is encapsulated in a stainless-steel cylinder. The radiation source size is typically about 1 cm in diameter and 1 cm in height, depending on the strength required. When not in use, this cylinder is placed in a lead housing to shield the gamma rays. When therapy is required, the source is brought to an opening in the housing and the photons exit from the housing through a beam-collimating mechanism. When cobalt-60 is used as an interstitial implant, it is usually in the form of a wire placed inside a sheath of stainless steel.

Besides these radioactive sources, x-ray photons of different energies can be produced by a variety of machines that generate high-energy x-rays on demand. An obvious advantage of this approach is the convenience of choosing any photon energy to meet the requirements of specific applications.

To produce x-ray photons, a stream of electrons must be accelerated to a very high energy level. These electrons are then directed onto a target of high-Z material, such as tungsten ($Z = 74$). When the electrons penetrate the target, they lose energy through interactions with other electrons and nuclei to produce a spectrum of x-ray radiation. Some of the x-rays can have energies as high as those of the incident electrons.

A conventional diagnostic x-ray machine accelerates electrons simply as a result of the difference in electrical potential between the anode and the cathode ends of the x-ray tube. In radiation therapy in which x-rays of very high energy and intensity are needed, the electrons are accelerated by electromagnetic fields. When electrons are accelerated in a straight line by a high-radio-frequency electromagnetic wave, the accelerator is called a *linear accelerator*—probably the most popular type of x-ray machine used in radiation therapy today. The electron energies from these machines are generally 4 to 18 MeV but can be as high as 35 MeV. When electrons are accelerated in a circular orbit by a changing magnetic field, the accelerator is called a *betatron*; this machine can produce electron energies above 40 MeV. The average x-ray energy from a 4-MeV electron acceleration system is slightly above 1 MeV, which is similar to that of cobalt-60. A medium-energy linear accelerator is comparable in size to a gantry-mounted cobalt-60 teletherapy unit, which is about 8 feet high.

## INTERACTIONS OF RADIATION AND MATTER

When a high-energy electron penetrates a target material, it undergoes many types of interactions in the medium before all its energy is dissipated. Most of the interactions occur between the incoming electron and the atomic electrons. Occasionally, the incident electron interacts with the nucleus of the atom.

### Electron-Electron Collisions

In collisional energy losses, the incoming energetic electron interacts with the outer-shell electrons of the target atom. Electrons from the target atom are moved to an outer shell and form an "excited atom," which loses its excess energy as heat. Some electrons may be ejected from the atom, thus rendering it positively charged or ionized. When an inner-shell electron is ejected, an electron from one of the outer shells will fill the inner vacancy, and the atom will emit characteristic x-ray photons of energy equal to the difference between the binding energies of the inner- and outer-shell electrons. Thus, an incoming electron may lose all or part of its energy through multiple collisions with other electrons.

## Bremsstrahlung

When an electron travels close to the atomic nucleus, its path may be altered by the large positive charge of the nucleus. If this happens, the electron will be decelerated, and all or part of its energy will be given off as x-rays, conventionally known as *bremsstrahlung*. If an incoming electron is brought to rest in a single nuclear interaction, all of its kinetic energy will be converted to bremsstrahlung. For example, if an electron is accelerated through a potential of 10 million volts (10 MV), it will have a kinetic energy of 10 MeV, and the resulting photon can also have a maximum energy of 10 MeV. However, the probabilistic nature of the interaction permits portions of the electron's energy to be converted to bremsstrahlung during multiple interactions, producing photons of lower energies. These interactions result in a continuous x-ray spectrum, with energies ranging from zero to the energy of the incident electron.

This is the principal source of x-ray photons for medical use. Thus, x-ray photons are produced by accelerating a beam of electrons which is then focused to strike a target, typically tungsten, resulting in x-rays called bremsstrahlung. These x-rays are filtered by various metals to remove undesirable low-energy components, including the characteristic x-rays that result from the electron-electron collision process. The filtered spectrum is then collimated to produce consistent beam characteristics for radiation treatments.

## Ionization Process

Whenever one or more electrons are ejected from the atomic configuration, ionization of an atom can occur. The remaining atom is then a positively charged ion. Radiation sources cause both direct and indirect ionizations. *Directly* ionizing radiations are charged particles that change the atomic structure of the material through which they pass by collision. Examples of charged-particle radiations are high-energy electrons, π-mesons, protons, and heavy ions. *Indirectly* ionizing radiations are uncharged particles, electromagnetic radiations, and neutrons, all of which can produce directly ionizing particles secondarily through interactions with the medium they traverse.

The ionization and excitation of atoms by heavy charged particles going through a medium occur mostly along the track of the particles. In general, the amount of ionization depends on the mass and the kinetic energy of the charged particle, which has a defined range of penetration. The ionization ability of various charged particles can be compared using the concept of *linear energy transfer* (*LET*). The LET of charged particles in a medium is the ratio of the average energy locally imparted to the medium by a charged particle of specified energy to the length of the path the particle traverses. The unit for the LET is usually keV per micrometers ($\mu$m) of the medium. For cobalt-60, the average

LET is about 0.3 keV/$\mu$m, while for heavily charged particle tracks it may be 100 to 200 keV/$\mu$m in water.

The process of ionization is important in understanding both biologic damage and radiation dosage. Ionization in tissue causes physiochemical changes in living matter. These changes occur in a fraction of a second (range = $10^{-12}$ to $10^{-1}$ second) and lead to biologic changes such as breaks in DNA strands, genetic damage (mutation), and cell death (which requires much longer time periods to become manifest). Since the origin of biologic damage is ionization, radiation can damage both normal and malignant cells. Thus, the goal of radiation treatment planning is the selective deposition of radiation energy into cancer cells while sparing normal ones.

Ionization in air is of fundamental importance in radiology and radiotherapy, since it forms the basis for dose specification as well as for dosimetric measuring systems. These formalisms are discussed later, under "Radiation Exposure and Absorbed Dose."

## SPECIFIC PHOTON INTERACTIONS IN MATTER

Because x-rays in the megavoltage range (1.0 MeV or more) are most commonly used in radiation therapy, it is important to understand in detail their interactions in a medium. The three main interactive processes are the photoelectric effect, Compton scattering, and pair production (Fig. 7-2). The relative occurrence of these processes in a medium generally depends on the energy of the incident photons, the atomic number, and the density of the medium.

## Photoelectric Effect

To achieve the photoelectric effect, the incident photon interacts with the atom and transfers all of its energy to an inner-shell electron of the atom (Fig. 7-2A). This electron will be ejected from the atom with kinetic energy equal to the difference between the incident photon energy and the binding energy of the ejected electron. Loss of the ejected electron creates an inner-shell vacancy that will be filled by electrons from the outer shells. Excess energy from these electron transitions will be emitted as characteristic x-rays that may also interact with the medium subsequently. The ejected electron then loses its energy primarily through collision interactions in the medium.

The photoelectric process is an important mode of interaction in tissue for photons of low energy (less than 0.05 MeV). The probability that the photoelectric effect will occur per gram of medium varies approximately as $Z^3$. Thus, bones with an effective Z of about 11.6 can attenuate low-energy photons to a dramatically greater extent than can tissue with an effective Z of 7.4. This attenuation differential in media with different atomic numbers is the basis for the use of low-energy x-rays in diagnostic radiology.

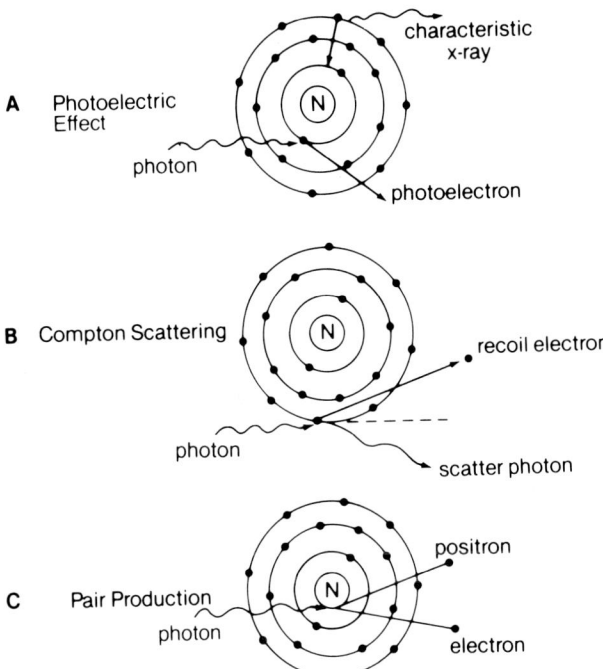

FIGURE 7-2 The three main photon interaction processes in matter. (A) *Photoelectric effect:* An incident photon interacts with an atom to eject an electron from the K shell, producing a photoelectron. An outer-shell electron fills this vacancy, and the excess energy is emitted as characteristic x-rays. (B) *Compton scattering:* An incident photon is scattered by an outer-shell electron. Part of the incident photon energy is transferred to the recoil electron, and the rest is carried by the scatter photon. (C) *Pair production:* An incident photon interacts with the nucleus of the atom, and a positron-electron pair is produced.

## Compton Scattering

When the energy of the incident photon is between 0.10 and about 5 MeV, the predominant interaction in tissue is Compton scattering. In this process, the incoming photon interacts with outer-shell electrons in the medium. These electrons can essentially be considered free electrons, since their binding energies are small compared with the energy of the incident photon. Such a collision causes the partial transfer of energy from the incident photon to the electron and creates a lower-energy photon. The electron set in motion is called the *recoil electron*, and the lower-energy photon is called the *scatter photon* (Fig. 7-2B). For an incident photon energy on the order of a few megavolts, the recoil electron acquires most of the incident photon energy. The recoil electron from this interaction then loses its energy, as discussed above, through collisions with other atomic electrons. The scattered photon subsequently interacts by Compton scattering or photoelectric processes, depending on its energy. The probability that the Compton process will take place is almost independent of the atomic number. This provides a distinct advantage in megavoltage treatment, since the presence of a bone in the path of the beam will not significantly alter the dose to the patient.

## Pair Production

The process of pair production starts to occur at an incident photon energy greater than 1.02 MeV. During this process, the incident photon interacts with the nucleus of the atom and undergoes conversion into mass in the form of two particles—an electron and a *positron* (a positively charged particle with the mass of an electron) (Fig. 7-2C). Since the mass of an electron or a positron at rest is equivalent to 0.511 MeV, the minimum photon energy required for pair production is 1.02 MeV. When the photon energy is greater than this, energy in excess of 1.02 MeV becomes the kinetic energy of the electron and the positron, which lose their energy and produce ionization and excitation in the medium.

The positron does not normally exist in nature. After losing all of its kinetic energy, it comes to a virtual halt. When it meets an electron, the two particles annihilate each other and produce two photons, each having an energy of 0.511 MeV. These photons, known as *annihilation radiation*, further interact with matter as outlined above. The probability that the pair production process will occur per unit mass of the medium varies linearly with Z.

In summary, the energy of the incident photons determines which of these processes is most likely to occur. The probability that pair production will occur begins when the incident photon energy is above 1.02 MeV and increases with increasing photon energy; the photoelectric effect is more likely to occur when the incident photon energy is below 0.05 MeV and decreases with increasing photon energy; Compton scattering predominates at photon energies of 0.10 to 5.00 MeV for almost any medium. Figure 7-3 shows the relative at-

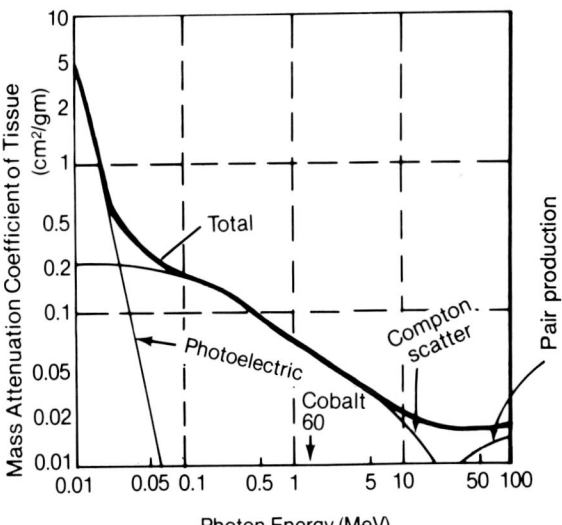

FIGURE 7-3 The mass attenuation coefficient of soft tissue as a function of photon energy. The relative components of the three photon interaction processes are plotted. Most of the high-energy linear accelerators operate at an effective energy between 1 and 5 MeV. Therefore, most of the interactions are Compton scattering.

tenuation coefficient in soft tissue as a function of photon energy. For megavoltage radiation therapy, the predominant interaction is Compton scattering.

# RADIATION DOSIMETRY

## Attenuation

When photons interact with a medium, they are attenuated by the medium. At each point in the medium, the fractional decrease in photon intensity per unit thickness due to attenuation is proportional to the photon intensity at that point. Mathematically, this phenomenon can be translated into the following exponential equation:

$$I = I_0 e^{-\mu x} \qquad (1)$$

where $I$ is the photon intensity at thickness $x$, $I_0$ is the initial photon intensity, $e$ is the base of the natural logarithm, $\mu$ is the linear attenuation coefficient specific to the medium and photon energy under study, and $x$ is the thickness through which the photons penetrate. The attenuation coefficient represents the total probability of interaction from all three photon interactive processes. This relationship is fundamental to photon interactions in a medium.

Photon intensity can be reduced or attenuated simply by using various intervening absorbing materials. It is customary to use the term *half-value layer* (*HVL*) to describe the penetrating ability or quality of the incident photons. HVL is defined as that thickness of attenuating medium required to reduce the original photon intensity by half. In mathematical terms, HVL equals the thickness $x$ when $I/I_0 = 0.5$. Substituting this value in Equation 1 yields

$$HVL = \frac{0.693}{\mu} \qquad (2)$$

Thus, the larger the HVL, the greater the amount of material required to attenuate photon intensity. After penetrating seven HVLs, the original photon intensity will be reduced to less than 1%. HVL is always defined in terms of both the specific photon energy and the attenuating medium. For example, an x-ray beam produced at 200 kilovolts peak (kVp) has an HVL of 1.5 millimeters of copper (mm Cu).

## Inverse Square Law

Another factor that reduces the intensity of the photon is the distance between the radiation source and the point of observation. It is a purely geometric factor, unrelated to the interaction of radiation and matter. Consider a point photon source emitting $N$ photons per second uniformly in all directions from the center of a sphere with a radius of $r_1$. The number of photons reaching the surface of the sphere per unit area per second is $N/4\pi r_1^2$. If the radius of this sphere is increased to $r_2$, the number of photons reaching the larger spherical surface per unit area per second is $N/4\pi r_2^2$.

Thus, the ratio of the intensity at distance $r_1$ to the intensity at distance $r_2$ is

$$\frac{I_1}{I_2} = \frac{(r_2)^2}{(r_1)^2} \qquad (3)$$

This is the inverse square law, which states that radiation intensity varies inversely as the square of the distance from the source. This law, together with the exponential attenuation relationship, describes the intensity of a given photon source at any point in space.

## Radiation Exposure and Absorbed Dose

The products of ionization are ion pairs, i.e., electrons and positively charged ions. The total number of ion pairs produced is proportional to the energy deposited in the medium. Of particular importance in radiation dosimetry is the formation of ion pairs in air. The definition of radiation exposure is based on the collection of the total charge (negative or positive) that is formed when x-rays or gamma rays interact in air. Thus, if $Q$ is the total charge produced in air when all the electrons liberated from the photon interactions in a small volume of air of mass ($m$) are stopped completely in air, then the radiation exposure ($X$) at the location of the small volume is

$$X = \frac{Q}{m} \qquad (4)$$

The unit of exposure is the roentgen (R), which equals $2.58 \times 10^{-4}$ C/kg of air at standard temperature and pressure (STP).

In practice, the definition of exposure is applicable only to photon radiation less than about 3 MeV because the large electron range would require an impractical charge collection volume. Furthermore, it is not applicable to charged-particle radiation. For these reasons, the term *rad* (radiation absorbed dose) was adopted. It is the most useful unit for radiobiologic purposes because it is a measure of the radiation energy absorbed by the medium. In this sense, it is applicable to any type of radiation passing through any type of medium. The unit of rad is defined as follows:

$$1 \text{ rad} = 100 \text{ ergs/gm} \qquad (5)$$

Using the definitions of roentgen and rad, an x-ray exposure of 1 R in air is equivalent to the absorbed dose of 0.869 rad in air. More recently, the International Commission on Radiation Units and Measurements adopted the SI (Système Internationale) system of units, in which the Gray (Gy) is the unit designated for absorbed dose: 1 Gy = 1 joule/kg = 100 rads and 1 centigray (cGy) = 1 rad.

## Measurement of Radiation Dose

Although the rad is the most useful unit in radiation therapy, its actual measurement in a biologic medium can be difficult. To measure the absorbed dose in a medium, one must determine the total amount of energy deposited while the medium is irradiated. Since this energy eventually generates heat, the most direct method of measuring the absorbed dose is to detect the rise in temperature of the medium. Usually, the increase in temperature of an isolated mass of the medium is detected by calorimetric techniques. Although this method is direct, it is a rather involved procedure to be carried out on a routine basis. The most popular method for obtaining routine dose measurements involves the use of an *ionization chamber*. In this case, the amount of ionization collected inside a known volume of gas within the chamber correlates with the absorbed dose according to empirically established quantities of the gas and the medium exposed to a given type of radiation.

An ionization chamber typically contains a small volume of gas (usually air) surrounded by a wall constructed of either tissue-equivalent or air-equivalent material. Two electrodes inside the chamber are maintained at a fixed electric potential difference. When radiation produces ionizations in the chamber, the electrodes collect the charged particles and generate a measurable electric current. By integrating the current over the period of irradiation, the total charge and therefore the total amount of ionization produced can be determined. On the basis of this measured quantity, one can calculate the absorbed dose delivered to the medium. However, because many technical and empirical data are involved, most ionization chambers used for practical applications are calibrated at the US National Bureau of Standards for a specific radiation. For example, ionization chambers for megavoltage radiation therapy are usually calibrated for a cobalt-60 beam under specific irradiation conditions. Once calibration is done, the same chamber can be used for other photon energies provided that proper correction factors are included.

*Film and thermoluminescent dosimetric (TLD) techniques* are often used in radiation therapy. Photographic film emulsions consist of microscopic silver halide crystals or grains embedded in a gelatin base. As these crystals are irradiated, they are activated and become more sensitive to chemical changes. The irradiated film then contains a latent image. When the film is developed, the chemical process precipitates the activated crystals to form grains of metallic silver, while the unaffected crystals are dissolved and washed away. The area exposed to a higher dose will contain more silver after the process, and this will appear as the darker area on the film. *Thermoluminescence* refers to the ability of certain materials to absorb and store energy that can be released later in the form of light photons when the material is heated. The amount of light detected is proportional to the absorbed dose. Although many materials exhibit thermoluminescence, the ones commonly used in radiation therapy are lithium fluoride and lithium borate. Usually the material is embedded in a small Teflon disk that can be used repeatedly. Both film dosimetry and TLD are good for relative-dose measurements, but they must be carefully calibrated before they can be used for absolute-dose measurements.

## RADIATION TREATMENT PLANNING

### Beam Characteristics

Regardless of their source, photons must be collimated to produce well-defined fields or beams for radiation treatments. For low-energy photons, collimation is usually achieved by placing a lead cone between the source and the patient. For high-energy photons, such as those from cobalt-60 or high-energy linear accelerators, photons are collimated by four movable jaws or shielding blocks. These jaws are usually made of lead and/or tungsten. When they are closed, photon transmission is on the order of 0.1%. Thus, the size of a beam is defined by the extent to which the jaws are opened.

In the patient, the dose absorbed by various tissues is a function of a large number of beam characteristics, tissue type, and photon energy. It would be extremely inefficient and impractical to measure the dose at various points in the patient for each treatment. To permit efficient and reliable treatment planning on a routine basis, a "phantom" (usually a tank of water) is used to simulate the patient because water is an excellent tissue-equivalent material radiologically. Doses measured in the water phantom for different but well-defined beam geometries will then form the data base for patient dose calculations.

Figure 7-4 shows the geometric parameters of an incident beam directed toward a water phantom. Those of major importance are the radiation source size (S),

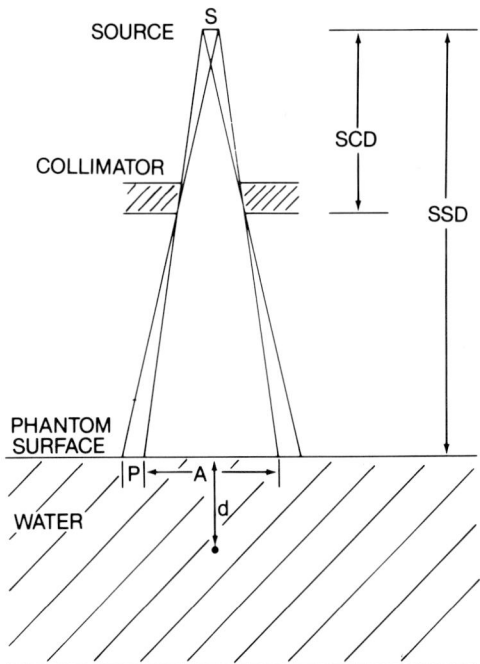

**FIGURE 7-4** Geometric parameters of a radiation treatment beam. S = size of radiation source; SCD = distance from source to collimator; SSD = distance from source to surface of the patient or a water phantom used to simulate the patient; A = field size at the surface; d = depth from surface to point where radiation dose is to be calculated; P = penumbra area exposed to only part of the radiation source.

source-to-surface distance (SSD), source-to-collimator jaw distance (SCD), field size (A), and the depth (d) at which the dose is calculated. The SSD directly affects the radiation intensity at a point of interest; the intensity follows the inverse square law. The field area defined by A in Figure 7-4 is irradiated fairly uniformly, since this area "sees" the entire radiation source. The diameter of the radiation source of a modern accelerator is very small (about 2 mm) but is not really a point source. This finite source size produces the penumbra region (P) at the edge of the beam. The dose across this area is smaller than the dose inside region A, since P "sees" only part of the radiation source. The dose decreases dramatically across this region. Typically, the dose decreases by 80 to 90% across a distance of 1 cm in area P for a modern accelerator. Geometrically, the size of P is inversely proportional to SCD for a given SSD.

Since S and SCD are fixed parameters, a typical data base specifies dose as a function of field size A, depth d, and source-to-surface distance SSD. These systematic measurements are usually obtained with an ionization chamber and the data are normalized to a reference-beam geometry. This normalization procedure enables one to calculate absolute doses, since the dose at any point in the reference beam can be accurately determined by using a calibrated ionization chamber. This calibration procedure essentially relates the dose administered to the patient to the radiation output from the linear accelerator. Once the reference beam is calibrated, the absolute dose at any other geometry can be determined from the tabulated data.

When a large number of point doses are required, a computer is needed to calculate them. Although there are many models of dose computation, probably the most versatile one requires the separation of the measured dose into two doses: that from the primary beam and that resulting from scatter radiation in the medium. The primary dose is a function of attenuation and the inverse square law, while the scatter component is a function of energy, field size, depth, and SSD. Although this distinction is not absolutely necessary, it does offer a clearer physical understanding of the contributions to the dose and allows more flexible manipulation of computerized data for treatment planning.

Perhaps the most important data base is the *percent depth dose* (PDD). PDD is a ratio expressed as a percentage of two doses measured in a phantom and is defined as follows:

$$\text{PDD (A, SSD, d)} = \frac{D(A, \ SSD, \ d)}{D(A, \ SSD, \ d^{max})} \qquad (6)$$

where D(A, SSD, d) is the dose at a point along the central axis of the beam at depth d below the surface, and D(A, SSD, $D_{max}$) is the dose at a point where the maximum dose occurs along the central axis (Fig. 7-4). The location of the maximum dose ($d_{max}$) is sometimes called the *depth of maximum electronic buildup.*

The $d_{max}$ is a unique and important quantity in radiotherapy. It is the depth in tissue at which electrons generated by the incident photons reach electronic equilibrium. These electrons have a finite range and deposit their energy along their tracks through the medium. At the point of electronic equilibrium, the electrons deposit as much energy as they carry away during the course of their motions. The $d_{max}$ does not exist at the interface of two different media for photon energies of about 1 MeV or greater, and it accounts for the "skin-sparing" effect of megavoltage radiation. Because the $d_{max}$ for orthovoltage radiation (usually 200 to 300 kV) is at the skin surface, marked skin reactions were observed in the days before cobalt-60 and linear accelerator radiation therapy. The distance required for this equilibrium to occur increases with increasing photon energy.

Figure 7-5 shows the $d_{max}$ for different photon energies. The $d_{max}$ increases from the surface for a 140-kV beam to 3 cm for a 15-MV beam. Higher-energy photon beams not only have greater PDD characteristics but also have a greater $d_{max}$ and, consequently, an increased capacity to spare the skin and subcutaneous region. For a static beam, the skin dose is reduced from about 128% (140 kV) to about 25% (6 MV) relative to a 100% dose prescribed at d = 1.5 cm. Moreover, the PDD at a depth of 10 cm is only 20% (140 kV) compared with 65% (6 MV). Obviously, low kilovolt x-rays (HVL less than a few millimeters of copper) are of value only in the treatment of superficial lesions, whereas the high-energy x-rays are more efficient for treating deep-seated tumors and have a significant skin-sparing effect.

## Isodose Representation

When many dose points have been measured or calculated, it is often easier to represent the dose distribution by a set of isodose lines. An *isodose line* is a line connecting all the points receiving a particular dose level of interest. Figure 7-6 compares the isodose curves of beams from a low-kilovolt x-ray machine, a cobalt-60 unit, and a 22-MV betatron. Doses along the central axis of the beam are the PDDs. The isodose distributions for the high-energy photon beams show the flattest profiles across the beams. The accelerators producing these beams have special flattening filters designed to modify the intensity across the beam, thereby achieving a flat profile at typical treatment depths.

Doses outside the beam are also lowest at high-photon energy. This is because the scatter photons and electrons are more forward-directed when the incident photon energy increases. The rate of dose decrease outside the beam is therefore slower for low-energy x-rays.

At the edge of the beam, the isodose curves for low-kilovolt x-rays exhibit sharp demarcation curves. This is because of the small effective focal spot and the short distance between the surface of the phantom and the beam-collimating cones. This kind of discontinuity disappears, however, with cobalt-60 and linear accelerator isodoses because the source size is finite and the distance between the surface of the phantom and the collimating jaws is large (Fig. 7-4). The geometric penumbra for linear accelerators is a few millimeters because of the small focal spot; the penumbra effect can be considerably larger for cobalt-60 beams, however, where the diameter of the source is often 1 cm or greater.

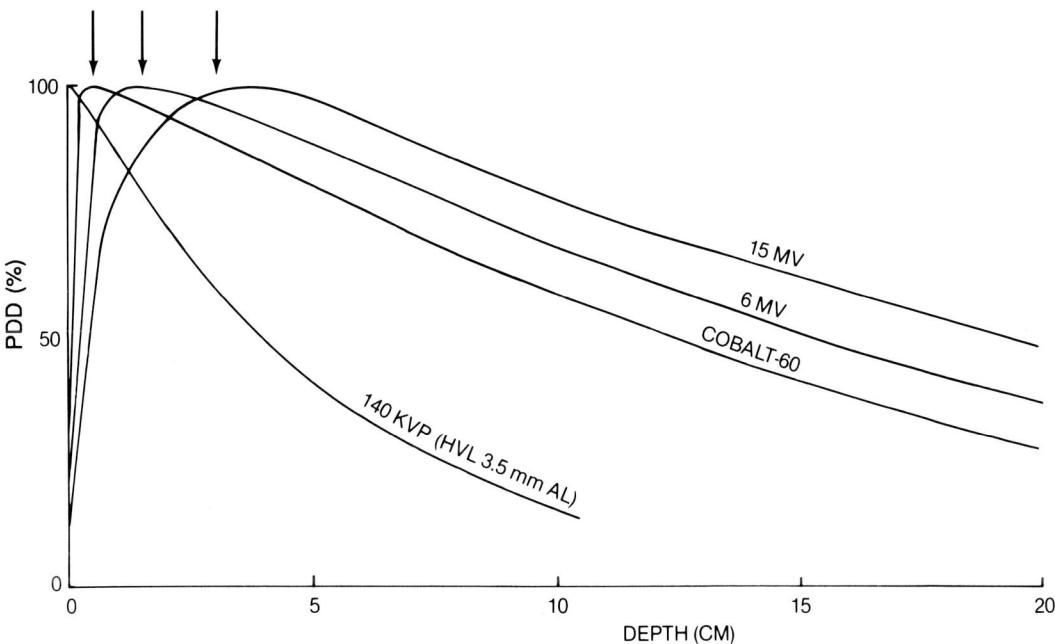

**FIGURE 7-5** Percent depth dose (PDD) plotted as a function of depth for various photon energies. The depth of maximum buildup for each energy is indicated by the arrow of each curve. The field size is 10 × 10 cm at the surface for all the beams. The SSD is 50 cm for the 140-kV beam and 100 cm for the cobalt-60, 6-MV, and 15-MV beams. (HVL = half-value layer.)

## Graphic Treatment Plan

A basic problem in the clinical application of radiation in cancer treatment is defining as accurately as possible the tumor to be irradiated as well as the critical normal tissues to be spared. The tumor, along with an adequate margin, is often referred to as the *target volume*. This is the volume to be irradiated up to a specific dose according to a specified time-dose schedule. Once the target volume and the adjacent normal tissues are defined, an optimal treatment plan is designed to meet the specific requirements of the patient. An optimal plan is one that can deliver a high and uniform dose to the

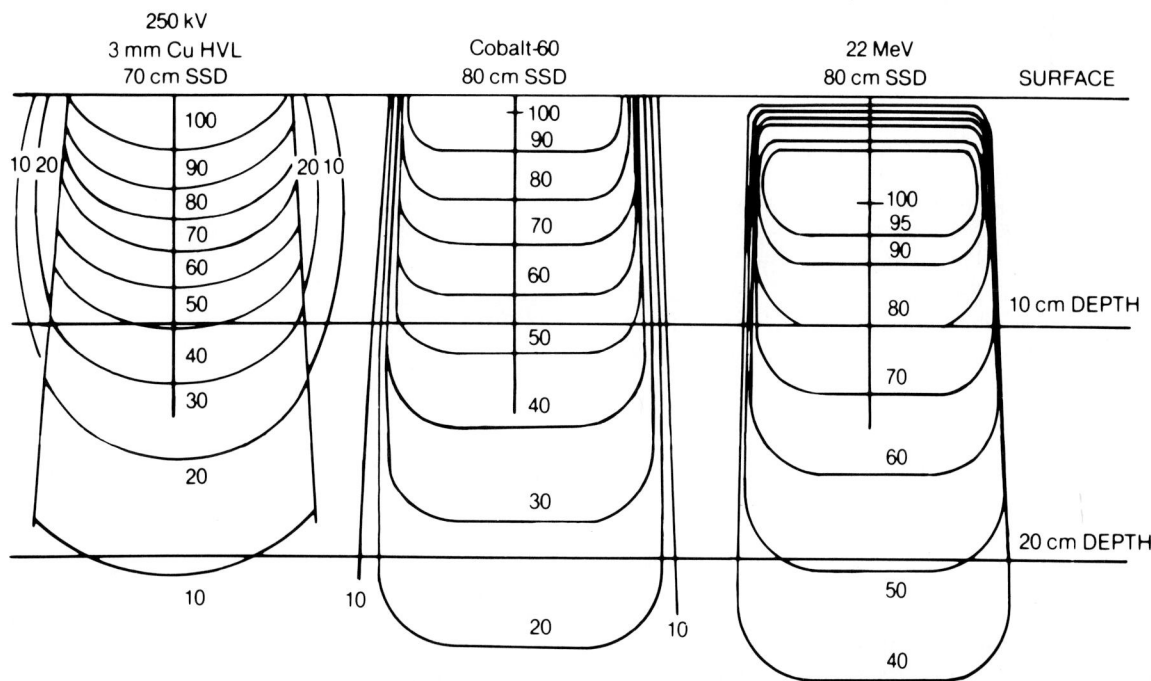

**FIGURE 7-6** Comparison of isodose distributions of 250-kV, cobalt-60, and 22-MV linear accelerator beams. The field size is 10 × 10 cm at the surfaces for all the beams; respective SSDs are indicated. Note the sharp dose gradient of the high-energy beam at the beam edge (the penumbra region).

target volume while keeping the surrounding normal tissues below their level of radiation tolerance. This goal can often be accomplished by the judicious selection of the radiation source, energy, and the geometric configuration of the beam.

Before dose distributions are planned for different photon-beam combinations, data relevant to radiation treatment planning must be collected and analyzed. The objective is to integrate all the diagnostic data obtained by various tests in order to assess the extent of tumor and delineate normal tissues. Routine diagnostic x-ray procedures are used in treatment planning together with computed tomography (CT), lymphoscintigraphy, lymphangiography, and ultrasonography. Contrast diagnostic radiographs are excellent means of localizing major normal anatomic structures and tumor volumes. CT is invaluable in providing cross-sectional anatomic data. Lymphoscintigrams and lymphangiograms are used to localize lymph nodes. Ultrasound is sometimes employed to detect the lung-tissue interface.

A simulation of the actual radiation treatment is part of this integration process. The patient is positioned under a simulator as if he or she were actually being prepared for therapy. The simulator is constructed much like the actual treatment machine except that the radiation source is a diagnostic x-ray tube. Fluoroscopic studies and radiographs from selected positions are obtained to define the treatment-beam parameters.

Computer-assisted techniques can be used to integrate all the diagnostic data into coordinates of the actual treatment position. When a consistent set of patient data is defined in the treatment geometry, a dose calculation program can be used to generate radiation beams that will produce the optimal dose distribution.

## Opposed Fields

The simplest way to distribute the radiation dose uniformly is to use a pair of opposed photon beams. Figure 7-7A illustrates the typical features of parallel opposed beams. Because the isodoses along the beam edges are usually rounded, the combination of two opposing beams causes the higher isodose lines to have an hourglass appearance. The degree of bowing-in depends on the photon energy, patient thickness, and size of the irradiation field. The physician must take this hourglass effect into account when selecting a field size and dose. Usually the 90% isodose line relative to 100% at the midpoint of the patient is reasonably straight along the beam edge and is used as a guide to define field size and dose. The 50% isodose line usually defines the geometric field size of the radiation beam. Figure 7-7A represents a distribution that has been normalized to the 90% line, so that the dose to the midplane of the patient is 111%. The minimum target dose is then prescribed to the 100% isodose line, which is slightly larger than the target volume laterally.

When such a simple treatment plan is used, the high-dose regions are always in the subcutaneous tissues, and the magnitude also depends on the photon energy, patient thickness, and field size. Dose uniformity can be

markedly improved if higher photon energies are used. If the tumor is centrally located in the pelvis and one wants to minimize the dose to the bladder and rectum, multiple stationary beams or a rotating-beam technique offers a better dose distribution than do parallel opposed high-energy photon beams (Figs. 7-7B and 7-7C).

## Multiple Stationary Beams

A common radiation technique for target volumes centrally located in the pelvis is the four-field or "box" technique. This requires two pairs of opposed beams crossing one another orthogonally at the center of the target (Fig. 7-7B). The term *box* is derived from the appearance of the uniform rectangular high-dose region. Dose inhomogeneity inside the target with this type of treatment plan is low—about 5 to 8% above the 100% isodose line encompassing the target volume. Moreover, the subcutaneous doses are distributed around the pelvis, in contrast to the use of parallel opposed beams, in which the undesirable high doses are concentrated in the anterior and posterior areas. The additional pair of opposing beams simply distributes the subcutaneous dose over four areas rather than two.

## Full and Partial Rotations

A full 360-degree rotational field represents the summation of an infinite number of stationary beams. If the tumor volume is elliptical in cross section, this type of treatment plan may not be optimal (Fig. 7-7C). However, when the target volume is round in cross section, or when the subcutaneous doses should be even lower than those delivered with the four-field technique, rotational beams may be optimal. Figure 7-8A shows a full 360-degree rotation to cover a target volume that is a circular cylinder. A uniform dose is achieved at the center and the subcutaneous dose is spread over a larger volume of the patient. Variations of a full rotation are partial arcs, as shown in Figure 7-8B. Arc rotations work well with oval-shaped target volumes in the pelvis and provide maximum sparing of normal tissues located anteriorly and posteriorly along the patient's midline.

## Shrinking Field Technique

Theoretically, all tumor cells can be sterilized if they are irradiated with a large enough dose. In practice, however, a tumor-controlling dose can be delivered less often because of normal tissue tolerance. Due to factors such as tumor size and lack of oxygenation, the central core of a tumor is often more resistant to irradiation than are the microscopic extensions into surrounding normal tissues. Subclinical microscopic disease can be controlled with a lower dose than that required for control of the gross tumor. The rationale for a shrinking field technique is to deliver a dose sufficient to sterilize microscopic disease in a volume containing both microscopic and gross tumor. Then a smaller field is used to irradiate only the primary tumor to a higher dose.

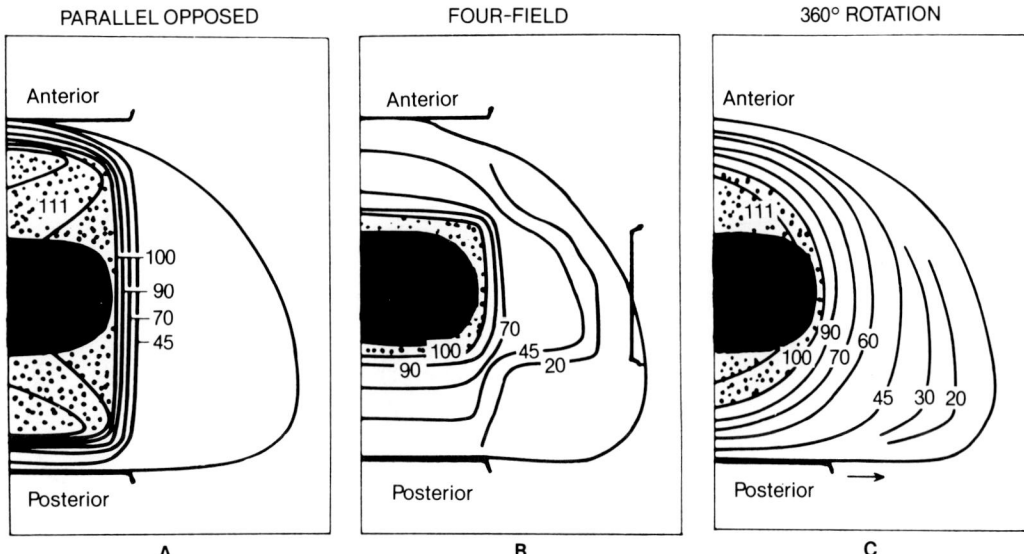

PARALLEL OPPOSED                FOUR-FIELD                360° ROTATION

A                              B                          C

FIGURE 7-7  Comparison of three high-energy photon treatment plans for a target volume with an elliptical cross section. The plans were normalized so that the target receives 100% of the prescribed dose. Plan A is clearly not optimal, since a large volume of normal tissue (stippled area) outside the target (blackened) area also receives a dose higher than 100%. By simply adding a pair of opposed lateral beams to Plan A, the 100% isodose conforms well to the target volume, and the transit doses through normal tissue are rel-atively low (Plan B). Plan C is a 360-degree rotation and is not optimal to cover an elliptical target, since the field width must be larger than the longer axis of the ellipse. A 360-degree rotation is better suited for circular target volumes. Source: From Dritschillo A, Chaffey JT, Bloomer WD, Marck A: The complication probability factor: A method for selection of radiation treatment plans. *Br J Radiol* 51:371, 1978.

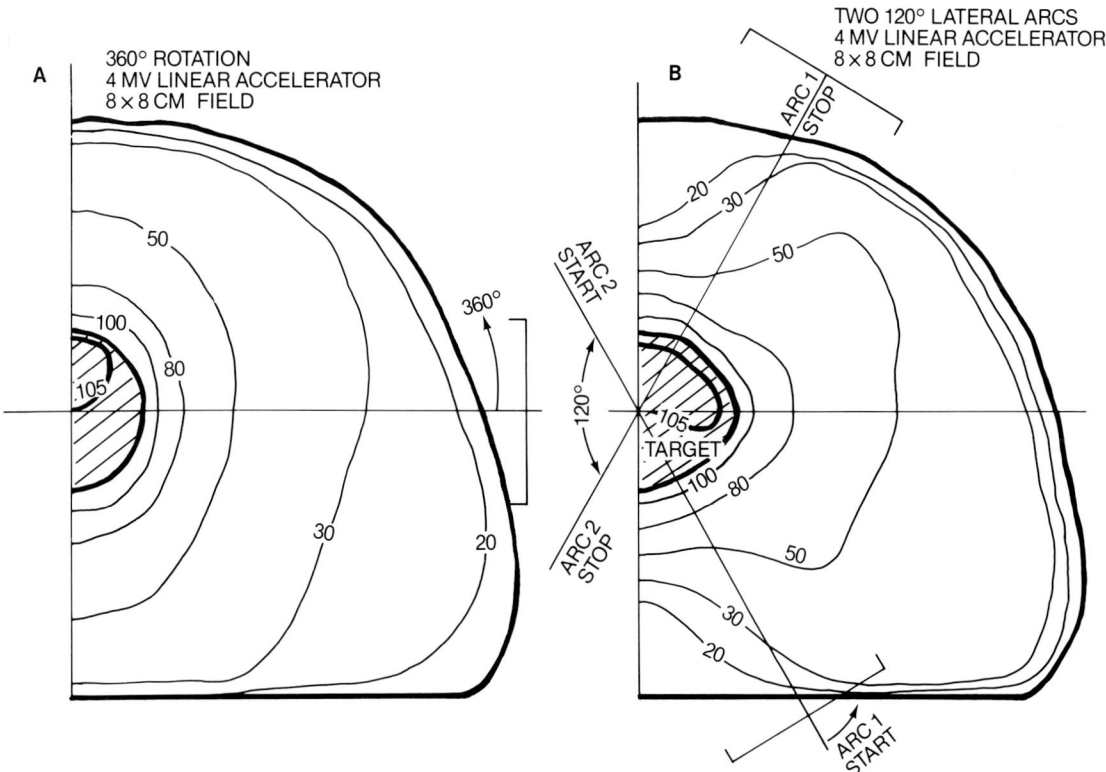

FIGURE 7-8  Characteristics of a 360-degree rotation (Plan A). Rotational beams are useful for treating centrally located target volumes that have circular cross sections. A high uniform dose can be delivered to the target, and the dose outside the target is spread around the patient. Characteristics of partial arcs (Plan B). This example consists of two 120-degree lateral arcs. These are useful to cover targets that have elliptical cross sections and when anterior and posterior structures are to be spared, as in pelvic treatments.

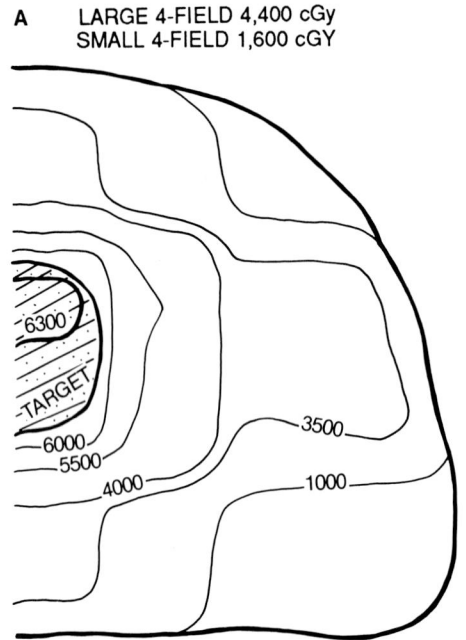

**A**     LARGE 4-FIELD 4,400 cGy
         SMALL 4-FIELD 1,600 cGY

**B**     8 MV LINEAR ACCELERATOR
         LARGE 4-FIELD 4,400 cGy
         SMALL FIELD 360° ROTATION

**FIGURE 7-9** Comparison of cumulative treatments. Treatment A consists of two four-field plans. After 4,400 cGy have been delivered with the first-course four-field plan (15 × 15 cm and 9 × 15 cm fields), an additional 1,600 cGy are delivered by the second-course four-field plan (8 × 10 cm fields). The target will receive a total of 6,000 cGy. This composite plan is to be compared with Treatment B, in which the second course is replaced by a 360-degree rotation (8 × 10 cm field). Although there is no significant change in doses above the 4,000-cGy level, the rotation clearly brings the 3,500-cGy isodose closer to the center.

Smaller fields are used in the second part of the treatment to spare more of the normal tissues.

Figure 7-9 illustrates two typical cumulative dose distributions using the shrinking field technique. In Treatment A, the four-field technique is used to cover the whole pelvis, including the pelvic nodes. It is followed by a smaller four-field box to include only the cervix. In Treatment B, a large four-field box is followed by a rotation with a smaller field.

### Normal Tissue Shielding

Radiation fields are initially defined by the collimator jaws and are square or rectangular in shape. Such fields often encompass normal tissues that should not be irradiated. To shield these structures, lead blocks are made and placed in the beam to stop the radiation (2 to 3% transmission) from reaching these volumes. Using special metal alloys, these blocks are often customized—i.e., they are individually molded so that when they are mounted in the treatment beam, the block projections will match the size and shape of the shielded areas specified on the simulation films.

### BRACHYTHERAPY

Placement of sealed radioactive sources to deliver gamma radiation at a distance of up to a few centimeters is very effective in delivering a highly localized dose to the tumor while sparing adjacent normal tissues. This technique is known as *interstitial/intracavitary radiation* or *brachytherapy*. The radioactive sources are encapsulated so that almost all the particulate radiations are stopped and only the gamma rays penetrate the capsule.

Historically, radium has been the most frequently used source. Recently, however, other radionuclides have been used as replacements. The most popular of these are cesium-137 and iridium-192. For gynecologic applications, radium-226 and cesium-137 are most commonly used. They are applied as either interstitial or intracavitary implants. Interstitial implants require the insertion of sealed sources directly into the tumor. These sealed sources are in the form of needles or small seeds embedded in a polyethylene strand or implanted directly. Intracavitary implants require the placement of sealed sources within a body cavity; these sources are usually in the form of tubular capsules.

### Radium Sources

The physics of radium was previously discussed. If radium-226 is sealed in a container so that the decay products cannot escape, a state of equilibrium will be reached within approximately 1 month. At that time, these products will decay with the same half-life as the parent (1,622 years). The container will absorb all of the alpha and almost all of the beta radiation emitted.

Radium comes in the form of a salt and is sealed in cylindrical cells. The walls of these cells are made of gold and are about 0.1 mm thick. Depending on the physical length of the source, one or more cells are then encapsulated by a platinum (Pt) wall reinforced with iridium (Ir). This wall is 0.5 to 1.0 mm thick and only slightly attenuates the gamma rays. This double encapsulation is necessary not only because of the alpha and beta radiations but also because of the need to prevent gaseous radioactive radon daughter products from escaping and causing a serious radiation contamination problem. The amount of radon will increase over the years, and it is important to monitor it periodically to ensure that radon is not leaking from the capsules.

Specifications of each radium source for brachytherapy usually include the active length of the source (i.e., the length defined by the ends of the radioactive material), the actual physical length, the activity or strength, the diameter of the cylindrical container, and the thickness or filtration of the source. For clinical applications, the exposure rate from a radium source is always specified in terms of activity, size and shape of the source, wall filtration, and distance from the source.

Many different photons are emitted during the radium decay process. After encapsulation, the average photon energy is about 0.8 MeV. The quantity of radium in a sealed source is specified in milligrams (mg) of radium. For radionuclides other than radium, activity is commonly expressed in *"milligram radium-equivalent."* At equilibrium, the radioactivity from 1 mg of radium is equivalent to 1 millicurie (mCi) of radon. A millicurie is defined as a unit of activity that yields $3.7 \times 10^7$ disintegrations per second. Thus, a tube containing 1 mCi of radon will have the same activity as a 1-mg radium needle.

## Cesium-137 Source

Cesium-137 is a fission product and can be encapsulated in needles or tubes similar to those used with radium. The physical half-life of cesium-137 is about 30 years, which makes the decay correction easy to manage (the activity is reduced by 2% per year). There is only one gamma ray per disintegration, and its energy is 0.662 MeV—slightly lower than the average energy of radium (0.800 MeV). Unlike radium, however, which emits some gamma rays greater than 1 MeV, the monoenergetic gamma rays from cesium-137 are more effectively attenuated by high-Z materials. Thus, for cesium-137, it is easier to design shields as parts of the ovoids or colpostats to protect the bladder and rectum. Obviously, use of the lower-energy photons should reduce personnel exposure as well. Another advantage of cesium-137 is that it does not have any gaseous daughter products in its decay, eliminating the possibility of the potential radiation hazard associated with damaged radium sources.

Cesium-137 source strengths can be specified in millicuries and wall filtration. More often, however, the strength or activity is specified in terms of the milligram radium-equivalent. Under these circumstances, the cesium-137 source is used as if it were radium, and all the distribution rules and dose tables prepared for radium will apply. However, some caution must be used when cesium-137 sources are used in gynecologic applications originally designed for radium. Attenuation by the walls and shielding materials used in the various applicators can be quite different for the two radioactive sources due to differences in their energy spectra.

# PRINCIPLES OF RADIOBIOLOGY APPLIED TO RADIOTHERAPY

## Tumor Radiosensitivity

Based on early experience in radiotherapy, it was inferred that certain tumor types are either more or less sensitive to radiation than others. For example, a malignant lymphoma will often completely and rapidly disappear following a dose as low as 20 Gy given over 2 weeks, whereas a melanoma of similar size may not appear to respond to doses that would exceed normal tissue tolerance. Such observations gave rise to an impression that the property of radiosensitivity could be predicted if one knew the cell of origin. However, extensive experimental studies have clearly shown that intrinsic cellular radiosensitivity is relatively constant throughout a wide range of normal and malignant cell types.

Therefore, observed differences in response to treatment must be explained by additional processes known to affect cell survival. These processes are often referred to as the four R's of radiobiologic response—*repair, repopulation, redistribution, and reoxygenation*—and are described fully in Chapter 6. Since all these processes tend to work adversely in large, bulky tumors, it is often assumed that removing bulk from a tumor, by either surgery or chemotherapy, will significantly improve its radiosensitivity. However, owing to the exponential nature of cell killing by radiation, the removal of 99% of a tumor cell population that initially contains approximately 10 billion cells may reduce the tumor lethal dose by only a few Grays. Also, even this small benefit may be lost if the remaining cells are poorly oxygenated or are able to proliferate more rapidly during therapy.

## Normal Tissue Tolerance

It has long been known that there is a limit of radiation dose that can be delivered to a normal tissue or organ beyond which the risk of severe, irreversible, and possibly fatal injury is high. Because of the primitive nature of available equipment, early radiotherapy was limited by severe skin and mucosal reactions. Conventional techniques of fractionation have since evolved to allow delivery of tumoricidal doses that will not exceed the tolerance of these acutely reacting tissues.

With modern equipment and techniques, acute reactions are rarely dose-limiting. However, doses must still be limited in order to minimize the risk of chronic or late-appearing injuries that may involve any tissue or organ, independent of the severity of its acute response. Some organs once thought to be radioresistant because they exhibited no acute clinical or pathologic changes are now known to be extremely radiosensitive with regard to late reactions. For example, doses that exceed 20 Gy to the kidneys and 30 Gy to the liver are associated with a significant risk for fatal radiation nephritis and hepatitis, respectively. Recent research indicates that the radiobiology of such late-occurring reactions differs significantly from that of acute reactions.

Of clinical relevance, tolerance of a late-reacting tissue may be greatly improved by reducing the individual treatment doses to less than the conventional value of 200 cGy. At present, doses to individual organs are limited by accepted values for tolerance based on available clinical data (Rubin and Cassarett, 1968).

## Therapeutic Ratio

The relative sensitivity of a tumor and the associated normal tissue gives rise to the concept of therapeutic ratio for a given clinical situation. Consider the dose-response curves for tumor control and normal tissue damage (Fig. 7-10). In general, the curves are relatively close, so that a high probability of cure is not possible without significant risk of injury. In a situation in which the curves are widely separated, so that the probability of cure without complication is high (e.g., treatment of a small, localized carcinoma of the cervix), a large therapeutic ratio is said to apply. Conversely, if the curves are so close that there is little or no likelihood of cure without complication, a small therapeutic ratio applies and the role of radiotherapy would be palliative at best. Such a case might be treatment of a bulky ovarian carcinoma that extends throughout the peritoneal cavity. Thus, any manipulation of treatment that alters the dose-response curve for either tumor or normal tissue will alter the therapeutic ratio.

At present, the most effective way known to maximize the therapeutic ratio is to deliver radiation as multiple, small, daily fractions over a period of several weeks (presumably to allow for maximal recovery of normal tissues and reoxygenation of the tumor) combined with progressive shrinking of the treatment field to reduce the dose to critical organs while allowing the maximal dose to be delivered to the primary tumor site.

## RADIOTHERAPY FOR GYNECOLOGIC CANCERS

### Carcinoma of the Cervix

The role of radiotherapy in cervical carcinoma was established in the early part of this century. The anatomy of the cervix is uniquely suitable for intracavitary radium therapy. By placing sources in a line (i.e., in tandem) within the cervical canal as well as in the lateral fornices (usually contained in structures called colpostats), extremely large doses of radiation can be delivered to the cervix and medial parametrial regions without exceeding the tolerance of the normal bladder and rectum. The earliest techniques were developed in Paris and Stockholm, and employed applicators having a wide range of shapes and sizes. Doses were usually prescribed by simply multiplying the number of milligrams of radium inserted by the total number of hours for which the patient was exposed. This product, known as milligram-hours (mghr), provides a rough estimate of actual radiation dose to various pelvic structures and, if a standardized technique is routinely used, still has clinical usefulness.

The *Paris technique* was characterized by the use of colpostats made of cork separated by a spring designed to place the radium as far laterally into the fornices as possible, thus increasing the dose to the parametria relative to the dose to the surface of the cervix and vagina. Relatively small amounts of radium (approximately 60 mg) were used, with the result that exposure times were long; it was typical for the applicator to be left in place for 6 to 8 days.

In contrast, the *Stockholm technique* utilized small boxes or plaques that allowed the radium to be placed close to the external surface of the cervix. Relatively large amounts (approximately 120 to 160 mg) of radium were used, and applications typically consisted of short exposures (1 or 2 days) repeated weekly two or three times. Because this technique delivers very high doses to the external cervix, exposures must be kept short, with time allowed for recovery before treatment is repeated in order to avoid severe, intolerable acute reactions.

The intracavitary treatment of cervical cancer was subsequently rationalized by the Manchester group in the 1930s (Paterson and Parker, 1934). In the *Manchester system*, the size and shape of the applicators were standardized and the colpostats were replaced with ovoids. A small, medium, or large applicator could be selected based on the patient's anatomy. Only two ovoids were used, separated by either a washer (small separation) or a spacer (large separation). Once the appropriate applicator was chosen, it could be loaded with predetermined amounts of radium to deliver a standard dose at a standard rate (e.g., 50 cGy/hr) to a given point related to the cervix.

For prescribing purposes, two points are defined (Fig. 7-11): point A, located 2 cm superior to the mucous membrane of the lateral fornix and 2 cm lateral to the cervical canal, and point B, located on the same transverse axis as point A but 5 cm lateral to the cervical canal. Although these points have no precise anatomic significance, they are still clinically useful for defining doses to the lateral cervix and obturator nodes, respectively.

Many other applicators and techniques have been described for the treatment of cervical cancer, all of which essentially represent modifications of the Paris and Stockholm methods. One such device is the *Ernst applicator*, which allows several small radium sources to be placed close to the cervix and held in place by a fixture to the tandem (Fig. 7-12).

Currently, the most popular intracavitary system is that developed at the M.D. Anderson Hospital by Fletcher and Suit (Fig. 7-13). The *Fletcher-Suit device* incorporates the advantages of the Paris and Manchester systems with the added advantage that the radioactive sources (either radium or cesium-137) can be loaded after the applicators have been inserted and the patient has been returned to her hospital bed. Prior to loading, localizing radiographs can be used to generate isodose curves that indicate the proper dose rates for any desired reference point in the pelvis and for any choice of sources (Fig. 7-14). Typically, a loading will be chosen to provide a dose rate of 50 to 80 cGy/hr to point A, with maximum rectal and bladder dose rates kept as low as possible with respect to this value. The

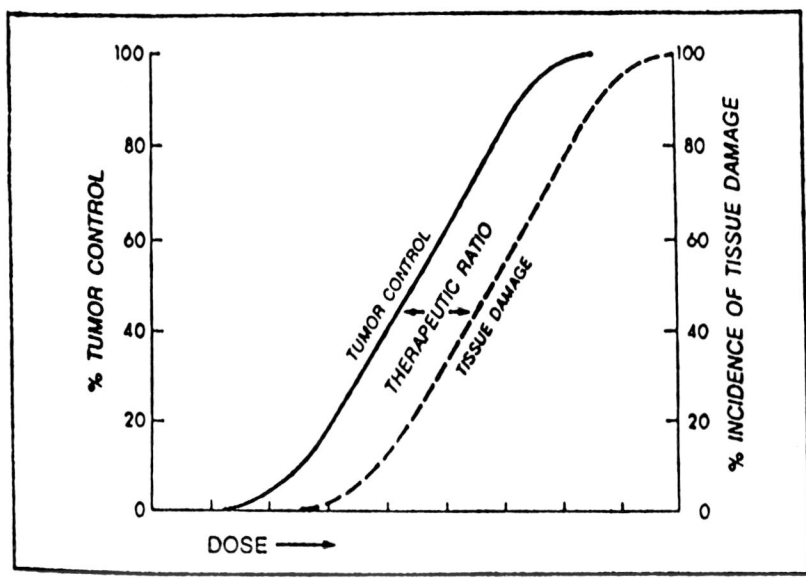

FIGURE 7-10 Dose-response curves for tumor control and normal tissue damage. The relative separation of the curves determines the therapeutic ratio.

choice of total dose from the application will be determined by the amount of external-beam radiation delivered prior to the implant as well as consideration of the therapeutic ratio.

Most centers limit treatment by estimating maximal doses to the rectum and bladder, as identified on the localizing films; others continue to rely on the estimate of milligram-hours, which, although not necessarily a good estimate of maximal rectal and bladder dose, does give an estimate of integral dose, or the total energy absorbed by critical pelvic structures. In practice, if a standard technique is used, it is reasonable to assume a correlation between mghr and tolerance. However, if the technique is suboptimal or varied, the mghr estimate should be used with caution, and an equivalence between mghr and absorbed dose should never be assumed.

For small tumors—i.e., lesions confined to but not expanding the cervix—intracavitary treatment alone is sufficient to control the primary disease. Treatment generally consists of two (occasionally three) insertions separated by 2 to 3 weeks, delivering a total dose of 70 to 90 Gy to point A, with rectal and bladder doses kept below 70 Gy and total mghr below 10,000. If the pelvic lymph nodes are at risk to contain metastatic disease, additional external-beam therapy may be given, so that the combined intracavitary and external-beam dose to those nodes will reach a value of 50 to 55 Gy. This dose is sufficient to sterilize microscopic disease in the majority of cases and will not exceed the limits of tolerance of the small bowel.

For larger tumors, treatment will usually consist of a combination of external-beam pelvic therapy followed by one or two intracavitary placements. The pelvic fields will cover at least the cervix, upper vagina, and parametria plus internal, external, and (for larger tumors) common iliac nodes. For optimal use of the two modalities, the dose of pelvic radiation must be sufficient to (1) shrink the primary tumor, so that residual tumor is likely to be encompassed by the high-dose region of the implant; and (2) control subclinical disease in the parametrial and nodal regions. In addition, the dose should be low enough to avoid exceeding the tolerance of normal tissues and to prevent the application of less than 3,000 mghr from the implant.

Examples of typical treatment prescriptions for various stages of cervical carcinoma are given in Table 7-1. Note that the stage, and tumor histopathology are less important than bulk and anatomic localization of tumor in determining the choice of treatment.

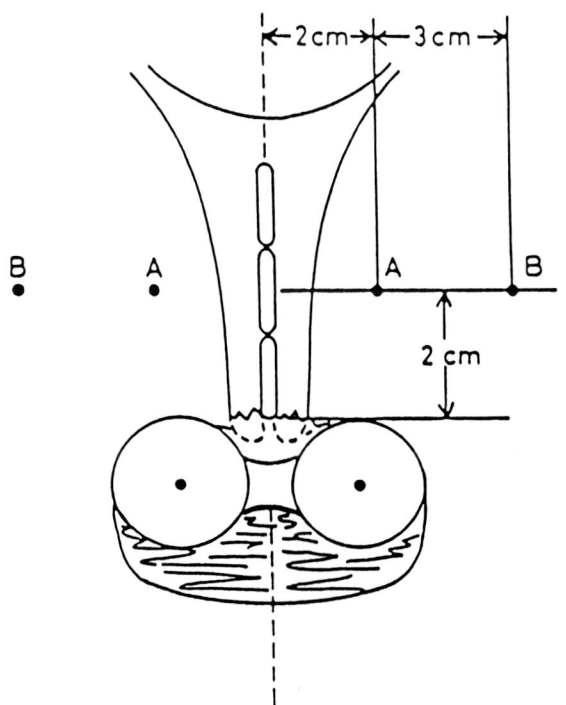

FIGURE 7-11 Locations of points A and B. (See text for explanation.)

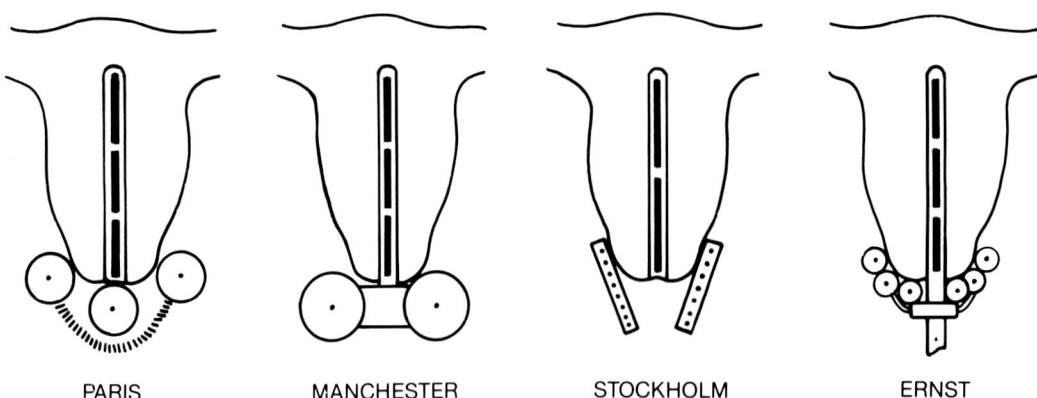

PARIS MANCHESTER STOCKHOLM ERNST

FIGURE 7-12 Gynecologic applicators with various radioactive source configurations. Both the Paris and Manchester applicators use relatively smaller amounts of radium, and the vaginal sources are located at a distance from the cervix through use of larger colpostats or spacers. The Stockholm applicator uses a large amount of radium, and all the sources are close to the cervix. The Ernst applicator represents a hybrid of the Manchester and Stockholm applicators.

Very large tumors that significantly alter normal pelvic anatomy may never be suitable for intracavitary implantation. Such disease may be treated with external-beam techniques only, in which the treatment volume is significantly reduced after 50 Gy to include only gross residual disease. Because of limitations of tolerance, the total dose can rarely exceed 70 Gy and is therefore not likely to control bulky disease permanently. Small tumors, however, can be controlled with such doses, and external-beam radiation may be appropriate for patients who for medical reasons are unable to tolerate intracavitary implantation.

An alternative when the patient's anatomy is not suitable for the placement of intracavitary devices but she is otherwise medically fit is interstitial implantation, in which radioactive sources are placed directly into the tumor bed. Historically, radium and more recently cesium-137 needles have been used for this purpose. Although high radiation doses can be delivered with these sources, the distribution of dose is generally nonho-

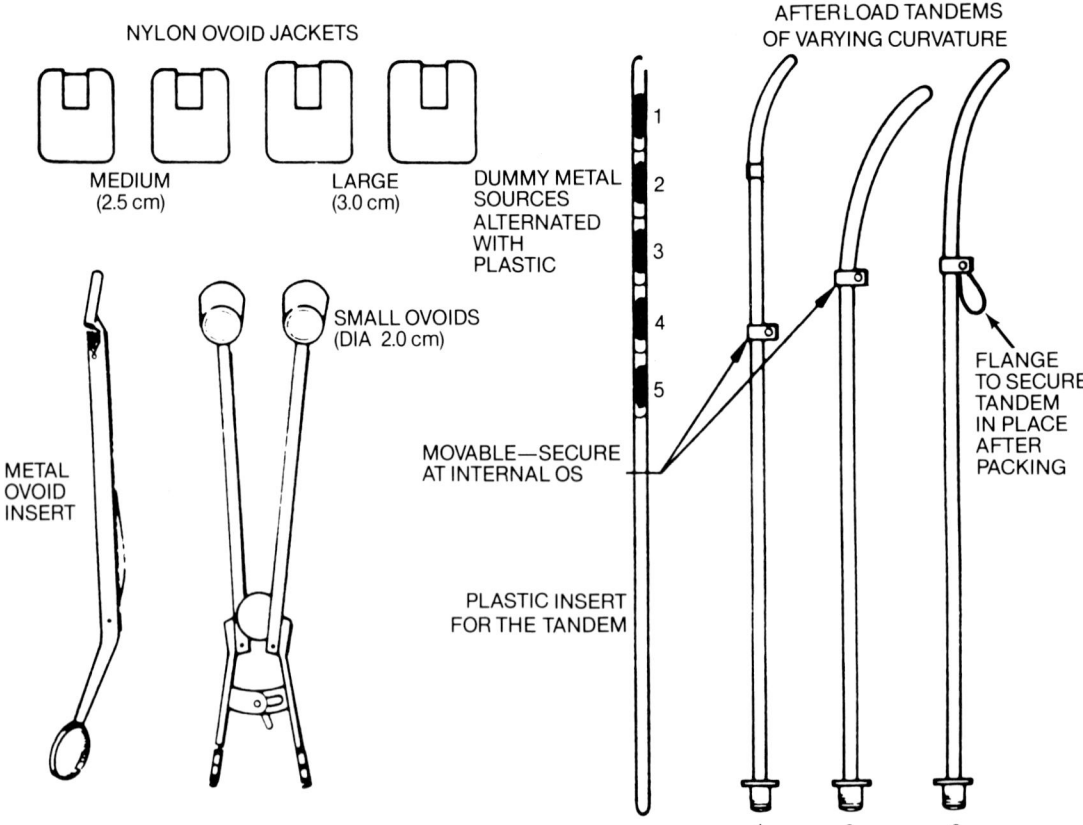

FIGURE 7-13 Fletcher-Suit afterloading applicators. Different sizes and shapes of tandems and ovoids are shown.

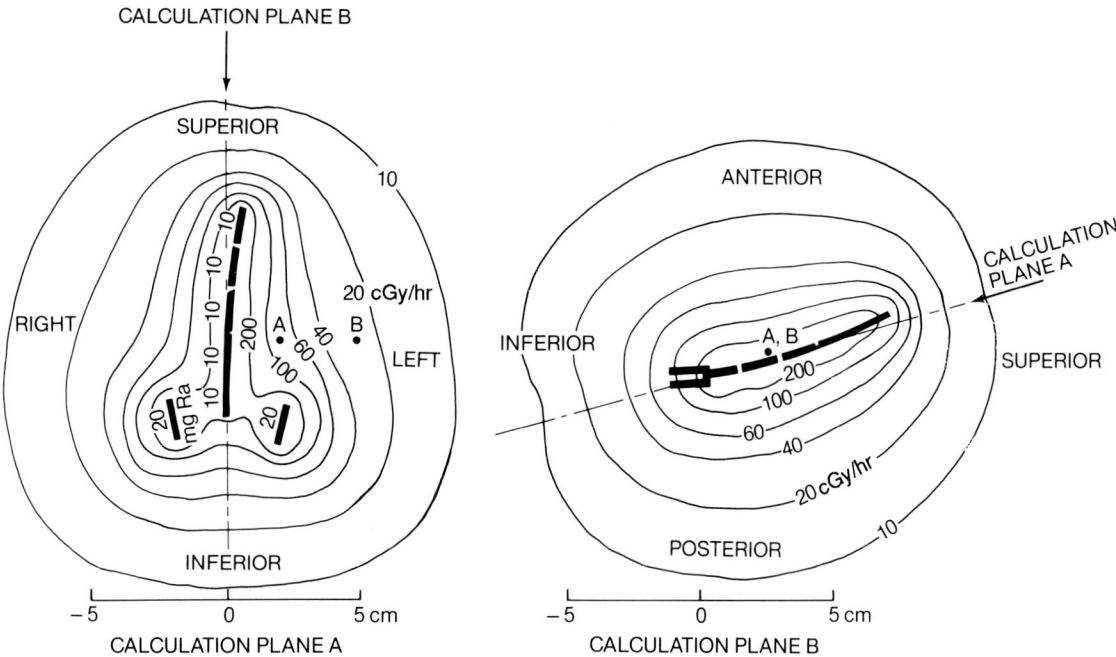

FIGURE 7-14 Example of a Fletcher-Suit tandem and ovoid after-loading application. The tandem has five radium sources loaded with 10 mg each (active length = 0.6 cm, physical length = 1.0 cm, filtration = 0.5 mm Pt [Ir]), and each ovoid has 20 mg (active length = 1.6 cm, physical length = 2.0 cm, filtration = 0.5 mm Pt [Ir]). Point A receives 78 cGy/hr and Point B receives 25 cGy/hr.

mogeneous because source strengths are limited and it is difficult to place the needles in an ideal distribution. Recently, much improved techniques have been developed by which a variety of radioactive source types can be afterloaded into hollow plastic catheters. These techniques also employ a predrilled plastic template that can be attached to the cervix and perineum, ensuring optimal placement of catheters as determined by computerized dosimetric preplanning. With such techniques, it is now possible to deliver large, homogeneous doses to many bulky tumors without hazardous exposure of the patient and the clinical staff (Martinez et al, 1985).

## Carcinoma of the Vagina

The principles of treatment for vaginal carcinoma are similar to those for cervical cancer, with external-beam radiation used to treat the primary tumor and regional nodes (including inguinal nodes) to a dose of approximately 50 Gy, followed by an implant boost. Small, superficial tumors can be satisfactorily boosted with a vaginal cylinder containing radioactive sources placed along its central axis. A plastic cylinder (of a size that will fit the vaginal lumen as closely as possible) is inserted into the vagina and secured with packing or occasionally suture. Sources are loaded along the central axis to provide a dose rate at the surface of the cylinder of 60 to 100 cGy/hr. Total dose is prescribed to a depth that will encompass the thickness of any residual tumor and should be in the range of 60 to 70 Gy.

Because the rate of dose fall-off with this technique is rapid, the treatment of tumors more than a few millimeters in thickness will deliver extremely large doses to the entire vaginal mucosa, posing the risks of chronic

TABLE 7-1    Treatment Recommendations for Carcinoma of the Cervix

| Extent of Tumor | Pelvic XRT (Gy) | Intracavitary Dose | | XRT Boost (Total Gy) |
|---|---|---|---|---|
| | | Minimum (Gy) | Maximum (mghr × 1,000) | |
| Microinvasive | — | 65 to 85 | 8 to 10 | — |
| Gross, not bulky | — | 65 to 85 | 8 to 10 | 45 to 55 to nodes |
| Gross, cervix only | 40 | 70 to 90 | 6.5 | — |
| Parametria involved | 40 | 70 to 90 | 6.5 | 55 to 60 to involved side |
| Sidewall involved | 50 | 70 to 90 | 5 | 60 to 65 to involved side |
| Lower vagina or sidewall involved | 50 | 70 to 80 | Minimum tumor dose via interstitial implant | — |

XRT = external-beam irradiation.

mucosal injury, interference with sexual function, and fistula formation. Larger tumors should therefore be boosted with an interstitial, preferably template-guided, technique that will ensure adequate coverage of the tumor volume but will keep the maximal dose to the vaginal mucosa below 85 Gy (Perez et al, 1977).

## Cancer of the Endometrium

Total abdominal hysterectomy is the cornerstone of treatment for all resectable endometrial carcinomas. However, for inoperable or unresectable tumors, radiotherapy may still be curative. The principles and techniques are similar to those described above for cervical cancer, although the uterine cavity should be packed with radioactive sources in order to ensure that an adequate dose of radiation will be delivered to the entire uterus.

The original packing technique was developed in Stockholm by Heyman using relatively bulky, preloaded radium capsules. Currently, the same objective can be achieved with smaller, flexible containers known as *Simon applicators*, which can be afterloaded with cesium-137. Tandems and colpostats are also generally employed to ensure adequate coverage of the cervix and parametria.

With computerized dosimetry and anatomic imaging, it may be possible to estimate the minimal dose to the entire uterine wall. In such a case, treatment is planned to deliver at least 60 Gy to the uterus with consideration of a supplementary pelvic boost to deliver total nodal doses of approximately 50 Gy. If complete dosimetric information is not available, treatment may be prescribed as 4,000 to 5,000 mghr radium-equivalent (Grigsby et al, 1987).

Radiotherapy is often given either before or after hysterectomy to patients known to be at risk for pelvic or vaginal recurrence. Pelvic treatment generally comprises delivery of a dose of 45 to 50 Gy over a period of approximately 5 weeks using a four-field box technique that encompasses the iliac nodes and vagina. Patients at increased risk for vaginal recurrence may receive an intracavitary boost to deliver an additional 20 to 40 Gy to the vaginal mucosa by means of a cylinder. Patients at low risk for nodal involvement may be treated with a vaginal cylinder only, receiving 50 to 70 Gy to the mucosa over a period of 2 to 4 days.

## Carcinoma of the Ovary

Radiotherapy in ovarian carcinoma is hindered by the fact that treatment must encompass the entire peritoneal cavity. Consequently, total doses are severely limited by the tolerance of critical organs such as the kidney and liver. However, if patients with only microscopic disease are considered, doses on the order of 20 to 30 Gy may be sufficient to achieve cure (Dembo, 1985).

Many techniques have been developed that permit maximally tolerated doses to be delivered to the whole abdomen. In general, high-energy photons should be used with opposed fields encompassing the abdomen and pelvis, from the diaphragms to the pelvic floor. This entire volume receives approximately 30 Gy, with daily doses limited to 120 to 150 cGy to minimize the risk of acute and chronic bowel injury. Blocks are placed to protect the kidneys after they have received approximately 20 Gy. If indicated, pelvic and paraaortic regions may be boosted to receive total doses of 45 to 60 Gy.

Patients who have undergone minimal prior abdominal surgery and chemotherapy will generally tolerate whole abdominal radiotherapy well, with only a low risk for significant chronic injury. On the other hand, those who have undergone extensive and repeated cytoreductive surgery will be predisposed to chronic radiation enteritis, small bowel obstruction, and fistula (Schray et al, 1989).

## RADIATION PROTECTION

When living cells are exposed to ionizing radiation, energy will be transferred to individual molecules in the volume through which the radiation passes. This transferred energy can disrupt the normal molecular structures and affect normal cellular functions. Some cells will suffer irreparable damage and die; others may undergo malignant transformation. Ionization is the underlying process leading to cell damage. Fortunately, the probability that a single interaction will cause significant damage is small. However, the degree and probability of damage increase as the amount of radiation received increases.

The effects of radiation depend on the total absorbed dose, type of radiation, dose rate, and type of tissue irradiated. The most conservative viewpoint regarding radiation effects is to assume that there is some risk of genetic damage or cell transformation with any radiation exposure. However, the obvious beneficial uses of radiation in medicine and technology must be counterbalanced by a reasoned approach to the potential attendant risks. In general, the potential benefits of diagnostic and therapeutic irradiation far outweigh the potential risks when radiation is safely applied.

While we can sense light, heat, and sound easily and respond to them, we cannot sense exposure to ionizing radiation immediately. The three key words in radiation protection are time, distance, and shielding. *Time* is simply the duration of exposure, which should be as short as possible. Maintaining *distance* from the radiation sources is a very effective method of reducing radiation exposure. Radiation intensity generally follows the inverse square law, i.e., if we increase the distance from 1 to 2 m from the source, the intensity will decrease to $(1/2)^2$ or 25% of what it was at 1 m. *Shielding* is another effective safety measure. If possible, personnel should work behind radiation shields. All beta particles can be stopped by a shield with a thickness greater than their penetration range in that material. Although it is more difficult to stop x-rays or gamma rays, shielding always reduces the intensity of radioactivity from the source. A high-Z material is often used for photon shielding, e.g., 1.7 cm of lead will reduce the intensity of radium-226 by about 50%.

The *rem* (Roentgen equivalent man) is a quantity used for radiation protection purposes. It is defined as the product of absorbed dose and certain modifying factors, accounting for differences in the nature of the radiation and its biologic effects.

In the 1960s, the International Commission on Radiological Protection (ICRP) defined the concept of *maximum permissible dose (MPD)*—i.e., that dose which is not expected to produce body injury to a person during his or her lifetime. Values of MPD for specific organs and the whole body are based on the currently known radiation risks in causing genetic damage and cancer (Table 7-2) (National Council on Radiation Protection and Measurements, 1971). Although these values have been adopted by many government agencies as legal limits, the ICRP strongly recommends that exposures be justified on the basis of risk and benefit analyses and that all exposures be kept "as low as reasonably achievable" (International Commission on Radiological Protection, 1977); this is known as the ALARA principle of radiation protection.

For occupational workers (individuals whose normal occupational duties involve the likelihood of exposure to radiation), the MPD equivalent to the whole body should not exceed 5 rems per year. Limits for specific organs are listed in Table 7-2. Although these limits should include the sum of total irradiation from all sources, exposure resulting from necessary medical and dental procedures need not be included. Occupational exposures are usually monitored.

Nonoccupational workers are persons who work in a hospital but who do not work with radiation. The MPD equivalent to nonoccupationally exposed workers should not exceed 0.5 rem per year to the whole body. This is the same limit recommended for the general public. To achieve this, shielding, containment of airborne radioactivity, and proper monitoring of radiation are necessary.

Laws and regulations have been written to ensure proper control and uses of radiation sources. The objective is to prevent radiation accidents, minimize population exposure, and institute corrective measures if accidents occur. To this end, individual and/or institutional users of radiation sources must obtain authorization from a government agency at the federal or state level.

In most institutions, the radiation safety officer (RSO), a specialist in radiation protection, is responsible for all aspects of radiation safety. His or her duties include preparing regulations, administering a radiation safety program, advising on radiation protection problems, keeping accounts of all radioactive materials from procurement to disposal, monitoring personnel radiation exposures, surveying environmental radiation levels, and instituting corrective measures in case of accidental radiation exposures or emergencies related to the use of radiation.

Monitoring of personnel exposure to radiation is required by law, and records must be kept for radiation workers. The RSO develops and implements such a monitoring program. The most common devices used for long-term personnel monitoring are the film badge

**TABLE 7-2** Maximum Permissible Doses of Radiation (rems/yr)

| Exposed Part of Body | Occupationally Exposed Persons (> age 18) (rems/yr) | General Public (rems/yr) |
|---|---|---|
| Whole body, blood-forming organs, gonads | 5 | 0.5 |
| Bone, thyroid, skin | 30 | 3.0 |
| Hands, forearms, feet, and ankles | 75 | 7.5 |
| All other organs | 15 | 1.5 |

and the thermoluminescent dosimeter, which are used to measure radiation exposure for a 1- to 3-month period. In high-risk areas where it may be desirable to have immediate knowledge of radiation exposure, direct-reading pocket dosimeters are worn.

Personnel monitoring is very useful in radiation control, since it ensures that normal and unexpected exposures will be recorded. To be effective in monitoring the radiation exposures, these devices must be worn by the worker consistently and should be positioned on the trunk between the waist and the shoulder; the location should represent the area of highest exposure that the body may receive. These records constitute legal evidence of the actual exposure of the worker and are periodically reviewed by government agencies.

In treating gynecologic disease with radiation, two types of treatments must be monitored and surveyed by the RSO. The first is treatments using external radiation beams. The irradiation facility must be designed so that the maximum permissible limits for occupational workers, nonoccupational personnel, and the general public will most likely not be exceeded. The ALARA principle is often applied in the shielding design of irradiation facilities, since in most instances a significant reduction in dose can be achieved without major difficulties. Once the facility has been designed and a careful radiation survey has been made to verify the acceptable radiation level, it is then a matter of routine radiation safety monitoring of the personnel to make certain that their exposure levels are not exceeded.

The second area is related to intracavitary or interstitial applications of radiation sources. In this case, the source of radiation originates from the radioactive material inserted in the patient, and the types of radiation, strength of the sources, and environment of the patient are more variable. Protection is of special concern for nurses and others who care for patients undergoing interstitial or intracavitary therapy.

## Radiation Safety Procedures in Intracavitary Applications

Specific guidelines have been written regarding radiation safety in intracavitary applications (National Council on Radiation Protection and Measurements, 1970). For example, the RSO should always be informed before the use of any therapeutic application in order to coordinate the activities of physicians, nurses, and other personnel. The RSO makes sure that radiation sources are correctly loaded and safely transported. Usually, the patient is assigned to a room designed specifically for brachytherapy applications. After the sources are loaded, the RSO is responsible for surveying the room, the adjacent rooms, and the hallway to make sure that radiation levels are acceptable. In particular, he or she calculates or measures the exposure rate at 1 m from the patient. The RSO issues any special nursing instructions and limitations on visitors. A "Radioactivity Precaution" label is attached to the chart of each patient who receives interstitial or intracavitary therapy, and similar tags are attached to the patient, the bed, and the door of the patient's room. The tag attached to the patient's chart specifies the radiation source, activity (in millicuries) at the time of administration, the exposure rate at 1 m, and the date on which the radioactive sources will be removed.

### Nursing Care and Precautions with Intracavitary/ Interstitial Implants

All personnel providing direct care to patients should wear a radiation monitor badge while at work. When sealed sources are used, there is no danger of direct radioactive contamination unless the source is damaged or lost. As noted earlier, the main issues to be considered in radiation protection are time, distance, and shielding. The nurse should limit the amount of time spent in various activities related to patient care. Whenever possible, the nurse should keep as far away from the sources as possible and work behind mobile lead shields.

During intracavitary or interstitial implants, changing of surgical bandages, dressings, or perineal pads should be undertaken only by trained personnel. If dislodged, the radioactive sources should be picked up with forceps and placed in a special lead container provided by the RSO.

As an example, a typical intracavitary application has 60 to 70 mg of radium in the tandem and ovoids. This will yield a potential exposure rate of about 50 mR/hr at 1 m distance from the sources. The exact exposure rate depends on the position of measurement and the thickness of the patient. A study of radiation exposure among nursing personnel working with brachytherapy patients in several hospitals indicated that the average annual dose recorded per nurse ranged from 25 to 150 mrem, which is well below the MPD of 5 rems per year (Cobb et al, 1978). The study also found that the radiation exposure per nurse was proportional to

the total potential exposure and did not correlate with the size of the nursing staff. Thus, it is possible to minimize personnel exposure by providing a good training program in the management of these patients and by applying the ALARA principle.

### Protection of Other Patients and Visitors

Other patients and visitors who may be in close proximity to a radioactive patient are not considered to be occupationally exposed. Limiting the duration of visits and isolating the patient in a private room or a specially designed room are necessary measures to minimize such exposure. It is unlikely that visitors will exceed the exposure dose limit if they stay at least 2 m or more from the patient. However, pregnant women, women of childbearing age, and children should not be allowed to visit a radioactive patient because the risk of genetic effects is higher in these groups.

## REFERENCES

Cobb PD, Kase KR, Bjarngard BE: Radiation exposure of nursing personnel to brachytherapy patients. *Health Physics* 34:661-665, 1978.

Dembo AJ: Abdominal pelvic radiotherapy in ovarian cancer. *Cancer* 55:2285-2290, 1985.

Grigsby PW, Kuske RR, Perez CA, Waltz BJ, Camel MH, Kao MS, Galakatos A: Medically inoperable Stage 1 adenocarcinoma of the endometrium treated with radiotherapy alone. *Int J Rad Oncol Biol Phys* 13:483-488, 1987.

Martinez A, Edmunson GK, Cox R, Gunderson LL, Howes AE: Combination of external beam irradiation and multiple site perineal applicator (MUPIT) for treatment of locally advanced gynecologic malignancies. *Int J Rad Oncol Biol Phys* 11:391-398, 1985.

International Commission on Radiological Protection: *Recommendations of the International Commission on Radiological Protection*. ICRP Publ No 26. Oxford, Pergamon Press, 1977.

National Council on Radiation Protection and Measurements: *Basic Radiation Protection Criteria*. NCRP Report No 39. Washington, DC, 1971.

National Council on Radiation Protection and Measurements: *Precautions in the Management of Patients Who Have Received Therapeutic Amounts of Radionuclides*. NCRP Report No 37. Washington, DC, 1970.

Paterson R, Parker HM: A dosage system for gamma ray therapy. *Br J Radiol* 7:592-612, 1934.

Perez CA, Korba A, Sharma S: Dosimetric considerations in irradiation of carcinoma of the vagina. *Int J Rad Oncol Biol Phys* 2:639-649, 1977.

Rubin P, Cassarett GW: *Clinical Radiation Pathology*, Vols 1 and 2. Philadelphia, WB Saunders Co, 1968.

Schray MF, Martinez A, Howes AE: Toxicity of open-field whole abdominal irradiation as primary postoperative treatment in gynecological malignancy. *Int J Rad Oncol Biol Phys* 16:397-403, 1989.

# Chapter 8 | Epidemiologic Aspects of Gynecologic Oncology

*Daniel W. Cramer,*

In this chapter, cancer occurrence and survival statistics will be considered under the heading descriptive epidemiology, while risk factors for cancer will be considered under the heading etiologic epidemiology and in greater detail for individual types of gynecologic cancer. Under both headings, methodology as well as specific findings will be discussed. The chapter will conclude with comments on how epidemiologic findings may contribute to cancer prevention.

## DESCRIPTIVE EPIDEMIOLOGY

The basic measures of cancer occurrence are incidence, cumulative incidence, and prevalence.

### Incidence

The incidence rate (IR) of cancer is defined as the number of new cases per population per time:

$$IR = \text{new cases/population/time}$$

In general, cancer incidence is stated as cases per 100,000 population per year (or cases per 100,000 person-years) and must be measured in a specific population over a specified time period. Cancer incidence rates generally come from cancer registries, which count the number of new cancer cases diagnosed during a calendar year among residents of a specific geographic area and then divide by the population of that area, as estimated by the Census Bureau. In particular, the National Cancer Institute has assembled 11 registries to define cancer incidence in the United States (US Department of Health and Human Services, 1989). Worldwide incidence can be obtained from the International Agency for Research on Cancer, which assembles incidence data from over 40 national registries (Muir et al, 1987).

*Crude incidence* is the number of new cases per population per time without regard to age, whereas *age-specific incidence* is the number of new cases that develop in a particular age group per time. The age-specific incidence rates for the gynecologic cancers for all women in the United States are shown in Figure 8-1. Invasive cervical cancer rates increase sharply between ages 25 and 35, followed by a broad plateau, with a peak occurrence of about 20 cases per 100,000 woman-years. For in situ cervical cancer, the peak occurrence is between ages 25 and 35 at about 130 cases per 100,000 women-years. Both endometrial and ovarian cancers show a sharp increase during the perimenopau-

sal years and a peak occurrence around age 75 of about 115 cases per 100,000 for endometrial and 55 cases per 100,000 for ovarian cancer. Vulvar and the more rare vaginal cancers gradually increase during the woman's life in a pattern similar to that of nonmelanoma skin cancers, with a combined peak occurrence after age 80 at about 25 cases per 100,000.

*Mortality rate* is a type of incidence in which the number of deaths is counted. Age-specific mortality rates for all US women are shown in Figure 8-2. These mortality data offer a somewhat different perspective on the relative importance of the female cancers. For example, cervical cancer emerges as a greater threat to life than does endometrial cancer, and ovarian cancer emerges as a greater threat than both cervical and endometrial cancer combined.

While age-specific incidence or mortality rate is the best way to describe the occurrence of cancer in a population, it is difficult to use these measures to compare cancer occurrence among many different populations. Although crude incidence may be used, it may be misleading if the populations differ in regard to their age distribution. An "old" population would have a higher crude incidence of endometrial cancer and a lower crude incidence of in situ cervical cancer than a "young" population, even though both populations might have identical age-specific incidences for these two cancers. Techniques that may be used to summarize age-specific incidence curves using a single number include age adjustment and calculation of the cumulative incidence.

*Age adjustment* is performed by multiplying the incidence rate for each age stratum ($IR_i$) by the proportion of individuals in that age stratum from a "standard" population ($W_i$) and summing these over the entire age range:

$$\text{Age-adjusted rate} = \frac{\Sigma IR_i(W_i)}{\Sigma W_i}$$

The age-adjusted rate will differ from the crude rate if the age distribution of the study population differs from that of the standard population.

### Cumulative Incidence

Cumulative incidence (CI) is another summary measure of disease occurrence and may be defined as the proportion of a fixed population that becomes ill during a specified time interval (Rothman, 1986). The CI from age 0 to 80, or the lifetime risk for disease, may be inferred from age-specific incidence rates using a for-

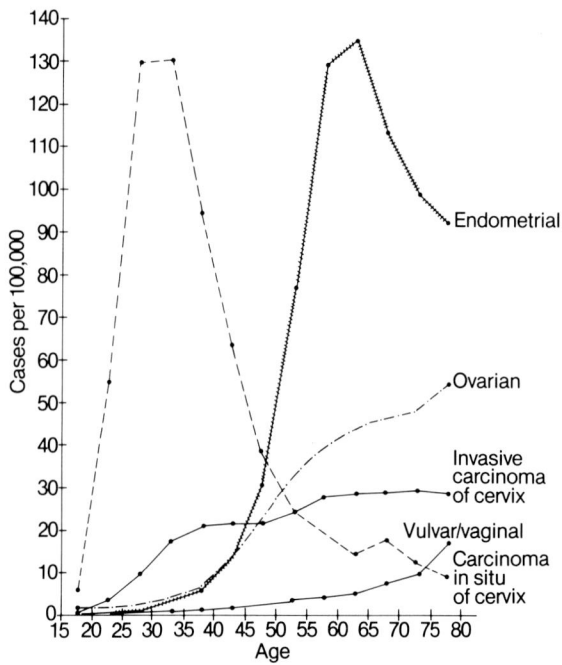

FIGURE 8-1 Age-specific incidence curves for gynecologic cancers in women in the United States.

mula that basically calculates the area under the age-specific incidence curve:

$$CI = 1 - \exp(-\Sigma IR_i t_i)$$

where $IR_i$ and $t_i$ are the age-specific incidence rate and size of age interval in the ith interval.

Another example of CI is the *case-fatality rate*, which is the cumulative incidence of death among those who develop an illness. The annual case-fatality rate may be estimated by the ratio of annual mortality to annual

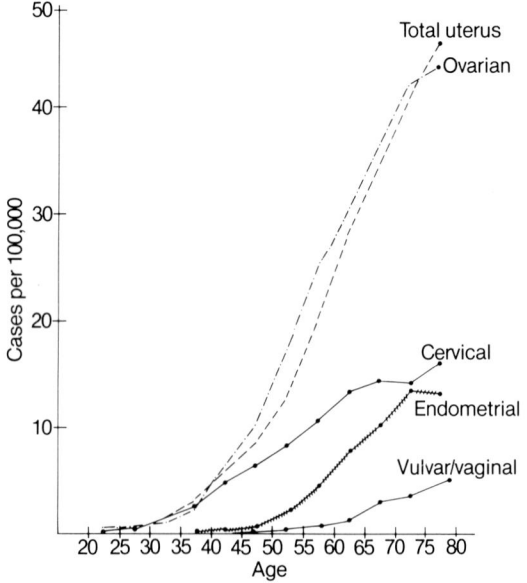

FIGURE 8-2 Age-specific mortality curves for gynecologic cancers in women in the United States.

incidence. A measure of survival perhaps more familiar to clinicians is the *5-year survival rate*, which is often taken as a measure of the number of patients potentially cured of their cancer.

Table 8-1 shows the cumulative incidences, annual case-fatality rates, and 5-year survival rates for the period 1982 to 1986 for white and black women in the United States. For white females, the lifetime risks for cervical, endometrial, and ovarian cancer are 1.0%, 3.7%, and 2.2%, respectively, with corresponding annual case-fatality rates of 30%, 9%, and 58%. For black females, the lifetime risks of cervical, endometrial, and ovarian cancer are 2.4%, 2.7%, and 1.6%, respectively, with corresponding annual case-fatality rates of 40%, 20%, and 57%. The 5-year survival rates for cervical, endometrial, and ovarian cancers are 67%, 83%, and 38% among white women and 59%, 52%, and 38% among black women. Whether the generally poorer survival rates in blacks reflect more aggressive disease, later stage at presentation, or lack of access to medical care is not clear. The incidence and survival rates in vulvar and vaginal cancers considered together are similar among white and black women; when considered separately, however, vulvar cancers are more common in whites and vaginal cancers are more common in blacks.

Lifetime risks for female cancers worldwide vary widely and are compared in Table 8-2. Geographic and ethnic variation often provides clues about disease etiology in ecologic studies that correlate disease rates with various characteristics of the populations. Lifetime risks for cervical cancer vary from 0.4% in Israel to 5.3% in Cali, Colombia, where cervical cancer is the most common malignancy in women. Although no formal ecologic studies have been published, cervical cancer would most likely be inversely correlated with various measures of socioeconomic status, including per capita income. Lifetime risks for endometrial cancer vary from a low of 0.2% in India to a high of 3.3% among white women in California. Endometrial cancer is positively correlated with per capita fat consumption (Armstrong and Doll, 1975). Lifetime risks for ovarian cancer vary from a low of 0.5% in Japan to a high of 1.7% in Sweden. Ovarian cancer is positively correlated with per capita milk consumption and lactase persistence, i.e., the ability to digest milk after infancy (Cramer, 1989). The significance of these correlations is discussed later under Risk Factors for the Gynecologic Cancers.

## Prevalence

Cumulative incidence (discussed above) should not be confused with disease prevalence, which is the proportion of a population affected by disease at a given point in time. Prevalence is often estimated by multiplying the incidence rate (IR) by the average duration (D) of the disease:

$$Prevalence = IR(D)$$

This association between prevalence and incidence has been used to estimate the duration of carcinoma in situ (CIS) of the cervix, which could not otherwise be ob-

Table 8-1  Cumulative Incidence, Annual Case-Fatality Rates, and 5-year Survival Rates for White and Black Women in the United States, 1982-1986

| Site | Cumulative Incidence (Lifetime Risk) Whites | Blacks | Annual Case-Fatality Rate Whites | Blacks | 5-Year Survival Whites | Blacks |
|---|---|---|---|---|---|---|
| Cervix (invasive) | 1.0% | 2.4% | 30% | 40% | 67% | 59% |
| Endometrial | 3.7% | 2.7% | 9% | 22% | 83% | 52% |
| Ovary | 2.2% | 1.6% | 58% | 57% | 38% | 38% |
| Vagina | 0.1% | 0.3% | 33% | 33% | 55% | 66% |
| Vulva | 0.4% | 0.2% | 19% | 18% | 74% | 67% |

*Source:* US Department of Health and Human Services: Cancer Statistics Review 1973-1986, NIH Publ No 89-2789, Bethesda, MD, 1989.

served, since it is unethical to permit CIS to be watched and not treated. The first application of cytologic screening in a previously unscreened population would yield the prevalence of CIS. After several cytologic evaluations in women previously screened and found to have negative results, the incidence of CIS could be estimated. By dividing the sum of the age-specific prevalences by the sum of the age specific-incidences, the average duration of carcinoma in situ was found to be at least 10 years (Kashgarian and Dunn, 1970).

## ETIOLOGIC EPIDEMIOLOGY

In contrast to descriptive epidemiologic studies, etiologic epidemiologic studies attempt to identify exposures that are either preventive or causal. These etiologic studies may be either experimental or, more commonly, nonexperimental. Types of experimental studies include clinical trials, field trials, and community intervention trials, while nonexperimental epidemiologic studies consist of cohort and case-control studies.

### Experimental Studies

Because an investigator must assign exposure according to a strict protocol, human experimental studies are limited to the study of measures that will prevent disease or the consequences of disease. *Clinical trials* generally evaluate new treatments for disease. The process of randomization is the cornerstone of a good clinical trial, since it minimizes bias that can result from the preferential assignment of treatment based on patient characteristics. *Field trials* generally evaluate measures that may prevent disease in well people. Large numbers of subjects are needed, and usually the disease must have serious consequences to warrant the expense of such studies. When the intervention is assigned on a community-wide basis, such as the fluoridation of water,

Table 8-2  Cumulative Incidence of Cervical, Endometrial, and Ovarian Cancer Worldwide (About 1980)

| Country (Location) | Cervical | Endometrial | Ovarian |
|---|---|---|---|
| Australia (Queensland) | 0.99% | 1.30% | 0.97% |
| Canada (Quebec) | 1.22% | 2.16% | 1.28% |
| China (Shanghai) | 1.09% | 0.35% | 0.54% |
| Colombia (Cali) | 5.31% | 0.67% | 0.87% |
| Denmark | 1.93% | 1.89% | 1.67% |
| France (Doubs) | 1.38% | 1.14% | 1.03% |
| Fed. Rep. Germany (Hamburg) | 2.05% | 1.40% | 1.41% |
| India (Bombay) | 2.22% | 0.24% | 0.75% |
| Israel | 0.43% | 1.22% | 1.37% |
| Italy (Varese) | 1.09% | 1.50% | 1.11% |
| Japan (Osaka) | 1.83% | 0.27% | 0.47% |
| Phillipines | 1.84% | 0.39% | 0.79% |
| Puerto Rico | 1.63% | 0.97% | 0.67% |
| Sweden | 1.01% | 1.58% | 1.73% |
| U.K. (Birmingham) | 1.27% | 1.10% | 1.25% |
| U.S. (Calif, Bay—Whites) | 0.89% | 3.28% | 1.47% |
| U.S. (Calif, Bay—Blacks) | 1.38% | 1.39% | 1.12% |
| U.S. (Calif, Bay—Chinese) | 1.34% | 1.58% | 0.91% |
| U.S. (Hawaii—Japanese) | 0.62% | 1.96% | 0.81% |
| Yugoslavia (Slovenia) | 1.40% | 1.40% | 1.08% |

*Source:* Muir C, Waterhouse J, Mack T, Powell J, Whelen S: Cancer incidence in five continents. International Agency for Research on Cancer, Lyon, France, 1987.

the experimental study is called a *community intervention trial*.

## Nonexperimental Studies

We have already discussed one type of nonexperimental study, the ecologic study, in which characteristics of populations are correlated with disease risk. More commonly, nonexperimental studies involve observing individuals and taking advantage of "natural experiments" in which individuals are exposed to possible carcinogens by virtue of their diet, occupation, lifestyle, or prior medical therapy. Nonexperimental epidemiologic studies are essentially the only way to obtain information about cancer risk associated with suspected carcinogens in humans, although inferences may sometimes be drawn from animal studies. Cohort and case-control studies are the primary types of nonexperimental studies (Table 8-3).

**The Cohort Study** In a cohort study, the groups (cohorts) are defined according to exposures that occurred prior to the disease of interest. Subjects are followed over time to determine the frequency with which the disease developed in the exposed and unexposed cohorts, and it is possible to calculate the incidence or prevalence of disease in each cohort. In the *retrospective* cohort study, exposures and outcomes have already occurred by the time the study is begun. For example, studies of the relationship between radiation and female cancer are based on records of women previously irradiated for cervical cancer, with medical records being used to identify them and death certificates being used to determine which women later died from cancers other than those of the cervix. In the *prospective* cohort study, the exposure may or may not have occurred by the time the study is begun, but the outcome of interest has not yet occurred. After the cohorts are selected, the investigator must wait for the disease or outcome to appear in the cohort members.

In cohort studies, the association between an exposure and an illness may be characterized by either the relative or the attributable risk. The *relative risk* divides the occurrence of disease in those exposed by the occurrence in the nonexposed group. If the number is not significantly different from one, there is no association; a number significantly lower than one indicates that the exposure has a protective effect, while a number significantly greater than one indicates that exposure may increase risk. The *attributable risk* is the difference between occurrence rate in the exposed and unexposed populations. A number significantly greater than zero indicates that the exposure may cause disease, whereas a number significantly lower than zero may indicate protection (in which case the attributable risk is called the "preventive fraction").

Advantages of the cohort study are (a) it is less susceptible to selection bias and (b) it allows both relative and attributable risks to be calculated. Disadvantages include their high costs in terms of time and money. Such studies are most suitable for identifying disease risks associated with unique or rare exposures (e.g., followup of atomic bomb survivors to determine the risks of cancer from radiation). When an investigator is dealing with a rare exposure, rates in the general population may be used to represent the nonexposed group. In this instance, the observed number of cases in the exposed cohort is compared with the number of cases that would be expected if the general population rates prevailed in the exposed cohort. This comparison is called the *standardized mortality or morbidity ratio* (SMR) and is equivalent to the relative risk.

---

**Table 8-3  Comparison of Cohort and Case-Control Studies**

| | | Cohort | | | Case-Control | |
|---|---|---|---|---|---|---|
| | | Exposed | Unexposed | | Exposed | Unexposed |
| Design | Diseased cases | $a$ | $b$ | Cases | $a$ | $b$ |
| | Person-time | $N_1$ | $N_0$ | Controls | $c$ | $d$ |
| Yield | Rate difference (attributable risk) | $\dfrac{a}{N_1} - \dfrac{b}{N_0}$ | | Not obtainable directly | | |
| | Relative risk (RR) | $\dfrac{a/N_1}{b/N_0}$ | | Exposure odds ratio (RR) | $\dfrac{a/b}{c/d} = \dfrac{ad}{bc}$ | |
| Cost/feasibility | | Generally costly; more feasible for well-defined exposures and common outcomes. Not efficient for rare outcomes. | | | Generally lower in cost; more efficient for rare disease but not for rare exposure. | |
| Biases | | Selection bias less common, but subject to misclassification and confounding. | | | Subject to selection, misclassification, and confounding. | |

***The Case-Control Study*** In case-control studies, the groups are selected on the basis of the presence (cases) or absence (controls) of a particular disease. In these two groups, exposures of interest are determined from records or interview, and the odds of exposure among the cases is compared with the odds of exposure among the controls. The resulting term is the *exposure odds ratio*, which is equivalent to the relative risk. If an entire population could be characterized by its exposure and disease status, the exposure odds ratio would be identical to the relative risk. Although this is rarely the case, the odds ratio will approximate the relative risk as long as the sampling of cases and controls was not influenced by their exposure status. The attributable risk is not directly obtainable in the case-control study, which is one of its disadvantages, as are the possibilities for selection and misclassification biases. The advantages of the case-control study are that it is generally low in cost and easy to conduct.

## Judging an Epidemiologic Study

Because patients frequently ask doctors their opinion about new studies linking certain exposures with cancer, it behooves the clinician to have some way of judging whether the conclusion of a particular study is believable. Criteria that should be taken into consideration in judging such associations include validity, dose response, consistency, and biologic credibility. The appropriateness of the statistical test(s) performed and its significance are also important and are discussed in Chapter 9.

***Validity*** Validity means freedom from *bias*, which is any systematic error in the design, conduct, or analysis of a study that leads to a mistaken conclusion. The major categories of bias include observation, selection, and confounding.

*Observation bias* (or misclassification) occurs when subjects have been incorrectly classified with respect to exposure or disease because (a) the criteria for exposure or disease were not clearly defined, (b) records were incomplete, or (c) different methods were employed for collecting information from the study groups. Random misclassification would generally mask a true association, whereas differential misclassification may cause a false association to be observed.

A frequent criticism of case-control studies linking exogenous hormones and female cancer is that women with such cancers may more readily recall past use of such hormones, whereas control subjects may not. One way to assess this bias would be independent verification of exposures reported at interview using pharmacy or physician records. Whenever possible, the researcher who is to record whether or not disease occurred among subjects in a cohort study should be unaware of the subjects' exposure status or, if possible, should be unaware of the subjects' disease status when recording exposure. "Blindness" of observation and strict criteria for classifying outcome are also important in clinical trials, since an enthusiastic researcher might be inclined to look for success when a new therapy is introduced.

Epidemiologic studies generally involve a comparison between two groups for disease or exposure frequency, and those groups are usually subsets of a larger population. *Selection bias* may occur when correlates of the exposure or outcome influence sampling from the larger population. For example, if we recruited subjects by asking, "Would you participate in a study of uterine cancer and birth control pills?" it is likely we might recruit a larger percentage of patients with uterine cancer who had used pills than if we had asked, "Would you participate in a study of uterine cancer in relation to your menstrual and pregnancy history?" Bias due to self-selection is possible in any study that requires sampling and informed consent for participation. Selection bias may also occur if the study involves patients who were diagnosed many years in the past and survival has been influenced by exposure. Using incident cases, from a defined geographic area, obtaining high participation rates, and attempting to describe nonparticipants are several means of reducing (or at least estimating) selection bias.

*Confounding* means that some other factor not considered in the design or analysis accounts for an association because the factor is correlated with both exposure and disease. For any study of cancer, obvious confounders include age, race, and socioeconomic status, since we have indicated previously how cancer risk can vary with these characteristics. One can control for confounding during the design of a study by limiting the subjects selected to a specific racial or age group or by matching each case to a specific control subject who is similar to the case with respect to the confounder. If confounders are not controlled for during the design of the study, they may be controlled for at the analysis stage by means of stratification or multivariate analysis, which effectively allows the association to be investigated in groups that are homogeneous with respect to the confounder.

***Dose Response*** Some exposures, such as a family history of cancer, can be treated only as a dichotomous (yes/no) variable. However, variables that can be ranked, such as pack-years of smoking, allow the investigator to look for a dose response. Evidence of an increase in risk with increasing levels of exposure often provides support for a biologic interpretation for the association. In addition, such information may be helpful in making public health recommendations about safe or unsafe levels of exposure.

***Consistency and Credibility*** Issues of consistency and credibility require the researcher to look beyond his or her own data to review other relevant studies. Agreement among different investigators, particularly if they have used different study methodologies, may suggest a real association. Credibility means that an association is plausible, taking into consideration all aspects of what is known about the natural history or demographics of the disease or what has been observed in relevant experimental models. This process is perhaps easier to illustrate than to explain:

In the 1970s, a number of reports linked the use of

menopausal hormones with endometrial cancer (Smith et al, 1975; Ziel and Finkle, 1975; Mack et al, 1976; Shapiro et al, 1980). The associations were statistically significant, and a dose response was observed. These additional observations supported the credibility of this association:

1. Women with granulosa–theca cell tumors as a source of endogenous estrogen develop endometrial cancer (Salerno, 1962).
2. Women with decreased degradation of estrogen secondary to liver failure may develop endometrial cancer (Spert, 1949).
3. Women who are obese and have excessive peripheral conversion of androstenedione to active estrogen are at increased risk for endometrial cancer (MacDonald and Siiteri, 1974).
4. The perimenopausal period is characterized by anovulatory cycles with unopposed estrogen, and this is the same age group in which the age-specific incidence of endometrial cancer increases rapidly.
5. Unopposed estrogen administration may cause endometrial hyperplasia, which can be prevented or reversed by the administration of progesterone (Whitehead et al, 1980).

This collection of epidemiologic and biologic observations not only supports the credibility of an association between unopposed exogenous estrogen and endometrial cancer but also suggests a biologic framework for viewing endometrial cancer as a consequence of states that lead to an excess of estrogen relative to progesterone.

## RISK FACTORS FOR SPECIFIC GYNECOLOGIC CANCERS

In the previous section, we emphasized the desirability of constructing a framework within which to view epidemiologic associations for a particular cancer. In this section, underlying pathogenetic models are suggested. Although no claim is made that these models have been proven or that all the details are complete, the reader may find them useful for ordering the diverse and sometimes confusing risk factors reported for these cancers.

### Cervical Cancer

The framework for viewing invasive squamous cell carcinoma of the cervix is that it is the end stage of cervical intraepithelial neoplasia (CIN), progressing from dysplasia to carcinoma in situ to invasive disease. Thus, risk factors for cervical cancer will be those that relate to the initiation of CIN and those that relate to its progression to invasive disease (Table 8-4).

CIN is believed to arise during the process of squamous metaplasia—the transformation of columnar to squamous mucosa (Coppleson and Reid, 1967). Factors linked to atypical transformation appear to be overwhelmingly associated with sexual history (Terris et al, 1967; Martin, 1967; Rotkin, 1967). Early age at first intercourse appears to be an important risk factor and

---

**Table 8-4** Risk Factors for Cervical Cancer Relative to Proposed Pathogenetic Model

*Model:* Cervical cancer arises as an aberration of squamous metaplasia and progresses through various stages of intraepithelial neoplasia.

A. Factors affecting atypical transformation:
 1. Periods of heightened squamous metaplasia, such as early adolescence, offer greater opportunity for atypical transformation.
 2. Venereal infections, especially papillomavirus infection with types 16/18, are probably the major cause of atypical transformation.
 3. Chemicals such as coal tars, to which women were exposed through douching, may also cause atypical transformation. Tobacco smoke components absorbed in the blood and secreted in the cervical mucus could have a similar effect.

B. Factors affecting progression of intraepithelial disease:
 1. Access to and use of cervical cytologic examination.
 2. Possible micronutrient deficiency, including folic acid and vitamin A deficiencies.

---

may relate to the fact that adolescence is a period of heightened squamous metaplasia and that intercourse during such times may increase the risk for atypical transformation and subsequent CIN (Singer, 1976). Agents that specifically cause atypical transformation are likely to be one or more sexually transmitted diseases, as indicated by the importance of intercourse with multiple partners or with a "high-risk male"—i.e., one who has himself had contact with multiple partners or prostitutes (Skegg et al, 1982). The relevance of the male's sexual history to his consort's cervical cancer is suggested by the occurrence of marital "clusters" of cervical cancer in which men whose first wives died of cervical cancer remarried and their second wives got cervical cancer (Kessler, 1976). Risk for cervical neoplasia is also high in women who have had contact with males who have penile condylomas (Campton et al, 1985).

Sexuallly transmitted diseases that might cause atypical transformation include *Trichomonas* infection (Patten et al, 1963); cytomegalovirus infection (Melnick et al, 1978); herpes genitalis (Aurelian et al, 1981); and human papillomavirus (HPV) infection, especially with HPV types 16 and 18 (Kurman et al, 1983; Reeves et al, 1989). The papillomavirus is undoubtedly the most likely candidate so far, although interactions between various infections such as herpes and HPV are possible (zur Hausen, 1982). Regardless of which specific agent is eventually found to be the cause of atypical transformation, a woman can decrease her risk for cervical cancer by safe sexual practices. Use of barrier methods of contraception (condoms or diaphragms) offers some protection against cervical cancer (Terris and Oalmann, 1960). In addition, women members of ethnic or religious groups that encourage monogamy are known to have low rates of cervical cancer (Martin, 1967).

Our focus on sexual factors does not preclude noncoital factors in this disease. Chemical carcinogenesis may be suggested by the observation that douching with coal-tar substances, as practiced earlier in this century, was found to be a strong risk factor for cervical cancer (Smith, 1931). Although such products are no longer available, douching should probably be discouraged among adolescents during the stage of active squamous metaplasia. It appears that components of tobacco smoke may be secreted in the cervical mucus, raising the possibility that smoking may be either an independent risk factor or perhaps a cofactor in this disease (Trevathan et al, 1983).

In terms of factors related to the progression of CIN, a key factor is the woman's access to and use of cervical cytologic examination. Declining mortality from cervical cancer in various populations is correlated with the use of such screening (Miller et al, 1976). Case-control studies demonstrate that the risk for invasive cervical cancer in women who have Pap tests at least every 3 years is one-tenth that of women who have never had a Pap test (La Vecchia et al, 1984a). The progression of CIN may be more rapid in women who use oral contraceptives (Stern et al, 1977); one investigator attributed this risk to a derangement in folic acid metabolism and suggested supplementation with this vitamin (Butterworth et al, 1982), while another study suggests that vitamin A is the key dietary factor in this association (La Vecchia et al, 1984b).

## Endometrial Cancer

In a model already discussed, the framework for viewing endometrial adenocarcinoma is the finding that risk is mediated through states that lead to an excess of estrogen relative to progesterone as a result of increased production, decreased degradation, or exogenous intake (Table 8-5).

Estrogen-producing tumors of the ovary, such as granulosa cell tumors, are one example of endometrial cancers caused by increased production. A more important risk factor, via this mechanism, is obesity (Wynder et al, 1966). Obesity is associated with increased peripheral conversion of androstenedione into active estrogens in fat (MacDonald and Siiteri, 1974). Alternatively, lean body mass and exercise (Frisch et al, 1985) and smoking (Lesko et al, 1985) are associated with lower levels of endogenous estrogens and lower risk for

endometrial cancer, although smoking cannot be encouraged as a preventive measure. It is also known that women who underwent oophorectomy at an early age with retention of the uterus are at reduced risk (Jansen and Ostergaard, 1954).

Endometrial cancer as a consequence of decreased degradation of estrogen is illustrated by the previously noted case report of this cancer associated with cirrhosis (Spert, 1949). Alcohol use may retard the degradation of estrogen and could be predicted according to this model to be a risk factor for endometrial cancer just as it has been noted for breast cancer (Willett et al, 1987).

Finally, increased risk is associated with exogenous intake of estrogen via unopposed menopausal hormones (as noted previously) or through the use of estrogen-dominant sequential birth control pills (Silverberg and Makowski, 1975). Alternatively, the use of combination birth control pills appears to decrease the risk for endometrial cancer (Weiss and Sayvet, 1980).

## Ovarian Cancer

The framework for viewing the epidemiology of ovarian cancer is that this disease may be a consequence of *hypergonadotropic hypogonadism*—i.e., high levels of gonadotropins consequent to failing ovaries or ovaries otherwise incapable of exerting feedback control on the pituitary (Table 8-6). The basis for this assertion lies in certain parallel findings in animal models in which ovarian tumors were induced through mechanisms that caused premature depletion of follicles, including irra-

---

**Table 8-5   Risk Factors for Endometrial Cancer Relative to Proposed Pathogenetic Model**

*Model*: Endometrial cancer is a consequence of states that lead to an excess of estrogen relative to progesterone.
A. Estrogen excess through increased production:
  1. Estrogen-producing tumors of ovary or adrenal gland.
  2. Enhanced peripheral conversion of estrogen precursor in fat occurring in the obese.
  3. Factors that decrease endogenous estrogen (surgical castration, exercise, smoking) are protective.
B. Estrogen excess through decreased degradation:
  1. Liver failure or factors that affect the metabolism of estrogen in the liver.
C. Estrogen excess through exogenous exposure:
  1. Unopposed estrogen during menopause increases risk.
  2. Use of sequential oral contraceptives.

---

**Table 8-6   Risk Factors for Ovarian Cancer Relative to Proposed Pathogenetic Model**

*Model*: Ovarian cancer is a consequence of hypergonadotropic hypogonadism. Whether a stromal or an epithelial tumor is observed may depend upon the degree of stromal-epithelial admixture.
A. Factors that predispose to stromal-epithelial admixture:
  1. Factors such as "incessant" ovulation or foreign body exposure (talc) may predispose to greater stromal-epithelial admixture and may be risk factors for epithelial tumors.
B. Environmental factors that induce hypogonadism:
  1. Radiation if received premenopausally, if sufficient to induce menopause, and after a long latency.
  2. Viruses, possibly mumps.
  3. Chemicals toxic to oocytes, such as polycyclic hydrocarbons.
  4. Dietary factors such as galactose, shown to be an oocyte toxin in rodents.
C. Genetic factors that induce hypogonadism:
  1. Deficiency of galactose 1-phosphate uridyl transferase.
D. Factors that operate at the enterohepatic or pituitary level to raise or lower gonadotropins:
  1. Phenobarbital or halogenated hydrocarbons may enhance estrogen degradation and raise gonadotropin levels in a functional counterpart of the intrasplenic ovary.
  2. Case reports link the use of fertility drugs that raise gonadotropin levels with development of ovarian tumors.
  3. Oral contraceptives lower gonadotropin levels and are protective.

diation of the gonads (Furth and Butterworth, 1936) and the use of polycyclic hydrocarbons toxic to oocytes (Howell et al, 1954), and the use of animal strains predisposed to congenital deficiency of germ cells (Murphy and Russell, 1963). It is believed that such mechanisms were mediated through high levels of gonadotropins that resulted from depletion of the oocytes, since hypophysectomy prevented tumor development when it was included in the experimental model (Marchant, 1961)—hence the term hypergonadotropic hypogonadism.

It has been argued that these animal models are not relevant to human tumors because the interventions produced primarily stromal tumors, whereas humans develop epithelial-type tumors. However, human ovaries differ from rodent ovaries in the degree of stromal-epithelial admixture. Inclusion cysts, which are islands of surface epithelium entrapped with the stroma from which the epithelial tumors are thought to originate, are rarely seen in rodent ovaries. That stromal stimulation (in response to gonadotropins) may lead to epithelial differentiation and proliferation is suggested by elegant experiments that have shown the importance of the stromal-epithelial interaction (Cunha et al, 1985).

It is possible that factors predisposing to greater stromal-epithelial interaction might increase the risk for ovarian cancer independent of any effect on gonadotropins, such as uninterrupted ovulation (Fathalla, 1983) or perhaps foreign body exposure in women who use talc in genital hygiene (Cramer et al, 1982). However, the primary risk factors probably operate through the induction of hypergonadotropic hypogonadism comparable to the animal models. That *radiation* is a risk factor for human ovarian cancer has been demonstrated in cohort studies of women treated with radiation therapy for cervical cancer and those exposed to the effects of the atomic bomb blasts (Day and Boice, 1983; Darby et al, 1984). Such studies show that radiation exposure is associated with increased risk for ovarian cancer when exposure occurs at an early age (when the ovaries are still functioning), when the dose is sufficient to induce menopause, and after a long latency period (at least 10 years).

That *chemical exposures* may also cause premature depletion of follicles and ovarian cancer is suggested by the animal models involving polycyclic hydrocarbons. Women may be exposed to such agents through tobacco smoke, and one study has suggested an excess risk for ovarian cancer among smokers (Doll et al, 1980). As is the case for radiation, the risk may be greater in women exposed at an early age and after a long latency period.

A "chemical" to which women may be exposed through their diet is *galactose*, a sugar that is generally consumed in its disaccharide form, lactose. The potential importance of galactose as an oocyte toxin is shown by the fact that female rodents fed diets high in galactose developed ovulatory dysfunction and produced offspring with oocyte deficiency (Swartz and Mattison, 1988; Chen et al, 1981). It is also known that galactosemic women with a severe deficiency of galactose 1-phosphate uridyl transferase (transferase) may develop hypergonadotropic hypogonadism (Kaufman et al,

1981*a*) and the possible relationship of galactose consumption and metabolism to the risk for ovarian cancer has been investigated (Cramer et al, 1989). The patients with ovarian cancer more frequently consumed dairy products with a high content of prehydrolyzed lactose, such as yogurt, in which galactose is more readily digestible, and had lower levels of transferase.

Figure 8-3 shows the distribution of ovarian cancer cases and controls by the *lactose/transferase* (L/T) ratio—i.e., a woman's estimated daily lactose consumption divided by transferase activity. There was a highly significant difference in the distribution of cases compared with controls, indicating that the affected women had consumed more galactose relative to their ability to metabolize it than had the controls. Further epidemiologic evidence for the importance of galactose consumption is suggested by the observation that, internationally, ovarian cancer risk is strongly correlated with per capita milk consumption and with the ability to absorb lactose in adulthood (*lactase persistence*) (Cramer, 1989).

The model for ovarian cancer as a consequence of hypergonadotropic hypogonadism may explain other risk factors for this cancer. It has been found that women with ovarian cancer are less likely to recall having had *mumps* that affected the parotid gland (Cramer et al, 1983*a*), yet such patients have similar levels of mumps antibodies (Menczer et al, 1979). This may mean that ovarian cancer patients have had mumps infections that were not perceived as parotitis, namely mumps oophoritis. Menopause as a consequence of

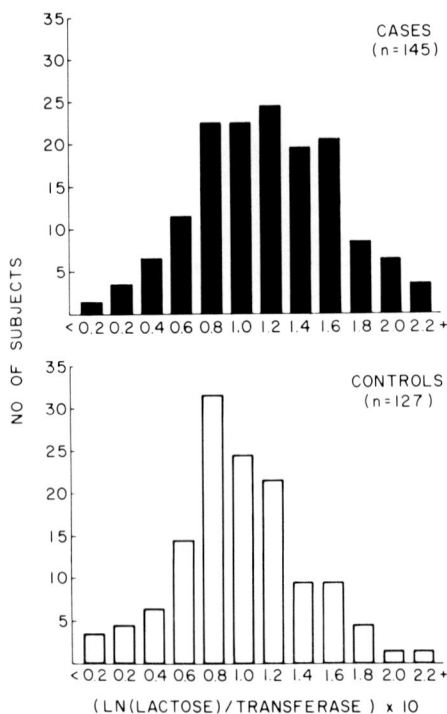

**FIGURE 8-3** Distribution of the ratio of lactose consumption to transferase activity in ovarian cancer cases and controls. (From Cramer DW, et al: Galactose consumption and metabolism in relation to the risk of ovarian cancer. *Lancet* 2:66, 1989.)

documented mumps oophoritis has been described (Morrison et al, 1975). Thus, mumps could be an example of a viral cause of hypergonadotropic hypogonadism that could lead to ovarian cancer.

*Hypogonadism* as a precursor fits with clinical manifestations of hypogonadism as risk factors for ovarian cancer. The increased risk for this disease among nulliparous compared with parous women may therefore be partly explained by infertility as a marker for hypogonadism (Cramer et al, 1983b). However, pregnancy itself might have a protective effect perhaps through its ability to alter the secretion of tropic hormones in later life; this could explain the additional protective effect exerted by subsequent pregnancies. That the hypogonadism must be accompanied by the increased secretion of gonadotropins may explain the importance of birth control pills in lowering the risk for ovarian cancer (Centers for Disease Control, 1983). It may be safely predicted that women at greatest risk for hypergonadotropic hypogonadism will benefit most from using the pill. As women age, gonadotropin secretion increases (Reyes et al, 1977), so that women who use the pill after age 30 would be expected to show greater benefit as a result.

It is important to emphasize that the risk for ovarian cancer may have a genetic component. If a patient has a primary relative with ovarian cancer, the patient's risk for ovarian cancer may be increased up to 11-fold (Cramer et al, 1983b).

Finally, other factors operating at either the pituitary or the enterohepatic level to raise gonadotropins may also be risk factors for the disease. Case reports suggest that ovarian cancer may be associated with *clomiphene therapy* (Ben-Hur et al, 1986). Chemicals that enhance the metabolism of estrogen in the liver, such as phenobarbital (Fahim et al, 1968), might also be risk factors for ovarian cancer as functional counterparts of the intrasplenic ovary animal models for ovarian cancer (Biskind and Biskind, 1944).

### Vaginal and Vulvar Neoplasms

Other than clear cell adenocarcinomas of the vagina associated with the use of diethylstilbestrol (DES) (Herbst et al, 1972), vaginal carcinoma is primarily a disease of women over age 50, with an age distribution nearly identical to that for vulvar carcinoma. Like cervical neoplasms, vulvar and vaginal cancers may be preceded at an earlier age by an in situ phase; however, the natural history of these lesions is debated. Vulvar and vaginal neoplasms frequently occur in the same patient and in asssociation with epithelial neoplasms of other anogenital sites, including the cervix, the anus, and even the urethra and bladder (Newman and Cromer, 1959; Marcus, 1960; Stern and Kaplan, 1969).

From the standpoint of developing a framework for pathogenesis, the "cloacal field theory" concerning a common origin of anogenital neoplasms is appealing. Thus, risk factors known to exist for cervical neoplasms—especially the sexually transmitted diseases herpes and condyloma—have also been shown to be pertinent in the development of vulvar and vaginal neoplasms (Kaufman et al, 1981b; Crum et al, 1982). Another possible risk factor for vulvar neoplasms is smoking (Newcomb et al, 1984). Further study of dietary factors, especially the carotenoids, would likely be worthwhile.

### Gestational Trophoblastic Neoplasia

Neoplasms of the trophoblast include complete and partial hydatidiform moles, invasive moles, and choriocarcinoma. The epidemiology of hydatidiform mole is better understood than is that of the other two forms of the disease; however, it is likely to be relevant to them, since invasive moles and choriocarcinoma are commonly preceded by molar pregnancy. The prevalence of molar pregnancy varies from 1 per 100 pregnancies in Asia to 1 per 1,000 or 1,500 pregnancies in the United States (Table 8-7). The risk for molar pregnancy increases with maternal age, but it is less clear whether adolescents are also at increased risk (Stone and Bagshawe, 1979; Hayashi et al, 1982). Possible gynecologic factors include prior miscarriage (Insler et al, 1981) or twin pregnancies (DeGeorge, 1970) and the use of birth control pills. The peculiar cytogenetic patterns of complete and partial hydatidiform moles may indicate the importance of aberrant germ cells in the origin of these disorders.

A possible dietary factor for molar pregnancy is a protective effect of vitamin A or its precursor, carotene, as reported in two epidemiologic studies (Berkowitz et al, 1985, Parazzini et al, 1988). Vitamin A deficiency causes fetal wastage and aberrations of epithelial development in female animals as well as degeneration of seminiferous epithelium with poor gamete development in male animals (O'Toole et al, 1974; Evans et al, 1934; Kim et al, 1981). A relationship between vitamin A deficiency and trophoblastic diseases is compatible with the observation that in regions where molar pregnancy is common, there is also a high incidence of night blindness (McLaren, 1966).

## PREVENTION OF GYNECOLOGIC CANCERS

Prevention of morbidity and mortality for the gynecologic cancers may take place on several levels. *Primary prevention* consists of identifying and eliminating causal factors or in some way preventing such factors from exerting their effect. *Secondary prevention* refers to the identification of disease at earlier, presumably more treatable stages through the use of cancer screening. *Tertiary prevention* refers to effective treatment methods. In this section, we will discuss the present and future role of epidemiology in the prevention of gynecologic cancers on the primary and secondary levels.

### Primary Prevention

The role of epidemiology in the primary prevention of gynecologic cancer is to identify modifiable risk factors. The association between smoking and lung cancer is perhaps the premier example of an epidemiologic finding that could serve as a basis for primary prevention

| Table 8-7 Prevalence of Hydatidiform Mole Worldwide | |
| --- | --- |
| Area | Rate/1,000 Pregnancies |
| Taiwan | 8.3 |
| India | 6.3 |
| Philippines | 5.8 |
| Mexico | 5.0 |
| Iraq | 4.5 |
| Hong Kong | 4.1 |
| Australia | 1.2 |
| Uganda | 1.0 |
| United Kingdom (Belfast) | 0.8 |
| Israel | 0.8 |
| Sweden | 0.6 |
| United States (Boston) | 0.5 |

if doctors could motivate patients to alter their smoking habits. With regard to cervical cancer, links between this disease and smoking provide an additional reason for gynecologists to encourage patients to enter smoking cessation programs. Even though the principal infection that causes cervical cancer is not known with certainty, the avoidance of multiple partners and the use of barrier methods of contraception are key factors that could serve in the primary prevention of cervical cancer.

General advice offered by the National Cancer Institute to reduce the use of animal fats and increase the intake of vegetables high in carotene would likely be beneficial in the primary prevention of endometrial cancer and trophoblastic disease. If estrogen replacement therapy is to be instituted during menopause, regimens that include a progestogen would be advisable. Dietary factors and exogenous hormones may ultimately prove important in the prevention of ovarian cancer as well. For ovarian cancer, it is possible that the avoidance of lactose-rich foods may be of value. In addition, the use of oral contraceptives is probably an important factor in prevention; as discussed earlier, the ability of oral contraceptives to prevent ovarian cancer is probably related to the lowering of gonadotropin levels and is therefore most beneficial in those women at greater risk for hypergonadotropism. Since gonadotropin levels increase with age, it would be more beneficial to use birth control pills at a later age (say after 30) than at an earlier age.

### Secondary Prevention

Secondary prevention of disease morbidity and mortality can be achieved for those diseases in which a preclinical stage can be identified through screening and for which the prognosis is more favorable when the disease is identified and treated during its preclinical stage. The premier example of a disease for which morbidity and mortality have been reduced through screening is cervical cancer. The efficacy of cervical cancer screening can be further improved if epidemiologic information on high-risk groups is used to target screening efforts. In this connection, women who have multiple partners, have had condylomas, have had a prior ab-

normal Pap smear, are smokers, or are using oral contraceptives must be encouraged to continue to have annual Pap tests despite the recent advice that longer interscreening intervals may be appropriate in some women. Gynecologists should also be familiar with the quality-control measures employed by the cytology laboratory to assure that the specimens obtained are properly interpreted.

Screening methods that can be applied to all women are not yet available for endometrial or ovarian cancer. Women who are obese, who have a late menopause, and who use unopposed estrogen are at risk for endometrial cancer and are appropriate candidates for endometrial biopsy. No screening method has been established for ovarian cancer; however, in view of the poor prognosis for this disease, it seems reasonable to consider ultrasound screening of the pelvis or measurement of serum CA 125 (see Chapter 14) in those women who have a first-degree relative with the disease when such women enter their late 30s or 40s.

## CONCLUSIONS

We have discussed the epidemiology of the gynecologic cancers from the standpoint of how these cancers vary according to age, race, geography, and personal risk factors. The epidemiology of squamous cell cervical cancer is dominated by socioeconomic and sexual factors. Prevention might be achievable through avoidance of harmful exposures and sexually transmitted diseases and through identification and treatment of the disease in its intraepithelial stage. The epidemiology of endometrial cancer is dominated by nutritional or medical factors that contribute to a hyperestrogenic state. Prevention might be achievable through maintenance of a lean body mass, avoidance of high-fat diets, or hormonal means using progestins. The epidemiology of ovarian cancer is dominated by environmental and genetic factors that may induce hypergonadotropic hypogonadal states. Environmental factors may include radiation, polycyclic hydrocarbons, and dietary galactose, while genetic factors may include enzymes affecting the absorption and metabolism of galactose. Ovarian cancer might be prevented through the avoidance of exposure to substances toxic to oocytes or through hormonal manipulation that will lower gonadotropin levels.

## REFERENCES

Armstrong B, Doll R: Environmental factors and cancer incidence and mortality in different countries with special reference to dietary practices. *Int J Cancer* 15:617, 1975.

Aurelian L, Manak MM, McKinlay M, et al: "The herpes hypotheses"—are Koch's postulates satisfied? *Gynecol Oncol* 12:556, 1981.

Bagshawe KD, Lawler SD: Choriocarcinoma. In Schottenfeld DF, Frauemeni JF (eds): *Cancer Epidemiology and Prevention.* Philadelphia, WB Saunders Co, 1982, pp 909-924.

Ben-Hur H, Dgani R, Lancet M, Katz Z, Nissim F, Rosenman D:

Ovarian carcinoma masquerading as ovarian hyperstimulation syndrome. *Acta Obstet Gynaecol Scand* 65(7):813, 1986.

Berkowitz RS, Cramer DW, Bernstein MR, et al: Risk factors for complete molar pregnancy from a case-control study. *Am J Obstet Gynecol* 152:1016, 1985.

Biskind MS, Biskind GR: Development of tumors in the rat ovary after transplantation into the spleen. *Proc Soc Exp Biol Med* 55:176, 1944.

Butterworth CE, Hatch KD, Gore H, et al: Improvement in cervical dysplasia associated with folic acid therapy in users of oral contraceptives. *Am J Clin Nutr* 39:73, 1982.

Campton MJ, Singer A, Clarkson PK, McCance DJ: Increased risk of cervical neoplasia in consorts of men with penile condylomata acuminata. *Lancet* 1:943, 1985.

Centers for Disease Control: Cancer and Steroid Hormone Study: Oral contraceptives and the risk of ovarian cancer. *JAMA* 249:1596, 1983.

Chen VT, Mattison DR, Feigenbaum L, et al: Reduction in oocyte number following prenatal exposure to a diet high in galactose. *Science* 214:1145, 1981.

Coppleson M, Reid B: *Preclinical Carcinoma of the Cervix Uteri: Its Nature, Origin and Management.* New York, Pergamon Press, 1967.

Cramer DW: Lactase persistence and milk consumption as determinants of ovarian cancer risk. *Am J Epidemiol* 130:904, 1989.

Cramer DW: Harlow BL, Willett WC, et al: Galactose consumption and metabolism in relation to the risk of ovarian cancer. *Lancet* 2:66, 1989.

Cramer DW, Welch WR: Determinants of ovarian cancer risk. II. Inferences regarding pathogenesis. *J Natl Cancer Inst* 71:717, 1983.

Cramer DW, Welch WR, Cassells S, Scully RE: Mumps, menarche, menopause, and ovarian cancer. *Am J Obstet Gynecol* 147:1, 1983a.

Cramer DW, Welch WR, Hutchison GB, et al: Determinants of ovarian cancer risk. I. Reproductive experiences and family history. *J Natl Cancer Inst* 71:711, 1983b.

Cramer DW, Welch WR, Scully RE, Wojciechowski CA: Ovarian cancer and talc: A case-control study. *Cancer* 50:372, 1982.

Crum CP, Fu YS, Levine RU, et al: Intraepithelial squamous lesions of the vulva: Biologic and histologic criteria for the distinction of condylomas from vulvar intraepithelial neoplasia. *Am J Obstet Gynecol* 144:77, 1982.

Cunha GR, Bigsby RM, Cooke PS, Sugimura Y: Stromal-epithelial interaction in adult organs. *Cell Differ* 17:137, 1985.

Darby SC, Nakashima E, Kato H: A parallel analysis of cancer mortality among atomic bomb survivors and patients with ankylosing spondylitis given x-ray therapy. Radiation Effects Research Foundation, Technical Report 4-84, Hiroshima, 1984.

Day NE, Boice JD: *Second Cancer in Relation to Radiation Treatment for Cervical Cancer.* International Agency for Research on Cancer, Publication 52. World Health Organization, 1983.

DeGeorge FV: Hydatidiform moles in other pregnancies of mothers of twins. *Am J Obstet Gynecol* 108:369, 1970.

Doll R, Gray R, Hafner B, et al: Mortality in relation to smoking: 22 years' observation on female British doctors. *Br Med J* 1:967, 1980.

Evans HM, Lepkovsky S, Murphy EA: Vital need of the body for certain unsaturated fatty acids. VI. Male sterility on fat-free diets. *J Biol Chem* 106:445, 1934.

Fahim MS, King TM, Hall DG: Induced alterations in the biologic activity of estrogen. *Am J Obstet Gynecol* 100:171, 1968.

Fathalla MF: Incessant ovulation—a factor in ovarian neoplasia? *Lancet* 1:717, 1983.

Frisch RE, Wyshak G, Albright NL, et al: Lower prevalence of breast cancer and cancers of the reproductive system among former college athletes compared to non-athletes. *Br J Cancer* 52:885, 1985.

Furth J, Butterworth JS: Neoplastic diseases occurring among mice subjected to general irradiation with x-rays. *Am J Cancer* 28:66, 1936.

Hayashi H, Bracken MB, Freeman DH, et al: Hydatidiform mole in the United States (1970-1977): A statistical and theoretical analysis. *Am J Epidemiol* 115:1238, 1982.

Herbst AL, Kwiman RJ, Scully RE, Poskanzer DC: Clear cell adenocarcinoma of the genital tract in young females. *N Engl J Med* 287:1259, 1972.

Howell JS, Marchant J, Orr JW: The induction of ovarian tumors in mice with 9-10 dimethyl 1:2-benzanthracene. *Br J Cancer* 8:635, 1954.

Insler V, Meizner I, Kahane A, et al: Long term follow-up in 109 women with gestational trophoblastic disease. *Excerpta Med Int Cong Sci* 551:405, 1981.

Jacobs PA, Hunt PA, Matsuura J, et al: Complete and partial hydatidiform mole in Hawaii: Cytogenetics, morphology and epidemiology. *Br J Obstet Gynaecol* 89:258, 1982.

Jansen D, Ostergaard E: Clinical studies concerning the relationship of estrogens to the development of cancer of the corpus uteri. *Am J Obstet Gynecol* 67:1094, 1954.

Jones RW, McLean MR: Carcinoma in situ of the vulva: A review of 31 treated and 5 untreated cases. *Obstet Gynecol* 68:499, 1986.

Kashgarian M, Dunn JE: The duration of intraepithelial and preclinical squamous cell carcinoma of the uterine cervix. *Am J Epidemiol* 92:211, 1970.

Kaufman FR, Kogut MD, Donnell GN, et al: Hypergonadotropic hypogonadism in female patients with galactosemia. *N Engl J Med* 304:994, 1981a.

Kaufman RH, Dreesman GR, Burek J, et al: Herpes virus–induced antigens in squamous cell carcinoma in situ of the vulva. *N Engl J Med* 305:483, 1981b.

Kessler I: Human cervical cancer as a venereal disease. *Cancer Res* 36:783, 1976.

Kim HL, Picciano MF, O'Brien W: Influence of maternal dietary protein and fat levels on fetal growth in mice. *Growth* 45:8, 1981.

Kurman FJ, Jenson AB, Lancaster WD: Papillomavirus infections of the cervix. II. Relationship to intraepithelial neoplasia based on the presence of specific viral structural proteins. *Am J Surg Pathol* 7:39, 1983.

La Vecchia C, DeCarli A, Gentile A, et al: Pap smear and the risk of cervical neoplasia: Quantitative estimates from a case-control study. *Lancet* 2:779, 1984a.

La Vecchia C, Franceschi S, DeCarli A, et al: Dietary vitamin A and the risk of invasive cervical cancer. *Int J Cancer* 34:319, 1984b.

Lesko MS, Rosenberg L, Kaufman DW, et al: Cigarette smoking and the risk of endometrial cancer. *N Engl J Med* 313:593, 1985.

MacDonald PC, Siiteri PK: The relationship between the extraglandular production of estrone and the occurrence of endometrial neoplasia. *Gynecol Oncol* 2:259, 1974.

Mack TM, Pike MC, Henderson BE, et al: Estrogens and endometrial cancer in a retirement community. *N Engl J Med* 294:1262, 1976.

Marchant J: The effect of hypophysectomy on the development of ovarian tumors in mice treated with dimethylbenzanthracene. *Br J Cancer* 15:821, 1961.

Marcus SL: Multiple squamous carcinomas involving the cervix, vagina and vulva: The theory of multicentric origin. *Am J Obstet Gynecol* 80:802, 1960.

Martin CE: The epidemiology of cancer. II. Marital and coital factors in cervical cancer. *Am J Public Health* 57:815, 1967.

McLaren DS: Present knowledge of the role of vitamin A in health and disease. *Trans Roy Soc Trop Med Hyg* 60:436, 1966.

Melnick JL, Lewis R, Wimberly I, et al: Association of cytomegalovirus (CMV) infection with cervical cancer: Isolation of CMV from cell cultures derived from cervical biopsies. *Intervirology* 10:115, 1978.

Menczer J, Mordon M, Ranon L, Golan A: Possible role of mumps virus in the etiology of ovarian cancer. *Cancer* 43:1375, 1979.

Miller AB, Lindsay J, Hill GB: Mortality from cancer of the uterus in Canada and its relationship to screening for cancer of the cervix. *Int J Cancer* 17:602, 1976.

Morrison JC, Gwens JR, Wiser WL, Fish SA: Mumps oophoritis: A cause of premature menopause. *Fertil Steril* 29:655, 1975.

Muir C, Waterhouse J, Mack T, Powell J, Whelen S: Cancer incidence in five continents. International Agency for Research on Cancer, Lyon, France, 1987.

Murphy ED, Russell ES: Ovarian tumorigenesis following genic deletion of germ cells in hybrid mice. *Acta Un Int Cancer* 19:779, 1963.

Newcomb PA, Weiss NS, Daling JR: Incidence of vulvar carcinoma in relation to menstrual, reproductive, and medical factors. *J Natl Cancer Inst* 73:391, 1984.

Newman W, Cromer JK: The multicentric origin of carcinomas of the female anogenital tract. *Surg Gynecol Obstet* 108:272, 1959.

O'Toole BA, Fradkin R, Warkay J, et al: Vitamin A deficiency and reproduction in rhesus monkeys. *J Nutr* 104:1513, 1974.

Parazzini T, La Vecchia C, Mangili G, Caminiti C, Negri E, Cecchetti G, Fasoli M: Dietary factors and risk of trophoblastic disease. *Am J Obstet Gynecol* 158:93, 1988.

Patten SF, Hughes CP, Reagan JW: An experimental study of the relationship between *Trichomonas vaginalis* and dysplasia in the uterine cervix. *Acta Cytol [Balt]* 7:187, 1963.

Radisavljevic SV: The pathogenesis of ovarian inclusion cysts and cystomas. *Obstet Gynecol* 49:424, 1977.

Reeves WC, Brenton LA, Garcia M, et al: Human papillomavirus infections and cervical cancer in Latin America. *N Engl J Med* 320:1437, 1989.

Reyes FI, Winter J, Faiman C: Pituitary-ovarian relationships preceding the menopause. *Am J Obstet Gynecol* 129:557, 1977.

Rothman KJ: *Modern Epidemiology.* Boston, Little, Brown and Co, 1986.

Rotkin ID: The epidemiology of cancer of the cervix. III. Sexual characteristics of a cervical cancer population. *Am J Public Health* 57:815, 1967.

Salerno LJ: Feminizing mesenchymomas of the ovary: An analysis of 28 granulosa–theca cell tumors and their relationship to coexistent carcinoma. *Am J Obstet Gynecol* 84:731, 1962.

Shapiro S, Kaufman DW, Slone D, et al: Recent and past use of conjugated estrogens in relation to adenocarcinoma of the endometrium. *N Engl J Med* 303:485, 1980.

Silverberg SG, Makowski EL: Endometrial carcinoma in young women taking oral contraceptive agents. *Obstet Gynecol* 45:503, 1975.

Singer A: The cervical epithelium during puberty and adolescence. In Jordan JA, Singer A (eds): *The Cervix.* London, WB Saunders Co, 1976.

Skegg DCG, Corwin PA, Paul C: Importance of the male factor in cancer of the cervix. *Lancet* 2:581, 1982.

Smith DC, Prentice R, Thompson DJ, Herrmann WL: Association of exogenous estrogens and endometrial carcinoma. *N Engl J Med* 293:1164, 1975.

Smith FR: Etiologic factors in carcinoma of the cervix. *Am J Obstet Gynecol* 21:18, 1931.

Spert H: Endometrial cancer and hepatic cirrhosis. *Cancer* 2:597, 1949.

Stern BD, Kaplan L: Multicentric foci of carcinomas arising in structures of cloacal origin. *Am J Obstet Gynecol* 104:255, 1969.

Stern E, Gorsythe AB, Youkeles L, Coffelt CF: Steroid contraceptive use and cervical dysplasia: Increased risk of progression. *Science* 196:1460, 1977.

Stone M, Bagshawe KD: An analysis of the influence of maternal age, gestational age, contraceptive method, and the primary mode of treatment of patients with hydatidiform mole and the incidence of subsequent chemotherapy. *Br J Obstet Gynaecol* 86:782, 1979.

Swartz WJ, Mattison DR: Galactose inhibition of ovulation in mice. *Fertil Steril* 49:522, 1988.

Terris M, Oalmann MC: Carcinoma of the cervix. An epidemiologic study. *JAMA* 1174:1847, 1960.

Terris M, Wilson F, Smith H, et al: The epidemiology of cancer of the cervix. *Am J Public Health* 57:815, 1967.

Trevathan E, Layde P, Webster LA, et al: Cigarette smoking and dysplasia and carcinoma in situ of the uterine cervix. *JAMA* 250:499, 1983.

United States Department of Health and Human Services: Cancer Statistics Review 1973-1986. NIH Publ No 89-2789. Bethesda, MD, 1989.

Vessey MP, McPherson K, Lawlers M, Yeates D: Neoplasia of the cervix uteri and contraception: A possible adverse effect of the pill. *Lancet* 2:930, 1983.

Weiss NS, Sayvet TA: Incidence of endometrial cancer in relation to the use of oral contraceptives. *N Engl J Med* 302:551, 1980.

Whitehead MI, Townsend PT, Pryse-Davies J, et al: Effects of estrogens and progestins on the biochemistry and morphology of the postmenopausal endometrium. *N Engl J Med* 305:1599, 1980.

Willett WC, Stampfer MJ, Colditz GA, Rosner BA, Hennekens CH, Speizer FE: Moderate alcohol consumption and the risk of breast cancer. *N Engl J Med* 316:1174, 1987.

Wynder EL, Escher GC, Mantel NP: An epidemiological investigation of cancer of the endometrium. *Cancer* 19:489, 1966.

Ziel HK, Finkle WD: Increased risk of endometrial carcinoma among users of conjugated estrogens. *N Engl J Med* 293:1167, 1975.

zur Hausen H: Human genital cancer: Synergism between two virus infections or synergism between a virus infection and initiating events? *Lancet* 2:1370, 1982.

# Chapter 9 | Clinical Trials in Gynecologic Oncology: Biostatistics Issues

## *Philip T. Lavin*

As described in other chapters, research in gynecologic oncology involves diagnostic and surgical procedures, chemotherapeutic drugs, radiation therapy, immunotherapy, and tumor markers. In this chapter, we will summarize current strategies for evaluating disease-directed therapy as well as tumor markers for diagnosis and monitoring and will review basic biostatistic issues in the design and conduct of clinical studies in gynecologic oncology. In this way, readers can be alerted to problems that may arise as they review the medical literature and the results of medical research.

*Clinical therapeutic trials* comprise three phases: The Phase I study seeks to determine how a new drug's dose,

scheduling, and adverse outcomes are related. The Phase II study seeks to identify those diseases in which the new treatment exhibits antitumor activity. The Phase III study seeks to establish whether a new treatment is superior to standard therapy in terms of survival, response, or toxicity. Phase III studies are always comparative, that is, two or more treatments are being evaluated.

In studies of *tumor markers*, the study phases are generally less well defined compared with their therapeutic counterparts. In Phase I, both radioimmunoassays and ELISA-based assays require an initial evaluation of calibrators, precision, accuracy, recovery, drift, and interfering substances before clinical testing can begin, and the intra- and interassay coefficients of variation need to be sufficiently low. (These topics will not be further discussed here.) In Phase II, sensitivity and specificity need to be estimated prospectively in well-defined populations; however, such parameters are often assessed retrospectively based on poorly defined populations. The disease status must be known in order to have a gold standard for estimation of sensitivity and specificity. Phase III studies must also demonstrate prospectively how tumor markers improve the diagnostic accuracy, stage shift, treatment timing, outcome prediction, and improvement of good outcomes both alone or in optimal sequence with other diagnostic tests. Tumor marker studies are now developing the type of research structure already extant in therapeutic trials. Such a structure is necessary for planning clinical studies of diagnostics, therapeutics, and tumor markers.

This chapter begins with a review of the history of clinical trials and presents the basic terminology used in such trials. Guidelines for writing a protocol are provided along with some basic study design options and sample size calculations. In addition, specific requirements for gynecologic oncology studies are discussed and specific problems that can arise in the reporting of clinical trials are addressed. More general requirements regarding data management and computing are also covered.

## HISTORICAL BACKGROUND

The concept of the clinical trial has been around for centuries. In tracking the evolution of clinical trials up through modern times, Bull (1959) and Lilienfeld (1982) reported an account of a planned experiment involving a 10-day diet, with evaluation at baseline and followup, that appeared in the Book of Daniel (verses 12–15). Around 1600, it was reported that lemon juice effectively prevented scurvy, and in 1747, the daily consumption of oranges and lemons was declared advantageous in preventing scurvy when compared with other diets and concurrent controls. The concept of randomization as a means of assigning treatments was introduced by Fisher in agricultural experiments in 1923. Amberson et al (1931) was among the first to randomize patients in a clinical trial of tuberculosis, while Diehl et al (1938) were the first to report on the use of a double-blind procedure treating the common cold. Multicenter trials examining the treatment of pulmonary tuberculosis were first carried out by Mount and Ferebee in the United States in 1952. A milestone in the modern era of clinical trials was the publication in 1962 of *Statistical Methods in Clinical and Preventive Medicine* by Sir Austin Bradford Hill. During the 1960s, the Veterans Administration provided support for clinical trials of chemotherapeutic agents for tuberculosis.

The National Cancer Institute, founded in 1937, funded the largest number of clinical trials of any governmental agency, focusing particularly on chemotherapy in patients in advanced stages of cancer. Recognizing that a multisite approach would allow drugs to be tested more rapidly, cancer cooperative groups were formed in the 1960s. The Eastern Cooperative Oncology Group (ECOG) was initially founded to test Phase I and II agents specifically for cancer. Under the leadership of Gordon Zubrod and Emil Frei in the 1960s and Paul Carbone and Marvin Zelen in the 1970s and 1980s, procedures were established for designing and conducting clinical trials and for analyzing and reporting the results. An Operations Office and Statistical Center were staffed with full-time personnel responsible for protocol development, centralized patient registration and randomization, coordination of modality and disease committee activities, semiannual interim reports, institutional evaluation, investigator audits, community outreach programs, and continuing medical education programs (Carbone et al, 1978). ECOG has become a model for other cancer cooperative groups such as the Gynecology Oncology Group, the Gastro-Intestinal Tumor Study Group, and the Ludwig Group, among others.

Clinical trials are regulated by the Food and Drug Administration (FDA). The Federal Register defines general design and standards of conduct for trials carried out under an FDA Investigational New Drug Application (INDA) and New Drug Application (NDA) (Food and Drug Administration, 1969*a* and *b* and 1970*a* and *b*). Informed consent guidelines help protect the rights of human subjects, as initially defined by the Helsinki Agreement.

## TERMINOLOGY

Appendix I contains an extensive list of definitions developed by the ECOG.

### Clinical Trials

The word *trial* is used as a synonym for "study," with the adjective *clinical* being used to designate a study involving human subjects. The term *randomized* refers to a clinical trial in which more than one treatment is under study and the treatments are assigned by "chance." In a randomized clinical trial, there is a *control* group and one or more *experimental* groups; the existing treatment program constitutes the control, whereas the innovation(s) to be compared with the control constitute the experimental treatment(s). In a *double-blind clinical trial*, neither the investigator nor the patient is aware of the treatment assignment or which treatment is being administered to the patient. The conduct of a *controlled clinical trial* is directed by a written document called a *protocol*, which dictates specifics about patient eligibility, study objectives, experimental design, treatment plan, end points, standardization, statistical considerations, informed consent, and management. Study *end points* are the specific variables being evaluated in order to demonstrate a treatment effect or advantage. The *experimental design* is the type of study being used to evaluate the treatments and describes the treatment allocation plan. *Standardization* describes the efforts to treat, evaluate, and manage patients in a uniform manner within each treatment group. The *sample size* is the number of patients needed to complete the study. *Historical controls* provide comparison data collected in advance of the clinical trial. Data collected for one purpose and then later used for another purpose are called *retrospective* data, whereas data gathered according to a protocol after it has begun are designated as *prospective*.

Clinical trials are not the only means of gathering data. A *registry* is a prospective collection of patients who meet specific eligibility criteria and are followed to determine subsequent outcomes without a defined treatment plan. A *survey* is a written plan for gathering data in order to ascertain the characteristics of a defined population. A *case-control study* is a retrospective evaluation of a series of patients (*cases*) who have a preselected clinical condition and matched patients (*controls*) who do not have this condition to determine those factors (*relative risks*) associated with the condition under study. (The reader is referred to Chapter 8, "Epidemiologic Aspects of Gynecologic Oncology," for a discussion of case-control studies and for definitions of sensitivity, specificity, and predictive values.)

Specific names are used for clinical trials and for the individuals who manage these studies. A *pilot study* is a short-term clinical trial conducted to gain the experience and information needed to plan a subsequent clinical trial. A *pre-post study* evaluates the same patient before and after a specific treatment intervention. A *crossover study* evaluates the patient given two or more separate treatments with an adequate recovery interval between the successive treatments. The pre-post and crossover studies use the patients as their own controls. A *dose-finding study* establishes the proper dose and schedule of a specific treatment for further study. A *dose-response study* evaluates a particular treatment at different doses or schedules. A *multisite trial* is a clinical trial performed at two or more sites, as opposed to a *single-site trial*. The *investigator* is the individual responsible for the study at a particular site, while the *principal investigator* is responsible for the multisite study. The *clinical coordinating center* manages the trial, while the *data coordinating center* manages and analyzes the data for the trial.

## Biostatistics

Biostatistics as a discipline evolved from the need to design and analyze clinical trials objectively. All well-designed clinical trials contain an experimental design, sample size rationale, analysis schedule, and analysis plan. At the conclusion of the study, *significance tests* are performed to evaluate the study findings.

**Assessing Significance** The significance test is necessary to compare outcomes for treatment groups. Initially, an end point of interest is selected, after which an underlying *statistical model* is selected for that end point. Survival, disease-free interval, and time to progression typically obey an exponential model. Tumor response and the occurrence of toxicity are modeled using a binomial distribution. In the comparison of two treatment groups, a *test statistic* is formed to compare the differences in observed outcomes between treatment groups. The *p-value* is the probability of getting a difference at least as large as would be observed if the treatments were equivalent and a chance mechanism were operating. The p-value is also called the *significance level*. If the theoretical direction of the treatment difference may favor either treatment, the test is called a *two-sided test*. If the direction must be in favor of one of the treatments, the test is called a *one-sided test*. The two-sided test allows for either of the treatments to be superior, while the one-sided test assumes that, in advance, a designated treatment will be better (e.g., standard treatment versus observation). The two-sided test is more conservative than the one-sided test and will yield a p-value approximately twice that for the one-sided test. A p-value less than or equal to 0.05 is called *significant*.

**Hypothesis Testing** The formal structure for computing p-values is derived from Neyman and Pearson (1928). Initially, before the study is conducted, a *null hypothesis* is defined as the hypothesis that the two treatments are equivalent in terms of the end point of interest; the *alternative hypothesis* is defined as the hypothesis that the two treatments differ. The idea of hypothesis testing is to test for *rejection* of the null hypothesis; it is not possible to prove the null hypothesis. In the decision-rule framework of hypothesis testing, the *type I error* is the percentage of time that the null hypothesis is rejected when it is really true, while the *type II error* is the percentage of time that the alternative hypothesis would be rejected when really true. Often the type II error is restated in terms of the *power* of a study, e.g., the probability of rejecting the null hypothesis when the alternative hypothesis is true. The type II error equals 1 − power. The type II error and the power both depend on the choice of the alternative hypothesis. Thus, upon collection of the data, the decision rule is applied, and the null hypothesis is either rejected or not. In formal hypothesis testing, the type II error does not influence the test of the null hypothesis.

In study design application, the probability limit for a type I error is often set at 0.05 and the type II error should be no larger than 0.20 (0.80 power) in selecting sample size. (Examples of sample size calculations are provided later in this chapter.) In the interpretation of study results, the null hypothesis is rejected when the p-value is less than or equal to 0.05. Thus, the same significant test outcome can be expected whether a formal hypothesis test or p-value calculation is done.

## PROTOCOL COMPONENTS

The protocol is a prerequisite for any clinical study. It should describe the literature relevant to both the population and the treatments under study, the purpose of the investigation, patient eligibility, study design, patient registration process, treatment details relating to doses and schedules, clinical and laboratory data to be collected, data forms and a completion timetable, standardized evaluation criteria for effectiveness and toxicity, treatment modifications in case of toxicity, statistical considerations, the names and telephone numbers of key study personnel, a procedure for informed consent, and a bibliography. The document should be internally consistent and self-contained. The protocol should defend the choice of the treatment and should indicate the exact degree of improvement sought for the experimental treatment. The protocol should be written jointly by the study chairperson, study coordinator, statistician, data manager, and patient-care provider(s). It must address all standardization issues concerning eligibility verification, pathology review, end point definition, timetable for submission of forms, sample size accrual target and defense, and interim analysis timetable. The protocol should be reviewed periodically by the human subjects committee and other peer-review groups and can be amended as the study progresses. Written amendments should be issued if the protocol is changed. If properly prepared, the introduction and the materials and methods section of ensuing publications can be taken from the protocol.

Appendix II contains a guideline for writing a protocol adapted from the Dana-Farber Cancer Institute.

## Study Objectives

The study objectives should be explicit in the protocol and should be influenced by other studies in the same disease setting. The treatments should be structured so as to facilitate comparisons with previous studies, and the study should be designed to investigate a series of well-focused hypotheses that can answer specific questions as opposed to diffusely stated ones. Study objectives can include both efficacy, safety, and tolerance. Improved quality of life and reduced cost of care are also worthy study objectives. Study objectives should be realistic, and, whenever possible, should parallel those from similar studies. The objectives of the study should allow for a clinically meaningful gain to be detected.

## Eligibility

Patient eligibility needs to specify histologically proven disease, proof of stage, normal hematologic and chemistry tests, time since prior therapy (including surgery), age and physical status requirements (performance status), allowable concurrent diseases and medications, and prior drug therapy allowed. Some care must be taken to exclude patients who cannot hope to benefit from therapy (e.g., ECOG 4 patients). Strict eligibility criteria have an up side and a down side. The investigator must balance the rigidness of the entrance criteria and thus the gain in patient homogeneity against delays in completing accrual and the ability to apply the study results to a larger, more general population. Sometimes more broad eligibility criteria will mask the ability to detect a difference because the population has been "diluted" by the inclusion of poor-risk patients. Often it is wise to test the eligibility criteria retrospectively against a series of consecutive patients who have the

disease in question as a means of testing the reasonableness of the criteria before the protocol is activated. Loss of momentum in case accrual can jeopardize study completion.

## End Points

The number of study end points is relatively finite for a cancer clinical trial. Typical end points include response and toxicity for both Phase II and Phase III studies and survival, disease-free interval, and time to recurrence for Phase III studies. Recently, quality-of-life end points have been introduced to evaluate the perception of patient benefit. In cancer trials, survival is regarded as the premier indication of success.

Defining end points is essential for internal consistency as well as for promoting comparisons across studies. The *complete response rate* remains the most definitive way to show antitumor effect. ECOG has developed toxicity and response criteria that are now used across protocols involving chemotherapy (Oken et al, 1983). Criteria for body system *toxicity* have been developed for complications of chemotherapy and include a 6-point scale for grading severity of the toxic effect. In contrast, *response* criteria are subject to considerable misinterpretation because of variable access to measurable tumors and errors in estimating tumor size (Lavin and Flowerdew, 1980). Other investigators have also concluded that response rates may be misleading (Moertel and Hanley, 1976; Gurland and Johnson, 1965). Response criteria can be replaced with analyses of actual tumor cross-sectional areas (Lavin, 1981). For response criteria to be valid, all patients must be seen at scheduled visits and disease evaluations must be consistent for all patients. Otherwise, the onset time of a partial response may be missed. Measures such as time to response and duration of response are difficult to measure consistently, since visit timing is very critical.

One problem that often arises is the claim that a response is associated with *survival*. Comparisons between responders and nonresponders are biased for two major reasons (Weiss et al, 1983): First, responders have a guaranteed survival advantage because they live long enough to respond. Second, responders may have more favorable prognostic factors at the time of entry into the study. Comparing survival between responders and nonresponders is not necessary to prove that a treatment is beneficial. To overcome this problem, a landmark analysis has been proposed to test for survival advantage (Anderson et al, 1983).

Another end point measure is *quality of life*. This can pertain to the physical status, validated instruments, or summary measures related to other study end points. Serial performance status, need for pain medication, and days lost from work are examples of *physical measures* that can be used as end points. A vast array of *validated instruments* to assess health perceptions and sickness inventory profiles has been reported in the literature (Tchekmedyian, 1990). *Summary measures* have also been developed; for example TWIST (i.e., time without symptoms of disease and toxicity of treatment) was developed to evaluate long-term Phase III survival studies (Gelber et al, 1989). These end points deserve more consideration in the reporting of Phase III study outcomes.

## Controls

The rationale for including a control group in a clinical trial is well accepted. The need for a control depends on the experimental setting and is minimal when a new treatment is being tested for a uniformly fatal, rare disease. For a disease with a potential for cure, the existence of standard treatments begs for a control when one is testing the activity of a new, experimental treatment. Here, the choice of a control treatment is essential for comparison with an experimental treatment. The control is the standard to be tested, and the end points allow one to determine the precise advantage of the new therapy relative to the control group. A control group can be either historical or concurrent. Concurrent controls, collected prospectively, are the optimal way to test an experimental treatment.

A *historical control* represents a retrospective data base and has several disadvantages. It can come from the literature, a registry, or prior studies in which data were collected at an earlier time, under possibly different experimental conditions, and were subject to variable patient selection biases and referral patterns. Rules for eligibility and exclusions may be unknown or undocumented (Zelen, 1977) and prognostic factors may not be known or accounted for in a standard manner. Outcome data may have been subjected to differential followup patterns for different purposes, and end points may not have been collected in a standardized manner. When Pocock (1977) identified 19 situations in which data were collected over consecutive studies to test the validity of historical controls, he concluded that even in the best of situations, where data were collected and reviewed in a uniform manner by the same investigators using the same protocol, four of the 19 comparisons resulted in significant differences. Thus, prerequisites for using historical controls do not exist at levels that are reliable, so that historical controls should generally be avoided in Phase II and III evaluations.

Ideally, *concurrent controls* should be collected through randomization in order to minimize systematic bias and promote comparable treatment groups (Lasagna, 1955; Ingelfinger, 1972; Chalmers et al, 1972). The randomization plan should be described in the Phase II and III protocol and should not allow the investigator to know the next available treatment assignment. The specific time after eligibility verification when randomization is to take place should be addressed. Although the process of randomization does not determine which patients will ultimately agree to enroll in the study, it does help guarantee that those enrolled in each treatment group will be homogeneous in terms of prognostic factors. If successful, this will result in balanced treatment groups with regard to both known and unknown prognostic factors (Simon, 1984). It also helps to avoid the pitfalls of treatment assignment and lack of knowledge of prognostic factors.

The timing of randomization is also important. It should be done just prior to the randomized intervention (Peto et al, 1977). In a surgical adjuvant situation in which postoperative treatment is to be tested against observation alone, randomization should take place after the surgery and pathology reviews are performed. Otherwise, surgical complications might prevent certain patients from receiving subsequent adjuvant therapy. This situation is in contrast to trials in which preoperative radiotherapy is compared with observation alone; in this situation, randomization must take place before the surgery. Another situation involves use of a standard induction therapy followed by different maintenance therapies; it is advisable to register patients prior to the induction phase and then to randomize the patients as they are ready to begin maintenance. It is important to register patients in order to have a valid denominator.

## STUDY DESIGN OPTIONS

Separate designs and treatment allocation strategies can be devised for Phase I, Phase II, and Phase III studies. For the Phase III studies, choices include the randomized, crossover, optional control, and factorial designs. Here, we will present the role and advantages of randomization for Phase II and Phase III studies.

Before describing these design options, it is appropriate to consider the advantage of these randomized designs compared with observational studies, such as a survey or registry. Investigators are often tempted to draw inferences from accessible databases, since these databases may represent a convenient sample and may be touted as being "readily available." Such databases, while they may ideally serve the purpose for which they were collected, are not adequate for use in a clinical trial. Consider the case of the tumor registry. The state-mandated registry may be an excellent source of incidence data but would be of limited use in evaluating specific surgical treatments for breast cancer, since investigators differ widely in their rationale for treatment choices, subsequent monitoring, and followup care. As stressed by Byar (1980), patient selection biases limit the usefulness of registry data for treatment evaluation.

## Phase I Studies

Before a drug can be tested for its antitumor effect or its ability to prolong survival, an optimum dose and schedule must be selected. This is the objective of a Phase I study. Usually, treatment is begun with a low dose that is then increased in increments if no serious toxicity is observed in three patients at the dose level being studied. As many as five dose levels may be studied in a single Phase I study. Carter et al (1977) advise that six patients be treated at each dose level above the initial level, which is often based on animal toxicology models (Homan, 1972). If no short-term toxic effects are noted, the dose can be increased. Dose escalation plans have been based on a modified Fibonacci series (i.e., 10, 20, 30, 50, and 80 mg), as suggested by Schneiderman (1967). Other methods have been described by Gottlieb (1974) to achieve a more rapid escalation of dose. Criteria for modifying the dose based on toxicity must be defined in advance, and both acute and long-term toxicities need to be rigorously monitored, even after Phase I therapy has ended.

The concept of dose escalation studies can also be used to evaluate different schedules and routes of administration. In such cases, patients should be randomized to the different schedules or routes in order to reduce selection bias when patients are being assigned to treatment groups.

Dose-finding studies are also applicable when evaluating a patient who is receiving a series of incremental doses. Such an analysis must distinguish between patients and therapy dose. Because the sample size of this design may be too small to separate out cumulative drug effect from the effect due to higher dose levels, it is easier to evaluate one dose per patient.

## Phase II Studies

The objective of a Phase II study is to establish the antitumor activity of a specific drug—a difficult task, since patients who are eligible for these studies usually have not responded to earlier disease-directed therapy and are not likely to achieve a tumor response. When disease stabilization is of interest, Lavin (1985) has advised that the cross-sectional area of the tumor be used as a more sensitive measure of antitumor activity than the response outcome. For the randomized Phase II study, Peto (1978) and Lee et al (1981) advise that randomization to a new drug versus an existing drug occur in a ratio of 2 to 1, respectively, in order to confirm any lack of activity due to poor patient selection. Ideally, ambulatory, previously untreated patients should be assessed so as to improve the probability of seeing a response or stabilizing disease.

In the cooperative group setting, Phase II drugs are evaluated according to a master protocol, which promotes standardized eligibility and response criteria. Randomization is advised to control for selection bias in assigning patients to Phase II drugs in master protocols.

## Phase III Stratified Randomization

Most randomized Phase III clinical trials also include stratification based on key prognostic factors. This will result in more balanced treatment groups with respect to these factors and thus facilitate the comparison (Zelen, 1975*a* and 1975*b*). Prognostic factors might include initial performance status, disease stage, menopausal status, or interval since diagnosis of the disease.

The mechanics of stratified randomization involve the choice of one to three prognostic factors and appropriate levels for each factor and as well as the generation of a random list of treatment assignments within each possible combination of levels across the list of prognostic factors. Generally, a minimum of 5 to 10 patients per stratum is advised. If there are too many strata combinations, the benefit of stratification will be lost because some strata will not contain enough patients. The idea of stratification can be illustrated by a Phase III study of ovarian cancer involving treatments A and B, where the strata might be defined as the size of the primary before debulking surgery (largest dimension below or above 10 cm) as well as the extent of disease after surgery (largest dimension below or above 2 cm). In this situation, there would be four strata combinations. It is best to limit stratification factors to leading prognostic factors. Ideally, these strata factors should not be correlated so that the number of entries in each stratum can be better balanced.

Random treatment assignments can be generated from a random-number table. Assume that the study involves two treatments to be assigned with equal probability. To proceed, select a column of digits. These digits will be transformed into the treatment assignment order by simply assigning the odd numbers to treatment A and the even numbers to treatment B. Although this method generates a list of random treatment assignments, statisticians often apply the principle of "blocking" to insure balance between treatment groups. In blocking, the random digits determine enumerations of possible letter strings. For example, for a block size of four, the possible enumerations are AABB, ABAB, ABBA, BBAA, BABA, and BAAB. Each enumeration would be assigned one number. This process has the advantage of insuring that the number of treatments assigned will be no more than two apart for a block size of four. In a list of random numbers, there is no guarantee that the number of treatments will be out of balance by no more than two. For this reason, blocking is popular. Block size should not be stated in the protocol or told to the investigators. The concept of stratification easily generalizes to more than two treatments and to more than two strata.

For the example cited above, a block size of two has been used to illustrate a list of random assignments for each stratum combination as shown below:

| Largest Tumor Dimension (cm) | | |
|---|---|---|
| Before Surgery | After Surgery | Random Assignments |
| Under 10 | Under 2 | A,B,B,A,A,B,A,B,B,A |
| Under 10 | Over 2 | B,A,B,A,A,B,B,A,A,B |
| Over 10 | Under 2 | B,A,A,B,A,B,A,B,B,A |
| Over 10 | Over 2 | A,B,A,B,B,A,B,A,B,A |

Randomization assignments should be prepared by a statistician and set up as a closed-envelope system or administered at a central office. In multicenter trials, an operations office or data coordinating center provides the randomization assignments, and the use of institution balancing helps to ensure that the number of treatment assignments is comparable within each institution (Zelen, 1974). Other plans for stratification have been summarized by Simon (1979).

An alternative to stratification at the time of randomization is poststratification. However, this can be misleading if a large number of covariates are being considered. In the latter case, poststratification can lead to false-positive covariates because of repeated significance testing. If the sample size warrants, randomized stratification is advised.

## Crossover Design

The crossover design allows one to evaluate more than one treatment in the same patient. Typically, the patient is randomized to a designated treatment sequence. For two treatments, half the patients would be randomized to the AB sequence while the other half would be randomized to the BA sequence. In a crossover study, the length of the treatment interval and the washout period between treatments must be specified. Classic methods for analyzing crossover studies have been developed by Hills and Armitage (1979) and by Koch (1972). One approach is to use the same baseline for both periods, with no adjustment for the washout period.

Use of a crossover design is controversial for a variety of reasons. While using the patient as his or her own control is an accepted method of evaluation, it has been discouraged by the FDA because the relative effectiveness of the treatments may differ for the two different phases or the second treatment may be influenced by the outcome of the first treatment (Brown, 1980). The test for such an interaction may require as many patients as a randomized design. Moreover, the condition of the patient changes with time, and the effect of the treatment may depend, in an unknown manner, on prior treatments. Since the crossover design almost always represents a nonstandard approach to patient management, it requires a subsequent clinical study to confirm any treatment advantage in more practical settings.

## Factorial Designs

In planning clinical trials that involve two or more therapeutic modalities, factorial designs are used to evaluate the contributions of the individual treatments. In a surgical adjuvant study, the individual effects of chemotherapy and radiation therapy can be tested using the following four treatment programs:

Treatment 1—Surgery followed by observation
Treatment 2—Surgery followed by radiation therapy
Treatment 3—Surgery followed by chemotherapy
Treatment 4—Surgery followed by both radiation therapy and chemotherapy

The experimental design is called a 2 x 2 factorial design because there are two levels for each therapeutic modality. The design is attractive because, in the absence of an interaction between treatment modalities, half the patients would be randomized to receive chemotherapy, while the remainder would not receive chemotherapy. A similar situation exists for the evaluation of radiation therapy. However, if the advantage for chemotherapy depends on whether radiation therapy is given, an interaction may exist. Then treatments must be evaluated by simultaneous comparisons of the four

treatments. This requires an adjustment for the p-values, which negates any advantage gained by pooling the data into treatment-group pairs. Data pooling may not be allowable due to an interaction.

## REPORTING DIFFICULTIES IN CLINICAL TRIALS

Reports of results from clinical trials must be read critically. The reader should recognize that such publications can contain errors in design, methods of conduct, and analysis. In a series of papers on this subject, Hawkins (1980, 1981, 1982, 1983) has identified some common mistakes made by researchers.

The following eight situations are representative of frequently encountered problems.

*1. Patient Exclusions* Reasons for exclusions can vary considerably across studies. In almost all situations, exclusion promotes bias (Peto et al, 1977; Peto, 1978). Exclusion may be made on the basis of eligibility, compliance, and outcome, with all exclusions reported in the final analysis. Uniform rules and the limits for exclusions should be clearly stated in the paper.

*Eligibility violations* are reasons for excluding a patient from the analysis. Losses due to ineligibility should always be reported. In no way should reasons for ineligibility be related to treatment outcome. For example, in a study involving two chemotherapy regimens, the history of hematologic requirements may differ for the two treatments. It constitutes bias to apply different eligibility requirements to different treatments in a randomized clinical trial, since this exclusion may well favor one of the two treatments.

Sometimes *deviations from protocol* are used to exclude cases from analysis. Typical reasons cited are the patient received only one course of therapy, the dose or schedule was incorrect, the patient did not tolerate the therapy, the doctor removed the patient from the study, or the patient refused to return. These exclusions introduce biases because an unexpected outcome resulted in the loss of cases from analysis. It is always advisable to include all patients who were randomized in the final analysis. A subgroup analysis of those patients who did not deviate from protocol is useful only in that it supports the analysis of all randomized patients. Moreover, the proportion of protocol deviations should be reported, and, if high, may suggest that the treatments cannot be delivered as planned. Variations between patients with and without protocol deviations may also suggest that the results of the study may not be readily extended to a larger population of patients to be treated.

Another type of exclusion relates directly to *study outcome*. Survival minimums are sometimes included as an eligibility requirement. Typically, the expected survival should exceed the planned treatment interval. A way around this problem (i.e., to avoid the appearance of a guaranteed survival time) is to include a Karnofsky or ECOG criteria requirement at study entry. Exclusions represent a measure of credibility for a study; a study with an ineligibility rate above 10% should be viewed with some caution. During analysis of a study, cases are often excluded from particular analyses. When one is reporting safety and laboratory data, it makes sense to report on all treated patients. If more than 10% never started treatment, it is advisable to present results for the subgroup who received any treatment. Dropout due to toxicity or withdrawal of consent should be reported as a measure of treatment feasibility.

A review of the literature shows that exclusions can be found in the majority of clinical trials. Sometimes excluded cases are analyzed separately in an attempt to show that results would be the same either way. However, results should be considered with caution if the conclusions of a study depend on exclusions. In all studies, all registered cases should be reported to allow readers to reach their own opinions.

**2. Classification of Deaths** "Disease-free interval" needs to be carefully defined in clinical trials. In Phase II studies in which response is an end point, the case should be counted as a failure for survival and response if death was related to disease or treatment. If death was unrelated to disease or treatment, then death and response can be considered as being censored. For Phase III studies, the same rules can apply for survival and disease-free interval; however, a distinction should be made between death from all causes and death related to disease. Reporting deaths related only to disease always leads to estimates of longer median survival than median disease-free interval. Reporting deaths from all causes can result in confusion when the median disease-free interval exceeds the median survival. Consequently, definitions of disease-free interval and death should be clearly and consistently stated in any study involving these measures.

**3. Multiple End Points, Covariates, and Outcome Measurements** The desire to evaluate multiple study objective arises in studies having multiple study end points. For example, when one wishes to evaluate quality-of-life data when there is no overall measure of quality of life, typical instruments can include up to 30 outcome measures. In this situation, repeated tests of significance will lead to false-positive claims due to an overinflated type I error. Development of a global test statistic or correction of the p-value has been advised to solve this problem (Pocock et al, 1987). A global test statistic can be developed using an analysis of principal components to reduce the dimension of end points.

Other problems often accompany studies having multiple end points when applied to selected subgroups or strata. This situation frequently arises when a large data base is collected at baseline and is subjected to repeated univariate analyses within subgroups. Simon (1982) has developed methods for performing subset analyses. The proper solution is to use a multivariate regression technique to control for prognostic factors as well as any variables for which there is an imbalance between the treatment groups being compared.

Another mistake is to compare treatments at the end of each observation interval during the study. If observations take place at fixed times and few observations

are missing, a multivariate analysis of variance should be used. One approach is to use a Bonferroni adjustment to adjust for repeated tests. Another way to approach this problem of multiple comparisons is to first form patient summary measures like the slope of the outcome and then perform statistical tests on the summary measures. Finally, average levels can be defined over distinct study phases, such as induction and maintenance, to reduce the number of possible statistical tests.

**4. Inadequate Sample Size** All studies should report the underlying type I and type II errors as well as the null and alternative hypotheses being tested. In a review of the literature, Freiman et al (1978) found that most studies did not have adequate power to claim that two treatments were equal. The power of a study should be at least 80% to rule out a treatment difference, and most comparative studies are too small to establish a claim of "no difference." It is not well understood that statistical significance can be reached with many fewer patients than would be needed to rule out a clinically meaningful difference.

A variation of this problem would be when the study population contains distinct subgroups. Take, for example, a comparison of two Phase III treatments. Because the chance of a response is much lower in non-ambulatory than in ambulatory patients, the nonambulatory patient really does not count as much as an ambulatory patient when one is evaluating the rate of response. Thus, a study can be diluted by the inclusion of patients who would be unlikely to respond to treatment. Analogous reasoning suggests that it is always advisable to separate out patients who have previously received chemotherapy from those with no prior chemotherapy.

**5. Poorly Designed Hypotheses** The selection of treatments requires coordination to test a hypothesis that involves the addition of a new therapeutic modality to an existing modality. For example, to test a Phase III hypothesis involving radiotherapy as an adjuvant to chemotherapy, it is advisable to have one treatment program involving chemotherapy alone while the other treatment includes both modalities. It is also preferable, but not essential, to have the same chemotherapy drug, dose, and schedule in order to isolate any contribution made by the radiotherapy. If the chemotherapy regimen must be modified because of concerns about toxicity, the modification should be limited to either dose or schedule. In a study in which the dose and schedule differ, and a claim of significant difference can be made, it will not be known whether the advantage was due to the additional radiotherapy or the dose and schedule change. In addition, if a study has a nonstandard control, a claim of significance for the experimental group may not be interpretable. Thus, coordination is needed in selecting a valid control group and a new treatment to test a specific hypothesis.

**6. Effects of Interim Analysis** The interim analysis plan should be clearly stated in the protocol as well as in the publication. With the advent of computing, it is theoretically possible for interim analyses to be performed every week and for a study to be terminated owing to a chance fluctuation in the score statistic that determines significance. Fortunately, cost and time considerations limit this possibility. The major cooperative groups schedule interim reports at least annually, while studies conducted at a single hospital may undergo more frequent analyses for progress reports and institutional review. The effect of interim analyses is to enhance the chances of seeing a significant p-value (Armitage et al, 1969; McPherson, 1974). In the comparison of two treatments, the type I error increases from 5% with repeated interim analyses (Peto et al, 1977). Unless measures are taken to preserve blinding of results and the consequences of the interim analysis are considered, a p-value adjustment will be needed.

Repeated evaluation of clinical trials can have advantages. An interim evaluation allows sample size assumptions to be checked. Using a two-stage design, an evaluation of underlying standard deviations without looking at the mean values can result in a sample size adjustment without a large change in the experiment-wide type I error. Another advantage is the evaluation of compliance and safety. Accrual rates can be monitored to see whether the study assumptions regarding sample size were valid.

Disadvantages involve the generation of informal hypotheses based on the "bad news first" phenomenon. In reporting a clinical trial, it is usual for the first interim analysis to overrepresent early deaths and toxic complications. Bad outcomes can be explained by the inclusion of patients with poor prognostic factors, who may dominate the early reports (Pocock, 1978). Unfavorable interim reports may, in turn, make the study less attractive to investigators. Moreover, repeated interim analyses require adjustments of the type I error for sequential evaluations (Armitage, 1975). The type I error for the overall experiment must be adjusted upward, as will be discussed later.

Cancer clinical trial groups have developed procedures for reporting interim analyses. First, in interim reports, treatments are always blinded until all patients have completed protocol therapy. Adverse experiences and safety data are not blinded. Second, efficacy data are not analyzed until more than half the target accrual objective is met. Third, major analyses at meetings leading to decisions to stop treatment are not done until treatment is completed and desired followup has been carried out for all patients. Another approach used in multicenter clinical trials is to have a data monitoring and safety review committee make independent judgments about safety and efficacy.

Often a sequential plan is included in the protocol to define the timing of interim analyses. These can be geared to fixed times or to fixed numbers of failures. The key measure affected is the type I error, which depends on how frequently the data are analyzed, the nature of the decision rule, and the sequence of possible outcomes that might have resulted from earlier interim looks at the data. Armitage (1975) developed monitoring plans that bound the overall type I error to 0.05. His methods have been extended to apply to evaluations

of survival data (Jones and Whitehead, 1979) and response (Pocock, 1982; O'Brien, 1979) at a finite number of interim looks. One net effect of sequential monitoring is that if the treatment difference is similar, sequential monitoring plans generally need more patients than a one-time evaluation, since the chances of falsely stopping the study at each look must be considered. Tukey (1977) has recommended the use of sequential monitoring with only two or three interim looks, while other authors have indicated valid approaches that have allowed up to five interim looks.

The concept of fixed interim looks has been adopted by the cancer cooperative groups. Peto (1978) advised that interim evaluations be performed at fixed times, with termination when the p-value reaches a sufficiently low level (0.001) in order to protect against extreme outcomes. If no interim looks result in significance, the study is terminated as originally planned. The final analysis is then done without regard for the interim analyses because the type I error is not affected much under this monitoring plan. This helps to explain the rationale for the fixed interim analyses of cancer clinical trials groups.

**7. Study Termination** A study can be terminated when accrual and followup objectives have been met or when the treatment difference is significant. All protocols should state the accrual and followup objectives, interim analysis plans, and the principal end point to be used for the purposes of study termination. The decision to terminate a clinical trial must be properly imbedded in the protocol.

Stochastic curtailment has been developed to help make decisions regarding study termination (Lan and Wittes, 1988). The idea of stochastic curtailment is to look at the conditional power to see what would happen if the null hypothesis of no difference were to apply for the remainder of the study. Thus, a study showing an early difference could be stopped prematurely with a sufficiently high conditional power (over 80%) because it could withstand the null hypothesis until the prescribed followup interval for the study. Conversely, a study with no difference could be stopped prematurely if the conditional power were sufficiently low (under 20%) when the alternative hypothesis is assumed to apply for the remainder of the study. Also, stochastic curtailment applies if the underlying assumptions behind sample size did not apply, e.g., higher than expected recruitment of low-risk cases.

**8. Followup Variations** Monitoring patients being followed for disease-free interval and time to progression can introduce a followup bias. In clinical trials involving long-term survival, followup is generally good during the treatment interval and may become more difficult after treatment is completed. The bias arises because patients developing positive symptoms are likely to return for medical evaluation, whereas asymptomatic patients may miss visits. Missed visits can translate into being lost to followup, resulting in a loss of favorable survival and disease-free interval results. In reviewing of long-term studies involving survival and disease-free interval, investigators should look for some measure of frequency of followup among the groups being reported. It is also advisable to look for a distinction between the numbers of patients whose disease was discovered during scheduled visits compared with unplanned visits.

## CALCULATING THE SAMPLE SIZE

All investigators who have ever designed and conducted clinical trials have faced the question of sample size. The typical investigator wants to conduct the study as economically and as rapidly as possible. Upon completion of the study, they seek acceptance of their findings by peer groups who are sensitive to the internal and external validity of the study. There is a need to design a study with an optimal study design, clearly stated hypotheses (null and alternative), corresponding end points to test the hypotheses, type I and type II errors, and following interval. The number of patients follows from a precise statement of design, hypotheses, end points, and error specifications. These elements constitute the means to determine sample size.

Surveys of published clinical trials have identified inadequate sample size as a major problem. Since most clinical trials are planned with a 5% type I error, it is reasonable to assume that in 5% of all published reports the results are false-positives, that is, there is no treatment difference even though the difference between treatments was significant. Moreover, many clinical trials that did not report a treatment difference did not have a large enough sample size to ensure adequate power. This is the leading flaw of single-center studies. Thus, as described by Staquet et al (1979) and Zelen (1982), literature reports can include false claims of treatment difference as well as missed claims of treatment difference. The bias of study reporting favors the publication of these positive claims and does not favor the reporting of these claims of no difference (Berlin et al, 1989). Thus, the proportion of false claims is probably much greater than 5%. The cancer cooperative groups perform a valuable service in verifying claims of treatment effect and in designing clinical trials with adequate power.

The task of study planning begins with choosing of a proper design. The distinction between Phase I, II, and III clinical trials is usually very clear. For Phase II and III studies, the need for a control group was discussed earlier. The sample size cannot be selected until the experimental design has been chosen (Lachin, 1981; Ellenberg, 1989). Part of this thinking process should include the selection of appropriate type I and type II errors. Although the type I error selected is usually 0.05, performing multiple comparisons when more than two treatments are under study can lead to increases in the type I error. If two experimental treatments are to be compared to a control, the type I error is set to 0.025 to allow for the two comparisons to control. The type II error is often set between 0.10 and 0.20 but would not be adjusted for multiple comparisons. A decrease in the type I or type II error leads to larger sample sizes.

The choice of hypotheses is the most negotiable aspect of sample size calculation. The null hypothesis is always defined as the hypothesis of no difference. Choosing the alternative hypothesis allows some latitude in the selection of sample size. Common sense dictates that the further the alternative hypothesis diverges from the null hypothesis, the smaller the sample size will be. This choice is limited by practicality. It is unlikely that a new treatment will have a median survival or disease-free interval that is more than two times the control. For response, a gain of more than 30% versus the control would also be unlikely. This reasoning can translate into the selection of placebo controls or minimal intervention controls. At the other extreme lies the selection of two treatments with trivial differences. In either case, a proper balance must be struck among the ethical choice of a control group, the willingness of patients to enroll in the study, and the desire to finish the study as quickly as possible.

The study end points to test the hypotheses of interest are usually dictated by conventions adopted in previous studies of the same disease population. Standardization of end points such as tumor response, toxicity, and recurrence allow comparisons with other studies. Generally, there is little flexibility in the choice of study end points with regard to sample size calculation. Moreover, this will immediately define an underlying statistical distribution to model the end point under study. Time-dependent data such as survival, disease-free interval, and time to response are modeled as an exponential distribution, while data such as proportions responding, those with life-threatening toxicity, or those alive at a given study milestone are modeled as a binomial distribution. The choice of these distributions then allows the statistician to compute the sample size.

In practice, three situations exist for sample size calculation:

1. The investigator is studying a treatment that has been previously evaluated with respect to the hypotheses and end points under study. Existing data allow the investigator to choose the experimental design and the alternative hypothesis in a manner to be consistent with previous studies. In this situation, the investigator is faced with the straightforward calculation of sample size.

2. The investigator is studying a treatment that has not been previously evaluated in the experimental setting of interest. If pilot study data exist, the estimates from these data can be used as a surrogate for previous studies, but the investigator should plan to perform an interim data analysis to ensure that the assumptions based on the pilot data are valid.

3. The investigator may be looking at a series of new end points, such as experimental biochemical or physiologic measures. Planning a study can be blocked by not knowing reasonable options for the alternative hypotheses. In this last situation, investigators will select a fixed sample size in terms of what is an attainable sample size and then will work backward to find the alternative hypotheses that can be detected for each end point for the type II error of interest. This situation also arises when a

series of known biochemical markers are being studied, but each would have a different sample size in the absence of one definitive marker. This choice of a fixed sample size for a family of end points also introduces a repeated significance testing problem that can be addressed through adjustment of the type I error.

## Methods for Computing Sample Size

The following questions are often used to determine the information needed for calculating sample size:

1. What are the purposes of and hypotheses for the study?
2. Is there anything unique about the study population?
3. Is there a need for randomization?
4. What treatments are to be studied (or compared)?
5. What previous data are available regarding the efficacy of the treatments?
6. What is the motivation behind the study design?
7. What are the primary study end points?
8. What distributions best describe these primary study end points?
9. What data will be collected and when will it be collected?
10. What kind of changes in the primary study end points will be clinically or operationally meaningful?
11. What do these changes mean in terms of null and alternative hypotheses?
12. Are these one- or two-sided tests of hypothesis?
13. What type I error (alpha) and type II error (beta) are acceptable?
14. What cost and time limitations exist?
15. How will the findings be used?

The following methods for sample size determination are featured for the comparison of two treatments:

1. T-tests involving means.
2. Binomial tests involving proportions.
3. Exponential tests involving failure rates with incomplete followup.

All involve tests of hypotheses involving the mean of the underlying distribution. Each requires an exact specification of the null and alternative hypotheses as well as choices for alpha and beta. All tests apply to studies with two treatment groups. Hsieh (1987) has provided sample size adjustment formulas for treatment comparisons involving unequal sample sizes. All generalize to the case of an unbalanced k:1 randomization by simply multiplying the sample size needs for balanced randomization by the quantity $(k + 1)^2/4k$.

## T-tests

T-tests are useful for comparing two treatment groups at baseline (unpaired comparison), changes during treatment (paired comparison), or changes during treat-

ment for the two treatments. The t-test is amenable to the analysis of continuous outcome measures such as blood chemistries, tumor volume, or tumor marker changes. The t-test fits naturally with the use of the patient as his or her own control.

To design a study using these end points, Figure 9-1 has been developed. The figure requires an estimate of the means ($\mu_o$ and $\mu_a$) under the null and the alternative hypotheses, respectively; the standard deviation ($\sigma$) of the end point being measured (use the standard deviation of the difference if a pre-post comparison is being made); and the type I and type II errors. In the graphs, d equals the difference of the means divided by the standard deviation. A large effect (d = 1.00), medium effect (d = 0.80), and small effect (d = 0.50) correspond to a measure of the relative difference between the null and alternative hypothesis.

Follow these steps to determine sample size:

1. Determine the means under the null and alternative hypotheses.
2. Determine the standard deviation of the mean under the null hypothesis.
3. Compute the standardized difference (std) by dividing the difference of the means by the standard deviation.
4. Find the sample size from the graph for the given type I and type II errors and the choice of a one-sided or two-sided test.

## Binomial Tests Involving Proportions

When success or failure outcomes apply, the binomial distribution is used. A binomial model is used to analyze outcomes such as response rate, incidence of life-threatening adverse events, and recurrence or death at a fixed time point, because each of these events can be considered to be a binary outcome. Each patient represents an independent observation in the analysis of treatment differences. To design a study to compare two treatments using these end points, a series of graphs have been developed (Aleong and Bartlett, 1979) that require an estimate of the proportions under the null and the alternative hypotheses as well as the type I and type II errors.

Follow these steps to determine sample size:

1. Determine the response rate under the null hypothesis.
2. Determine the response rate difference under the alternative hypothesis.
3. Find the sample size from the graph for the given type I and type II errors and the choice of a one- or two-sided test.

## Exponential Tests

The analysis of survival, disease-free interval, time to progression, and time to response share the use of the exponential distribution to model time to failure or death. To design a study to compare two treatments using these end points, a series of nomograms have been

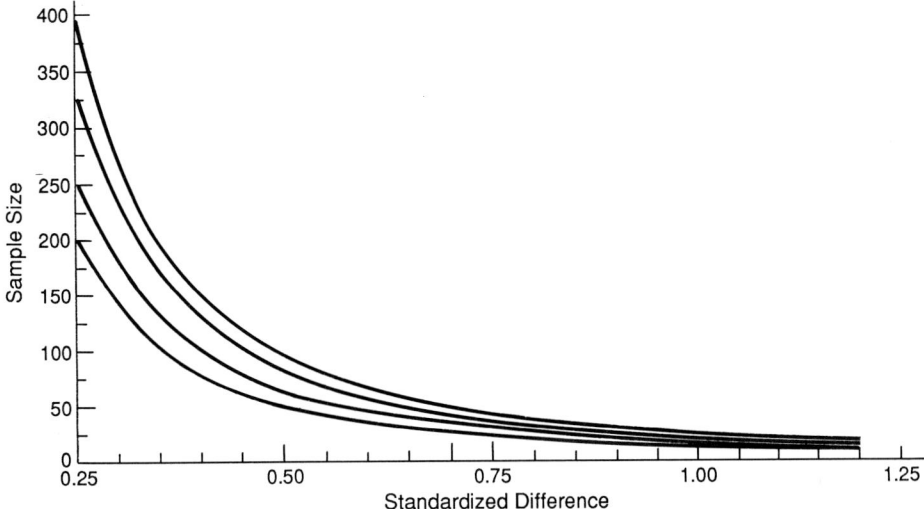

**Figure 9-1** Sample-size needs per group are based on the standardized difference between two groups being compared. The standardized difference is defined as the difference in means under the alternative hypothesis divided by the pooled standard deviation. From top to bottom, the four curves shown correspond to alpha = 0.01, 0.02, 0.05, and 0.10 for a two-sided test of hypothesis with 0.80 power.

developed (Schoenfeld and Richter, 1982) that require an estimate of the median time to failure or death under the null and the alternative hypotheses, the accrual and followup intervals, and the type I and type II errors.

Follow these steps to determine sample size:

1. Determine the median survival ratios under the alternative hypothesis of the two treatments under the hypothesis alternative.
2. Divide the accrual period by the average of the median survivals.
3. Divide the followup period by the average of the median survivals.
4. Find the sample size from the nomogram for the given type I and type II errors and the choice of a one- or two-sided test.

## Other Calculations

Sample size calculation can extend far beyond our discussion here. Charts have been constructed for the single treatment situation involving the mean of normal distributions and proportions as well as for tests of equality involving the standard deviation or variance (Zar, 1984); sample size tables have also been generated for planning pilot studies (Schoenfeld, 1980) for only one treatment. Cohen (1977) has published extensive tables for the computation of sample sizes for correlations and proportions for both one- and two-sample cases and has provided analyses of variance tables when the differences between the null and alternative hypotheses are measured as effect sizes. Donner (1988) and Lachin (1981) summarized methods for sample size calculation for comparative studies. Makuch and Simon presented calculations for comparisons with a conservative treatment (1978) and with historical controls (1980). Nam (1980) provided methods for calculating sample sizes for linear trends in proportions.

The extension of results to more than two treatments is best addressed by adjusting the type I error. In this case, the starting type I error (usually 0.05) is divided by the number of meaningful treatment comparisons. For example, the type I error involving a Phase III study involving a control and two experimental treatments can be adjusted to 0.025 if meaningful comparisons are limited to the new treatments versus the control.

The following examples illustrate the computation of sample sizes and the preparation of statistical considerations sections for a range of Phase II and Phase III studies involving both treatments and tumor markers.

### Example 1: Phase II Drug Study

This Phase II evaluation of carboplatinum plus VP-16 (etoposide) plus granulocyte-macrophage colony-stimulating factor (GM-CSF) will evaluate the complete and partial response rates in separate subgroups of patients with ovarian cancer who have relapsed or are refractory to therapy. A 30% response rate or a 5% complete response rate would indicate the need for further study. An accrual rate of 30 patients per year (both groups combined) is anticipated.

The sample size can be determined using the two-stage accrual plan for Phase II studies proposed by Gehan (1961). If no responses are seen in the first 14 patients (in each subgroup of interest), further testing would not be advised because the null hypothesis of a 20% activity level could be rejected with a 5% type I error. If the type I error were raised to 10%, a 20% activity level could be rejected if no responses were seen in 11 patients. For the first case (5% type I error), if any responses were seen, 11 additional patients would be needed in the second stage if the standard error of the response rate were to be 10%. For the second case (10% type I error), then 14 additional patients would be needed if the standard error of the response rate were to be 10%.

The table on the next page gives the 95% confidence limits on response rates for various sample size outcomes in the first stage of the study.

| 95% Lower Confidence Limits on Observed Response Rates | | | | | |
|---|---|---|---|---|---|
| Study End Point | Sample Size | | | | |
| | 10 | 15 | 20 | 25 | 30 |
| Number of responses required to establish >5% CR rate | 3 | 3 | 4 | 4 | 4 |
| Number of responses required to establish >30% CR + PR rate | 6 | 8 | 10 | 12 | 14 |
| Number of responses required to rule out <30% CR + PR rate | 0 | 1 | 2 | 3 | 4 |
| CR = complete response; PR = partial response. | | | | | |

Regarding toxicity as an end point for this example, it may be appropriate to pool data across the refractory and relapsed subgroups. For example, if no grade 4 myelosuppression was noted in 30 patients, a 95% upper confidence limit on the true complication rate would be 10% for a 5% type I error.

## Example 2: Phase III Survival and Response Study

A randomized clinical trial of standard combination chemotherapy with cyclophosphamide, doxorubicin (Adriamycin), and cisplatin (CAP) is to be compared with a new combination chemotherapy regimen for treating Stage IV ovarian cancer after initial debulking surgery. Patients are to be stratified according to initial tumor volume and remaining tumor volume postoperatively. Standard CAP therapy is associated with a 60% response rate (no clinical evidence of disease) and an 11-month median survival. The investigators plan to recruit patients for 1 year, with a 2-year followup phase once accrual is complete.

The regimen would be considered to represent a clinically meaningful gain if median survival were increased by 50%. A sample size of 110 patients per group would be required to test the one-sided hypothesis of a 50% gain in median survival according to a test of equality of the hazard rates for the two treatments. These calculations assume 80% power and a 5% type I error. With 110 patients per group, the investigators could also detect a 17% gain in response rates from 60 to 77% according to a one-sided test of hypothesis on the equality of the response rates.

The effect of a two-sided test can also be demonstrated with this example. Suppose that the new regimen were associated with life-threatening toxicity; in that case, a two-sided test might be considered more appropriate. Then, under the same experimental design conditions, a sample size of 150 patients per group would be required to test the two-sided hypothesis of a 50% change in median survival according to a test of equality of the hazard rates for the two treatments. These calculations assume 80% power and a 5% type I error. With 150 patients per group, the investigators could also detect a difference in response rates from 60% to 76% or from 60% to 43% according to a two-sided test of hypothesis on the equality of the response rates for the two treatments under study.

## Example 3: Phase III Psychological Intervention Study

This prospective, randomized study was designed to test the hypothesis that survival in patients with Stage II and Stage IV metastatic breast cancer is prolonged when patients participate in more intense behavioral intervention programs (intervention) compared with no such participation (control). This study will examine one control group receiving traditional medical support compared with two intervention groups determined by randomization as described in the methods section.

In this study, a subgroup will be randomized between two interventions while another hospital will enroll concurrent controls. Separate randomization will occur for Stage II and Stage IV patients. At least two separate hospitals will be participating in the randomized part of this study. Randomization will be blocked by hospital. Patients will be stratified by menopausal status (no, peri, yes) to help achieve balanced treatment groups.

Two hospitals will initially enroll patients into the randomized phase, while another hospital will enroll patients into an observation phase (concurrent controls). Yearly case entry projections for the randomized patients include both incident and prevalent breast cancer cases. Annual case contact with incident breast cancer patients for the disease stages are 118 Stage I cases, 110 Stage II cases, 33 Stage III cases, and 27 Stage IV cases. Year 1 prevalence contact for randomized breast cancer patients is projected to be 500 Stage I cases, 400 Stage II cases, and 100 Stage III cases. Patients in Stages I to III may develop Stage IV if recurrence is observed during the first 3 years. The chances of recurrence in patients with Stage I, II, and III disease are assumed to be 4%, 12%, and 15% per year, respectively. A 25% acceptance rate is assumed across all stages. Based on these assumptions, after 3 years of accrual, 181 Stage II patients and 69 Stage IV patients will be enrolled in the randomized portion of the study, with the majority of patients recruited during the first year (from prevalent diagnoses). For concurrent controls, annual accrual projections of incident cases are 33 Stage I, 30 Stage II, 21 Stage III, and 20 Stage IV cases, with no prevalent cases available. Assuming a 50% study acceptance rate and similar Stage IV conversion rates from Stages I to III, there will be 45 Stage II cases and 33 Stage IV cases for the concurrent controls analysis. In total, there will be 226 Stage II cases and 102 Stage IV cases after 3 years of followup.

For the 226 Stage II patients, comparisons can be made between the concurrent controls and the pooled randomized groups as well as between the two intervention groups. For comparing the two intervention groups, the sample size would be adequate to detect a 10% versus 25% 5-year failure rate with 80% power after 3 years of accrual and 5 years of followup according to binomially distributed failure rates. A one-sided test of hypothesis with 5% type I error was assumed. If there was no difference between the randomized groups, comparisons to the concurrent controls could be performed as a sequential test of hypothesis. The power would be 80% to detect a 10% versus a 30% difference in failure rates between the concurrent controls and either of the two intervention groups because the size of the control sample is smaller than that of either intervention group. Heterogeneity considerations may not allow for data pooling or tests of comparison without the need for rate adjustment.

For the 102 Stage IV patients, comparisons can also be made between the concurrent controls and the pooled randomized groups as well as between the two intervention groups. For the comparison of the two intervention groups, the sample size is adequate to detect a doubling in median survival (18 months vs. 36 months) according to an exponential model with 80% power after 3 years of accrual and 3 years of followup according to a one-sided test of equality of the medians with 5% type I error. If there was no difference between the randomized groups, comparisons to the concurrent controls could be performed as a sequential test of hypothesis. The power would be 80% to detect a doubling in median survival between the concurrent controls and either of the two intervention groups. Heterogeneity considerations may not allow for data pooling or tests of comparison without the need for rate adjustment.

Thus, the investigators project that 5 years of additional followup will be needed for Stage II and 3 extra years for Stage IV to test for an intervention effect.

Psychological outcomes will also be compared before and after intervention. The pre-post differences for each study group will be compared separately within the Stage II and Stage IV subgroups. The intent of this analysis will be to see whether there are treatment differences and whether the differences are the same for the two stages. The Stage II sample sizes are adequate to detect standardized differences of 0.38 between the two randomized groups and 0.51 for the concurrent control versus one of the intervention groups for a one-sided test of hypothesis on the equality of the mean changes. For Stage IV, the samples sizes are adequate to detect standardized differences of 0.64 between the two randomized groups and 0.70 for the concurrent control versus one of the intervention groups for a one-sided test of hypothesis on the equality of the mean changes.

### Example 4: Phase II Retrospective Marker Study

Since metastatic progenitor cells produce metastases, their presence and relative frequency must first be established a posteriori through both retrospective and prospective studies of available primary and possibly available metastatic tissue. The goal is to show that the phenotype profiles are different in primary tissue with no evidence of metastases compared with primary tissue with accompanying metastases. This study would require at least 50 primaries with no metastases as well as at least 50 primaries with accompanying metastatic tissue. The phenotypic expression rates would be compared in primary tissues with and without metastatic tissue using an exact test (Mehta et al, 1961) to establish a training hypothesis of increased phenotypic expression in primaries that metastasized. With 50 per group, a difference in expression rates from 75% to 95% (or 40% to 65%) could be detected with 80% power according to a one-sided significance test with 5% type I error using a binomial model. The phenotypic expression rates in the metastatic tissue could be compared with those in primary tissue in the same patient using McNemar's paired comparison test to test for the equality of the probability of specific phenotype expression. Discordant pairs of (0,6) or (1,9) would be significant (p < 0.05) (McNemar, 1947). The most favorable outcome would be a significantly higher expression in metastases compared with matched primaries,

which in turn would have significantly higher expression than in primaries with no metastases.

### Example 5: Phase II Prospective Marker Screening Study

This pilot study will evaluate the consistency of a new marker in women with pelvic masses who are observed over a 3-month interval. Thirty premenopausal, 30 perimenopausal, and 30 postmenopausal patients will be recruited. A group of 30 normal controls for each pelvic mass group will be selected with the aim of recruiting age-matched controls. All study participants will have blood drawn at monthly intervals over the 3-month study interval.

Prior studies of the marker in 11 premenopausal patients with pelvic masses noted significantly elevated levels (mean = 3.14, standardized difference = 4.03) versus normal premenopausal controls (mean = 0.79, standardized difference = 0.80). A 95th percentile for normal premenopausal controls is estimated to be 2.4. The marker distribution is thought to be independent of menopausal studies in normal control.

With a total of 30 patients per subgroup and 30 matched controls per subgroup, the following can be achieved:

1. A standardized difference of 0.85 can be detected with 80% power between each subgroup with adnexal masses and corresponding controls according to a one-sided test of hypothesis on the equality of means for the two matched groups for a test with 1% type I error. A 1% type I error is used because five apriori paired comparisons between groups are planned.
2. Using the estimate of the 95th percentile from the normal controls, there would be 80% power to detect a 45% elevation rate (proportions with a level above the 95th percentile) according to a one-sided test of hypothesis of the equality of the proportions of elevations in the two matched groups for a test with 1% type I error.

### Example 6: Phase II Prospective Marker Study

Once specific progenitor cells with the potential for predicting metastases are identified, a prospective clinical study will be conducted to test the value of these markers for predicting recurrence and time to recurrence. The size of the sample required to detect differences between marker expression rates in patients who do and do not develop metastases within 3 years of resection for cure will vary depending on the marker frequencies in the two groups. For a test of equality of recurrence, percentages for the marker+ subgroup versus the marker− subgroup versus the alternative hypothesis of an increased percentage of patients with recurrence in the

| % with Hypothetical Recurrence | | Total Sample Size Needed to Detect 25% Gain (Marker −/+ Ratio) | | | | Resulting Specificity/Sensitivity (%) | | | | | | | |
| --- | --- | --- | --- | --- | --- | --- | --- | --- | --- | --- | --- | --- | --- |
| | | | | | | P[ −|NR] (Marker −/+ Ratio) | | | | P[ +|R] (Marker −/+ Ratio) | | | |
| Marker − | Marker + | 4 | 3 | 2 | 1 | 4 | 3 | 2 | 1 | 4 | 3 | 2 | 1 |
| 0 | 25 | 109 | 93 | 79 | 70 | 84 | 80 | 73 | 57 | 100 | 100 | 100 | 100 |
| 10 | 35 | 133 | 113 | 96 | 85 | 85 | 81 | 73 | 58 | 47 | 54 | 64 | 78 |
| 20 | 45 | 156 | 133 | 113 | 100 | 85 | 81 | 74 | 59 | 36 | 43 | 53 | 69 |
| 30 | 55 | 175 | 149 | 126 | 112 | 86 | 82 | 76 | 61 | 31 | 38 | 48 | 65 |
| 40 | 65 | 188 | 160 | 135 | 120 | 87 | 84 | 77 | 63 | 29 | 35 | 45 | 62 |
| 50 | 75 | 175 | 149 | 126 | 112 | 89 | 86 | 80 | 67 | 27 | 33 | 43 | 60 |

P[ −|NR] = probability of negative marker given no recurrence.
P[ +|R] = probability of a positive marker given a recurrence.

marker + subgroup, the following table gives the total sample size requirements to detect a 25% gain (20% vs. 45%) in the recurrence + subgroup versus the recurrence − subgroup. It is assumed that 50% of the patients will have recurrence during a 3-year followup. These calculations were made by first picking the percentages of marker − and marker + subgroups with recurrence under the assumed percentage in the first two columns of the table and then computing sample size need based on the difference in recurrence proportions to be detected using various marker −/marker + sample ratios.

### Example 7: Phase II Marker Study of Treatment and Marker Relationship

The comparison of marker expression before and after treatment will be analyzed using a linear regression model where post-treatment marker level will be the dependent variable and pre-treatment marker level (and specific clinical factors) will be the independent variables. With 40 patients in this study, a standardized difference of 0.40 could be detected with 80% power under the assumption of a one-sided significance test with 5% type I error. A one-sided test is assumed in anticipation of a positive association between marker change and treatment benefit.

### Example 8: Phase II Predictive Value Study

This study will evaluate the predictive value of preoperative ultrasound prior to ovarian cancer surgery in the prognosis of FIGO staging alone and in combination with preoperative level of CA-125 assay (CA-125). A series of 70 patients will

125 levels, the equality of the sensitivities for CA-125 level and ultrasound would be rejected (p = 0.03) according to McNemar's test for paired comparisons.

### Example 9: Phase I Evaluation of New Biochemical Markers

The sample size for the normotensive study is motivated by the results of a pilot study that evaluated five normal subjects for platelet adenylate cyclase (AC) measures. Calculations were based on five platelet AC measures. Platelet AC measures before and after a physical stress phase were used to help justify the sample size. Given the multiplicity of study end points, a 1% type I error and 80% power were used in the calculations. Tests of hypothesis were based on two-sided tests on the equality of the means. Three possible tests were formulated:

1. Detection of a paired change in mean platelet AC levels at rest and after stress at Day 28 (within) using subjects as their own controls.
2. Detection of a difference between intervention groups at Day 28 (between) in mean platelet AC levels at rest and during stress.
3. Detection of a change in the paired differences (Day 28 minus baseline) in mean platelet AC levels between intervention groups at Day 28 (paired between).

With a total of 60 normotensives (30 per intervention group), the following differences can be detected with 80% power for a two-sided significance test with 1% type I error:

| Platelet AC Measure | Relaxed State | | | Stressed State | | |
|---|---|---|---|---|---|---|
| | Within | Between | Paired Between | Within | Between | Paired Between |
| Basal | 2.0 | 3.6 | 1.8 | 2.3 | 3.1 | 3.1 |
| Prostaglandin $E_2$ | 30.0 | 40.1 | 18.9 | 30.0 | 36.5 | 31.9 |
| Prostaglandin $D_2$ | 23.7 | 17.8 | 22.0 | 10.0 | 23.8 | 25.7 |
| Epinephrine suppression | 13.3 | 13.4 | 20.5 | 13.3 | 10.7 | 9.5 |
| Guanosine-5-C3-0-thio-triphosphate | 10.0 | 18.5 | 5.3 | 10.0 | 15.4 | 10.9 |

be enrolled over 2 years and followed for another 2 years for recurrence. All patients will undergo surgery and evaluation at the same hospital.

With a total of 70 patients, the study will allow the following:

1. For negative CA-125 versus positive CA-125 subgroups, the detection of a threefold difference in 2-year failure rates (25% vs. 75%) for recurrence with 80% power and 5% type I error under a binomial distribution assumption.
2. For an estimated 24 patients with a positive ultrasound prior to surgery, if 75% were to have subsequent recurrence, the 95% confidence interval for the predictive value (true value) of a positive test would be 55% to 90%.
3. For an estimated 50 patients with recurrence after 2 years of followup, if 45 patients had a positive ultrasound prior to surgery, the 95% confidence interval for the sensitivity would be 76% to 95%.
4. For an estimated 50 patients with recurrence after 2 years of followup, if there were two patients with elevated CA-125 levels and negative ultrasounds as compared with seven patients with positive ultrasounds and normal CA-

For correlational studies of platelet AC measures with diastolic blood pressure changes during stress, we expect correlations between 0.40 and 0.80 for the hypertensive patients. Adjusting for multiple comparisons, we set the alpha level (type I error) at 0.01 for a two-sided test. For a test with 80% power, the sample size requirements would be 67, 41, 27, and 18 subjects for correlation coefficients of 0.40, 0.50, 0.60, and 0.70, respectively, according to Cohen (1977). Thus, the sample size of 60 normotensive subjects should be adequate to detect correlations above 0.40.

## STUDY COORDINATION

The organizational structure of a clinical trial includes a medical investigator, data coordinator, data manager, and biostatistician. This group may also include an external review panel for review of pathology, surgery, and radiology data. The cancer cooperative groups have an Operations Office and a Statistical Center to run series of studies as well as disease committees to design and interpret protocols and modality committees to provide standardization across protocols. The mechanics of planning and managing clinical trials have been summarized for single-site and multicenter trials by Lavin (1983). Comprehensive texts on the management and conduct issues for clinical trials have been written by Mienert (1986), Buyse et al (1984), Pocock (1983), and Shapiro and Louis (1983).

The following rules should be adhered to in the planning and management of a clinical trial:

1. Data forms should be pretested prior to study activation.
2. Data forms should be organized into precollated notebooks or data screens according to visit and form sequences.
3. Data forms should be self-coding to allow for data entry or scanning.
4. Data forms should be critically reviewed before the study is activated to ensure that key prognostic factors are included and that all hypotheses can be tested as planned.
5. Separate manuals should be prepared to describe how to complete forms as well as how to check forms.
6. A confirmation of registration form is needed to identify patients at the time of study entry.
7. Case-record review should be both timely and prospective to detect toxicities and to check for misinterpretations in data recording.
8. Data on the forms should be verified against both the medical record and the computerized data base.
9. Computers should be used to track patient entry, schedule visits and form submissions, check for inconsistent data, and update data files.
10. Only validated software should be used for data management and analyses.
11. A summary and evaluation form is advised to document the review of completed cases with respect to eligibility, compliance, and outcome evaluation by the principal investigator.
12. Timing and consequence of interim analyses should be stated in the protocol.

Advances in microcomputing hardware and software now allow for the registration, remote data entry, scheduling, tracking, and analysis of patients from multicenter trials involving geographically distant sites. The 80386 microcomputer with sufficient RAM, hard drive, cache, and clock speed can meet the needs of most clinical trials. Scanners exist for cost-effective data entry. Modems and communications software packages allow for remote data capture and communications with distant sites. The use of SQL-based data management software allows rapid update and correction of data. Other software exists for rapid conversion of these relational data bases into analysis data files. Moreover, both analytic software output and graphics output can be integrated into word processing files to simplify the generation of tables and reports. Considerable benefit can be gained from careful planning of the study and designing of the forms as well as the selection of a proper computing environment.

## OVARIAN CANCER STUDIES: SPECIFIC NEEDS

The research needs in ovarian cancer have many parallels with other malignancies. However, the specific application of clinical trials to ovarian cancer studies presents unique challenges and requirements, as follows:

*1. Cost-Effective Screening Interventions* In screening for ovarian cancer, the incidence of the disease must be considered when one is developing a cost-effective strategy. Each year in the United States, 8,000 new cases are diagnosed among 130 million women. If each woman underwent a $100 evaluation every year, the cost per detected case would be $1,625,000 before it could be demonstrated that any lives were saved as a result of early diagnosis. Thus, it becomes clear that screening resources must be allocated to detect multiple conditions or, if disease specific, should be limited to women at higher risk. Suppose a screening program were limited to 10 million nulliparous women over 40 years of age (who account for 5,000 new cases each year). This would reduce the cost per detected case to $200,000. It is important to realize that these calculations do not include cost provisions for medical evaluation when results are false-positive. This illustrates the challenge of developing a cost-effective screening strategy for any style malignancy with a relatively low incidence.

The problem of cost-effective screening is further complicated by the stage of the cases detected. Ideally, a cost-effective screening program could result in a shift toward detecting disease at an earlier stage. However, to detect a shift from 20% Stage I to II for historical controls to 30% Stage I to II for a prospectively controlled series, approximately 130 new diagnoses of ovarian cancer would have to be made as a result of the screening program in order to detect this 10% shift with 80% power according to a one-sided test of hypothesis with 5% type I error. To detect this favorable shift, 260,000 nulliparous women over age 40 would have to be screened, which would represent an enormous project.

Even if a shift in stage were detected, it remains to be proved whether a survival advantage would be gained. The survival experience of the 130 new ovarian cancer diagnoses would also need to be evaluated by stage relative to historical controls. This sample size would be adequate to detect a shift in cure rates from 70% to 80% with 80% power according to a one-sided test of hypothesis with 5% type I error. The comparison would also be complicated by the comparison of costs to achieve the projected 13 additional cures among the 260,000 women under study.

In conclusion, a disease-specific screening study is unlikely to be cost-effective unless prevalence can be increased. Moreover, the cost of false-positives and the demonstration of improved survival are also important considerations. However, it is likely that cost-effective screening strategies can be achieved for pelvic mass diagnosis of malignancy.

**2. *Standardized Staging Definitions, Surgical Procedures, and Disease Evaluations*** Standardized definitions and procedures are essential for the success of multicenter trials as well as for the consistent interpretation of results across studies. The FIGO staging criteria help in comparisons of different patient series, and their value is greatest when interventions are begun at the time of the staging. For example, in a randomized clinical trial of adjuvant therapy for Stage II ovarian cancer involving observation as the control group, investigators would be able to compare informally results from this trial with other FIGO Stage II series in the literature. The value of FIGO staging decreases as the interval increases between staging and the start of the study. Consequently, FIGO staging would be of limited value in a Phase II evaluation of two chemotherapeutic agents after results of second-look surgery were found to be positive.

The example of surveillance or second-look surgery can also be used to illustrate variations in surgical procedures. The timing and extent of these surgeries vary between hospitals. Although no definitive study has so far been performed to determine the optimal timing and extent of these surgeries, it is clear that more extensive procedures (laparotomy) would be more likely to uncover disease than would less extensive procedures (laparoscopy). Thus, it could be hypothesized that disease discovered on second-look laparoscopy might be underrepresented compared with that in patients enrolled in studies in which disease status was determined by laparotomy. A smaller volume of disease found on second-look surgery might translate into improved survival, which could be misinterpreted as being the result of the treatments being studied.

Similar biases can be introduced during evaluation of the disease. The advent of magnetic resonance imaging, computed tomography, and tumor markers constitute a major source of variation. Bias arises because these imaging methods for diagnosing new disease are not 100% sensitive and 100% specific in determining disease status. False-positive and false-negative results lead to possible misclassification errors. For the patient with a false-positive result (i.e., said to have disease when none was present) survival is prolonged, while for the patient with a false-negative result (i.e., said to be disease-free when disease was present) survival or the disease-free interval is shortened. One solution is to require a positive biopsy for studies that require clinical evidence of disease and to require that all diagnostic evaluations be negative to confirm that a patient is disease-free. All studies should pay careful attention to the diagnostic and monitoring methodologies used in documenting disease status, since these methodologies will probably differ across studies, thus limiting the ability to interpret results.

**3. *Use of Tumor Markers in Diagnosis and Monitoring***
With the emergence of tumor markers such as CA-125 one can now assess gains in diagnostic and monitoring accuracy associated with current medical practice. In evaluating new information, it is of key importance to collect the new information prospectively for each pa-

tient, to blind the results from the primary care provider, and to evaluate the results independently. The key measure of interest is the gain in information provided by the new diagnostic or monitoring procedure, when added to existing procedures.

For diagnosing of pelvic masses based on clinical impression and ultrasound, the additional effect of CA-125 has been evaluated (Finkler et al, 1988). Initially, patients were stratified on the basis of menopausal status. For the subgroup with a diagnosis of benign disease, sensitivity and specificity of a CA-125 level below 35 U/ml were compared separately with serum CA-125 levels of 35 U/ml or more for possible combinations of clinical and ultrasound assessments. The CA-125 assessments offered significant gains in diagnostic accuracy among the postmenopausal subjects. These gains were not apparent until the data were stratified according to menopausal status.

For monitoring disease status after surgical debulking and subsequent chemotherapy for management of Stage IV ovarian cancer, the level of CA-125 at 3 months was examined as a predictor of subsequent clinical status at the completion of therapy (Lavin et al, 1987). Serial CA-125 levels were not used to direct management. After controlling for the initial extent of disease before and after debulking, CA-125 levels below 35 U/ml were associated with a significantly higher probability of being clinically free of disease at the completion of therapy.

In monitoring disease status, a serial trend in marker levels can be useful in detecting recurrences and in confirming disease-free status. This problem is complicated by the irregular interval between consecutive assays as well as the assumption that serial observations are statistically independent. Serial marker evaluation should use patients as their own controls, identify possible laboratory errors, and suggest possible recurrences for clinical confirmation. In the analysis of clinical tumor marker data, the problem of detecting recurrence is often translated into a threshold level algorithm that depends on the number and frequency of serial assays in the presence of serial correlations. This general problem is complex, and no easy solution has been developed to deal with these constraints.

Recently, Jones (1985, 1987) has identified a statistical procedure for testing for steady-state changes using a Kalman filter for a first-order autoregressive model. The model estimates the serial correlation, compensates for irregular serial observations, and produces statistically independent recursive residuals to test for departures from steady state (bad test values, disease recurrences), allows for the patient to be a random effect, and lets covariates into the model. This Kalman filter, when applied to a continuous, first-order autoregressive model (CAR[1]) with observation error, can be used to adjust for serial correlation, unequal intervals, and random patient effects. The Kalman filter assumes that each patient has a steady state marker level over time after resection for cure. As more data are collected for a specific patient, the estimate of steady state for that patient improves. As more patients are added to the model, the estimates also improve. At each data time point, the CAR(1) model can predict the marker value at any future point in time. The differences between predicted and actual marker levels (innovations) are scaled by their standard errors and become recursive residuals. The recursive residuals are statistically independent and, for large samples, are normally distributed with mean 0 and standard deviation 1. Exact maximum likelihood is used to estimate the unknown parameters in the model. Parameters might include baseline factors like FIGO stage, or initial tumor size, or baseline CA-125 level. The patient can be included as a random effect in the model to obtain more accurate initial parameter estimates for that patient with just one to two serial measurements. The model can be readily applied to adjuvant or advanced disease settings for individual markers or combinations of other tumor markers.

The recursive residuals with absolute values in excess of 3.5 signal a shift from steady state. The model can fit using a forward or backward order to detect shifts occurring at the start or end of the serial sequence. A high level in the first month of monitoring might be due to a bad test; reversing the data order allows subsequent observations to be used to evaluate earlier marker observations retrospectively.

The model includes a second stage in which a Cusum quality-control scheme is used to evaluate the residuals corresponding to the difference between actual and predicted marker levels. Cumulative sums of the recursive residuals detect slow trends that might not be picked up by a single recursive residual. This methodology may help overcome problems with irregularly spaced monitoring intervals and patient-specific trends.

# REFERENCES

Aleong J, Bartlett D: Improved graphs for calculating sample size when comparing two independent binomial distributions. *Biometrics* 35:875-881, 1979.

Amberson JB Jr, McMahon BT, Pinner M: A clinical trial of sanocrysin in pulmonary tuberculosis. *Am Rev Tuberc* 24:401-435, 1931.

Anderson JR, Cain KC, Gelber RD: Analysis of survival by tumor response. *J Clin Oncol* 1:710-719, 1983.

Armitage P: *Sequential Medical Trials*, 2nd ed. New York, John Wiley & Sons, 1975.

Armitage P, McPherson CK, Rowe BC: Repeated significance tests on accumulating data. *J R Stat Soc A* 132:235-244, 1969.

Berlin JA, Begg CB, Louis TA: An assessment of publication bias using a sample of published clinical trials. *JASA* 84: 381-392, 1989.

Brown BW Jr: The crossover experiment for clinical trials. *Biometrics* 36:69-79, 1980.

Bull JP: The historical development of clinical therapeutic trials. *J Chron Dis* 10:218-248, 1959.

Buyse ME, Staquet MJ, Sylvestor RJ (eds): *Cancer Clinical Trials: Methods and Practices*. New York, Oxford University Press, 1984.

Byar DP: Why data bases should not replace randomized clinical trials. *Biometrics* 36:337-342, 1980.

Carbone PP, Davis TE, Zelen M, Lavin PT: Eastern Cooperative Oncology Group: Progress report of activities and plans. *Cancer Clin Tr* 1:65-75, 1978.

Carter SK, Selawry O, Slavik M: Phase I clinical trials. In Saunders JP, Carter SK (eds): Methods of development of new anti-cancer drugs. *Natl Cancer Inst Monogr* 45:75-80, 1977.

Chalmers TC, Block JB, Lee S: Controlled studies in clinical cancer research. *N Engl J Med* 287:75-78, 1972.

Cohen J: *Statistical Power Analysis for the Behavioral Sciences*. New York, Academic Press, 1977.

Diehl HS, Baker AB, Cowan DW: Cold vaccines: An evaluation based on a controlled study. *JAMA* 111:1168-1173, 1938.

Donner A: Approaches to sample size estimation in the design of clinical trials—A review. *Statistics in Med* 3:199-214, 1984.

Ellenberg SS: Determining sample sizes for clinical trials. *Oncology* 8:39-46, 1989.

Finkler NJ, Benacerraf B, Lavin PT, Wojciechowski C, Knapp RC: Comparison of CA-125, clinical impression and ultrasound in the preoperative evaluation of ovarian masses. *Obstet Gynecol* 72: 659-664, 1988.

Fisher RA, MacKenzie WA: Studies in crop variation. II. The manurial response of different potato varieties. *J Agric Sci* 13:311-320, 1923.

Food and Drug Administration: Hearing procedure for refusal or withdrawal of approval of new drug applications and for issuance, amendment or repeal of antibiotic drug regulations: Interpretative description of adequate and well controlled clinical investigations. *Fed Register* 34:14596-14598, Sept 19, 1969a.

Food and Drug Administration: Novobiocin-tetracycline combination drugs: Calcium novobiocin-sulfamethizole tablets. Final order repealing regulations and working certificates. *Fed Register* 34: 14598-14599, Sept 19, 1969b.

Food and Drug Administration: Hearing requests on refusal or withdrawal of new drug applications and issuance, amendment or repeal of antibiotic drug regulations and describing scientific content of adequate and well-controlled clinical investigations. *Fed Register* 35:3073-3074, Feb 17, 1970a.

Food and Drug Administration: Hearing regulations describing scientific content of adequate and well-controlled clinical investigations. *Fed Register* 35:7250-7253, May 8, 1970b.

Freiman JA, Chalmers TC, Smith H Jr, Kuebler RR: The importance of beta, the type II error, and sample size in the design and interpretation of the randomized control trial: Survey of 71 "negative" trials. *N Engl J Med* 299:690-694, 1978.

Gehan EA: The determination of the number of patients required in a preliminary and follow-up trial of a new chemotherapeutic agent. *J Chron Dis* 13:346-353, 1961.

Gelber RD, Gelman RS, Goldhirsch AA: A quality of life oriented endpoint for comparing therapies. *Biometrics* 45:781-796, 1989.

Gottlieb JA: Phase I and II clinical trials: A critical reappraisal. In *The Pharmacological Basis of Cancer Chemotherapy*. Baltimore, William & Wilkins, 1974, pp 485-498.

Gurland J, Johnson RO: How reliable are tumor measurements? *JAMA* 29:973-978, 1965.

Hawkins BS: Perusing the literature. *Controlled Clin Tr* 1:71-74, 181-185, and 269-274, 1980.

Hawkins BS: Perusing the literature. *Controlled Clin Tr* 2:51-57, 257-265, and 327-333, 1981.

Hawkins BS: Perusing the literature. *Controlled Clin Tr* 3:371-383, 1982.

Hawkins BS: Perusing the literature. *Controlled Clin Tr* 4:75-86, and 239-253, 1983.

Hill AB: *Statistical Methods in Clinical and Preventive Medicine*. New York, Oxford University Press, 1962.

Hills M, Armitage P: The two-period cross-over clinical trial. *Br J Clin Pharmacol* 8:7-20, 1979.

Homan ER: Quantitative relationships between toxic doses of antitumor chemotherapeutic agents in animals and man. *Cancer Chemother Rep* 3:13-19, 1972.

Hsieh FY: A simple method of sample size calculation for unequal sample size designs that use the log-rank or t-test. *Statistics in Med* 6:577-581, 1987.

Ingelfinger FJ: The randomized clinical trial. *N Engl J Med* 287:100-101, 1972.

Jones D, Whitehead J: Sequential forms of the log rank and modified Wilcoxon tests for censored data. *Biometrika* 66:105-113, 1979.

Jones RH: Time series analysis with unequally spaced data. In Hannan EJ, Krishnaian PR, Rao MM (eds): *Handbook of Statistics*, Vol 5. New York, Elsevier Science Publishers, 1985, pp 157-177.

Jones RH: Serial correlation in unbalanced mixed models. Proceedings of the 46th Session, Tokyo, Book 4. *Bull Int Statistical Inst* 1987, pp 105-112.

Koch GG: The use of non-parametric methods in the statistical analysis of the two-period change-over design. *Biometrics* 28:577-584, 1972.

Lachin JM: Introduction to sample size determination and power analysis for clinical trials. *Controlled Clin Tr* 2:93-113, 1981.

Lan KKG, Wittes J: The B-value: A tool for monitoring data. *Biometrics* 44:579-585, 1988.

Lasagna L: The controlled clinical trials: Theory and practice. *J Chron Dis* 1:353-367, 1955.

Lavin PT: Alternative measures of anti-tumor activity in the evaluation of solid tumors. *Cancer Clin Tr* 4:451-459, 1981.

Lavin PT: Practical considerations in the coordination of clinical trials: In Louis TA, Shapiro SH (eds): *Issues in the Conduct of Clinical Trials*. New York, Marcel Dekker, 1983, pp 129-153.

Lavin PT: Problems with tumor response criteria: In Mastromarino A (ed): *Biology and Treatment of Colorectal Cancer Metastases*. Boston, Martinus Nijhoff, 1985, pp 211-214.

Lavin PT, Flowerdew G: Studies in variation associated with the measurement of solid tumors. *Cancer* 46:1286-1290, 1980.

Lavin PT, Knapp RC, Malkasian G, Whitney CW, Berek JC, Bast RC: CA-125 for the monitoring of ovarian carcinoma during primary therapy. *Obstet Gynecol* 69:223-227, 1987.

Lee YJ, Wesley RA: Statistical considerations to phase II trials in cancer: Interpretation, analysis and design. *Semin Oncol* 8:403-416, 1981.

Lilienfeld AM: Ceteris paribus: The evolution of the clinical trial. *Bull Hist Med* 56:1-18, 1982.

Lucas JM: Combined Shewhart-Cusum quality control schemes. *J Quality Technol* 14(2):51-58, 1982.

Makuch R, Simon R: Sample size requirements for evaluating a conservative therapy. *Cancer Treat Rep* 62:1037-1040, 1978.

Makuch RW, Simon R: Sample size considerations for non-randomized comparative studies. *J Chron Dis* 33:171-175, 1980.

McNemar Q: Note on the sampling error of the difference between correlated proportions or percentages. *Psychometrica* 12:153-157, 1947.

McPherson K: Statistics: The problem of examining accumulating data more than once. *N Engl J Med* 290:501-502, 1974.

Mehta CR, Patel NR, Tsiatis AA: Exact significance testing to establish treatment equivalence for ordered categorical data. *Biometrics* 40:819-825, 1984.

Mienert CL: *Clinical Trials: Design, Conduct and Analysis*. New York, Oxford University Press, 1986.

Moertel CG, Hanley JA: The effect of measuring error on the results of therapeutic trials in advanced cancer. *Cancer* 38:388-394, 1976.

Mount FW, Ferebee SH: Control study of comparative efficacy of isoniazid, streptomycin-isoniazid, and streptomycin-para-aminosalicylic acid in pulmonary tuberculosis therapy. I. Report on twelve-week observations on 526 patients. *Am Rev Tuberc* 66:632-635, 1952.

Nam J: A simple approximation for calculating sample sizes for detecting linear trends in proportions. *Biometrics* 43:701-706, 1987.

Neyman J, Pearson ES: On the use and interpretation of certain test criteria. *Biometrika* 20A:175-240, and 263-294, 1928.

O'Brien PC, Fleming TR: A multiple testing procedure for clinical trials. *Biometrics* 35:549-556, 1979.

Oken MM, Creech RH, Tormey D, Horton J, Davis TE, McFadden ET, Carbone PP: Toxicity and response criteria of the Eastern Cooperative Oncology Group. *Am J Clin Oncol* 5:649-655, 1983.

Peto R: Clinical trial methodology. *Biomedicine* 28:24-36, 1978.

Peto R, Pike MC, Armitage P, et al: Design and analysis of randomized clinical trials requiring prolonged observation of each patient. I. Introduction and design. *Br J Cancer* 34:585-612, 1976; II. Analysis and examples. *Br J Cancer* 35:1-39, 1977.

Pocock SJ: Randomized clinical trials (Letter). *Br Med J* 1:1161, 1977.

Pocock SJ: Size of cancer clinical trials and stopping rules. *Br J Cancer* 38:757-766, 1978.

Pocock SJ: Allocation of patients to treatment in clinical trials. *Biometrics* 35:183-197, 1979.

Pocock SJ: *Clinical Trials: A Practical Approach*. New York, John Wiley and Sons, 1983.

Pocock SJ, Geller NL, Tsiatis AA: The analysis of multiple endpoints in clinical trials. *Biometrics* 43:487-498, 1987.

Schneiderman MA: Mouse to man: Statistical problems in bringing a drug to clinical trial. In Proc Fifth Berkeley Symp Math Statis Prob, University of California 4:855-866, 1967.

Schoenfeld D: Statistical considerations for pilot studies. *Int J Radiat Oncol Biol Phys* 6:371-374, 1980.

Schoenfeld DA, Richter J: Nomograms for calculating the number of patients needed for a clinical trial with survival as an endpoint. *Biometrics* 38:162-170, 1982.

Shapiro SH, Louis TA (eds): *Clinical Trials: Issues and Approaches*. New York, Marcel Dekker, 1983.

Simon R: Restricted randomization designs in clinical trials. *Biometrics* 35:503-512, 1979.

Simon R: Patient subsets and variation in therapeutic efficacy. *Br J Clin Pharmacol* 14:473-482, 1982.

Simon R: The importance of prognostic factors in cancer clinical trials. *Cancer Treat Rep* 68:185-192, 1984.

Staquet MJ, Rozencweig M, Von Hoff DD, et al: The delta and epsilon errors in the assessment of the cancer clinical trials. *Cancer Treat Rep* 63:1917-1921, 1979.

Tchekmedyian NS, Cella DF: Quality of life in current oncology practice and research. *Oncology* 4:1-232, 1990.

Tukey, JW: Some thoughts on clinical trials, especially problems of multiplicity. *Science* 198:679-684, 1977.

Weiss GB, Bunce H, Hokanson JA: Comparing survival of responders and non-responders after treatment: A potential source of confusion in interpreting cancer clinical trials. *Controlled Clin Tr* 4:43-52, 1983.

Zar JH: *Biostatistical Analysis*. Englewood Cliffs, Prentice-Hall, 1984.

Zelen M: The randomization and stratification of patients to clinical trials. *J Chron Dis* 27:365-375, 1974.

Zelen M: Aspects of the planning and analysis of clinical trials in cancer. In Srivastava JN (ed): *A Survey of Statistical Design and Linear Models*. New York, Elsevier, North Holland, 1975a, pp 629-645.

Zelen M: Importance of prognostic factors in planning therapeutic trials. In Staquet MJ (ed): *Cancer Therapy: Prognostic Factors and Criteria of Response*. New York, Raven Press, 1975b, pp 1-6.

Zelen M: Statistical options in clinical trials. *Semin Oncol* 4:441-446, 1977.

Zelen M: Strategy and alternate randomized designs in cancer clinical trials. *Cancer Treat Rep* 66:1095-1100, 1982.

# *Appendix I*
# Glossary of Terms for Clinical Trials

**Accrual**   The number of subjects entered into a study.

**Adjuvant**   Therapy used to enhance the effectiveness of the primary mode of treatment (e.g., surgery).

**Administrative listing**   A summary of the basic record status for patients under study.

**Affiliate**   An institution that participates in a collaborative study.

**Analysis**   A study of the data.

**Analyzable case**   A term used in reference to a case record that indicates whether the case record has been included in the analysis.

**Arm**   A specific therapy program under study. (Often used synonymously with treatment program, treatment regimen, treatment arm, or treatment.)

**Balanced**   A statistical term used to describe a study in which all treatments are to be assigned with equal probability.

**Baseline**   Time of initial study entry.

**Blocking:**   Division of a population into subpopulations that are on average similar in composition.

**Canceled**   A term applied to patients withdrawn from a protocol prior to the commencement of protocol therapy.

**Case record**   The completed forms that document the medical history and protocol results for a particular patient.

**Censored observation**   An incomplete observation relating to a time-dependent end point (e.g., survival, time to progression, disease-free interval). A patient still alive is said to be a censored observation for survival.

**Clinical**   A term used to describe a study based upon observation and treatment.

**Clinical trial**   A study of two or more treatment programs according to a protocol to detect differences in treatment programs with respect to study end points.

**Complete response**   A term used to describe the complete disappearance of all disease(s).

**Confirmation of registration (form)**   A term used to describe a form that registers a patient into a particular protocol.

**Contingency tables analysis**   An analytic procedure for a given table or series of tables of data frequency presented by levels for each factor in which the probability of all less likely tables are calculated. Examples of analytic procedures include Fisher's exact test, chi-square tests, and log-linear tests.

**Control**   A term used to describe a standard for comparison. (A control is always recommended in a clinical trial.)

**Controlled**   A term used to describe a clinical trial that is based upon a written protocol.

**Cooperative group**   An independent research team funded by grants composed of:
1. Group chairperson
2. Operations office
3. Statistical center
4. Institutions, with the intent of conducting a controlled evaluation of protocol treatments on groupwide collaborative basis.

**Covariate**   A term used to describe an ancillary variable under consideration.

**Cox model**   A statistical modeling of the hazard function associated with the elapsed time to an event that incorporates covariates and strata as explanatory variables. This model is often used to correct for imbalances within treatment groups.

**Crossover**   A term used to describe a study with two or more specific phases or steps of therapy.

**Data base**   A term used to describe a computerized representation of case records.

**Data file**   The computerized portion of the case records for a particular patient.

**Data manager, statistical center**   An individual responsible for
1. Requesting data
2. Collecting data
3. Checking data for consistency and accuracy
4. Entering data into computerized data files
5. Obtaining data clarification.

**Disease-free interval**   The time from resection for cure or complete response to the time of recurrence or relapse or death.

**Duration of response**   A term (used in studies in which response is an end point) that refers to the time from date of onset of partial or complete response to date of progression.

**Eligible**   A patient who meets all protocol entrance criteria.

**End point**   A defined study objective for a protocol (e.g., survival, objective tumor response, toxicity, time to relapse, time to progression).

**Factor**   A term used to describe a variable under consideration

**Final analysis**   A term used to describe a detailed study report for which followup is essentially complete and all major end points can be explored in depth.

**Flow sheets**   A collection of forms completed by the patient care team that documents the details of treatment administration, resulting toxicities, and laboratory chemistries.

**Followup**   The monitoring of a patient enrolled in a protocol.

**Forms**   A collection of documents that record and document essential data (e.g., on-study form, pathology form, radiotherapy form, flow sheet, measurement sheets, interim forms, summary and evaluation form, case evaluation form).

**Group chairperson**   A scientist with overall responsibility for
1. Group leadership
2. Group organization
3. Group direction

**Hazard function**   The force of mortality or instantaneous failure rate.

**Human Subjects Committee**   A team of individuals who approve a study for ethical conduct within a particular institution.

**Induction**   The initial phase or step of therapy that is to be automatically followed by a second treatment phase or step.

**Ineligible**   A term used to describe a patient that did not meet all the eligibility criteria for study entry.

**Informed consent**   A legal document signed by the patient to be treated that gives consent to be treated, explains patient's rights, and summarizes major risks.

**Initial treatment**   The initial phase or step of therapy that represents the first therapy received while the patient is on study.

**Institution**   A hospital that enrolls patients into protocols.

**Institution balancing**   A statistical term used to describe a treatment allocation rule effected at the time of randomization to ensure that no institution has an imbalance of patients assigned to a particular treatment program.

**Institutional Review Board (IRB)**   A team of health care personnel, scientists, administrators, and laypersons concerned with reviewing scientific and ethical principles prior to activation of a study. Specific guidelines with respect to IRB member composition and documentation of review must be filed with the Department of Health and Human Services, National Institutes of Health.

**Interim record**   A term used to describe a case record that is not complete.

**Kaplan-Meier method**   A statistical method used to generate life-tables based on a conditional analysis of patients dead, alive, and at risk.

**Key**   A computing term used to describe an identifying variable that references a collection of items.

**Level**   A possible factor outcome.

**Level of significance**   The probability of rejecting a null hypothesis when it is true; often called type I error.

**Life-table method**   A statistical method used to display actuarial curves relative to time-dependent end points (e.g., survival, time to progression).

**Log**   A register for recording entry of patients into the study or receipt of forms.

**Log-rank test**   A statistical test devised by Peto that makes no assumption on the distribution of the underlying data.

**Logical check**   A computerized or manual check of two of more data items to check for consistency (e.g., date of birth, date of randomization, age at study entry).

**Logistic model**   A statistical model of the probability of a discrete outcome that incorporates covariates as explanatory variables in describing the probabilities of the possible outcomes. It is used in models of objective tumor response to determine the prognostic level of the covariates.

**Lost to followup**   A patient who was last reported as being alive but can no longer be located.

**Maintenance treatment**   A specific phase or step of therapy that follows induction therapy or which follows initial therapy which has induced a complete or partial response.

**Measurement sheets**   A collection of forms that document quantitative measures serially for all measurable indicators.

**Modality**   A term used to describe oncology specializations (e.g., pathology, immunology, chemotherapy, radiotherapy, surgery, or immunotherapy).

**No change**   A term used to describe stable disease.

**Objective response**   A term used to describe disease status (i.e., complete response, partial response, no change, progression).

**Off study**   A term used to describe a patient who has completed protocol-specific treatment.

**On study**   A term used to describe a patient still receiving protocol-specified treatment.

**On-study form**   A form used to record patient history prior to study entry, collecting the following data:
1. Demographic characteristics
2. Prior treatment
3. Associated diseases and medications
4. Signs and symptoms
5. Disease involvement
6. Pathology findings
7. Laboratory findings

**Operations office**   An organization in the cooperative group composed of administrators, clerical staff, and secretaries responsible for
1. Conducting randomization and registrations
2. Planning meetings
3. Preparing and distributing protocols
4. Amending protocols
5. Distributing and collecting forms
6. Distributing study reports
7. Keeping the group informed

**Partial response**   A term used to describe a partial disappearance of disease, as defined by the protocol.

**Performance status**   The physical status of a patient (e.g., Karnofsky scale, ECOG scale) that represents his or her level of activity.

**Phase I**   A study of a treatment regimen to determine optimal dosages and schedules.

**Phase II**   A study of one or more treatment regimens to determine antitumor activity.

**Phase III**   A comparative study of one or more treatment regimens to determine which programs or combinations of those with proven Phase II activity are best.

**Privacy Act**   A law that provides for the privacy of the patient so that his or her identification will not be disclosed without permission.

**Prognostic factor**   A factor such as performance status that influences a study end point (e.g., response, survival, time to progression).

**Progression**   Advance of disease.

**Prospective**   A term used to describe data collected in an ongoing fashion.

**Protocol**   A formal document written by the protocol study chairperson that details the exact patient population, treatment selection rationale, hypotheses under study, method of treatment, method of observation, and data to be reported.

**Protocol office**   An organization in the institution composed of administrators, computer specialists, and secretaries responsible for
1. Protocol preparation and distribution
2. Patient entry
3. Institution Review Board and Human Subjects Committee coordination
4. National Cancer Institute report coordination
5. Liaison activities

**Protocol study chairperson**   A scientist in charge of a protocol responsible for
1. Planning the protocol
2. Monitoring the protocol
3. Reviewing patient records
4. Conducting record evaluation
5. Publishing results

**Quality of life**   The evaluation of the disease and treatment effect of daily activities.

**Randomization**   A statistical plan by which treatments are allocated by chance to patients under study. (Randomization is the cornerstone of the statistical methodology used in the clinical trial setting.)

**Recurrence**   Disease that has reappeared.

**Registration**   The act of entering the patient into the study.

**Relapse**   Disease that has progressed after involvement had once been reduced.

**Remission**   Disappearance of disease.

**Request**   A call for data for the purpose of updating patient data files.

**Retrospective**   A term used in data analysis to describe a data set that is already complete and will be analyzed for a new purpose other than the one for which it was originally collected.

**Review procedure**   A term used to describe critical examination of a document in draft form.

**Significant (clinically)**   An outcome that is considered to be important from a clinical point of view (e.g., important increase in response rate).

**Significant (statistically)**   An outcome that could have occurred as a result of random variation only with very low probability.

**Statistical center**   An organization composed of statisticians, computer scientists, data base administrators, data managers, and secretaries responsible for
1. Scientific collaboration
2. Statistical research
3. Statistical consulting
4. Software development
5. Protocol development
6. Forms design
7. Data processing
8. Data collection
9. Statistical computing
10. Data analysis

**Statistician**   A scientist responsible for
1. Scientific collaboration
2. Statistical research
3. Statistical consulting
4. Protocol development
5. Data analysis
6. Biostatistical coordination

**Step**   A term synonymous with "phase," used to describe a specific treatment program.

**Stratification**   A statistical tool used at the time of randomization to ensure that the treatment groups under study are homogeneous with respect to variables thought to have important bearing upon study end points.

**Survival**   A term used to describe the length of survival measured from some specified starting point (e.g., date of surgery or date of randomization).

**Tables**   A multidimensional data display technique.

**Toxicity**   A quantifiable side effect of therapy.

**Toxicity audit**   A special survey of all study participants to determine the extent of toxicity associated with a certain treatment program.

**Type I error**   The percentage of time that the null hypothesis is rejected when it is really true.

**Type II error**   The percentage of time that the alternative hypothesis would be rejected when really true.

**Unevaluable**   A term used to describe a patient that cannot be evaluated.

**Update**   A term used to describe the addition of new data to an existing file.

**Workshop**   A meeting of study participants who complete forms with those who process the forms to review basic principles and problem areas related to forms completion.

# *Appendix II*
# Outline for Writing a Protocol

## GENERAL REQUIREMENTS

1. Schema and summary of tests
2. Table of contents
3. Numbered pages (with protocol number on each page)
4. Treatment programs (Section 5.0)
5. Statistical considerations (Section 9.0)

## BODY OF PROTOCOL

Schema
1.0 Introduction
2.0 Objectives
3.0 Selection of patients
4.0 Patient entry
5.0 Treatment programs
    5.1 Drug formulation and procurement
    5.2 Description of treatment program
    5.3 Administration of drug
    5.4 Anticipated major toxicities/adverse reactions
    5.5 Management of toxicity/adverse reactions
    5.6 Dose modifications
    5.7 Supportive therapy
    5.8 Therapy duration
    5.9 Additional therapy
6.0 Study end points
7.0 Required data
8.0 Modality review procedure
9.0 Statistical considerations
10.0 Patient consent and peer judgment
11.0 References

## INFORMED CONSENT

1. Scientific and clinical rationale
2. Description of treatment or procedure (listing each drug with its side effects)
3. Costs
4. Benefits
5. Risks, side effects
6. Route of administration; duration of treatment
7. Alternatives
8. Statements of voluntary participation, confidentiality, and FDA inspection
9. Standard paragraphs and signature page

## OUTLINE FOR WRITING A PROTOCOL

### SCHEMA

This diagrammatic representation should have sufficient detail so that someone not familiar with the protocol can grasp the main details of the study.

### 1.0 INTRODUCTION

The introduction should give the background and rationale for initiating the study. Earlier related studies and data should be quoted in detail along with appropriate references.

### 2.0 OBJECTIVES

The objectives should give a concise statement of the experimental hypothesis to be investigated. Typically, these hypotheses can be expressed in the following terms:

2.1 Toxicity
2.2 Dose and schedule
2.3 Objective tumor response
2.4 Survival
2.5 Time to progression or relapse
2.6 Tumor-free survival
2.7 Therapy completion status
2.8 Effect of regimen on markers such as suppressor cells, carcinoembryonic antigen, myeloma protein, etc.
2.9 Cross resistance between single drugs or drug combinations.

### 3.0 SELECTION OF PATIENTS

This section shall delineate the study population in which the protocol therapies are to be tested. The following will help to define the patient population:

3.1 Conditions for patient eligibility
    3.11 Histologic confirmation of disease
    3.12 Documentation of specific disease stage (x-ray, scans, surgical staging, etc.)
    3.13 Adequate hepatic, renal, or bone marrow function (e.g., bilirubin $\leq$ 1.5 mg%, SGOT $\leq$ 60 IU, BUN $\leq$ 20 mg%, creatinine $\leq$ 1.0 mg%, WBC, $\geq$ 4,000/mm$^3$, platelets $\geq$ 100,000/mm$^3$) (Hematologic limits may vary if drug is non-myelosuppressive)
    3.14 Time since completion of prior therapy (if applicable)
    3.15 Other specific features for a given protocol
    3.16 Informed consent
3.2 Conditions for patient ineligibility
    3.21 For example, the following (if applicable):
    (a) Prior therapy with study agents
    (b) Any prior chemotherapy
    3.22 A disease process that might be exacerbated by use of a specific drug, such as doxorubicin (congestive heart failure) or bleomycin (significant lung disease)
    3.23 Patients with acute intercurrent complications such as infection or postsurgical complications
    3.24 Patients above a certain age and/or performance status (e.g., 75 years old or completely bedridden)
    3.25 Patients with a second malignancy, excluding skin cancer

## 4.0 PATIENT ENTRY

This section outlines methods of patient registration or randomization. It should include

4.1 A statement that the study chairperson must contact the Protocol Office in order to register or randomize patient

4.2 Details of registration or randomization procedure, including required patient identification and, if randomized, any other information (e.g., stratification factors)

4.3 Parameters in patient condition to check
  (a) Laboratory tests: creatinine, hematocrit, etc.
  (b) Physical condition: vital signs, urine output, etc.
  (c) When to hold drug

4.4 Consideration of ancillary study before onset of main study

## 5.0 TREATMENT PROGRAMS

5.1 Drug Formulation and Procurement (Phase I and II Agents)
  5.11 Description: chemical formula and molecular weight
  5.12 Description of form supplied: color and appearance, powder or liquid, etc.
  5.13 Method of procurement
  5.14 Method of storage: temperature, shelf-life, etc., as specified by the manufacturer
  5.15 Instruction for mixing and stability of reconstituted solutions and solutions that are diluted further
    5.151 Primary dilution: NS, $H_2O$, special diluents with or without bacteriostatic agents, and amount of diluent
    5.152 Second dilution: amount (in ml) (If variable, specify range and type [e.g., D5W, NS, lactated Ringer's])
  5.16 Other pertinent information: filtration, pumps, light sensitivity, line protection, etc.
  5.17 Type of line required (If separate lines must be used, specify requirements)

5.2 Description of Treatment Program
  5.21 Timing (prior notice, lead time, preparation time, etc.)
  5.22 Dose parameters (e.g., body weight, surface area) on which calculations are based
  5.23 Schedule
  5.24 Route (e.g., IV, PO, etc.)
  5.25 Prerequisites (e.g., premedical; physical; prehydration; additional medication to be given before, during, and after investigational drug administration; lab tests; x-rays; transfusions, etc.)
  5.26 Additional requirements (e.g., posthydration, "rescue," lab tests, vital signs, pulmonary function tests, ECGs, arterial blood gases [ABGs], etc.)
    Time and frequency of pulmonary function tests and interventions, *if critical*, should be specified

5.3 Administration of Drug
  5.31 Route (e.g., PO)
  5.32 For drug administration by vein, state the mode of IV administration with respect to time (e.g., IV push over 10 minutes, constant infusion over 24 hours, etc.); also state preferred order of administration if regimen involves multiple drugs administered sequentially
  5.33 Specify if drug filtration is or is not required during administration; also state size of filter to be utilized if one is required
  5.34 IV drugs: specify if a known vesicant or if high potential for skin irritation or extravasation
  5.35 Indicate when first x-ray must be taken once line is inserted for vesicant
  5.36 Instructions for multiple drug administration through a single IV (e.g., "piggybacking")

5.4 Anticipated Major Toxicities and Adverse Reactions Include nature (e.g., local or systemic) and timing of toxicity (e.g., leukopenia—usual nadir between 9 to 14 days after discontinuation of therapy); leukopenia—onset 10 days, thrombocytopenia—onset 10 to 15 days

5.5 Management of Toxicity/Adverse Reactions
  5.51 Local and systemic management of acute toxicity or overdose—indicate whether management is specific (e.g., if antidote is known, specify type and dosage), symptomatic, or supportive

5.6 Dose Modifications—Drug- or Treatment Program-Specific
  5.61 Treatment deescalation (termination, suspension, reduction)
  5.62 Treatment escalation (dose, schedule)
    If applicable, consider as examples:

Hematologic

| | Dose Modification | | |
|---|---|---|---|
| | WBC Nadir | | |
| Platelet Nadir | >4,000/mm$^3$ | 2,000 to 4,000/mm$^3$ | <2,000/mm$^3$ |
| >100,000/mm$^3$ | 100% | 50% | 0% |
| 75 to 100,000/mm$^3$ | 50% | 50% | 0% |
| <75,000/mm$^3$ | 0% | 0% | 0% |

Renal
For example, stop administration of methotrexate until creatinine reduced to less than 1.0 mg/100 ml.
Hepatic
For example, decrease doxorubicin dose by 50% until liver function tests return to normal.

Mucositis

For example, stop methotrexate until mucosa has completely healed.

5.7 Supportive Therapy
5.8 Therapy Duration
   5.81 Progression, relapse, recurrence
      5.811 Define a stopping point to treatment administration in individual patients
      5.812 Define subsequent treatment programs to be administered
   5.82 Stable disease, response
      5.821 Define what is to be done with the patient after maximum total dose or dose-limiting toxicity has been reached (e.g, doxorubicin, bleomycin, etc.)
5.9 Additional Therapy (radiotherapy, surgical treatment, or other therapy)

## 6.0 STUDY END POINTS
Define (state criteria for)
   6.1 Toxicity
   6.2 Objective response(s)
      6.21 Complete response
      6.22 Partial response
      6.23 Stable disease
      6.24 Progression
   6.3 Recurrence or relapse

## 7.0 REQUIRED DATA
   7.1 Summarize the data set in tabular form:

| Data Set | At Study Entry | Once Weekly | Once Monthly | At Progression |
|---|---|---|---|---|
| Age | X | | | |
| Sex | X | | | |
| WBC | X | X | | |
| Platelets | X | X | | |
| Bilirubin | X | | X | |
| ECG | X | | | |
| PFT | X | | | |
| ABG | X | | | |
| SGOT | X | X | | |
| Tumor measurements | X | X | X | |
| Disease involvement | X | X | X | |
| Progression | | | X | X |
| Survival | | | X | X |

The test data above are intended to serve as a representative example and may be modified as required by the clinical situation or the investigator's judgment.
   7.2 Indicate the data collection plan:
      7.21 What records are required (e.g., on-study form, confirmation of registration form, flow sheets, measured sheets, summary statement)
      7.22 When records are to be submitted
      7.23 Who will receive these records

## 8.0 MODALITY REVIEW PROCEDURE
If applicable, give clear directions as to how this is to be done (e.g., pathology, radiotherapy materials review, etc.)

## 9.0 STATISTICAL CONSIDERATIONS
Every protocol should contain a statistical considerations section that summarizes the statistical plan and reasoning behind the study. The considerations should include (if applicable):
   (a) Specification of control group
   (b) Treatment allocation plan (stratification, dynamic allocation, play the winner, randomized consent, etc.)
   (c) Statement of statistical precision (level of significance, power, etc.). Statistical consultation is encouraged at the earliest stage of study design.
   (d) Sample size requirements (entry, followup, etc.)
   (e) Statistical model used to compute sample size
   (f) Indication of projected losses for ineligibility or exclusions
   (g) Special subgroup analyses to be justified a priori
   (h) Adjustments for multiple comparisons or repeat significance testing
   (i) Firming of interim analyses
   (j) Analysis plan

## 10.0 PATIENT CONSENT AND PEER JUDGMENT
Statement that all institutional, National Cancer Institute, state, and federal regulations concerning informed consent and peer judgment will be fulfilled.

## 11.0 REFERENCES

## 12.0 INFORMED CONSENT
   A. *General:* Informed consent may be defined as consent freely given by a participant in a research project based upon full disclosure of the procedures that the individual will undergo. The consent form should be written in terms comprehensible to the layperson and should include all information about the study that any reasonable person needs and wants to know. It should honestly express the realistic expectations of such participation and carefully avoid inducement by raising false hopes.

Of all aspects of clinical investigation, informed consent is one of the most troublesome and, at the same time, most important. Since informed consents can be the subject of differences of opinion regarding wording and terminology, staff are encouraged to seek advice and assistance from the hospital protocol coordinator.

The informed consent used for research programs is not a legal document in the sense that either the form or the language has been circumscribed by judicial decisions or legal procedures. However, it should be pointed out that severely defective informed consents have been the basis of adverse legal decisions.

Informed consent is to be obtained from every person

who agrees to participate in a program falling under the jurisdiction of the Human Subjects Committee. The consent form for each study is to be submitted to the Committee with the protocol and approved prior to the commencement of any activity. If it appears that patients, parents, or guardians are incapable of understanding the information contained in the informed consent form due to such factors as mental incompetence or language difficulties, the Human Subjects Committee should be contacted to seek aid in attempts to assist the physician in obtaining informed consent. In cases of a language barrier, an attempt should be made to obtain the assistance of a person knowledgeable in that language to translate the informed consent or act as interpreter during the explanation.

B. *Written Informed Consent*: An informed consent should be written using the standardized format and should contain the following elements:

1. A statement that the study involves research, an explanation of the purposes of the research, the expected duration of the procedures to be followed, and identification of any procedures that might be experimental.
2. A description of any reasonably foreseeable risks or discomforts to the subject.
3. A description of any benefits to the subject or to others that may reasonably be expected from the research.
4. A disclosure of appropriate alternative procedures or courses of treatment, if any, that might be advantageous to the subject.
5. A statement describing the extent, if any, to which confidentiality of records identifying the subject will be maintained.

6. For research involving more than minimal risk, an explanation concerning any compensation and any other medical treatments due to injury.
7. An explanation of whom to contact for answers to pertinent questions about the research and research subjects' rights and of whom to contact in the event of a research-related injury to the subject.
8. A statement that participation is voluntary, refusal to participate will involve no penalty or loss of benefits to which the subject is otherwise entitled, and the subject may discontinue participation at any time without penalty or loss of benefits to which the subject is otherwise entitled.

## PARTICIPATION OF CHILDREN IN THE CONSENT PROCESS:

Many states classify anyone under 18 as a minor, but there are no federal or state laws pertaining to minors consenting to participation in research. Whenever appropriate or feasible, children should be involved in the consent process, should be as fully informed as possible about the research project depending on age, and should be given the right to refuse participation. When there is a conflict between parent and child regarding participation, it is recommended that the child not be used as a subject in research unless there is some clear potential benefit to the child. It is advised that children under the age of 18 who are capable of understanding a procedure and its ramifications, and who agree to participation, sign the consent form along with the parent or guardian. This process is left to the discretion of the investigator and the wishes of the child and parent concerned. In some instances, a minor may be required to sign the form together with the parent or guardian.

# UNIT II

## Sites

# Chapter 10 | Intraepithelial Squamous Lesions of the Cervix

*Christopher P. Crum*

*Peyton T. Taylor*

## ANATOMY

The uterus and endocervix arise from the müllerian ducts, which distally meet with the vaginal epithelium to form the ectocervix (Krantz, 1973). The ectocervix merges with the endocervical canal near the external os, and the point at which the endocervical canal joins the isthmus is termed the internal os. Originally, the squamocolumnar junction is located in the region of the external os, where the squamous epithelium of the portio joins the mucus-secreting columnar epithelium of the endocervix. The anatomic position of this junction varies among different patients and during different phases of life in the same patient. During the childbearing years, the "original" squamocolumnar junction shifts to the ectocervix owing to *eversion*, or protrusion, of the cervical lips. This process occurs as a consequence of hormonal factors that influence the conformation of the cervix during fetal life, puberty, and particularly pregnancy. Eversion of the anterior cervix is more extensive and occurs twice as often as eversion of the posterior lip (Ferenczy, 1982). The endocervix is composed of stromal papillae lined with mucinous epithelium, and the recesses between the papillae (crypts) are termed "glands," although they are not true glands.

During the reproductive years, the endocervical columnar epithelium is "transformed" and replaced by squamous epithelium. This process occurs in the region of the original squamocolumnar junction, delineating an irregular, circular zone around the os that varies in width and is termed the *transformation zone*, or *T zone*. It is found principally on the anterior and posterior cervical lips, in parallel with the most prominent sites of cervical eversion. This transformation occurs either by ingrowth of portio epithelium into the region of the columnar epithelium or by replacement of the columnar cells from beneath by reserve cells that have undergone squamous metaplasia, the latter event being characteristic of the dual potential of these reserve cells to differentiate into either squamous or glandular components. Squamous epithelium gradually replaces the endocervical columnar cells, bridging the endocervical papillae and changing the irregular surface of the grapelike papillae to a smooth surface. When this process

Supported by grants from the National Cancer Institute (CA 47676) and the American Cancer Society (MV-395). Dr. Crum is a recipient of a Physician Scientist Award from the National Institute of Allergy and Infectious Disease (A100628).

involves the necks (entrance) of the endocervical crypts, distention of the crypt (or "gland") will result in the formation of nabothian cysts distally.

The process of transformation begins with menarche and is considered a consequence of the acidic vaginal pH produced by the action of bacteria on the glycogen-containing squamous cells. Chronic inflammation and repair produced by infectious or other stumuli also contribute to squamous metaplasia and development of the T zone. The gradual reduction of cervical eversion combined with advancement of the T zone eventually results in a squamocolumnar junction that is located deep within the endocervical canal by the time of menopause (Richart, 1973).

The T zone is where the vast majority of precancerous lesions and invasive squamous cell carcinomas of the cervix originate. Predictably, these neoplasms most commonly occur on the anterior and posterior lips of the cervix (Richart, 1973).

## VIRAL PATHOGENESIS AND EPIDEMIOLOGY

*Human papillomavirus* (HPV) is closely associated with both cervical intraepithelial lesions (precursors) and invasive cancer (Broker and Botchan, 1986). As discussed in Chapter 3, one of several specific HPV types, such as types 16, 18, 31, 33, 35 and others, are found in up to 90% of precancerous and invasive cervical neoplasms (Boshart et al, 1984; Durst et al, 1983; Crum et al, 1984; Crum et al, 1984). In contrast, HPV types 6, 11, and others are found predominantly in the increasingly frequent vulvovaginal condylomas and in the relatively uncommon exophytic condylomas of the cervix (Gissman et al, 1983; Mortality and Morbidity Weekly Report, 1983; Willett et al, 1989). Presumably, this relatively strong link between HPV and sexual transmission explains the strong association observed between cervical neoplasia and either the number of male sexual partners or the sexual history of those partners (Brinton et al, 1989; Kessler, 1974; Kjaer et al, 1989; Slattery et al, 1989).

Inapparent or occult infection with HPV occurs in up to 28% of women (Koutsky et al, 1988; Schneider et al, 1987). Still the relationship between infection and neoplastic transformation is not straightforward, and the mechanisms by which occult infection evolves into an HPV-*related* intraepithelial lesion and subsequently

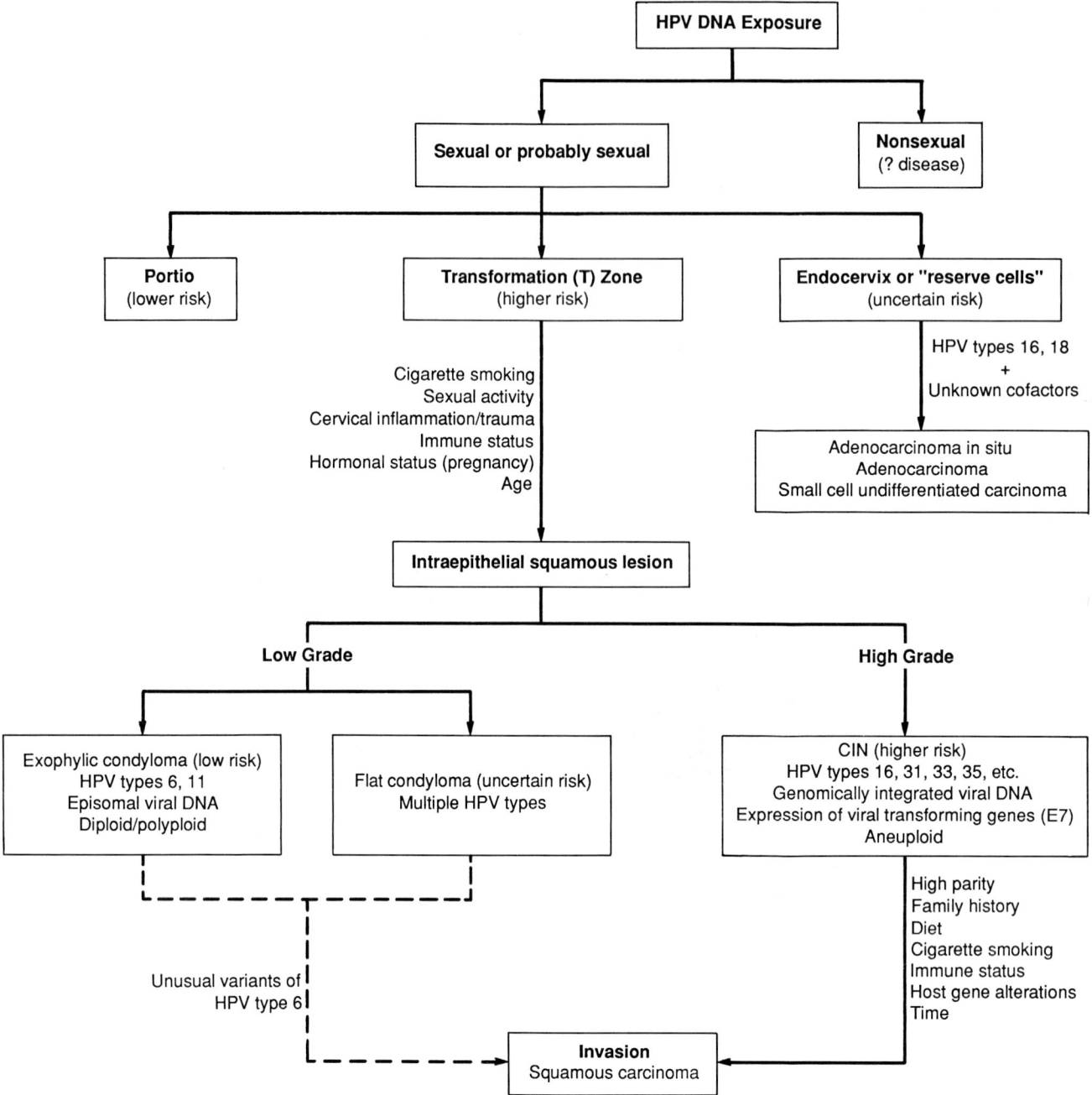

FIGURE 10-1 Evolution of cervical neoplasia and potential role(s) of specific risk factors. (See text for relevant references.)

progresses to invasive cancer (in some patients) are not clear (Koutsky et al, 1988). Factors influencing the development and natural history of HPV-related intraepithelial lesions may include HPV type (Reid et al, 1987), immune status (Koutsky et al, 1988), cigarette smoking (Hellberg et al, 1986; Layde, 1989; Layde and Broste, 1989), hormonal status (Verreault et al, 1989), status of the T zone, and age (Coppelson and Brown, 1975); these and other factors, such as parity (Brinton et al, 1989), family history (Furgyik et al, 1986), and nutritional status (Vessey and Grice, 1989), may also

influence the likelihood of a precursor lesion progressing to invasive cancer (Fig. 10-1).

There is some disparity between the epidemiologic profiles of women with "occult" HPV infection, which is detected by the presence of the HPV *DNA* only, and those of women with HPV-related cervical intraepithelial and invasive lesions. As noted previously, cervical neoplasia is associated strongly with number of sexual partners (Kessler, 1974; Kjaer et al, 1989) and smoking (Layde, 1989; Layde and Broste, 1989). In contrast, the number of sexual partners alone correlates poorly with the frequency of detecting HPV DNA in the genital tract (Burkett et al, in press; Kiviat et al, 1989). Likewise, smoking has yet to be correlated with an increased chance of detecting HPV DNA (Kiviat et al, 1989). Predictably, the risk of invasive cancer correlates poorly with the *prevalence* of HPV DNA in the population (Acs et al, 1989; Kjaer et al, 1988). In a study of two populations having different degrees of risk for invasive cervical cancer, Kjaer et al (1988) demonstrated that the prevalence of occult infection with HPV types 16 and 18 was higher in the low-risk group, underscoring the complex factors involved in the stepwise progression to cancer and apparent need for multiple cofactors.

The genesis of a precancerous squamous cervical lesion involves several events, and potential mechanisms are detailed in Figure 10-1. Exposure to HPV type 16 or similar viruses probably produces initial infection of the squamous epithelium in the T zone, followed by morphologic and biologic alterations that depend upon the HPV type involved. Lower-grade lesions (flat condyloma or cervical intraepithelial neoplasia [CIN] Grade I) are less commonly associated with "cancer-associated" HPV types and, depending upon the population studied, comprise approximately one-third of the lesions detected (Franquemont et al, 1989; Gissman et al, 1983; Willett et al, 1989). In contrast, higher-grade lesions (CIN Grade II or III) frequently contain HPV type 16 and other cancer-associated HPV types (Crum et al, 1984; Crum et al, 1984; Wright, 1988). Although the interaction between HPV and cellular genes in this process is unclear, experimental evidence supports the need for oncogene involvement in addition to HPV nucleic acids to produce invasive cancer (Di-Paolo et al, 1989). Evidently, specific types of HPV (such as type 16) have a tendency to integrate into the cellular genome in precancers and to possess genes (such as E7) that preferentially transform epithelial cells in culture and may alter host gene products (Dyson et al, 1987; Lehn et al, 1988; Phelps et al, 1988).

## NATURAL HISTORY

Traditionally, the various intraepithelial lesions have been considered part of a continuum of change rather than morphologically or biologically distinct steps that progress inevitably from one to the next (Richart, 1973). This view has been modified somewhat by the discovery that specific HPV types are generally associated with higher-grade lesions. Moreover, with techniques such as morphometry and DNA microspectrophotometry, lower-grade lesions have been found to have a principally diploid or polyploid DNA content, which in turn correlates with their tendency to regress (Bibbo et al, 1989; Fu et al, 1981; Fu et al, 1983; Fu et al, 1988). In contrast, higher-grade lesions are frequently biologically aneuploid, demonstrate greater degrees of cytologic atypia, and are more likely (as a group) to persist or progress (Bibbo et al, 1989; Fu et al, 1981; Fu et al, 1983; Fu et al, 1988; Wilbanks et al, 1967). Notwithstanding the value of the techniques

mentioned above in segregating lesions into general groups (Taylor et al, 1987), it is accepted that one cannot consistently distinguish true precancerous lesions from cytologically and histologically similar lesions that are benign. As outlined in Figure 10-1, the variability in natural history of histologically (and biologically) similar lesions may well be influenced by a multitude of factors.

Nasiell et al (1983, 1986) found that approximately two-thirds of mildly dysplastic lesions and one-third of moderately dysplastic lesions regressed during followup. Problems encountered in most studies, however, include length of followup, arbitrary criteria for determining the grade of an individual lesion, and the potential alteration of the natural history of a lesion as a result of biopsy (Nasiell et al, 1983; Nasiell et al, 1986; Richart and Barron, 1969).

The time required for a lesion to evolve from a low grade to a high grade or to progress eventually to invasive cancer is not known and impossible to determine by direct observation. Obviously, it would not be ethically permissible nor pragmatically possible to take a large group of women who have what is believed to be a potentially dangerous and progressive epithelial lesion, allow the lesion to run its course without biopsy or treatment, and follow them over many years to see what will happen. In order to try to understand what *might* happen, mathematical models have been developed based on data from several studies involving women of different ages who have different epidemiologic risk factors. Barron and Richart (1968) have calculated that the mean time it takes for intraepithelial lesions to progress from one grade to the next is approximately 5 years. The mean time required for high-grade intraepithelial lesions (CIN III) to progress to invasive disease is also uncertain but has been estimated to range from 1 to 30 years, with a reasonable average figure being 10 to 13 years (Barron et al, 1978; Coppelson and Brown, 1975; Gustafsson and Adami, 1989).

## CONCEPTS IN DIAGNOSIS AND MANAGEMENT

The Papanicolaou smear (Pap test) is an effective screening tool, identifying those women who need colposcopic examination, biopsy, and further study. By combining and correlating findings on colposcopy, guided cervical biopsies, and cytologic examination, it is possible to sort patients into distinct groups:

1. Those with unsuspected invasive cancer.
2. Those with lesions amenable to office/outpatient treatment.
3. Those who require diagnostic (and often therapeutic) conization.

The approach used to categorize these patients involves the following steps: (1) the selection of women for colposcopic analysis based on an abnormal Papanicolaou smear, (2) the colposcopic exam itself, (3) his-

TABLE 10-1 Comparison of Cytologic Classifications for Cervical Intraepithelial Lesions

| | Classification System | | |
| --- | --- | --- | --- |
| Finding on Pap Smear | Group | Grade | Bethesda |
| Negative | Group I | Negative | Negative |
| Uncertain | Group II | Narrative* | Narrative* |
| Abnormal | Group III | CIN | Abnormal |
| | IIIa | CIN I/Condyloma† | Low-grade SIL |
| | IIIb | CIN II | |
| | IIIc | CIN III | High-grade SIL |
| | Group IV | CIN III | |
| | Group V | Cancer | Cancer |

SIL = Squamous intraepithelial lesion.
*Description and explanation of why smear is considered borderline.
†Flat or exophytic.

tologic confirmation of the grade and extent of the lesion, and (4) exclusion of invasive cancer.

## Patient Selection

The process of diagnosing precursor lesions begins with analysis of the *Papanicolaou smear*. This test has proved to be an effective tool for screening the population and reducing the risk of cancer through early detection of its precursor lesions. The efficacy of Pap testing lies in the practice of sampling of the cervix at regular intervals (Guzick, 1978). It has been estimated that with screening every 3 years, mortality from cervical cancer can be reduced by at least 70% (Mortality and Morbidity Weekly Report, 1989; National Cancer Institute, 1986). Although there is controversy over what the accepted interval should be, this realistically depends upon the population and the availability of medical care. For example, the goals of screening in developing countries with limited resources may be modest compared with those in the United States, where sampling every 1 to 3 years is feasible in a population of which only 5% of women have never had a Pap test (Makuc et al, 1989); however, it is estimated that 37% of women with in-

vasive cancer come from that 5% (Mortality and Morbidity Weekly Report, 1989). Approximately one-third of women with invasive cancer have had a negative Pap smear in the past 5 years (Dunn et al, 1984). It is assumed that sampling error or reader error contributes to this lack of correlation in most cases, although it is possible that a subset of invasive cancers develop rapidly in the absence of a precursor lesion of long standing (Kurman et al, 1988; Mortality and Morbidity Weekly Report, 1989).

False-negative rates due to sampling have been reduced by the use of both the Ayers spatula and endocervical sampling, such as cervical os aspiration (Richart and Vaillant, 1964). More recently, the endocervical brush has become the preferred method for obtaining specimens, reducing the rate of inadequate smears to less than 2% (Townsend et al, 1970). Determining the laboratory "false-negative" rate depends upon the parameters used in its calculation. For example, if errors are calculated based upon total smears processed, false-negative rates are usually less than 1%, however, if the calculation consists of dividing the false-negatives by the total number of positives (including false-negatives), in the course of processing a large volume of smears the

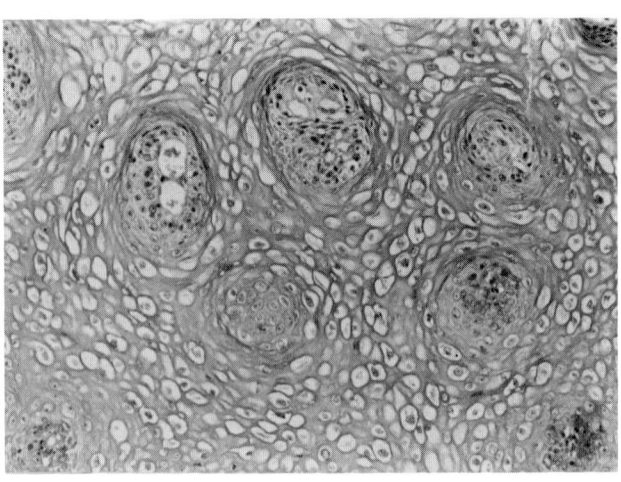

**A**

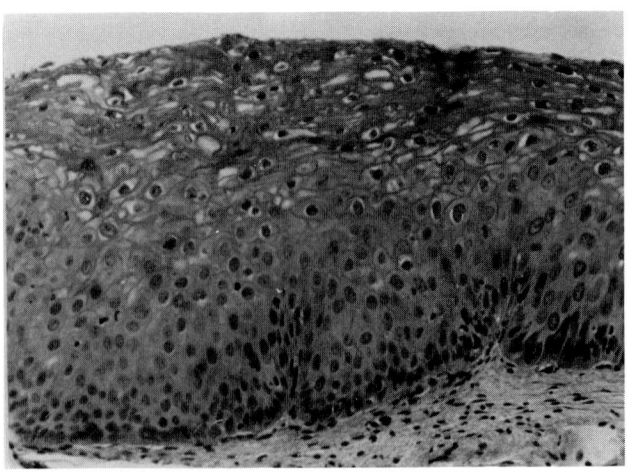

**B**

FIGURE 10-2 Histology of cervical squamous intraepithelial lesions (SIL) (*A* to *D*). *A*, Exophytic condyloma (low-grade SIL). *B*, Flat condyloma (low-grade SIL). *(Continued on p. 183.)*

proportion of positive smears that are incorrectly diagnosed as negative rises to 11 to 23% (Editorial, 1989).

Classification of Pap smear abnormalities has traditionally included normal (group I), uncertain (group II), abnormal consistent with precancer (group III), high-grade CIN (group IV), and invasive cancer (group V). Recently, this has been replaced by the *Bethesda classification*, in which groups II to V are divided into nonspecific atypia and abnormal (National Cancer Institute Workshop, 1988), as outlined in Table 10-1. The latter category includes three subdivisions: abnormal, of uncertain significance; low-grade intraepithelial lesion; and high-grade intraepithelial lesion. This approach is useful in clearly segregating nonspecific abnormalities and reducing the number of classifications for intraepithelial lesions. The Bethesda terminology is designed to avoid use of the term "intraepithelial neoplasia," which has been increasingly difficult to define in the face of HPV-related changes and condylomas. However, such terms as CIN or dysplasia may be included to clarify the message. This classification conforms loosely to the concept that there are low- and high-risk intraepithelial lesions, as defined above. However, it must be stressed that it is impossible to make these distinctions consistently based on cytologic findings alone (National Cancer Institute Workshop, 1988).

## Colposcopic Analysis

Patients with Pap smears that contain high- or low-grade lesions or those for which two consecutive smears show an abnormality of unknown significance should be referred for colposcopy. The intention is to define the nature and extent of the lesion as predicted from the screening Pap smear and to exclude invasive cancer. If invasive cancer cannot be excluded, a cone biopsy may be required.

The techniques of colposcopy are summarized elsewhere (Kolstad and Stafl, 1982). Briefly, the Pap smear is obtained, relevant samples are removed as needed for microbial analysis, and the cervix is examined after 5%

acetic acid has been applied by either swab or spray. The T zone must be analyzed in its entirety, particularly the squamocolumnar junction. The position of the latter will depend upon the conformation of the cervix and the patient's age and hormonal status. Precursor lesions are distinguished from surrounding metaplastic or native squamous epithelium by differences in whiteness, thickness, color, and vascular changes. Comparisons of colposcopic pattern and lesion grade have shown that it is possible to predict the histologic grade (within limits) based on the colposcopic pattern (Reid et al, 1984). However, predicting HPV DNA type by colposcopy alone is more difficult (Follen et al, 1987). Once the lesion has been identified, the colposcopist maps its extent, determining the degree of portio involvement and whether there is extension into the endocervical canal. The latter may require evaluation with an endocervical speculum. Endocervical curettage is performed, in which case the endocervical canal is sampled beyond the limits of visibility. The lesion is then biopsied repeatedly. Both the biopsy specimens and curettage material are placed on squares of absorbent paper (not gauze) and are fixed immediately in buffered formalin or Bouin's solution (Richart et al, 1981). Owing to the deleterious effect of prolonged Bouin's fixation on the stability of nucleic acids (Nuovo and Richart, 1989), buffered formalin is recommended if subsequent analysis of HPV nucleic acids is anticipated.

## Histologic Confirmation

Histologic diagnosis can, within limits, be correlated with the Bethesda cytologic classification system. Lesions in the low-grade category (condyloma or CIN I) include exophytic and flat condylomas and occasional immature variants thereof (Fig. 10-2, *A* and *B*) (Crum et al, 1983; Meisels and Morin, 1981; Purola and Savia, 1977). Virtually all exophytic condylomas contain HPV type 6 or 11 nucleic acids, but the flat lesions are less well characterized, and approximately 15% contain HPV type 16 nucleic acids (Franquemont et al, 1989; Reid et al, 1987; Wright, 1988). The low-grade group

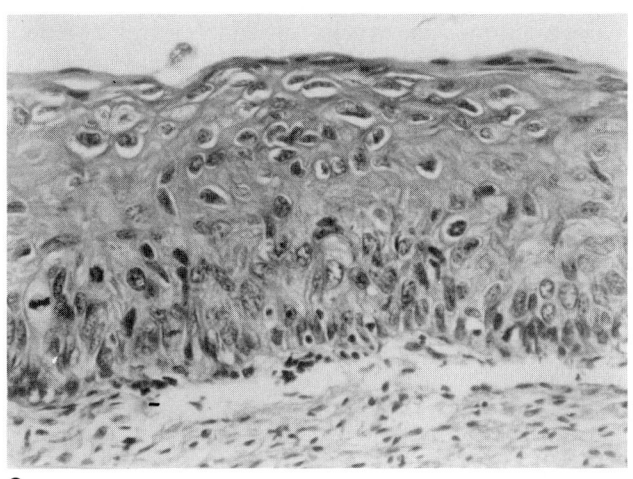

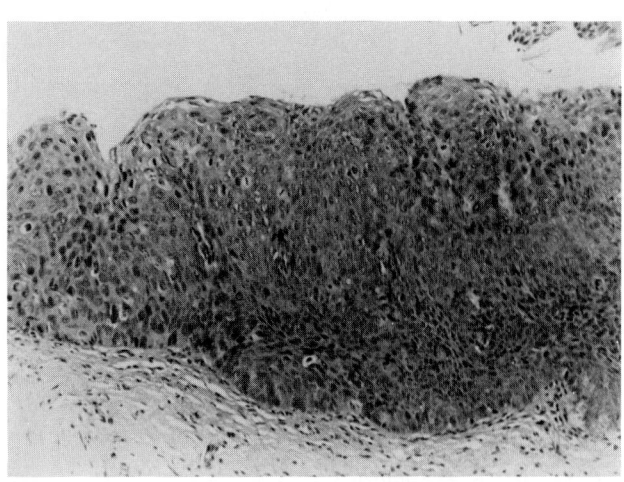

C                                                                        D

FIGURE 10-2 (continued) *C,* CIN II (high-grade SIL). *D,* CIN III (high-grade SIL).

comprises approximately 30% of the intraepithelial cervical lesions seen in our clinic (Franquemont et al, 1989). In the high-grade category are lesions conforming to the definitions of CIN II and CIN III. Approximately 70% of the lesions in this category contain HPV type 16–related nucleic acids, and this category comprises about 70% of all lesions encountered in our colposcopic practice (Franquemont et al, 1989). The designation of a high-grade lesion is based on the presence of nuclear atypia in all layers of the epithelium in at least a portion of the lesion, which is characterized by anisonucleosis, abnormal mitotic figures, a high mitotic index, nuclear crowding, and loss of cell polarity (Fig. 10-2, *C* and *D*) (Crum and Nuovo, 1989). The distinction between CIN II and CIN III is based on the degree of maturation, the latter lesion comprising a full-thickness population of immature abnormal cells (Fig. 10-2D).

The histologic differential diagnosis includes lesions that might be overdiagnosed as low grade (i.e., mild, nonspecific atypias) and those which may mimic high-grade disease. The former consist of minor epithelial abnormalities with perinuclear halos but without sufficient nuclear atypia to justify a diagnosis of low-grade lesion (Fig. 10-3). Studies analyzing such lesions for HPV nucleic acids have demonstrated HPV DNA in approximately 15% of cases (Nuovo et al, 1988). Abnormalities that may mimic high-grade disease include severe inflammatory atypia and repair and atrophy.

## Exclusion of Invasive Cancer

The exclusion of invasive cancer, or the decision to perform a cone biopsy, requires that all parameters of the triage agree (Richart et al, 1981).

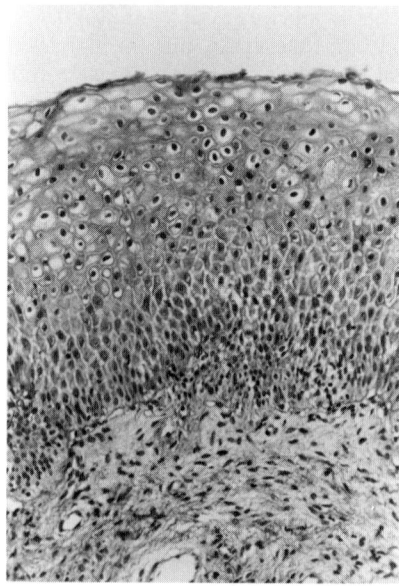

**FIGURE 10-3** Cervical lesion showing cytoplasmic halos and minimal nuclear abnormality. These histologic changes correlate poorly with the presence of HPV nucleic acids and are not diagnosed as intraepithelial lesions.

***Cytologic-Histologic Correlation*** The cytology must correlate, within limits, with the histology. It is not uncommon for the cytology to demonstrate a low-grade lesion while biopsy shows a high-grade abnormality. The critical issue is that both analyses combine to identify the lesion and rule out invasive cancer. If the cytology suggests a high-grade lesion and the biopsy specimen is negative or contains minor abnormalities, the cytology must be reexamined and correlated with the biopsy. If a high-grade cytology is confirmed, the patient must be reexamined and may require cone biopsy if the lesion cannot be found. On the other hand, low-grade cytologic abnormalities or squamous atypias of uncertain significance coexisting with normal findings on colposcopy and biopsy must be approached more conservatively, since the tissue changes may not be related to a cervical precursor. Repeatedly low-grade lesions on Pap smear are best evaluated with repeat examinations, particularly if the abnormality appears to arise from the cervix portio.

***Colposcopic Correlation*** Of primary importance is the identification of the entire T zone or entire lesion on colposcopy. The former may be hampered if the patient is perimenopausal or postmenopausal and the cervical os is narrow or occluded. If this occurs, the colposcopic examination should be considered unsatisfactory.

***Status of the Patient*** Personal factors related to the individual patient contribute to the decision to perform cone biopsy. If the patient is not compliant or considered unreliable, some authors recommend cone biopsy. Likewise, if the patient is particularly concerned about the risk of cancer, specifically if she is older, cone biopsy may be considered.

***Criteria for Therapy*** In summary, according to the American College of Obstetricians and Gynecologists, the following criteria must be met before one considers outpatient/office therapy for a precursor lesion: (a) there must be adequate cytologic, histologic, and colposcopic correlation; (b) the entire lesion must be visible on colposcopy; (c) there should be no suspicion of microinvasion or invasion on cytologic examination or biopsy; (d) there should be no endocervical extension of a precursor lesion—i.e., results of endocervical curettage must be "negative"; and (e) the patient must be reliable and compliant.

## SPECIFIC ISSUES IN MANAGEMENT
### Terminology

Once a histologic diagnosis of papillomavirus infection or CIN has been made, it is generally agreed that the lesion should be removed. Although many conventional flat condylomas will probably regress, a proportion will progress to higher grades of CIN, and it is virtually impossible to clearly distinguish all "benign" papillomavirus-related lesions from those which are going to be associated with progression. In this context, the precise distinction of one grade from the other (i.e., low

**Table 10-2  Selection of Criteria for Cervical Diagnosis**

| Cytologic Findings | Diagnosis | Management |
|---|---|---|
| Negative, no transformation zone seen | Descriptive | Repeat if indicated |
| Acanthosis, parakeratosis, nonspecific halos, atropy | Descriptive | Follow |
| Severe inflammation, reparative atypia | Descriptive | Culture and follow |
| Koilocytosis, maturation, minimal basal atypia | Low-grade squamous intraepithelial lesion (flat or exophytic condyloma, CIN I) | Remove |
| Koilocytosis, maturation, diffuse atypia | High-grade squamous intraepithelial lesion (CIN II) | Remove |
| Minimal koilocytosis or maturation, diffuse atypia | High-grade squamous intraepithelial lesion (CIN III) | Remove |
| Neoplastic epithelium in the ECC | Strips of neoplastic squamous epithelium | Cone biopsy |
| Condyloma in the ECC | Descriptive | Optional* |
| Very scant condyloma or neoplastic epithelium in the ECC | Descriptive | Optional* |

*Management will depend on clinical assessment of the endocervical canal and lesion.
E = endocervical curettage.

versus high) is not as important as (1) determining whether a distinct lesion is present and (2) ruling out invasive cancer. If a lesion is not recognized on biopsy, the pathologist must ensure that the biopsy specimen was taken from the region of the cervix containing the T zone. If metaplastic epithelium or endocervical glands are not identified, it cannot be assumed that the biopsy was adequate and the pathologist should note on the report that the T zone is not present (Table 10-2) (Richart et al, 1981).

## Management of Inflammation

When confronted with a smear containing inflammation and equivocal biopsy results, the pathologist should review the biopsy specimen and the Pap smear and determine whether the atypia on the smear can be explained by the biopsy. Depending on the interpretation, empiric treatment with an antibiotic followed by a repeat exam or repeat colposcopy and biopsies is rec-

ommended. Ideally, this approach will resolve may cytologic- histologic discrepancies and minimize the number of cases requiring repeat biopsy. We have found that the single most important factor in resolving discrepancies between the Pap smear and the biopsy is an active dialogue between the gynecologist and cytopathologist.

## Management of Subtle Lesions

An unsettled issue is the precise morphologic threshold for the diagnosis of HPV infection. As noted above and illustrated in Figure 10-3, a spectrum of subtle changes exists in the cervix, which may contain perinuclear halos and have features resembling a low-grade lesion (condyloma), most of which represent nonspecific abnormalities (Nuovo et al, 1988). If the pathologist is not certain whether a low-grade lesion is present, such patients should be followed with Pap smears and reexamined if there is evidence of a clear-cut lesion. Likewise, in the postmenopausal patient with abnormal Pap smears and a negative colposcopic exam, 4 to 6 weeks of intravaginal estrogen therapy may make it possible to distinguish atrophy from a bona fide intraepithelial lesion or worse.

## The Role of HPV DNA Testing

As technologies for detecting and classifying HPV DNA in the genital tract have developed, interest has grown in the feasibility of HPV DNA testing as an adjunctive technique for diagnosing HPV-related diseases of the cervix. Such testing can be used (1) to reduce the "false-negative" rate of screening Pap smears; (2) to evaluate screening smears that show squamous atypia of uncertain significance; (3) to detect occult or latent HPV infection; or (4) to modify treatment of patients with morphologically distinct HPV-related lesions.

*Reducing false-negative Pap smears*: As described above, the Pap smear clearly carries a significant false-negative rate, and the most preventable component of false-negatives is the misreading of the smear. Adding HPV DNA testing to reduce this would involve rescreening of negative smears that were HPV DNA–positive. Studies indicate that approximately 20% of such smears will be found to contain abnormal cells that were missed on the first analysis (Lorincz et al, 1986; Ward and Crum, 1990). However, it is not clear (1) how efficiently routine viral testing would reduce false-negative rates for Pap smear interpretation, (2) what the impact of such a program would be on morbidity and mortality related to cervical cancer, and (3) what the cost would be of achieving an incremental reduction in morbidity and mortality. On the one hand, approximately one-third of the nearly 7,500 women who die of cervical cancer–related causes each year have had a negative Pap smear in the past 5 years prior to diagnosis and conceivably might have benefitted from more intensive screening (Dunn and Schweitzer, 1981). On the other, the cumulative cost of delivering this test indiscriminately would be extremely high and its value to women who already receive regular examinations is questionable.

*HPV DNA testing to evaluate borderline Pap smears*: In this scenario, HPV DNA testing would be used to "fine tune" the management of women with Pap smear abnormalities of uncertain significance. In a recent study of "nondiagnostic" squamous atypias, it was found that those associated with HPV DNA were more likely to remain abnormal on followup and correlate with the presence of a distinct cervical lesion (Nuovo, personal communication). However, the principal objections to using HPV DNA testing to resolve these borderline abnormalities are (1) the inherent false-negative rate of HPV DNA sampling and (2) the requirement that any persistent cytologic abnormality be evaluated by colposcopy whether or not HPV DNA is detected.

*Detecting occult or latent HPV infection*: By definition, programs aimed at detecting occult infection would necessitate sampling large populations. Unlike the approach outlined above regarding the use of HPV DNA testing to reduce false-negative rates, HPV-positive patients would be notified that they carried the infection and be counseled to return for routine cytologic followup. However, at present, the significance of HPV DNA in the absence of cytologic or histologic abnormalities is unknown. Furthermore, the rate of conversion from subclinical infection to clinical disease and the factors influencing this conversion are not clear. There is also the risk of considerable emotional morbidity inherent in the knowledge that one carries occult HPV infection with no alternative but to adhere to the currently accepted practice of undergoing regular Pap testing.

*HPV DNA testing to modify therapy*: Because the accepted approach to cervical intraepithelial lesions is to remove them, HPV DNA testing has little value in the management of women prior to ablative therapy. When lesions are extensive or the patient is receiving concomitant immunosuppressive therapy, HPV DNA testing may be useful for identifying extensive infections with "low-risk" HPV types, possibly supporting an approach centering on a period of followup rather than proceeding directly to extensive ablation. However, there is no evidence that such a decision requires more than careful histologic interpretation. Moreover, most commercially available techniques for HPV DNA detection categorize HPV DNA positives using groups of more than one probe (i.e., 6/11, 16/18, 31/33/35, etc.). Depending on the hybridization conditions specified by the detection technique, specifying precisely which HPV DNA is present may be impossible. Because there is no evidence that the probe types in some groups identify infections with the same natural history, the "prognostic" value of categorizing lesions as positive for "6/11," "16/18," or "31/33/35" is questionable.

In summary, HPV DNA testing remains an experimental technique that has provided insights into the distribution of papillomaviruses in the population and their association with neoplasia. At the same time, questions have surfaced concerning the relationship between HPV DNA and risk of disease. The ultimate impact of viral testing on the incidence of cancer is still uncertain, given the complex nature of cervical carcinogenesis.

## Positive Endocervical Curettage

The concept of effective office/outpatient management of squamous intraepithelial lesions in lieu of conization assumes that the colposcopic impression, the colposcopically guided biopsy, *and* the predictable absence of endocervical disease are extremely accurate. The routine use of the endocervical curettage was initially described as an essential component of the colposcopic exam (Shingleton et al, 1976; Townsend et al, 1970). Moreover, in an analysis of patients who developed cancer after treatment for precursors, Townsend et al (1981) reported that a proportion had not undergone endocervical curettage. However, the precise contribution of endocervical curettage to management—particularly in the majority of women for whom the limits of the lesion are easily visualized—has been questioned (Drescher et al, 1983; Krebs and Wheelock, 1985).

We advocate use of endocervical curettage in all patients unless a focal lesion is seen and normal villous columnar epithelium is proximal to the lesion. A simplified system of reporting on the curettings, as suggested by Richart et al (1981), includes (1) inadequate or insufficient tissue, (2) adequate fragments of negative endocervix, (3) strips of neoplastic epithelium, and (4) (possibly) invasive cancer. Determining the adequacy of a sample is subjective, although it may be possible to quantify the amount of material in the sample in a semiobjective fashion (Andersen et al, 1988).

Results on endocervical curettage should corroborate the colposcopic impression. If the sample contains numerous free strips of neoplastic squamous epithelium or confirms the suspicion of canal involvement, cone biopsy is necessary (Richart et al, 1981). If the curetting contains strips of "condyloma" or very low-grade disease, conization should be seriously considered, but only after the clinician and pathologist have excluded the possibility of either a microscopic misdiagnosis or inadvertent sampling of a large lesion in the cervical os. Another possible exception would be if the sample contains very small amounts of neoplastic or condylomatous epithelium in the context of a clinically negative endocervical canal. In such a case, inadvertent sampling of an otherwise clearly visualized lesion must also be ruled out (Richart et al, 1981).

Another concern is the value of endocervical curettage for followup after ablative therapy (Krebs and Wheelock, 1985). Although this procedure has been traditionally recommended to ensure that occult therapeutic failures will be detected, endocervical brushing may be more sensitive and should be equally efficacious in the followup of women treated with cryosurgery or laser (Taylor et al, 1987).

## The Pregnant Patient

The incidence of HPV infection, either clinical or occult, in pregnant women ranges from 10 to 29% (Koutsky et al, 1988). The primary goal of management is to exclude invasive cancer, which is achieved by sequential Pap testing, colposcopic examination, and (when necessary) directed cervical biopsies. A limited cone biopsy will occasionally be necessary when lesions extend deeply into the endocervix *and* the Pap smear suggests cancer. In such cases, it is useful to review the results of the Pap test before proceeding to cone biopsy. This will minimize the possibility of misdiagnosing an inflammatory atypia, which may mimic cancer when associated with high-grade CIN. If invasive cancer is not suspected, a complete colposcopic reevaluation with colposcopic examination and cytology can be performed 2 months post partum.

Cone biopsy may be required during pregnancy but should be considered only after consultation, repeat examination, and a review of the parameters do not satisfactorily rule out cancer. Excessive bleeding and premature labor can be minimized by performing the procedure during the second trimester (Jones, 1980).

## THERAPEUTIC ALTERNATIVES
### Selection of Modality

The principal techniques for removing cervical lesions include cryosurgery, laser therapy, and cone biopsy. In general, cryotherapy and laser are considered comparably effective for removing most cervical lesions. In fact, from a large number of studies cryotherapy appears slightly superior (Table 10-3). However, extensive lesions, including those involving the portio, are usually treated by laser ablation, and lesions of uncertain biology or extending into the endocervical canal are most effectively managed by cone biopsy.

If the Pap smear, cervical biopsy, endocervical curettage, and colposcopic examination all indicate a flat condyloma or CIN, most investigators feel the lesion should be removed. An alternative approach for a patient with colposcopically confirmed exophytic condyloma is a period of followup, particularly because these lesions invariably contain the HPV DNA types associated with genital warts and may be associated with multiple lesions in the vagina or elsewhere. The rationale for conservative management is twofold: First, lesions of the vagina and vulva often regress and are infrequently associated with progression to cancer in those sites. Second, there is concern (although not rigorously documented) that treating lesions in the T zone without ablating the vaginal or vulvar lesions may in-

crease the risk of recurrence at those sites. Therefore, for women with multiple asymptomatic exophytic lesions on the vagina and cervix, a period of followup may be preferable to attempted laser ablation or the intravaginal application of 5-fluorouracil. However, followup is mandatory to exclude persistence of the genital lesion.

### Cryotherapy

This technique has evolved as an alternative to electrocautery, the latter being an effective but painful approach to ablating the T zone (Chanen and Rome, 1983). A cryoprobe of variable size is applied to the cervix, and freezing is achieved by a nitrous oxide refrigerant forced through a small orifice at the base of the probe tip. Tissue destruction is achieved by tissue and cellular dehydration; the formation of ice crystals, with cell membrane rupture; cellular protein denaturation; thermal shock; and vascular stasis (Charles and Savage, 1980). The extent of freezing is determined by the size of the lesion, and the goal is to produce an ice ball that extends at least 4 mm beyond the lesion. Currently, two consecutive applications with an interim period of partial thawing are recommended. For larger lesions, multiple applications may be necessary.

The success of the technique is linked to several factors. General causes of failure include inadequate freezing (produced by poor contact, short duration of freeze, and low tank pressure) and the freezing of lesions that are too large for complete coverage (Charles and Savage, 1980). The size of the lesion is of considerable importance, with cure rates dropping substantially for lesions greater than 1 centimeter in diameter (Townsend, 1974). In addition, deep gland (or crypt) involvement may influence therapeutic success. The efficacy of conventional cryosurgery in destroying lesions within cervical clefts ("glands") has been disputed. Although it is generally accepted that cryotherapy will produce tissue necrosis to a depth that will destroy all crypt involvement, Stafl et al (1977) noted that gland crypts may remain in up to 25% of cases, and Savage et al (1982) found that 18% of lesions involving glands recurred following cryotherapy. The chance that invasive cancer may develop as a result of inadequate destruction of disease within clefts and may be "covered over" by regenerating epithelium appears remote. Rather, these cases appear to be related to improper colposcopic triage (i.e., unsuspected intracanal involvement) or may simply represent lesions that were missed owing to their subtle appearance.

As with any other destructive or ablative modality, success after cryosurgery is defined by three negative Pap smears over one year of followup. An abnormal smear during the first year is presumed to result from treatment failure (Richart et al, 1981). A summary of failure rates associated with cryotherapy is listed in Table 10-4. The higher failure rates for high-grade CIN are principally attributable to the larger size of these lesions.

Complications of cryotherapy are generally minimal

| TABLE 10-3 Comparison of Modalities for Removing Cervical Precursor Lesions | | |
| --- | --- | --- |
| Modality | No. of Cases | Cured |
| Cryosurgery (5 studies) | 2,944 | 2,677 (91%) |
| Laser (8 studies) | 987 | 788 (80%) |

TABLE 10-4   Comparison of Failure Rates as a Function of Lesion Grade

| Modality | CIN I | | CIN II | | CIN III | |
|---|---|---|---|---|---|---|
| | No. | % Cured | No. | % Cured | No. | % Cured |
| Cryosurgery (5 Studies | 1,152 | 94.0% | 1,297 | 93.0% | 1,650 | 86.6% |
| Laser (5 studies) | 132 | 88.7% | 240 | 88.0% | 109 | 72.0% |

and include a moderate (rarely severe) degree of pain and cramping during the procedure. This can be minimized by pretreatment with ibuprofen. After treatment, a sometimes troublesome watery discharge will ensue and last approximately 2 to 3 weeks. Healing takes place in approximately 1 month. Pap smears must be taken at least 3 months after therapy to avoid false-positive results due to epithelial repair (Richart et al, 1991). To minimize cervical stenosis, shallow conical or flat cryoprobes can be used. Cryoprobes with long narrow tips are not recommended because of potential complications such as stenosis, incomplete freezing of the endocervical clefts, and shifting of the new squamocolumnar junction so that it is deep within the cervical canal.

## Carbon Dioxide Laser Therapy

A laser, an acronym for "*l*ight *a*mplified by *s*timulated *e*mission of *r*adiation," produces electromagnetic radiation that is coherent, collimated, and monochromatic. These characteristics produce a beam of light that can be focused on tissue to produce vaporization and necrosis on contact. The wavelength of the light depends on the gas being used, which in turn determines the effects of the light beam on the tissue. The energy beam produced by the carbon dioxide laser is absorbed by water, and its contact with tissue produces steam and thermal necrosis. The heat produced will seal small blood vessels, producing hemostasis. At high-power densities there is little thermal injury, and epithelial repair has been shown to cover the wound within 10 days (Baggish, 1983; Wright, 1988).

The two approaches to cervical disease include *laser vaporization* and *laser excision*. The former is recommended for uncomplicated lesions when invasive cancer has been clearly ruled out. The entire T zone is ablated to a depth of 6 to 8 mm peripherally and 4 to 5 mm centrally (Baggish, 1983; Baggish, 1980). When invasive cancer has not been completely excluded, or when the lesion can be seen to extend deeper into the canal, the laser may be used to remove a cylinder of intact tissue for pathologic analysis (McIndoe et al, 1981). A combination of vaporization and excision may be feasible when the lesion extends onto the portio and into the canal. In this case, a cylinder can be removed centrally for pathologic examination, and the well-visualized peripheral lesion can be ablated.

Complications resulting from laser surgery primarily include bleeding and pain. Bleeding is usually minimal, and bleeding requiring sutures was reported by Baggish et al to have occurred in only 1.34% of 3,070 patients treated by laser vaporization (Baggish, 1983; Baggish, 1980). Cervical stenosis (1.1%) and pelvic infection (0.05%) were likewise minimal (Baggish, 1983; Baggish, 1980). Laser ablation is more uncomfortable than cryotherapy, and effective ablation will usually require a paracervical block or direct infiltration of the cervix with a local anesthetic. Regional or general anesthesia are generally required for laser excision.

## Cone Biopsy

Prior to the era of colposcopy, cone biopsy was the standard approach to cervical precursor lesions. With colposcopy, the gynecologist can now visualize the entire cervix, so that fewer patients will require the removal of tissue to rule out invasive cancer. Cone biopsy is indicated when (a) the endocervical limits of a lesion cannot be determined, (b) the results of endocervical curettage are clearly positive, (c) a high-grade lesion on Pap smear cannot be confirmed on biopsy, (d) invasion is suspected based on one parameter, or (e) the colposcopist is concerned about patient compliance or does not feel sufficiently experienced to rule out cancer in a given case (Jones, 1983; Jones and Butler, 1980). In practice, only about 10% of patients referred with abnormal Pap smears will need to undergo conization (Jones and Butler, 1980).

Conization is a surgical procedure not suited for the office or clinic setting and requires a surgical facility and anesthesia. Complications following cone biopsy vary. The most common is bleeding, which can occur during or immediately after conization, or secondary hemorrhage, occurring 5 to 14 days after the procedure. In one study, 2% of patients eventually required transfusion (Jones, 1983). The risk for an incompetent cervix varies. Some studies report no difference in cervical competence between patients who have undergone cone biopsy and control subjects, whereas others demonstrate a significantly greater risk for premature delivery, which appears related to the size of the cone specimen (Jones and Butler, 1980). At present, in view of the increasing use of the carbon dioxide laser, laser conization may provide results comparable or superior to cold-knife conization. However, the latter approach is still required by many practitioners who are not familiar with use of the carbon dioxide laser.

## Other Management Techniques

Two additional techniques for conservative management of cervical precursors include *cold coagulation* and *large-loop excision* of the T zone (Carter, 1984; Duncan, 1983; Prendiville et al, 1989). Contrary to its name, cold coagulation employs a thermocouple that delivers heat via a thermosound in the range of 50 to 120° C. Tissue destruction is achieved by boiling, in which case the epithelium is "blistered off," with thermal destruction of the underlying crypt epithelium. Failure rates have been reported to be approximately 5% over 12 months (Duncan, 1983). Large-loop excision employs a wire loop of variable size that functions as a diathermy electrode, allowing excision (paring off) of the T zone with minimal tissue damage (Cartier, 1984). Proponents of this technique point out that it is easy to apply and leads to a tissue diagnosis while removing the lesion. As the instrument containing the wire is drawn across the tissue, the current produces a cutting effect. Loops of different sizes are used to remove larger portions of tissue. Prendiville et al (1989) reported a 2% failure rate with this technique.

Although recommended principally for extensive vaginal lesions, *intravaginal 5-fluorouracil* may be useful for treating multiple exophytic low-grade cervical warts, usually when they are associated with vaginal lesions (Krebs, 1987). However, the adjunctive value of this approach in treating cervical disease and the risk/benefit ratio inherent in using this compound in young women with uncomplicated warts is unknown.

## LONG-TERM FOLLOWUP

Abnormal findings on Pap smear after ablative therapy indicate either treatment failure or recurrence. For practical purposes, *failure* is defined as a lesion recurring in the first 12 months of followup, preferably after three Pap smears have been obtained. After one year, cervical abnormalities are presumed to be persistent lesions or lesions that have developed directly from occult virus adjacent to the treatment field (Ferenczy et al, 1985; Richart et al, 1980; Richart et al, 1981). *Recurrences* are defined as lesions detected after three negative Pap smears over the first year of followup. Richart et al (1980) found the long-term (after one year) recurrence rate to be 0.44%/year, which according to their calculations approached the level of risk of populations known to be at risk. In a study of cone biopsies, Bjerre et al (1976) reported a recurrence rate of 0.5% for 749 women who initially had negative smears after conization. Kolstad and Klem (1976) reported a 2.4% recurrence rate following cone biopsy, but only 0.8% of these lesions developed after 2 years of followup (Baggish, 1983).

With cone biopsy, a primary concern is the status of the cone margins and their relationship to recurrent disease and the risk of missed cancer. Ostergaard (1980) reported that 30% of 516 cone biopsies were found to have disease in the margins. However, the reliability of this information is unclear. For example, in Ostergaard's study, 84% (21/25) of patients with positive margins with long-term followup did not suffer a recurrence. Similarly, Bjerre et al (1976) found that 60% of women whose cone biopsy specimens had positive margins had negative Pap smears for at least 5 years. Conversely, Ostergaard found that 16% of 268 women with negative margins on cone biopsy had residual disease at subsequent hysterectomy.

Thus, the management of women after cone biopsy is based primarily on the use of repeated cytologic evaluation of the cervical os and canal. The actual risk of invasive cancer is not certain. Ostergaard reported microinvasion in the endocervical canal in 2 of 26 women with positive apical cone margins. In practice, determining which women should proceed to hysterectomy to confirm this should be based upon postoperative cytology, careful analysis of the specimen to rule out invasion, and the amount of disease adjacent to the endocervical margin when this margin is deemed positive.

## REFERENCES

Acs J, Hildescheim A, Reeves WC, Brenes M, Brinton L, Lavery C, de la Guardia ME, Godoy J, Rawls WE: Regional distribution of human papillomavirus DNA and other risk factors for invasive cervical cancer in Panama. *Cancer Res* 49:5725, 1989.

Andersen WA, Frierson H, Barber S, Tabbarah S, Taylor P, Underwood PB: Sensitivity and specificity of endocervical curettage and the endocervical brush for the evaluation of the endocervical canal. *Am J Obstet Gynecol* 159:702, 1988.

Baggish MS: Laser management of cervical intraepithelial neoplasia. *Clin Obstet Gynecol* 26:968, 1983.

Baggish MS: High-power density carbon dioxide laser therapy for early cervical neoplasia. *Am J Obstet Gynecol* 136:117, 1980.

Barron BA, Richart RM: A statistical model of the natural history of cervical carcinoma based on a prospective study of 557 cases. *J Natl Cancer Instit* 41:1343, 1968.

Barron BA, Cahill MC, Richart RM: A statistical model of the natural history of cervical neoplastic disease: The duration of cervical carcinoma-in-situ. *Gynecol Oncol* 6:196, 1978.

Bellina JH, Wright VC, Voros JI, Riopelle MA, Hottenschutz V: Carbon dioxide laser management of cervical intraepithelial neoplasia. *Am J Obstet Gynecol* 141:828, 1981.

Benedet JL, Nickerson KG, White GW: Laser therapy for cervical intraepithelial neoplasia. *Obstet Gynecol* 58:188, 1981.

Bibbo M, Dytch SB, Alenghat E, Bartels PH, Wied GL: DNA ploidy profiles as prognostic indicators in CIN lesions. *Am J Clin Pathol* 92:261, 1989.

Bjerre B, Eliasson G, Linell F, Soderberg H, Sjoberg N-O: Conization as only treatment for carcinoma in situ of the uterine cervix. *Am J Obstet Gynecol* 125:143, 1976.

Boshart M, Gissman L, Ikenberg H, Kleinheinz A, zur Hausen H: A new type of papillomavirus DNA and its presence in genital cancer biopsies and in cell lines derived from cervical cancer. *EMBO J* 3:1151, 1984.

Brinton LA, Reeves WC, Brenes MM, Herrero R, Gaitan E, Tenorio F, de Britton RC, Garcia M, Rawls WE: The male sexual factor in the etiology of cervical cancer among sexually monogamous women. *Int J Cancer* 44:199, 1989.

Brinton LA, Reeves WC, Brenes MM, Herrero R, de Britton RC, Gaitan E, Tenorio F, Garcia M, Rawls WE: Parity as a risk factor for cervical cancer. *Am J Epidemiol* 130:486, 1989.

Broker TR, Botchan M: Papillomaviruses: Retrospectives and prospectives. In Botcham M, Grodzicher T, and Sharp PA (eds): *Cancer Cells, Vol 4, DNA Tumor Viruses.* Cold Spring Harbor Laboratory, New York, 1986, pp 17-35.

Burke L, Covell L, Antonioli D: Carbon dioxide laser therapy of cervical intraepithelial neoplasia: Factors determining success rate. *Lasers Surg Med* 1:113, 1980.

Burkett B, Peterson C, Ward BE, Nuckols M, Burch L, Brennan C, Crum CP: The relationship between contraceptives, sexual practices, and cervical human papillomavirus infection among a college population. *J Clin Epidemiol* (in press).

Carter R, Krantz KE, Hava GS, Lin F, Masterson BJ, Smith S: Treatment of cervical intraepithelial neoplasia with the carbon dioxide laser beam. *Am J Obstet Gynecol* 131:831, 1978.

Cartier R: *Practical Colposcopy*, 2nd ed. Laboratoire Cartier, 20 rue des Cordelieres, F75013 Paris, 1984.

Chanen W, Rome RM: Electrocoagulation diathermy for cervical dysplasia and carcinoma in situ: A 15 year survey. *Obstet Gynecol* 61:673, 1983.

Charles EH, Savage EW: Cryosurgical treatment of cervical intraepithelial neoplasia. *Obstet Gynecol Surv* 35:539, 1980.

Coppelson LW, Brown B: Observations on a model of the biology of carcinoma of the cervix. *Am J Obstet Gynecol* 122:127, 1975.

Creasman WT, Parker RT: Management of early cervical neoplasia. *Clin Obstet Gynecol* 18:233, 1975.

Creasman WT, Clark-Pearson DL, Weed JC: Results of outpatient therapy of cervical intraepithelial neoplasia. *Gynecol Oncol* 12(suppl):S306, 1981.

Crum CP, Egawa K, Fu YS, Barron BA, Levine RU, Fenoglio CF, Richart RM: Atypical immature metaplasia (AIM): A subset of human papillomavirus infection of the cervix. *Cancer* 51:2214, 1983.

Crum CP, Ikenberg H, Richart RM, Gissman L: Human papillomavirus type 16 in early cervical neoplasia. *N Engl J Med* 310:880, 1984.

Crum CP, Mitao M, Levine RU, Silverstein S: Cervical papillomaviruses segregate within morphologically distinct precancerous lesions. *J Virol* 54:675, 1984.

Crum CP, Nuovo G: The cervix. In Sternberg SS (ed): *Diagnostic Surgical Pathology*. New York, Raven Press, 1989, pp 1557-1589.

DiPaolo JA, Woodworth CD, Popescu NC, Notario V, Doniger J: Induction of human cervical squamous cell carcinoma by sequential infection with human papillomavirus 16 DNA and viral Harvey ras. *Oncogene* 4:395, 1989.

Drescher CW, Peters WA, Roberts JA: Contribution of endocervical curettage in evaluating abnormal cervical cytology. *Obstet Gynecol* 62:343, 1983.

Duncan ID: The Semm cold coagulator in the management of cervical intraepithelial neoplasia. *Clin Obstet Gynecol* 26:996, 1983.

Dunn JE, Schweitzer V: The relationship of cervical cytology to the incidence of invasive cervical cancer and mortality in Alameda County, California 1960 to 1974. *Am J Obstet Gynecol* 139:868, 1981.

Dunn JE, Crocker DW, Rube IF, Erickson CC, Coleman SA: Cervical cancer occurrence in Memphis and Shelby County, Tennessee, during 25 years of its cervical cytology screening program. *Am J Obstet Gynecol* 150:861, 1984.

Durst M, Gissman L, Ikenberg H, zur Hausen H: A papillomavirus DNA from a cervical carcinoma and its prevalence in cancer biopsy samples from different geographic regions. *Proc Natl Acad Sci USA* 80:3812, 1983.

Dyson N, Howley PM, Munger K, Harlow E: The human papillomavirus-16 E7 oncoprotein is able to bind to the retinoblastoma gene product. *Science* 243:934, 1989.

Editorial: Toward optimal laboratory use. Quality assurance in cervical cytology: The Papanicolaou smear. Report by the Council on Scientific Affairs. *JAMA* 262:1672, 1989.

Ferenczy A: Anatomy and histology of the cervix. In Blaustein A (ed): *Pathology of the Female Genital Tract*. New York, Springer-Verlag, 1982, pp 119-135.

Ferenczy A, Mitao M, Nagai N, Silverstein S, Crum CP: Latent papillomavirus and recurring genital warts. *N Engl J Med* 313:784, 1985.

Follen M, Levine RU, Carillo E, Richart RM, Nuovo G, Crum CP: Colposcopic correlates of cervical papillomavirus infection. *Am J Obstet Gynecol* 157:809, 1987.

Franquemont DW, Ward BE, Andersen WA, Crum CP: Prediction of "high risk" cervical papillomavirus infection by biopsy morphology. *Am J Clin Pathol* 92:577, 1989.

Fu YS, Reagan JW, Richart RM: Definition of precursors. *Gynecol Oncol* 12(Suppl):S220, 1981.

Fu YS, Braun L, Shah KV, Lawrence KD, Robboy SJ: Histologic, nuclear DNA and human papillomavirus study of cervical condylomas. *Cancer* 52:1705, 1983.

Fu YS, Huang I, Beaudenon S, Ionesco M, Barrasso R, de Brux J, Orth G: Correlative study of human papillomavirus DNA, histopathology, and morphometry in cervical condyloma and intraepithelial neoplasia. *Int J Gynecol Pathol* 7:297, 1988.

Furgyik S, Grubb R, Kullander S, Sandahl B, Wingerup L, Eydal A: Familial occurrence of cervical cancer, stages 0-IV. *Acta Obstet Gynecol Scand* 65:223, 1986.

Gissman L, Wolnick L, Ikenberg H, Koldovsky K, Schnurch HG, zur Hausen H: Human papillomavirus type 6 and 11 DNA sequences in genital and laryngeal papillomas and in some cervical cancers. *Proc Natl Acad Sci USA* 80:560, 1983.

Gustafsson L, Adami H-O: Natural history of cervical neoplasia: Consistent results obtained by an identification technique. *Brit J Cancer* 60:132, 1989.

Guzick DS: Efficacy of screening for cervical cancer: A review. *Am J Public Health* 68:125, 1978.

Hellberg D, Valentin J, Nilsson S: Smoking and cervical intraepithelial neoplasia. An association independent of sexual and other risk factors? *Acta Obstet Gynecol Scand* 65:625, 1986.

Jones HW: Cone biopsy in the management of cervical intraepithelial neoplasia. *Clin Obstet Gynecol* 26:968, 1983.

Jones HW III, Butler RE: The treatment of cervical intraepithelial neoplasia by cone biopsy. *Am J Obstet Gynecol* 137:882, 1980.

Kessler II: Perspectives on the epidemiology of cervical cancer with special reference to the herpes virus hypothesis. *Cancer Res* 34:1091, 1974.

Kiviat NB, Koutsky LA, Paavonen JA, Galloway DA, Critchlow CW, Beckmann AM, McDougall JK, Peterson ML, Stevens, Lipinski CM, Holmes KK: Prevalence of genital papillomavirus infection among women attending a college student health clinic or a sexually transmitted disease clinic. *J Infect Dis* 159:293, 1989.

Kjaer SK, de Villers EM, Haugaard BJ, Christenson RB, Teison C, Moller KA, Poll P, Jensen H, Vestergaard BF, Lynge E: Human papillomaviruses, herpes simplex virus and cervical cancer incidence in Greenland and Denmark. A population-based cross-sectional study. *Int J Cancer* 41:518, 1988.

Kjaer SK, Teison C, Haugaard BJ, Lynge E, Christenson RB, Moller KA, Jensen H, Poll P, Vestergaard BF, de Villiers E-M, Mensen OM: Risk factors for cervical cancer in Greenland and Denmark: A population-based cross-sectional study. *Int J Cancer* 44:40, 1989.

Kolstad P, Klem V: Long-term followup of 1121 cases of carcinoma-in-situ. *Obstet Gynecol* 48:125, 1976.

Kolstad P, Stafl A: *Atlas of Colposcopy*, 3rd ed. Oslo, Universitets Forlaget 1982.

Koutsky LA, Galloway DA, Holmes KK: Epidemiology of genital human papillomavirus infection. *Epidemiol Rev* 10:122, 1988.

Krantz KE: The anatomy and the human cervix, gross and microscopic. In Blandau RJ, Moghissi K (eds): *The Biology of the Cervix*. Chicago, University of Chicago Press, 1973 pp 57-69.

Krebs HB: The use of topical 5-fluorouracil in the treatment of genital condylomas. *Obstet Gynecol Clin N Amer* 14:559, 1987.

Krebs HB, Wheelock JB: Endocervical curettage after cryotherapy for cervical intraepithelial neoplasia. *Obstet Gynecol* 30:379, 1985.

Kurman RJ, Shiffman RM, Lancaster WD, Reid R, Jenson AB, Temple GF, Lorincz AT: Analysis of individual human papillomavirus types in cervical neoplasia: A possible role for type 18 in rapid progression. *Am J Obstet Gynecol* 159:293, 1988.

Layde PM: Smoking and cervical cancer: Cause or coincidence. *JAMA* 261:1631, 1989.

Layde PM, Broste SK: Carcinoma of the cervix and smoking. *Biomed Pharmacother* 43:161, 1989.

Lehn H, Villa LL, Marziona F, Hilgarth M, Hillemans HG, Sauer G: Physical state and biological activity of HPV genomes in precancerous lesions of the female genital tract. *J Gen Virol* 69:187, 1988.

Levine RU, Carillo EJ, Crum CP: Outpatient management of cervical intraepithelial neoplasia. A summary of 279 cases. *J Reprod Med* 30:351, 1985.

Lorincz AT, Temple GF, Patterson JA, Jenson AB, Kurman RJ, Lancaster WD: Correlation of cellular atypia and human papillomavirus DNA sequences in exfoliated cells of the uterine cervix. *Obstet Gynecol* 68:508, 1986.

Makuc DM, Fried VM, Kleinman JC: National trends in the use of preventive health care by women. *Am J Public Health* 79:21, 1989.

Masterson BJ, Krantz K, Calkins JW, Magrina JF, Carter RP: The carbon dioxide laser in cervical intraepithelial neoplasia, a five year experience in treating 230 patients. *Am J Obstet Gynecol* 139:565, 1981.

McIndoe GAJ, Robson MS, Tidy JA, Mason WP, Anderson MC: Laser excision rather than vaporization: The treatment of choice for cervical intraepithelial neoplasia. *Obstet Gynecol* 74:165, 1989.

Meisels A, Morin C: Human papillomavirus and cancer of the uterine cervix. *Gynecol Oncol* 12(Suppl):S111, 1981.

*Mortality and Morbidity Weekly Report* 23:306, 1983, and 38:650 and 659, 1989.

Nasiell K, Nasiell M, Vaclavinkova V: Behavior of moderate cervical dysplasia during long term follow-up. *Obstet Gynecol* 61:609, 1983.

Nasiell K, Roger V, Nasiell M: Behavior of mild cervical dysplasia during long term followup. *Obstet Gynecol* 67:665, 1986.

National Cancer Institute: Cancer control objectives for the nation: 1985-2000. Bethesda MD, US Department of Health and Human Services, Public Health Service, 1986. NIH Pub No 86-2880 (NCI monograph No 2).

National Cancer Institute Workshop: The 1988 Bethesda System for Reporting Cervical/Vaginal Cytologic Diagnoses. *JAMA* 262:931, 1988.

Nuovo GJ, Nuovo MA, Cottral S, Gordon S, Silverstein SJ, Crum CP: Histological correlates of clinically occult papillomavirus infection of the uterine cervix. *Am J Surg Pathol* 12:198, 1988.

Nuovo G, Richart RM: A comparison of buffered formalin and other fixatives for the detection of human papillomavirus DNA by in-situ hybridization. *Lab Invest* 60:67A, 1989.

Ostergaard DR: Prediction of clearance of cervical intraepithelial neoplasia by conization. *Obstet Gynecol* 56:77, 1980.

Phelps WC, Yee CL, Munger K, Howley PM: The human papillomavirus type 16 E7 gene encodes transactivation and transformation functions similar to those of adenovirus E1A. *Cell* 53:539, 1988.

Prendiville W, Cullimore J, Norman S: Large loop excision of the transformation zone (LLETZ). A new method of management for women with cervical intraepithelial neoplasia. *Br J Obstet Gynecol* 96:1054, 1989.

Purola E, Savia E: Cytology of gynecologic condyloma accuminatum. *Acta Cytol* 21:26, 1977.

Popkin DR, Scali V, Ahmed NW: Cryosurgery for the treatment of cervical intraepithelial neoplasia. *Am J Obstet Gynecol* 130:551, 1978.

Rando RF, Groff DE, Chirkjian JG, Lancaster WD: Isolation and characterization of a novel human papillomavirus type 6 DNA from an invasive vulvar carcinoma. *J Virol* 57:353, 1986.

Reid R, Stanhope CR, Herschman BR, Crum CP, Agronow SJ: Genital warts and cervical cancer: A colposcopic index for differentiating subclinical papillomavirus infection from cervical intraepithelial neoplasia. *Am J Obstet Gynecol* 149:815, 1984.

Reid R, Greenberg M, Jenson AB, Husain M, Willett J, Daoud Y, Temple G, Stanhope CR, Sherman AI, Phibbs GD, Lorincz AT: Sexually transmitted papillomaviral infection. I. The anatomic distribution and pathological grade of neoplastic lesions associated with different viral types. *Am J Obstet Gynecol* 156:212, 1987.

Richart RM: Cervical intraepithelial neoplasia. In Sommers SC (ed): *Pathol Annu.* New York, Appleton-Century-Crofts, 1973, pp 301-328.

Richart RM, Vaillant HM: An evaluation of the "true" false-negative rate in cytology. *Am J Obstet Gynecol* 89:723, 1964.

Richart RM, Barron BA: A followup study of patients with cervical dysplasia. *Am J Obstet Gynecol* 105:386, 1969.

Richart RM, Townsend DE, Crisp W, DePetrillo A, Ferenczy A, Johnson G, Lickrish G, Roy M, Villa Santa K: An analysis of "long term" follow-up results in patients with cervical intraepithelial neoplasia treated by cryotherapy. *Am J Obstet Gynecol* 137:823, 1980.

Richart RM, Crum CP, Townsend DE: Workup of the patient with the abnormal Papanicolaou smear. *Gynecol Oncol* 12(Suppl):S265, 1981.

Roman A, Fife K: Human papillomaviruses: Are we ready to type? *Clin Microbiol Rev* 2:166, 1989.

Savage EW, Matlock DL, Salem FA, Charles EH: The effect of endocervical gland involvement on the cure rates of patients with cervical intra-epithelial neoplasia undergoing cryosurgery. *Gynecol Oncol* 14:194, 1982.

Schneider A, Hotz M, Gissman L: Increased prevalence of human papillomaviruses in the lower genital tract of pregnant women. *Int J Cancer* 40:198, 1987.

Shingleton HM, Gore H, Austin JM: Outpatient evaluation of patients with atypical Papanicolaou smears: Contribution of endocervical curettage. *Am J Obstet Gynecol* 126:122, 1976.

Slattery ML, Overall JC, Abbott TM, French TK, Robison LM, Gardner J: Sexual activity, contraception, genital infections, and cervical cancer: Support for a sexually transmitted disease hypothesis. *Am J Epidemiol* 130:248, 1989.

Stafl A, Wilkinson EJ, Mattingly RF: Laser treatment of cervical and vaginal neoplasia. *Am J Obstet Gynecol* 128:128, 1977.

Stoler MH, Walder AN, Mills SE: Small cell neuroendocrine carcinoma of the cervix: A human papillomavirus type 18 associated cervix cancer. *Lab Invest* 60:92A, 1989.

Tase T, Okagaki T, Clark BA, Twiggs LB, Ostrow RS, Faras AJ: Human papillomavirus DNA in adenocarcinoma in situ, microinvasive adeno-carcinoma of the uterine cervix and coexisting cervical squamous intraepithelial neoplasia. *Int J Gynecol Pathol* 8:8, 1989.

Taylor PT, Andersen WA, Barber SR, Covell JL, Smith EB, Underwood PB: The screening Papanicolaou smear: Contribution of the endocervical brush. *Obstet Gynecol* 70:734, 1987.

Townsend DE, Ostergaard DR, Mishell OR, Hirose FM: Abnormal Papanicolaou smears—evaluation by colposcopy, biopsies and endocervical curettage. *Am J Obstet Gynecol* 108:429, 1970.

Townsend DE: Cryosurgery for cervical intraepithelial neoplasia. *Obstet Gynecol Surv* 34:828, 1974.

Townsend DE, Richart RM: Cryotherapy and carbon dioxide laser management of cervical intraepithelial neoplasia. A controlled comparison. *Obstet Gynecol* 61:75, 1983.

Townsend DE, Richart RM, Marks E, Nielson J: Invasive cancer following outpatient evaluation and therapy for cervical disease. *Obstet Gynecol* 57:145, 1981.

Verreault R, Chu J, Mandelson M, Shy K: A case-control study of diet and invasive cervical cancer. *Int J Cancer* 43:1050, 1989.

Vessey M, Grice D: Carcinoma of the cervix and oral contraceptives: Epidemiological studies. *Biomed Pharmacother* 43:157, 1989.

Ward BE, Crum EP: Unpublished data, 1990.

Wilbanks GD, Richart RM, Terner JY: DNA content of cervical intraepithelial neoplasia studied by two-wavelength Feulgen cytophotometry. *Am J Obstet Gynecol* 98:792, 1967.

Willett GD, Kurman RJ, Reid R, Greenberg M, Jenson AB, Lorincz AT: Correlation of the histological appearance of intraepithelial neoplasia of the cervix with human papillomavirus types. *Int J Gynecol Pathol* 8:18, 1989.

Wright VC: Carbon dioxide laser surgery for the cervix and vagina: Indications, complications and results. *Comprehensive Ther* 14:54, 1988.

# Chapter 11 | Invasive Cervical Cancer

## J. R. VAN *Nagell*    R. V. *Higgins*
## D. E. *Powell*

With the increasing use of regular cervical cytologic screening, most patients with cervical neoplasia will be diagnosed while the disease is still confined to the epithelium. Nevertheless, invasive cervical cancer continues to occur with alarming frequency in certain rural areas of the United States and in the developing countries. Unfortunately, early cervical cancer produces few symptoms, so that patients who have never been screened often present with disease in an advanced stage. It has been estimated that in 1992 there will be 13,500 new cases of invasive cervical cancer in the United States and that 4,400 women will die of this disease.

Clearly, the most important factor in decreasing cervical cancer mortality is regular cervical cytologic screening. In fact, several investigators have reported that the death rate from cervical cancer is inversely proportional to the frequency of such screening in a population (Christopherson et al, 1976; Johannesson et al, 1978). As technologies to evaluate cellular function have grown more sophisticated, it has become apparent that cervical cancers vary widely in terms of their biologic behavior. For this reason, it is important to evaluate all prognostically important histologic and clinical variables so that therapy can be properly individualized.

## ETIOLOGY AND EPIDEMIOLOGY

The etiology of cervical intraepithelial neoplasia (CIN) was discussed in detail in Chapter 10, and there is little evidence to suggest that agents which cause invasive cervical cancer are different from those which cause CIN. Risk factors for invasive cervical cancer are listed in Table 11-1, and risk has been shown to be related directly to the number of sexual partners and inversely to the woman's age at first intercourse (Kessler, 1976; Chamberlain, 1981). Cervical cancer tends to be more common in women who marry at an earlier age and who have had several sexual partners. Also, the incidence is significantly higher among women whose husbands were previously married to women with cervical cancer (Kessler, 1976). Such data clearly implicate a venereally transmitted agent in the genesis of this disease.

The infectious agent most directly associated with cervical cancer is the *human papillomavirus* (HPV) (zur Hausen et al, 1974). Since papillomavirus DNA was first isolated in cervical cancer cells by Durst and co-workers in 1983, numerous investigators have confirmed the role of HPV in cervical oncogenesis (Crum et al, 1984; Lorincz et al, 1987; Reeves et al, 1989).

Over 70 types of HPV have now been identified, about one-third of which have been detected in the genital tract. Under nonstringent hybridization conditions, DNA sequences from two types, HPV-16 and HPV-18, have been detected in 90% of cervical carcinomas (Beaudenon et al, 1986). Venereal transmission of the virus was studied by Barrasso and colleagues (1987), and penile viral lesions were noted in 64% of men whose sexual partners had cervical condylomas; papillomavirus DNA sequences were isolated in 60% of these lesions. A high degree of concordance was noted between the viral type found on the penis and that found in the female genital tract. Finally, the presence of HPV-16/18 DNA in cells of the cervix is associated with an increased risk for cervical cancer (risk ratio = 2.1 to 9.1) (Reeves et al, 1989).

The other viral agent associated with the genesis of invasive cervical cancer is *herpes simplex virus type 2* (HSV-2). This association is based on (1) retrospective seroepidemiologic studies showing a significantly higher incidence of HSV-2–associated antigens in the sera of patients with cervical cancer than in age-matched controls, (2) the ability of HSV-2 to cause malignant transformation of embryonic cells in tissue culture, (3) the known sexual transmission of HSV-2, and (4) a significant increase in the incidence of CIN in patients followed prospectively after genital herpes infection (Nahmias and Sawanabori, 1978; Nahmias et al, 1974). In addition, HSV-2 viral proteins and HSV-2 nucleic acid sequences have been identified in a high percentage of cervical cancer biopsy specimens (Aurelian et al, 1981; McDougall et al, 1981). Although most investigators believe that HPV is more directly related to cervical oncogenesis than is HSV-2, infection with either of these viruses is associated with a significantly higher risk for cervical neoplasia.

Cigarette smoking, particularly for a long period of time (over 20 years), has also been reported to be an independent risk factor for invasive squamous cell cancer of the cervix and may act as a cocarcinogen (Brinton et al, 1986).

## DETECTION

In the majority of patients, the diagnosis of cervical cancer is first suggested by abnormal cervical cytology. There is little doubt about the value of cervical cytologic screening in reducing mortality from this disease. In the United States, the annual death rate from cervical cancer has decreased from over 30 per 100,000 in 1930 to less

TABLE 11-1 Risk Factors for Invasive Cervical Cancer

| | Relative Risk |
|---|---|
| Coitarche before age 15 | 16.1 |
| ≥ 3 sexual partners | 3.5 |
| Genital warts (≥ 2 episodes) | 5.0 |
| Cigarette smoking (> 4 years) | 4.0 |

*Source:* Peters RK, Thomas D, Hagan DG, Mack TM, Henderson BE: Risk factors for invasive cervical cancer among Latinas and non-Latinas in Los Angeles County. *J Natl Cancer Inst* 77:1063, 1986.

than 6 per 100,000 at the present time (Silverberg and Lubera, 1989). Since patients with CIN and early invasive cervical cancer are essentially asymptomatic, cervical cytology is invaluable in detecting cervical neoplasia at a time when it is still highly curable. Accuracy of the results depends upon the thoroughness with which the sample is taken, the sampling method utilized, and the quality of the laboratory. A scraping of the ectocervix combined with a sample from the canal provides the lowest false-negative rate and the highest predictability. Since adenocarcinoma or adenosquamous cancer now represents over 15% of all cervical cancers (Artman et al, 1987), an endocervical sample must be obtained. With vaginal pool samples, false-negative rates approach 50%, so these samples are not acceptable for screening (Nelson et al, 1989).

Although the appropriate interval between Pap smears has been a matter of controversy, recent data support the use of annual screening. The mean age at diagnosis of patients with invasive cervical cancer varies from 50 to 55, depending on the population studied (van Nagell et al, 1982b; Silverberg and Lubera, 1989). Although the mean age of patients with CIN III is at least 10 years less than the age of patients with invasive disease, it should not be concluded that it takes that amount of time for intraepithelial neoplasia to progress to invasive cancer. Recent evidence suggests that selected intraepithelial lesions, particularly those associated with HPV-18, are biologically aggressive and may progress rapidly. In addition, epidemiologic data indicate that an interval between Pap smears of 2 or more years conveys a significantly higher risk for the development of invasive cervical cancer than does a screening interval of less than 2 years (Peters et al, 1986; Day, 1986).

It is important to note that about 10% of women in the United States have never had a Pap test; in certain rural areas of Appalachia, this figure may be as high as 30%. The prevalence of cervical cancer screening is also directly related to the educational status and mean income of the population. Nearly 20% of women with a grade-school education have never had a Pap test, whereas this figure is only 4% for college graduates. The most recent recommendation for cervical cytologic screening by the American Cancer Society is as follows: "All women who are, or have been, sexually active or have reached the age of 18 years should have an annual Pap test and pelvic examination. After a woman has had three or more satisfactory normal annual examinations, the Pap smear may be performed less frequently at the discretion of her physician" (Fink, 1988). The authors strongly support this recommendation.

Although the diagnosis of invasive cervical cancer is usually first suggested by abnormal cervical cytology, histologic confirmation of invasive cancer is necessary before proceeding to a more detailed evaluation of the patient. In this regard, colposcopic examination of the cervix may be helpful in directing biopsies of the specific area of invasion. Colposcopic findings suggestive of invasive cancer include abnormal blood vessels, irregular surface contour, and erosion of the epithelium. For a biopsy to be adequate, the tissue specimen must be large enough so that the predominant cell type, depth of invasion, and lymph vascular space invasion can be evaluated. A cervical curettage should also be performed to rule out an occult endocervical lesion. Although cervical conization is generally not necessary to establish the diagnosis of invasive cervical cancer, this procedure is indicated if (1) no abnormalities are visible on colposcopy and the lesion is thought to be located in the endocervix, (2) the entire lesion cannot be visualized with the colposcope and the biopsies show only intraepithelial neoplasia, (3) there is a persistent discrepancy between the cervical cytologic findings and the findings on colposcopically directed biopsy, (4) a diagnosis of microinvasive carcinoma is made on colposcopically directed biopsy, or (5) adenocarcinoma in situ is diagnosed on cervical biopsy.

## EVALUATION

Once the diagnosis of invasive cervical cancer has been established histologically, the patient should be thoroughly evaluated to establish the biologic behavior and anatomic extent of the tumor prior to therapy. Recently, it has become apparent that certain histomorphologic variables are prognostically important in cervical cancer. These include cell type, the presence of lymph vascular space invasion, and the depth of stromal invasion.

### Cell Type

Although many histologic classifications have been used in cervical cancer, the system proposed by Reagan and coworkers (1957) has the greatest prognostic significance. According to this classification, cervical cancer is divided into large cell nonkeratinizing cancer (Fig. 11-1A), keratinizing squamous cell cancer (Fig. 11-1B), small cell cancer (Fig. 11-1C), and adenocarcinoma (Fig. 11-2). Stage for stage, patients with *large cell nonkeratinizing squamous cell cancers* have a better prognosis than do those with *keratinizing cancers* when treated with irradiation (van Nagell et al, 1977a; Randall et al, 1988); no such prognostic difference is noted when patients with these two cell types are treated with radical surgery. Therefore, the poorer survival of patients with keratinizing tumors appears to be related to the

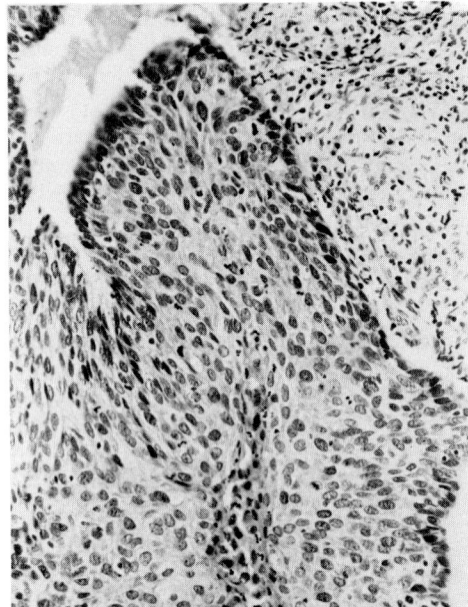

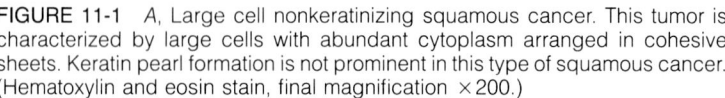

FIGURE 11-1  *A,* Large cell nonkeratinizing squamous cancer. This tumor is characterized by large cells with abundant cytoplasm arranged in cohesive sheets. Keratin pearl formation is not prominent in this type of squamous cancer. (Hematoxylin and eosin stain, final magnification ×200.)

*B,* Large cell keratinizing squamous cancer. This tumor demonstrates prominent keratin pearl formation (arrow) in addition to cytoplasmic keratinization. (Hematoxylin and eosin stain, final magnification ×132.)

*C,* Small cell cervical cancer infiltrates the cervical stroma in a diffuse pattern. Individual tumor cells have scant cytoplasm and indistinct cytoplasmic borders and do not exhibit prominent nucleoli. (Hematoxylin and eosin stain, final magnification ×160.)

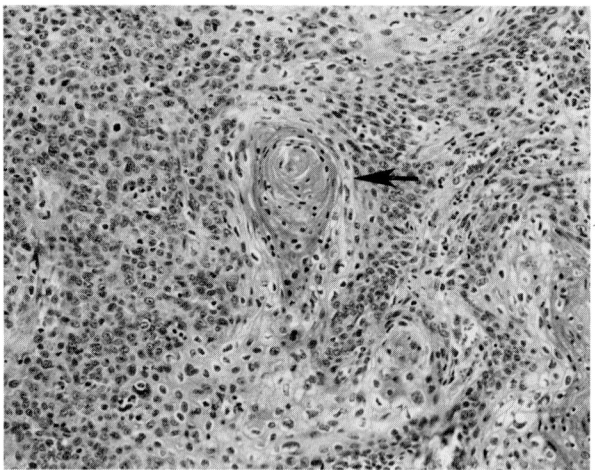

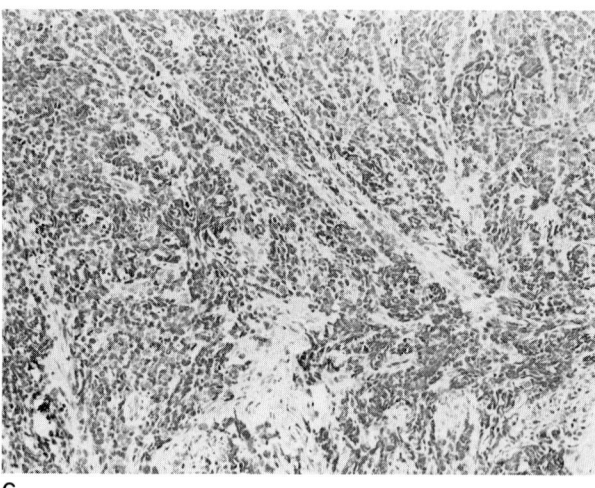

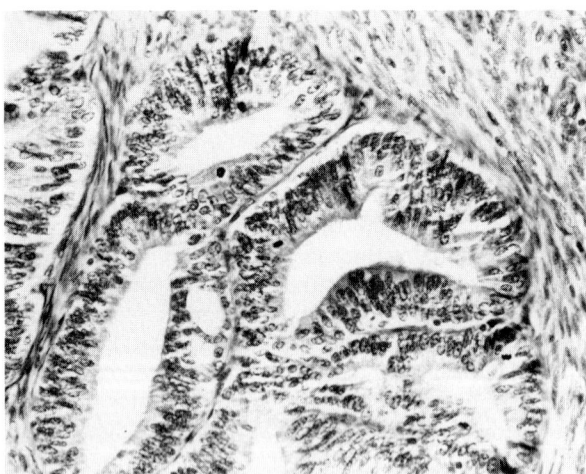

FIGURE 11-2  Endocervical adenocarcinoma exhibits different types of growth patterns. In this example, the tumor invades as discrete but closely crowded glands with obvious cytologic atypia and loss of cytoplasmic mucin. (Hematoxylin and eosin stain, final magnification ×320.)

intrinsic resistance of these tumors to radiation rather than to their biologic aggressiveness.

In contrast, the prognosis in *small cell cancers* is poor regardless of the therapeutic method employed (van Nagell et al, 1988). These tumors are characterized morphometrically by their small nuclear size ($< 160 \ \mu^2$) and their propensity for vascular invasion and extra-pelvic metastases. Some of these small cell tumors have a neuroendocrine origin and stain positively for neuron-specific enolase and chromogranin.

*Adenocarcinomas of the cervix* appear to be increasing in frequency relative to squamous cancers. In earlier studies, approximately 5% of all cervical cancers were found to be adenocarcinomas (Mikuta and Celebre, 1969; Rutledge et al, 1975), whereas more recent investigations indicate that adenocarcinomas constitute as many as 15 to 20% of all cases (Tamimi and Figge, 1982; Berek et al, 1985). Although cervical adenocarcinomas have been reported to have a poorer prognosis than squamous cancers of a similar stage (Pettersson, 1988), this difference in survival may be attributable to

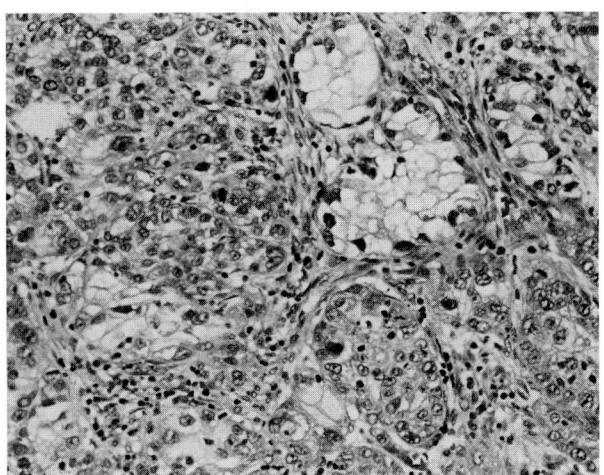

FIGURE 11-3 Adenosquamous carcinoma is characterized by a biphasic growth pattern of both adenocarcinoma and squamous cancer. In this photomicrograph, sheets of large cell nonkeratinizing squamous cancer are mixed with tumor cell clusters containing abundant cytoplasmic mucins. (Hematoxylin and eosin stain, final magnification ×264.)

the growth patterns of these tumors. Characteristically, adenocarcinomas grow endophytically and expand into the lower uterine segment. As a result, tumor volume is much larger than would be appreciated on clinical examination. Several recent studies have indicated that the prognosis in adenocarcinoma is highly dependent on the depth of stromal invasion and the degree of cellular differentiation (Berek et al, 1985; Hopkins et al, 1988*b*). When these variables are matched to those of squamous cell carcinomas, survival is similar for both types (Shingleton et al, 1981). Patients with early-stage adenocarcinomas should undergo computed tomographic (CT) scanning or magnetic resonance imaging (MRI) of the pelvis to define more accurately the depth

of stromal invasion and the total volume of these lesions.

Histologic subtypes of adenocarcinoma include adenosquamous carcinoma (Fig. 11-3), glassy cell carcinoma (Fig. 11-4), and clear cell carcinoma (Fig. 11-5). There is some controversy concerning the prognostic implications of *adenosquamous carcinoma*. Tamimi and Figge (1982) noted that survival was poorer in patients with cervical adenosquamous carcinomas than in those with pure adenocarcinomas. However, Randall and colleagues (1988) reported similar rates of survival when these tumors were treated with radiation therapy alone. Likewise, Kilgore and associates (1988) could find no statistically significant difference in survival rates when other prognostically significant variables were controlled.

A rare histologic variant of cervical adenosquamous cancer is the *glassy cell carcinoma* (Fig. 11-4) initially described by Glucksman and Cherry (1956). Glassy cells have a moderate amount of cytoplasm with a groundglass appearance, a distinct cell wall, and large nuclei with prominent nucleoli (Littman et al, 1976). These tumors are poorly differentiated and biologically aggressive, with a propensity to develop extrapelvic metastases (Tamimi et al, 1988).

Two additional histologic subtypes of cervical cancer are *adenoid cystic carcinoma* and *clear cell carcinoma*. Adenoid cystic carcinoma of the cervix was first described by Poolman and Counsellor (1949) and is characterized histologically by small basal cells with hyperchromatic nuclei surrounding a central area of amorphous material (Fig. 11-6). In general, these tumors have a high mitotic rate and exhibit vascular invasion and nodal spread early in the disease process (Ferry and Scully, 1988, King et al, 1989) (Fig. 11-5). Although less common than vaginal clear cell carcinomas, clear cell carcinomas of the cervix are associated with in utero exposure to diethylstilbestrol (DES) during the first trimester of pregnancy. Recent epidemiologic

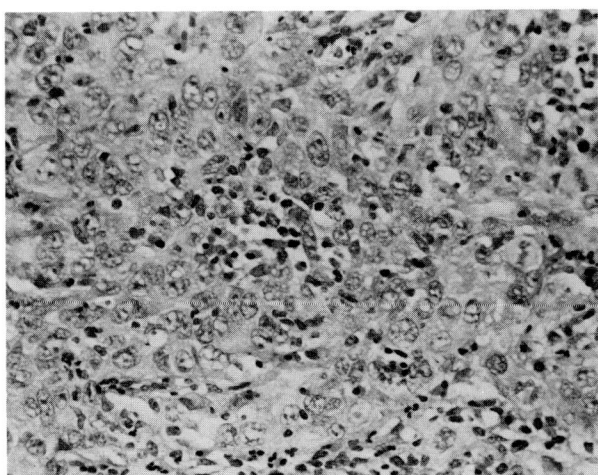

FIGURE 11-4 Glassy cell carcinoma. This unusual type of adenosquamous carcinoma is characterized by large cells with prominent nucleoli. Cytoplasm is abundant, and there is frequently an associated inflammatory infiltrate containing eosinophils as shown in this photomicrograph. (Hematoxylin and eosin stain, final magnification ×400.)

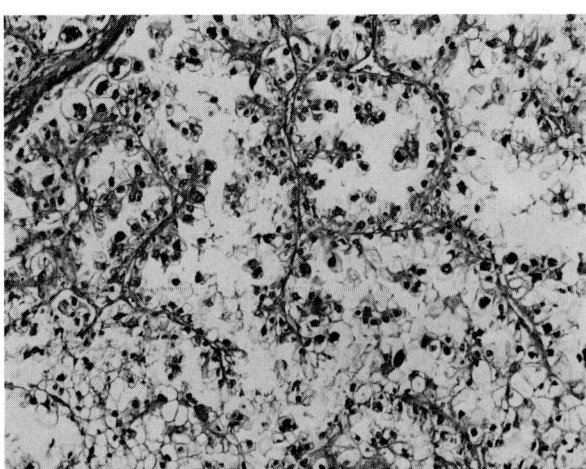

FIGURE 11-5 Clear cell carcinoma commonly forms microcystic spaces. Tumor cells are of two types: clear cells and hobnail cells. The former have a clear glycogen-filled cytoplasm, while the latter have large protruding and hyperchromatic nuclei. (Hematoxylin and eosin stain, final magnification ×200.)

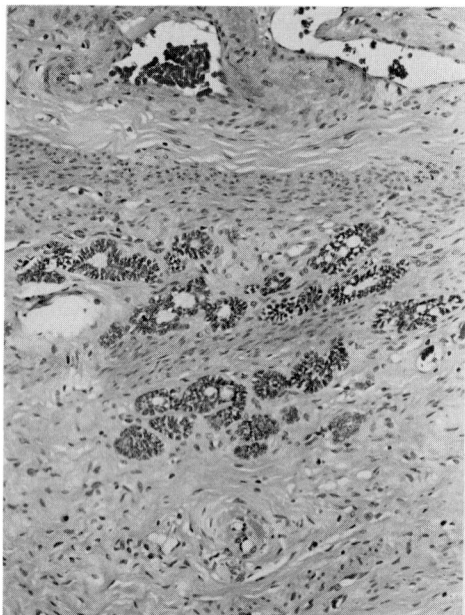

FIGURE 11-6 Adenoid cystic carcinoma. Small nests of hyper-chromatic basaloid tumor cells infiltrate the cervical stroma. These tumor cells are frequently arranged around a central mass of pale-staining amorphous material. (Hematoxylin and eosin stain, final magnification ×200.)

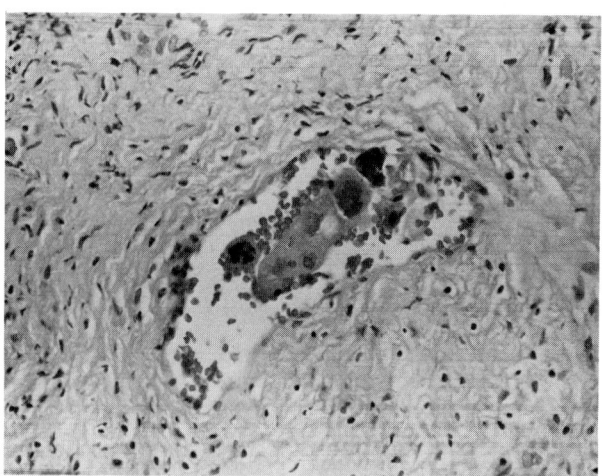

FIGURE 11-7 Lymph vascular space invasion in cervical cancer. Tumor cells are identified within the lumen and adhere to the wall of an endothelial-lined vascular structure that also contains erythrocytes. (Hematoxylin and eosin stain, final magnification ×200.)

data suggest that the risk for cervical or vaginal clear cell carcinoma in women exposed to DES in utero is less than 1 per 1,000 (Melnick et al, 1987). Histologically, these tumors are characterized by clear cells in hobnail, solid, or tubulocystic patterns (Robboy et al, 1984).

### Lymph Vascular Space Invasion

A second feature that should be evaluated is lymph vascular space invasion by tumor cells. The depth of stromal penetration at which access to lymph vascular spaces first occurs is unknown. Nevertheless, it has been clearly established that lymph vascular space invasion can occur with minimal stromal invasion. van Nagell and coworkers (1983), for example, reported invasion in 17 of 145 patients (11.7%) with tumors penetrating the cervical stroma to a depth of 3.0 mm or less. Once such invasion has occurred, the risk of extracervical spread is greater. Both pelvic and extrapelvic metastases occur more frequently in patients with tumors demonstrating lymph vascular space invasion than in patients without this finding (van Nagell et al, 1978; Barber et al, 1977). Lymph vascular space invasion is diagnosed when tumor cells are seen within or attached to the wall of capillary or lymphatic spaces lined by flattened endothelial cells (Fig. 11-7).

### Depth of Stromal Invasion

Cervical cancers invading the cervical stroma to a depth of 1.5 cm or more have been shown to recur significantly more often than do more superficial lesions after treatment by radical surgery (Gauthier et al, 1985).

Often, it is difficult to assess the depth of tumor invasion prior to therapy. Nevertheless, preliminary studies indicate that MRI can accurately determine the depth of stromal invasion by cervical cancer (Angel et al, 1987). If these early findings are confirmed in studies involving larger numbers of patients, MRI should become a valuable means of assessing tumor volume and depth of stromal invasion in patients with cervical cancer.

## ANATOMIC PATHWAYS OF SPREAD

Cervical cancer spreads by direct invasion into the cervical stroma and adjacent pelvic organs (Fig. 11-8). It also gains access to lymph vascular spaces and spreads to regional lymph nodes. The three major pathways of spread of invasive cervical cancer are as follows:

1. *Lateral spread.* The major pathway of cervical cancer spread is laterally through the paracervical lymphatics into the parametria and, ultimately, to the structures of the lateral pelvic wall. This pattern of spread often causes extrinsic compression of the ureter, with resulting ureteral obstruction and progressive loss of renal function.

2. *Inferior spread.* Inferiorly, cervical cancer spreads by direct extension into the vaginal stroma and eventually replaces the adjacent epithelium of the upper vagina. With progressive involvement of the subvaginal lymphatics by tumor cells, there is further spread into the lower vagina from which metastases to the inguinal lymph nodes can occur.

3. *Superior spread.* Cervical cancer can also spread superiorly to involve the proximal endocervix and the lower uterine segment. Although this pattern of spread is not recognized in the current staging system formulated by the International Federation of Gynecology and Obstetrics (FIGO), tumors that involve the lower uterine segment are often quite large and may extend beyond the curative isodose of radiation. Uterine involve-

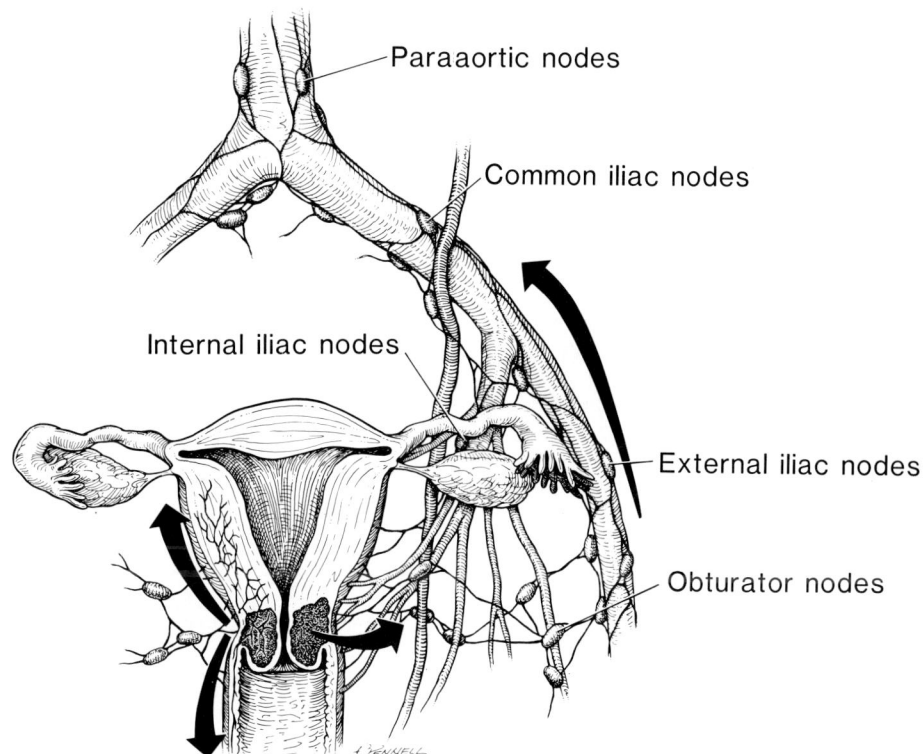

Paraaortic nodes

Common iliac nodes

Internal iliac nodes

External iliac nodes

Obturator nodes

FIGURE 11-8 Anatomic pathways of spread in invasive cervical cancer.

ment can be diagnosed by hysteroscopy or MRI and confirmed by endometrial curettage, and its incidence may be as high as 20%. Patients with this finding have a poorer prognosis, stage for stage, than do those without it (Perez et al, 1975).

The four primary regional lymph node groups to which cervical cancer metastasizes are the internal iliac, obturator, external iliac, and common iliac nodes. According to Plentyl and Friedman (1971), the anatomic distribution of nodal metastases in 700 patients with cervical cancer was as follows: external iliac 23%, obturator 19%, internal iliac 17%, and common iliac 12%. An additional 21% of patients had metastatic involvement of the parametrial or paracervical lymph nodes. The frequency of pelvic lymph node metastases is related directly to tumor volume and varies from 18% in patients with stage IB disease to 55% in patients with stage IVA disease (Table 11-2). After involvement of the primary regional lymph node groups, cervical cancer spreads beyond the pelvis to the paraaortic nodes and eventually to the supraclavicular nodes.

## STAGING

Once the diagnosis of invasive cervical cancer has been confirmed histologically, the lesion should be staged. Staging can be defined as the clinical estimation of the extent of disease and should be performed in all patients prior to definitive therapy. The clinical stage is important in that it relates directly to prognosis and provides an approximation of tumor size and configuration for treatment planning. Under no circumstances should

clinical staging be postponed or changed at a later date. It is never permissible to alter the stage on the basis of surgical or postmortem findings, even if it is obviously incorrect. When the stage to which a particular case should be allotted is in doubt, the earlier stage should be chosen. The current FIGO staging system for cervical cancer is presented in Table 11-3 and further illustrated in Figure 11-9.

Procedures allowed by FIGO for staging cervical cancer are summarized in Table 11-4. Although CT scanning and MRI are useful in determining the extent of tumor spread, these techniques are not yet accepted as part of the FIGO clinical staging system for cervical cancer. Because ureteral obstruction remains a major

TABLE 11-2  Pelvic Lymph Node Metastasis by Stage (N = 1,891)

| Stage | No. of Patients | Positive Pelvic Nodes |
|-------|-----------------|------------------------|
| IB | 1,341 | 18% |
| IIA | 90 | 27% |
| IIB | 341 | 36% |
| III | 96 | 43% |
| IVA | 23 | 55% |

*Sources:* Averette et al (1975), Ballon et al (1981), Berman et al (1984), Buchsbaum et al (1979), Chung et al (1980), Delgado et al (1977), DePriest et al (in press), Gauthier et al (1985), Hughes et al (1980), Inoue (1984), Lagasse et al (1980), LaPolla et al (1986), Martinbeau et al (1982), Rubin et al (1984), van Nagell et al (1979b), Welander et al (1981), Wharton et al (1977).

TABLE 11-3   Clinical Stages in Carcinoma of the Cervix Uteri (FIGO System)

| Stage | Description |
|---|---|
| Stage 0 | Carcinoma in situ, intraepithelial carcinoma. |
| Stage I | The carcinoma is strictly confined to the cervix. (Extension to the corpus should be disregarded.) |
| Stage IA | Preclinical carcinomas of the cervix—i.e., those diagnosed only by microscopy. |
| Stage IA1 | Minimal microscopically evident stromal invasion. |
| Stage IA2 | Lesions detected microscopically that can be measured. The upper limit of the measurement should not show a depth of invasion of more than 5 mm taken from the base of the epithelium, either surface or glandular, from which it originates, and a second dimension, the horizontal spread, must not exceed 7 mm. Larger lesions should be staged as IB. |
| Stage IB | Lesions of greater dimension than stage IA2, whether seen clinically or not; preformed space involvement should not alter the staging but should be specifically recorded to determine whether it should affect future treatment decisions. |
| Stage II | The carcinoma extends beyond the cervix but has not extended to the pelvic wall. The carcinoma involves the vagina but not as far as the lower third. |
| Stage IIA | No obvious parametrial involvement. |
| Stage IIB | Obvious parametrial involvement. |
| Stage III | The carcinoma has extended to the pelvic wall. On rectal examination, there is no cancer-free space between the tumor and the pelvic wall. The tumor involves the lower third of the vagina. All patients with hydronephrosis or a nonfunctioning kidney are included. |
| Stage IIIA | No extension to the pelvic wall. |
| Stage IIIB | Extension to the pelvic wall and/or hydronephrosis or a nonfunctioning kidney. |
| Stage IV | The carcinoma has extended beyond the true pelvis or has clinically involved the mucosa of the bladder or rectum. A bullous edema as such does not permit a case to be allotted to stage IV. |
| Stage IVA | Spread to adjacent organs. |
| Stage IVB | Spread to distant organs. |

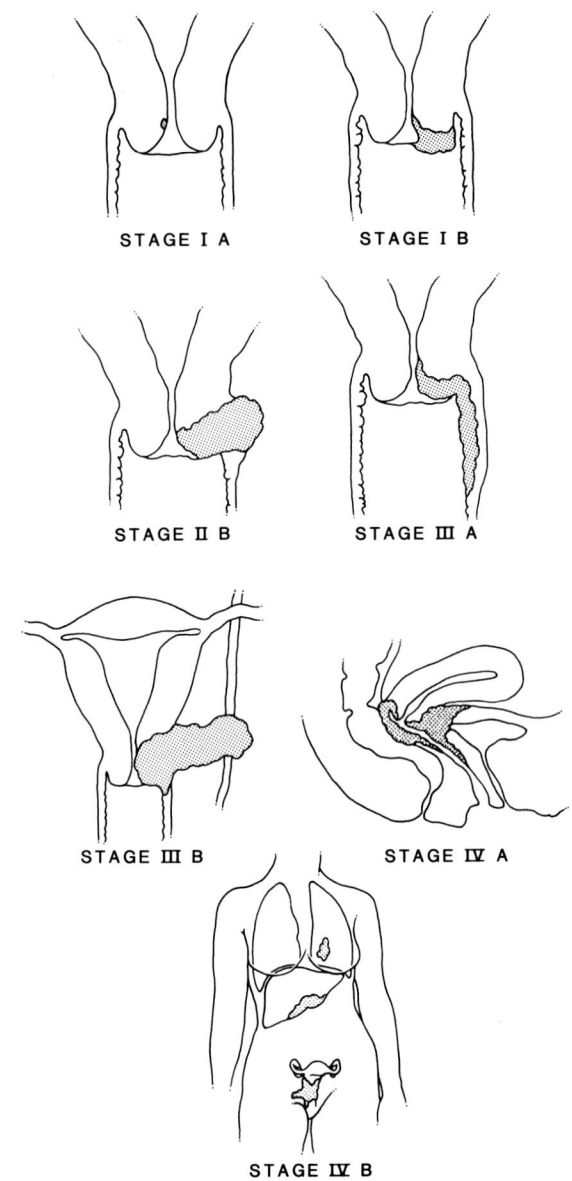

FIGURE 11-9   FIGO staging system for cervical cancer. This is a clinical staging system and cannot be changed by operative findings.

prognostic variable in cervical cancer, an intravenous pyelogram should be obtained for every patient prior to therapy. Patients with ureteral obstruction are considered to have stage IIIB disease and have a significantly poorer prognosis than do those without obstruction. The results of intravenous pyelography for a large number of cervical cancer patients are given in Table 11-5. Approximately 5% of patients are reclassified to a higher stage because of the finding of ureteral obstruction. The most common site of obstruction in cervical cancer is the distal third of the ureter or the ureterovesical junction.

Although histologic confirmation of bladder mucosal invasion by cervical cancer is necessary for inclusion in stage IVA, the role of cystoscopy in the routine evaluation of patients with invasive disease is less clear. Some investigators advocate the use of cystoscopy in all pa-

tients, whereas others favor its use only when there is palpable or visible extension of tumor toward the bladder. Cystoscopic findings in 583 patients with cervical cancer were reported by van Nagell and coworkers (1975) and are presented in Table 11-6. Bladder biop-

TABLE 11-4   Procedures for Staging Cervical Cancer (FIGO)

History
Physical examination
Complete blood cell count
Liver function studies
Chest x-ray
Intravenous pyelography
Cystoscopy
Sigmoidoscopy

TABLE 11-5   Ureteral Obstruction Related to Stage in Cervical Cancer

| Stage Prior to IVP | No. of Patients | Ureteral Obstruction | |
|---|---|---|---|
| | | Unilateral | Bilateral |
| I | 181 | 4 (2.2) | 0 |
| IIA | 40 | 0 | 0 |
| IIB | 159 | 12 (7.5) | 0 |
| IIIA | 9 | 1 (11.1) | 1 (11.1) |
| IIIB | 115 | 32 (27.8) | 6 (5.2) |
| IV | 79 | 24 (30.4) | 6 (7.6) |

*Source:* van Nagell JR Jr, Greenwell N, Powell DE, Donaldson ES, Hanson MB, Gay EC: Microinvasive carcinoma of the cervix. *Am J Obstet Gynecol* 145:981, 1983.
IVP = intravenous pyelography.

sies were performed in 120 patients, with histologic confirmation of invasion of the bladder mucosa in 45. The only patients with cystoscopic evidence of invasive cancer involving the bladder mucosa were those with clinical evidence of stage IIIB or IVA disease. For this reason, cystoscopy is recommended only for patients with stage III or IV disease or for those with clinical signs or symptoms that suggest bladder involvement.

Likewise, sigmoidoscopy should be limited to patients with a history of rectal bleeding or large cervical tumors found to invade the rectovaginal septum on clinical examination. Biopsies should be taken from any suspected lesions through the sigmoidoscope, since histologic evidence of rectal mucosal tumor is necessary for inclusion into stage IVA.

Within each stage of cervical cancer, the anatomic extent and biologic behavior of a tumor can vary widely. Patient survival is directly related to tumor volume, and it is helpful to know the size and anatomic locations of each tumor in planning treatment, particularly for patients with stage IB disease. Several investigators have shown that stage IB squamous cell cancers 3 cm or less in diameter have a significantly better prognosis than do larger lesions. Piver and Chung (1975), for example, reported that the 5-year survival of patients with stage IB cervical cancers 3 cm or less in diameter was 88%

as opposed to 65% for larger lesions. In a more recent investigation, DePriest and colleagues (in press) reported a 97% 5-year survival rate after stage IB large cell squamous cancers 3 cm or less were treated with radical hysterectomy and pelvic lymphadenectomy. Finally, observation of lesion size during radiation therapy provides an important means of evaluating the response of the tumor to such therapy (Marcial and Bosch, 1970; Hardt et al, 1982).

Tumor configuration is also important for treatment planning. Barrel-shaped stage IB tumors often extend beyond the curative isodose of radiation and contain areas of poorly perfused hypoxic cells that are resistant to photon therapy (O'Quinn et al, 1980). The addition of extrafascial hysterectomy following radiation therapy has improved survival rates for these patients (Gallion et al, 1985). For these reasons, lesion size and anatomic configuration should be accurately recorded prior to treatment in all cases.

One of the most important prognostic variables in cervical cancer is the presence of *lymph node metastases.* Paraaortic metastasis is of particular concern, since traditional therapeutic methods are designed to include only the primary tumor and those regional (pelvic) lymph node groups to which it first spreads. In general, the frequency of paraaortic lymph node metastases is directly related to tumor volume and stage of disease (Table 11-7). In addition, small cell cancers and tumors with lymph vascular space invasion have demonstrated a propensity for extrapelvic spread (van Nagell et al, 1988). With the recent success of extended-field radiation in the treatment of paraaortic metastases, the diagnosis of occult nodal spread is even more important (Horii et al, 1988; Lovecchio et al, 1989).

Methods most commonly used for diagnosing lymph node spread are lymphangiography, CT scanning, and paraaortic lymphadenectomy and biopsy. Reports of the accuracy of *lymphangiography* in detecting node metastases in cervical cancer vary widely. A filling defect in a lymph node is the most reliable diagnostic criterion for metastasis. However, the sensitivity of lymphangiography is only 60%, and up to 15% of patients with normal lymphangiograms actually have histologic evidence of microscopic metastases (van Nagell and Hig-

TABLE 11-6   Cystoscopic Findings in Patients with Cervical Cancer

| Stage Prior to Cystoscopy | No. of Patients | Invasive Cancer | Mass Elevating Bladder | Bullous Edema | Bladder Inflammation | Vesicovaginal Fistula |
|---|---|---|---|---|---|---|
| I | 177 | 0 | 0 | 1 | 4 | 0 |
| IIA | 40 | 0 | 2 | 0 | 0 | 0 |
| IIB | 147 | 0 | 6 | 5 | 3 | 0 |
| IIIA | 7 | 0 | 1 | 0 | 0 | 0 |
| IIIB | 133 | 27 | 41 | 6 | 0 | 0 |
| IV | 79 | 18 | 5 | 1 | 0 | 2 |
| Totals | 583 | 45 | 55 | 13 | 7 | 2 |

*Source:* van Nagell JR Jr, Donaldson ES, Gay EC: Urinary tract involvement by invasive cervical cancer. In Buchsbaum HJ, Schmidt JD (eds): *Gynecologic and Obstetric Urology.* Philadelphia, WB Saunders Co, 1982, pp 410-421.

TABLE 11-7  Paraaortic Lymph Node Metastasis by Stage (N = 3,420)

| Stage | No. of Patients | Positive Paraaortic Nodes |
|---|---|---|
| IB | 1,922 | 5.3% |
| IIA | 245 | 11.4% |
| IIB | 621 | 9.3% |
| III | 552 | 27.5% |
| IVA | 80 | 31.3% |

*Sources:* Averette et al (1975), Ballon et al (1981), Berman et al (1984), Buchsbaum et al (1979), Chung et al (1980), Delgado et al (1977), Gauthier et al (1985), Hughes et al (1980), Inoue (1984), Lagasse et al (1980), LaPolla et al (1986), Lovecchio et al (1989), Martinbeau et al (1982), Rubin et al (1984), Twiggs et al (1984), Welander et al (1981), Wharton et al (1977).

gins, 1989). Fine-needle aspiration or excisional biopsy of the involved node must be performed in patients with an abnormal lymphangiogram.

*CT scanning* of the pelvic and paraaortic lymph nodes has replaced lymphangiography in many centers. The accuracy of CT-directed fine-needle biopsy for detecting paraaortic metastases from cervical cancer is approximately 85% (van Nagell and Higgins, 1989). Nevertheless, since access to a specific lymph node can be difficult in a given patient, open biopsy is required in patients with an abnormal lymphangiogram or CT scan when the results of fine-needle biopsy are negative.

The most accurate way to assess paraaortic metastases is selected *lymph node biopsy.* Two surgical approaches to the paraaortic nodes have been used. The intraperitoneal approach involves a midline incision that is extended to expose the abdominal aorta. Lymph nodes anterior and lateral to the aorta are then removed en bloc from the aortic bifurcation superiorly to the level of the left renal vein. This technique provides excellent exposure of the common iliac and paraaortic nodes, although it was initially associated with significant postirradiation enteric complications (Wharton et al, 1977; Piver et al, 1981). The extraperitoneal approach is made through a left lateral incision and the peritoneum is reflected anteriorly, exposing the paraaortic lymph node chain. These lymph nodes are removed

en bloc superiorly. Exposure of the right pelvic lymph nodes is often more difficult through this type of incision. However, the incidence of radiation-related enteric complications following extraperitoneal paraaortic lymphadenectomy is significantly reduced compared with that following intraperitoneal surgery (Twiggs et al, 1984; Weiser et al, 1989).

Unfortunately, retroperitoneal selected lymph node biopsies as a routine method for evaluating lymph node spread in cervical cancer is often impractical. This procedure involves major surgery and may be associated with significant morbidity in patients already compromised by an extensive tumor burden. Furthermore, radiation therapy must be delayed several weeks until the operative site is completely healed. At the present time, the authors recommend CT evaluation of the pelvic and paraaortic lymph nodes prior to treatment in all patients with cervical cancer. Fine-needle biopsy or, in selected cases, open biopsy should be performed when the findings suggest metastatic lymph node disease.

Patients with histologically confirmed paraaortic lymph node metastases in the absence of systemic disease should undergo a *left scalene fat pad biopsy.* A transverse incision is made approximately 2 cm above the heads of the sternocleidomastoid muscle (Fig. 11-10). This muscle is then retracted laterally, and the fat pad and lymph nodes are exposed. All nodal tissue is then removed from the triangular space bordered by the internal jugular vein, the subclavian vein, and the omohyoid muscle. Approximately 15% of patients with positive paraaortic nodes will be found to have scalene lymph node metastases and will require some form of systemic therapy (van Nagell and Higgins, 1989).

Although cervical cancer commonly spreads systematically from regional to paraaortic lymph node groups, lymph vascular metastases to extrapelvic sites also occur. In patients with untreated cervical cancer, the most common sites of extrapelvic metastases are the liver, lung, and bone (Hendrikson, 1949). Therefore, liver function tests (serum glutamic oxaloacetic transaminase, glutamic pyruvic transaminase, and alkaline phosphatase) and chest radiography should be performed for all patients with cervical cancer as part of their initial evaluation. Bone scans should be obtained only in those patients with elevated alkaline phosphatase or bone

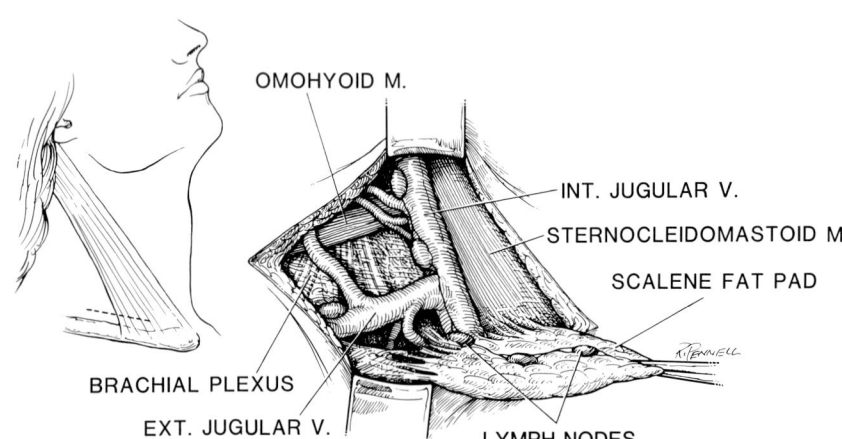

FIGURE 11-10  Anatomic landmarks in scalene fat pad biopsy. An incision is made 2 cm above the clavicle, and the sternocleidomastoid muscle is reflected medially. The exposed fat pad and lymph nodes are then removed.

TABLE 11-8   Evaluation of Patients with Invasive Cervical Cancer

History
Physical examination
—Lesion size
—Tumor configuration
Staging
Histomorphology of lesion
Complete blood cell count, liver function studies
Chest x-ray
Intravenous pyelography
CT of abdomen/pelvis based on stage
Cystoscopy, sigmoidoscopy based on stage

pain. The most common site of bone metastases is the vertebral bodies nearest an area of paraaortic spread (Matsuyama et al, 1989). Other sites of bone involvement in order of decreasing frequency are the ilium, the skull, and the long bones of the lower extremities. A CT scan of the involved area is often helpful in differentiating bone metastasis from osteoporosis or inflammation in patients with abnormal bone scans.

The role of *tumor markers* in cervical cancer has not been fully defined. The squamous cell carcinoma (SCC) antigen, initially described by Kato and Torigoe (1977), has been isolated in the serum of a high percentage of patients with cervical cancer. Although this antigen is not specific for invasive cervical cancer, it has provided a useful means of monitoring response to therapy and predicting occult tumor recurrence (Maiman et al, 1989; Patsner and Mann, 1989). Similarly, carcinoembryonic antigen (CEA) has been a clinically useful marker in patients with mucin-producing adenocarcinomas of the endocervix (van Nagell et al, 1979*a*). Immunohistochemical staining of biopsy specimens can be employed to establish the antigen profile of each tumor and to identify those markers which should help to assess response to treatment. A baseline measurement of the appropriate marker in serum should be obtained prior to therapy when the tumor stains positively for that marker.

In summary, all patients with cervical cancer should undergo a thorough and standardized evaluation, as outlined in Table 11-8. In this way, therapy can be properly individualized.

## THERAPY

### Microinvasive Cervical Cancer

Based on available data, there appears to be a group of invasive cervical cancers with early stromal invasion that present virtually no risk of lymph node metastases and can therefore be treated by conservative hysterectomy. Although a number of different definitions of microinvasion have been proposed, the authors favor that adopted by the Society of Gynecologic Oncologists (SGO) in 1974. According to the SGO definition, a microinvasive lesion is one that invades the cervical stroma to a depth of 3.0 mm or less below the base of the epithelium with no evidence of lymph vascular space

invasion (Fig. 11-11). This diagnosis can be made only after thorough examination of an adequately sectioned conization specimen in which the depth of stromal invasion is measured using an ocular micrometer. At a minimum, each conization specimen should be divided into 12 sections, and three step sections should be examined from each section. Depth of invasion is measured from the basement membrane to the point of maximal stromal penetration by tumor cells. Likewise, the presence of lymph vascular space invasion must be evaluated by a pathologist experienced in making this diagnosis.

The frequency of lymph node metastases in a large number of patients with early invasive cervical cancer treated by radical hysterectomy and pelvic lymphadenectomy is shown in Table 11-9. Among over 500 patients with stromal invasion to 3.0 mm or less and no evidence of lymph vascular space invasion, no lymph node metastases were found. In contrast, approximately 9% of patients with tumors demonstrating stromal invasion of 3.1 to 5.0 mm had metastases. According to the SGO definition, the presence of lymph vascular space invasion precludes the diagnosis of microinvasive cervical cancer. Numerous investigators have confirmed the presence of lymph node metastases in patients whose tumors demonstrate lymph vascular space invasion in spite of minimal (less than 3.0 mm) stromal penetration (Nelson et al, 1989; Tsukamoto et al, 1989).

Since van Nagell and coworkers (1983) initially reported that vaginal or abdominal hysterectomy was as effective as radical hysterectomy in treating lesions with stromal invasion of 3.0 mm or less and no evidence of lymph vascular space invasion, this observation has been confirmed in many centers. There is a small but

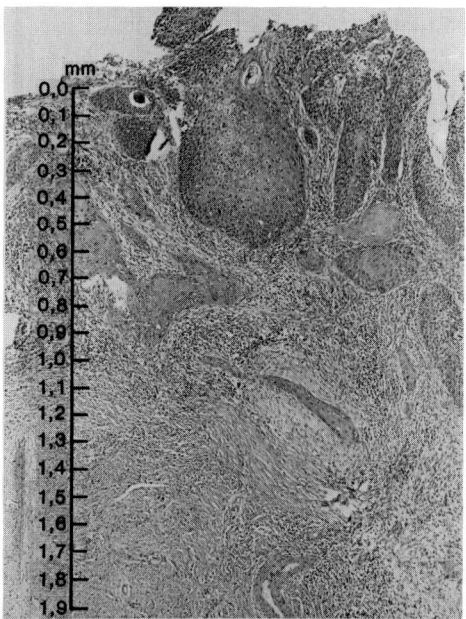

FIGURE 11-11   Microinvasive carcinoma of the cervix. An ocular micrometer is used to measure the depth of stromal invasion beneath the basement membrane. (Hematoxylin and eosin stain, final magnification ×53.)

TABLE 11-9 Frequency of Lymph Node Metastases Related to Stromal Invasion in Patients with Stage IA Cervical Cancer (N = 695)

| Depth of Stromal Invasion* | No. of Patients | No. of Patients with Positive Nodes |
|---|---|---|
| ≤ 1.0 mm | 162 | 0 |
| 1.1 to 3.0 mm | 407 | 0 |
| 3.1 to 5.0 mm | 124 | 9 |

*Measured by ocular micrometer from conization specimen.
Sources: Averette et al (1976), Fouchee et al (1969), Leman et al (1976), Roche and Norris (1975), Seski et al (1977), Simon et al (1986), Taki et al (1979), Tsukamoto et al (1989), van Nagell et al (1983), Yajima and Noda (1979).

definite risk for an area of intraepithelial neoplasia extending to the vagina in patients with early stromal invasion. For this reason, every patient with microinvasive cervical cancer should undergo colposcopy prior to surgery. If an area of vaginal extension is identified, it can be removed at the time of surgery. At present, there is no evidence to suggest that routine excision of a wide vaginal cuff is indicated in the treatment of microinvasive cervical cancer. As to whether certain patients with microinvasive cancer can be treated by cervical conization alone, we must await the results of controlled clinical trials. Unfortunately, the FIGO definitions of early invasive cervical cancer (stages IA1 and IA2) do not take into consideration the presence of lymph vascular space invasion. Therefore, it is more difficult to relate specific types of therapy to these definitions.

## Invasive Cervical Cancer

The basic requirement for any therapeutic modality for invasive cervical cancer is that it effectively treat not only the primary lesion but also the regional lymph node groups to which the tumor may metastasize. As has been mentioned previously, these groups include the internal iliac, obturator, sacral, external iliac, and common iliac lymph nodes. Treatment methods for primary invasive cervical cancer include radical surgery, radiation therapy, or a combination thereof. In addition, experimental protocols are in progress to evaluate the combination of chemotherapy with both radical surgery and radiation therapy.

Few randomized trials have compared radiation therapy and radical surgery as treatment methods in patients with various stages of cervical cancer. Consequently, analytical methods applied to retrospective data have been used to identify patients who would be best treated by radical surgery. These methods are based on the general concept that radical surgery is most effective when cervical cancer has not spread beyond the cervix to involve the parametrium or regional lymph nodes. Inoue and Okumura (1984) reported that the 5-year survival of patients treated with radical surgery decreased from 95% to 69% when the parametrium was involved. Similarly, Webb and Symmonds (1979) noted

that in the presence of lymph node metastases, 5-year survival decreased from 83% to 59% in patients treated with radical surgery. As expected, the recurrence rate was directly related to the number of lymph nodes involved by metastatic cancer.

The histomorphologic variables most useful in predicting lymph node status in patients with stage IB cervical cancer are lesion size, cell type, lymph vascular space invasion, and depth of stromal penetration. Several investigators have studied the relationship between *lesion size* and the frequency of lymph node metastases. For example, Piver and Chung (1975) reported that 35% of patients with stage IB lesions greater than 3 cm in diameter had metastatic disease in the pelvic lymph nodes as opposed to only 21% of patients with smaller lesions. Similarly, van Nagell and colleagues (1979*b*) noted that only 6% of patients with stage IB cervical cancers less than 2 cm in diameter had positive pelvic lymph nodes compared with 18% of those with larger lesions.

*Cell type* is also useful in determining the optimal method of therapy for each patient. Small cell cancers, although rare, are highly aggressive tumors that respond poorly to radical surgery. For example, the frequency of lymph node metastases in patients with stage IB small cell carcinomas less than 3 cm in diameter is 40%, and the majority of these patients die within a short time from metastatic disease (van Nagell et al, 1988). Obviously, there is a need for prospective multiinstitutional trials to determine the efficacy of adjuvant chemotherapy in these tumors.

Although the presence of *lymph vascular space invasion* by tumor cells is not an absolute contraindication to radical surgery, patients with this finding are more likely to have lymph node metastases and extrapelvic spread (van Nagell et al, 1978).

Unfortunately, *depth of stromal penetration* is often not known prior to therapy and hence cannot be used routinely to select patients for a specific type of treatment.

## Radical Hysterectomy

Radical hysterectomy with pelvic lymphadenectomy is therefore the treatment of choice in relatively healthy patients with stage IB large cell squamous cancers or adenocarcinomas 3 cm or less in diameter. All candidates for radical hysterectomy must undergo a thorough medical evaluation prior to surgery. This includes clinical staging and CT scanning to rule out paraaortic lymphadenopathy or occult ureteral obstruction. Since dehydration and decreased intravascular volume are of particular concern, patients should receive preoperative hydration and nutritional supplementation. The purpose of this operation is to remove the primary cervical tumor, uterus, parametria, and upper vagina en bloc along with the internal iliac, external iliac, common iliac, obturator, and lateral sacral lymph nodes (Fig. 11-12, *A* and *B*).

Since its initial description by Clark (1895) and Ries (1895), this operation has benefited from several technical advances. These include vaginal vault closure with reperitonealization of the bladder base and, more recently, the use of retroperitoneal suction drainage and suprapubic bladder catheterization. Reperitonealization of the bladder base combined with *retroperitoneal suction drainage* in radical hysterectomy was initially reported by Symmonds and Pratt (1961), who noted that this approach significantly reduced the frequency of postoperative urinary tract fistulas and lymphocyst formation. Since then, these observations have been confirmed by a number of institutions, and retroperitoneal suction drainage of the pelvis is now employed routinely after radical pelvic surgery.

Hemovac drains are usually placed in the paravesical space after the surgical specimen has been removed and the vaginal vault closed. The drains are then brought out through stab wounds in both lower abdominal quadrants and are connected to intermittent wall suction (Fig. 11-12, *C* and *D*). When Roddick and colleagues (1973) examined volume, protein concentration, and electrolyte content of retroperitoneal suction drainage fluid following radical hysterectomy and pelvic lymphadenectomy, they reported that the protein and electrolyte concentrations closely approximated those of serum. Retroperitoneal suction drainage was greatest on the first postoperative day (200 to 400 ml) and decreased to less than 50 ml by the fifth postoperative day. By measuring retroperitoneal suction drainage, one can replace the daily losses of protein and electrolytes following radical surgery and thus prevent electrolyte imbalance and abnormalities in intravascular colloid oncotic pressure.

The use of *suprapubic bladder drainage* has decreased the frequency of urinary tract complications and patient discomfort following radical hysterectomy. The extensive dissection of the bladder base and transection of the uterosacral ligaments associated with this operation often interrupt the sympathetic beta-adrenergic nerve supply to the bladder, resulting initially in increased myogenic tone and bladder hypertonicity (Low et al, 1981; Scotti et al, 1986). This hypertonic phase is followed by a hypotonic phase secondary to interruption of parasympathetic nerve fibers (Forney, 1980). As a result, bladder sensation is usually diminished and overdistention can occur, increasing the risk for fistula formation. van Nagell and coworkers (1972) initially reported the efficacy of suprapubic bladder drainage in patients undergoing radical hysterectomy with pelvic lymphadenectomy.

After the surgical specimen has been removed, the bladder is filled with 300 ml of sterile saline and carefully inspected for any evidence of surgical injury. A cystotomy is then carried out through the anterior bladder wall, and a No. 18 French Silastic catheter is placed in the bladder. The catheter is brought out through the anterior vesical space and sutured to the skin (Fig. 11-13), and the patient is instructed to begin clamping the suprapubic catheter approximately 5 days after surgery so that postvoiding residual urine volumes can be measured. The catheter is removed when these volumes are consistently less than 50 ml. In a recent large series of patients who underwent radical hysterectomy and suprapubic bladder drainage, the mean time to normal

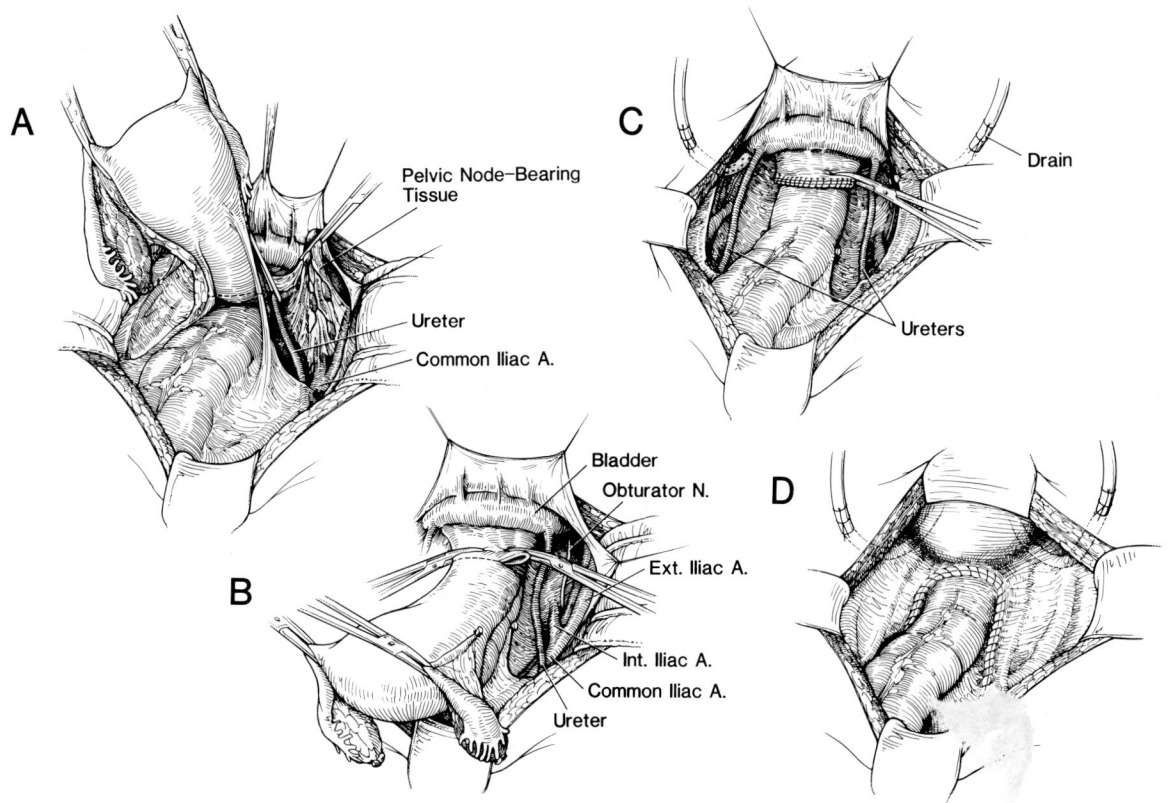

FIGURE 11-12 Radical hysterectomy with pelvic lymphadenectomy. The uterus, parametria, and pelvic lymph nodes are removed en bloc (*A* and *B*). Hemovac drains are placed in the paravesical spaces (*C*), and the pelvis is reperitonealized (*D*).

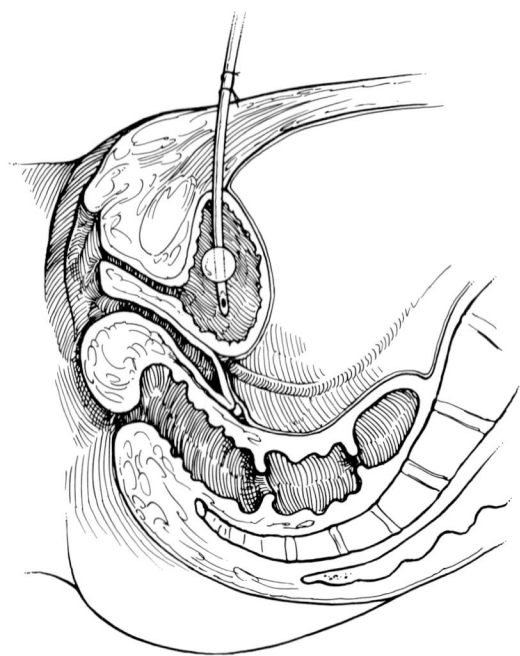

**FIGURE 11-13** Suprapubic bladder drainage following radical hysterectomy and pelvic lymphadenectomy. A Silastic catheter is introduced into the bladder using a cystotomy incision and is brought out through the anterior vesical space.

voiding was 25 days (range = 4 to 77 days) (DePriest et al, in press). Forney (1980) has reported that incomplete transection of the cardinal ligaments at the time of radical hysterectomy is associated with more rapid return of bladder function; spontaneous voiding occurred significantly earlier (20 vs 51 days) with incomplete transection. Unfortunately, incomplete removal of the cardinal ligament at the time of radical hysterectomy may increase the risk for microscopic residual disease and persistence of tumor.

The most common complications of radical hysterectomy with pelvic lymphadenectomy continue to be related to the urinary tract (Table 11-10). *Urinary tract*

*infection* has been reported to occur in as many as 15% of patients. The aforementioned increase in bladder residual volumes after radical hysterectomy predisposes to such infection, so that patients should receive antibacterial prophylaxis until the suprapubic catheter has been removed.

The frequency of *urinary tract fistulas* following radical hysterectomy has progressively declined over the past decade. Although ureterovaginal fistulas are still more common than vesicovaginal fistulas, the combined fistula rate in most recent series is less than 3% (Lee et al, 1989; Artman et al, 1987). This reduction in the rate of fistula formation is attributable largely to careful intraoperative inspection of the bladder and ureter after the specimen has been removed, immediate repair of any observed abnormality, and continuous suprapubic bladder drainage. Should bladder or ureteral damage go undetected, urinary tract fistulas may appear during the postoperative period. In patients suspected of having a vesicovaginal or ureterovaginal fistula, cystoscopy and retrograde ureteral dye studies can be performed in order to locate the fistula. Ureteral fistulas should be repaired immediately to prevent obstruction and subsequent loss of renal function. Unfortunately, vesicovaginal fistulas often cannot be repaired at the time of diagnosis because of necrosis and infection at the fistula site. The patient should be placed on antibiotics and vaginal peroxide washes prior to surgical repair. Cystoscopy will determine the relationship of the fistulous tract to the ureteral orifices. When these recommendations are followed, primary fistula repair is usually successful, and urinary diversion or nephrectomy can be avoided.

The most serious life-threatening complication following radical hysterectomy with pelvic lymphadenectomy is *pulmonary embolism*. Although this complication is rare, the associated mortality is so high that many investigators have sought ways to prevent it. The most extensively studied methods for preventing venous thromboembolism are prophylactic low-dose heparin and external pneumatic calf compression. At present,

| Authors | Year | No. of Patients | Urinary Fistula (%) | | Bladder Atony (%) | Thrombo-phlebitis (%) | Pulmonary Embolism (%) | Lympho-cysts (%) | Intestinal Obstruction (%) |
| | | | Vesico-vaginal | Uretero-vaginal | | | | | |
|---|---|---|---|---|---|---|---|---|---|
| Hoskins et al | 1976 | 224 | 0.4 | 1.3 | — | — | 0.4 | — | — |
| Christensen and Foglmann | 1976 | 670 | 0.4 | 5.7 | 6.9 | 1.9 | 0.3 | — | — |
| Webb and Symmonds | 1979 | 423 | 0.7 | 1.4 | — | 5.0 | 2.1 | 4.3 | 0.5 |
| Sall et al | 1979 | 349 | 0.9 | 2.0 | 0.9 | 1.1 | 0.3 | 1.7 | 0.9 |
| Underwood et al | 1979 | 178 | 1.1 | 2.8 | — | — | — | — | — |
| Langley et al | 1980 | 284 | 1.4 | 5.6 | 3.5 | — | — | — | — |
| Lerner et al | 1980 | 108 | — | 0.9 | 5.6 | 0.9 | 0.9 | 0.9 | 1.9 |
| Powell et al | 1984 | 255 | 1.6 | 0.8 | 2.7 | 2.7 | 2.0 | 0.8 | 1.2 |
| Artman et al | 1987 | 153 | 1.3 | 1.3 | — | 0.7 | 1.3 | 1.3 | — |
| Lee et al | 1989 | 954 | 1.3 | 1.3 | — | 0.2 | — | — | 1.0 |
| Kenter et al | 1989 | 213 | 2.8 | 3.3 | 6.1 | 1.4 | 0.47 | 6.6 | — |
| Totals | | 3,811 | 1.1 | 2.4 | 4.3 | 1.7 | 1.0 | 2.6 | 1.1 |

TABLE 11-10  Complications of Radical Hysterectomy (N = 3,811)

over 15 randomized prospective trials are under way to compare low-dose heparin with placebo or no treatment as a means of preventing venous thrombosis in patients undergoing general thoracoabdominal surgery. The majority of these studies have demonstrated a significant reduction in venous thrombosis as detected by $^{125}$I-labeled fibrinogen leg scanning in patients treated with low-dose heparin prophylaxis (Genton and Turpie, 1980). In these studies, heparin in doses of 5,000 units is given prior to operation and every 12 hours thereafter until the patient is fully ambulant. There have been no randomized trials specifically to determine whether low-dose heparin prevents pulmonary emboli in patients undergoing radical pelvic surgery. However, in general surgical patients, such trials have demonstrated that prophylactic low-dose heparin reduces the frequency of fatal pulmonary embolism (Genton and Turpie, 1980; International Multicentre Trial, 1975).

External pneumatic calf compression has also proved successful in reducing the frequency of postoperative venous thromboembolism. Clarke-Pearson and colleagues (1984) reported that pneumatic calf compression decreased the incidence of deep venous thrombosis in patients undergoing radical pelvic surgery from 34 to 13% (p ≤ 0.005). Calf compression was applied intraoperatively and for the first 5 postoperative days. At present, it is our policy to administer prophylactic low-dose heparin and external pneumatic calf compression to all patients undergoing radical hysterectomy with pelvic lymphadenectomy.

Postoperative *vaginal cuff or pelvic cellulitis* has been reported in as many as 25% of patients (Miyazawa et al, 1987). Prospective double-blind studies have clearly demonstrated that prophylactic antibiotics significantly decrease the frequency of pelvic infection in this group of patients. Therefore, antibiotic prophylaxis with either a broad-spectrum cephalosporin or a semisynthetic penicillin is in order for all patients undergoing radical hysterectomy with pelvic lymphadenectomy.

### Radiation Following Radical Hysterectomy and Pelvic Lymphadenectomy

Data are limited concerning the efficacy of postoperative radiation in patients with pelvic lymph node metastases at the time of radical hysterectomy. The number of patients with pelvic lymph nodal metastases is relatively small, and no prospective randomized trials have been reported. In 1979, representatives from several institutions served on a panel of the SGO to determine the effect of postoperative radiation therapy in these patients. Recurrence and survival rates of patients with positive pelvic lymph nodes who received radiation were compared with rates among similar patients who received no additional therapy. Although the survival rates of the two groups were not significantly different, there was a trend toward improved survival with radiation, particularly in patients with more than three positive lymph nodes. In addition, the incidence of the pelvic recurrence was reduced in those who received radiation (Morrow, 1980).

Both these findings have been confirmed in a more recent retrospective study by Kinney and coworkers (1989), who evaluated the effect of postoperative radiation therapy on the rate of recurrence in 185 patients with stage IB or IIA cervical cancer and positive pelvic lymph nodes. Patients were matched according to lesion size and the location and number of positive lymph nodes. Although long-term survival was essentially the same in both groups, adjuvant radiation therapy improved short-term survival and reduced the frequency of local recurrence.

It is our policy to recommend adjuvant radiation at the time of radical hysterectomy in patients with pelvic lymph nodal metastases. This consists of 5,000 cGy of external-beam radiation delivered to a standard pelvic field at a rate of 180 to 200 cGy/day. A prospective multiinstitutional trial is needed to compare the benefits of adjuvant chemotherapy with those of adjuvant radiation therapy in patients with histologically confirmed pelvic lymph node metastases.

### Combined Radiation and Extrafascial Hysterectomy

During the past decade, interest has increased in the combination of radiation therapy and surgery to treat bulky stage IB cervical cancer. These lesions contain a large volume of poorly perfused hypoxic tumor cells that are characteristically in the noncycling phase of the cell cycle and therefore resistant to radiation therapy. In addition, many of these tumors spread superiorly into the lower uterine segment and therefore extend beyond the curative isodose for radiation therapy (Fig. 11-14). Thus, there are obvious theoretical advantages to adding extrafascial hysterectomy to radiation therapy for these lesions. Durrance and coworkers (1968) were the first to report improved results using combination therapy for bulky stage IB cervical cancers. Briefly, 4,000 cGy of external-beam radiation and one intracavitary implant were followed after 6 weeks by extrafascial hysterectomy. Utilizing this protocol, Rutledge and coworkers (1976) reported a 5-year survival of 93% in patients with bulky stage I disease. In a more recent study, Gallion and colleagues (1985) reported a reduction in the recurrence rate of patients with bulky barrel-shaped stage IB tumors (> 4 cm in diameter) from 47% to 16% with the addition of extrafascial hysterectomy. Since these large-volume tumors have a high incidence of lymph node metastases, paraaortic lymph node sampling is routinely performed at the time of surgery. Patients with paraaortic metastases are treated with additional extended-field radiation.

Another indication for postirradiation extrafascial hysterectomy is the failure of a stage IB tumor to regress during radiation therapy. Marcial and Bosch (1970) related regression patterns of cervical tumors during radiation to prognosis. Patients whose tumors had disappeared by the completion of radiation therapy had a 96% 3-year survival rate compared with only 2% in patients whose tumors never regressed during treatment. These observations were confirmed by Hardt and coworkers (1982) in a subsequent investigation. Patients with no palpable or visible evidence of a cervical tumor one month after completing radiation therapy had a 95% 5-year survival rate. In contrast, patients with obvious disease in the cervix at this time had a recurrence rate of 80%.

For this reason, the regression of cervical tumors should be carefully evaluated at regular intervals throughout radiation therapy. Patients with stage IB disease whose tumors do not respond by the time radiation therapy is completed should be considered candidates for extrafascial hysterectomy provided that there is no evidence of extracervical spread on CT scan. Preliminary data indicate that this procedure can be performed safely at this time and the frequency of central pelvic recurrence can be decreased.

### Radiation Therapy

Radiation therapy is an effective treatment method for patients with all stages of cervical cancer. Specifically, it is the treatment of choice in patients with stage IB cervical cancer who are not candidates for radical surgery and in all patients with disease at a more advanced stage. Modern radiation therapy is a sophisticated science, the principles of which were reviewed in Chapter 7. Of particular interest, is the recent use of radiation in combination with surgery or chemotherapy in the treatment of specific stages or anatomic configurations of cervical cancer. Optimal therapeutic results have been achieved in centers where there is close cooperation between the gynecologic oncologist, radiation oncologist, and pathologist, so that a specific type of treatment can be matched to the histologic and anatomic features of each tumor.

In addition to the standardized evaluation system for cervical cancer previously presented, patients who are candidates for radiation therapy should be questioned carefully to determine the presence of factors that may predispose to radiation-related complications. Pelvic inflammation has been shown to produce reactive vasculitis and fibrin thrombosis within small vessels of the bowel and bladder (van Nagell et al, 1977b). Radiation-induced vascular endothelial proliferation can cause localized hypoperfusion and hypoxia within these organs, and the combination of radiation therapy and pelvic inflammatory disease has been associated with a high incidence of enteric complications. A history of prior abdominal surgery is also of note, since adhesions may fix loops of bowel within the pelvis at sites that receive abnormally high doses of radiation. Likewise, the frequency of radiation-related enteric complications is increased in patients with preexisting vascular disease. Patients with a history of diabetes mellitus or hypertension should be thoroughly evaluated to determine the extent of underlying small vessel disease so that radiation fractionation can be adjusted accordingly. Finally, the patient's nutritional status is related to the incidence of radiation complications. Nutritional status should be evaluated, particularly in patients with a history of recent weight loss, so that enteral or parenteral supplementation can be provided during radiation therapy.

Radiation therapy for patients with invasive cervical cancer is given as a combination of external and intracavitary therapy. Definitions for a number of important terms in pelvic radiation are presented in Table 11-11. Generally, the goal of effective treatment planning is to maximize the radiation dose to the tumor while not exceeding the tissue tolerance of normal pelvic and abdominal structures. The radiation tissue tolerance of normal pelvic organs is presented in Table 11-12.

External-beam irradiation is usually delivered from a linear accelerator. The higher the energy of the linear accelerator, the greater the depth-dose distribution of radiation in the patient. This is particularly important in the obese patient, in whom the tumor may be a significant distance from the skin. The purpose of external therapy is to decrease the tumor volume and reduce the anatomic distortion produced by the tumor, which has the effect of optimizing the dose from intracavitary therapy. For this reason, it is preferable to deliver external-beam irradiation prior to implant therapy, particularly when gamma radiation is being used.

In patients with stage IB or IIA disease, 4,000 to 4,500 cGy are delivered at a rate of 180 to 200 cGy/day. Patients with more advanced disease receive 4,000 to 5,000 cGy of external-beam irradiation over a period of 4 to 6 weeks. Those with severe vascular disease receive the same dose but over a larger number of fractions, with a lower dose per fraction, since some of the normal tissues may be relatively hypoxic secondary to vascular disease and will require more time to repair sublethal radiation damage. Although the dimensions of the radiation field are individualized, they usually approximate 16 cm x 16 cm (256 cm$^2$). Thin patients

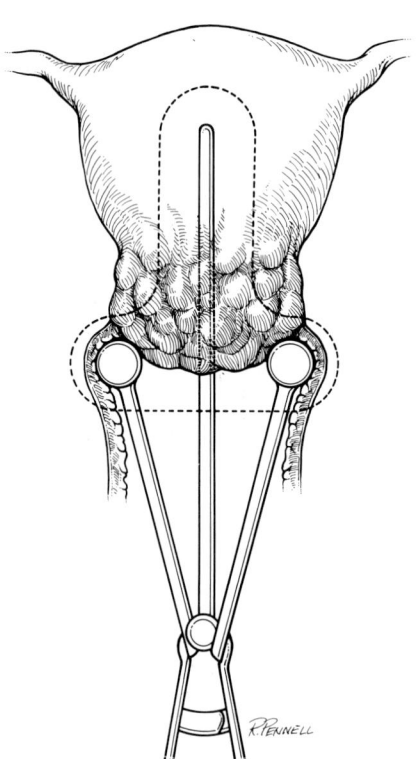

**FIGURE 11-14** Tandem and ovoid radioactive implants placed in a barrel-shaped cervical cancer. The superior lateral aspects of the tumor extend beyond the curative isodose (broken line).

TABLE 11-11  Terms Used in Radiation Therapy of Cervical Cancer

| | |
|---|---|
| Intracavitary therapy | Therapy in which radiation source is inside the patient (e.g., intracervical or intravaginal). |
| External-beam therapy | Therapy in which radiation source is outside the patient. |
| Source-skin distance (SSD) | Distance along the central ray between radiation source and patient's skin. |
| Field size | Size of irradiated field measured at the stated source-skin distance. |
| Centigray (cGy) | Unit of absorbed dose (equal to 1 rad). |
| Point A | A point 2 cm lateral and 2 cm superior to the external cervical os. |
| Point B | A point 3 cm lateral to point A, corresponding to the pelvic sidewall. |
| Half-life | Time necessary for half the atoms from a radioactive source to disintegrate. |
| Inverse square law | A dose of radiation at a given point is inversely proportional to the square of the distance from the source of radiation. |
| Isodose curve | Lines of equal absorbed dose. |
| Linear energy transfer (LET) | Energy lost by a particle per micron of path length. |
| Oxygen enhancement ratio (OER) | The ratio of maximum sensitivity in oxygen, as compared with hypoxic conditions. |
| Relative biologic effectiveness (RBE) | Ratio of dose of test radiation to 250 KeV radiation in producing an equal biologic effect. |

with an anteroposterior (AP) diameter of less than 20 cm are treated with two opposing AP ports; larger patients are most often treated with two opposing AP ports and two lateral ports to achieve an optimal distribution of dose within the pelvis. In selected patients with large AP diameters, rotational fields are also beneficial.

Once external therapy has been completed, one or two intracavitary implants are inserted. Radionuclide

TABLE 11-12  Radiation Tissue Tolerance of Normal Pelvic and Abdominal Structures

| Organ | Radiation Tissue Tolerance (cGy) |
|---|---|
| Kidney | 2,000 |
| Liver | 3,000 |
| Small bowel | 4,500 |
| Colon | 6,000 |
| Rectum | 6,000 |
| Bladder | 7,000 |
| Ureter | 7,500 |

*Source:* Maruyama Y, van Nagell JR Jr: Radiation therapy in the treatment of invasive cervical cancer. In van Nagell JR Jr, Barber HRK (eds): *Modern Concepts of Gynecologic Oncology.* Chicago, Illinois, Mosby-Year Book, 1982, pp 91-158.

sources used for *intracavitary or interstitial therapy* in cervical cancer are summarized in Table 11-13. Radium-226 has largely been replaced by cesium-137 because of its shorter half-life and more defined gamma energy. In addition, breakage of a radium source can produce radon gas, which is hazardous and difficult to contain. Recently, heavy-particle radiation has been employed (Maruyama et al, 1987). Californium-252, a source of both gamma radiation and fast neutrons, has been used in intracavitary therapy for cervical cancer. The theoretical advantages of neutron therapy are its lower oxygen enhancement ratio (OER) and its higher relative biologic effect (RBE) compared with conventional gamma radiation. Consequently, californium-252 is advantageous for treating bulky cervical tumors that are poorly perfused and contain a high proportion of hypoxic cells. The higher RBE of neutron therapy also allows for a shorter implant time compared with gamma radiation.

van Nagell and coworkers (1986) have described the use of intracavitary neutron therapy in patients with bulky, barrel-shaped stage IB cervical cancer. Extrafascial hysterectomy and paraaortic lymph node biopsies were performed 6 weeks after the completion of radiation therapy. Tumor was completely cleared from the cervix in 72% of the patients, and the 5-year survival in these cases was 94%. Intracavitary neutron therapy was well tolerated, and all implants were inserted on an outpatient basis. The combination of external gamma radiation and intracavitary neutron therapy has also been reported to be effective in patients with stage IIIB cervical cancer (Gallion et al, 1987).

## Invasive Cancer Found at Simple Hysterectomy

When invasive cervical cancer is found on hysterectomy performed for apparently benign disease, patients may be treated with either reoperation or radiation therapy. Young patients with minimally invasive disease can be treated successfully by radical surgery, which includes removal of the parametria, bilateral pelvic lymphadenectomy, and upper vaginectomy. Orr and coworkers (1986) treated 23 such patients with radical reoperation, three of whom had lymph node metastases while another three had persistent disease in the vagina or parametria. Reoperation was well tolerated in all cases, and only one patient has died of recurrent cancer.

Radiation has been the predominant method of ad-

TABLE 11-13  Radionuclides Used in Intracavitary or Interstitial Therapy for Cervical Cancer

| Isotope | Gamma Energy (MeV) | Half-Life (yr) |
|---|---|---|
| Radium-226 | 0.8 (0.04-2.4) | 1,620 |
| Cesium-137 | 0.66 | 30 |
| Cobalt-60 | 1.1, 1.3 | 5.3 |
| Californium-252 | 0.4 to 1.0 (fast neutrons) | 2.65 |
| Iridium-192 | 0.32-0.61 | 74 days |

TABLE 11-14  Five-Year Survival After Simple Hysterectomy and Radiation Therapy for Invasive Cervical Cancer

| Author(s) | Year | No. of Patients | 5-Year Survival (%) | |
|---|---|---|---|---|
| | | | Tumor-Free Surgical Margin | Tumor at Surgical Margin |
| Cosbie | 1963 | 86 | 71 | 20 |
| Green and Morse | 1969 | 27 | 0 | 27 |
| Andras et al | 1973 | 118 | 89 | 59 |
| Davy et al | 1977 | 64 | 77 | 38 |
| Papavasiliou et al | 1980 | 36 | 89 | 0 |
| Perkins et al | 1984 | 36 | 72 | 40 |

juvant therapy in patients found to have invasive cancer on examination of the hysterectomy specimen. Dosimetry regimens usually include external-beam therapy (4,500 to 5,000 cGy) followed by one intracavitary implant that will provide a surface dose of 7,000 cGy to the vagina. Prognosis has been shown to be related to the depth of stromal invasion and to the cell type of the lesion. Andras and coworkers (1973) reported a 5-year survival rate of 96% when microscopic disease was confined to the cervix; in contrast, patients whose tumors were deeply invasive had a 5-year survival rate of 85%. In a more recent study, Hopkins and coworkers (1990) noted a 5-year survival rate of 96% when cervical stromal penetration was less than 50% as opposed to only 68% in patients with deeper stromal invasion ($p < 0.02$). The presence of tumor cells at the margin of surgical resection reduces the 5-year survival rate from 80% to less than 40% (Table 11-14).

In most studies, survival rates have been worse in patients with undiagnosed adenocarcinoma than in those with squamous cell carcinoma. This may be explained by the endocervical location of adenocarcinoma and the possibility that these lesions may attain a significant volume without having a visible component. In the aforementioned series (Hopkins et al, 1990) the 5-year survival rate for patients with stage I squamous cell carcinoma was 80% compared with only 41% in those with stage I adenocarcinoma.

A final prognostic factor in all series has been the time between surgery and the initiation of adjuvant radiation therapy. Survival rates are highest when radiation is started as soon as possible after surgery. Durrance (1968) reported tumor recurrence only in patients whose radiation therapy had been delayed for more than 6 months following hysterectomy.

## Radiation Therapy Combined With Chemotherapy

The use of chemotherapy with radiation therapy is based on the theory of "synergistic cell kill"—i.e., cell kill will be greater if two therapeutic modalities are combined than if the effects of the two modalities individually are simply added together. Specific chemotherapeutic agents that have been combined with radiation to treat cervical cancer are 5-fluorouracil (5-FU), hydroxyurea, and, more recently, cisplatin.

The efficacy of combining 5-FU and radiation ther-

apy was initially suggested by Cummings and associates (1984) in the treatment of squamous cell carcinoma of the anus. These investigators reported primary tumor control rates of 93% in anal cancer treated by 5-FU plus radiation compared with 60% in similar patients treated with radiation alone. In order to achieve the conditions required for radiation sensitization, cells must be exposed to 5-FU constantly for at least 24 hours after radiation therapy is begun (Byfield, 1986). Consequently, most protocol studies are designed to initiate a 5-day infusion of 5-FU at the time of radiation exposure. The higher the concentration of drug per given time period, the more likely the tumor will respond. In patients with advanced cervical cancer, the combination of 5-FU and radiation, when given after an initial bolus of mitomycin C, appears to result in local tumor clearance rates of 80% (Evans et al, 1988). Currently, the Gynecologic Oncology Group (GOG) is comparing hydroxyurea with 5-FU infusion and bolus cisplatin as an adjunct to radiation therapy, but the results of this trial have not yet been published.

A second chemotherapeutic agent that has been used extensively with radiation therapy in the treatment of advanced-stage cervical cancer is hydroxyurea. The sensitivity of tumor cells to radiation therapy is lowest during the S phase of the cell cycle. Hydroxyurea preferentially kills cells in the S phase and causes surviving cells to accumulate at the $G_1$-S interphase, when they are highly sensitive to radiation therapy. In a prospective randomized trial of patients with surgical stage IIIB cervical cancer with no paraaortic metastases, the combination of hydroxyurea and radiation produced a 5-year progression-free survival rate of 91% compared with 60% in the group given placebo plus radiation (Piver et al, 1987).

The beneficial effect of combining cisplatin and radiation therapy was initially suggested by animal and cell culture studies that showed a synergism between these two therapeutic modalities (Douple and Richmond, 1978). To test the hypothesis that adding platinum chemotherapy to radiation in cervical cancer could improve local and regional tumor clearance while achieving distant control by eliminating micrometastases, Choo and colleagues (1986) randomized patients with stage IIB, IIIA, and IIIB disease to receive cisplatin plus radiation versus radiation alone. Cisplatin was given in a dose of 25 mg/m$^2$ intravenously on day 1 of radiation therapy and was repeated at weekly intervals during the period of irradiation. A complete response—defined as no evidence of tumor on colposcopy, clinical examination, and cervical biopsies—was observed in 55% of patients in the combined-therapy arm as opposed to only 20% of the patients treated with radiation therapy alone. Although the exact mechanism of radiation potentiation by cisplatin is unknown, available evidence suggests that cisplatin inhibits the repair of radiation damage in mammalian cells (Coughlin and Richmond, 1989). At present, the GOG and several other institutions are carrying out phase III studies to determine the most effective radiopotentiating agents in cervical cancer.

### Extended-Field Radiation

The frequency of paraaortic lymph node metastases varies from approximately 5% in patients with stage IB cervical cancer to 30% in patients with stage III and IV disease. When paraaortic metastases are histologically confirmed, extended-field radiation therapy is indicated, with the dimensions of the field dependent on the location of the metastases. In patients with metastatic disease in the common iliac nodes, the radiation field is elevated to the level of the third lumbar vertebra. Patients with paraaortic metastases are treated to the level of the twelfth thoracic vertebra. Clips are used to identify areas from which positive lymph nodes are removed so that they can be included in the extended field of radiation. The width of the extended field usually varies from 8 to 10 cm.

Numerous investigators have attempted to determine the proper dose and fractionation for extended-field therapy. Initially, doses as high as 5,500 cGy were delivered to a paraaortic field at dose rates of 200 cGy/day. However, the rate of complications associated with these doses was unacceptable. Often, the stomach and small bowel are located within the extended field, and radiation-induced gastric ulceration and small bowel perforation were observed (Wharton et al, 1977). More recent evidence suggests that 4,500 to 5,000 cGy given at a rate of 160 to 170 cGy/day is sufficient to control paraaortic metastases, provided that these nodes are not markedly enlarged and fixed to adjacent structures. Survival rates for cervical cancer patients with paraaortic lymph node metastases treated by extended-field radiation are summarized in Table 11-15. Five-year survival rates ranged from 14 to 50% (mean = 25%). Doses of 4,000 to 5,000 cGy have been well tolerated, and major enteric complications have been rare (Lovecchio et al, 1989).

### Complications Related to Radiation

The biologic effects of radiation are related to total dose, field size, dose fractionation, and the normal-tissue tolerance of structures within the radiation field (see Table 11-12). Computer methodology is utilized in treatment planning, and dosimetry is optimized so that the radiation tolerance of normal tissues will not be exceeded. As a result, radiation complications have been steadily decreasing for the past 20 years.

Complications of radiation can generally be divided into acute (those which occur during or immediately after therapy) and chronic (those which occur as late as 12 to 18 months after therapy). One immediate complication is *perforation of the uterus* at the time of tandem insertion for intracavitary therapy. If unrecognized, uterine perforation may cause blood loss and severe radiation damage. When perforation is suspected, ultrasound or CT scanning should be employed to verify the position of the tandem. If perforation cannot be excluded based on noninvasive studies, laparoscopy should be performed. Patients with uterine perforation should be placed on a broad-spectrum antibiotic and observed closely, and the implant therapy should be terminated and rescheduled as soon as uterine healing permits.

The most common acute radiation reactions include sigmoiditis and hemorrhagic cystitis (Table 11-16). *Proctosigmoiditis* occurs in approximately 8% of patients undergoing pelvic irradiation and is noted most often in those who receive more than a 5,000-cGy dose of external-beam radiation or in those with relative fixation of the sigmoid colon close to the implant system. Symptoms associated with sigmoiditis include abdominal pain, diarrhea, and occasional nausea. In most patients, sigmoiditis can be treated with antispasmodics, a low-gluten and low-lactose diet, and cortisone enemas. However, severe cases may require hospitalization with hyperalimentation and electrolyte replacement. Colostomy is almost never required unless sigmoiditis continues to worsen despite medical therapy.

*Acute hemorrhagic cystitis* has been reported in approximately 3% of patients following radiation therapy for cervical cancer. This complication is best treated by

TABLE 11-15  Five-Year Survival after Extended-Field Radiation for Cervical Carcinoma with Paraaortic Nodal Metastases

| Authors | Year | No. of Patients | Radiation Dose (cGy) | 5-Year Survival (%) |
|---|---|---|---|---|
| Hughes et al | 1980 | 38 | 4,500 to 5,100 | 30 |
| Piver et al | 1981 | 21 | 6,000 | 14 |
| Tewfik et al | 1982 | 23 | 5,000 to 5,500 | 22 |
| Rubin et al | 1984 | 14 | 4,000 to 5,000 | 43 |
| Nori et al | 1985 | 27 | 5,000 to 5,200 | 30 |
| Gaspar et al | 1989 | 18 | 4,000 to 6,000 | 17 |
| Lovecchio et al | 1989 | 36 | 4,500 | 50 |

**TABLE 11-16** Acute and Chronic Complications of Radiation Therapy in Patients Treated for Cervical Cancer

| Authors | Year | No. of Patients | Sigmoiditis | Recto-vaginal Fistula | Rectal Stricture | Small Bowel Obstruction | Vesico-vaginal Fistula | Ureteral Stricture |
|---|---|---|---|---|---|---|---|---|
| van Nagell et al | 1974 | 271 | — | 4 (1.5) | — | 8 (3.0) | 2 (0.7) | — |
| Punnonen et al | 1976 | 279 | 18 (6.5) | 2 (0.7) | 3 (1.0) | 1 (0.4) | — | 2 (0.7) |
| Bosch and Frias | 1977 | 1,129 | 86 (7.5) | 9 (0.8) | 9 (0.8) | 5 (0.4) | 3 (0.3) | 1 (0.1) |
| Alert et al | 1980 | 2,248 | 4 (0.8) | 28 (4.3) | — | 13 (2.5) | 8 (1.5) | — |
| Hamberger et al | 1983 | 325 | 4 (1.2) | 10 (3.1) | 1 (0.3) | 5 (1.5) | 2 (0.6) | 2 (0.6) |
| Perez et al | 1984 | 811 | 17 (2.1) | 7 (0.9) | 8 (1.0) | 12 (1.5) | 9 (1.1) | 13 (1.6) |
| Combes et al | 1985 | 581 | 18 (3.1) | 8 (1.4) | — | 23 (4) | — | — |
| Montana et al | 1987 | 197 | 17 (8.6) | 1 (0.5) | — | — | 1 (0.5) | 3 (1.5) |
| Totals | | 5,841 | 164 (2.9) | 69 (1.2) | 21 (0.8) | 67 (1.2) | 25 (0.5) | 20 (0.7) |

Values in parentheses are percentages.

bladder irrigation and appropriate antibiotics. Rarely, cystectomy is required to prevent continued bladder hemorrhage unresponsive to medical treatment. Prompt management of acute radiation reactions may prevent more serious chronic complications, since it has been shown that patients who experience acute radiation reactions are at increased risk for severe enteric or urinary tract injury (Buchler et al, 1974).

The most frequent chronic complications of radiation therapy are vaginal stenosis, vesicovaginal or rectovaginal fistulas, and small bowel obstruction. *Vaginal stenosis* has been observed in approximately 70% of patients treated with radiation for cervical cancer (Abitbol and Davenport, 1974). This complication can be minimized by encouraging the patient to continue sexual activity during and immediately after radiation therapy. Patients who are not sexually active should use vaginal dilators to decrease narrowing and fibrosis of the vaginal tissues. Oral or intravaginal conjugated estrogens have also been advocated as a means of limiting radiation-induced vaginal stenosis. However, because estrogens can be rapidly absorbed across irradiated vaginal mucosa (Greenberg et al, 1984), estrogen should be combined with cyclic progesterone when given for this purpose.

*Rectovaginal or vesicovaginal fistulas* each occur in approximately 1% of patients undergoing radiation therapy for cervical cancer. Rectal ulceration usually occurs on the anterior wall at the site where the dose from the intracavitary implant is greatest. If the dose to the rectum is above normal-tissue tolerance or if the patient has underlying vascular disease, localized fibrosis, hypoxia, and necrosis can occur, with subsequent fistula formation. Proctoscopy should be performed in order to visualize the fistula site, and biopsy specimens should be taken from the edge of the fistula to rule out tumor recurrence. Usually, a temporary colostomy is performed to divert the fecal stream and facilitate healing. Before surgical correction is attempted, the margins of the fistula must be clean and have a reasonably good blood supply. The fistula tract should be excised and the rectal defect closed. When possible, an omental flap should be constructed and transposed to the operative site to provide a new blood supply. After the repair has healed, the colostomy can be reversed.

The same surgical principles apply to repair of radiation-related vesicovaginal fistulas. Small vesicovaginal fistulas can often be surgically corrected through a combined vesical and vaginal approach provided that pedicle flaps or omentum can be used to provide a blood supply. However, the failure rate in surgical repair of large radiation-related fistulas is high, often necessitating urinary diversion.

*Small bowel obstruction* is a severe complication that occurs in approximately 2% of patients undergoing definitive radiation therapy for cervical cancer. It is most common in those who have vascular disease or who have undergone abdominal surgery. Radiation-induced damage to the small arterioles in the mesentery often produces segmental hypoperfusion, with subsequent necrosis, obstruction, and perforation. Patients with intermittent partial small bowel obstruction present with a history of postprandial crampy abdominal pain, nausea, and weight loss. The diagnosis of obstruction is confirmed by the presence of dilated loops of small bowel on flat and upright films of the abdomen. Since patients are typically anemic and volume-depleted, blood, electrolyte, and colloid replacement should be instituted prior to surgical intervention. Patients with mild degrees of partial small bowel obstruction may be treated conservatively by nasogastric suction and total parenteral nutrition. However, surgery is required in more severe cases. The most common site of small bowel obstruction is the terminal ileum, which is relatively fixed in the radiation field by the cecum.

At present, there is some controversy concerning optimal surgical procedures to correct small bowel obstruction. A side-to-side ileocolonic bypass is the easiest and quickest procedure to perform (Wheeless, 1973). However, the bypassed segment may undergo further necrosis, with perforation and fistula formation between adjacent loops of bowel or between the small bowel and the skin. More recently, resection of the obstructed segment of small bowel with anastomosis of the small bowel to the ascending colon has been shown to be effective (Schmitt and Symmonds, 1982). When the terminal ileum is the site of obstruction, Smith and co-workers (1985) advocate resection of the involved small bowel segment and the cecum. The normal small bowel is then reanastomosed to the ascending colon in an end-to-end fashion. When these authors compared the complication rate in small bowel bypass with that in bowel resection with primary reanastomosis, the rate of enteric fistula formation was reduced in the patients who underwent primary resection, and mortality was decreased when resection rather than bypass was performed in cases of small bowel perforation.

## INVASIVE CERVICAL CANCER IN PREGNANCY

The incidence of invasive cervical cancer associated with pregnancy is approximately 1 per 2,200 pregnancies (Hacker et al, 1982), and 3% of all cases of cervical carcinoma occur in pregnant women (Donegan, 1983). All women should have a Pap test as part of their initial evaluation for pregnancy; those in whom cervical cytology is abnormal should undergo the same type of evaluation as nonpregnant patients. Histologic specimens of all areas found to be abnormal on colposcopy should be obtained using directed biopsies. Conization should be reserved for patients found to have microinvasive cancer on biopsy and preferably should be performed in the second trimester, since the reported risk for abortion after first-trimester conization is 15 to 33% (Moore et al, 1966; Averette et al, 1970). Conization during the third trimester is often associated with severe hemorrhage. Therefore, when microinvasive carcinoma is diagnosed on cervical biopsy during the third trimester, wedge biopsy may be preferable to conization to rule out frank invasion. Another alternative in this situation would be to allow vaginal delivery and then perform cervical conization post partum.

Patients with microinvasive carcinoma (less than 3 mm stromal invasion without lymph vascular space invasion) can continue the pregnancy, with repeat cytology and colposcopy every 2 months to assess tumor growth. Patients with normal cytology and colposcopy following conization can safely be allowed to deliver vaginally. Vaginal or abdominal hysterectomy should then be performed 2 to 3 months post partum. No cases of tumor recurrence have been reported in patients with microinvasive cervical cancer treated in this fashion (Hacker et al, 1982).

Optimal treatment for pregnant patients with cervical cancer depends on the stage of disease and the trimester at the time of diagnosis. Patients with non-bulky stage IB cervical cancer can usually be treated with radical hysterectomy and pelvic lymphadenectomy. If invasive cervical cancer is diagnosed during the first trimester, it is recommended that radical surgery be performed as soon as possible. If cervical cancer is diagnosed late in the second trimester, it may be possible to delay surgery for a short time until the fetal lungs have matured. Amniocentesis should be carried out at weekly or biweekly intervals, with surgery performed as soon as fetal lung maturity is confirmed. The surgical procedure of choice is cesarean section using a classic incision followed by radical hysterectomy and pelvic lymphadenectomy.

Radiation therapy is the therapeutic method of choice in pregnant patients with stage II to IV cervical cancer. This usually involves a combination of external and intracavitary therapy, and dosimetry is similar to that for the nonpregnant patient. If advanced-stage disease is diagnosed during the first trimester, radiation therapy should be started immediately and will often induce spontaneous abortion. In the second trimester, however, fetal tissues are less sensitive to radiation, and prolonged treatment-abortion intervals may be noted. Saunders and Landon (1988) reported a mean treatment-abortion interval of 43 days when radiation was initiated during the second trimester. For this reason, hysterotomy should be performed prior to radiation therapy when advanced-stage cervical cancer is diagnosed early in the second trimester.

The pregnancy can also be prolonged several weeks to assure fetal lung maturity if advanced-stage cervical cancer is diagnosed during the early third trimester. Cesarean section should be performed as soon as fetal lung maturity is established, with radiation therapy initiated shortly thereafter. Because of the increased risk for hemorrhage and infection, vaginal delivery through invasive cervical cancer continues to be contraindicated. Although there may be theoretical reasons why invasive cervical cancer should behave differently in the pregnant and nonpregnant patient, available data suggest that, stage for stage, the survival rates in these two groups are statistically similar (Hacker et al, 1982). Survival rates according to stage for pregnant patients with cervical cancer are summarized in Table 11-17.

## RECURRENT CERVICAL CANCER

The frequency of tumor recurrence is related to the stage of disease at the time of initial therapy. Before further therapy is initiated, histologic confirmation of tumor recurrence should be obtained in all cases. Treatment of recurrent cervical cancer depends upon such factors

TABLE 11-17  Five-Year Survival in Cervical Cancer During Pregnancy and Post Partum by Clinical Stage

| Stage | No. Treated | No. of Survivors (%) |
|---|---|---|
| IB | 367 | 273 (74.4) |
| II | 380 | 184 (48.4) |
| III/IV | 254 | 52 (20.8) |
| Totals | 1,001 | 509 (50.8) |

*Sources:* Bosch and Marcial (1966), Creasman et al (1970), Gorton (1965), Gustafsson and Kottmeier (1962), Jones and Osband (1960), McDuff et al (1956), Pratt and Malkasian (1964), Prem et al (1966), Sablinska et al (1977), Sall et al (1974), Stander and Lein (1960), Thompson et al (1975), Van Praagh et al (1965), Waldrop and Palmer (1963), Wanless (1971), Williams and Brack (1964).

as the method used for primary therapy, the site of recurrence, and the extent of disease.

*Radiation* can be effective in patients treated initially with radical surgery and usually involves a combination of a 4,500- to 5,000-cGy dose of radiation to a pelvic field followed by one intravaginal implant. CT scanning of the pelvis and paraaortic lymph nodes should be performed prior to radiation therapy to define the extent of disease. Fine-needle biopsy of enlarged paraaortic nodes will indicate whether extended-field radiation should be administered to patients with paraaortic metastases.

Krebs and coworkers (1982) reviewed the outcome of patients with recurrent cancer of the cervix after radical hysterectomy and node dissection. Radiation therapy was the most effective therapeutic method in these patients, yielding a 5-year survival rate of approximately 25%. Prognosis was better in patients with central pelvic recurrence than in those with more lateral disease.

When cervical cancer recurs after primary radiation, treatment can often be difficult. Most of these patients have received a full course of external and intracavitary therapy, and further radiation is of limited therapeutic benefit. Furthermore, radiation-induced fibrosis and arteriolar narrowing reduce tumor perfusion, so that chemotherapy is relatively ineffective. For this reason, radical surgery is the major treatment modality in such cases.

In selected patients with small-volume recurrence confined to the cervix itself, *radical hysterectomy and pelvic lymphadenectomy* can be performed (Van Dyke and van Nagell, 1975). Confirming the location of the tumor on CT scanning or MRI is imperative in these cases, so that tumor will not be encountered at the margins of surgical resection. In addition, vesicovaginal or rectovaginal fistulas following radical hysterectomy for recurrent cancer occur in as many as 25% of cases because of the proximity of the irradiated bladder and rectum to the cervix. In a report by Symmonds and coworkers (1964), 25 of 49 patients treated with radical hysterectomy and pelvic lymphadenectomy for recurrent carcinoma of the cervix were cured of disease, but the rate of fistula formation was 19%.

For these reasons, most oncologists recommend *pelvic exenteration* as the surgical procedure of choice in patients with recurrent cervical cancer. The one-stage method for cervical malignancy was first described by Alexander Brunschwig in 1948. Basically, there are three types of pelvic exenteration. Anterior pelvic exenteration, which combines radical cystectomy with radical hysterectomy and vaginectomy, is indicated in the treatment of recurrent disease limited to the cervix, anterior vagina, or bladder. Posterior pelvic exenteration combines abdominal perineal resection of the rectum with radical hysterectomy and vaginectomy; this procedure is indicated for lesions confined to the posterior fornix and rectovaginal septum. Total pelvic exenteration (Fig. 11-15), which involves the en bloc excision of the bladder, uterus, rectum, fallopian tubes, ovaries, and vagina, is most often required for recurrent cervical cancer.

Despite numerous surgical refinements, pelvic exenteration remains a formidable operation with a high complication rate. Therefore, every effort should be made to select the best candidates for whom cure can

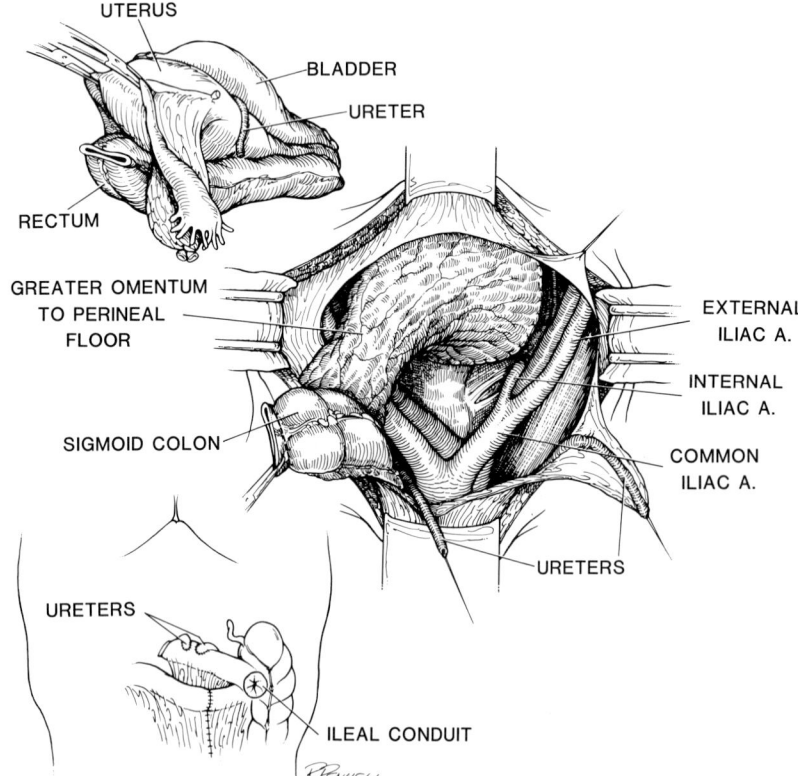

FIGURE 11-15 Total pelvic exenteration involving en bloc resection of the bladder, uterus, rectum, fallopian tubes, ovaries, and vagina. An omental graft is used to cover the defect in the pelvic floor and to provide a blood supply for low rectal anastomosis.

be achieved. A thorough investigation should be undertaken to rule out extrapelvic metastases, including a CT scan of the paraaortic lymph nodes. Any suspiciously enlarged lymph node should be sampled using fine-needle aspiration biopsy. Liver metastases can be identified on CT scan, and lung metastases are usually apparent on chest x-ray or tomographic scanning. In most recent series, approximately 25% of patients with recurrent cervical cancer are deemed satisfactory candidates for exenterative surgery.

Often, it is difficult to predict preoperatively which patients will have resectable lesions confined to the central pelvis. A number of contraindications to pelvic exenteration include:

1. Extrapelvic metastatic disease.
2. Metastases to the lateral pelvic lymph nodes.
3. Unilateral leg edema.
4. Ureteral obstruction by cervical cancer.
5. Sciatic pain suggesting neural involvement by recurrent cancer.

In addition, the patient's psychologic status is extremely important. Because of the extensive nature of the operation and the resultant physiologic alterations, the patient must have a stable personality and must be able to adjust to these changes. Although not an absolute contraindication to operation, psychologic instability or lack of a supportive family environment would be a reason to avoid pelvic exenteration.

When a patient with recurrent cervical cancer meets the above criteria, an exploratory laparotomy with intent to perform exenterative surgery is undertaken. Preoperatively, patients should be prepared for a major operative procedure, including mechanical and antibiotic bowel preparation and the administration of minidose heparin to prevent thromboembolic complications. During the past decade, interest in the nutritional status of patients undergoing pelvic exenteration has increased. As a result, total parenteral nutrition is usually begun prior to surgery and is continued during the postoperative period until normal bowel function returns. At the time of surgery, a thorough effort is made

to rule out lateral pelvic wall disease prior to committing the patient to exenteration. Lateral pelvic lymph nodes are inspected through a retroperitoneal approach, and appropriate biopsy specimens are obtained and sent for frozen-section examination. Likewise, careful inspection and selected sampling of the peritoneal surfaces of the upper abdomen should be carried out before proceeding with extirpative surgery.

The technique of pelvic exenteration has been modified in some ways since it was originally described. The first modifications involved methods of *urinary diversion*. In 1950, Bricker described the use of an isolated segment of terminal ileum as a urinary conduit (Fig. 11-16A). The subsequent use of ureteral stents has further protected ureteral-ileal anastomoses and has decreased the frequency of anastomotic leakage. Use of the sigmoid colon as a urinary conduit (Fig. 11-16B) was then proposed as an alternate method of urinary diversion (Schmitz et al, 1960; Symmonds and Gibbs, 1970). Although this method avoided reanastomosis of the small bowel, it was associated with a higher incidence of hyperchloremic acidosis than were ileal conduits (Symmonds and Jones, 1975). Schmidt and coworkers (1976) have recommended the transverse colon conduit as a preferred method of supravesical urinary diversion in patients undergoing pelvic exenteration. The advantage of this type of conduit is that the transverse colon and its mesentery are usually well outside the radiation field, and the frequency of ureteral-colonic anastomotic leaks is low. Since the transverse colon empties by mass action and not by peristalsis, either the proximal or the distal end can be used for the stoma. Most recently, a continent vesicotomy (Fig. 11-17) has been advocated. Following this procedure, the patient remains totally continent and performs intermittent self-catheterization to empty the conduit. Recently, Penalver and coworkers (1989) reported the results of continent urinary diversion using a colonic reservoir in nine patients undergoing pelvic exenteration. Postoperative urodynamic studies revealed that all patients were continent, with no evidence of urinary reflux.

A second technical advance in pelvic exenteration is

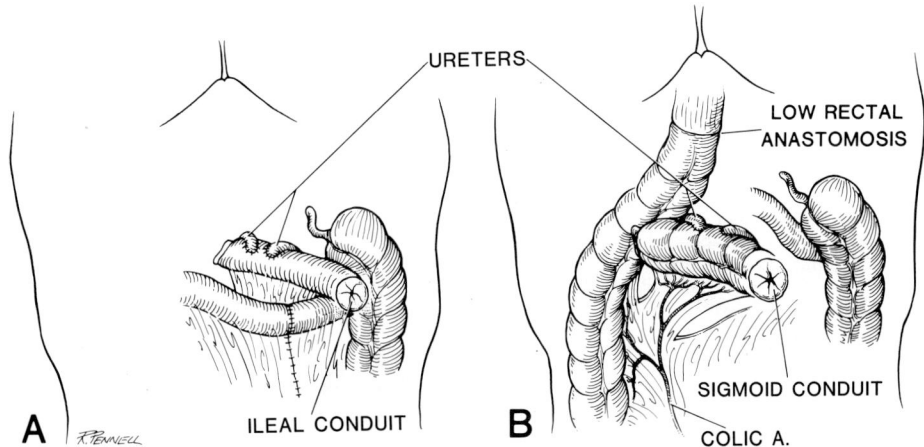

FIGURE 11-16 Two types of urinary diversion following pelvic exenteration. *A*, Segment of ileum is used as a urine conduit to the skin. *B*, Sigmoid colon conduit with low rectal anastomosis.

### Kock Ileal Reservoir

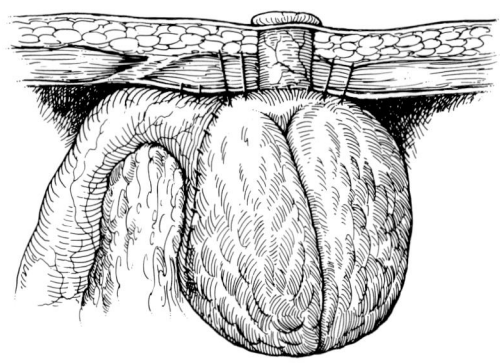

FIGURE 11-17  Continent vesicotomy. Two segments of ileum are anastomosed to form the pouch. The intussuscepted valve mechanism allows continence, and the patient performs periodic self-catheterization through the stoma.

the use of *low rectal anastomosis* (Fig. 11-18). The invention and refinement of the end-to-end circular stapling device has permitted low rectal anastomosis in patients who previously required sigmoid resection and colostomy. In a review of 20 patients undergoing low rectal anastomosis at the time of exenteration, Hatch

and coworkers (1988) reported that primary healing occurred in 70% of cases. Anastomotic leaks were more common when the rectal stump was less than 6 cm in length. These authors emphasized the importance of using an omental wrap to provide a blood supply to the anastomotic site. Bowel continence was excellent in over 60% of these patients. Recently, the use of a rectal J pouch has been proposed to decrease rectal tenesmus and fecal frequency in these patients (Wheeless and Hempling, 1989).

A third major development relates to *management of the pelvic floor*. Particularly after total pelvic exenteration, there is a major defect in the pelvic floor, which is often devoid of peritoneum. Consequently, the small bowel often adheres to the pelvis, resulting in obstruction or fistula formation. In 1976, Morley and Lindenauer reported the use of a free peritoneal graft to cover the denuded pelvic aperture following exenteration. Since then, these authors have reported using this procedure in 62 patients, and vaginal dehiscence or other complications related to reconstruction of the pelvic floor have not been observed (Morley et al, 1989). Several investigators have also reported excellent results using the omentum to cover the denuded pelvic floor after exenteration (see Fig. 11-15) (Buchsbaum and White, 1973; Webb and Symmonds, 1977). The right gastroepiploic artery is divided, and the omentum is

### Low Rectal Anastomosis

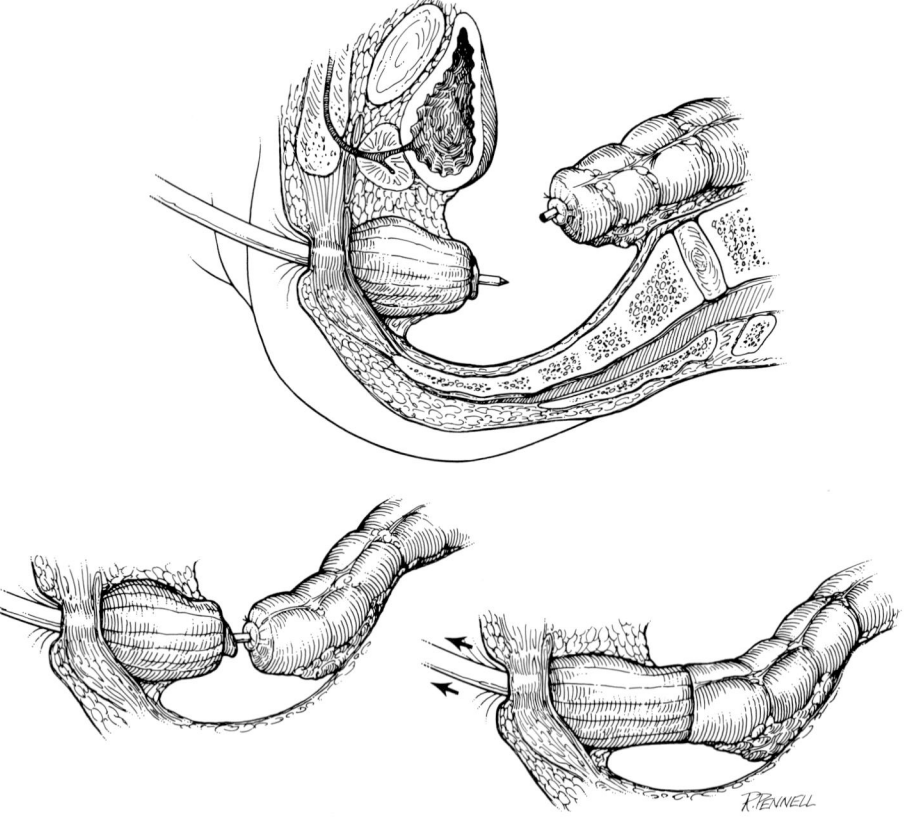

FIGURE 11-18  Low rectal anastomosis using end-to-end stapling device. When possible, an omental graft can be used to provide a blood supply to the suture line.

TABLE 11-18    Operative Mortality and 5-Year Survival After Pelvic Exenteration

| Author(s) | Year | Total Cases | Cases of Invasive Cervical Cancer | Operative Mortality (%) | 5-Year Survival (%) |
|---|---|---|---|---|---|
| Brunschwig | 1967 | 312 | 312 | 17.3 | 18 |
| Bricker | 1970 | 207 | 207 | 7.7 | 35 |
| Ketcham et al | 1970 | 162 | 162 | 7.4 | 38 |
| Symmonds et al | 1975 | 198 | 117 | 8.1 | 33 |
| Rutledge et al | 1977 | 296 | 196 | 13.5 | 37 |
| Averette et al | 1984 | 92 | 70 | 23.9 | 37 |
| Kraybill et al | 1988 | 99 | 66 | 14.1 | 45 |
| Shingleton et al | 1989 | 143 | 143 | 6.3 | 50 |
| Morley et al | 1989 | 100 | 66 | 2.0 | 61 |

detached from the stomach and transverse colon, passed along the left lateral paracolic space, and sutured to the pelvic floor. Hemovac drains are placed above the omental lid to remove lymphatic fluid from the pelvis, which may accumulate in volumes as high as 1,000 ml during the first 24 hours after surgery. Unfortunately, in some cases, the omentum may not be long enough to provide support to the pelvic floor. Recently, Vicryl mesh has been used to reconstruct the pelvic floor after exenterative surgery. This mesh, which is sutured across the pelvic brim to support the small bowel, successfully prevents small bowel adhesions but may be associated with a slight increase in the frequency of postoperative pelvic infection (Hoffman et al, 1989).

The final area of technical improvement in pelvic exenteration relates to *vaginal reconstruction.* Many patients are sexually active prior to surgery, and every effort must be made to maintain sexual function following exenteration. Split-thickness skin grafts can be used to create a neovagina; however, this technique requires a base of granulation tissue, which is difficult to achieve after total pelvic exenteration. Wheeless (1989) has reported the successful construction of a neovagina using an omental cylinder to form the base for split-thickness

skin grafts. However, most surgeons now favor the use of bilateral myocutaneous gracilis pedicle grafts to construct a neovagina following pelvic exenteration. These grafts not only form a functional vagina but also provide excellent pelvic support (Berek et al, 1984).

These technical modifications have significantly decreased operative mortality from pelvic exenteration over the past decade (Table 11-18). In the two most recent large series of patients undergoing pelvic exenteration, for example, operative mortality was less than 7% and the 5-year survival rate exceeded 50% (Shingleton et al, 1989; Morley et al, 1989).

Since isolated pelvic recurrence occurs infrequently after modern radiation therapy, the number of suitable candidates for pelvic exenteration continues to decline. Nevertheless, this operation remains an effective therapeutic method for properly selected patients with recurrent cervical cancer.

## CHEMOTHERAPY

Chemotherapy is the therapeutic method of choice for patients with extrapelvic metastases as well as for those

TABLE 11-19    Response of Squamous Cell Cervical Cancer to Single-Agent Chemotherapy

| Author(s) | Year | Drug | No. of Patients | Complete Response (%) | Partial Response (%) |
|---|---|---|---|---|---|
| Malkasian et al | 1964 | Fluorouracil | 22 | 0 | 23 |
| Smith et al | 1967 | Cyclophosphamide | 91 | 0 | 20 |
| Moore et al | 1968*a* | Mercaptopurine | 18 | 0 | 5 |
| Moore et al | 1968*b* | Chlorambucil | 26 | 4 | 23 |
| Mathe | 1970 | Bleomycin | 18 | 5 | 28 |
| Stolinsky and Bateman | 1973 | Hexamethylmelamine | 21 | 0 | 38 |
| Slavik | 1975 | Doxorubicin | 20 | 0 | 15 |
| Krakoff | 1977 | Bleomycin | 32 | 6 | 25 |
| Cavins and Geisler | 1978 | Doxorubicin (Adriamycin) | 18 | 6 | 33 |
| Thigpen et al | 1981 | Cisplatin | 34 | 9 | 30 |
| Potter et al | 1989 | Cisplatin | 68 | 16 | 24 |
| McGuire et al | 1989 | Carboplatin | 175 | 8 | 7 |
| | | Iproplatin | 177 | 4 | 7 |
| Totals | | | 720 | 4 | 22 |

TABLE 11-20　Response of Squamous Cell Cervical Cancer to Combination Chemotherapy

| Author(s) | Year | Drug Combination | No. of Patients | Complete Response (%) | Partial Response (%) |
|---|---|---|---|---|---|
| Papavasiliou | 1969 | Methotrexate and cyclo-phosphamide | 23 | 13 | 30 |
| Piel et al | 1973 | Methotrexate and bleomycin | 8 | 37 | 25 |
| Barlow et al | 1973 | Doxorubicin and bleomycin | 25 | 0 | 13 |
| Conroy et al | 1976 | Methotrexate and bleomycin | 20 | 0 | 60 |
| Day et al | 1978 | Doxorubicin-methyl CCNU | 31 | 29 | 16 |
| Baker et al | 1978 | Bleomycin, mitomycin, and vincristine | 50 | 16 | 44 |
| Greenberg et al | 1982 | Bleomycin and mito-mycin | 18 | 0 | 11 |
| Trope et al | 1986 | Doxorubicin and cis-platin | 31 | 7 | 10 |
| Alberts et al | 1987 | Mitomycin, vincristine, bleomycin, and cisplatin | 54 | 7 | 15 |
| Alberts et al | 1987 | Mitomycin and cisplatin | 51 | 4 | 51 |
| Rustin et al | 1987 | Vincristine, methotrexate, bleomycin, and cisplatin | 19 | 11 | 37 |
| Giannone et al | 1987 | Mitomycin, vincristine, bleomycin, and cisplatin | 16 | 13 | 31 |
| Rustin and Newlands | 1988 | Carboplatin, vincristine, methotrexate, and bleo-mycin | 19 | 0 | 26 |
| Buxton et al | 1989 | Bleomycin, ifosfamide, and cisplatin | 49 | 20 | 49 |
| Totals | | | 414 | 11 | 28 |

previously treated with surgery and irradiation who have recurrent tumor. The responses of squamous cell cervical cancers to single-agent chemotherapy are summarized in Table 11-19. In these studies, total disappearance of tumor was considered a complete response, whereas partial response was defined as a reduction in the measurable perpendicular tumor dimensions of at least 50% for 1 month or more. The best results were obtained with cisplatin, which led to a partial response in 24% of cases and a complete response in 16% in patients with advanced squamous cell cancer of the cervix (McGuire et al, 1989). This is similar to the GOG experience, in which 800 patients were treated with cisplatin, and the response rate was 23% (Thigpen et al, 1987). In these trials the usual dose of cisplatin was 50 mg/m$^2$ every 3 weeks. In a subsequent study, the GOG compared low-dose cisplatin (50 mg/m$^2$) given every 3 weeks to high-dose cisplatin (100 mg/m$^2$) given every 3 weeks. Although response rates improved approximately 10% among patients who received the higher dose regimen, this difference was not statistically significant.

At present, interest is focused on several cisplatin analogues that cause less nephrotoxicity than the parent

TABLE 11-21　Results of Chemotherapy for Adenocarcinoma of the Cervix

| Authors | Year | No. of Patients | Agents | Partial Response (%) | Complete Response (%) | Median Survival (mo) |
|---|---|---|---|---|---|---|
| Slayton et al | 1984 | 19 | Etoposide | 5 | — | — |
| Thigpen et al | 1986 | 14 | Piperazinedione | — | 14 | 2.0 |
| | 1986 | 20 | Cisplatin | 15 | 5 | 7.3 |
| Kavanagh et al | 1987 | 24 | FDC | 17 | 25 | 18.0 |

FDC = 5-fluorouracil, doxorubicin, and cisplatin.

compound. The GOG conducted a randomized trial of two of these analogues, iproplatin (CHIP) and carboplatin (CBDCA), in patients with squamous cell carcinoma of the cervix. Both these analogues showed some activity against squamous cell carcinoma, but both were inferior to cisplatin (McGuire et al, 1989). In most studies, the response of cervical cancer to cisplatin has been short-lived (3 to 6 months). However, in isolated cases complete responses have lasted longer than one year.

Data on the efficacy of combination chemotherapy in the treatment of squamous cell carcinoma of the cervix are presented in Table 11-20. To date, the most effective regimens all contain cisplatin. However, there is little objective evidence to suggest that any one of these regimens is superior to single-agent therapy with cisplatin, so that large prospective randomized trials to compare these combinations with cisplatin alone are needed. Although the reported number of patients with adenocarcinoma of the cervix receiving chemotherapy is small, available data indicate that platinum-based combination chemotherapy is also the most effective treatment in these cases (Table 11-21). As in squamous cell carcinoma, there is little objective evidence to suggest that combination chemotherapy is superior to platinum alone.

## SURVIVAL AND FOLLOWUP

The 5-year survival rates for patients with invasive cervical cancer treated at various centers throughout the world are summarized in the FIGO Annual Report on the Results of Treatment in Gynecological Cancer (Pettersson, 1988) (Table 11-22). Since the contributing centers represent widely divergent geographic and socioeconomic areas, results of treatment often vary significantly from one institution to another. In general, survival rates are highest in centers where there is a standardized evaluation system and multidisciplinary consultation, allowing therapy to be individualized.

Among the patients with recurrent cervical cancer, lesions recur within 12 months of therapy in about 50% and within 2 years in 75% (van Nagell et al, 1979*b*; Fuller et al, 1989). Because over 70% of women with pelvic recurrence will have abnormal cervical cytology, patients should be examined at least every 2 months

after therapy for one year and every 6 months thereafter. Cervical cytologic specimens should be obtained at the time of these regular examinations. Since ureteral obstruction by tumor still remains the most common cause of death in cervical cancer, intravenous pyelography should be performed at yearly intervals to rule out occult recurrence. In addition, an annual chest x-ray is indicated in order to detect pulmonary metastases. Should these tests be abnormal, CT scanning or MRI with directed biopsies should be performed to confirm tumor recurrence histologically.

## REFERENCES

Abitbol M, Davenport JH: The irradiated vagina. *Obstet Gynecol* 44:249, 1974.

Alberts DS, Mason-Liddil N: The role of cisplatin in the management of advanced squamous cell cancer of the cervix. *Semin Oncol* 16:66, 1989.

Alberts DS, Kronmal R, Baker LH, Stock-Novak D, Surwit E, Boutselis J, Hannigan E: Phase II randomized trial of cisplatin chemotherapy regimens in the treatment of recurrent or metastatic squamous cell cancer of the cervix. A Southwest Oncology Group study. *J Clin Oncol* 5:1791, 1987.

Alert J, Jimenez J, Beldarrain L, Montalvo J, Roca C: Complications from irradiation of carcinoma of the uterine cervix. *Acta Radiol* 19:13, 1980.

American Cancer Society: *Cancer Facts and Figures—1988*. New York, NY, 1988.

Andras EJ, Fletcher GH, Rutledge F: Radiotherapy of carcinoma of the cervix following simple hysterectomy. *Am J Obstet Gynecol* 115:647, 1973.

Angel C, Beecham J, Rubens D: Magnetic resonance imaging and pathologic correlation in stage IB cervix cancer. *Gynecol Oncol* 27:357, 1987.

Artman LE, Hoskins WJ, Bibro MC, Heller PB, Weiser EB, Barnhill DR, Park RC: Radical hysterectomy and pelvic lymphadenectomy for stage IB carcinoma of the cervix: 21 years experience. *Gynecol Oncol* 28:8, 1987.

Aurelian L, Kessler II, Rosenshein NB, Barbour G: Viruses and gynecologic cancers: Herpes-virus protein. A cervical tumor antigen that fulfills the criteria for a marker of carcinogenicity. *Cancer* 48:455, 1981.

Averette HE, Ford JH Jr, Dudan RC, Girtanner RE, Hoskins WJ, Lutz MH: Staging of cervical cancer. *Clin Obstet Gynecol* 18:215, 1975.

Averette HE, Lichtinger M, Sevin BU, Girtanner RE: Pelvic exenteration: A 15-year experience in a general metropolitan hospital. *Am J Obstet Gynecol* 150:179, 1984.

Averette HE, Nasser N, Yankow SL: Cervical conization in pregnancy. *Am J Obstet Gynecol* 106:543, 1970.

Averette HE, Nelson JH, Ng AG, Hoskins WJ, Boyce JG, Ford JH Jr: Diagnosis and management of microinvasive (stage IA) carcinoma of the uterine cervix. *Cancer* 38:414, 1976.

Baker LH, Opipari M, Wilson H: Mitomycin C, vincristine and bleomycin therapy for advanced cervical cancer. *Obstet Gynecol* 52:146, 1978.

Ballon SC, Berman ML, Lagasse LD, Petrilli ES, Castaldo TW: Survival after extraperitoneal pelvic and paraaortic lymphadenectomy and radiation therapy in cervical carcinoma. *Obstet Gynecol* 57:90, 1981.

Barber HRK, Sommers SC, Rotterdam H, Kwon T: Vascular invasion as a prognostic factor in stage IB cancer of the cervix. *Obstet Gynecol* 52:343, 1977.

Barlow J, Piver M, Chuang J: Adriamycin and bleomycin alone and in combination in gynecologic cancers. *Cancer* 32:735, 1973.

Barrasso R, DeBrux J, Croissant O, Orth G: High prevalence of papillomavirus-associated penile intraepithelial neoplasia in sexual partners of women with cervical intraepithelial neoplasia. *N Engl J Med* 317:916, 1987.

Beaudenon S, Kremsdorf D, Croissant O, Jablonska S, Wain-Hobson

TABLE 11-22   Five-Year Survival of Patients with Cervical Cancer According to Stage

| Stage | No. of Patients | 5-Year Survival (%) |
|-------|-----------------|---------------------|
| I     | 10,933          | 79.4                |
| II    | 12,561          | 58.2                |
| III   | 9,139           | 31.4                |
| IV    | 1,461           | 8.4                 |

*Source:* Pettersson F (ed): International Federation of Gynecology and Obstetrics (FIGO) Annual Report on the Results of Treatment in Gynecological Cancer. Stockholm, Panorama Press AB, 1988.

S, Orth G: A novel type of human papillomavirus associated with genital neoplasias. *Nature* 321:246, 1986.

Berek JS, Hacker NF, Lagasse LD: Vaginal reconstruction performed simultaneously with pelvic exenteration. *Obstet Gynecol* 63:318, 1984.

Berek JS, Hacker NF, Fu YS, Sokale JR, Leuchter RC, Lagasse LD: Adenocarcinoma of the uterine cervix: Histologic variables associated with lymph node metastasis and survival. *Obstet Gynecol* 65:46, 1985.

Berman ML, Keys H, Creasman W, DiSaia P, Bundy B, Blessing J: Survival and patterns of recurrence in cervical cancer metastatic to para-aortic lymph nodes. *Gynecol Oncol* 19:8, 1984.

Bosch A, Frias Z: Complications after radiation therapy for cervical carcinoma. *Acta Radiol Ther Phys Biol* 16:53, 1977.

Bosch A, Marcial VA: Carcinoma of the uterine cervix associated with pregnancy. *Am J Roentgenol* 96:92, 1966.

Bricker EM: Bladder substitution after pelvic evisceration. *Surg Clin NA* 30:1511, 1950.

Bricker EM: Pelvic exenteration. In *Advances in Surgery*, Vol 4. Chicago, Year Book Medical Publishers, 1970.

Brinton L, Haenszel W, Stolley P, Schairer C, Lehman HF, Levine R, Savitz R: Cigarette smoking and invasive cervical cancer. *JAMA* 255:3265, 1986.

Brunschwig A: Complete excision of the pelvic viscera for advanced carcinoma. *Cancer* 1:177, 1948.

Brunschwig A: Surgical treatment of carcinoma of the cervix, recurrent after irradiation or combination of irradiation and surgery. *Am J Roentgenol* 99:365, 1967.

Buchler DP, Kline JC, Carr WF: Intracavitary dosimetry for carcinoma of the cervix and subsequent complications. *Am J Obstet Gynecol* 120:83, 1974.

Buchsbaum HJ: Extrapelvic lymph node metastases in cervical carcinoma. *Am J Obstet Gynecol* 133:814, 1979.

Buchsbaum HJ, White AJ: Omental sling for management of the pelvic floor following exenteration. *Am J Obstet Gynecol* 117:407, 1973.

Buxton EJ, Meanwell CA, Hilton C, Mould JJ, Spooner D, Chetiyawardana A, Latief T, Paterson M, Redman CW, Luesley DM, Blackledge GR: Combination bleomycin, ifosfamide, and cisplatin chemotherapy in cervical cancer. *J Natl Cancer Inst* 81:359, 1989.

Byfield JE: Theoretical basis and clinical applications of 5-fluorouracil as a radiosensitizer. In Rosenthal CJ, Rotman M (eds): *Clinical Applications of Continuous Infusion Chemotherapy and Concomitant Radiation Therapy*. New York, Plenum Press, 1986, pp 113-125.

Cavins JA, Geisler HE: Treatment of advanced unresectable, cervical carcinoma already subjected to complete irradiation therapy. *Gynecol Oncol* 6:256, 1978.

Chamberlain G: Etiology of gynecological cancer. *J Roy Soc Med* 74:246, 1981.

Choo YC, Choy TK, Wong LC, Ma HA: Potentiation of radiotherapy by cis-dichlorodiammine platinum (II) in advanced cervical carcinoma. *Gynecol Oncol* 23:94, 1986.

Christensen A, Foglmann R: Cervical carcinoma stage I and II treated by primary radical hysterectomy and pelvic lymphadenectomy: 320 cases by the method of Meigs-Taussig and 350 by the method of Okabayashi. *Acta Obstet Gynecol Scand Suppl* 58:1, 1976.

Christopherson WM, Lundin FE, Mendez WM, Winifred M, Parker JE: Cervical cancer control: A study of morbidity and trends over a twenty-one year period. *Cancer* 38:1357, 1976.

Chung C, Nahhas W, Stryker J, Curry S: Analysis of factors contributing to treatment failures in stage IB and IIA carcinoma of the cervix. *Am J Obstet Gynecol* 138:550, 1980.

Clark JG: A more radical method of performing hysterectomy for cancer of the uterus. *Johns Hopkins Bull* 53:120, 1895.

Clarke-Pearson DL, Synan I, Henshaw M, Coleman E, Creasman W: Prevention of postoperative venous thromboembolism by external pneumatic calf compression in patients with gynecologic malignancy. *Obstet Gynecol* 63:92, 1984.

Combes PF, Daly NJ, Horiot JC, Achille E, Keiling R, Pigneux J, Pourquier R, Rozan R, Schraub S, Vrousos C: Results of radiotherapy alone in 581 patients with stage II carcinoma of the uterine cervix. *Int J Radiat Oncol Biol Phys* 11:463, 1985.

Conroy J, Lewis G, Brady L: Low dose bleomycin and methotrexate in cervical cancer. *Cancer* 37:550, 1976.

Cosbie WG: Radiotherapy following hysterectomy performed for or in the presence of cancer of the cervix. *Am J Obstet Gynecol* 85:332, 1963.

Coughlin CT, Richmond RC: Biologic and clinical developments of cisplatin combined with radiation: Concepts, utility, projections for new trials, and the emergence of carboplatin. *Semin Oncol* 16:31, 1989.

Creasman WT, Rutledge FN, Fletcher GH: Carcinoma of the cervix associated with pregnancy. *Obstet Gynecol* 36:495, 1970.

Crum C, Ikenberg H, Richart RM, Gissman L: Human papillomavirus type 16 and early cervical neoplasia. *N Engl J Med* 310:880, 1984.

Cummings B, Keane T, Thomas G, Harwood A, Rider W: Results and toxicity of the treatment of anal canal carcinoma by radiation therapy or radiation therapy and chemotherapy. *Cancer* 54:2062, 1984.

Davy M, Bentzen H, Jahren R: Simple hysterectomy in the presence of invasive cervical cancer. *Acta Obstet Gynecol Scand* 56:105, 1977.

Day NE: The epidemiological basis for evaluating different screening policies. *IARC Sci Publ* 76:199, 1986.

Day T, Wharton J, Gottlieb JA, Rutledge FN: Chemotherapy for squamous carcinoma of the cervix: Doxorubicin-methyl CCNU. *Am J Obstet Gynecol* 132:545, 1978.

Delgado G, Chun B, Caglar H, Bepko F: Para-aortic lymphadenectomy in gynecologic malignancies confined to the pelvis. *Obstet Gynecol* 50:418, 1977.

DePriest PD, Gallion HH, van Nagell JR Jr: The efficacy of radical hysterectomy with pelvic lymphadenectomy as a treatment method in patients with stage IB cervical cancer 3 cm in diameter. *Gynecol Oncol* (in press).

Donegan WL: Cancer in pregnancy. *CA—A Cancer Journal for Clinicians* 33:5, 1983.

Douple EB, Richmond RC: Platinum complexes as radiosensitizers of hypoxic mammalian cells. *Br J Cancer* 37:98, 1978.

Durrance FY: Radiotherapy following simple hysterectomy in patients with stage I and II carcinoma of the cervix. *Am J Roentgenol Radiat Th Nucl Med* 116:165, 1969.

Durrance FY, Fletcher GH, Rutledge FN: Analysis of central recurrent disease in stages I and II squamous cell carcinomas of the cervix on intact uterus. *Am J Roentgenol Radiat Th Nucl Med* 106:831, 1969.

Durst M, Gissmann L, Ikenberg H, zur Hausen H: A papillomavirus DNA from a cervical carcinoma and its prevalence in cancer biopsy samples from different geographic regions. *Proc Natl Acad Sci [USA]* 80:3812, 1983.

Evans LS, Kersh CR, Constable WC, Taylor PT: Concomitant 5-fluorouracil, mitomycin-c, and radiotherapy for advanced gynecologic malignancies. *Int J Radiat Oncol Biol Phys* 15:901, 1988.

Ferry JA, Scully RE: Adenoid cystic carcinoma and adenoid basal carcinoma of the uterine cervix. *Am J Surg Pathol* 12:134, 1988.

Fink DJ: Change in American Cancer Society check-up guidelines for detection of cervical cancer. *Cancer* 38:127, 1988.

Forney JP: The effect of radical hysterectomy on bladder physiology. *Am J Obstet Gynecol* 138:374-382, 1980.

Fouchee JH, Greiss FC, Loch FR: Stage IA squamous cell carcinoma of the uterine cervix. *Am J Obstet Gynecol* 105:46, 1969.

Fuller AT, Elliott N, Kosloff C, Hoskins WJ, Lewis JL: Determinants of increased risk for recurrence in patients undergoing radical hysterectomy for stage IB and IIA carcinoma of the cervix. *Gynecol Oncol* 33:34, 1989.

Gallion HH, Maruyama Y, van Nagell JR Jr, Donaldson ES, Rowley KC, Yoneda J, Beach JL, Powell DE, Kryscio RJ: Treatment of stage IIIB cervical cancer with californium-252 fast neutron brachytherapy and external photon therapy. *Cancer* 59:1709, 1987.

Gallion HH, van Nagell JR Jr, Donaldson ES, Hanson MB, Powell DE, Maruyama Y, Yoneda J: Combined radiation therapy and extrafascial hysterectomy in the treatment of stage IB barrel-shaped cervical cancer. *Cancer* 56:262-265, 1985.

Gaspar LE, Cheung AY, Allen H: Cervical carcinoma: Treatment results and complications of extended-field irradiation. *Radiology* 172:271, 1989.

Gauthier P, Gore I, Shingleton HM, Soong SJ, Orr JW, Hatch KD: Identification of histopathologic risk groups in stage IB squamous cell carcinoma of the cervix. *Obstet Gynecol* 66:569, 1985.

Genton E, Turpie AGG: Venous thromboembolism associated with gynecologic surgery. In Pitkin RM (ed): *Clinical Obstetrics and*

*Gynecology.* Hagerstown, Maryland, Harper & Row, 1980, pp 209-241.

Giannone L, Brenner DE, Jones HW, Greco FA, Burnett LS: Combination chemotherapy for patients with advanced carcinoma of the cervix: Trial of mitomycin-c, vincristine, bleomycin, and cisplatin. *Gynecol Oncol* 26:178, 1987.

Glucksman A, Cherry C: Incidence, histology and response to radiation of mixed carcinomas (adenoacanthomas) of the uterine cervix. *Cancer* 9:971, 1956.

Gorton G: Carcinoma of the uterine cervix in pregnancy. *Acta Obstet Gynecol Scand* 44:71, 1965.

Green TH, Morse WJ: Management of invasive cervical cancer following inadvertent simple hysterectomy. *Obstet Gynecol* 33:763, 1969.

Greenberg BR, Hannigan J, Gerretson L: Sequential combination of bleomycin and mitomycin in advanced cervical cancer: An American experience. A Northern California Oncology Group Study. *Cancer Treat Rep* 66:163, 1982.

Greenberg H, Penney LL, Smith ML: Transvaginal absorption of estrogens through irradiated mucosa. *Gynecol Oncol* 17:301, 1984.

Gustafsson DC, Kottmeier HL: Carcinoma of the cervix associated with pregnancy. *Acta Obstet Gynecol Scand* 41:1, 1962.

Hacker NF, Berek JS, Lagasse LD, Elseworth HC, Savage E, Moore G: Carcinoma of the cervix in pregnancy. *Obstet Gynecol* 58:735, 1982.

Hamberger AD, Unal A, Gershenson DM, Fletcher GH: Analysis of the severe complications of irradiation of carcinoma of the cervix: Whole pelvis irradiation and intracavitary radium. *Int J Radiat Oncol Biol Phys* 9:367, 1983.

Hardt N, van Nagell JR Jr, Hanson MB, Donaldson ES, Yoneda J, Maruyama Y: Radiation-induced tumor regression as a prognostic factor in patients with invasive cervical cancer. *Cancer* 49:35, 1982.

Hatch KD, Shingleton HM, Potter ME, Baker VV: Low rectal resection and anastomosis at the time of pelvic exenteration. *Gynecol Oncol* 32:262, 1988.

Hendriksen E: The lymphatic spread of carcinoma of the cervix and the body of the uterus, a study of 420 necropsies. *Am J Obstet Gynecol* 58:924, 1949.

Henk JM: The role of radiosensitizers. In Hope-Stone HF (ed): *Radiotherapy in Clinical Practice.* London, Butterworths, 1986, pp 19-26.

Hoffman MS, Roberts WS, LaPolla JP, Cavanaugh D: Use of Vicryl mesh in the reconstruction of the pelvic floor following exenteration. *Gynecol Oncol* 35:170, 1989.

Hopkins MP, Peters WA, Anderson W, Morley GW: Invasive cervical cancer treated initially by standard hysterectomy. *Gynecol Oncol* 36:7, 1990.

Hopkins MP, Schmidt RW, Roberts JA, Morley GW: Gland cell carcinoma (adenocarcinoma) of the cervix. *Obstet Gynecol* 72:789, 1988*a*.

Hopkins MP, Schmidt RW, Roberts JA, Morley GW: The prognosis and treatment of stage I adenocarcinoma of the cervix. *Obstet Gynecol* 72:915, 1988*b*.

Horii T, Mitsumoto T, Noda K: Significance of paraaortic node irradiation in the treatment of cervical cancer. *Gynecol Oncol* 31:371, 1988.

Hoskins WJ, Ford JH, Lutz MH, Averette HE: Radical hysterectomy and pelvic lymphadenectomy for the management of early invasive cancer of the cervix. *Gynecol Oncol* 4:278, 1976.

Hreshchyshyn MM, Aron BS, Boronow RC, Franklin EW, Shingleton HM, Blessing JA: Hydroxyurea or placebo combined with radiation to treat stages IIIB and IV cervical cancer confined to the pelvis. *Int J Radiat Oncol Biol Phys* 5:317, 1979.

Hughes RR, Brewington KC, Hanjani P, Photopulos G, Dick D, Votava C, Moran M, Coleman S: Extended field irradiation for cervical cancer based on surgical staging. *Gynecol Oncol* 9:153, 1980.

Inoue T: Prognostic significance of the depth of invasion relating to nodal metastases, parametrial extension, and cell types. *Cancer* 54:3035, 1984.

Inoue T, Okumura M: Prognostic significance of parametrial extension in patients with cervical carcinoma stages IB, IIA, and IIB. A study of 628 cases treated by radical hysterectomy and lymphadenectomy with or without postoperative irradiation. *Cancer* 54:1714, 1984.

International Multicentre Trial: Prevention of fatal postoperative pulmonary embolism by low doses of heparin. *Lancet* 2:45, 1975.

Johannesson G, Geinsson G, Day N: The effect of mass screening in Iceland 1965-1974 on the incidence and mortality of cervical cancer. *Int J Cancer* 21:418, 1978.

Jones WN, Osband R: Cancer of the cervix in pregnancy. *South Med J* 53:199, 1960.

Karlan BY, Byfield JE, Lagasse LD: Multimodality therapy for gynecologic malignancies. *Contemp Ob Gyn,* 33:27, 1989.

Kato H, Torigoe T: Radioimmunoassay for tumor antigen of human cervical squamous cell carcinoma. *Cancer* 40:1621, 1977.

Kavanagh JJ, Gershenson D, Copeland L, Roberts WS: Combination chemotherapy for metastatic or recurrent adenocarcinoma of the cervix. *Clin Oncol* 5:1621, 1987.

Kenter GG, Ansink AC, Heintz AP, Aartsen EJ, Delemarre JF, Hart AA: Carcinoma of the uterine cervix stage I and IIA. Results of surgical treatment: Complications, recurrence and survival. *Eur J Surg Oncol* 15:55, 1989.

Kessler II: Human cervical cancer as a venereal disease. *Cancer Res* 36:783, 1976.

Kessler II: Venereal factors in human cervical cancer: Evidence from marital clusters. *Cancer* 39:1912, 1977.

Ketcham AS, Deckers PJ, Sugarbaker EV, Hoye RC, Thomas LB, Smith RR: Pelvic exenteration for carcinoma of the uterine cervix. *Cancer* 26:513, 1970.

Kilgore LC, Soong SJ, Gore H, Shingleton HM, Hatch KD, Partridge EE: Analysis of prognostic features in adenocarcinoma of the cervix. *Gynecol Oncol* 31:137, 1988.

King LA, Talledo E, Gallup DG, Melhus O, Otken LB: Adenoid cystic carcinoma of the cervix in women under the age of 40. *Gynecol Oncol* 32:26, 1989.

Kinney WK, Alvarez RD, Reid GC, Schray MF, Soong SJ, Morley GW, Podratz KC, Shingleton HM: Value of adjuvant whole-pelvis irradiation after Wertheim hysterectomy for early-stage squamous carcinoma of the cervix with pelvic nodal metastasis: A matched-control study. *Gynecol Oncol* 34:258, 1989.

Krakoff IH: Clinical, pharmacologic, and therapeutic studies of bleomycin given by continuous infusion. *Cancer* 40:2027, 1977.

Kraybill WG, Lopez M, Bricker EM: Total pelvic exenteration as a therapeutic option in advanced malignant disease of the pelvis. *Surg Gynecol Obstet* 166:259, 1988.

Krebs HB, Helmkamp BF, Sevin B-U, Poliakoff SR, Nadji M, Averette H: Recurrent carcinoma of the cervix following radical hysterectomy and pelvic node dissection. *Obstet Gynecol* 59:422, 1982.

Lagasse LD, Creasman WT, Shingleton HM, Ford JH, Blessing JA: Results and complications of operative staging in cervical cancer experience of the Gynecologic Oncology Group. *Gynecol Oncol* 9:90, 1980.

Langley II, Moore DW, Tarnasky JW, Roberts PH: Radical hysterectomy and pelvic lymph node dissection. *Gynecol Oncol* 9:37, 1980.

LaPolla JP, Schlaerth JB, Gaddis O Jr, Morrow CP: The influence of surgical staging on the evaluation and treatment of patients with cervical carcinoma. *Gynecol Oncol* 24:194, 1986.

Lee YN, Wang KL, Lin MH, Liu CH, Wang KG, Lan CC, Chuang JT, Chen AC, Wu CC: Radical hysterectomy with pelvic lymph node dissection for treatment of cervical cancer: A clinical review of 954 cases. *Gynecol Oncol* 32:135, 1989.

Leman MH, Benson WL, Kurman RJ, Park RC: Microinvasive carcinoma of the cervix. *Obstet Gynecol* 48:571, 1976.

Lerner HM, Jones HW III, Hill EC: Radical surgery for the treatment of early invasive cervical carcinoma (stage IB): Review of 15 years' experience. *Obstet Gynecol* 56:413, 1980.

Littman P, Clement PB, Henriksen B, Wang CC, Robboy SJ, Taft PD, Ulfelder H, Scully RE: Glassy cell carcinoma of the cervix. *Cancer* 37:2238, 1976.

Lorincz AT, Temple GF, Kurman RJ, Jenson AB, Lancaster WD: Oncogenic association of specific human papillomavirus types with cervical neoplasia. *J Natl Cancer Inst* 79:671, 1987.

Lovecchio JL, Averette HE, Donato D, Bell J: Five-year survival of patients with periaortic nodal metastases in clinical stage IB and IIA cervical carcinoma. *Gynecol Oncol* 34:43, 1989.

Low JA, Mauger GM, Carmichael JA: The effect of Wertheim hysterectomy upon bladder and urethral function. *Am J Obstet Gynecol* 139:826, 1981.

Maiman M, Feurer G, Boyce J: Value of squamous cell carcinoma antigen levels in invasive cervical carcinoma. *Gynecol Oncol* 32:96, 1989.

Malkasian GD, Decker D, Muney E: Preliminary observations of carcinoma of the cervix treated with 5-fluorouracil. *Am J Obstet Gynecol* 88:82, 1964.

Marcial VA, Bosch A: Radiation-induced tumor regression in carcinoma of the uterine cervix: Prognostic significance. *Am J Roentgenol* 108:113, 1970.

Martinbeau PW, Kjorstad KE, Iversen T: Stage IB carcinoma of the cervix, the Norwegian Hospital. II. Results when pelvic nodes are involved. *Obstet Gynecol* 60:215, 1982.

Maruyama Y, van Nagell JR Jr: Radiation therapy in the treatment of invasive cervical cancer. In van Nagell JR Jr, Barber HRK (eds): *Modern Concepts of Gynecologic Oncology.* Littleton, Massachusetts, John Wright Publisher, 1982, pp 91-158.

Maruyama Y, van Nagell JR Jr, Yoneda J, Donaldson E, Gallion H, Rowley K, Kryscio R, Beach JL: Phase I-II clinical trial of californium-252. Treatment of stage IB carcinoma of the cervix. *Cancer* 59:1500-1505, 1987.

Mathe G: Study of the clinical efficacy of bleomycin in human cancer. *Br Med J* 2:243, 1970.

Matsuyama T, Tsukamoto N, Imachi M, Nakano H: Bone metastases from cervix cancer. *Gynecol Oncol* 32:72, 1989.

McDougall JK, Galloway DA, Crum C, Levine R, Richart R, Fenoglio CM: Detection of nucleic acid sequences in cervical tumors. *Gynecol Oncol* 12:S42, 1981.

McDuff HC Jr, Carney WI, Waterman GW: Cancer of the cervix and pregnancy. *Obstet Gynecol* 8:196, 1956.

McGuire WP, Arseneau J, Blessing JA, DiSaia PJ, Hatch KD, Given FT, Teng NH, Creasman WT: A randomized comparative trial of carboplatin and iproplatin in advanced squamous carcinoma of the uterine cervix: A Gynecologic Oncology Group study. *J Clin Oncol* 7:1462, 1989.

Melnick S, Cole P, Anderson D, Herbst A: Rates and risks of diethylstilbestrol-related clear cell adenocarcinoma of the vagina and cervix. *N Engl J Med* 316:514, 1987.

Micha J, Kucera P, Birkett J, Chambers G, Sheets EE, DiSaia PJ: Prophylactic mezlocillin in radical hysterectomy. *Obstet Gynecol* 69:251, 1987.

Mikuta JJ, Celebre JA: Adenocarcinoma of the cervix. *Obstet Gynecol* 33:753, 1969.

Miyazawa K, Hernandez E, Dillon MB: Prophylactic topical cefamandole in radical hysterectomy. *Int J Obstet Gynecol* 25:133, 1987.

Montana GS, Fowler WC, Varia MA, Walton LA, Mack Y: Analysis of results of radiation therapy for stage IB carcinoma of the cervix. *Cancer* 60:2195, 1987.

Moore G, Bross I, Austman R: Effects of 5-mercaptopurine in 290 patients with cancer. *Cancer Chemother Rep* 52:655, 1968a.

Moore G, Bross I, Austman R: Effects of chlorambucil in 374 patients with advanced cancer. *Cancer Chemother Rep* 52:661, 1968b.

Moore JG, Wells RG, Morton DG: Management of superficial cervical cancer in pregnancy. *Obstet Gynecol* 27:307, 1966.

Morley GW, Lindenauer J: Pelvic exenterative surgery for gynecologic malignancy. *Cancer* 38:581, 1976.

Morley GW, Hopkins MP, Lindenauer SM, Roberts JA: Pelvic exenteration, University of Michigan: 100 patients at 5 years. *Obstet Gynecol* 74:934, 1989.

Morrow CP: Panel Report: Is pelvic radiation beneficial in the postoperative management of stage IB squamous cell carcinoma of the cervix with pelvic node metastasis treated by radical hysterectomy and pelvic lymphadenectomy? *Gynecol Oncol* 10:105, 1980.

Nahmias AJ, Sawanabori S: The genital herpes–cervical cancer hypothesis—10 years later. *Prog Exp Tumor Res* 21:117, 1978.

Nahmias AJ, Naib ZM, Josey WE: Epidemiological studies relating genital herpes to cervical cancer. *Cancer Res* 34:1111, 1974.

Nelson JH, Averette HE, Richart RM: Cervical intraepithelial neoplasia and early invasive cervical carcinomas. *Cancer* 39:157, 1989.

Nigro ND, Vaitkericins CB: Combined therapy for cancer of the anal canal: A preliminary report. *Dis Colon Rectum* 17:354, 1974.

Nori D, Valentine E, Hilaris BS: The role of paraaortic node irradiation in the treatment of cancer of the cervix. *Int J Radiat Oncol Biol Phys* 11:1469, 1985.

O'Quinn AG, Fletcher GH, Wharton JT: Guidelines for conservative hysterectomy after irradiation. *Gynecol Oncol* 9:68, 1980.

Orr JW, Ball GC, Soong SJ, Hatch KD, Partridge EE, Austin JM: Surgical treatment of women found to have invasive cervix cancer at the time of total hysterectomy. *Obstet Gynecol* 68:353, 1986.

Pak HY, Yokota SB, Paladugu RR, Agliozzo CM: Glassy cell carcinoma of the cervix. *Cancer* 52:307, 1983.

Papavasiliou C, Angelaskis P, Gouvalis P: Treatment of cervical carcinoma by methotrexate combined with cyclophosphamide. *Cancer Chemother Rep* 52:225, 1969.

Papavasiliou C, Yivgarakis D, Pappas J, Keramopoulous A: Treatment of cervical carcinoma by total hysterectomy and postoperative external irradiation. *Int J Radiat Oncol Biol Phys* 6:871, 1980.

Patsner B, Mann WJ: Does preoperative serum squamous cell carcinoma (SCC) antigen level predict occult extracervical disease in patients with stage IB invasive squamous cell carcinoma of the cervix? *Gynecol Oncol* 32:95, 1989.

Penalver MA, Bejany DE, Averette HE, Donato DM, Sevin BU, Suarez G: Continent urinary diversion in gynecologic oncology. *Gynecol Oncol* 34:274, 1989.

Perez CA, Breaux S, Bedwinek JM, Madoc-Jones H, Camel HM, Purdy JA, Walz BJ: Radiation therapy alone in the treatment of carcinoma of the uterine cervix. II. Analysis of complications. *Cancer* 54:235, 1984.

Perez CA, Zivnuska F, Askin F, Kumar B, Camel HM, Powers WE: Prognostic significance of endometrial extension from primary carcinoma of the uterine cervix. *Cancer* 35:1493, 1975.

Perkins PL, Chau AM, Jose B, Achino E, Tobin DA: Posthysterectomy megavoltage irradiation in the treatment of cervical carcinoma. *Gynecol Oncol* 17:340, 1984.

Peters RK, Thomas D, Hagan DG, Mack TM, Henderson BE: Risk factors for invasive cervical cancer among Latinas and non-Latinas in Los Angeles County. *J Natl Cancer Inst* 77:1063, 1986.

Pettersson F (ed): International Federation of Gynecology and Obstetrics (FIGO) Annual Report on the Results of Treatment in Gynecological Cancer. Stockholm, Panorama Press AB, 1988.

Piel I, Slayton R, Perlia CP: Combination chemotherapy with bleomycin and disseminated cervical carcinoma: A preliminary study. *Gynecol Oncol* 1:184, 1973.

Piver MS, Chung WS: Prognostic significance of cervical lesion size and pelvic node metastases in cervical carcinoma. *Obstet Gynecol* 46:507, 1975.

Piver MS, Barlow JJ, Krisnamsetty R: Five-year survival in patients with biopsy confirmed aortic node metastasis from cervical carcinoma. *Am J Obstet Gynecol* 139:575, 1981.

Piver MS, Barlow JJ, Vongtama V, Blumenson L: Hydroxyurea as a radiation sensitizer in women with carcinoma of the uterine cervix. *Am J Obstet Gynecol* 129:379, 1977.

Piver MS, Vongtama V, Emrich LJ: Hydroxyurea plus pelvic radiation versus placebo plus pelvic radiation in surgically staged stage IIIB cervical cancer. *J Surg Oncol* 35:129, 1987.

Plentyl AA, Friedman E: *The Morphologic Basis of Oncologic Diagnosis and Therapy,* Vol 2. Philadelphia, WB Saunders Co, 1971, pp 85-115

Poolman RJ, Counsellor VS: Cylindroma of the cervix with procidentia. *Am J Obstet Gynecol* 58:184, 1949.

Potter ME, Hatch KD, Potter MY, Shingleton H, Baker VV: Factors affecting the response of recurrent squamous cell carcinoma of the cervix to cisplatin. *Cancer* 63:1283, 1989.

Powell JL, Burrell MO, Franklin EW III: Radical hysterectomy and pelvic lymphadenectomy. *South Med J* 77:596, 1984.

Pratt JH, Malkasian GD: The treatment of invasive carcinoma of the cervix during pregnancy. *Ann NY Acad Sci* 114:868, 1964.

Prem KA, Makowski EL, McKelvey JL: Carcinoma of the cervix associated with pregnancy. *Am J Obstet Gynecol* 95:99, 1966.

Punnonen R, Gronroos M, Rauramo M, et al: Complication following radiation therapy in gynaecological carcinoma: Comparison between x-ray and megavoltage therapy. *Ann Chir Gynaecol Fenn* 65:62, 1976.

Randall ME, Constable WC, Hahn SS, Kim JA, Mills SE: Results of radiotherapeutic management of carcinoma of the cervix with emphasis on the influence of histologic classification. *Cancer* 62:48, 1988.

Reagan JW, Hamonic MJ, Wentz WB: Analytical study of cells in cervical squamous cell cancer. *Lab Invest* 5:241, 1957.

Reeves WC, Brinton LA, Garcia M, Brenes MM, Herrero R, Gaitan E, Tenorio F, de Britton RC, Rawls WE: Human papillomavirus infection and cervical cancer in Latin America. *N Engl J Med* 320:1437, 1989.

Ries E: Extended hysterectomy for cervical cancer. *Chicago Med Rec* 9:284, 1895.

Robboy SJ, Young RH, Welch WR, Truslow GY, Prat J, Herbst AL, Scully RE: Atypical vaginal adenosis and cervical ectropion. Association with clear cell adenocarcinoma in diethylstilbestrol-exposed offspring. *Cancer* 54:869, 1984.

Roche WD, Norris HJ: Microinvasive carcinoma of the cervix: The significance of lymphatic invasion and confluent patterns of stromal growth. *Cancer* 36:180, 1975.

Roddick JW, van Nagell JR, Bell RM: Protein and electrolyte content of retroperitoneal suction drainage after radical hysterectomy and pelvic lymphadenectomy. *Gynecol Oncol* 1:149, 1973.

Rubin SC, Brookland R, Mikuta JJ, Mangan C, Sutton G, Danoff B: Para-aortic nodal metastases in early cervical carcinoma: Long-term survival following extended field radiotherapy. *Gynecol Oncol* 18:213, 1984.

Rustin GJS, Newlands ES: Phase I-II study of carboplatin, vincristine, methotrexate, and bleomycin (COMB) in carcinoma of the cervix. *Br J Cancer* 58:818, 1988.

Rustin GJS, Newlands ES, Southcott BM, Singer A: Cisplatin, vincristine, methotrexate, and bleomycin (POMB) as initial or palliative chemotherapy for carcinoma of the cervix. *Br J Obstet Gynaecol* 94:1205, 1987.

Rutledge FN, Galakatos AE, Wharton JT, Smith JP: Adenocarcinoma of the uterine cervix. *Am J Obstet Gynecol* 122:236, 1975.

Rutledge FN, Smith JP, Wharton JT, O'Quinn AG: Pelvic exenteration: Analysis of 296 patients. *Am J Obstet Gynecol* 129:881, 1977.

Rutledge FN, Wharton JT, Fletcher GH: Clinical studies with adjunctive surgery and irradiation therapy in the treatment of carcinoma of the cervix. *Cancer* 38:596, 1976.

Sablinska R, Tarlowska L, Stechmachow J: Invasive carcinoma of the cervix associated with pregnancy. *Gynecol Oncol* 5:363, 1977.

Sall S, Pineda A, Calanog A, Heller P, Greenberg H: Surgical treatment of stages IB and IIA invasive carcinoma of the cervix by radical abdominal hysterectomy. *Am J Obstet Gynecol* 135:442, 1979.

Sall S, Rini S, Pineda A: Surgical management of invasive carcinoma of the cervix in pregnancy. *Am J Obstet Gynecol* 118:1, 1974.

Saunders N, Landon CR: Management problems associated with carcinoma of the cervix diagnosed in the second trimester of pregnancy. *Gynecol Oncol* 30:120, 1988.

Scotti RJ, Bergman A, Bhatia N, Ostergard DR: Urodynamic changes in urethrovesical function after radical hysterectomy. *Obstet Gynecol* 68:111, 1986.

Schmidt JD, Buchsbaum HJ, Jacobo EC: Transverse colon conduit for supravesical urinary tract diversion. *Urology* 8:542, 1976.

Schmitt EH, Symmonds RE: Surgical treatment of radiation induced injuries of the intestine. *Surg Gynecol Obstet* 153:896, 1982.

Schmitz RL, Schmitz HE, Smith CJ, Molitor JJ: Details of pelvic exenteration evolved during an experience with 75 cases. *Am J Obstet Gynecol* 80:43, 1960.

Seski JC, Abell MR, Morley GW: Microinvasive squamous carcinoma of the cervix: Definition, histologic analysis, late results of treatment. *Obstet Gynecol* 50:410, 1977.

Sevin B, Ramos R, Lichtinger M, Girtanner RE, Averette H: Antibiotic prevention of infections complicating radical abdominal hysterectomy. *Obstet Gynecol* 64:539, 1984.

Shingleton HM, Gore H, Bradley DH, Soong SW: Adenocarcinoma of the cervix. I. Clinical evaluation and pathologic features. *Am J Obstet Gynecol* 139:799, 1981.

Shingleton HM, Soong SJ, Gelder MS, Hatch KD, Baker VV, Austin JM: Clinical and histopathologic factors predicting recurrence and survival after pelvic exenteration for cancer of the cervix. *Obstet Gynecol* 73:1027, 1989.

Silverberg E, Lubera JA: Cancer statistics 1989. *Cancer* 39:3, 1989.

Silverberg E, Boring CC, Squires TS: Cancer statistics—1990. *Ca—A Cancer Journal for Clinicians.* 40:9, 1990.

Simon NL, Gore H, Shingleton HM, Soong SJ, Orr JW, Hatch KD: Study of superficially invasive carcinoma of the cervix. *Obstet Gynecol* 68:19, 1986.

Slavik M: Adriamycin activity in genitourinary and gynecologic malignancies. *Cancer Chemother Rep* 6:297, 1975.

Slayton RE, Blessing JA, Homesley HD: Phase II trial of etoposide in the management of advanced or recurrent non–squamous cell carcinoma of the cervix: A Gynecologic Oncology Group study. *Cancer Treat Rep* 68:1513, 1984.

Smith JP, Rutledge F, Burns B: Systemic chemotherapy for carcinoma of the cervix. *Am J Obstet Gynecol* 97:800, 1967.

Smith ST, Seski JC, Copeland LJ, Gershenson DM, Edwards CL, Heron J: Surgical management of irradiation-induced small bowel damage. *Obstet Gynecol* 65:563, 1985.

Sorbe B, Frankendal B: Bleomycin-Adriamycin-cisplatin combination chemotherapy in the treatment of primary advanced and recurrent cervical carcinoma. *Obstet Gynecol* 63:167, 1984.

Stander RW, Lein JN: Carcinoma of the cervix and pregnancy. *Am J Obstet Gynecol* 79:164, 1960.

Stolinsky D, Bateman J: Further experience with hexamethyl-melamine in the treatment of carcinoma of the cervix. *Cancer Chemother Rep* 57:497, 1973.

Symmonds RE, Gibbs CP: Urinary diversion by way of sigmoid conduit. *Surg Gynecol Obstet* 131:687, 1970.

Symmonds RE, Jones IV: Sigmoid conduit urinary diversion after exenteration. In Taymor ML, Green TH Jr (eds): *Progress in Gynecology*, Vol VI. New York, Grune and Stratton, 1975, p 729.

Symmonds RE, Pratt JH: Prevention of fistulas and lymphocysts in radical hysterectomy. *Obstet Gynecol* 17:57, 1961.

Symmonds RE, Pratt JH, Webb MJ: Exenterative operations: Experience with 198 patients. *Am J Obstet Gynecol* 121:907, 1975.

Symmonds RE, Pratt JH, Welch JS: Extended Wertheim operation for primary, recurrent, or suspected recurrent carcinoma of the cervix. *Obstet Gynecol* 24:15, 1964.

Taki I, Sugimori H, Matsuyama T, Kashimura Y, Yoshins T: Treatment of microinvasive carcinoma. *Obstet Gynecol Surv* 34:839, 1979.

Tamimi HK, Figge DC: Adenocarcinoma of the uterine cervix. *Obstet Gynecol* 13:335, 1982.

Tamimi HK, Marit EK, Hesla J, Cain JM, Figge DC, Greer BE: Glassy cell carcinoma of the cervix—redefined. *Obstet Gynecol* 71:837, 1988.

Tewfik HH, Buchsbaum HJ, Latourette HB, Lifshitz SG, Tewfik FA: Para-aortic lymph node irradiation in carcinoma of the cervix after exploratory laparotomy and biopsy proven positive aortic nodes. *Int J Radiat Oncol Biol Phys* 8:13, 1982.

Thar TL, Million RR, Daly JW: Radiation treatment of carcinoma of the cervix. *Semin Oncol* 9:299, 1982.

Thigpen T, Blessing JA, Fowler WC, Hatch K: Phase II trials of the cisplatin and piperazinedione as single agents in the treatment of advanced or recurrent non–squamous cell carcinoma of the cervix: A Gynecologic Oncology Group study. *Cancer Treat Rep* 70:1097, 1986.

Thigpen T, Shingleton H, Homesley H, Lagasse L, Blessing J: Cisplatinum in treatment of advanced or recurrent squamous cell carcinoma of the cervix: A phase II study of the Gynecologic Oncology Group. *Cancer* 48:889, 1981.

Thigpen T, Vance R, Lambuth B, Balducci L, Khansur T, Blessing J, McGehee R: Chemotherapy for advanced or recurrent gynecologic cancer. *Cancer* 60:2104, 1987.

Thomas G, Pembo A, Beale F, Bean H, Bush R, Herman J, Prigle J, Rawlings G, Sturgeon J, Fine S, Black B: Concurrent radiation, mitomycin-c, and 5-fluorouracil in poor prognosis carcinoma of the cervix: Preliminary results of a phase I-II study. *Int J Radiat Oncol Biol Phys* 10:1785, 1984.

Thompson JD, Caputo TA, Franklin EW III, Dale E: The surgical management of invasive cancer of the cervix in pregnancy. *Am J Obstet Gynecol* 121:853, 1975.

Trope C, Horvath G, Haadem K, Gudmundsson T, Simonsen E: Doxorubicin-cisplatin combination chemotherapy for recurrent carcinoma of the cervix. *Cancer Treat Rep* 70:1325, 1986.

Tsukamoto N, Kaku T, Matsukuma K, Matsuyama T, Kamura T, Saito T, Suenaga T: The problem of stage Ia (FIGO, 1985) carcinoma of the uterine cervix. *Gynecol Oncol* 34:1, 1989.

Twiggs LB, Potish RA, George RJ, Adcock LL: Pretreatment extraperitoneal surgical staging in primary carcinoma of the cervix uteri. *Surg Gynecol Obstet* 158:243, 1984.

Underwood PB Jr, Wilson WC, Kreutner A, Miller MC III, Murphy E: Radical hysterectomy: A critical review of twenty-two years' experience. *Am J Obstet Gynecol* 134:889, 1979.

Van Dyke AH, van Nagell JR Jr: The prognostic significance of ureteral obstruction in patients with recurrent carcinoma of the cervix uteri. *Surg Gynecol Obstet* 141:371, 1975.

van Nagell JR Jr, Higgins RV: Invasive cancer of the cervix: Clinical features and pretreatment evaluation. In Coppleson M (ed): *Gynecologic Oncology*. London, Churchill Livingstone, 1991, pp 209-240.

van Nagell JR Jr, Donaldson ES, Gay EC: Urinary tract involvement by invasive cervical cancer. In Buchsbaum HJ, Schmidt JD (eds): *Gynecologic and Obstetric Urology.* Philadelphia, WB Saunders Co, 1982a, pp 410-421.

van Nagell JR Jr, Donaldson ES, Gay EC, Hudson S, Sharkey RM, Primus J, Powell DF, Goldenberg DM: Carcinoembryonic antigen in carcinoma of the uterine cervix. Part 2. Tissue localization and correlation with plasma antigen concentration. *Cancer* 44:944, 1979a.

van Nagell JR Jr, Donaldson ES, Parker JC, Van Dyke AH, Wood EG: The prognostic significance of cell type and lesion size in patients with cervical cancer treated by radical surgery. *Gynecol Oncol* 5:142, 1977a.

van Nagell JR Jr, Donaldson ES, Wood EG, Parker JC: The significance of vascular invasion and lymphoplasmacytic infiltration in invasive cancer of the uterine cervix. *Cancer* 41:228, 1978.

van Nagell JR Jr, Gay EC, Powell DE, Maruyama Y: Invasive cervical cancer. In van Nagell JR Jr, Barber HRK (eds): *Modern Concepts of Gynecologic Oncology.* Littleton, Massachusetts, John Wright Publisher, 1982b, pp 57-90.

van Nagell JR Jr, Greenwell N, Powell DE, Donaldson ES, Hanson MB, Gay EC: Microinvasive carcinoma of the cervix. *Am J Obstet Gynecol* 145:981, 1983.

van Nagell JR Jr, Maruyama Y, Yoneda J, Donaldson ES, Hanson MB, Gallion HH, Powell DE, Kryscio RJ: Treatment of bulky stage IB and IIB cervical cancers with outpatient neutron brachytherapy, external pelvic radiation and extrafascial hysterectomy. *Nuc Sci Appl* 2:483, 1986.

van Nagell JR Jr, Parker JC, Maruyama Y: The effect of pelvic inflammatory disease on enteric complications following radiation therapy for cervical cancer. *Am J Obstet Gynecol* 128:767, 1977b.

van Nagell JR Jr, Penny R, Roddick JW Jr: Suprapubic bladder drainage following radical hysterectomy. *Am J Obstet Gynecol* 113:849, 1972.

van Nagell JR Jr, Powell DE, Gallion HH, Elliott DG, Donaldson ES, Carpenter, AE, Higgins RV, Kryscio R, Pavlik EJ: Small cell carcinoma of the uterine cervix. *Cancer* 62:1586, 1988.

van Nagell JR Jr, Rayburn W, Donaldson ES, Hanson MB, Gay EC, Maruyama Y, Yoneda J, Powell D: Therapeutic implications of patterns of recurrence in cervical cancer. *Cancer* 44:2354, 1979b.

van Nagell JR Jr, Sprague AD, Roddick JW Jr: The effect of intra-

venous pyelography and cystoscopy on the staging of cervical cancer. *Gynecol Oncol* 3:87, 1975.

Van Praagh IGL, Harvey MH, Vernon CP: Carcinoma of the cervix associated with pregnancy. *J Obstet Gynecol Br Commonw* 72:74, 1965.

Waldrop GM, Palmer JP: Carcinoma of the cervix associated with pregnancy. *Am J Obstet Gynecol* 86:202, 1963.

Wanless JF: Carcinoma of the cervix in pregnancy. *Am J Obstet Gynecol* 110:173, 1971.

Webb MJ, Symmonds RE: Management of the pelvic floor after pelvic exenteration. *Obstet Gynecol* 50:166, 1977.

Webb MJ, Symmonds RE: Wertheim hysterectomy: A reappraisal. *Obstet Gynecol* 54:140, 1979.

Weiser EB, Bundy BN, Hoskins WJ, Heller PB, Whittington RR, DiSaia PJ, Curry SL, Schlaerth J, Thigpen T: Extraperitoneal versus transperitoneal selective para-aortic lymphadenectomy in the pretreatment surgical staging of advanced cervical cancer (A Gynecologic Oncology Group Study). *Gynecol Oncol* 33:283, 1989.

Welander CE, Pierce VK, Nori D, Hilaris BS, Kosloff C, Clark DG, Jones WB, Kim WS, Lewis JL Jr: Pretreatment laparotomy in carcinoma of the cervix. *Gynecol Oncol* 12:336, 1981.

Wharton JT, Jones HW, Day TG, Rutledge FN, Fletcher GH: Preirradiation celiotomy and extended field irradiation for invasive carcinoma of the cervix. *Obstet Gynecol* 49:333, 1977.

Wheeless CR: Small bowel bypass for complications related to pelvic malignancy. *Obstet Gynecol* 92:661, 1973.

Wheeless CR: Neovagina constructed from omental J-flap and a split thickness skin graft. *Gynecol Oncol* 35:224, 1989.

Wheeless CR, Hempling RE: Rectal J pouch reservoir to decrease the frequency of tenesmus and defecation in low coloproctostomy. *Gynecol Oncol* 34:379, 1989.

Williams TJ, Brack CB: Carcinoma of the cervix in pregnancy. *Cancer* 17:1486, 1964.

Yajima A, Noda K: The results of treatment of microinvasive carcinoma (stage IA) of the uterine cervix by means of simple and extended hysterectomy. *Am J Obstet Gynecol* 135:685, 1979.

zur Hausen H, Meinhof W, Scheiber W, Bornkamm GW: Attempts to detect virus-specific DNA in human tumors. I. Nucleic acid hybridizations with complementary RNA of human wart virus. *Int J Cancer* 13:650, 1974.

# Chapter 12 | Adenocarcinoma of the Uterine Corpus

*William T. Creasman*   *Gary L. Eddy*

## INCIDENCE AND ETIOLOGY

Cancer of the uterine corpus is the most common malignancy of the female pelvis. According to the American Cancer Society, cancer of the uterus will develop in approximately 34,000 women this year in the United States. This malignancy is almost twice as common as carcinoma of the ovary and almost three times more common than cervical cancer. It is generally agreed that the incidence of endometrial cancer has increased, particularly in the industrialized countries. In reviewing the predicted incidence for the decade beginning in 1970,

the American Cancer Society noted a 1.5-fold increase in the number of patients with endometrial cancer. The incidence apparently peaked in the early 1980s, when approximately 39,000 new cases were identified, but it has since slowly declined to a figure of 34,000.

It is interesting to note that during the interval in which the frequency of endometrial cancer increased, the predicted number of deaths from this malignancy actually decreased. Explanations for this apparent increase in frequency include a longer-lived population and more precise identification of the pathologic criteria for diagnosing endometrial cancer, although the reason most commonly cited has been the increase in the use of unopposed estrogen replacement therapy (ERT). Nevertheless, researchers in Norway and Czechoslovakia have reported a 50 to 60% increase in the rate of endometrial cancer despite the fact that estrogens are rarely prescribed or not generally available in those countries. The now decreasing incidence may well be due to the standard use of the combination of a progestin and estrogen for ERT when the uterus is in situ. Progestins counteract the cancer-promoting effect of estrogen on the endometrium.

It is generally accepted that endometrial cancer is an estrogen-dependent neoplasm (Smith et al, 1975). When an adenocarcinoma is present in a woman receiving ERT, it is usually well-differentiated, limited in extent, and highly curable. In fact, studies have shown that women taking estrogen who develop cancer live just as long as—if not longer than—their contemporaries who neither took estrogen nor developed adenocarcinoma of the endometrium (Chu et al, 1982).

## FACTORS AFFECTING RISK

Endometrial carcinoma develops during the reproductive years and after menopause, with the peak incidence between ages 50 and 69 (median age = 61). About 5% of women will be found to have adenocarcinoma before age 40, and approximately one-fourth will be diagnosed before the menopause.

Multiple risk factors have been identified and divided into three general categories (MacMahon, 1974): (1) variants of normal anatomy and physiology, (2) frank abnormality or disease, and (3) exposure to external carcinogens.

*Obesity, nulliparity,* and *late menopause* are all variants of normal anatomy or physiology that have classically been associated with endometrial carcinoma. Risk for developing endometrial cancer is 10 times greater in women who are more than 50 pounds overweight. This risk is three times higher in the nullipara compared with women who have had 5 or more children. In women whose menopause occurs after age 52, the chance of developing endometrial cancer is 2.5 times greater than that in women with earlier menopause. If a patient is nulliparous, is obese, and reaches menopause at age 52 or later, there appears to be a fivefold increase in the risk for endometrial cancer over women who do not satisfy these criteria.

Apparently, the use of *combination oral contraceptives* (OC) decreases a woman's risk for endometrial cancer. The Centers for Disease Control compared cases of endometrial cancer in women 20 to 54 years of age from eight population-based cancer registries with control subjects selected at random from the same centers (Centers for Disease Control, 1983). Among those women who used OC at some time, the relative risk of developing endometrial cancer was 0.5 compared with women who had never used OC. This protection was evident in women who used OC for at least 12 months and persisted for at least 10 years after OC were discontinued. In addition, such protection appeared to be most notable for the nulliparous patient. These investigators estimated that past or current OC use prevents as many as 2,000 cases of endometrial cancer each year in the United States.

As previously mentioned, replacement therapy with unopposed exogenous *estrogen* (ERT) appears to be associated with risk for endometrial neoplasia. Similarly, the increased risk in the obese patient is attributed to an increase in the endogenous production of estrogen. After menopause, the major circulating estrogen is estrone, derived through the peripheral aromatization of androstenedione in fat. The increased availability of estrogen in obesity is not unique to endometrial cancer but rather is a function of the patient's weight. Probably the basis for considering estrogen as an etiologic agent is the fact that hyperplasia of the endometrium is frequently associated with carcinoma, and such hyperplasia has been widely recognized in patients on prolonged unopposed estrogen. The validity of this association has, however, been disputed. It is now appreciated that only those patients with atypical hyperplasia (cytologic abnormalities) are at increased risk for endometrial cancer.

Experiments of nature have also implicated estrogen as a possible contributing factor in the development of endometrial cancer since it has been known for years that this neoplasm may develop in patients with *hormone-secreting tumors.* Some studies have shown a high correlation between endometrial cancers and the so-called "feminizing" ovarian tumors. Among 115 patients studied by Gusberg and Kardon (1971), 31% were found to have cancer of the uterine corpus and 43% had suspected precursors of this disease, such as endometrial hyperplasia and carcinoma in situ. However, these authors were unable to draw any firm conclusion about the possible carcinogenicity of estrogen in humans. When Norris and Taylor (1968) evaluated 203 patients with granulosa-theca cell tumors at the Armed Forces Institute of Pathology, they found that only 9% also had adenocarcinoma of the uterus.

Another condition in which endogenous estrogen might contribute to the development of endometrial cancer is in patients with *polycystic ovary syndrome* (Stein-Leventhal syndrome). Endometrial cancer has been reported to be as high as 25% in patients with this syndrome. If the effects of unopposed estrogen in such cases can be alleviated by either wedge resection or the administration of clomiphene citrate, the stimulation of the endometrium by estrogen and the potential for premalignant changes may be reversed. Patients with *ovarian dysgenesis* have also been reported to be at high risk for endometrial cancer because of their need for long-term supplemental estrogen beginning at an early age.

Over the last 15 years, numerous retrospective studies have correlated the use of exogenous estrogen in postmenopausal women with the increasing incidence of endometrial cancer. It is generally agreed that there may be a fourfold increase in endometrial cancer in patients who received estrogen alone as replacement therapy. In addition, women who develop endometrial cancer while on estrogen usually differ phenotypically from the typical obese, diabetic, hypertensive women commonly affected. Based upon several studies, including the large retrospective evaluation by Gambrell (1982), standard protocols now recommend the use of estrogen plus progesterone in the management of the postmenopausal patient with an intact uterus who is receiving ERT.

*Cigarette smoking* appears to decrease the risk for endometrial cancer, with the level of risk decreasing as the amount of smoking increases. The greatest reductions noted in this regard were in the heaviest women. Although the risk of developing early-stage endometrial cancer may appear to decrease with smoking, this advantage is strongly outweighed by the increased risk of lung cancer and other major health hazards associated with this habit.

The frequent association between endometrial cancer and *diabetes mellitus* or *hypertension* has been evident for years. Risk appears to be increased among patients with a history of diabetes even after study results are controlled for age, weight, and socioeconomic status. High blood pressure, on the other hand, does not appear to be a significant factor by itself even though as many as one-fourth of patients with endometrial cancer have hypertension or arteriosclerotic heart disease.

## DIAGNOSIS

*Uterine bleeding* in the postmenopausal patient mandates an evaluation for endometrial cancer. Only 20% of such patients will have a genital malignancy, although the risk is greater as the time since menopause increases. It is important to remember that in the perimenopausal patient with irregular bleeding, endometrial cancer may very well be the cause. In many cases the patient and even the physician may consider this aberrant bleeding to be a "normal" consequence of the menopause. However, these patients should be evaluated in the same way as the postmenopausal patient with bleeding. The pattern of bleeding during menopause should be lighter and lighter menses that occur farther and farther apart. In young patients with endometrial cancer, prolonged and heavy menstrual periods may result from endometrial cancer. By and large, the premenopausal patient who develops endometrial cancer may be quite obese with anovulatory menstrual cycles.

Historically, fractional dilatation and curettage has been the definitive diagnostic procedure in evaluating patients with bleeding problems. Today, *endometrial biopsy* is frequently used, so that the need for a formal D and C has decreased considerably. Several studies have indicated that diagnosis based on office biopsies using the apparatuses now available are highly accurate. It should be noted that when the endometrial biopsy is negative but the patient continues to bleed, a D and C should be seriously considered. Also, the patient found to have atypical endometrial hyperplasia on biopsy should probably undergo D and C, since adenocarcinoma is a possibility in association with the hyperplasia. Historically, the endocervical canal has routinely been evaluated in patients with adenocarcinoma of the endometrium, since the findings may affect staging as well as management. More recently, as information from

surgical staging protocols has accrued, and has led to a new staging classification for endometrial cancer, endocervical involvement can also be assessed on evaluation of the uterine specimen.

Routine cervical Papanicolaou smears have been of little value in endometrial cancer. Several studies have indicated that only one-third to one-half of patients with adenocarcinoma of the endometrium have abnormal findings on routine cytologic evaluation, although specimens obtained directly from the endometrial cavity are more likely to be abnormal compared with those taken from the cervix or vaginal pool.

*Hysteroscopy* and *hysterography* have both been suggested as adjuvant techniques for diagnosing endometrial carcinoma and establishing the extent of disease. Findings on hysterography correlate fairly well with surgical findings. Tumor volume and origin, the extent of disease within the uterine cavity and the shape of the cavity, and cervical involvement can be determined using this technique. Hysteroscopy has been used more frequently to evaluate patients with abnormal uterine bleeding. If a focal lesion is present, direct biopsy can be performed. Hysteroscopy can also be used to evaluate the endocervical canal. However, as use of a primary surgical approach to treating endometrial carcinoma increases, the information gained from these diagnostic methods will no longer be needed.

## PATHOLOGY

*Adenocarcinoma* of the endometrium as a histologic entity has been recognized for decades, with variants of this neoplasm noted in the literature for almost half a century. In the 1940s, mixed adenocarcinomas and squamous cell carcinomas (*adenosquamous carcinomas*) of the uterus were being described. Subsequently, *adenoacanthomas* were identified and are now well-recognized entities.

It has been suggested that adenoacanthoma (squamous metaplasia) is usually associated with well-differentiated cancers and has characteristics similar to those of pure adenocarcinomas (Fig. 12-1). As a result, the prognosis appears to be good, with survival dependent on the degree to which the adenocarcinoma component is differentiated.

The significance of adenosquamous carcinoma of the endometrium (Fig. 12-2) has not been entirely determined. It has been suggested that these tumors have increased in incidence, occur at an older age, have a shorter symptomatic period, and are more advanced at the time of detection. Also, they appear to be associated with a less differentiated glandular element, are seen more commonly with extrauterine disease and increased vascular invasion, and as a result carry a poorer prognosis than do pure adenocarcinomas (Ng et al, 1973). It has been suggested, however, that it is the degree of differentiation of the adenocarcinoma that determines the final prognosis and not the squamous component per se (Silverberg et al, 1972). Alberhasky et al (1982), in their extensive experience, noted that patients with mixed adenosquamous carcinoma had a considerably poorer prognosis than did those with pure adenocarci-

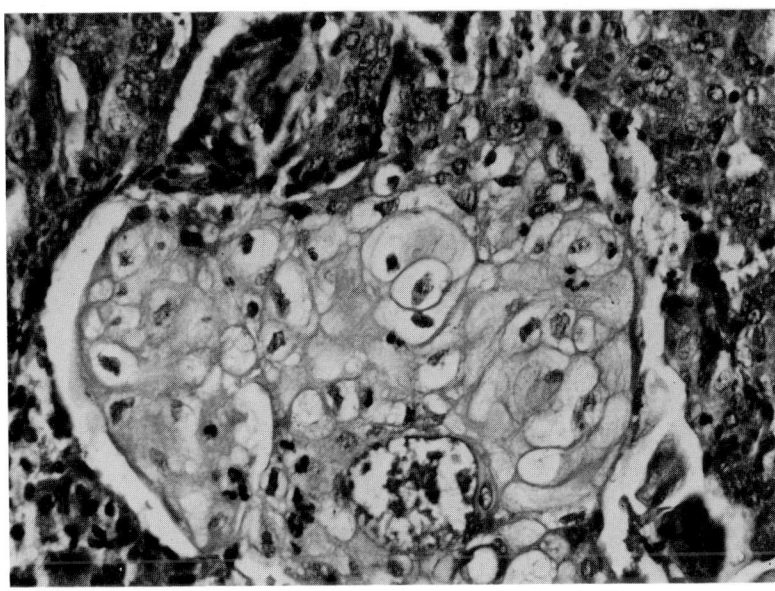

FIGURE 12-1 Adenoacanthoma with prominent squamous metaplasia. The squamous component is benign and the adenoacanthoma is usually well-differentiated. (Courtesy of Dr. Ted Gansler, Department of Pathology, Medical University of South Carolina.)

noma; they did not believe that the grade of the glandular component influenced survival. In general, patients with adenosquamous carcinoma tend to have a more poorly differentiated adenocarcinoma component. Obviously, further evaluation is needed to resolve the controversy concerning this variant.

More recently, two additional histologic variants of adenocarcinoma, clear cell carcinoma and papillary adenocarcinoma, have been described and appear to be distinct entities. The *clear cell carcinomas* are recognized by large epithelial cells that may be admixed with typical non–clear cell carcinoma. In some instances, the mesonephric-type "hobnail" cells are part of this pattern, although some authorities feel that it is inappropriate to include this subset in the clear cell category (Fig. 12-3). Several investigators have suggested a worse prognosis with clear cell adenocarcinoma than with pure adenocarcinoma. Apparently, neither the FIGO classification nor the nuclear grading correlated with survival. Because of the low incidence, the final word concerning the significance of this cell type has not been written.

*Papillary adenocarcinoma* of the endometrium has been recognized for many years but has only recently received more attention. The tumor is papillary, with a central stalk containing multiple lobules (Fig. 12-4). Survival does not appear to be as good as with pure adenocarcinoma, although according to Christopherson (1982), papillary adenocarcinoma is associated with a better survival rate than are mixed adenosquamous and clear cell carcinomas. Chen et al (1985) have suggested that there may be two clinical pathologic types of papillary adenocarcinoma. The so-called papillary *serous* adenocarcinomas seemed to be present in significantly older patients, showed deep myometrial invasion, and involved the peritoneal surface, and mortality was higher than in patients with the more common type of adenocarcinoma. On the other hand, *well-differentiated*

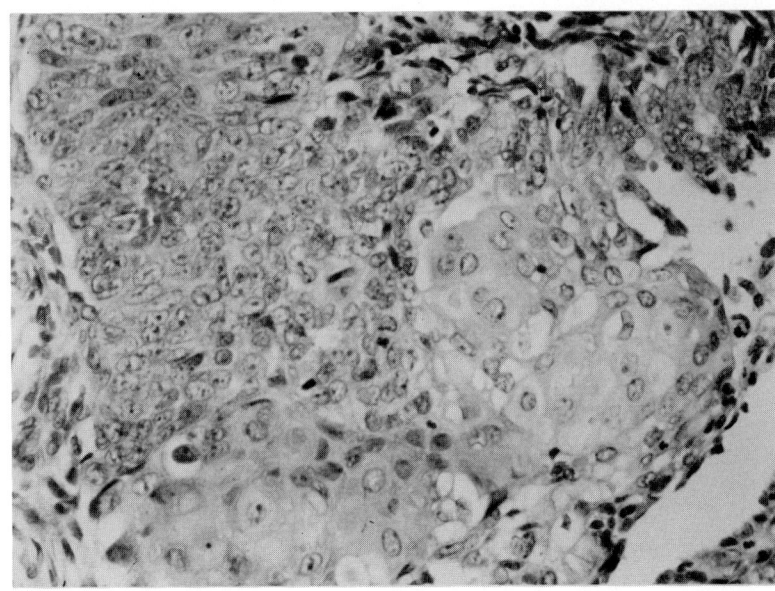

FIGURE 12-2 Adenosquamous carcinoma with both squamous and adenocarcinoma components poorly differentiated. (Courtesy of Dr. Ted Gansler, Department of Pathology, Medical University of South Carolina.)

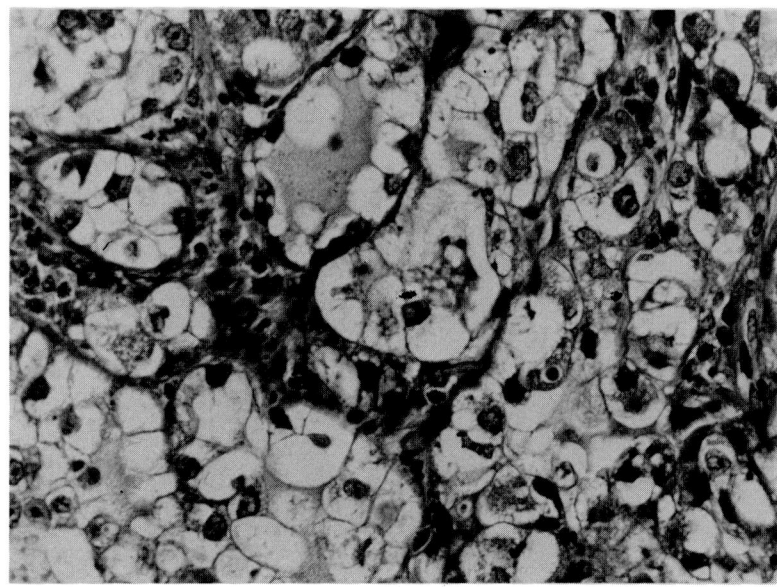

FIGURE 12-3 Clear cell carcinoma of the endometrium showing characteristic cells. (Courtesy of Dr. Ted Gansler, Department of Pathology, Medical University of South Carolina.)

papillary adenocarcinomas were similar to common adenocarcinomas with regard to tumor characteristics and survival.

Finally, *secretory adenocarcinoma* is an uncommon type of endometrial cancer that is difficult to differentiate from secretory endometrium and may be more of a histologic curiosity than a significant subset. Survival is quite good and comparable to that of patients with pure adenocarcinomas.

## PROGNOSTIC FACTORS

### Histologic Differentiation

Histologic differentiation has long been recognized as one of the most sensitive indicators of prognosis in endometrial cancer (Figs. 12-5 to 12-7). As a tumor

loses its differentiation, the chance for survival decreases. Many studies have substantiated this impression. In the Gynecologic Oncology Group (GOG) pilot study of 222 surgically evaluated clinical Stage I endometrial cancers, 42% were Grade 1 with a recurrence rate of only 4% compared with rates of 15% and 41% for Grade 2 and 3 cancers, respectively (Boronow et al, 1985). The latest FIGO (1988) Annual Report notes the following 5-year survival rates for patients with Stage I endometrial carcinoma: 76.9% for Grade 1 lesions, 73.1% for Grade 2, and 58.0% for Grade 3 (Table 12-1) (Pettersson, 1988). The degree of differentiation also correlates with other factors of prognosis, such as the depth of myometrial invasion—i.e., as the tumor becomes less differentiated, the chances of deep myometrial invasion increase. There are, however, notable exceptions to this rule.

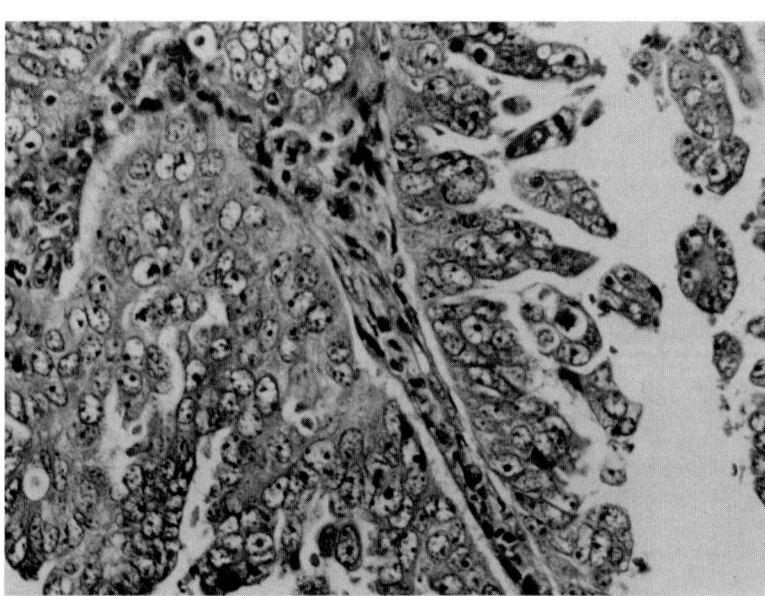

FIGURE 12-4 Papillary adenocarcinoma. (Courtesy of Dr. Ted Gansler, Department of Pathology, Medical University of South Carolina.)

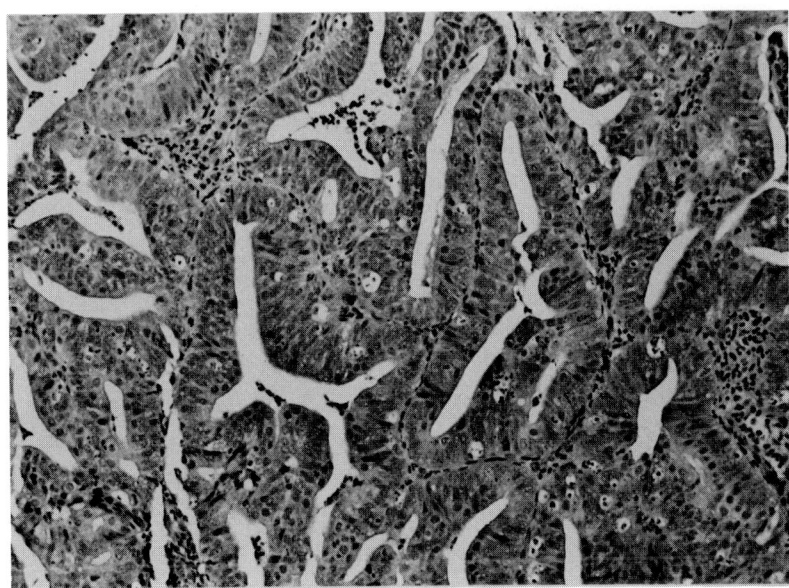

FIGURE 12-5   Well-differentiated adenocarcinoma of the endometrium. (Courtesy of Dr. Ted Gansler, Department of Pathology, Medical University of South Carolina.)

## Uterine Size and Cervical Involvement

For almost two decades, the size of the uterus (as determined by uterine sound) has been incorporated in the FIGO substaging process for endometrial cancer. Most researchers who have evaluated this factor with regard to survival agree that a larger uterine cavity is associated with poorer survival rate; however, some investigators have suggested that this might not be the case. In a survey by Jones (1975), women with a normal-size uterus survived longer than those with an enlarged uterus. Certainly all enlarged uteri are not the result of an increase in the extent of cancer. Other conditions such as fibromas and adenomyosis may contribute to this enlargement. In evaluating the hysterectomy specimens of 100 patients with endometrial cancer, Javert (1952) noted that about half were enlarged but in only eight was cancer the cause.

The location of the tumor within the endometrial cavity also appears to be significant. Tumors low in the cavity may be expected to involve the uterine cervix earlier than fundal lesions. In a study by the GOG of 621 patients with Stage I endometrial cancer, those with disease in the lower uterine segment had a higher incidence of pelvic lymph node metastases (16%) than did those with only fundal disease (8%); a similar pattern was observed for paraaortic node metastases (Creasman et al, 1987).

Cervical involvement is important, since this would result in a Stage II classification. Historically, such involvement has been determined by fractional dilatation and curettage or endocervical curettement in the office. Survival data from the FIGO Annual Report indicate that patients with Stage II disease have a considerably worse prognosis than those with Stage I endometrial

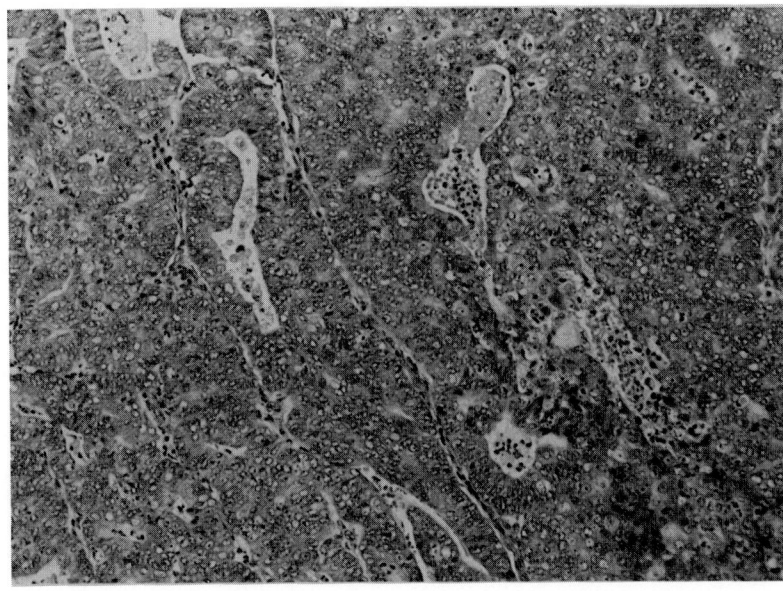

FIGURE 12-6   Moderately differentiated adenocarcinoma of the endometrium. (Courtesy of Dr. Ted Gansler, Department of Pathology, Medical University of South Carolina.)

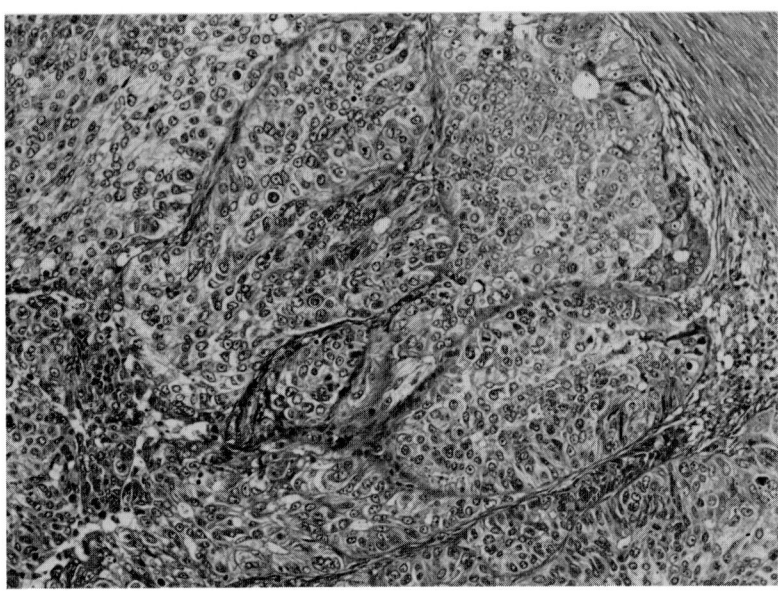

FIGURE 12-7 Poorly differentiated adenocarcinoma of the endometrium. (Courtesy of Dr. Ted Gansler, Department of Pathology, Medical University of South Carolina.)

cancer (56.4% vs 72.3%) (Table 12-2) (Pettersson, 1988). The accuracy of determining occult endocervical involvement using traditional techniques has been brought into question. Several studies have indicated that patients thought to have disease in the endocervix preoperatively were found at hysterectomy to have disease limited to the fundus. In many instances, this overdiagnosis is due to "contamination" from the uterine lesion and not true disease in the canal. Several studies have suggested that the rate of overdiagnosis may be as high as 50%. It also appears that the extent of cervical disease is of prognostic importance. Surwit et al (1979) and associates noted that the survival rate at 3 years was much lower in patients with stromal invasion of the cervix (47%) than in those in whom only the endocervical glands were involved (74%). Several other studies report the same findings.

With the new staging protocol as adopted by FIGO in 1988, preoperative evaluation of the endocervical canal may be considered unnecessary, since final staging is now based on examination of the hysterectomy specimen, which allows a complete evaluation of the endocervix as well as the extent of endocervical involvement (glands or stroma).

## Myometrial Invasion

It is well appreciated that the degree of myometrial invasion is an indicator of tumor virulence and volume. In a review of the literature, Jones (1975) found a decrease in the survival rate as myometrial penetration increased. Lutz et al (1978) felt that a more accurate determination of myometrial penetration was the proximity of the invading tumor to the uterine serosa. Patients whose tumor had invaded to within 5 mm of the serosa had a 65% 5-year survival rate compared with a rate of 97% for those with tumors more than 10 mm away from the serosa. As a general rule, *depth of myometrial invasion correlates with degree of differentiation*—i.e., the depth of penetration is greater for poorly differentiated tumors. It is, however, appreciated that patients with well differentiated cancers can have deep myometrial invasion and those with poorly differentiated cancers can have only superficial involvement of the endometrium. Irrespective of the grade of the tumor, the depth of invasion does appear to be an independent prognostic factor, as noted by DiSaia et al (1985). They found that patients with Stage I carcinoma with only endometrial involvement had an 8% recurrence rate, whereas those with superficial or medium myometrial involvement had recurrence rates of 13% and 12%, respectively; this rate increased to 46% when deep muscle (the outer one-third) was involved.

## Peritoneal Cytology

It has been suggested that findings in cytologic evaluation of peritoneal fluids or washings are an important prognostic factor in several pelvic malignancies. Creasman and Rutledge (1971) reported positive washings in 12% of patients with corpus cancer, although many of the latter patients had gross metastatic disease outside the uterus. In a preliminary study of 167 patients with clinical Stage I carcinoma of the endometrium treated primarily with surgery, 26 (15%) had malignant cells on peritoneal cytology (Creasman et al, 1981). Recurrences were more frequent in these patients than in

TABLE 12-1 Relationship Between Level of Tumor Differentiation and 5-Year Survival in Stage I Endometrial Cancer

| Grade | Survival Rate |
|---|---|
| 1 | 2,796/3,637 (76.9%) |
| 2 | 1,791/2,451 (73.1%) |
| 3 | 583/1,006 (58.0%) |

From Pettersson F (ed): Annual Report on the Results of Treatment in Gynecologic Cancer, Vol 20. International Federation of Gynecology and Obstetrics, Stockholm, 1988, FIGO.

Table 12-2   5-Year Survival in Endometrial Cancer

| Stage | No. of Patients<br>(% Survival) |
|-------|---------------------------------|
| I | 7,976/11,035 (72.3%) |
| II | 1,135/2,014  (56.4%) |
| III | 290/921  (31.5%) |
| IV | 43/409  (10.5%) |

From Pettersson F (ed): Annual Report on the Results of Treatment in Gynecologic Cancer, Vol 20. International Federation of Gynecology and Obstetrics, Stockholm, 1988, FIGO.

patients with negative peritoneal cytology (34% vs. 10%). Thirteen of these 26 patients had disease outside the uterus at the time of surgery, seven of whom (54%) have died from the disease. Malignant cells were found on peritoneal cytology in 13 patients with no disease outside the uterus, six of whom (46%) have died of disseminated intraabdominal carcinomatosis. In the GOG study of 621 patients, malignant cells were identified on cytologic examination of the peritoneal washings in 76 (12%) (Creasman et al, 1987); 25% of these patients had positive pelvic nodes compared with only 7% of the patients with no malignant cells on peritoneal cytology. It is true that the results of peritoneal cytology to a certain degree mimic other known prognostic factors; however, peritoneal cytology may be important as an independent factor as well.

Treatment with intraperitoneal phosphorus-32 in patients with malignant cytologic specimens appears to be effective. In a report of the Duke University experience, Soper et al (1985) utilized $^{32}P$ in 65 patients with malignant peritoneal cytology, 53 of whom had clinical Stage I disease. The rate of disease-free survival beyond 24 months was 89% for clinical Stage I patients and 94% for surgical Stage I patients. Significant acute and chronic complications of this treatment were not seen except when it was combined with external-beam radiation.

Peritoneal specimens should be obtained immediately after the peritoneal cavity is opened. If any ascitic fluid is present, it is removed and sent for cytologic evaluation. If no appreciable fluid is present, 100 or 125 ml of saline is instilled into the pelvis admixed with the small amount of fluid and withdrawn for cytologic evaluation. Quantitation of malignant cells has been reported to correlate well with prognosis; however, this method is probably not practical in everyday practice.

## Lymph Node Metastases

For decades the hallmark of therapy for endometrial cancer has been total abdominal hysterectomy and bilateral salpingo-oophorectomy. For many years the significance of lymph node metastases was not appreciated nor evaluated. A review of the literature reveals that a significant number of women with endometrial cancer, even Stage I disease, will have pelvic lymph node metastases. Morrow et al found that in a collected series of 369 patients with Stage I endometrial carcinoma, 39 had metastases to the pelvic lymph node area (1973).

In 1976, Creasman et al reported on an additional 140 patients, 16 of whom had positive pelvic nodes. In the pilot study of the GOG, which involved 222 patients, as well as a subsequent groupwide protocol (621 patients), it was noted that 81 of the 843 patients (9.6%) had pelvic node metastases (Boronow et al, 1984).

Unlike cervical cancer, in which lymph nodes are in many instances large and fixed, the diagnosis of metastases in lymph nodes in endometrial cancer is made almost exclusively under the microscope. Thus, it is unusual to find clinical evidence of lymph node metastases in endometrial cancer. In reporting results of long-term followup in the pilot study of the GOG, DiSaia et al (1985) noted a recurrence rate of 10.5% for patients with negative pelvic nodes (21 of 200) compared with a rate of 56% for those with pelvic node metastases (13 of 22). Most of the patients with positive pelvic nodes received postoperative pelvic irradiation. Certainly, the finding of micrometastases in patients with clinical Stage I carcinoma of the endometrium carries a poor prognosis.

Although it had been suggested that paraaortic lymph nodes could be involved in endometrial cancer, until recently there were few data to support this except from autopsy studies. In the GOG pilot study, Boronow et al (1984) reported metastases in 16 of 156 patients with Stage I disease in whom paraaortic nodes were removed. The rate of recurrence among those with negative paraaortic nodes was 10% (15 of 140) as opposed to 59% (10 of 16) when paraaortic nodes were positive. In the subsequent GOG study, Creasman et al (1987) noted that 34 of the 621 patients with surgical Stage I disease had positive nodes in the paraaortic area. In many instances, patients had both pelvic and paraaortic metastases, while a small number of these patients had metastases to the paraaortic nodes but negative pelvic nodes. Of the 621 patients, 11% had metastasis to either pelvic or paraaortic nodes or both. Most of the patients with paraaortic node metastases underwent radiation therapy to this area, and preliminary followup indicates that approximately 50% have survived long-term.

Lymph node metastases occur more often in patients with Stage II carcinoma of the endometrium than in patients with Stage I disease. Among 85 patients in whom pelvic nodes were evaluated, Morrow et al (1973) found that 31 (36%) showed metastatic disease. An analysis of metastases using the large data base for surgical Stage II patients collected by the GOG has yet to be reported.

## Adnexa

Endometrial cancer can and often does metastasize to the adnexa. For several decades the finding of a palpable adnexal mass indicated clinical Stage III disease. As many as 10% of patients will have metastases to the adnexa even though they may be considered to have clinical Stage I adenocarcinoma of the endometrium. In the GOG analysis of 222 patients with clinical Stage I carcinoma of the endometrium, 16 (7%) had metastasis to the adnexa (Boronow et al, 1984). This finding correlated with many of the other prognostic factors assessed. The depth of invasion appeared to be significant in that only 4% of patients with endometrial involvement alone had adnexal disease, whereas adnexal metastases were present in 24% of those with deep muscle involvement.

In contrast, tumor grade did not appear to be prognostically important, since 6% of patients with Grade 1 tumors had adnexal disease compared with 10% of those with poorly differentiated carcinoma. When tumor was limited to the uterine fundus, 5% of the patients had disease in the adnexa; however, when the lower uterine segment or endocervix was involved, the adnexa was involved in one-third of cases. On peritoneal cytology, malignant cells were present in 60% of patients with adnexal metastases compared with only 11% when the adnexa was not involved. Adnexal metastasis was also associated with a higher recurrence rate (38%) in contrast to a rate of 14% when the adnexa was free of disease. Only 34 of the 621 (5%) patients in the most recent GOG study showed metastases to the adnexa (Creasman et al, 1987), and the patients were also more likely to have metastases to both the pelvic and the paraaortic node areas.

## Other Prognostic Factors

**Tumor Size** It has been suggested that the size of the tumor is an important indicator of lymph node status. Schink et al (1987) evaluated 91 patients with Stage I endometrial carcinoma with regard to tumor size. When the tumor was less than 2 cm in size, fewer than 6% of the patients had lymph node metastases. When the tumor was greater than 2 cm, 21% had nodal metastases, and this number increased to 40% when the entire endometrium was involved. Those patients who had small lesions (<2 cm in size) and invasion to less than one-half the myometrium had no nodal metastasis. Tumor size was found to be an independent and significant prognostic factor on multivariate analysis.

**Hormonal Receptor Status** In a multivariate analysis of hormone receptor status, Creasman et al (1985) noted that for Stage I and II cancers, positive progesterone-receptor status was a highly significant independent prognostic factor in endometrial cancer. When progesterone-receptor status was eliminated from the model and estrogen-receptor status was evaluated in its place, the latter became an independent prognostic factor but was not as predictive as positive progesterone-receptor status.

**Capillary-Like Space (CLS) Involvement** In 111 patients with Stage I endometrial cancer, Hansen et al (1985) found CLS involvement in 16. It occurred most often in patients with poorly differentiated tumors that showed deep invasion. The rate of recurrence was 44% in patients with CLS involvement compared with 2% when the CLS was not involved. In the GOG study of 621 patients, 93 (16%) had CLS involvement (Creasman et al, 1987), and the incidence of pelvic and paraaortic metastases was 27% and 19%, respectively.

When there was no CLS involvement, the incidence of pelvic node metastases was 7% and 3% for paraaortic metastases.

## Correlation of Prognostic Factors

As has been discussed, multiple prognostic factors appear to be important in endometrial cancer. Several of these have been known for many years—even decades; however, it was not until the results of the initial GOG study along with preliminary data from the subsequent study that all known or suggested prognostic factors were evaluated using the same data base.

In the second GOG study, 621 patients with Stage I carcinoma of the endometrium underwent primary TAH-BSO, peritoneal cytologic examination, and pelvic and paraaortic selective lymphadenectomy (Creasman et al, 1987). The size of the uterus, histology, tumor grade, depth of myometrial invasion, adnexal involvement, peritoneal cytology, and extrauterine disease (intraabdominal) were assessed relative to both pelvic and paraaortic lymph node metastases. Patients with poorly differentiated cancer made up 25% of the patients and 22% had deep muscle involvement. Metastases were found in the pelvic area in 58 (9%) patients and in the paraaortic area in 34 (6%). Uterine size, grade of the tumor, and depth of muscle involvement all correlated with nodal metastases (Tables 12-3 to 12-5). Adnexal metastases were discovered on exploratory laparotomy in 35 patients (5%). The likelihood of having disease in the adnexa increased with depth of invasion and when the lower uterine segment or endocervix was involved. The chance of lymph node metastases was greater among patients with disease in the lower uterine segment or endocervix than among those with disease limited to the fundus. On cytologic evaluation, malignant cells were found in 76 patients (12%). When the six substages of clinical Stage I were evaluated, lymph node metastases increased with tumor grade and uterine size (Table 12-6).

The correlation between prognostic factors and survival was fully evaluated using data from the GOG pilot study (n = 222) in the hope that patients at high or low risk for recurrence could be identified and subsequent therapy (if needed) could be planned accordingly (DiSaia et al, 1985). At the time of analysis, the patients had been followed for 3 to 6 years. Since recurrence in endometrial cancer most often appears within 24 months, the researchers estimated that subsequent recurrence would not be likely. Sixty-eight patients (31%) were treated with surgery only and an additional 97

TABLE 12-3   Pelvic and Paraaortic Node Metastases Relative to Stage (GOG Results)

| Stage | Pelvic | Paraaortic |
|---|---|---|
| IA (n = 346) | 23 (7%) | 11 (3%) |
| IB (n = 275) | 35 (13%) | 23 (8%) |

Modified from Creasman WT, et al: Surgical pathological spread patterns of endometrial cancer. *Cancer* 60:2035, 1987.

TABLE 12-4  Pelvic and Paraaortic Node Metastases Relative to Grade (GOG Results)

| Grade | Pelvic | Paraaortic |
|---|---|---|
| G1 (n = 180) | 5 (3%) | 3 (2%) |
| G2 (n = 288) | 25 (9%) | 14 (5%) |
| G3 (n = 153) | 28 (18%) | 17 (11%) |

Modified from Creasman WT, et al: Surgical pathological spread patterns of endometrial cancer. *Cancer* 60:2035, 1987.

(44%) received radiation therapy prior to surgery. In all those who received preoperative radium, surgery was carried out during the same hospitalization. Recurrence rates were 9% for patients treated with surgery alone and 8% for those treated with surgery plus radiation. Only 25% of the patients were thought to have disease significant enough to require external-beam irradiation, and of these 35% had a recurrence. If postoperative radiation therapy were applied only to those patients thought to be at high risk, risk levels, as determined by the rate of recurrence, could probably be adequately determined. The fact that only 25% of these patients were considered eligible for postoperative radiation therapy indicates a rather marked deviation from accepted protocols as practiced in many institutions. Prior to the recording of this data base, virtually all patients with endometrial cancer received some form of radiation therapy as part of their primary treatment, even for Stage I disease.

When the sites of recurrence were evaluated for this data base, only two patients (1%) had an isolated recurrent lesion of the vaginal vault: one patient had been treated with surgery only and the other with surgery plus preoperative radium. Based on this study and other reports in the recent literature, we seem to succeed in achieving local control (i.e., vagina) in Stage I carcinoma of the endometrium, irrespective of the form of therapy. Therefore, since the vaginal vault does not appear to be at high risk for recurrence, the value of preoperative or postoperative brachytherapy must be questioned. In only five patients was recurrence identified in the pelvis only, and 79% of the recurrences were at distant sites outside the treatment field. This study did not address the issue of control of distant disease.

Thus, it would appear that prognostic factors do identify patients at high risk for recurrence in endometrial cancer. As a result, it would be best to select

adjuvant therapy during the postoperative period, when the status of the disease has been determined. Based on the literature, patients do not seem to be at a disadvantage if they receive postoperative as opposed to preoperative radiation. Certainly, it would be more efficacious to identify the patients at high risk and to treat them appropriately than to treat them all the same preoperatively, since 75% of the patients in this study did not need any type of adjunctive radiation therapy. Obviously, if disease is limited to the uterus, patients fare much better. Only 7% of the patients with disease limited to the uterus suffered a recurrence compared with 43% when extrauterine disease was present at the time of surgery.

## TREATMENT

Although many institutions, both in the United States and abroad, adopted a primary surgical approach to endometrial cancer even before 1988, when FIGO revised the staging classification, the role of preoperative radiation remains controversial. This is particularly true for patients with poorly differentiated lesions. According to the most recent FIGO Annual Report, only 40% of patients with Stage I carcinoma of the endometrium were treated with primary surgery (Pettersson, 1988). It should be remembered that this data base represents the period from 1979 to 1981, before the impact of the results of the GOG and other studies was appreciated.

Of course, therapy for adenocarcinoma of the endometrium has varied considerably since the turn of the century. As early as 1900, Cullen stated that the treatment of choice for patients with endometrial cancer was hysterectomy and bilateral salpingo-oophorectomy, and this remains the hallmark of therapy for this disease today. For most of this century, it has been readily apparent that carcinoma of the endometrium occurs in older patients and is therefore often inoperable because of concurrent medical conditions. As a result, when radium and external-beam radiation became available, surgery was in many instances abandoned altogether. At one point, staging for endometrial carcinoma included the category "inoperable," and these patients were evaluated separately. That designation has not been used for at least 2 decades, since improved monitoring techniques and anesthesia have made it possible

TABLE 12-5  Pelvic and Paraaortic Node Metastases Relative to Maximal Invasion (GOG Results)

| Maximal Invasion | Pelvic | Paraaortic |
|---|---|---|
| Endometrium only (n = 87) | 1 (1%) | 1 (1%) |
| Superficial muscle (n = 279) | 15 (5%) | 8 (3%) |
| Intermediate muscle (n = 116) | 7 (6%) | 1 (1%) |
| Deep muscle (n = 139) | 35 (25%) | 24 (17%) |

Modified from Creasman WT, et al: Surgical pathological spread patterns of endometrial cancer. *Cancer* 60:2035, 1987.

TABLE 12-6  Pelvic and Paraaortic Node Metastases Relative to Stage I Subsets (GOG Results)

| Stage I Subset | Pelvic | Paraaortic |
|---|---|---|
| IAG1 (n = 101) | 2 (2%) | 0 (0%) |
| IAG2 (n = 69) | 13 (4%) | 6 (4%) |
| IAG3 (n = 76) | 8 (11%) | 5 (7%) |
| IBG1 (n = 79) | 3 (4%) | 3 (4%) |
| IBG2 (n = 119) | 12 (10%) | 8 (7%) |
| IBG3 (n = 77) | 20 (26%) | 12 (16%) |

Modified from Creasman WT, et al: Surgical pathological spread patterns of endometrial cancer. *Cancer* 60:2035, 1987.

for many of these elderly patients to undergo surgical procedures safely.

Although adjunctive radiation, even in the form of brachytherapy or external-beam radiation, has been used as adjuvant therapy, all agree that, when possible, hysterectomy is the procedure of choice in this disease. In the 1930s, Heyman recommended packing the uterus with multiple capsules of radium before hysterectomy, particularly as a means of decreasing local recurrence. These initial reports showed a 5-year survival rate of about 60% in Stage I disease. In the 1940s, interest was renewed in radical surgery for carcinoma of the endometrium. Javert (1956) advocated this procedure and felt that preoperative radiation added nothing to the surgical procedure. Rutledge (1974), in his excellent review, concluded that the role, if any, of radical hysterectomy and pelvic lymphadenectomy in Stage I carcinoma of the endometrium was extremely limited. However, he noted that if positive nodes were present in patients treated with radical hysterectomy and pelvic lymphadenectomy, survival was not as good as in those patients with negative nodes.

Data concerning the role of radiation therapy in carcinoma of the endometrium have varied. Most studies have not evaluated multiple prognostic factors, particularly tumor grade and myometrial involvement, with regard to treatment. Patients found to have a poorly differentiated lesion would likely be treated with combined therapy. As a result, overall survival might be prejudiced in this group. The last two FIGO Annual Reports have listed survival in Stage I endometrial carcinoma with regard to grade and treatment. Interestingly, survival is essentially the same for patients treated with surgery alone and those given combined therapy when the grade of the tumor is evaluated; this was also true when the depth of myometrial invasion was evaluated in the two treatment groups. In some studies, patients who received preoperative and postoperative radiation appeared to have a slightly lower incidence of vaginal vault recurrence, although for Grades 1 and 2 there was no difference. Vaginal vault recurrence alone did not appear to affect survival.

The role of preoperative radium in patients with endometrial cancer has been addressed by several authors. de Waal and Lochmuller (1982) compared results after preoperative intracavitary radiotherapy and after primary operation without radiation in patients with Stage 1 and 2 disease. There was no difference in 5-year survival rates or in the incidence of vaginal, pelvic sidewall, or distant metastases in the two treatment groups. Patterson et al (1982) attempted to individualize treatment based on the grade of the tumor and the depth of myometrial invasion. Primary TAH and BSO were performed in patients with Grade 1 and 2 tumors. If less than one-third of the myometrium was involved, brachytherapy was utilized. Patients with greater myometrial involvement were treated with external-beam irradiation of the whole pelvis. In the latter group, 5-year survival was 96% and 92% of patients were free from recurrence. These authors believed that radiation therapy could be applied individually, since only 20%

of these patients required some form of radiation therapy.

Onsrud, Kolstad, and Normann (1976) carried out a prospective randomized study to evaluate the role of external-beam radiation and radium versus radium alone in addition to surgery in patients with Stage I endometrial carcinoma. Among patients who received external-beam radiation, 5-year survival was 88%, whereas this rate was 90% among those who did not receive external-beam radiation. When histologic grade and myometrial involvement were considered, there was no difference in recurrence or survival rates with regard to therapy. It appears that those patients who receive external irradiation had better local control; however, distant metastasis was more common in those who had received external-beam radiation.

Most would agree that there is probably no role for preoperative irradiation in patients with Stage I, Grade 1 lesions. These patients should be treated primarily with hysterectomy and bilateral salpingo-oophorectomy. If disease is found outside the uterus at the time of surgery, appropriate adjunctive therapy can be applied on an individual basis. However, there is no agreement regarding optimal therapy for patients with Grade 2 or 3 disease. Some authors prefer to deliver preoperative radiation either by packing plus vaginal ovoids or by tandem and ovoids if the uterus is small. TAH and BSO are then carried out 6 weeks later. Some clinicians still elect preoperative external-beam radiation followed by TAH and BSO. It appears, however, that a considerable number of patients with Grade 2 disease and even some with Grade 3 have only superficial myometrial invasion. In patients with no lymph node metastases, there is no evidence to suggest that preoperative external-beam radiation is of benefit. If this could be determined preoperatively, these patients could be saved the time and expense of adjuvant therapy. It is only with a primary surgical approach that this determination can be made.

In an evaluation of 703 patients with Stage IA or IB adenocarcinoma treated with or without vaginal irradiation after hysterectomy, Bond (1985) found fewer vaginal recurrences in those who received postoperative vaginal therapy (0 vs 3% for noninvasive lesions and 4.3% vs 8.3% for invasive tumors). The vagina was the first site of recurrence in only 3.4% of cases, whereas four times as many individuals developed pelvic or metastatic disease. The author concluded that postoperative vaginal irradiation was of limited value in only a small percentage of patients and that it did not influence survival rates or the incidence of pelvic or paraaortic disease in any histologic group and could therefore not be recommended for routine use.

For many years, the MD Anderson group and others have suggested that patients with enlarged uteri or poorly differentiated carcinomas be treated preoperatively with external-beam irradiation (4,000 to 5,000 rads to the whole pelvis) followed by radium and 6 weeks later by TAH and BSO. A significant number of patients with Grade 3 neoplasms will have disease outside the treatment field. Because there can be a significant delay between the diagnosis and surgery, it may be more prudent to do the surgery first and then apply optimal directed radiation postoperatively to the sites of metastasis or the areas at risk for recurrent disease.

## Primary Surgical Management

Obviously, when adjuvant therapy is undertaken for a patient with carcinoma of the endometrium, potential patterns of spread must be considered. To a large degree, this can be determined by evaluating prognostic factors. Patients with a poor prognosis may then undergo radiation therapy. Currently, the grade of the tumor can be determined before surgery as can potential sites of metastasis, such as the vagina, adnexa, or lungs. The depth of myometrial invasion, however, cannot be known until the time of hysterectomy and pathologic evaluation. Certainly some patients can have a well-differentiated cancer in conjunction with deep myometrial invasion, while others can have a poorly differentiated tumor yet disease may be limited to the endometrium or only superficially involve the myometrium. Apparently, the former patient is at greater risk for metastases and potential recurrence than is the latter. Of course, these situations are exceptions to the rule; however, such findings would significantly affect adjuvant therapy.

Looking at the surgical pathologic data base, which depends on the correlation of multiple prognostic factors, one would expect it to provide criteria for selecting therapy. If the tumor grade is high, lymph node metastases as well as deep invasion and recurrence can be predicted with some certainty (Table 12-7). In patients with Stage I, Grade 1 disease, the surgical intervention can be limited to peritoneal cytology and TAH and BSO. Only a small number of patients with Grade 1 disease will have deep myometrial invasion; such patients can be evaluated intraoperatively, and if deep invasion is present, selective lymphadenectomy would be advocated by some investigators. Patients with Grade 2 or 3 disease are considered to be at higher risk for lymph node metastases, and it has been suggested that pelvic and paraaortic selected lymphadenectomy be added to the surgical procedure described for Grade 1 disease.

It is appreciated that lymphadenectomy in Grade 2 adenocarcinomas is controversial, and further data are needed to clarify the applicability of lymphadenectomy in this group of patients. If necessary, postoperative adjunctive therapy can then be planned, depending mainly on whether there is intrauterine or extrauterine disease. In patients with *intrauterine disease* only, those with Grade 1 or 2 disease had only a 4% recurrence rate; those with grade 3 and superficial invasion had a 14% recurrence rate, with all lesions at distant sites. It would appear that surgery alone may be adequate for Grades 1 and 2 as well as for Grade 3 and superficial disease. In patients with Grade 3 disease and significant myometrial invasion, the recurrence rate was 40%, with the majority of lesions at distant sites. It is in this small group of patients with disease limited to the uterus that one could probably justify the use of postoperative ex-

| | TABLE 12-7 Grade and Risk Factors in Stage I Cancer | | |
|---|---|---|---|
| Grade | Lymph Node Metastases | Deep Muscle Invasion | Recurrence Rate |
| 1 | 2% | 4% | 4% |
| 2 | 11% | 15% | 15% |
| 3 | 27% | 39% | 42% |

ternal-beam radiation to the pelvis as well as consider progestins or chemotherapy. Although the latter recommendation appears prudent, it may have limited practicality. To be responsive to progestins, tumors are usually considered to need positive receptors and, as a general rule, Grade 3 tumors tend to have few detectible receptors. Doxorubicin is now considered the drug of choice in recurrent adenocarcinoma; however, only about 10% of patients with advanced or recurrent disease will respond completely to this drug. Its role, if any, as an adjunct remains to be defined. One can say this about any single therapeutic agent at the present time.

When *extrauterine disease* is present (i.e., metastasis to adnexa, or lymph nodes, intraperitoneally or presence of malignant cells in the peritoneal cytologic specimens), the rate of recurrence is quite high. Most of these patients have recurrent lesions at distant sites. The need to develop adjunctive therapy to prevent such metastases is apparent. As mentioned earlier, adjunctive therapy in the form of chemotherapy has been unsuccessful to date and its role is still undetermined. When disease is limited to the pelvic and/or paraaortic lymph nodes, irradiation of these areas can be given, with a long-term survival of about 50%.

Patients with Stage II carcinoma of the endometrium will have a greater propensity for lymph node metastases because disease is present in the cervix. With the increased incidence of lymph node metastases, radical hysterectomy and pelvic lymphadenectomy might be appropriate therapy, as suggested by several reports. Others prefer to use preoperative external-beam radiation to the whole pelvis with at least one radium application prior to TAH and BSO performed 6 weeks later. Another option that appears to be gaining favor is that noted for patients with Stage I, Grade 2 or 3 cancers (TAH, BSO, and lymphadenectomy). This is certainly true if disease appears to be limited to the endocervix. Because of the high false-positive rate (overdiagnosis) in Stage II, the latter option may obviate preoperative radiation, particularly when the surgical specimen shows no disease in the endocervix. Because of the frequency of overdiagnosing in Stage II disease, the latter option would seem prudent. Onsrud et al (1982) address this problem in a retrospective review, noting that only 96 of 174 patients (56%) originally thought to have Stage II carcinomas did in fact have disease in the endocervix. Those patients who were overdiagnosed had survival rates similar to those of patients with Stage I disease. Of those patients with true Stage II disease, the use of radiation therapy did not seem to improve survival compared with results in patients who did not receive external-beam radiation therapy.

For the small number of patients unfortunate enough to have Stage III and IV disease, therapy must be individualized. One can make a good case for hormonal treatment or chemotherapy or both, in addition to surgery plus radiation therapy.

Extrafascial hysterectomy is considered the technique of choice in endometrial carcinoma. Removing the upper portion of the vagina does not appear to reduce vault recurrences. Immediately after the peritoneal cavity is opened, peritoneal cytology should be obtained if ascitic fluid is not present. If selective lymphadenectomy is to be performed, the retroperitoneal spaces in the pelvis should be opened in the routine fashion. The vessels are outlined, and any enlarged lymph nodes are removed separately and sent for histologic evaluation. It should be noted that, unlike cervical cancer, it is unusual to have enlarged lymph nodes secondary to metastasis. External iliac nodes from the bifurcation to the inguinal ligament are removed as is lymphatic tissue anterior to the obturator nerve in the obturator fossa. Lymph nodes over the common iliac are also removed. The small intestine is then retracted into the upper abdomen, and the peritoneum over the major vessels is incised. The main vessels are outlined and the ureters are retracted laterally. Tissue overlying the vena cava and aorta is removed en bloc, beginning at the bifurcation and extending usually to the level where the second portion of duodenum crosses the vessels retroperitoneally.

As has already been mentioned, adjunctive systemic therapy appears to be needed in high-risk patients with endometrial cancer, since most recurrences are outside the treatment field. The GOG evaluated Stage I and occult Stage II endometrial cancer patients at high risk (Morrow et al, 1990). Treatment consisted of TAH and BSO with peritoneal cytology, and selective pelvic and paraaortic lymphadenectomy. Patients then received external-beam radiation to the pelvis with or without paraaortic radiation and were randomized to receive either doxorubicin, 60 mg/m$^2$, every 3 weeks for 8 doses or no further therapy. Of 181 patients entered into this protocol, 22% of those given doxorubicin and 26% of

those who did not receive chemotherapy suffered a recurrence. Among those with recurrence, the risk for metastases to the abdomen was greater in the patients who received chemotherapy than in those not treated (40% vs 17%). However, distant metastases occurred more often in the patients who did not receive chemotherapy (56% vs 18%).

Based on the data derived from the surgical staging protocols, FIGO decided that endometrial cancer should be surgically staged and in 1988 changed the staging classification for this disease (Table 12-8).

## RECURRENCE

Only about 10% of patients with endometrial cancer will die from the disease, but approximately half of these deaths will occur in patients with Stage I disease. Some recurrences, especially those in the vagina, can be successfully treated with surgery or radiation therapy or a combination of the two. Many of these patients do well and become long-term survivors. As mentioned earlier, the vast majority of recurrent lesions are located outside the treatment field and thus are not amenable to surgery or radiation. For this reason, hormonal therapy or chemotherapy is the treatment of choice in many cases.

Several large prospective randomized studies have evaluated the use of progestins as adjunctive therapy in adenocarcinoma of the endometrium in the hope of preventing recurrence. Recurrences developed in patients with Stage I disease who are so treated, and no difference in survival has been noted between the groups who did and did not receive adjuvant progestins (DePalo et al, 1985).

Progestins have been used for several decades to treat patients with recurrent disease, and objective responses have been noted in many cases. It has been stated that as many as one-third will respond to these hormones, and those with well differentiated tumors have a higher rate of response than do those with moderately or poorly differentiated lesions. In a large study conducted by the GOG, patients with advanced or recurrent endometrial cancer were treated with medroxyprogesterone acetate, 50 mg 3 times a day (Thigpen et al, 1985b). Of the 219 patients with objective measurable disease, only 17 responded completely (8%) and 13 showed partial response (6%). More than half the patients remained stable and one-third progressed. Median survival was 10.5 months. Grade 1 lesions did respond more frequently than did the poorly differentiated carcinomas.

It is well established that adenocarcinomas of the endometrium bear specific estrogen-progesterone receptors, and there are more of both receptors in well-differentiated lesions than in poorly differentiated ones. In one small group of patients, about one-third of those with recurrent cancer had positive results on receptor analysis for both estrogen and progesterone. Perhaps receptor status may someday be used to correlate responsiveness to treatment with progesterone, since preliminary data support this hypothesis. If receptor anal-

| TABLE 12-8 Staging of Cancer of the Uterine Corpus | |
|---|---|
| Stage IA G123 | Tumor limited to endometrium |
| IB G123 | Invasion to < 1/2 myometrium |
| IC G123 | Invasion to > 1/2 myometrium |
| IIA G123 | Endocervical glandular involvement only |
| IIB G123 | Cervical stromal invasion |
| IIIA G123 | Tumor invades serosa and/or adnexa and/or positive peritoneal cytology |
| IIIB G123 | Vaginal metastases |
| IIIC G123 | Metastases to pelvic and/or paraaortic lymph nodes |
| IVA G123 | Tumor invasion of bladder and/or bowel mucosa |
| IVB | Distant metastases including intraabdominal and/or inguinal nodes |

ysis is positive for both estrogen and progesterone, the chances of responding to progesterone are good even if the lesion is poorly differentiated. If, on the other hand, the receptor analysis is negative, those patients would benefit more from cytotoxic chemotherapy. In at least one small study (Kauppila, 1980), results suggested that cytotoxic chemotherapy should be the first line of therapy in receptor-negative patients.

Progesterone therapy can be administered by a variety of routes and in different doses. Neither the type of progestin nor its dosage seems to affect the response rate. At present, the GOG is carrying out a prospective randomized study of medroxyprogesterone acetate given in two different daily doses, 200 mg or 1,000 mg. Only time will tell whether or not response to progesterone appears to be dose-dependent.

Cytotoxic therapy in endometrial cancer has historically been given only to those individuals who have not responded to a progestin. Doxorubicin appears to have been used most often, possibly as many as one-third of these patients might respond to this drug (Thigpen et al, 1979). In a small group of patients reported by the GOG, the complete response rate was only 10%, and the responses lasted only 7 months (Thigpen et al, 1985a). The Eastern Oncology Group achieved only a 19% response rate in a trial of doxorubicin (Horton et al, 1978); however, they used a lower dose than that used by the GOG. The MD Anderson group reported their experience with cisplatin as a single agent, which led to a 42% objective response rate (10 partial responses and one complete response in 26 patients) (Seski et al, 1982). The mean duration of response was only 5 months, with a complete response lasting 8 months. The same authors have noted a 30% response rate in patients treated with doxorubicin and cyclophosphamide (Seski et al, 1981). In the GOG trial, only 1 of 23 patients treated with cisplatin responded (Thigpen et al, 1980). Almost all these patients had previously been treated with other cytotoxic agents. A subsequent study of the GOG using cisplatin as a first line drug resulted in a higher response rate (Thigpen et al, 1989).

The one large prospective randomized study (GOG) evaluated multiple agents for recurrent endometrial cancer (Cohen et al, 1984). Melphalan and 5-FU were compared with doxorubicin, 5-FU, and cyclophosphamide. Medroxyprogesterone acetate was also used. Approximately one-third of both groups achieved an objective response, and there was no difference in the progression-free interval nor the median response rate between the two groups. Median survival was approximately 10 months in both groups; however, complete responders had a median survival of 18.3 months. Toxicity was considerably tolerable with both regimens.

The GOG also evaluated 336 patients with advanced recurrent adenocarcinoma who were treated with doxorubicin with or without cyclophosphamide (Thigpen, 1985a). All these patients had been previously treated with progestin. Only 7 (5.4%) of those treated with doxorubicin had a complete or partial response compared with 18 (12.5%) who received doxorubicin plus cyclophosphamide. Median survival was 7 months for both groups, and there was no difference in survival

between the two groups. Piver et al (1987) treated 50 patients with melphalan, 5-FU, and medroxyprogesterone acetate with or without tamoxifen as first-line chemotherapy. They noted a 20% complete response rate and a 48% total response rate. The median progression-free survival was only 5 months for the whole group, although the complete responders had a median progression-free interval of 24 months.

# REFERENCES

Alberhasky RC, Connely PJ, Christopherson WN: Carcinoma of the endometrium. IV. Mixed adenosquamous carcinoma. *Am J Clin Pathol* 77:655, 1982.
Bond WH: Early uterine body carcinoma: Is postoperative vaginal irradiation of any value? *Clin Radiol* 36:619, 1985.
Boronow RC, Morrow CP, Creasman WT, et al: Surgical staging in endometrial cancer: Clinical pathological findings of a prospective study. *Obstet Gynecol* 63:825, 1984.
Centers for Disease Control: Cancer in Steroid Hormone Study: Oral contraceptive use and the risk of endometrial cancer. *JAMA* 249:1600, 1983.
Chen JL, Tros DC, Wilkinson EJ: Endometrial papillary carcinoma: Two clinical pathological types. *Int J Gynecol Pathol* 4:279, 1985.
Christopherson WN, Alberhasky RC, Connely PJ: Carcinoma of the endometrium. II. Papillary adenocarcinoma: A clinicopathological study of 46 patients. *Am J Clin Pathol* 77:534, 1982.
Chu J, Schweid AL, Weiss NS: Survival among women with endometrial cancer: A comparison of estrogen users and nonusers. *Am J Obstet Gynecol* 143:569, 1982.
Cohen CJ, Bruckner HW, Deppe GE, et al: A randomized study comparing multiple agent chemotherapeutic regimens in the treatment of advanced and recurrent endometrial carcinoma. A Gynecologic Oncology Group study. *Obstet Gynecol* 63:719, 1984.
Creasman WT, DiSaia PJ, Boronow RC, et al: Adenocarcinoma of the endometrium: Its metastatic lymph node potential: A preliminary report. *Gynecol Oncol* 4:239, 1976.
Creasman WT, Rutledge FN: The prognostic value of peritoneal cytology in gynecologic malignant disease. *Am J Obstet Gynecol* 110:773, 1971.
Creasman WT, DiSaia PJ, Blessing J, et al: Prognostic significance of peritoneal cytology in patients with endometrial cancer and preliminary data concerning therapy with intraperitoneal radiopharmaceuticals. *Am J Obstet Gynecol* 141:921, 1981.
Creasman WT, Soper JT, McCarty KS Jr, et al: Influence of cytoplasmic steroid receptor content on prognosis of early stage endometrial carcinoma. *Am J Obstet Gynecol* 151:922, 1985.
Creasman WT, Morrow CP, Bundy L, et al: Surgical pathological spread patterns of endometrial cancer. *Cancer* 60:2035, 1987.
de Waal JC, Lochmuller H: Preoperative radium insertion in the management of carcinoma of the endometrium. *Geburtshilfe Frauenheilkd* 42:394, 1982.
DePalo G, et al: Adjuvant treatment with medroxyprogesterone acetate in pathological stage I endometrial cancer with myometrial invasion. In Volla, Racine, and Vrousos (eds): *Endometrial Cancers,* 5th Cancer Research Workshop, Grenoble, France. Basel, S. Karger, 1985, p 209.
DiSaia PH, Creasman WT, Boronow RC, et al: Risk factors in recurrent patterns in stage I endometrial carcinoma. *Am J Obstet Gynecol* 151:1009, 1985.
Gambrell RD Jr: Role of hormones in the etiology and prevention of endometrial and breast cancer. *Acta Obstet Gynecol Scand (Suppl)* 106:37, 1982.
Gusberg SB, Kardon P: Proliferative endometrial response to thecal granulosa cell tumors. *Am J Obstet Gynecol* 3:633, 1971.
Hanson NB, Van Nagell JR, Powell DE, et al: Prognostic significance of lymph-vascular space invasion in stage I endometrial cancer. *Cancer* 55:1753, 1985.
Heyman J: The so-called Stockholm method and the results of treatment of uterine cancer at the Radiumhemmet. *Acta Radiol* 16:129, 1935.

Javert CT, Douglas R: Treatment of endometrial carcinoma. *Am J Roentgenol* 75:580, 1956.

Javert CT: The spread of benign and malignant endometrium in the lymphatic system with a note on co-existing vascular involvement. *Am J Obstet Gynecol* 64:780, 1952.

Jones HW: Treatment of adenocarcinoma of the endometrium. *Obstet Gynecol Surv* 30:147, 1975.

Kauppila A, Janne O, Kujansuu E, et al: Treatment of advanced endometrial adenocarcinoma with combined cytotoxic therapy. *Cancer* 46:2162, 1980.

Horton J, Begg CB, Arseneault J, et al: Comparison of Adriamycin with cyclophosphamide in patients with advanced endometrial cancer. *Cancer Treat Rep* 62:159, 1978.

Lutz MH, Underwood PB, Kreutner A, et al: Endometrial carcinoma: A new method of classification of therapeutic and prognostic significance. *Gynecol Oncol* 6:83, 1978.

MacMahon B: Risk factors for endometrial cancer. *Gynecol Oncol* 2:122, 1974.

Morrow CP, DiSaia PJ, Townsend DE: Current management of endometrial carcinoma. *Obstet Gynecol* 42:399, 1973.

Morrow CP, Bundy BN, Homesly HD, et al: Doxorubicin as an adjuvant following surgery and radiation therapy in patients with high-rate endometrial carcinoma, stage I and occult stage II: A Gynecologic Oncology Group Study. *Gynecol Oncol* 36:166, 1990.

Morrow CP, et al: A randomized study of Adriamycin adjuvant chemotherapy for patients with high risk stage I and II (occult) endometrial carcinoma. Presented at International Gynecologic Cancer Society, Amsterdam, October, 1987.

Ng ABP, Reagan JW, Storaasli JP, et al: Mixed adenosquamous carcinoma of the endometrium. *Am J Clin Pathol* 59:765, 1973.

Norris HJ, Taylor HG: Prognosis of granulosa thecal tumor of the ovary. *Cancer* 21:255, 1968.

Onsrud M, Kolstad P, Normann T: Postoperative external pelvic irradiation in carcinoma of the corpus stage I: A controlled clinical trial. *Gynecol Oncol* 4:222, 1976.

Onsrud N, Aalders J, Abeler V, Taylor P: Endometrial carcinoma with cervical involvement (stage II): Prognostic factors in value of combined radiological surgical treatment. *Gynecol Oncol* 13:76, 1982.

Patterson E, Spratt D, Tenkiewicz Z, et al: Management of stage I carcinoma of the uterus. *Obstet Gynecol* 59:755, 1982.

Pettersson F (ed): Annual Report on the Results of Treatment in Gynecological Cancer, Vol 20. International Federation of Gynecology and Obstetrics, Stockholm, 1988, p 75-96.

Piver MS, Lele SB, Patsner B, et al: Melphalan, 5-FU, and medroxyprogesterone acetate in metastatic endometrial carcinoma. *Obstet Gynecol* 67:261, 1987.

Rutledge FN: The role of radical hysterectomy in adenocarcinoma of the endometrium. *Gynecol Oncol* 2:331, 1974.

Schink JC, Lurain JR, Wallemark MS, et al: Tumor size in endometrial cancer: A prospective factor for lymph node metastases. *Obstet Gynecol* 70:216, 1987.

Seski JC, Edwards CL, Gershenson DM, et al: Adriamycin and cyclophosphamide chemotherapy for disseminated endometrial cancer. *Obstet Gynecol* 58:88, 1981.

Seski JC, Edwards CL, Herson J, Rutledge FN: Cisplatin chemotherapy for disseminated endometrial cancer. *Obstet Gynecol* 59:225, 1982.

Silverberg SG, Bolin MG, DeGiorgi LS: Adenoacanthoma and mixed adenosquamous carcinoma of the endometrium. *Cancer* 30:1307, 1972.

Smith DC, et al: Association of exogenous estrogen and endometrial carcinoma. *N Engl J Med* 293:1164, 1975.

Soper JT, Creasman WT, Clarke-Pearson DL, et al: Intraperitoneal chromic phosphate P-32 suspension therapy in malignant peritoneal cytology and endometrial carcinoma. *Am J Obstet Gynecol* 153:191, 1985.

Thigpen JT, Buchsbaum HJ, Mangan C, Blessing JA: Phase II trial of Adriamycin in treatment of advanced or recurrent endometrial carcinoma. *Cancer Treat Rep* 63:21, 1979.

Thigpen JT, Blessing J, DiSaia P, Ehrlich C: A randomized comparison of Adriamycin with or without Cytoxan in the treatment of advanced recurrent adenocarcinoma. *American Society of Clinical Oncology* #C-448, 1985a.

Thigpen JT, Blessing J, DiSaia P, Ehrlich C: Treatment of advanced or recurrent endometrial cancer with medroxyprogesterone acetate. *Gynecol Oncol* 20:250, 1985b.

Thigpen JT, Shingleton H, Homesley H, et al: Cisplatinum in the treatment of advanced or recurrent cervix and uterine cancer. In Prestayka AW, Cooke ST, Carter SK (eds): *Cis-platin: Current Status and New Developments.* New York Academic Press, 1980.

Thigpen JT, Blessing JA, Homesley H, et al: Phase II trial of cisplatin as first-line chemotherapy in patients with advanced or recurrent endometrial cancer: A Gynecologic Oncology Group Study. *Gynecol Oncol* 33:68, 1989.

# Chapter 13 | Uterine Sarcomas

*Karen H. Antman*

One per cent of gynecologic malignancies are sarcomas. While sarcomas represent 1.2 to 6% of all *uterine* malignancies (Bartsich et al, 1968; Crawford and Tucker, 1959; Forney and Buchsbaum, 1981; Kaether et al, 1980), primary sarcomas of the ovaries, vagina, and labia are relatively rare.

Sarcomas had already been distinguished from carcinomas at the time of Hippocrates. Derived from the root *sarc* (flesh) joined to the suffix *oma* (tumor), fleshly sarcomas were contrasted to "crablike" carcinomas. ("Sarcasm," or a flesh-tearing criticism, is derived from the same Greek root.) These tumors can be conveniently divided into two groups: those arising in bone and those of the soft tissues. The latter are further subdivided into the classic somatic visceral soft tissue sarcomas, generally of the extremities and retroperitoneum, and sarcomas of parenchymal organs, including gastrointestinal and gynecologic sarcomas.

## ETIOLOGIC FACTORS

Prior radiotherapy appears to be the only clearly documented etiologic factor in the development of gynecologic sarcomas. Nevertheless, overall, a minority of these tumors are radiation associated, as reported in various series (Mantravadi et al, 1981; Salazar et al, 1978a) (Table 13-1). Thirteen to 26% of mixed müllerian sarcomas (Gilbert et al, 1975; Norris et al, 1966), 13% of carcinosarcomas (Norris and Taylor, 1966b), 2 to 8% of leiomyosarcomas (Aaro et al, 1966; Gallup and Cordray, 1979; Gilbert et al, 1975), and a few anecdotal cases of endometrial stromal sarcoma (Mantravadi et al, 1981; Norris and Taylor, 1966a) have occurred after radiation, which generally had been administered 7 to 26 years earlier for benign uterine bleeding (Aaro et al, 1966; Gallup and Cordray, 1979). In addition, sarcomas have developed in a few patients previously treated with radiation for cervical or ovarian cancer (King and Kramer, 1980; Norris et al, 1966; Norris and Taylor, 1966b).

Nongynecologic sarcomas have also occurred after exposure to vinyl chloride, agent orange (Sarma and Jacobs, 1982), arsenic, and asbestos and after the use of thorium dioxide as a roentgenographic contrast agent (Table 13-1). Proclivity for sarcoma appears to be genetically determined in some cases. Von Recklinghausen's disease is associated with a 10% lifetime incidence of sarcoma, developing either de novo or in a previously existing neurofibroma. A small percentage of persons with Paget's disease (0.2%) develop osteogenic sarcoma. Up to 7% of patients with familial retinoblastoma are at risk for osteogenic sarcoma that will

arise not only within cranial radiotherapy ports but also in the long bones of the extremities—obviously distant from any sites of radiation delivery.

Species-specific sarcoma viruses exist, including simian sarcoma and avian sarcoma RNA viruses, and a uterine leiomyosarcoma was experimentally induced in a rabbit after herpes virus type 2 inoculations (Gallup and Cordray, 1979). Associations have been observed between cytomegalovirus (CMV) and Kaposi's sarcoma in homosexuals (Centers for Disease Control, 1982) and between human T-cell leukemia virus (HTLV) and the acquired immune deficiency syndrome (AIDS) (Essex et al, 1983). Certainly these patients with multiple infections are compromised immunologically; CMV and perhaps HTLV may be opportunistic pathogens rather than causally related to Kaposi's sarcoma.

Case reports also include a man who developed a sarcoma within 6 months of the diagnosis of a uterine sarcoma in his wife. Although the authors suggested that this was a chance occurrence, a viral etiology for human sarcomas cannot be disregarded (Gallup and Cordray, 1979). Huth et al (1981, 1982) have detected a common cross-reacting antigen in sarcomas of different histologic types (including uterine leiomyosarcoma), a finding that suggests a viral etiology. Furthermore, a high incidence of antisarcoma antibodies has been noted among close relatives of sarcoma patients. As yet, however, there is no conclusive evidence of a causal association between any virus and the development of human soft tissue sarcomas (Gallup and Cordray, 1979).

There is no known association between the use of birth control pills or postmenopausal estrogens and subsequent development of uterine sarcoma.

## STAGING AND CLASSIFICATION OF UTERINE SARCOMAS

As can be seen in the previous chapters, Salazar and the Gynecologic Oncology Group (GOG) have advocated the application of the FIGO staging classification used for carcinoma of the uterine corpus to stage uterine sarcomas (Salazar et al, 1978a). However, these authors did not subdivide Stage I into Stages IA and IB, which are based on uterine depth less than and greater than 8 cm, respectively, since there was no difference in prognosis between these two groups (Salazar et al, 1978a, 1978b).

A criticism of the use of FIGO staging in the classification of uterine sarcomas is that it divides patients into only two prognostic groups: those with Stage I disease and those with Stages II to IV. Five-year survival for patients with Stage I disease is approximately 50%

TABLE 13-1    Etiology of Sarcomas

| Etiologic Agent | % Associated | Associated Sarcoma |
|---|---|---|
| Radiation | 13-26 | Mixed müllerian sarcoma |
| | 13 | Carcinosarcoma |
| | 2-8 | Leiomyosarcoma of the uterus |
| | Anecdotal | Endometrial stromal sarcoma |
| Chemical | | |
| Asbestos | 50 | Mesothelioma |
| Thorotrast | Rare | Angiosarcoma |
| Vinyl chloride | Rare | Angiosarcoma |
| Arsenic | Rare | Angiosarcoma |
| Dioxide (agent orange) | | No specific histology |
| Genetic | | |
| Von Recklinhausen's disease | | Neurofibroma or fibrosarcoma |
| Retinoblastoma | | Osteogenic sarcoma |
| Chronic injury | | |
| Paget's disease | | Osteogenic sarcoma |
| Swollen extremity | | Lymphangiosarcoma |
| Scars | Rare | No specific histology |
| ? Viral | | |
| Cytomegalovirus in homosexuals* | | Kaposi's sarcoma |
| Avian and/or feline viruses | | Sarcoma in cats |
| Simian sarcoma virus | | Sarcoma in monkeys |

* Associated but not necessarily causally.

and that for the remaining stages is about 10%. A staging system that considers grade (as is currently used for nongynecologic soft tissue sarcomas) has the advantage of dividing patients into four prognostic stages (Eberl et al, 1980).

In 1970, Kempson introduced a simplified classification based on Ober's retrospective analysis of uterine sarcomas evaluated at Barnes Hospital in St. Louis (Table 13-2). Generally believed to be histogenically accurate, this classification has now gained considerable acceptance. Uterine sarcomas are first classified as either pure or mixed and then further divided into homologous or heterologous types (i.e., derived from mesenchymal tissue normally present in or absent from the uterus, respectively). Thus, leiomyosarcomas represent a pure homologous sarcoma of the uterus, since smooth muscle is a normal uterine component. Mixed sarcomas include more than one homologous or heterologous histologic type, while mixed müllerian sarcomas contain both carcinomatous and sarcomatous elements.

Although leiomyosarcomas predominate in some series (Dallenbach-Hellweg, 1980; Kenda et al, 1981), an overall review of the literature shows that the most common histologic types of uterine sarcoma are, in order of frequency, mixed müllerian sarcoma (50%), leiomyosarcoma (30%) and endometrial stromal sarcoma (15%) (Salazar et al, 1978a). Whereas Kempson and Bari (1970) advocate classifying carcinosarcomas (CS) within the mixed müllerian sarcomas (as they are here), Norris considers them separately on the basis of their better prognosis (Norris and Taylor, 1966b).

## PATHOLOGY AND PROGNOSIS

### Leiomyosarcomas (LMS)

The incidence of LMS ranges in various series from 0.2 to 6% of all uterine smooth muscle tumors. The same discrepancy can be found in 5-year survival figures, which range from 3 to 75% (Dinh and Woodruff, 1982). Both the incidence of LMS and the 5-year disease-free survival are substantially increased when significant numbers of cellular leiomyomas are included in an analysis.

TABLE 13-2    Classification of Uterine Sarcomas

*Pure sarcomas*
  Pure homologous
    Leiomyosarcoma (LMS)
    Endometrial stromal sarcoma (ESS)
    Endolymphatic stromal meiosis (ESM)
    Angiosarcoma
    Fibrosarcoma
  Pure heterologous
    Rhabdomyosarcoma (including sarcoma botryoides)
    Chondrosarcoma
    Osteosarcoma
    Liposarcoma
*Mixed sarcomas*
    Mixed homologous
    Mixed heterologous with or without homologous elements
*Malignant mixed müllerian tumors (mixed mesodermal tumors)*
*(MMS)*
    Homologous type: Carcinoma plus leiomyosarcoma, stromal sarcoma, or fibrosarcoma, or mixtures of these sarcomas
    Heterologous type: Carcinoma plus heterologous sarcoma with or without homologous sarcoma

*Source:* Modified from Kempson RL, Bari W: Uterine sarcomas. Classification, diagnosis, and prognosis. *Hum Pathol* 1:331-349, 1970.

***Gross Description*** LMS are whitish-gray or pale pink lesions with cystic, necrotic, or hemorrhagic areas and a diameter of up to 20 cm (Dinh and Woodruff, 1982). Multiple lesions may be present in almost half of the patients. About two-thirds are intramural and 10% are submucous (Dinh and Woodruff, 1982; Kempson and Bari, 1970). Spread to lymph nodes is distinctly unusual (Dinh and Woodruff, 1982; Salazar et al, 1978*b*).

Most hysterectomy specimens in LMS also contain smaller benign myomas (Aaro et al, 1966). LMS have been considered primary (arising de novo in the myometrium) or secondary (arising in a leiomyoma); the incidence of secondary LMS in various series has ranged from 0 to 80% (Aaro et al, 1966; Christopherson et al, 1972; Crawford and Tucker, 1959). Some investigators have concluded that malignant degeneration of benign fibroids does not occur (Gallup and Cordray, 1979), while others estimate the incidence of such degeneration to be up to 0.13% of all myomas. Patients with LMS originating in a leiomyoma are said to have a better prognosis (Gallup and Cordray, 1979).

***Microscopic Description*** Differentiating LMS from benign but cellular, bizarre, or parasitic leiomyomas is frequently challenging and requires evaluation by a pathologist experienced in the diagnosis of uterine sarcomas.

All authors accept a diagnosis of LMS if a lesion is histologically invasive, metastatic, or recurrent (Bartsich et al, 1968; Kempson and Bari, 1970). Truly invasive LMS must be distinguished from benign parasitic leiomyomas, which also grow into other organs. A more reproducible criterion for determining malignancy, which was proposed by Kempson and is now generally accepted, is based on the number of mitoses observed in histologic specimens, i.e., the mitotic index, with consideration also given to the presence of pleomorphism (Hannigan and Gomez, 1979; Kempson and Bari, 1970; Lanberge, 1962). Kempson advocates the designation *leiomyosarcomas* for tumors that show 10 or more mitoses per 10 high-power fields (HPF), with or without significant cellular atypia (Table 13-3) (Kempson and Bari, 1970). Those with 5 to 10 mitoses/10 HPF and substantial pleomorphism should also be considered malignant; in Kempson's series, five out of six of these patients died. Tumors with less than 5 mitoses/10 HPF can usually be considered benign lesions, although occasionally metastatic disease eventually develops.

Vascular invasion and the presence or absence of giant cells do not correlate with survival (Kempson and Bari, 1970). In contrast, pleomorphism tends to occur in tumors with a high mitotic index; tumors that show large numbers of mitoses but only minimal or moderate pleomorphism may also be seen occasionally. In these latter cases, patients frequently survive for considerable periods of time before relapsing (Dinh and Woodruff, 1982; Kempson and Bari, 1970). The presence of hyalinization may indicate a favorable prognosis (Dinh and Woodruff, 1982).

Independent of the mitotic index, the level of invasion correlates with prognosis (Aaro et al, 1966; Han-

**TABLE 13-3  Criteria for Differentiating Uterine Leiomyosarcoma from Other Lesions**

Leiomyosarcoma
  ≥10 mitoses/10 HPF
  5-10 mitoses/10 HPF and anaplasia, pleomorphism, or epithelioid histology
Lesions of uncertain malignant potential
  5-9 mitoses/10 HPF if well differentiated
  2-4 mitoses/10 HPF and anaplasia, pleomorphism, or epithelioid histology
Unusual (malignant-appearing) but benign leiomyomas
  Benign metastasizing leiomyomas
  Intravenous leiomyomatosis
  Bizarre leiomyomas
  Disseminated peritoneal leiomyomatosis
  Cellular leiomyomas
  Parasitic leiomyomas

nigan and Gomez, 1979). Seventy per cent of patients with tumor confined to the myometrium and half of those with tumor invading the endometrium or endocervix survive for 5 years. In contrast, only one of 9 patients with involvement of the serosa and only one of 12 with extension beyond the uterus (to the broad ligament) survive for 5 years (Aaro et al, 1966; Hannigan and Gomez, 1979).

***Lesions Considered Benign*** A biologic and pathologic continuum of abnormality exists, with benign leiomyomas at one end of the spectrum and the high-grade LMS at the other. An occasional tumor with less than 5 mitoses/10 HPF may be locally aggressive or fall into the category of benign metastasizing leiomyoma or intravenous leiomyomatosis (see below). Metastases from either entity may appear long after initial surgery, and surgical excision of a single recurrent lesion may result in prolonged disease-free survival (Kempson and Bari, 1970). These rare, histologically benign but biologically malignant tumors are impossible to separate prospectively from leiomyomas (Kempson and Bari, 1970). In contrast, histologically bizarre but biologically benign leiomyomas must also be correctly identified, and parasitic leiomyomas must be distinguished from truly invasive LMS.

*Benign metastasizing leiomyomas (BML)* generally arise in women 24 to 40 years of age and are apparently more common among black women. Metastasizing leiomyomas appear to be responsive to ovarian steroid hormones, since regression has occurred after both termination of pregnancy and oophorectomy (Cramer et al, 1980). The tumor seems to progress more rapidly in premenopausal women; thus, tamoxifen therapy has been suggested (Tomasian et al, 1982; Winter, 1981). BML may spread throughout the pelvis and peritoneum and may metastasize to lungs and lymph nodes. The percentage of tritiated-thymidine labeling in BML in vitro was near the upper limit of the range seen in seven ordinary uterine leiomyomas but was distinctly lower than that in LMS (Cramer et al, 1980). The number of cytosolic estrogen receptors has also been within the range seen in uterine leiomyomas. Although there have been reports of spontaneous regression of BML, other women have died of the disease (Cramer et al, 1980).

*Intravenous leiomyomatosis (IVL)*, first recognized in 1903, has now been described in almost 100 cases and is characterized by nodular masses of histologically benign smooth muscle growing within uterine and other pelvic veins. Patients have generally been white and premenopausal and in many cases pregnant. Extension of the tumor up the vena cava and into the right atrium may result in obstruction of venous return to the heart, in which case cardiac surgery is indicated (Tierney et al, 1980). IVL either originates in the uterus or arises from blood vessel walls. Some patients have survived for long periods of time after incomplete resection of the tumor, and subsequent resections have been associated with prolonged disease-free survival. Substantial levels of cytoplasmic estradiol and progesterone receptors are found in some tumors, and IVL frequently stabilizes or regresses after menopause. Metastases to the lung and retroperitoneal space have been reported (Tierney et al, 1980).

*Cellular or bizarre leiomyomas* are also seen. Pregnant patients or those taking large doses of steroid hormones that include synthetic progesterones may have highly cellular leiomyomas with hyperchromatic nuclei. Although rare mitotic figures are seen, these tumors can generally be distinguished histologically from the sarcomas which they mimic (Gallup and Cordray, 1979).

## Endometrial Stromal Sarcomas

Malignant tumors composed entirely of cells that resemble endometrial stroma are classified into two groups: (1) endolymphatic stromal meiosis and (2) endometrial stromal sarcoma.* A benign stromal nodule, a third entity with a low mitotic count, infiltrates neither lymphatic spaces nor myometrium.

*Endometrial stromal meiosis (ESM)*, a Grade 0 to 1 sarcoma with an indolent course, occurs in younger women (median age = 42; range = 18 to 69 years) (Hart and Yoonessi, 1977). Occasionally ESM may arise in extrauterine endometriosis (Hart and Yoonessi, 1977), and a single patient developed ESM after radiotherapy (Gloor et al, 1982). Histologically, ESM resembles proliferative endometrial stroma (typically without glands). The mitotic index is below 10 mitoses/10 HPF, and nuclear atypia and pleomorphism are absent. Invasion of lymphatics and veins does not indicate a poor prognosis (Gloor et al, 1982). While tumors with low mitotic counts were often seen to have pushing borders, the finding of an invasive border in a tumor with a low mitotic count did not indicate a poor prognosis.

Recurrences or metastases are rare (sometimes oc-

curring 20 to 30 years after the initial resection) and generally involve the vagina, pelvis, or peritoneal cavity or occasionally lymph nodes, lung, bone, and brain (Gloor et al, 1982). High numbers of estrogen-progesterone receptors have been reported. Shrinkage of metastatic lesions has occurred with oophorectomy and/or progesterone therapy (Gloor et al, 1982; Hart and Yoonessi, 1977).

*Endometrial stromal sarcoma (ESS)* (Grades 2 to 3), in contrast to ESM, infiltrates the myometrium, metastasizes widely, and is frequently lethal. Grossly, ESS is yellow to gray-white and contains hemorrhagic and necrotic areas. Measuring between 2 and 15 cm, it bulges into the endometrial cavity and invades the myometrium (Kempson and Bari, 1970). Microscopically, ESS is composed of monotonous sheets of cells with basophilic nuclei and indistinct cytoplasm (Kempson and Bari, 1970). Reticulum surrounds individual tumor cells or small clumps of cells. Tumor is generally found within lymphatics or lymphatic-like spaces.

The number of mitoses/10 HPF in the most active area of the tumor has proved to be reliable in determining the grade and predicting the prognosis (Norris and Taylor, 1966a). Metastases developed in nine of nine patients with >20 mitoses/10 HPF, while all seven patients with tumors showing ≤5 mitoses/10HPF were free of disease 3 to 15 years after surgery. In Kempson and Bari's series (1970) there were no tumors with 6 to 20 mitoses/10 HPF, thus facilitating the division between ESS and ESM, respectively. Pleomorphism appeared in both groups and did not correlate with the prognosis.

Differential diagnosis of these tumors includes malignant lymphoma or undifferentiated small cell carcinoma of the cervix. Reticulum staining readily distinguishes carcinomas from stromal sarcomas (Kempson and Bari, 1970).

## Mixed Mesodermal Sarcomas (MMS) (Including Carcinosarcomas and Adenosarcomas)

Between 15 and 60% of uterine sarcomas in various series are MMS (Crawford and Tucker, 1959; Salazar et al, 1978a). Between 1953 and 1969, the average yearly incidence of MMS was 0.5 per 100,000 women age 25 and older (Boram et al, 1972). MMS is believed to arise from either undifferentiated cell rests or the endometrial stroma. While cell rests have not been identified in hysterectomy specimens, the totipotentiality of endometrial stroma is supported by tissue culture studies.

Grossly, MMS are soft (77%) and polypoid (58%) or fungating, with areas of necrosis (58%) and hemorrhage (32%). The diameter ranges from 1.6 to 20 cm (median = 5.6 to 6.5 cm in various series) (Norris et al, 1966; Norris and Taylor, 1966b). In more than 90% of cases, MMS extends into the myometrium.

Histologically, a wide variety of patterns are encountered. Undifferentiated areas with tumor giant cells, sarcomatous stroma of fusiform cells (Norris et al, 1966), and abundant eosinophilic cytoplasm are common, as is lymphatic invasion. However, foci of recognizable

---

* The literature on these lesions is occasionally confusing. Some authors use the term *emdometrial stromal sarcoma* to refer to tumors generally considered to be endolymphatic stromal meiosis (seen in younger women, microscopically well-differentiated, having a low mitotic index) and the term *poorly differentiated endometrial sarcoma* to correspond to endometrial stromal sarcoma, as defined by other authors (Evans, 1982).

differentiated epithelial or stromal elements provide the diagnosis. These elements may be either homologous or heterologous. In homologous MMS, the sarcomatous component is stromal sarcoma in about 60% of the cases and LMS in most of the remaining 40%. Heterologous tumors include foci of chondrosarcoma, rhabdomyosarcoma, or osteogenic sarcoma.

In most series, homologous MMS are more common than the heterologous variant. However, when an assiduous search for striated rhabdomyosarcoma cells is undertaken, a high percentage (67%) of heterologous MMS are found (Kemson and Bari, 1970; King and Kramer, 1980; Norris et al, 1966). Adenocarcinomatous elements are three to four times more frequent than squamous elements (which may be either metaplastic or neoplastic) (Kempson and Bari, 1970). Rarely, tumors will contain both glandular and squamous areas. The presence of squamous elements seems to be associated with osteogenic sarcoma or chondrosarcoma histology (Kempson and Bari, 1970; King and Kramer, 1980). About half of the heterologous tumors also contain homologous elements (e.g., LMS or ESS).

Homologous MMS must be distinguished from adenocarcinomas of the endometrium that have not become sufficiently differentiated to form glands or glandlike spaces. Reticulum stains may be required, since single cells or small clumps of cells surrounded by reticulum fibers would indicate stromal sarcoma. A misleading diagnosis may also be made after hysterectomy if an inadequate number of tissue samples are submitted for histologic examination. MMS must also be differentiated from so-called collision tumors (two separate tumors arising within the uterus).

Heterologous MMS containing chondrosarcoma appear to be somewhat less virulent; on the other hand, the presence of osteosarcoma or rhabdomyosarcoma is generally associated with a lethal outcome (Kempson and Bari, 1970; King and Kramer, 1980; Norris et al, 1966). In Kempson's series, overall survival for those with homologous and heterologous MMS was 27 and 15%, respectively; however, in other series, heterologous tumors had a better prognosis (King and Kramer, 1980). Twenty per cent of Norris' patients survived; the remainder died of tumor 1 week to 3.1 years after diagnosis, and all but one of them died within 18 months (Norris et al, 1966). Median survival after surgical resection was only 6 months.

As with other sarcomas, survival with MMS appears to be related to the degree of uterine invasion. About half the patients with tumor confined to the inner half of the myometrium survive, while virtually all those with more extensive involvement succumb (Kempson and Bari, 1970). Long-term disease-free survivors as a group also have smaller tumors (less than 5 cm in the largest diameter), with a lower incidence of lymphatic invasion (Norris et al, 1966). A history of previous irradiation is associated with a poor prognosis (King and Kramer, 1980).

Forty-seven patients with MMS were treated at the University of Texas at Galveston by Dinh et al (1988). Patients ranged in age from 33 to 82 (median = 64), and three had undergone radiotherapy 6, 7, and 16 years prior to the diagnosis of MMS. Signs at presentation were vaginal bleeding 1 month to 2 years before the diagnosis in 83% and an abdominal mass in 45%. In 12 of 34 cases, Pap smears were suggestive of malignancy. Endometrial biopsy correctly identified MMS in 20 of 29 of the patients (68%), with diagnoses of adenocarcinoma or sarcoma in the remaining nine. In contrast to the observations reported by King and Kramer (1980), Dinh et al were unable to correlate survival with depth of uterine invasion by the tumor; there was also no correlation between survival and histologic type, tumor size, or uterine size within stage. Neither vascular invasion nor mitotic index was predictive of prognosis, although patients with radiation-associated MMS had a poor prognosis and died 6 to 7 months after the diagnosis. Homologous tumors were more common in white women than in the black women studied (67% vs 30%).

Nielsen et al (1989) described 60 patients with MMS who presented between 1959 and 1982. The 5-year survival rates were 58% when disease was confined to the uterus but only 15% when disease extended beyond the uterus. Surgical stage and depth of invasion, when stratified by stage, were significant additional prognostic determinants. No significant association was noted between survival and grade of the carcinoma, mitotic count of the sarcoma, histologic type of the sarcoma, amount of sarcoma necrosis, or capillary invasion. After stratification for tumor size, there was no significant survival advantage after surgery for the addition of radiotherapy or chemotherapy or for progression-free survival in those patients with complete resection of microscopic disease. When patients were stratified by stage, survival was not affected by the addition of radiotherapy.

In patients with recurrence, an adenocarcinomatous component was identified in the metastatic lesion in 40 to 87% of cases (Kempson and Bari, 1970; King and Kramer, 1980; Massoni and Hajdu, 1981). Sarcomatous histology was next in frequency, with mixed and undifferentiated tumor also observed.

***Carcinosarcomas (CS)*** These are generally considered a subset of homologous MMS. Norris advocates separating CS from MMS because of the better prognosis associated with the former (Norris and Taylor, 1966*b*). Since CS become MMS if any heterologous foci are found, the relative percentages of CS and MMS are a function of the care with which heterologous foci are sought. In Norris' series of 31 cases, the carcinomatous element was dominant in only five cases (Norris and Taylor, 1966*b*). Pelvic recurrence was common, occurring in three-fourths of patients with abdominal metastases. Metastatic lesions in six patients were generally the dominant element within the primary tumor and were histologically identified as adenocarcinoma in two, sarcoma in two, undifferentiated in one, and mixed in one. All long-term disease-free survivors (as well as two-thirds of those with relapses) had CS confined to the uterus at the time of primary treatment. In survivors the median tumor diameter was 3.6 cm, in contrast to 7 cm in those with recurrent tumor.

***Adenosarcomas*** These tumors are also uncommon variants of MMS with a benign glandular component. CS and mixed müllerian tumors differ from adenosarcoma in that the former have a malignant epithelial component, so that a thorough sampling of an adenosarcoma is required in order to rule out this component. Benign-appearing epithelium is distributed throughout an adenosarcoma, generally resembling inactive or proliferative endometrial glands. Squamous epithelium is found in less than half the patients (Zaloudek et al, 1981).

The most useful criterion for distinguishing adenofibromas from adenosarcomas is the frequency of mitotic figures found in the stroma. Adenofibromas have fewer than 4 mitoses/10 HPF in the most active areas, whereas adenosarcomas have 4 or more. Myometrial invasion, histologically malignant heterologous mesenchymal elements, and marked atypia of stromal cells are histologic features detected only in adenosarcoma.

Periglandular hypercellularity of the stroma is a characteristic feature in the vast majority. The range of mitotic activity of the sarcoma is 4 to 24 mitoses/10 HPF in the most active areas (average = 7.5 mitoses/10 HPF). The mesenchymal component is generally either a fibrous sarcoma or an ESS or a mix of these two patterns. Leiomyosarcomatous elements have been identified in 8%, and one-fourth of the tumors contained heterologous mesenchymal components, including cartilage, striated muscle, or lipoblasts. Deep myometrial invasion by the primary lesion is associated with recurrent tumor.

Twenty-five adenosarcomas were reviewed by the Armed Forces Institute of Pathology. Three of the 25 patients were adolescents and two were ages 37 and 39; the median age was 57 years, with a range of 14 to 79 years. None of the patients had undergone prior pelvic irradiation. Abnormal vaginal bleeding was the presenting complaint in 19 of the 25 patients. An enlarged uterus was felt in 7, and tumor protruded from the cervical os or from the posterior lip of the cervix in 11. Tumors were generally superficial and well circumscribed, ranging in size from 1.2 to 2 cm (median = 5 cm). Seven of the 25 tumors histologically invaded the myometrium. Multiple lesions occurred in five patients. Twenty of the 25 underwent total abdominal hysterectomy with bilateral salpingo-oophorectomy (TAH/BSO). The three teenage girls with adenosarcoma underwent TAH, amputation of the cervix, and an excisional biopsy followed by wide and deep curettage of the biopsy site, respectively. All three remained disease-free for 2 to 10 years. The third patient has subsequently carried a normal pregnancy.

Tumor recurred in 10 women (40%) 6 months to 7 years after initial treatment (median = 5 years). Six tumors recurred locally; four of the patients presented with metastatic spread to the lungs, lung and brain, mediastinum, and small bowel, respectively. After treatment for these recurrences, two of the 10 were rendered free of residual tumor. Histologic examination of the recurrent tumors revealed sarcomatous histology except for a single vaginal metastatic lesion, which contained a glandular epithelial component.

# CLINICAL PRESENTATION

Uterine sarcomas may develop in women of any age. While the median age at diagnosis of MMS, CS, and ESS (62, 62, and 63 years, respectively) is strikingly similar to that of endometrial carcinoma (62 years), women with LMS are a full decade younger, with mean ages of 44 to 57 reported and a range in age from 20 to 82 (Gallup and Cordray, 1979; Koll, 1980; Salazar et al, 1987a). When cellular and bizarre leiomyomas are specifically removed from analyses, however, the median age of patients with LMS does shift toward the older range. While patients with ESS and MMS are generally in their sixth or seventh decade, occasional pediatric patients have been reported (Aaro et al, 1966; Kempson and Bari, 1970).

Information on the parity of women with uterine sarcoma is lacking in reports from many centers; however, some authors have reported a high incidence (almost 30%) of nulligravidas (Aaro et al, 1966; Kempson and Bari, 1970; Norris and Taylor, 1966a and 1966b; Norris et al, 1966).

Sixty to 90% of patients with ESS and MMS initially seek medical attention for heavy, irregular, or postmenopausal vaginal bleeding (Crawford and Tucker, 1959; Kempson and Bari, 1970; Norris and Taylor, 1966a and 1966b; Norris et al, 1966; Salazar et al, 1978a). Blood loss in patients with ESS may occasionally be life-threatening (Kempson and Bari, 1970). From 20 to 30% complain of abdominal pain. An abdominal mass or increased abdominal girth is noted in approximately 10%. Bleeding is the presenting complaint in only 50% of ptients with LMS, however, and occurs more readily when the location is submucous (Gallup and Cordray, 1979). Pain, an enlarging abdomen, and an abdominal mass or discharge (in that order) account for the remainder and occur particularly with intramural LMS (Crawford and Tucker, 1959). The median duration of symptoms before diagnosis is about 2.7 months for all histologic types (Salazar et al, 1978a).

Pelvic examination reveals a normal uterus in up to 20% of patients with uterine sarcoma and an enlarged uterus in 45 to 90% (Norris and Taylor, 1966a and 1966b; Norris et al, 1966; Salazar et al, 1978a). Tumor protrudes from the cervical os in one-third of patients with MMS and in half of those with CS but in only 6% of patients with ESS (Norris and Taylor, 1966a and 1966b; Norris et al, 1966). Gross tumor may occasionally be passed per vagina or may be found in the vaginal vault (Crawford and Tucker, 1959; King and Kramer, 1980). Fibroids may be differentiated from a uterine LMS on physical examination by several characteristics. An increase in the size of a mass in a postmenopausal woman favors neoplastic origin, since fibroids remain stable or decrease in size after menopause. LMS are generally larger and softer than fibroids due to necrosis, cystic areas, and hemorrhage, and they tend to be difficult to separate from the surrounding myometrium because of their invasive nature. Fewer than one in 10 uterine sarcomas arises in the cervix (Atzinger et al, 1982).

Tumor extension beyond the uterus may be suspected during physical examination in about one-fourth of the patients. Extension into the pelvic structures or vaginal wall was detected in 15 and 5%, respectively (Norris and Taylor, 1966a and 1966b; Norris et al, 1966).

## DIAGNOSIS AND STAGING

A normal endometrial aspirate is obtained in 10 to 45% of the cases in which an attempt at cytologic diagnosis is made (Boran et al, 1972). The rare sarcoma involving the cervix as well as the more common tumor protruding from the cervical os can be easily biopsied. Dilatation and curettage will generally yield a definitive diagnosis of ESS but may be misleading in MMS, since only one type of tissue may be obtained (Boran et al, 1972). Results of dilatation and curettage will be negative in 60 to 75% of LMS—a fact that is not surprising, considering that 37% of LMS are located in the submucosa (Crawford and Tucker, 1959; Gallup and Cordray, 1979).

Preoperative staging for those patients with an established or suspected diagnosis of uterine sarcoma after dilatation and curettage should include a CT scan of the pelvis and abdomen (with a careful look at the liver) and chest tomograms or a CT scan of the lung. (Tomograms are generally preferred, since the incidence of false-positive results on CT scans in adults is significant.) A bone scan is indicated if the alkaline phosphatase level is abnormal. Several authors stress the role of surgical exploration, and if appropriate, TAH/BSO may be indicated both for staging and as a therapeutic procedure (Forney and Buchsbaum, 1981; Salazar et al, 1978b).

## TREATMENT OF LOCALIZED DISEASE

The optimal combination of surgery, radiation, and possibly chemotherapy is difficult to address, since each author reports relatively few patients. In general, the therapeutic procedure of choice for all uterine sarcomas clinically confined to the uterus is TAH/BSO. However, Aaro et al (1966) reported 5-year disease-free survival in seven of nine relatively young patients with LMS in whom at least one ovary was left intact. Dinh and Woodruff (1982) reported myomectomy only or hysterectomy only in 14% and 14% of his patients, respectively, although no survival figures for these patients were given. Several authors have concluded that adnexectomy does not alter survival for patients with LMS (Dinh and Woodruff, 1982; Teuffel et al, 1980).

Oophorectomy may be important in endometrial stromal meiosis; however, in a retrospective review of 78 cases of ESM, recurrences were seen in only 16% of the 37 cases treated with TAH/BSO but in 68% of the 41 cases with one or both ovaries left in situ. These data may indicate the hormonal dependency of ESM (Gloor et al, 1982). Because this tumor is so slow-growing, an attempt to debulk it should be made even if complete resection is impossible.

## Radiotherapy

In all series, the results of treatment stress the ineffectiveness of radiation alone in controlling sarcoma (Salazar et al, 1978a and 1978b). The role of pre- or postoperative radiotherapy remains controversial. Salazar advocates the use of adjuvant external pelvic radiation, i.e., 50 Grays (Gy)* to the pelvic axis, with further intracavitary irradiation using a vaginal cylinder to deliver 40 Gy to the vaginal surface if the cervix is involved or for vaginal cuff recurrence. He stresses that patients with a good prognosis will frequently be treated with surgery alone. Those with more extensive disease will undergo surgery and radiotherapy; poor surgical candidates and those with more advanced tumors will be treated with radiotherapy alone. Thus, one would expect patients undergoing surgery and radiotherapy to have poorer survival rates than those treated with surgery alone.

In a review of the literature by Salazar, the 5-year survival of patients with Stage I disease treated with surgery and radiotherapy was not significantly better than that with surgery alone (62 and 53%, respectively). For endometrial stromal sarcoma, the 5-year survival rates in these treatment groups were 88 and 47%, respectively, suggesting an advantage for the group who underwent radiotherapy (Salazar et al, 1978a, 1978b). Kempson and Bari (1970) also found no survival advantage for those treated with surgery and radiotherapy as opposed to surgery alone. Belgrad et al (1975), however, advocated preoperative radiotherapy for ESS and primary surgery for MMS and LMS. Gilbert et al (1975) would radiate MMS and ESS pre- or postoperatively but have found no evidence of benefit from radiotherapy for LMS.

The remainder of the data regarding the efficacy of radiation is anecdotal. In one series of patients with ESS treated with preoperative radiotherapy and surgery, there was usually an objective decrease in the size of the tumor mass after radiation (although all patients subsequently died of metastases). Other authors also report that in some instances ESS did not persist in preoperatively irradiated areas (Kempson and Bari, 1970; Norris and Taylor, 1966a). Thus, radiotherapy may be efficacious for ESS (Gilbert et al, 1975; Yazigi et al, 1979), although it is not generally utilized for patients with ESM.

Individual patients with homologous MMS or cervical CS were treated, respectively, with radiotherapy only or polypectomy, cervical fulguration, and x-irradiation; they survived free of disease (Kempson and Bari, 1970; Norris and Taylor, 1966b). In addition, one of nine patients treated with radiation alone in Salazar's series remained disease-free (Salazar et al, 1978a, 1978b). Significant amounts of stromal sarcoma in MMS may indicate that radiation may be beneficial.

When considering the timing of pelvic radiation, however, the physician must keep in mind that such treatment will severely compromise the use of any sub-

---

* 1 Gy = 100 rads.

sequent chemotherapy. High doses of chemotherapeutic agents are required for control of sarcomas, and these cannot be delivered after irradiation of a substantial portion of the pelvis because of myelosuppression. Therefore, when indicated, chemotherapy should be administered prior to pelvic irradiation.

## Adjuvant Chemotherapy

In a study by Omura et al (1985) from the GOG, patients with FIGO Stage I and II uterine sarcomas (stratified by stage and prior radiotherapy) were randomized after hysterectomy to either doxorubicin, 60 mg/m$^2$, or observation for eight treatment cycles. Pelvic irradiation (external or intracavitary) was optional prior to entry. Of 225 patients entered, 156 were evaluable. No significant differences in survival or disease-free survival were observed between the treatment groups. With a minimum followup of 24 months, disease-free and overall survival rates were 47% and 42%, respectively, for the observation arm and 59% and 45% for the chemotherapy arm (Table 13-4). Although pelvic radiotherapy reduced the rate of vaginal recurrence, overall survival and freedom from relapse were unaffected. Thus, adjuvant chemotherapy and radiotherapy is not helpful. In a previous GOG trial of metastatic uterine sarcoma by these investigators, the use of doxorubicin as a single agent resulted in a response rate of only 16% (Omura et al, 1983).

An earlier randomized trial of adjuvant doxorubicin was aborted when congestive heart failure developed in two of six women with uterine sarcomas who were treated with the drug (Piver et al, 1979).

In 1979, Buchsbaum et al reported the results of a historically controlled trial of actinomycin D, cyclophosphamide, and vincristine. Since five of the 17 patients with more than 5 mitoses/10 HPF survived for a median of 4 years after completing the chemotherapy regimen, the authors concluded that such treatment may be beneficial. However, nonrandomized studies, such as this one, are generally considered to be unreliable, since survival of the control groups in the randomized trials described below has proved significantly superior to that of historical controls from the same institution (Lindberg et al, 1977). Other randomized trials of adjuvant chemotherapy versus observation for soft tissue sarcomas are summarized in Table 13-5. Of the studies that included central and trunk sarcomas, none showed a significant advantage with adjuvant therapy overall.

Subset analysis of patients with sarcomas of the extremities treated at the National Cancer Institute (NCI) with a combination of doxorubicin, cyclophosphamide, and high-dose methotrexate showed a significantly longer disease-free (but not overall) survival (Baker et al, 1988; Chang et al, 1988; Rosenberg, 1984; Rosenberg, 1985; Rosenberg et al, 1983, 1985a and b, and 1987). Chemotherapy offered no advantage in terms of either disease-free or overall survival in patients with nonextremity sarcomas. Of 15 patients with primary retroperitoneal tumors, however, the 2-year actuarial survival was compromised in the chemotherapy arm of the study (100% vs 46% [p = 0.06]). Cardiotoxicity developed in two cases, cyclophosphamide-related cystitis in two, and severe bone marrow suppression in three (Glenn et a, 1985a and 1985b). Analysis of the 31 patients with primary lesions of the trunk or head and neck revealed a trend toward delayed recurrence but no difference in survival. Of the 22 patients with trunk lesions, 12 received chemotherapy, and time to recurrence was prolonged (3-year actuarial disease-free survival = 92% vs 47%); however, survival was not significantly altered (82% vs 61%). In the NCI trial, 14% of the patients experienced clinical doxorubicin-associated congestive heart failure, and an additional 56% had abnormal cardiac function on noninvasive testing after treatment (Dresdale et al, 1983). Up to 18% of the patients withdrew from the study because of gastrointestinal and hematologic toxicity. Response rates when high-dose methotrexate and cyclophosphamide are given as single agents are low (see below), and their contribution to doxorubicin-containing regimens in metastatic disease has been minimal (Baker et al, 1987; Bergsagel and Levin, 1960; Bramwell et al, 1987; Muss et al, 1985; Schenfeld et al, 1982).

## Followup and Prognosis

Because local recurrent lesions and pulmonary metastases may occasionally be resected to achieve a cure, patients with gynecologic sarcomas should be followed carefully after operation. A periodic history and pelvic examination, liver function studies, and a set of chest tomograms might be obtained every 3 to 4 months for the first 2 years and twice yearly thereafter for 2 years in patients at high risk.

The overall 5-year survival for all patients in Salazar's series was 48%, with the majority of deaths occurring early during the first 2 years (Salazar et al, 1978b). A striking observation was that there was no significant difference in survival among patients whose tumors were classified as FIGO Stages II, III, and IV. The 5-year survival of patients with Stage I tumors (64%) was significantly superior to that of patients with Stages II to IV (20%) (Salazar et al, 1978a, 1978b).

When one analyzes survival based on histologic type, the overall recurrence rates for LMS, MMS, and ESS in this series are found to be 35%, 75%, and 67%, respectively (Salazar et al, 1978a and 1978b), although

TABLE 13-4 Gynecologic Oncology Group Trial of Adjuvant Doxorubicin in Patients With Resected Stage I and II Uterine Sarcomas

| Type of Sarcoma | No. of Patients | % Failures | |
|---|---|---|---|
| | | Doxorubicin | Observation |
| LMS | 48 | 44 | 61 |
| MMS | 93 | 39 | 51 |
| Other | 15 | 50 | 44 |
| Total | 156 | 41 | 53 |

LMS = leiomyosarcoma; MMS = mixed mesodermal sarcoma.
*Source:* Omura GA, et al: A randomized clinical trial of adjuvant Adriamycin in uterine sarcomas. *J Clin Oncol* 3:1240-1245, 1985.

TABLE 13-5  Randomized Adjuvant Trials in Soft Tissue Sarcomas*

| Group | Drug(s) | Months of Followup (Median) | Stage(s) | No. of Patients | % Disease-Free Survival − | + | % Overall Survival − | + |
|---|---|---|---|---|---|---|---|---|
| ISSG | A | 20 | IIB-IVA | 92 | 53 | 73 | 55 | 76 |
| Scandinavian | A | 22 | III/IVA | 139 | 44 | 40 | 55 | 52 |
| UCLA | A | 28 | III | 119 | 52 | 56 | 70 | 80 |
| Rizzoli | A | 28 | III/IVA | 77 | 45 | 73 | 70 | 91 |
| NCI | ACM | | IIA-IVA | | | | | |
|   Retroperitoneal | | 24 | | 15 | 49 | 92 | 100 | 47 |
|   Trunk/Head and neck | | 36 | | 22 | 47 | 77 | 61 | 82 |
|   Extremities | | 60 | | 67 | 28 | 54 | 60 | 54 |
| Bordeaux | ACVD | 40 | IIB-IVA | 59 | 37 | 65 | 43 | 83 |
| EORTC | ACVD | 44 | I-IVA | 468 | 61 | 61 | 68 | 74 |
| DFCI/MGH | A | >46 | IIB-IVA | 45 | 68 | 69 | 72 | 74 |
| ECOG | A | >59 | IIB-IVA | 30 | 60 | 63 | 54 | 62 |
| GOG | A | 60 | FIGO I-II | 156 | 45 | 60 | 47 | 60 |
| Mayo | AVDAd | 64 | I-IVB | 61 | 68 | 65 | 70 | 70 |
| MDAH | ACVAd | >120 | IIB/IIIB | 47 | 83 | 76 | NA | NA |

* In order of months of followup. − = observation; + = chemotherapy.
A = doxorubicin (Adriamycin); Ad = actinomycin D; C = cyclophosphamide; D = dacarbazine (DTIC); V = vincristine. ISSG = The Intergroup Sarcoma Study Group (Antman et al, 1987); Scandinavian (Alvegard, 1986; Alvegard et al, 1989); UCLA = (Eilber et al, 1965, and Eilber et al, 1988) Rizzoli Institute (Picci et al, 1987) NCI = National Cancer Institute (Baker et al, 1988; Chang et al, 1988; Rosenberg, 1984 and 1985; Rosenberg et al, 1983, 1985a and 1985b, and 1987); Bordeaux (Bui et al, 1989); EORTC = European Organization for Research in the Treatment of Cancer (Bramwell et al, 1985 and 1988); DFCI/MGH = Dana-Farber Cancer Institute/Massachusetts General Hospital (Antman et al, 1984a and 1984b and 1985); ECOG = The Eastern Cooperative Oncology Group (Antman et al, 1984a and 1985); GOG = Gynecologic Oncology Group (Omura et al, 1985); Mayo = The Mayo Clinic (Edmonson, 1984; Edmonson et al, 1984); MDAH = MD Anderson Hospital, Houston (Benjamin et al, 1987; Lindberg et al, 1977).

in some series ESS was associated with a particularly bad prognosis (Salazar et al, 1978b; Yoonessi and Hart, 1977). LMS and CS appeared to be somewhat less extensive at the time of presentation, however, with two-thirds found to be Stage I at surgery (Gilbert et al, 1975; Norris and Taylor, 1966b; Salazar et al, 1978a and 1978b). Thus, stage for stage, there seemed to be no difference in prognosis among the histologic variants of uterine sarcoma. In other series, however, the survival in LMS was inferior to that in ESS or MMS (Kenda et al, 1981; Vongtama et al, 1976). The incidence and survival of LMS vary depending on whether cellular leiomyomas are included in the analysis—a fact which may explain the apparent discrepancy between the reported series.

At diagnosis, approximately 50% of all tumors are confined to the corpus (Stage I) (Kempson and Bari, 1970; Salazar et al, 1978a). Of those showing extrauterine extension or metastases, half extend to adnexal structures and 15% show intraabdominal metastases.

Uterine sarcomas progress rapidly. Almost 90% of those patients with recurrence die during the first 2 years (Salazar et al, 1978b). The average recurrence time for all patients in Salazar's series was 18.8 months, with a disease-free interval of 32 months for Stage I tumors compared with 9 months for Stages II to IV. About half the patients with Stage I disease (including all histologic types) survived for 5 years; however, only about 10% of those with Stage II to IV disease survived 5 years.

There appear to be no significant differences in recurrence sites among the major histologic types of uterine sarcoma: 13 to 14% recur in the pelvis alone, 51 to 60% recur in the pelvis and distantly, and 26 to 39% recur distantly only (Salazar et al, 1978b). MMS reportedly has a tendency to spread (like endometrial carcinoma) to adjacent pelvic organs, lymph nodes, and paraaortic lymphatics rather than hematogenously (like other sarcomas) (Norris et al, 1966). Salazar, however, failed to detect any significant difference in the patterns of dissemination of LMS and MMS; both tumors have a low incidence of nodal involvement (less than 25% of all recurrences) (Salazar et al, 1978b). Thus, when one analyzes the histologic types by stage, all these variants exhibit similar recurrence and survival rates and patterns of dissemination (Salazar et al, 1978b).

The time to recurrence was 3.4 months for patients treated with radiation therapy only. For patients with Stage I disease, the average recurrence time for those treated with surgery and radiotherapy was 41 months compared with 32 months for those treated with surgery alone (Salazar et al, 1978b).

Radiotherapy appeared to decrease the local recurrence rate. In 12 of 19 patients (63%) treated with surgery versus 7 of 20 patients (35%) treated with surgery plus radiotherapy, tumor recurred in the pelvis. However, survival was not affected, since isolated pelvic recurrences are rare, occurring in only 10% of patients who fail (Salazar et al, 1978b; Gilbert et al, 1975). From 90 to 96% of those with recurrences had metastases outside the pelvis (with or without pelvic recurrence). The most common sites of metastases were to the upper abdomen (69%), lung (60%), bone (24%) and brain (4%). Pulmonary metastases alone occurred in 10%. Simultaneous metastases to the upper abdomen and

TABLE 13-6   Single-Agent Chemotherapy for Uterine Sarcomas

| Institute | No. of Patients/No. of Responders (%) | Histologic Type | Drug | Dose (mg/m$^2$) |
|---|---|---|---|---|
| MDAH-1 | 9/0 (0) | MMS | Doxorubicin | 50 to 90 |
| GOG-1 | 41/4 (10) | MMS | Doxorubicin | 60 |
| GOG-1 | 28/7 (25) | LMS | Doxorubicin | 60 |
| RPMI | 17/1 (6) | All | Doxorubicin | 90 |
| Mississippi-1 | 19/1 (5) | LMS | Cisplatin | 50 |
| Mississippi-2 | 28/5 (18) | MMS | Cisplatin | 50 |
| MDAH-2 | 12/5 (42) | MMS | Cisplatin | 75 to 100 |
| GOG-2 | 28/9 (32) | MMS | Ifosfamide | 7,500 |

MDAH-1 = MD Anderson Hospital (Gershenson et al, 1987a); GOG-1 = Gynecologic Oncology Group (Omura et al, 1983); RPMI = Roswell Park Memorial Institute (Piver et al, 1979); Mississippi-1 (Thigpen et al, 1986b) and Mississippi-2 (Thigpen et al, 1986a); MDAH-2 (Gershenson et al, 1987b); GOG-2 (Sutton et al, 1989).

lungs occurred in 16 patients (36%). Spread to the omentum, peritoneum, and bowel were seen in over 50% of those patients with recurrences in the upper abdomen. Peritoneal and omental implants with bowel involvement resembling the spread of ovarian carcinoma was the rule rather than the exception, occurring in 50% of patients with upper abdominal metastases. Involvement of the liver, spleen, or paraaortic nodes occurred in 25% and was usually associated with widespread abdominal disease. Nodal involvement occurred in less than 20% of all recurrences.

The overall incidence of pelvic failures was 53% (with or without recurrences elsewhere), illustrating the need for better local control as well (Salazar et al, 1978b).

## TREATMENT OF RECURRENT OR METASTATIC DISEASE

### Resection of Pulmonary Metastases

If, after careful evaluation, pulmonary metastases are found to be the only form of spread, resection for cure should be considered. Most authors agree on the following criteria for patient selection:

1. The primary disease should be definitively controlled.
2. The patient should be an acceptable surgical candidate.
3. No extrapulmonary metastases should be present.

A tumor doubling time of more than 40 days has been advocated as an additional criterion for resection, with lesions having a shorter doubling time excluded from consideration. Morton has observed that the disease-free interval after resection of pulmonary metastases correlates with the tumor doubling time (with indolent tumors recurring later). The percentage of patients achieving long-term disease-free survival may not correlate as closely, however. Authors are also divided as to whether multiple, bilteral, or large metastases affect the prognosis after surgical resection.

### Palliative Chemotherapy for Metastatic Uterine Sarcoma

Doxorubicin appears to be the most effective single agent in the treatment of gynecologic, soft tissue, and osteogenic sarcomas, with response rates ranging from 0 to 25%. Results of single-agent studies in patients with uterine sarcomas are shown in Table 13-6.

TABLE 13-7   Response Rates for Combination Chemotherapy in Measurable Advanced Uterine Sarcomas—Randomized Trials

| | Drug(s) | No. of Patients | CR | RR |
|---|---|---|---|---|
| *Studies Comparing Doxorubicin With or Without DTIC Added:* | | | | |
| GOG (Omura et al, 1983) | A | 80 | 6% | 16% |
| | AD | 66 | 11% | 24% |
| ECOG (Lerner et al, 1983) | A | 34 | 3% | 18% |
| LMS only | AD | 32 | 3% | 44% |
| *Studies Comparing Doxorubicin With Cyclophosphamide Added:* | | | | |
| GOG (Muss et al, 1985) | A | 50 | 1% | 19% |
| | AC | 54 | 2% | 20% |

A = doxorubicin (Adriamycin); C = cyclophosphamide; CR = complete response; D = DTIC; RR = response rate.

TABLE 13-8 Response Rates for Combination Chemotherapy in Measurable Advanced Uterine Sarcomas—Non-Randomized Trials

| Group (Ref) | No. of Evaluable/ No. of Responders | Drug | Dose (mg/m²) | Histology | CR | CR + PR |
|---|---|---|---|---|---|---|
| Seattle (Peters et al, 1989) | 11/8 | Cisplatin Doxorubicin | 100 45 to 60 | Not specified | | |
| DFCI | 22/11 | Doxorubicin | 60 | 3 ESS | 1 | 3 |
| | | DTIC | 900 | 5 CS | 1 | 3 |
| | | Ifosfamide | 7,500 | 13 LMS | 0 | 5 |
| | | | | 1 MMS | 0 | 0 |

A = doxorubicin (Adriamycin); C = cyclophosphamide; CR = complete response; D = DTIC; PR = partial response.

***Combination of Chemotherapy in Uterine Sarcomas*** The addition of dacarbazine (DTIC) to single-agent doxorubicin has been evaluated in three randomized trials in patients with soft tissue sarcomas (Table 13-7). When the GOG and the Eastern Cooperative Oncology Group (ECOG) evaluated doxorubicin as a single agent versus doxorubicin plus DTIC for uterine sarcomas, the response rates were higher in both studies for the combination therapy, significantly so in the ECOG study (Borden et al, 1983; Lerner et al, 1983; Omura et al, 1983). In a third study, the Southwest Oncology Group (SWOG) compared doxorubicin, cyclophosphamide, and vincristine with the addition of either DTIC or actinomycin D and showed that the DTIC-containing arm was significantly more active (Benjamin et al, 1976). LMS appeared to be more responsive than MMS in the GOG study, a finding also observed by others (Lerner et al, 1983).

In contrast, the addition of cyclophosphamide to a doxorubicin-containing regimen did not prove advantageous in the ECOG, SWOG, and GOG studies (Baker et al, 1987; Muss et al, 1985; Schoenfeld et al, 1982). In fact, when the dose of doxorubicin was decreased from 70 to 50 mg/m² to accommodate the myelosuppression caused by cyclophosphamide in the ECOG study, the response to doxorubicin as a single agent at 70 mg/m² was significantly better than the response to the combination (Schoenfeld et al, 1982).

Four randomized studies addressed the role of dose and schedule (Baker et al, 1987; Bodey et al, 1981; Pinedo et al, 1984; Brennan et al, 1987). A SWOG study compared bolus and continuous-infusion doxorubicin and DTIC. The response rate was not affected by the schedule, but toxicity (particularly cardiotoxicity from doxorubicin and nausea and vomiting from DTIC) was substantially less severe with the continuous-infusion schedule (Baker et al, 1987). An adjuvant trial at Memorial Sloan-Kettering corroborated the decreased cardiotoxicity with continuous-infusion doxorubicin (Brennan et al, 1987). The EORTC studied full-dose versus alternating half-dose therapy (Pinedo et al, 1984), and the group at MD Anderson Hospital compared the combination of cyclophosphamide, vincristine, doxorubicin, and dacarbazine (CyVADIC) at high and intermediate doses (Bodey et al, 1981). These studies documented a correlation between dose and response.

Ifosfamide and doxorubicin were evaluated in the EORTC, with a response rate of 36% (Schutte et al, 1986), and in combination with DTIC at the Dana-Farber Cancer Institute (DFCI), with a response rate of 50% (Elias et al, 1989). The data for advanced uterine sarcomas from the DFCI study are shown in Table 13-8.

Thus, the regimen that now results in the highest response rates in soft tissue sarcomas consists of doxorubicin (70 mg/m²) and DTIC (1 g/m²), with doses preferably divided over 4 days to decrease the risk of cardiotoxicity and the severity of nausea and vomiting. Physicians may choose single-agent doxorubicin for palliation in patients who may not tolerate the combination. Ifosfamide is currently the most active salvage agent for patients who have not responded to a doxorubicin-containing regimen, and its role in a doxorubicin-based combination is now being evaluated in at least three randomized trials.

***Hormonal Therapy for Uterine Sarcomas*** Willson et al (1981) stressed the potential role for hormonal treatment of uterine sarcomas. Noting that a higher percentage of premenopausal compared with postmenopausal patients who developed uterine sarcomas survived for 5 years, these investigators have suggested that estrogen replacement may be efficacious in the treatment of postmenopausal women with sarcomas. Lantta et al (1984) have documented the presence of estradiol and progesterone receptors in two endometrial stromal sarcomas. One of the patients responded to hormonal therapy for a 2-year period. A case of endometrial stromal sarcoma (ESS) responding to medroxyprogesterone following failure of tamoxifen and combination chemotherapy was reported by O'Brien et al (1985). However, of 29 patients with uterine sarcomas treated with 20 mg/day of tamoxifen in a study by the Clinical Oncology Society of Australia, only one had an objective response (i.e., none of 19 with LMS, none of 3 with ESS, and 1 of 7 with MMS) (Rome et al, 1986). Anecdotal reports of complete responses to doxorubicin, vincristine, cyclophosphamide, and megestrol acetate in patients with ESS have also been reported (Lehrner et al, 1979).

# REFERENCES

Aaro LA, Symmonds RE, Dockerty MB: Sarcoma of the uterus. *Am J Obstet Gynecol* 94:101-109, 1966.

Alvegard T: Adjuvant chemotherapy with Adriamycin in high grade malignant soft tissue sarcoma: A Scandinavian randomized study. *Proc Am Soc Clin Oncol* 5:C-485, 1986.

Alvegard T, Sigurdsson H, Mouridsen H, Solheim O, et al: Adjuvant chemotherapy with doxorubicin in high grade soft tissue sarcoma: A randomized trial of the Scandinavian Sarcoma Group. *J Clin Oncol* 7:1504-1513, 1989.

Antman K, Amato D, Lerner H, Suit H, Corson J, Wood W, Proppe K, Carey R, Greenberger J, Wilson R, et al: Eastern Cooperative Oncology Group and Dana-Farber Cancer Institute/Massachusetts General Hospital Study. In Jones S, Salmon SE (eds): *Adjuvant Therapy of Cancer IV.* Orlando, Grune and Stratton, Inc, 1984a.

Antman KH, Suit H, Amato D, Corson J, Wood W, Proppe K, Harmon D, Carey R, Greenberger J, Blum R, Wilson R: Preliminary results of a randomized trial of adjuvant Adriamycin for sarcomas: Lack of apparent difference between treatment groups. *J Clin Oncol* 2:601-608, 1984b.

Antman K, Amato D, Lerner H, Suit H, Corson J, Wood W, Proppe K, Carey R, Greenberger J, Wilson R, et al: Adjuvant doxorubicin for sarcoma: Data from the ECOG and DFCI/MGH studies. *Cancer Treat Symp* 3:109-115, 1985.

Antman K, Amato D, Pilepich M, Lerner H, Balcerzak S, Borden E, Baker L: A preliminary analysis of a randomized intergroup (SWOG, ECOG, CALGB, NCOG) trial of adjuvant doxorubicin for soft tissue sarcomas. In Salmon SE (ed): *Adjuvant Therapy of Cancer V.* Orlando, Grune and Stratton, Inc, 1987.

Atzinger A, Ries G, Hötzinger H, Hermans M, Pfander K: Clinical presentation, therapy and prognosis of sarcomas of the uterus. *Strahlentherapie* 158:210-216, 1982.

Baker A, Chang A, Glatstein E, Rosenberg S: National Cancer Institute experience in the management of high-grade extremity soft tissue sarcomas. In Ryan JR, Baker LO (eds): *Recent Concepts in Sarcoma Treatment.* Dordrecht, Netherlands, Kluwer Academic Publishers, 1988, pp 123-130.

Baker L, Frank F, Fine G, et al: Combination chemotherapy using Adriamycin, DTIC, cyclophosphamide, and actinomycin D for advanced soft tissue sarcomas: A randomized comparative trial. *J Clin Oncol* 5:851-861, 1987.

Baker L, Green S, Rykan J, Rosenberg B, Balcerzak S: Combined modality therapy for disseminated soft tissue sarcoma, phase III. *Proc Am Soc Clin Oncol* 6:138, 1987.

Bartsich EC, Bowe ET, Moore JG: Leiomyosarcoma of the uterus. A 50 year review of 42 cases. *Obstet Gynecol* 32:101-105, 1968.

Belgrad R, Elbadawl N, Rubin P: Uterine sarcoma. *Radiology* 114:181-188, 1975.

Benjamin R, Gottlieb J, Baker L: CyVADIC vs CyVADACT—A randomized trial of cyclophosphamide, vincristine and Adriamycin, plus either dacarbazine or actinomycin D in metastatic sarcomas. *Proc Am Assoc Cancer Res* 17:256, 1976.

Benjamin R, Terjanian T, Fenoglio J, Barkley HT, et al: The importance of combination chemotherapy for adjuvant treatment of high-risk patients with soft-tissue sarcomas of the extremities. In Salmon SE (ed): *Adjuvant Therapy of Cancer V.* Orlando, Grune and Stratton, Inc, 1987, pp 735-744.

Bergsagel D, Levin W: A preclusive clinical trial of cyclophosphamide. *Cancer Chemother Rep* 8:120-134, 1960.

Bodey G, Rodriguez V, Murphy W, et al: Protected environment—Prophylactic antibiotic program for malignant sarcoma: Randomized trial during remission induction chemotherapy. *Cancer* 47:2422-2429, 1981.

Boram LH, Erlandson RA, Hajdu SI: Mesodermal mixed tumor of the uterus. *Cancer* 30:1295-1306, 1972.

Borden EC, Amato D, Enterline HT, Lerner H, Carbone PP: Randomized comparison of Adriamycin regimens for treatment of metastatic soft tissue sarcomas. *Proc Am Soc Clin Oncol* 2:231(C-902), 1983.

Bramwell V, Rouesse J, Santoro A, et al: European experience of adjuvant chemotherapy for soft tissue sarcoma: Preliminary report of randomized trial of cyclophosphamide, vincristine, doxorubicin, and dacarbazine (CyVADIC). *Cancer Treat Symp* 3:99-107, 1985.

Bramwell V, Mouridsen H, Santoro G, et al: Cyclophosphamide vs ifosfamide: Final report of randomized phase II trial in adult soft tissue sarcoma. *Eur J Cancer Clin Oncol* 23:311-321, 1987.

Bramwell V, Rouesse J, Steward W, Santoro A, Buesa J, Strafford-Koops H, Wagener T, Somers R, Ruka W, Markham D, Burgers M, Van Unnik J, Contesso G, Thomas D, Sylvester R, Pinedo H: European experience of adjuvant chemotherapy for soft tissue sar-

coma: Interim report of a randomized trial of CyVADIC versus control. In *Recent Concepts in Sarcoma Treatment.* Dordrecht, Netherlands, Kluwer Academic Publishers, 1988.

Brennan M, Friedrich C, Almadrones L, Magill G: Prospective randomized trial examining the cardiac toxicity of adjuvant doxorubicin in high-grade extremity sarcomas. In Salmon SE (ed): *Adjuvant Therapy of Cancer V.* Orlando, Grune and Stratton, Inc, 1987.

Buchsbaum HJ, Lifshitz S, Blythe JG: Prophylactic chemotherapy in stages I and II uterine sarcoma. *Gynecol Oncol* 8:346-348, 1979.

Bui NB, Maree D, Coindre JM, Bonichon F, Kantor G, Avril A, Ravaud A: First results of a prospective randomized study of CyVADIC adjuvant chemotherapy in adults with operable high-risk soft tissue sarcoma. *Proc Am Soc Clin Oncol* 8:318 (Abstract 1236), 1989.

Centers for Disease Control: Epidemiologic aspects of the current outbreak of Kaposi's sarcoma and opportunistic infections. *N Engl J Med* 306:248-252, 1982.

Chang A, Kinsella T, Glatstein E, Baker A, Sindelar W, Lotze M, Danforth DN, Sugarbaker P, Lack E, Steinberg S, White D, Rosenberg S: Adjuvant chemotherapy for patients with high-grade soft-tissue sarcomas of the extremity. *J Clin Oncol* 6:1491-1500, 1988.

Christopherson WM, Williamson EO, Gray LA: Leiomyosarcoma of the uterus. *Cancer* 26:1512-1517, 1972.

Cramer SF: Pulmonary lymphangiomyomatosis and metastasizing leiomyoma (letter). *N Engl J Med* 305:587, 1981.

Cramer SF, Meyer JS, Kraner JF, Camel M, Mazur MT, Tennenbaum MS: Metastasizing leiomyoma of the uterus. *Cancer* 45:932-937, 1980.

Crawford EJ, Tucker R: Sarcoma of the uterus. *Am J Obstet Gynecol* 77:286-291, 1959.

Dallenbach-Hellweg G: The stromal and myogenic sarcomas of the uterus. *Pathol Res Pract* 169:127-139, 1980.

Dinh TV, Woodruff JD: Leiomyosarcoma of the uterus. *Am J Obstet Gynecol* 144:817-823, 1982.

Dinh TV, Slavin RE, Bhagavan BS, Hannigan EV, Tiamson EM, Yandell RB: Mixed müllerian tumors of the uterus: A clinicopathologic study. *Obstet Gynecol* 74:388-392, 1988.

Dresdale A, Bonow R, Wesley R, Palmeri S, Barr L, Mathison D, D'Angelo T, Rosenberg S: Prospective evaluation of doxorubicin-induced cardiomyopathy resulting from postsurgical adjuvant treatment of patients with soft tissue sarcomas. *Cancer* 52:51-60, 1983.

Eberl M, Pfleiderer A, Teufel G, Bachmann F: Sarcomas of the uterus. Morphological criteria and clinical course. *Pathol Res Pract* 169:165-172, 1980.

Edmonson J: Role of adjuvant chemotherapy in the management of patients with soft tissue sarcomas. *Cancer Treat Rep* 68:1063-1066, 1984.

Edmonson JH, Fleming TR, Ivins JC, Burgert EO, Soule EH, O'Connell MJ, Sim FH, Ahmann DL: Randomized study of systemic chemotherapy following complete excision of nonosseous sarcomas: Interim report. *Proc Am Soc Clin Oncol* 1:182(C-709), 1982.

Edmonson J, Fleming T, Ivins J, et al: Randomized study of systemic chemotherapy following complete excision of nonosseous sarcomas. *J Clin Oncol* 2:1390-1396, 1984.

Eilber F, Giuliano A, Huth J, Mirra J, Rosen G, Morton D: Neoadjuvant chemotherapy, radiation, and limited surgery for high-grade soft tissue sarcoma of the extremity. Dordrecht, Netherlands, Kluwer Academic Publishers, 1988, pp 115-122.

Eilber F, Giuliano A, Huth J, Morton D: Adjuvant Adriamycin in high-grade extremity soft-tissue sarcomas—A randomized prospective trial. *Proc Am Soc Clin Oncol* 5:C-488, 1986.

Elias A, Ryan L, Sulkes A, Collins J, Aisner J, Antman K: Response to mesna, doxorubicin, ifosfamide, and dacarbazine in 108 patients with metastatic or unresectable sarcoma and no prior chemotherapy. *J Clin Oncol* 7:1-9, 1989.

Essex M, McLane MF, Lee TH, Falk L, Howe CWS, Mullins JL, Cabradilla C, Francis DP: Antibodies to human T-cell leukemia virus–associated cell membrane antigens (HTLV-MA) in patients with acquired immune deficiency syndrome (AIDS). *Science* 220:859-862, 1983.

Evans HL: Endometrial stromal sarcoma and poorly differentiated endometrial sarcoma. *Cancer* 50:2170-2182, 1982.

Forney JP, Buchsbaum HJ: Classifying, staging, and treating uterine sarcomas. *Contemp Obstet Gynecol* 18:47, 50, 55-56, 61-62, 64, and 69, 1981.

Gallup DG, Cordray DR: Leiomyosarcoma of the uterus: Case reports and a review. *Obstet Gynecol Surv* 34:300-311, 1979.

Gershenson D, Kavanagh J, Copeland L, Creighton L, Freedman RS, Wharton JT: High-dose doxorubicin infusion therapy for disseminated mixed mesodermal sarcoma of the uterus. *Cancer* 59:1264-1267, 1987*a*.

Gershenson D, Kavanagh J, Copeland L, et al: Cisplatin therapy for disseminated mixed mesodermal sarcoma of the uterus. *J Clin Oncol* 5:618-621, 1987*b*.

Gilbert HA, Kagan AR, Lagasse L, Jacobs MR, Tawa K: The value of radiation therapy in uterine sarcoma. *Obstet Gynecol* 45:84-88, 1975.

Glenn J, Kinsella T, Glatstein E, et al: A randomized, prospective trial of adjuvant chemotherapy in adults with soft tissue sarcomas of the head and neck, breast, and trunk. *Cancer* 55:1206-1214, 1985*a*.

Glenn J, Sindelar W, Kinsella T: Results of multimodality therapy of resectable soft-tissue sarcomas of the retroperitoneum. *Surgery* 97:316-325, 1985*b*.

Gloor E, Schnyder P, Cikes M, Hofstetter J, Cordray R, Burnier F, Knobel P: Endolymphatic stromal meiosis. *Cancer* 50:1888-1893, 1982.

Hannigan EV, Gomez LG: Uterine leiomyosarcoma. *Am J Obstet Gynecol* 134:557-564, 1979.

Hart WR, Yoonessi M: Endometrial stromatosis of the uterus. *Obstet Gynecol* 49:393-403, 1977.

Huth JF, Gupta RK, Morton DL: Development of an enzyme immunoassay to detect and quantitate tumor-associated antigens in the urine of sarcoma patients. *Cancer* 47:2856-2861, 1981.

Huth JF, Gupta RK, Morton DL: Relationship between circulating immune complexes and urinary antigens in human malignancy. *Cancer* 49:1150-1157, 1982.

Kaether M, Franz G, Schmidt U: Results of treatment on 56 sarcomas of the uterus between 1953 and 1977. *Pathol Res Pract* 169:179-184, 1980.

Kempson RL, Bari W: Uterine sarcomas. Classification, diagnosis, and prognosis. *Hum Pathol* 1:331-349, 1970.

Kenda R, DePalo G, Andreola S, Bandieramonte G, Lupi G, Musumeci E: A clinical and pathologic study of 34 sarcomas of the uterus. *Tumori* 67:341-348, 1981.

King ME, Kramer EE: Malignant müllerian mixed tumors of the uterus. *Cancer* 45:188-190, 1980.

Koll R: Report on 69 uterine sarcomas treated at the University Hospital for Women, Hamburg-Eppendorf, during 1953-1977. *Pathol Res Pract* 169:185-191, 1980.

Lanberge JL: Prognosis of uterine leiomyosarcomas based on histopathologic criteria. *Am J Obstet Gynecol* 84:1833-1837, 1962.

Lantta M, Kahanp K, Karkkainen J, Lehtovirta P, Wahlstrom T, Widholm O: Estradiol and progesterone receptors in two cases of endometrial stromal sarcoma. *Gynecol Oncol* 18:233-239, 1984.

Legha SS, Benjamin RS, Mackay B, Ewer M, Wallace S, Valdivieso M, Rasmussen SL, Blumenschein GR, Freireich EJ: Reduction of doxorubicin cardiotoxicity by prolonged continuous intravenous infusion. *Ann Intern Med* 96:133-139, 1982.

Lehrner LM, Miles PH, Enck RE: Complete remission of widely metastatic endometrial stromal sarcoma following combination chemotherapy. *Cancer* 43:1189-1194, 1979.

Lerner H, Amato D, Stevens C, Borden E, Enterline H: Leiomyosarcoma: The Eastern Cooperative Oncology Group experience with 222 patients. *Proc Am Assoc Cancer Res* 2:142, 1983.

Lindberg R, Murphy W, Benjamin R, Sinkovics J, Martin R, Jesse R, Romsdahl M, Russell W: Adjuvant chemotherapy in the treatment of primary soft tissue sarcomas: A preliminary report. In *Management of Bone and Soft Tissue Tumors*. Chicago, Year Book Medical Publishers, Inc, 1977, pp 343-352.

Mantravadi RV, Bardawil WA, Lochman DJ, Liebner EJ, Townsend EE, Chao JH, Chaudhuri B: Uterine sarcomas: An analysis of 69 patients. *Int J Radiat Oncol Biol Phys* 7:917-922, 1981.

Massoni EA, Hajdu SI: Cytology of primary and metastatic uterine sarcomas (meeting abstract). *Proc Am Soc Cytol* 1981, p 90.

Morton DL, Joseph WL, Ketcham AS, Geelhoed GW, Atkins PC: Surgical resection and adjunctive immunotherapy for selected patients with multiple pulmonary metastases. *Ann Surg* 178:360-366, 1973.

Muss H, Bundy B, DiSaia P, et al: Treatment of recurrent advanced uterine sarcoma—A randomized trial of doxorubicin vs doxorubicin and cyclophosphamide. *Cancer* 55:1648-1653, 1985.

Nielsen SN, Podratz KC, Scheithauer BW, O'Brien PC: Clinicopathologic analysis of uterine malignant mixed müllerian tumors. *Gynecl Oncol* 34:372-378, 1989.

Norris HJ, Taylor HB: Mesenchymal tumors of the uterus. I. A clinical and pathological study of 53 endometrial stromal tumors. *Cancer* 19:755-766, 1966*a*.

Norris HJ, Taylor HB: Mesenchymal tumors of the uterus. III. A clinical and pathologic study of 31 carcinosarcomas. *Cancer* 19:1459-1465, 1966*b*.

Norris HJ, Roth E, Taylor HB: Mesenchymal tumors of the uterus. II. A clinical and pathologic study of 31 mixed mesodermal tumors. *Obstet Gynecol* 28:57-63, 1966.

O'Brien AA, OBriain DS, Daly PA: Aggressive endometrial stromal sarcoma responding to medroxyprogesterone following failure of tamoxifen and combination chemotherapy. *Br J Obstet Gynaecol* 92:862-866, 1985.

O'Bryan RM, Baker LH, Gottlieb JE, Rivkin SE, Balcerzak SP, Grumet GN, Salmon SE, Moon TE, Hoogstraten B: Dose-response evaluation of Adriamycin in human neoplasia. *Cancer* 39:1940-1948, 1977.

Omura GA, Blessing JA: Chemotherapy of stage III, IV and recurrent uterine sarcomas: A randomized trial of Adriamycin versus AD + dimethyl triazeno imidazole carboxamide. *Cancer* 52:626-632, 1983.

Omura G, Major F, Blessing J, Sedlacek T, Thigpen J, Creasman W, Zaino R, et al: A randomized clinical trial of adjuvant Adriamycin in uterine sarcomas: A Gynecologic Oncology Group Study. *J Clin Oncol* 3:1240-1245, 1985.

Peters W III, Rivkin SE, Smith MR, Tesh DE: Cisplatin and Adriamycin combination chemotherapy of uterine stromal sarcomas and mixed mesodermal tumors. *Gynecol Oncol* 34:323-327, 1989.

Picci P, Bacci G, Gherlinzoni F, et al: Results of a randomized trial for the treatment of localized soft tissue tumors (STS) of the extremities in adult patients. In Ryan JR, Baker LO (eds): *Recent Concepts in Sarcoma Treatment*. Boston, Kluwer Academic Publishers, 1988, pp 144-149.

Pinedo H, Bramwell V, Mouridsen HT, et al: CyVADIC in advanced soft tissue sarcoma: A randomized study comparing two schedules. A study of the EORTC Soft Tissue and Bone Sarcoma Group. *Cancer* 53:1825-1832, 1984.

Piver MS, Barlow JJ, Shashikant BL, Yazigi R: Adriamycin in localized and metastatic uterine sarcomas. *J Surg Oncol* 12:263-265, 1979.

Presant CA, Lowenbraun S, Bartolucci AA, Smalley RV: Southeastern Cancer Study Group; Metastatic sarcomas: Chemotherapy with Adriamycin, cyclophosphamide, and methotrexate alternating with actinomycin D, DTIC, and vincristine. *Cancer* 47:457-465, 1981.

Rome RM, Campbell JJ, Cope TI, Hillcoat BL, Fortune DW, Planner RS, Morgan W: Tamoxifen in advanced and recurrent uterine sarcomas: A phase II study. *Cancer Treat Rep* 70:811-812, 1986.

Rosenberg S: Prospective randomized trials demonstrating the efficacy of adjuvant chemotherapy in adult patients with soft tissue sarcomas. *Cancer Treat Rep* 68:1067-1078, 1984.

Rosenberg S: Adjuvant chemotherapy of adult patients with soft tissue sarcoma. In DeVita VT Jr, Hellman S, Rosenberg S (eds): *Important Advances in Oncology*, 2nd ed. Philadelphia, JB Lippincott Co, 1985, pp 223-294.

Rosenberg S, Tepper J, Glatstein E, Costa J, Young R, Baker A, Brennan M, Demoss E, Seipp C, Sindelar W, Sugarbaker P, Wesley R: Prospective randomized evaluation of adjuvant chemotherapy in adults with soft tissue sarcomas of the extremities. *Cancer* 52:424-434, 1983.

Rosenberg S, Chang A, Glatstein E: Adjuvant chemotherapy for treatment of extremity soft tissue sarcomas: Review of National Cancer Institute experience. *Cancer Treat Symp* 3:83-88, 1985*a*.

Rosenberg S, Suit H, Baker L: Sarcomas of soft tissue. In DeVita VT Jr, Hellman S, Rosenberg S (eds): *Cancer: Principles and Practice of Oncology*, 2nd ed. Philadelphia, JB Lippincott Co, 1985*b*.

Rosenberg S, Lotze M, Muul L, et al: A progress report on the treatment of 157 patients with advanced cancer using lymphokine-activated killer cells and interleukin-2 or high-dose interleukin-2 alone. *N Engl J Med* 316:890-897, 1987.

Rosenberg SA, Tepper J, Glastein E, Costa J, Young R, Seipp C, Wesley R: Adjuvant chemotherapy for patients with soft tissue sarcomas. *Surg Clin NA* 61:1415-1423, 1981.

Salazar OM, Bonfiglio TA, Patten SF, Keller BE, Feldstein ML, Dunne

ME, Rudolph J: Uterine sarcomas: Natural history, treatment, and prognosis. *Cancer* 42:1152-1160, 1978*a*.

Salazar OM, Bonfiglio TA, Patten SF, Keller BE, Feldstein ML, Dunne ME, Rudolph J: Uterine sarcomas: Analysis of failures with special emphasis on the use of adjuvant radiation therapy. *Cancer* 42:1161-1170, 1978*b*.

Sarma PR, Jacobs J: Thoracic soft-tissue sarcoma in Vietnam veterans exposed to agent orange. *N Engl J Med* 306:1109, 1982.

Schoenfeld D, Rosenbaum C, Horton J, et al: A comparison of Adriamycin versus vincristine and Adriamycin, and cyclophosphamide for advanced sarcoma. *Cancer* 50:2757-2762, 1982.

Schutte J, Dombernowsky P, Santoro A, et al: Adriamycin and ifosfamide, a new effective combination in advanced soft tissue sarcomas. Preliminary report of a phase II study of the EORTC Soft Tissue and Bone Sarcoma Group. *Proc Am Soc Clin Oncol* 5:145, 1986.

Sutton G, Blessing JA, Rosenshein G, Photopulos G, DiSaia PJ: Phase II trial of ifosfamide and mesna in mixed mesodermal tumors of the uterus (A Gynecologic Oncology Group Study). *Am J Obstet Gynecol* 161:309-312, 1989.

Teufel G, Frauer A, Eberl M, Pfleiderer A, Neunhoeffer J: Sarcomas of the female genitalia. *Pathol Res Pract* 169:173-178, 1980.

Thigpen J, Blessing J, Orr J: Phase II trial of cisplatin in the treatment of patients with advanced or recurrent mixed mesodermal sarcomas of the uterus. *Cancer Treat Rep* 70:271-274, 1986*a*.

Thigpen J, Blessing J, Wilbanks G: Cisplatin as second-line chemotherapy in the treatment of advanced or recurrent leiomyosarcoma of the uterus. *Am J Clin Oncol* 9:18-20, 1986*b*.

Tierney W, Ehrlich CE, Bailey JC, King RD, Roth LM, Wann LS: Intravenous leiomyomatosis of the uterus with extension into the heart. *Am J Med* 69:471-475, 1980.

Tomasian A, Greenberg MS, Rumerman H: Tamoxifen for lymphangioleiomyomatosis (letter). *N Engl J Med* 306:745-746, 1982.

Vongtama V, Karlen JR, Piver SM, Tsukada Y, Moore RH: Treatment, results and prognostic factors in stage I and II sarcomas of the corpus uteri. *Am J Roentgenol Rad Ther Nucl Med* 126:139-147, 1976.

Willson JK, Ozols RF, Lewis BJ, Young RC: Current status of therapeutic modalities for treatment of gynecologic malignancies with emphasis on chemotherapy. *Am J Obstet Gynecol* 141:81-98, 1981.

Winter JA: Oophorectomy in lymphangioleiomyomatosis and benign metastasizing leiomyoma (letter). *N Engl J Med* 305:1416, 1981.

Yazigi R, Piver MS, Barlow JJ: Stage III uterine sarcoma: Case report and literature review. *Gynecol Oncol* 8:92-96, 1979.

Yoonessi M, Hart WR: Endometrial stromal sarcomas. *Cancer* 40:898-906, 1977.

Zaloudek CJ, McUsa MAJ, Norris HJ: Adenofibroma and adenosarcoma of the uterus: A clinicopathologic study of 35 cases. *Cancer* 48:354-366, 1981.

# *Chapter 14* | Ovarian Cancer

### M. Steven Piver    James Fanning    Kevin A. Craig*

## INCIDENCE, EPIDEMIOLOGY, AND ETIOLOGY

According to estimates from the National Cancer Institute's Surveillance, Epidemiology and End Results (SEER) Report, 20,000 new cases of ovarian cancer will be diagnosed in the United States in 1989, and 12,000 women will die of this disease (Silverburg, 1989). In this country, ovarian cancer is the sixth most common female cancer (4%), the fourth most common cause of female cancer death (5%), the most common cause of death from gynecologic cancer (52%), and the most common cancer to occur at an advanced stage (67%).

The incidence of this disease increases after age 40 and peaks between 50 and 59 years of age; the median age of patients with this disease is 61 years. Those at higher risk include middle and upper class women, nulliparous women, and women who have not used oral contraceptives, who have had difficulty conceiving, who have a family history of ovarian cancer, and who live in highly industrialized nations. Table 14-1 shows the high incidence of ovarian cancer in industrialized countries, Japan being the major exception. Although in most reports the median age is 52 to 58 years, the 1973-1982 SEER Report on 11,062 women diagnosed with ovarian cancer found a significantly higher median age—61. Moreover, the incidence increased significantly as women aged. In the 40- to 44-year-old age group, the incidence was 15.7 per 100,000 cases; after age 50, this rate more than doubled (35 per 100,000). The highest rates were reported in women between 65 and 85 years of age, with a peak of 54 per 100,000 women between 75 and 79 years of age (Yancik, 1986).

Although the cause or causes of ovarian cancer are unknown, a small subset of cases indicates a genetic link. Based on those factors which affect incidence or risk, possible causes include hereditary, reproductive and endocrine, environmental, dietary and viral agents.

### Hereditary Factors

A small percentage of cases of ovarian cancer appears to be related to heredity. As of December, 1989, the Familial Ovarian Cancer Registry had accessioned 310 families (725 cases) in which two or more first- and second-degree relatives had had ovarian cancer (Fig. 14-1) (Piver et al, 1984; Piver, 1989). An autosomal dominant inheritance (50% risk) with variable penetrance

---

* We would like to express our appreciation to Cheryl A. Blake for her important contributions to this chapter.

TABLE 14-1 Incidence of Ovarian Cancer

| Country | Cumulative Incidence (%) |
|---|---|
| Australia | 1.21 |
| Brazil | 0.94 |
| Canada | 1.58 |
| Colombia | 1.22 |
| Cuba | 0.58 |
| Czechoslovakia | 1.02 |
| Denmark | 2.03 |
| Finland | 1.44 |
| France | 0.75 |
| German Democratic Republic | 1.63 |
| Federal Republic of Germany | 1.81 |
| Hong Kong | 0.68 |
| Hungary | 0.84 |
| India | 0.85 |
| Israel | 1.66 |
| Italy | 1.47 |
| Jamaica | 0.91 |
| Japan | 0.43 |
| Netherlands Antilles | 0.55 |
| New Zealand (Maori) | 1.37 |
| Norway | 1.87 |
| Poland | 1.00 |
| Romania | 0.79 |
| Senegal | 0.38 |
| China (Shanghai) | 0.47 |
| Singapore (ethnic Chinese) | 0.69 |
| Spain | 0.63 |
| Sweden | 2.12 |
| Switzerland | 1.91 |
| United Kingdom (Scotland) | 1.50 |
| United States (Iowa) | 1.64 |
| Yugoslavia | 1.40 |

*Source:* Cramer DW: Lactase persistence and milk consumption as determinants of ovarian cancer risk. *Am J Epidemiol* 130:904, 1989.

dence of *c-ras-Ki* amplification in ovarian tumors, whereas van't Veer et al (1988) and Boltz et al (1989) reported that amplification of *c-ras-Ki* is rare, indicating that this abnormality probably does not play a fundamental role in the development of epithelial ovarian cancer. Loss or inactivation of normal growth regulatory genes (anti-oncogenes) could be involved in causing ovarian cancer. In a small series, Lee and coworkers (1989a) reported the loss of one *c-HA-ras-1* allele in 50% of DNA from an ovarian tumor.

Low serum levels of alpha-L-fucosidase are reportedly three times more prevalent among patients with ovarian cancer than in healthy controls (Barlow et al, 1981). Levels were also low in 153 serum samples from three families prone to ovarian cancer (Lynch et al, 1985). Therefore, since the serum level of alpha-L-fucosidase appears to be determined by heredity, the genetic predisposition to low levels may be associated with an increased risk for ovarian cancer and may be a cause of hereditary ovarian cancer.

## Reproductive and Endocrine Factors

Several studies have indicated that pregnancy and the use of oral contraceptives protect against the development of ovarian cancer. As a result, a plethora of theories have been proposed to explain this observation.

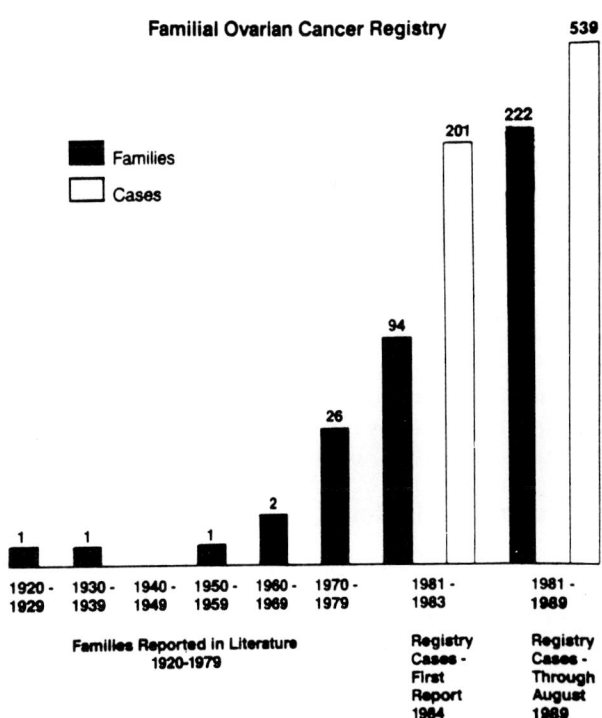

FIGURE 14-1 Number of families and cases with familial ovarian cancer registered in the Familial Ovarian Cancer Registry through August of 1989. As of December 31, 1989, the registry included 310 families with 725 cases. (From Piver MS, Mettlin CJ, Tsukada Y, et al: Familial Ovarian Cancer Registry. *Obstet Gynecol* 64:195, 1984; Piver MS, Malfetano J, Baker TR, et al: Adjuvant cisplatin based chemotherapy for stage I ovarian adenocarcinoma. A preliminary report. *Gynecol Oncol* 35:69, 1989.)

has been suggested. A less common form of familial ovarian cancer is seen in the hereditary breast/ovarian syndrome, in which there is a clustering of breast and ovarian cancers among family members (Lynch et al, 1974).

Several genetic syndromes are associated with an increased incidence of nonepithelial ovarian tumors, including gonadal dysgenesis (dysgerminoma) (Troche and Hernandez, 1986), Peutz-Jeghers syndrome (mucocutaneous pigmentation or gastrointestinal polyposis, granulosa cell tumor, and cystadenoma) (Dozois et al, 1970), and basal cell nevus syndrome (fibroma) (Berlin et al, 1966).

Although a specific genetic abnormality responsible for ovarian cancer has not been reported, alterations of protooncogenes—i.e., normal cellular genes that resemble retrovirus oncogenes—may be associated with the induction of a variety of human malignancies (including ovarian cancer) by amplification or by structural alterations in their coding sequences. Reports on the role of oncogene amplification in ovarian cancer are conflicting. Zhou and colleagues (1988) reported a high inci-

For example, when the Centers for Disease Control compared 546 women with ovarian cancer with 4,228 controls (1987), the use of oral contraceptives was found to have reduced the risk for ovarian cancer by 40% among the women 20 to 54 years of age. Wu et al (1988) compared 299 women who had ovarian cancer with 1,011 controls, and Kvale et al (1989) reported a prospective study of 60,565 women, of whom 445 developed ovarian cancer. Both studies showed a significant increase in the incidence of ovarian cancer among nulliparous women. Estrogen replacement therapy (Hoover et al, 1977), and long-acting progesterone (Liang et al, 1983) have not been associated with this disease.

Two theories have been offered to explain the decreased incidence of ovarian cancer associated with oral contraceptive use and multiparity or—conversely—why nulliparous women and, more significantly, women who have tried unsuccessfully to conceive are at higher risk. In 1948, Gardner proposed what Cramer and Welch (1983) named the "excess gonadotropin secretion theory." This theory held that ovarian cancer resulted from the effect on the ovary of persistently high levels of gonadotropin due to ovarian failure or the inability of the ovarian/pituitary feedback mechanism to inhibit excessive secretion of this hormone. According to the "incessant ovulation theory" of Fathala (1971), continuous ovulation repeatedly traumatizes the ovary and leads to malignancy, as evidenced by the finding that the risk for ovarian cancer increases with the number of times a woman ovulates during her lifetime.

More recently, Whittemore and colleagues (1989) reported that it was not the estimated number of years of ovulation, the number of pregnancies, or the use of oral contraceptives that affects the risk for ovarian cancer, but rather the inability to conceive among ovulating women who, unprotected by any type of contraception, had had sexual intercourse for 10 years or more. The risk for ovarian cancer was double that in women who became pregnant during 2 or more years of unprotected intercourse. Therefore, some other form of hormonal or endocrine abnormality must be responsible for inhibiting the ability to conceive, and this abnormal reproductive function is not related to parity, the number of years of ovulation, or the use of oral contraceptives.

## Environmental Factors

The increased incidence of ovarian cancer in industrialized nations, with the notable exception of Japan, suggests the possible etiologic role of environmental/industrial pollutants. Asbestos and talc (hydrous magnesium silicates) are the two main industrial chemicals implicated in this type of cancer (Longo and Young, 1979). Until recently, most cosmetic talcum powders contained asbestos. Conceptually, talcum powder on the perineum would reach the ovaries after being absorbed by the vagina or cervix. Despite the fact that after vaginal exposure these particulates have been recovered from the fallopian tubes (Egli and Newton, 1961) and that talc particles have been found embedded in both normal and malignant tissues (Henderson et al, 1979), reports

on the role of talc in causing ovarian cancer are conflicting. Cramer et al (1982) found that the use of talcum powder on the perineum or sanitary pads was associated with a relative risk of 1.9 (p < 0.03) for this disease, whereas Whittemore and colleagues (1988) could demonstrate no such association.

## Dietary Factors

The major dietary difference between persons living in industrialized as opposed to nonindustrialized nations is their high intake of meat and animal fat, which has been associated with an increased incidence of ovarian cancer in several studies (Cramer et al, 1984; Rose et al, 1986). No association has been found between ovarian cancer and the use of coffee, alcohol, or tobacco (Cramer et al, 1984). In 1989, Cramer and colleagues proposed that increased dietary galactose consumption and low serum levels of galactose 1-phosphate uridyl transferase, which prevents the degradation of galactose (a component of milk lactose) to glucose, may predispose to ovarian cancer. In a case-controlled study, these authors found that the incidence of ovarian cancer was three times higher in the women who consumed significantly more yogurt and cottage cheese—foods that contain high levels of lactose. Also, the serum levels of galactose 1-phosphate uridyl transferase were significantly lower among the patients with ovarian cancer compared with the control subjects. Whether these two observations are statistical aberrations or possible risk factors must await replication by other researchers. Cramer and associates (1989) reported that countries with the highest per capita milk consumption plus the highest percentage of women with an inability to digest lactose (galactose) have the highest incidence of ovarian cancer. These findings may provide a biological basis for the correlation between milk consumption and ovarian cancer.

However, Mettlin and Piver (1990) evaluated the association between ovarian cancer and milk in terms of the animal fat content of the milk. In their case-controlled study of 303 patients with ovarian cancer and 606 age-matched control subjects with nonmalignant disease, the relative risk for ovarian cancer was 3.1 for those who drank more than one glass of whole milk each day compared with those who never drank whole milk. Among persons who drank milk regularly, those who drank only whole milk were at increased risk compared with those who drank milk with 0% (skim) or 2% fat. Thus, the fat content of milk may explain the increase in risk.

## Viral and Blood Group Factors

Conflicting and highly speculative reports, unconfirmed by other investigators, have suggested an association between viral infections, including mumps (Cramer et al, 1983) and rubella (McGowan et al, 1979), and an increased risk for ovarian cancer. Bjorkholm (1984), for example, claims a statistically significant increase in the incidence of ovarian cancer in persons with blood group A; however, this probably reflects the large sample size

(1,930 ovarian cancer patients and 24,120 controls), since the actual difference in the frequency of blood group A was only 3%.

## SIGNS AND SYMPTOMS

Because ovarian cancer is often asymptomatic in its early stages, 70% or more patients present with widespread (stage III or IV) disease at the time of diagnosis. Not until the ovarian mass begins to encroach on other viscera or there is intraabdominal spread do symptoms occur. At that time, patients most commonly report vague abdominal pain, abdominal swelling, dyspepsia, urinary frequency, constipation, and weight change. Pelvic discomfort, low back pain, and vaginal (abnormal uterine) bleeding may also be noted.

This lack of significant symptomatology in the early stages of ovarian cancer accounts for an annual mortality rate in the United States that approximates 65% of the incidence rate—20,000 cases and 12,000 deaths/year. Ovarian cancer is the fourth leading cause of death from cancer among American women after lung, breast, and colon cancers and is the most lethal of all gynecologic malignancies.

Since 95% of ovarian cancers measure more than 5 cm in diameter at initial diagnosis, the finding of an ovarian mass of this size on pelvic examination, especially in women over 40 years of age, requires further evaluation. An exception to this dictum would be a 5 to 7 cm cystic mass in young menstruating females, since most of these masses will be functional and not malignant. Since only 5% of benign tumors are bilateral on initial presentation compared with 25% of malignant tumors, the presence of bilateral ovarian masses, even in the younger age group, requires immediate evaluation to rule out ovarian cancer. On pelvic examination, benign ovarian tumors tend to be smooth, cystic, mobile, unilateral, and no larger than 5 to 7 cm in diameter, whereas malignant tumors are nodular, semisolid, fixed, bilateral, and of any size. Ascites and nodularity of the rectovaginal septum may be present with malignant tumors. An adnexal mass should not be considered a functional ovarian cyst (follicular or corpus luteum cyst) unless it has the benign characteristics just described, persists for less than 4 to 6 weeks, occurs during the reproductive years and is primarily cystic (echogenic) on sonography.

## EARLY DIAGNOSIS

Clearly, physicians would welcome a noninvasive technique that would enable them to determine whether a pelvic mass is a benign uterine leiomyoma, an inflammatory condition of the fallopian tubes or ovaries, a benign ovarian cyst, an intestinal tumor, a pregnancy, or an ovarian malignancy. Unfortunately, state-of-the-art ultrasonography, computed axial tomography (CT), magnetic resonance imaging (MRI), and radiolabeled monoclonal antibody imaging are not sufficiently specific to distinguish between benign and malignant ovarian tumors.

## Ultrasound

Ultrasonography is 80 to 90% accurate in assessing the size, location, and consistency of ovarian tumors and in separating them from benign uterine leiomyomas. However, in evaluating the accuracy of ultrasonography in diagnosing pelvic masses (90%), Reeves et al (1980) found no significant difference between ultrasonography and pelvic examination in detecting masses or estimating their size and position. Ultrasonography was significantly more accurate, however, in determining the cystic or solid nature of the mass.

Recently, transvaginal ultrasonography has been introduced as a means of diagnosing pelvic masses. With a high-frequency transducer placed in the vagina near the pelvic structures, transvaginal ultrasonography eliminates the problems posed by the presence of bowel gas, inadequate bladder filling, or obesity. Disadvantages of this technique include the smaller field of view and its limitations in examining patients with large leiomyomas and in evaluating cephaloid or laterally displaced ovaries. In a retrospective study comparing transvaginal with transabdominal ultrasonography in 67 women with palpable pelvic masses, Leibman and colleagues (1988) reported that transvaginal ultrasonography provided more information about the internal architecture or anatomy of the mass in 76% (51) of the patients. They reported no diagnostic advantages for transabdominal ultrasonography. Since transvaginal color flow imaging combines ultrasound and images of blood flow to the ovarian tumor, it may reduce the false-positive rate associated with the use of ultrasound alone (Bourne et al, 1989).

Although ovarian masses larger than 5 cm in diameter detected on clinical examination, especially in women over age 40, should be considered ovarian cancer until proved otherwise, the more frequent use of ultrasonography has facilitated the detection of smaller ovarian cysts. In postmenopausal women, ovarian cysts cannot be functional in nature; therefore, even those measuring 5 cm or less were presumed to be ovarian cancer requiring laparotomy.

In a prospective study, Goldstein et al (1989) evaluated postmenopausal women in whom cysts diagnosed on ultrasound were unilateral, measured 5 cm or less in diameter, lacked septations or solid components, and were without ascites. Twenty-six women between ages 46 and 86 with ovarian cysts that fulfilled these criteria underwent laparotomy and all were found to have benign histopathology. In another study, Rulin and Preston (1987) evaluated 32 postmenopausal patients who had undergone surgery to remove ovarian cysts measuring less than 5 cm in diameter. Only one case proved to be ovarian carcinoma. In the same series, cysts larger than 5 cm were malignant in 11% of cases; the rate of malignancy for cysts larger than 10 cm was 63%. From among about 10,000 routine pelvic examinations, Flynt and Gallup (1981) reported nine postmenopausal patients who had ovarian masses measuring less than 5 cm in diameter, and none were diagnosed as malignant.

Based on the results of these three studies, the overall incidence of malignancy in unilocular, unilateral cysts measuring less than 5 cm in postmenopausal women is 2%. Therefore, Rulin and Preston (1987) conclude that such cases only rarely require immediate laparotomy, and this would also be true for postmenopausal women with palpable ovaries.

## CA 125 Screening

In the first report of a multimodal prospective study designed to screen apparently healthy postmenopausal women for ovarian cancer, Jacobs and colleagues (1988) evaluated 1,010 women in a program using CA 125 assays (see later) and pelvic examination for the initial evaluation. If results of both examinations were normal, patients were followed by questionnaire for one year after their initial visit. If either test was abnormal, patients underwent pelvic ultrasonography. Women with a normal ultrasound were followed at 3-month intervals with repeated ultrasound and CA 125 examinations. Of the 1,010 women, only one stage IA ovarian cancer was detected in a patient with a CA 125 level of 32 units/ ml and a palpable 10-cm adnexal mass.

Although the specificity of 97% from a single serum CA 125 measurement was high in this study, its predictive value would result in 74 cases of suspected ovarian cancer that turned out to be false-positive, all requiring laparotomy or laparoscopy. When ultrasonography and CA 125 assays were combined, the specificity was 99.6%, which would result in nine suspected cases of ovarian cancer that were false-positive and required laparotomy or laparoscopy. Therefore, these 74 (by CA 125) and nine (by CA 125 and ultrasonography) false-positive results do not justify the use of CA 125 or ultrasound for screening asymptomatic women for ovarian cancer, especially since the annual incidence of ovarian cancer for women over age 45 in the United States is about 40 per 100,000.

Even in patients with a known diagnosis of ovarian cancer, Jacobs and Bast (1989) documented that only 50% (48/96) of stage I ovarian cancer patients from 15 series had elevated levels of CA 125. Mann and colleagues (1988) reported elevated CA 125 levels in only 3 of 13 patients with surgical stage I ovarian cancer (23%).

## Computed Tomography

The value of computed axial tomographic (CT) scanning in detecting early-stage ovarian cancer has not been established. Drawbacks of this technique include radiation exposure, lack of clarity and detail in obese and very thin patients, and the small risk of a reaction to the contrast media.

In an attempt to avoid second-look laparotomy in patients known to have ovarian carcinoma but who were in complete clinical remission, Clarke-Pearson and colleagues (1986) evaluated CT of the abdomen and pelvis in 47 patients who had undergone second-look laparotomy. Preoperative CT detected only 7% of the nodules measuring less than 1 cm in diameter and only 37% of the nodules measuring greater than 1 cm found

at surgery. The authors concluded that because of the high false-negative rates (93% and 73%, respectively), a normal CT scan cannot replace second-look laparotomy for accurate assessment of residual tumor. A similar statement could be made concerning the value of CT for screening to detect early ovarian cancer.

## Magnetic Resonance Imaging

Although magnetic resonance imaging (MRI) can detect normal and abnormal structures, there are no MRI criteria to differentiate between benign and malignant masses. Also, a lack of bowel contrast agent makes it difficult to distinguish disease of the gastrointestinal tract from ovarian masses. Therefore, MRI does not appear to offer a significant advantage over ultrasound or CT in evaluating adnexal masses (Council of Scientific Affairs, 1989). In an evaluation of adnexal masses using MRI with ultrasound and CT correlation, ovarian cancer could not be distinguished from pelvic inflammatory disease or benign ovarian cysts in the series by Mitchell et al (1987).

## Monoclonal Antibodies

Radionuclide imaging in human ovarian cancer has involved primarily isotopes of iodine ($^{123}$I and $^{131}$I) and indium ($^{111}$In) conjugated to polyclonal and monoclonal antibodies that react with human milk globule protein (HMFG-2) (Granowska et al, 1986), placental alkaline phosphate (H17E2) (Epenetos et al, 1986), CA 125 (Chatal et al, 1987), and TAG-72 (Mansi et al, 1987). However, the immune response, the rapid clearance of mouse monoclonal antibodies, and the overall sensitivity and specificity rates (87% and 67%, respectively) (Fanning and Foon, 1989) have prevented the widespread clinical use of these techniques in the early diagnosis of ovarian cancer.

## CA 125 ASSAY

CA 125 is a high molecular weight glycoprotein antigenic determinant recognized by the murine monoclonal antibody OC 125. CA 125 is present in fetal tissue derived from coelomic epithelium (müllerian duct cells lining the fetal pleura, pericardium, and peritoneum) and amniotic epithelium (Kabawat et al, 1983); it has also been detected in adult coelomic epithelium (fallopian tube, endometrium, and endocervix) but not in the normal fetal or adult ovary. Although it is agreed that CA 125 is associated with a glycoprotein, its precise character is unknown, and it is variously reported to be an oligosaccharide (Hanisch et al, 1985) or proteinaceous (Davis et al, 1986).

Because CA 125 is not a pure preparation, measurements are expressed in arbitrary units. Not only do the results of CA 125 assays vary as much as 15% from day to day, but assay kits from different sources may produce variable results, prompting the recommendation that serial measurements be made using assay kits from the same source.

Bast et al (1983) originally reported that serum levels of CA 125 exceeded 35 μ/ml in 83% of patients with epithelial ovarian cancer compared with only 1% of health control subjects. CA 125 levels are increased in patients with different stages of epithelial ovarian cancer (stage I = 50%, stage II = 90%, stage III = 92%, and stage IV = 94%) and in patients with serous (80%), mucinous (69%), endometrioid (75%), clear cell (78%) and undifferentiated (80%) carcinomas of the ovary (Jacobs and Bast, 1989). Often, these levels are elevated in patients with carcinoma of the endometrium, fallopian tube, endocervix, and pancreas and less often elevated in patients with lung, breast, and colorectal cancer. Levels may also be elevated after laparotomy as well as in several nonmalignant conditions—i.e., menstruation, early pregnancy, endometriosis, pelvic inflammatory disease, adenomyosis, peritonitis, pancreatitis, hepatitis, and renal failure.

This assay may also be of prognostic significance. Moebus et al (1988) reported that patients with serum CA 125 levels less than 65 μ/ml preoperatively and postoperatively had a significantly better prognosis than those with CA 125 levels that were above 65 μ/ml preoperatively but decreased to less than 65 μ/ml postoperatively. All patients with optimal residual disease of (< 2 cm) following surgery but with CA 125 above 65 μ/ml postoperatively died within 42 months compared with a 48% survival rate at 74 months among patients with CA 125 levels below 65 μ/ml postoperatively. Lavin et al (1987) reported that when CA 125s did not drop to less than 35 μ/ml after 3 months of chemotherapy, the chance of finding persistent disease on clinical exam or at second-look laparotomy was significantly higher than when CA 125 levels fell to below 35 μ/ml after 3 months.

If CA 125 is used to monitor patients during therapy, an increasing level is almost universally associated with progression of disease. Elevated CA 125 is of value in predicting persistent disease after chemotherapy in patients with no clinical evidence of disease, whereas a normal CA 125 is not highly predictive of the presence or absence of disease. Jacobs and Bast (1989) found residual disease on second-look laparotomy in 96% of 243 patients with an elevated CA 125 preoperatively compared with only 46% of 336 patients with normal preoperative CA 125 levels, yielding an overall accuracy rate of 67% in 579 patients. Moreover, elevated CA 125 levels correlated with the size of residual disease: microscopic = 21%, < 1 cm = 38%, < 2 cm = 46%, > 1 cm = 79%, > 2 cm = 70%, and > 10 cm = 100%.

Although other monoclonal antibodies (CEA, CA 19-9, NB/70K, B72.3, and F36-22), immune complexes, and enzyme markers (placental alkaline phosphatase, galactosyltransferase) have been evaluated as markers for ovarian cancer, none is superior to CA 125 levels. Recent studies have suggested that combining measurements of plasma lipid–associated sialic acid with CA 125 levels may improve the sensitivity and specificity rates in monitoring women with epithelial ovarian cancer (Vardi et al, 1989).

## STAGING

In 1987, the International Federation of Gynecology and Obstetrics (FIGO) adopted a revised staging system (Table 14-2). Stages IAii, IBii, and IC in the original FIGO staging are now classified as stage IC. This does not change the criteria for stage I but rather places into stage IC those stage I cases considered to be more likely to recur compared with stages IA and IB. These include (1) tumors on the surface of the ovary, (2) tumors with a ruptured capsule, (3) tumors with malignant ascites, and (4) tumors with positive peritoneal washings. Recently, however, the prognostic significance of capsule rupture has been challenged in a report of 60 stage I patients in whom the 5-year survival rate (76%) was the same for patients with and without rupture of the ovarian capsule (Sevelda et al, 1989).

The prognostic significance of the newly adopted stage IIC is unclear, since, in stage II, there is already evidence of disease outside of the ovary.

Although a significant change has been adopted regarding stage III, the prognostic factor of residual disease *after* debulking or cytoreductive surgery is not taken into account. The prognostic value of debulking surgery was well documented in the seminal report of Griffiths and Fuller (1978) (see later, "Cytoreductive Surgery"). Moreover, most subsequent reports using the new stage III subclassification will include almost exclusively patients with stage IIIC and very few patients with stage IIIA or IIIB, lessening the value of having three subsections for this stage.

## PATHOLOGY

According to presupposed histogenesis, there are three predominant classes of ovarian tumors—common epithelial tumors (adenocarcinomas), germ cell tumors, and sex cord–stromal tumors. In the World Health Organization's (WHO) Classification (Table 14-3), the remaining ovarian tumors are separated from these three major classes because their histogenesis is undetermined, their histology is not specific, or they are metastatic to the ovary (Serov et al, 1973). Common epithelial tumors account for 90% of ovarian cancers, while germ cell and sex cord–stromal tumors account for 5% each.

### Common Epithelial Tumors

Common epithelial tumors are thought to evolve from the pelvic mesothelium (coelomic epithelium) as it reflects over the surface of the ovary. Consistent with the müllerian differentiation of the epithelial surface during the transformation to neoplasia, there are five major subtypes of common epithelial tumors: *serous* (50%), which are similar to fallopian tube epithelium; *endometrioid* (15%), which are similar to endometrial epithelium; *mucinous* (10%), which are similar to endocervical epithelium; *clear cell* (5%), which are similar to endometrial epithelium during pregnancy; and *Bren-*

TABLE 14-2 FIGO Stage Grouping for Primary Carcinoma of the Ovary

| | Current FIGO Stage Grouping |
|---|---|
| Stage I | Growth limited to the ovaries. |
| Stage IA | Growth limited to one ovary; no ascites. |
| Stage IAi | No tumor on the external surface and no capsule rupture. |
| Stage IAii | Tumor present on the external surface or capsule ruptured or both. |
| Stage IB | Growth limited to both ovaries; no ascites. |
| Stage IBi | No tumor on the external surface; capsule intact. |
| Stage IBii | Tumor present on the external surface or capsule ruptured or both. |
| Stage IC | Tumor either stage IA or IB but with ascites present or with positive peritoneal washings. |
| Stage II | Growth involving one or both ovaries with pelvic extension. |
| Stage IIA | Extension of metastases to the uterus or tubes. |
| Stage IIB | Extension to other pelvic tissues. |
| Stage IIC | Tumor either stage IIA or IIB but with ascites present or with positive peritoneal washings. |
| Stage III | Growth involving one or both ovaries with intraperitoneal metastases outside the pelvis or positive retroperitoneal nodes. Tumor limited to the true pelvis with histologically proved malignant extension to small bowel or omentum. |
| Stage IV | Growth involving one or both ovaries with distant metastases. If pleural effusion is present, there must be positive cytology to allot a case to stage IV. Parenchymal liver metastases indicate stage IV. |

| | Newly Adopted FIGO Stage Grouping* |
|---|---|
| Stage I | Growth limited to the ovaries. |
| Stage IA | Growth limited to one ovary; no ascites. No tumor on the external surface; capsule intact. |
| Stage IB | Growth limited to both ovaries; no ascites. No tumor on the external surface; capsules intact. |
| Stage IC† | Tumor either stage IA or IB but with tumor on the surface of one or both ovaries or with capsule ruptured or with ascites present containing malignant cells or with positive peritoneal washings. |
| Stage II | Growth involving one or both ovaries with pelvic extension. |
| Stage IIA | Extension and/or metastases to the uterus and/or tubes. |
| Stage IIB | Extension to other pelvic tissues. |
| Stage IIC† | Tumor either stage IIA or IIB but with tumor on the surface of one or both ovaries or with capsule(s) ruptured or with ascites present containing malignant cells or with positive peritoneal washings. |
| Stage III | Tumor involving one or both ovaries with peritoneal implants outside the pelvis and/or positive retroperitoneal or inguinal nodes. Superficial liver metastasis equals stage III. Tumor is limited to the true pelvis but with histologically verified malignant extension to small bowel or omentum. |
| Stage IIIA | Tumor grossly limited to the true pelvis with negative nodes but with histologically confirmed microscopic seeding of abdominal peritoneal surfaces. |
| Stage IIIB | Tumor of one or both ovaries with histologically confirmed implants of abdominal peritoneal surfaces, none exceeding 2 cm in diameter. Nodes negative. |
| Stage IIIC | Abdominal implants > 2 cm in diameter and/or positive retroperitoneal or inguinal nodes. |
| Stage IV | Growth involving one or both ovaries with distant metastasis. If pleural effusion is present, there must be positive cytologic test results to allot a case to stage IV. |

* Data from International Federation of Gynecology and Obstetrics: Changes in definitions of clinical staging for carcinoma of the cervix and ovary. *Am J Obstet Gynecol* 156:246, 1987.
† To evaluate the impact on prognosis of the different criteria for allotting cases to stage IC or IIC, it would be of value to know whether rupture of the capsule was spontaneous or caused by the surgeon and whether the source of malignant cells detected was peritoneal washings or ascites.

ner (1%), which are similar to urothelial epithelium. Approximately 20% of epithelial ovarian cancers are undifferentiated and cannot be categorized. Mixed epithelial tumors contain a significant component of a second or third of these subtypes.

Common epithelial tumors are further classified into three subtypes; two are based on architectural appearance and a third is based on degree of differentiation: (1) if the glandular component is largely cystic, the prefix "cyst" is used; (2) if the stromal component is predominant, the tumor is classified as an adenofibroma; and (3) borderline tumors or carcinomas have low malignant potential. These borderline tumors are characterized not by the absence of stromal invasion by tumor cells but by the presence of certain characteristics indicative of malignancy, such as an unusual degree of epithelial cell proliferation. Morphologic features include epithelial cell stratification (usually three layers or less), increased mitotic activity, nuclear abnormalities, cytologically atypical cells, and small cellular buds formed by the proliferating cells that may detach from the primary tumor. Borderline tumors are most often serous or mucinous and only rarely exhibit the characteristics of endometrioid, clear cell, or Brenner tumors.

Although histologic subtyping of common epithelial tumors is important, it is not an exact science. Cramer et al (1987) reported on the reproducibility of histologic subtyping of epithelial ovarian cancer. Fifty tumors were sent twice (under different code numbers) to seven ex-

**TABLE 14-3** World Health Organization (WHO) Histologic Classification of Ovarian Tumors

I. Common epithelial tumors
  A. Serous tumors
    1. Benign
      a. Cystadenoma and papillary cystadenoma
      b. Surface papilloma
      c. Adenofibroma and cystadenofibroma
    2. Of borderline malignancy (carcinomas of low malignant potential)
      a. Cystadenoma and papillary cystadenoma
      b. Surface papilloma
      c. Adenofibroma and cystadenofibroma
    3. Malignant
      a. Adenocarcinoma, papillary adenocarcinoma, and papillary cystadenocarcinoma
      b. Surface papillary carcinoma
      c. Malignant adenofibroma and cystadenofibroma
  B. Endometrioid tumors
    1. Benign
      a. Adenoma and cystadenoma
      b. Adenofibroma and cystadenofibroma
    2. Of borderline malignancy (carcinomas of low malignant potential)
      a. Adenoma and cystadenoma
      b. Adenofibroma and cystadenofibroma
    3. Malignant
      a. Carcinoma
        i. Adenocarcinoma
        ii. Adenoacanthoma
        iii. Malignant adenofibroma and cystadenofibroma
      b. Endometrioid stromal sarcomas
      c. Mesodermal (müllerian; mixed tumors, homologous and heterologous)
  C. Mucinous tumors
    1. Benign
      a. Cystadenoma
      b. Adenofibroma and cystadenofibroma
    2. Of borderline malignancy (carcinomas of low malignant potential)
      a. Cystadenoma
      b. Adenofibroma and cystadenofibroma
    3. Malignant
      a. Adenocarcinoma and cystadenocarcinoma
      b. Malignant adenofibroma and cystadenofibroma
  D. Clear cell (mesonephroid) tumors
    1. Benign
    2. Of borderline malignancy (carcinomas of low malignant potential)
    3. Malignant: carcinoma and adenocarcinoma
  E. Brenner tumors
    1. Benign
    2. Of borderline malignancy (proliferating)
    3. Malignant
  F. Mixed epithelial tumors
    1. Benign
    2. Of borderline malignancy
    3. Malignant
  G. Undifferentiated carcinoma
  H. Unclassified epithelial tumors
II. Sex cord–stromal tumors
  A. Granulosa–stromal cell tumors
    1. Granulosa cell tumor
    2. Tumors in the thecoma-fibroma group
      a. Thecoma
      b. Fibroma
      c. Unclassified
  B. Androblastomas, Sertoli–Leydig cell tumors
    1. Well-differentiated
      a. Tubular androblastoma, Sertoli cell tumor (tubular adenoma of Pick)
      b. Tubular androblastoma with lipid storage, Sertoli cell tumor with lipid storage (folliculome lipidique of Lecene)
      c. Sertoli–Leydig cell tumor (tubular adenoma with Leydig cells)
      d. Leydig cell tumor, hilus cell tumor
    2. Of intermediate differentiation
    3. Poorly differentiated (sarcomatoid)
    4. With heterologous elements
  C. Gynandroblastoma
  D. Unclassified
III. Lipid (lipoid) cell tumors
IV. Germ cell tumors
  A. Dysgerminoma
  B. Endodermal sinus tumor
  C. Embryonal carcinoma
  D. Polyembryoma
  E. Choriocarcinoma
  F. Teratomas
    1. Immature
    2. Mature
      a. Solid
      b. Cystic
        i. Dermoid cyst (mature cystic teratoma)
        ii. Dermoid cyst with malignant transformation
    3. Monodermal and highly specialized
      a. Struma ovarii
      b. Carcinoid
      c. Struma ovarii and carcinoid
      d. Others
  G. Mixed forms
V. Gonadoblastoma
  A. Pure
  B. Mixed with dysgerminoma or other form of germ cell tumor
VI. Soft tissue tumors not specific to ovary
VII. Unclassified tumors
VIII. Secondary (metastatic) tumors
IX. Tumor-like conditions
  A. Pregnancy luteoma
  B. Hyperplasia of ovarian stroma and hyperthecosis
  C. Massive edema
  D. Solitary follicle cyst and corpus luteum cyst
  E. Multiple follicle cysts (polycystic ovaries)
  F. Multiple luteinized follicle cysts and/or corpora lutea
  G. Endometriosis
  H. Surface epithelial inclusion cysts (germinal inclusion cysts)
  I. Simple cysts
  J. Inflammatory lesions
  K. Paraovarian cysts

*Source:* Serov SF, Scully RE, Sobin LH: *Histological typing of ovarian tumors. International Classification of Tumors #9.* World Health Organization, Geneva, 1973.

perienced pathologists with an academic interest in gynecologic pathology. In terms of reproducibility, the intraobserver rate was only 64% and the interobserver rate was only 52%. Therefore, treatment decisions in patients with common epithelial tumors should not be based on histologic subtype. Moreover, when controlled for stage and grade, histologic subtype is not a separate variable for response to therapy and disease-free survival.

In contrast, tumor grade is an essential prognostic variable with regard to response to therapy and disease-free survival in ovarian carcinoma. Tumor grading can be based on nuclear or architectural criteria. Nuclear grading depends on nuclear size, atypia, pleomorphism, and mitosis, while FIGO uses an architectural grading system based on the glandular pattern. Grade 1 tumors are well-differentiated and are predominantly glandular, grade 2 tumors are moderately differentiated and are 50% glandular, and grade 3 tumors are poorly differentiated and are predominantly solid.

Initial results of flow cytometric analysis indicate that DNA ploidy and relative DNA content are also significant prognostic factors for ovarian cancer. Aneuploid and multiploid tumors and tumors with a high DNA content are associated with decreased survival rates (Klemi et al, 1989).

**Serous Tumors** The epithelium of serous tumors varies from a flat mesothelioid to a tall columnar type, sometimes containing cilia, that resembles fallopian tube epithelium. Often calcified granules (psammoma bodies) are found and appear to result from degeneration of small papillae. In borderline and malignant serous tumors, the epithelium is arranged in multiple branching papillae with hyalinized cores and free cellular clusters. Unlike the other four subtypes of common epithelial tumors, which are endophytic tumors within the ovary, a small percentage of serous tumors are entirely exophytic and are designated *surface papillary serous tumors*.

**Endometrioid Tumors** Endometrioid tumors have the same morphology as endometrial adenocarcinomas, including adenoacanthomas, adenosquamous carcinomas, and secretory adenocarcinomas. The epithelium consists of oval or round branching glands lined by tall columnar epithelium with dense nuclei. Five percent of endometrioid tumors arise in endometriosis and one-third are associated with uterine adenocarcinomas.

**Mucinous Tumors** Mucinous tumors are lined by small columnar epithelium with basal nuclei and mucinous eosinophilic cytoplasm resembling endocervical epithelium. In malignant and borderline tumors, the epithelium is arranged in multiple papillary frons and mucin-secreting acini. By definition, borderline tumors have malignant characteristics, but the malignant glands do not invade the ovarian stroma. However, for some pathologists, the classification "borderline" includes tumors with areas of invasion into the stroma, although this invasion does not "destroy" the stromal part of the

tumor. Criteria for "destructive" invasion have not been agreed on and should therefore not be used to differentiate between borderline and invasive tumors. Moreover, for mucinous tumors, invasion of the stroma is often difficult to demonstrate.

For this reason, Hart and Norris (1973) defined mucinous ovarian tumors as "borderline" when the height of the atypical mucin cells lining the glandular cyst was three layers or less and as "invasive" when the height of these cells was four layers or more. Subsequently, Hart (1977) added the presence of a cribiform pattern to the criteria for invasive mucinous tumors. Although the Hart and Norris criteria differ from that used by the WHO, most pathologists use it for differentiating borderline from invasive mucinous tumors because the criteria separate prognostically borderline mucinous from invasive mucinous tumors.

Mucinous tumors may become large, weighing over 100 pounds in some reports. Although common epithelial tumors are classified based on the presumed histogenesis from müllerian duct differentiation exhibited by the surface epithelium, there are indications that mucinous tumors, although rare, evolve from monodermal differentiation of the germ cell tumor teratoma.

**Clear Cell Tumors** Clear cell tumors are lined by flattened or cuboidal polyhedral cells with clear cytoplasm. Often, hobnail cells with nuclei protruding into the glandular lumens are present. The epithelium of malignant or borderline tumors is arranged in a tubulocystic or papillary pattern. More often than any other tumor, clear cell tumors are associated with endometriosis. A recently described subtype of clear cell tumor is oxyphil clear cell carcinoma, which has an impressive component of cells with eosinophilic cytoplasm (Young and Scully, 1987). Misdiagnosis of clear cell carcinomas as endodermal sinus tumors of the ovary is a common but significant mistake.

**Brenner Tumors** Unlike other epithelial ovarian tumors, Brenner tumors are almost universally benign and are often found incidentally during surgery. They are thought to be of common epithelial ovarian origin based on the premise that they are derived from Walthard cell islands (rests) on the ovarian surface epithelium. Walthard cell islands are embryonic and share common characteristics with Brenner cells, including longitudinal grooving of the nuclei, cyst formation, and mucin secretion. Ultrastructurally, Brenner tumors closely resemble Walthard cell islands in that the two are derived from the coelomic epithelium of the ovary. Microscopically, Brenner tumors consist of small islands of transitional epithelium in abundant fibrous stroma. Several researchers believe that some Brenner tumors have a germ cell origin, while others believe they are derived from rete ovarii.

The rare borderline (or proliferative) Brenner tumors resemble noninvasive, grade 1 papillary transitional carcinoma of the bladder. In contrast, malignant Brenner tumors show definite areas of invasion by transitional cell or squamous cell carcinoma into the ovarian stroma. Recently, ovarian transitional cell carcinomas have been described. Histologically, these carcinomas are similar to transitional cell carcinoma of the urinary bladder and may be a component of malignant Brenner tumors or a distinct subtype of epithelial ovarian cancer (Robey et al, 1989).

***Undifferentiated Tumors*** Some epithelial ovarian cancers are so poorly differentiated that they cannot be classified. Most are probably poorly differentiated serous or endometrioid carcinomas.

## Germ Cell Tumors

Germ cell tumors consist of teratomas, dysgerminomas, endodermal sinus tumors, embryonal carcinomas, choriocarcinomas, and mixed germ cell tumors.

***Ovarian Teratomas*** Ovarian teratomas are germ cell tumors composed of tissues from all three germ cell layers (endoderm, ectoderm, and mesoderm); they may be either mature or immature.

*Mature teratomas* (the most common ovarian neoplasm) are also known as dermoid cysts or cystic teratomas. All three germ cell layers in mature ovarian teratomas consist of mature tissues only. Approximately 2% of mature teratomas have a malignant component, primarily squamous cell carcinoma but in rare cases other types, such as adenocarcinoma and sarcoma.

Before the 1973 WHO classification of ovarian tumors, *immature teratomas* were known as solid, malignant, or embryonal teratomas; teratocarcinomas; or teratoblastomas. Since immature teratomas are at least partially cystic, the term solid was considered inappropriate. The WHO formulated the term immature teratoma because the immaturity of the tissue determines its ability to metastasize. Like mature teratomas, immature teratomas consist of all three germ cell layers; however, one of the layers is immature or incompletely differentiated. Immature teratomas may include those tumors in which there is a predominance of a single tissue element, which is generally highly differentiated, such as thyroid (struma ovarii) and carcinoids or, very rarely, primary malignant melanomas, sebaceous gland tumors, retinal analogue tumors, and primitive neuroectodermal tumors (Aguirre and Scully, 1982).

There are four types of primary ovarian *carcinoids.* The most common is the insular carcinoid, which is similar to tumors that arise from the midgut of jejunum, the ileum, and the appendix. Histologically, insular carcinoids consist of small groups of acini. Trabecular carcinoids are the second most common type and are similar to tumors that arise from the hindgut or foregut. These tumors are characterized by anastomosing trabecular columns or a ribbon-type pattern. The third type, struma carcinoids, consist of an admixture of trabecular carcinoid and thyroid tissue. The least common type of ovarian carcinoid develops within a Sertoli-Leydig tumor.

Most insular carcinoids are associated with teratomatous elements (respiratory and gastrointestinal epithelium or cartilage), although occasionally they are the only element present. Insular carcinoids usually occur within a cystic teratoma or as a small part of a mature teratoma.

In 1970, Scully coined the term "struma carcinoid" for an ovarian tumor that consists of thyroid tissue intermixed with trabecular carcinoid. Previously, these tumors had been designated as mature teratoma, malignant struma ovarii, or, rarely, papillary adenocarcinoma of the thyroid within a stroma. Before this designation, many of these tumors were included with the cases of malignant struma ovarii. Because of the nonovarian tissue elements present within the tumor, struma carcinoids are considered to be of teratomatous origin. The term "struma ovarii" is used for ovarian tumors that consist of more than 50% thyroid tissue. Struma ovarii occur primarily within a benign cystic teratoma; however, they should not be confused with benign ovarian teratoma, in which a small foci of thyroid tissue is present.

***Dysgerminoma*** Dysgerminoma is morphologically and ultrastructurally consistent with, and in fact arises from, undifferentiated primordial germ cells. Dysgerminoma is the most common malignant germ cell tumor, occurring twice as often as endodermal sinus tumor. This tumor accounts for 1 to 2% of all ovarian tumors and 3 to 5% of all ovarian malignancies. Dysgerminoma is the female homologue of the seminoma of the testes. Histologically, germ cells in this tumor are easy to recognize but may be associated with syncytial giant cells, which may contain histochemically demonstrable human chorionic gonadotropin (HCG). Granulomatous or lymphocytic infiltration is seen in most dysgerminomas. A rare form of this tumor, referred to as anaplastic dysgerminoma because of its similarity to anaplastic seminoma of the testes, has the overall appearance of dysgerminoma but the germ cells appear anaplastic, and pleomorphism and increased mitotic activity are apparent.

***Endodermal Sinus Tumor/Embryonal Carcinoma of the Ovary*** Endodermal sinus tumor is the second most common malignant germ cell tumor of the ovary. Until 1959, when Teilum coined the term endodermal sinus tumor, this tumor had been referred to as embryonal carcinoma, extraembryonal teratoma, yolk sac tumor, immature mesonephroma, mesoblastoma vitellinum, extraembryonal mesoblastoma, and Teilum tumor. Teilum's classification lessened the confusion about germ cell tumors by separating them into tumors arising from extraembryonic structures such as the yolk sac and allantois (endodermal sinus tumor and choriocarcinoma) and those arising from the embryo (teratomas). Teilum selected the term endodermal sinus tumor because the tumor resembled the endodermal sinus of the rodent placenta, previously described by Duval.

Seen histologically, the endodermal sinus is referred to as the Schiller-Duval body and consists of layers of primitive germ cells with a central capillary; this pattern is seen in 75% of endodermal sinus tumors. The less common polyvesicular vitelline pattern consists of primitive cells surrounding a cystic space. The solid pattern is the least common pattern of endodermal sinus tumor.

In 1982, Pratt et al described the hepatoid variant of endodermal sinus tumor. This subtype is similar in appearance to hepatocellular carcinoma, which displays embryonic endodermal differentiation and forms mucinous glandular structures in cells resembling hepatocytes. The hepatoid variant should not be confused with hepatoid carcinoma of the ovary, described by Ishikura and Scully, 1987.

In 1976, Kurman and Norris (1976a) described 15 cases of an ovarian germ cell tumor that is now referred to as embryonal carcinoma. The authors separated these tumors histologically, immunohistochemically, and clinically from the more common endodermal sinus tumor of the ovary. Embryonal carcinoma of the ovary resembles the embryonal carcinoma of the adult testes, whereas the endodermal sinus tumor has the appearance of the same tumor of the infantile testes. The Schiller-Duval bodies of the endodermal sinus tumor are not seen in embryonal carcinoma, which is composed primarily of solid sheets of germ cells. Histologically, embryonal carcinoma lacks the excessive amount of hemorrhage and the syncytiotrophoblasts associated with ovarian choriocarcinoma. Syncytiotrophoblasts were not seen in any of the embryonal carcinomas described by Kurman and Norris; however, multinucleated giant cells that did resemble syncytial cells were scattered throughout the tumors.

***Ovarian Choriocarcinoma*** Similar to uterine choriocarcinoma, ovarian choriocarcinoma consists of an admixture of syncytiotrophoblasts and cytotrophoblasts. Ovarian choriocarcinoma can be a primary cancer resulting from an ovarian pregnancy (gestational) or can have no association with such a pregnancy (nongestational). It may also be one of the germ cell elements of a mixed germ cell tumor, which frequently contains areas of choriocarcinoma admixed with dysgerminoma, endodermal sinus tumor, embryonic carcinoma, and immature teratoma.

***Mixed Germ Cell Tumors*** At the Armed Forces Institute of Pathology, mixed germ cell ovarian tumors represented 8% of the germ cell tumors reported and ranked fourth in incidence behind dysgerminoma, pure endodermal sinus tumor, and immature teratoma and ahead of pure embryonal carcinoma, the rarest subtype (Kurman and Norris, 1976c). Histologically, dysgerminoma was the most common element, present in 70% of the cases, followed by immature teratoma (53%), ovarian choriocarcinoma (20%), and embryonal carcinoma (16%). Endodermal sinus tumor and dysgerminoma accounted for one-third of the mixed germ cell tumors and was the most common combination present.

## SEX CORD–STROMAL TUMORS

Sex cord–stromal tumors are thought to be derived from the sex cord and stromal elements of the embryonic gonad. Granulosa cell tumors can contain granulosa cells, theca cells, fibroblasts, and lutein cells, either alone or in combination. Sex cord–stromal tumors can be divided into four major categories: (1) female cell type, including granulosa cell tumors, thecomas, and thecoma-fibroma tumors; (2) male cell type, including Sertoli cell tumors, Leydig cell tumors and Sertoli–Leydig cell tumors; (3) male- and female-cell types, including gynandroblastoma (granulosa and Sertoli or Leydig cells); and (4) unclassified sex cord–stromal tumors, which include sex cord tumors with annular tubules and sclerosing stromal tumors.

***Granulosa Cell Tumors*** These tumors are composed of granulosa cells alone or combined with cells derived from the theca interna or externa. In over 50% of granulosa cell tumors, the granulosa cells form characteristic rosette arrangements referred to as *Call-Exner bodies*, similar to the arrangements seen in a graafian follicle. Granulosa cell tumors often have nuclear grooves (coffee bean nuclei) secondary to a "folded" nuclear membrane, a characteristic of sex cord–stromal tumors in general.

Granulosa cell tumors have been subdivided into three main histologic patterns: (1) follicular, (2) trabecular or insular, and (3) diffuse (formerly sarcomatoid). The follicular tumors are well-differentiated and either micro- or macrofollicular in character, with the microfollicular pattern characterized by the presence of Call-Exner bodies. The trabecular or insular pattern is well to intermediate in differentiation and does not form Call-Exner bodies. The diffuse pattern is poorly differentiated and is often confused with thecomas.

In addition, granulosa cell tumors may be either adult or juvenile, the latter occurring primarily during the first two decades of life. Granulosa cell tumors are characterized by a macrofollicular or diffuse pattern of growth and often by extensive luteinization of the granulosa, theca cells, and hyperchromatic nuclei, giving this tumor a more unusual appearance (Young, 1984a). Granulosa cell tumors are primarily estrogenic.

***Thecomas*** Thecomas are stromal tumors consisting of stromal cells, characteristic of theca cells or lutein cells. Diagnosis of benign thecomas is based on finding spindle or oval cells with reticulum fiber surrounding individual theca cells and demonstrating intracellular lipid. Whether malignant thecomas exist is problematic.

***Pure Sertoli Cell Tumors*** These rare tumors are primarily estrogenic; however, virilization can occur (Tavassoli and Norris, 1980). Pure Sertoli ovarian tumors of gonadal stromal origin are composed entirely of Sertoli cells. Previously, this tumor was classified as a Sertoli–Leydig cell tumor even though the features of such tumors—i.e., Leydig cells and primitive gonadal stroma—are absent.

***Sertoli–Leydig Cell Tumors*** Sertoli–Leydig cell tumors of the ovary contain Sertoli and Leydig cells with indifferent stroma, similar to that seen in the various phases of testicular development in males. They are the most common virilizing ovarian tumors but occur only one-fifth as often as granulosa cell tumors. Originally referred to as arrhenoblastoma (Myer, 1931) or androblastoma, Morris and Scully, in 1958, suggested replacing the term with Sertoli–Leydig cell tumor to avoid the connotation that all arrhenoblastomas and androblastomas were masculinizing. The WHO still uses both names.

The WHO classifies Sertoli–Leydig cell tumors in four categories: the most common are the well-differentiated Pick's adenomas, which consist of hollow tubules separated by Leydig cells. The intermediate-differentiated tumors contain primitive Sertoli cells arranged similarly to the cells of the sex cords of the embryonal testes. The poorly differentiated sarcomatoid tumors consist of cells resembling those in spindle cell sarcomas. The fourth type is the Sertoli–Leydig cell tumor with heterologous elements containing argentaffin cells, cartilage, skeletal muscle, or mucus-secreting epithelium. All four categories have well-differentiated Leydig cells identical to those seen in the male testes.

**Gynandroblastoma** This rare form of sex cord–stromal tumor contains granulosa and Sertoli or Leydig cells. Its malignant potential is similar to that of granulosa cell tumors.

**Sex Cord Tumor With Annular Tubules (SCTAT)** These tumors have patterns intermediate between granulosa cell and pure Sertoli cell tumors, are characterized by simple and complex ring-shaped tubules, are thought to be estrogenic (Scully, 1970b), and are often associated with Peutz-Jeghers syndrome. Their malignant potential is similar to that of granulosa cell tumors.

**Sclerosing Ovarian Stromal Tumors** In 10% of sex cord–stromal tumors, it is impossible to determine whether the cells are typical for the male or female gonad. Sclerosing ovarian stromal tumors are one rare distinct subtype, mainly owing to their characteristic feature of cellular areas undergoing collagenous sclerosis (Chalvardjian and Scully, 1973). These tumors are probably benign.

## Unclassified Tumors

Since the WHO classified ovarian tumors in 1973, several tumors have been described that do not fit into the established categories. One example is the ovarian tumor probably of Wolffian origin described by Young and Scully (1983), which is composed of nonmucin-secreting epithelial cells in cords or tubules or in a cystic, sievelike pattern. Another unclassified tumor is the small cell carcinoma, which consists of small cells that are epithelial in type and contain scanty cytoplasm (Dickersin et al, 1982). Their histogenesis is unknown and there is no effective treatment (Senekjian et al, 1989). Other unclassified ovarian tumors include lipid cell, hilar cell, and stromal Leydig cell tumors.

**Lipid Cell Tumors** Ovarian tumors with a preponderance of lipid-containing cells are designated lipid cell tumors, lipoid cell tumors, adrenal rest tumors, or adrenal-like tumors. Lipid cell tumors occur within the ovarian stroma and histologically consist of large, round, polygonal cells with a vacuolated, lipid-rich cytoplasm. Microscopically, lipid cell or steroid cell tumors resemble adrenal cortical, Leydig, or lutein cells. Since hilar cells, adrenal cortical cells, and luteinized ovarian stromal cells are cytologically similar, separation of these tumors into specific categories has often been impossible.

Before diagnosing lipid cell tumors, one must exclude the following conditions that are often associated with virilization: (1) stromal luteoma, a benign condition characterized by severe luteinization of the ovarian stroma in which the luteinized cells have a vacuolated lipid appearance; (2) nonhilar Leydig cells, which may also have a vacuolated lipid appearance; (3) pregnancy luteoma, a condition that is characterized by nodules of lutein cells containing little or no neutral lipid, is often present in both ovaries, and has increased numbers of mitoses, possibly leading to a mistaken diagnosis of malignancy; (4) luteinized granulosa cell tumors, which occur primarily during pregnancy and may be confused with lipid cell tumors; (5) metastatic carcinomas to the ovary with stromal luteinization, which may cause severe luteinization of the ovary and virilization, although a positive reaction for intracytoplasmic mucin in the metastatic carcinomas will separate these from lipid cell tumors; and (6) hilar cell tumors without the crystalloids of Reinke, which some authors believe cannot be specifically diagnosed as hilar cells and are therefore often included in the lipid cell category.

**Hilar Cell Tumors** Hilar cells are normally present in the ovarian hilus but may be located in any part of the ovary. Like lipid cell tumors, they contain intracytoplasmic lipid inclusions. However, hilar cell tumors are distinct from lipid cell tumors because 75% contain crystalloids of Reinke, eosinophilic, rod-shaped structures located in the cytoplasm that are a characteristic solely of hilar and Leydig cell tumors. When there is an increase in hilar cells without a distinctive tumor nodule, the condition is referred to as hilar cell hyperplasia; if a tumor is present, the term hilar cell tumor is used.

**Stromal Leydig Cell Tumors** Stromal Leydig cell tumors are rare and occur in the ovarian stroma. They consist of Leydig cells in nodular formation and contain crystalloids of Reinke. Sex cord–stromal elements, such as Sertoli and granulosa cells, are not present. In addition to the characteristic Leydig cells, spindle-shaped stromal cells are present, which are distinct from those in the stromal luteomas.

## TREATMENT OF STAGE I AND II OVARIAN CANCER

In the 1960s and 1970s, ovarian cancer that was clinically limited to FIGO stage I disease was treated primarily by surgical resection with or without postoperative radiation. However, the 5-year survival rate was

TABLE 14-4   Incidence of Subclinical Metastases in Apparent Stage I or II Ovarian Cancer

| Sites | Stage I | | Stage II | |
|---|---|---|---|---|
| | Piver | Buchsbaum | Piver | Buchsbaum |
| Diaphragm | 11.0% | 11.0% | 23.0% | 6.0% |
| Omentum | 3.0% | 0.0% | 7.0% | 19.0% |
| Paraaortic nodes | 13.0% | 4.0% | 10.0% | 19.5% |
| Pelvic nodes | 8.0% | 0.0% | — | 19.5% |
| Malignant peritoneal cytology | 33.0% | — | 12.5% | — |

*Source:* Piver MS, Barlow JJ, Lele SB: Incidence of subclinical metastasis in stage I and II ovarian carcinoma. *Obstet Gynecol* 52:100, 1978; Buchsbaum HJ, Brady MF, Delgado G, et al: Surgical staging of carcinoma of the ovaries. *Surg Gynecol Obstet* 169:226, 1989. By permission of *Surgery, Gynecology & Obstetrics.*

only 60 to 70% in this earliest stage, despite apparent curative surgery with or without radiation.

## Occult (Subclinical) Metastasis

When Bagley et al (1972) and Fuks (1977) reviewed the literature on survival rates independently, their results were nearly identical. Bagley's group reported a 67% survival rate for patients with stage I ovarian cancer treated with surgery alone and a 60% survival rate for those treated with the combination of surgery and radiation therapy. Fuks reported a 70% survival rate with surgery alone and 58% survival rate with a combination of surgery and primarily pelvic irradiation. The reasons for these poor survival rates were elusive until the 1970s, when it was discovered that five areas within the peritoneal cavity—the diaphragm, omentum, paraaortic lymph nodes, pelvic lymph nodes, and malignant cytologic peritoneal washings—harbored microscopic or unrecognized metastases from what appeared clinically to be localized ovarian cancer.

In 1978, Piver and colleagues reported a collective review of the incidence of such microscopic metastases in patients with stage I or II ovarian cancer. Of the women with presumed stage I disease, 11% were found to have diaphragmatic metastasis, 13% had paraaortic lymph node metastasis, 8% had pelvic lymph node metastasis, 3% had omental metastasis, and 33% had malignant peritoneal cytologic washings (Table 14-4). The findings were similar in patients with FIGO stage II disease. Thus, it became evident that surgical staging was required to truly define surgical stage I ovarian cancer.

The first prospective studies of such surgical staging in clinically localized ovarian cancer were reported by the Ovarian Cancer Study Group (OCSG), which was formed in 1976 and comprised of the Mayo Clinic, M.D. Anderson Tumor Institute, Roswell Park Cancer Institute, and the National Cancer Institute. Of the 100 women reported, 31% with presumed stage I or II ovarian cancer were upstaged as a result of exploration and surgical staging and 77% were reclassified as stage III (Young et al, 1983). Moreover, of the 100 patients who had had FIGO stage I or IIB ovarian cancer and were referred to member institutions within 4 weeks of their original surgery, 61 were considered to have no residual cancer after the initial operation. When restaging lap-

arotomy was performed at one of the four institutions within 4 weeks of the initial surgery, metastasis was present in the diaphragm (3%), in the omentum (11%), in abdominal tissues (9%), in other pelvic tissues (9%), in the cul-de-sac peritoneum (3%), in the paraaortic lymph nodes (12%), and in the pelvic lymph nodes (9%) of these supposedly disease-free patients (Table 14-5).

In a recent prospective study by the Gynecologic Oncology Group, (GOG), Buchsbaum and coauthors (1989) reported findings similar to those in the Piver et al (1978) and Young et al (1983) studies (Table 14-4). Therefore, complete surgical staging is required for apparent stage I and II ovarian cancer to identify those patients who truly have localized disease and to upstage the remaining patients to allow for appropriate treatment.

Surgical staging should include peritoneal cytologic sampling from the pelvis and right and left paracolic gutters, obtained immediately after the peritoneal cavity is entered to avoid the red cell contamination that interferes with cytologic interpretation; total abdominal hysterectomy and bilateral salpingo-oophorectomy, ipsilateral pelvic lymphadenectomy, paraaortic lymphadenectomy, right diaphragmatic biopsy, omentectomy, and biopsy of all adhesions and any suspicious areas.

## Adjuvant Therapy

Even before the discovery of the five primary sites of occult, or subclinical, metastasis from presumed local-

TABLE 14-5   Staging Laparotomy in 61 Patients With Early Stage I to IIB Ovarian Cancer*—Ovarian Cancer Study Group

| Sites | % Subclinical Metastasis |
|---|---|
| Diaphragm | 3 |
| Omentum | 11 |
| Other abdominal tissues | 9 |
| Other pelvic tissues | 9 |
| Cul-de-sac peritoneum | 3 |
| Paraaortic nodes | 12 |
| Pelvic nodes | 9 |

* Patients were apparently disease-free at time of referral.
Adapted from Young RC, Decker DG, Wharton JT, et al: Staging laparotomy in early ovarian cancer. *JAMA* 250:3072-3976, 1983. © American Medical Association.

ized stage I and II ovarian cancer, the need for adjuvant therapy to total abdominal hysterectomy and bilateral salpingo-oophorectomy was apparent because of the 30 to 40% death rate at 5 years in apparent stage I and a greater than 60% death rate at 5 years in apparent stage II disease.

A series of adjuvant therapies have been used as each became available: (1) pelvic radiation; (2) intraperitoneal radioactive gold ($^{198}$Au); (3) intraperitoneal chromic phosphate ($^{32}$P); (4) whole abdominal radiation by the open-field techniques; (5) whole abdominal radiation by the open-field technique, including the diaphragm; (6) whole abdominal radiation by the moving strip; (7) single-agent chemotherapy, primarily melphalan; and most recently (8) cisplatin-based chemotherapy.

### Intraperitoneal Chromic Phosphate and Radioactive Gold

Pelvic irradiation alone had fallen into disuse before the data on surgical staging were reported, after it was recognized that most recurrences were in the abdominal cavity. Subsequently, researchers employed first intraperitoneal gold-198 ($^{198}$Au) and then chromic phosphate ($^{32}$P) in patients not surgically staged.

Although the early results with $^{198}$Au appeared to be satisfactory, most institutions now use intraperitoneal $^{32}$P instead, owing in part to the significant complications associated with $^{198}$Au. These complications are believed to be due to differences in the characteristics of the two substances. $^{32}$P emits purely beta radiation, whereas $^{198}$Au emits both beta and gamma rays. The shorter half-life of $^{198}$Au of 2.7 days as opposed to 14.5 days for $^{32}$P results in irradiation of the tissues at a higher rate, which may be associated with a higher incidence of complications. Also, $^{32}$P is preferred to $^{198}$Au because (a) its higher beta energy allows deeper tissue penetration, (b) its long half-life makes it easier to order and use than $^{198}$Au (which must be used almost immediately), and (c) its pure beta emissions are not harmful to hospital personnel and obviate patient isolation.

Nevertheless, two preclinical studies have questioned the efficacy of intraperitoneal $^{32}$P. In the first study, Leichner et al (1981), using a rabbit model, estimated that 75 to 150 mCi of $^{32}$P would be required to produce a tumoricidal effect in human ovarian cancer. This dose is five to ten times greater than the dose used clinically. Currie et al, (1981) concluded that intraperitoneal $^{32}$P delivers a therapeutic dose to the superficial peritoneal surfaces (6,000 to 7,000 cGy) but not to the retroperitoneal lymph nodes.

$^{32}$P is administered intraperitoneally through a catheter that is placed during or after surgery. After proper catheter placement is confirmed by means of Hypaque peritoneography or technetium-99 scintigraphy, 15 mCi of $^{32}$P and 500 to 1,000 ml of sodium chloride are instilled into the peritoneal cavity. A significant volume of fluid must be administered and the patient must be turned frequently over the next several hours to ensure adequate distribution within the cavity. Although the rate of major complications with $^{32}$P is only about 5% (Piver et al, 1982), this form of therapy is associated

with significant life-threatening gastrointestinal complications (25%) if given concomitantly with pelvic radiotherapy (Klaassen et al, 1985).

Before the advent of surgical staging in ovarian cancer, three small series reported an overall survival rate of 92.7% using intraperitoneal $^{32}$P in presumed stage I ovarian cancer (Hester and White, 1969; Piver, 1972; Clarke et al, 1973). Subsequently, Piver et al (1988a) reported on 25 evaluable patients with FIGO stage I ovarian cancer treated with intraperitoneal $^{32}$P. All patients had undergone total abdominal hysterectomy and bilateral salpingo-oophorectomy, with (28%) or without (72%) omentectomy; none had undergone other surgical staging procedures at the time of referral. Patients were restaged by laparoscopy, with inspection of the diaphragm, abdomen and pelvis; biopsies of suspicious lesions; and cytologic peritoneal washings prior to $^{32}$P therapy. The estimated 5-year recurrence-free survival rate was 84% but was only 75% at 10 years. This long-term result (75%) still leaves open the question of the true effect of adjuvant $^{32}$P therapy on disease-free survival.

### Whole Abdominal Radiation

When whole abdominal radiation is used, only 2,250 to 3,000 cGy can be delivered to the whole abdomen and 4,500 to 5,000 cGy to the pelvis. The major drawback of this form of therapy is that only a limited dose (less than 2,500 cGy) can be delivered safely owing to the radiosensitivity of the intestine, liver, and kidney. Fletcher (1973) has shown that a dose of 5,000 cGy of external radiation therapy is needed to cure 90% of subclinical disease.

Clearly, if radiation was to play a major role in the treatment of ovarian cancer, a larger biologic effect was required. Patient tolerance to radiation is influenced by the total dose delivered, the volume of tissue irradiated, and the duration of each treatment. Therefore, it was theorized that the same dose delivered to a smaller area and given for a shorter period of time should have a much greater biologic effect.

To test this theory, the *moving-strip irradiation technique* was used in some institutions to overcome the two main disadvantages of open-field irradiation of the whole abdomen. Small areas (one 2.5-cm strip at a time) were irradiated over a shorter period of time to lessen intestinal reactions and to obtain a greater biologic effect. Each 2.5-cm strip is irradiated anteriorly and posteriorly for a total dose of about 2,250 to 2,500 cGy given in eight treatments over 10 calendar days; this was compared with approximately 8 weeks for delivery of the same dose using the open-field technique.

In a randomized trial comparing moving-strip and open-field whole abdominal irradiation, 5-year disease-free survival rates were identical (Dembo et al, 1983). However, the rate of bowel complications requiring surgery was significantly higher with the moving-strip technique. Moreover, Dembo (1985) reported a disease-free survival rate of only 73% in 79 patients with stage I (not staged) ovarian cancer treated by whole abdominal radiation and a rate of 65% in 108 patients with presumed stage II ovarian cancer with no residual disease. Finally, when Macbeth et al (1988) used the whole abdominal radiation techniques described by Dembo et al (1983) to deliver 2,500 cGy to surgically staged patients, they reported an estimated 5-year disease-free survival rate of 65% in 28 stage I ovarian cancer patients and of 39% in 25 stage II patients. The authors concluded that *these data do not seem to support a curative role for postoperative radiation of this dose in these patients.*

***Adjuvant Alkylating Agent (Melphalan) Chemotherapy*** Surgically staged patients from the Ovarian Cancer Study Group/Gynecologic Oncology Group (OCSG/GOG) study of presumed stage I and II ovarian cancer were entered into two prospective trials, protocols 7601 and 7602. (These trials were started in 1976, prior to the seminal report by Wiltshaw and Kroner [1976] on the effectiveness of cisplatin in ovarian cancer.)

Protocol 7601 included patients with stage IAi, IBi, grade 1 or 2 ovarian adenocarcinoma with no evidence of metastasis on complete surgical staging. Patients were randomized to either observation or treatment with melphalan for 12 cycles. With a median followup of over 6 years, the disease-free survival at 5 years was 95% for melphalan and 92% for observation, with no statistical difference (Young, 1987*b*; Young, 1989). Based on the exceedingly high cure rates, it was concluded that patients with stage IAi, IBi, G1, or G2 ovarian adenocarcinoma and no evidence of metastasis on complete surgical staging do not require adjuvant therapy.

Once the OCSG/GOG recognized that a subset of completely staged patients with stage I and II ovarian cancer could not be entered into protocol 7601 because of the high risk for recurrence should they be randomized to the observation arm, this subset (which included those with stage IG3, IAii, IBii, IC, IIA, B, and C disease) were placed on protocol 7602 and randomized to melphalan or intraperitoneal $^{32}P$ at a dose of 15 mCi. With a median followup of over 6 years, the 5-year disease-free survival rates were identical for both arms—80% (Young, 1989). Protocol 7602 was later updated to randomize these patients to either the control arm of $^{32}P$ or cisplatin, 100 mg/m², plus cyclophosphamide, 1,000 mg/m², every 21 to 35 days for three cycles.

Gallion et al (1989) reported on 50 patients with presumed stage I ovarian cancer treated with oral melphalan as adjuvant therapy. Patients were not surgically staged, with only 19 of the 50 patients operated on at the author's institution. Thirty-six patients underwent omentectomy, only five had paraaortic lymph node biopsy, apparently none had pelvic lymph node resection, and the number who underwent cytologic peritoneal washings was not stated. The authors concluded that the actuarial survival rate of 94% at 5 years indicates the efficacy of adjuvant melphalan. However, 36 of the 50 patients (72%) had stage IA or IB, grade 1 or 2 disease. Based on the randomized trial (protocol 7601) of the OCSG/GOG, the 5-year survival rate is 90% by observation alone, and these patients do not require adjuvant therapy. Of the remaining 14 stage I patients (12 stage IC and 2 stage IG3), the number is too small to draw any definitive conclusions.

***Cisplatin-Based Chemotherapy*** In a 1989 update of their 1987 study, Chiara and colleagues reported on 25 patients with stage I disease (completely surgically staged IAii, IBii, IA, BG3, and IC) treated with six courses of cisplatin (50 mg/m²) and cyclophosphamide (600 mg/m²). The disease-free survival rate was only 77% at 79 months (Fig. 14-2). Wils (1989) reported on a small

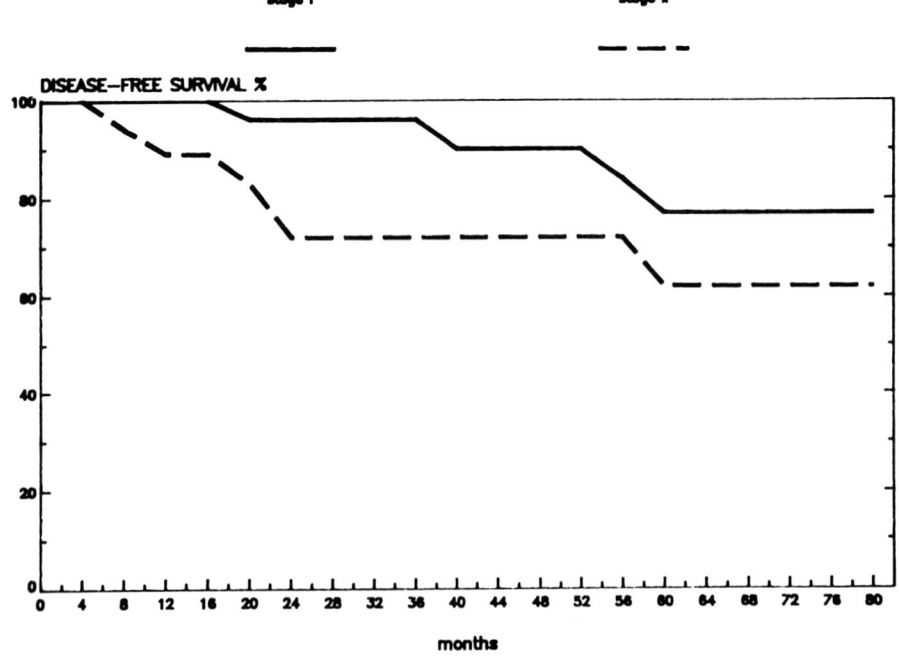

STAGE I—II OVARIAN CANCER: ADJUVANT CT

FIGURE 14-2 Disease-free survival in patients with stage I or II ovarian cancer treated with adjuvant cisplatin and cyclophosphamide. (From Chiara S, et al: Cisplatin and cyclophosphamide in early epithelial ovarian carcinoma. *Chemotherapie* 6:380, 1987.)

series of eight patients with stage IC disease not surgically staged with a median followup of 5 years. There was one relapse, and the disease-free survival rate was 87.5%.

In contrast to the report by Chiara et al, Piver and coauthors (1989) reported on 30 stage I patients, 47% of whom were not completely surgically staged, 60% of whom were considered stage IC, and 30% of whom had grade 3 tumors. These patients were treated with 6 months of adjuvant induction; weekly cisplatin (x4); and monthly cisplatin, doxorubicin, and cyclophosphamide (x5). Twenty-nine patients (97%) remain alive with no evidence of disease and 28 (93%) are progression-free with normal CA 125 levels after a median followup of 4 years (25 to 68 months).

Notwithstanding the excellent 93% disease-free survival rate with cisplatin-based chemotherapy in the latter study, longer followup is required, especially in patients with stage IAii, IBii, IA, BG3, and IC disease who were not surgically staged.

## CYTOREDUCTIVE SURGERY

By definition, cytoreductive or debulking surgery involves maximum tumor resection to enhance the likelihood of response to postoperative adjuvant treatment, primarily systemic chemotherapy. Griffiths and Fuller (1978) reported one of the first and most compelling studies on the benefit of cytoreductive surgery. They demonstrated a 40-month survival rate of about 30% in patients with stage III or IV ovarian cancer with postoperative tumor nodules measuring less than 1.5 cm at initial presentation. This compared to a similar survival rate of 30% at 40 months for those patients who had undergone cytoreductive surgery that resulted in residual tumor of less than 1.5 cm. In sharp contrast, no patients survived 40 months with residual disease greater than 1.5 cm after cytoreductive surgery (Fig. 14-3).

Therefore, it appears that it is not the percentage of the tumor removed, but the size of tumor at initial presentation or residual tumor (< 1.5 cm) after cytoreductive surgery that is the significant factor in improved survival. Of special importance is that this report was completed before the discovery of the effectiveness of cisplatin chemotherapy in epithelial ovarian cancer.

Models to explain the benefit of maximum cytoreductive surgery include resection of a preexisting resistant subclone (Skipper et al, 1978) and single random mutation (Goldie and Coldman, 1979). In the Skipper model, the presumption is that sensitive and resistant tumor cell populations are present at the initiation of chemotherapy, and resection may therefore remove a significant number of *denovo* resistant populations. The Goldie and Coldman model assumes an initially sensitive population of tumor cells with subsequent mutation causing treatment resistance to chemotherapy.

Notwithstanding the theoretical models for the benefit of cytoreductive surgery, clinical studies now confirm that response and survival rates are significantly better in patients with small tumor burdens prior to chemotherapy compared with those who have large re

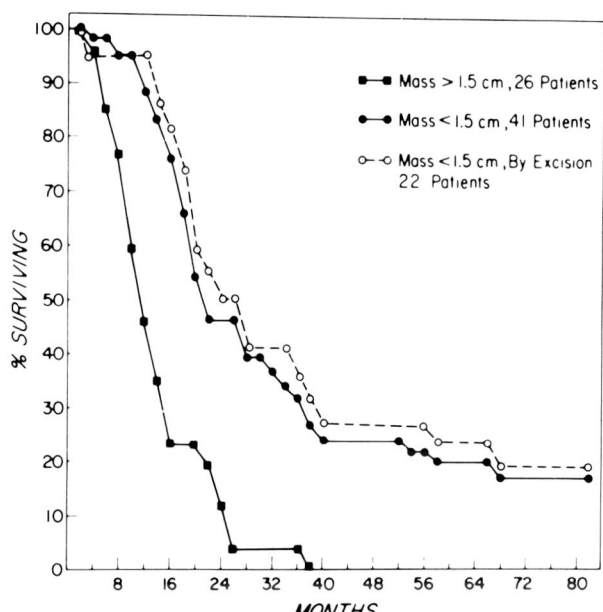

**FIGURE 14-3** Improved survival in patients with small residual metastatic ovarian carcinoma compared with those with larger disease. (From Griffiths CT, Fuller AF: Intensive surgical and chemotherapeutic management of advanced ovarian cancer. *Surg Clin N Amer* 58:131, 1978.)

sidual disease. This fact is clearly demonstrated in the long-term study by Wharton and colleagues (1984) of 395 patients with stage III and IV ovarian cancer treated with chemotherapy. Forty percent of the patients with less than or equal to 2 cm residual disease survived 4 years compared with only 14% of those with greater than 2 cm residual disease (p = 0.001). Moreover, patients with less than 2 cm residual disease after cytoreductive surgery have about a 40 to 50% chance of achieving complete remission with combination chemotherapy compared with less than 15% for those with larger disease.

However, in 10 large series of stage III and IV ovarian cancer patients, the median percentage of patients entered into these chemotherapy protocols with residual disease less than or equal to 2 cm was only 30% (range 18 to 43%) (Ehrlich et al, 1983; Louie et al, 1986; Williams et al, 1985; Wharton et al, 1984; Edwards et al, 1983; Vogl et al, 1983; Carmio-Pereira et al, 1981; Decker et al, 1982; Neijt et al, 1984; Steiner et al, 1985).

It is clear that many more patients with advanced ovarian cancer can undergo resection to achieve an optimal tumor size (≤ 2 cm) prior to chemotherapy—even those considered "inoperable"—prior to referral to a tertiary center. Piver and Baker (1986) conducted a prospective clinical trial to determine what percentage of patients with stage III and IV ovarian cancer referred to tertiary medical centers could undergo optimal cytoreduction. Of 50 consecutive patients, optimal cytoreduction was achieved in 76%, and in 77% of 18 patients referred as "inoperable." To achieve these results, six major operations were performed, including bilateral salpingo-oophorectomy (100%), hysterectomy (98%), omental resection (86%), peritoneal tumor re section (40%), intestinal resection (36%), and gastro-colic ligament resection (16%).

In a similar report, Hacker and colleagues (1983) were able to achieve optimal cytoreduction (≤ 1.5 cm) in 66% of patients (31/77); 12% required intestinal resection and 3.2% required resection of the lower urinary tract. Of importance, although 14 patients were referred as "inoperable," these authors were able to achieve optimal cytoreduction in 71%.

Even with most tertiary centers capable of performing cytoreductive surgery in a high percentage of patients, the long-term disease-free survival rate—although higher than it had been prior to the era of cytoreductive surgery and cisplatin-based chemotherapy—is not what was expected from these therapies. Piver et al (1988b) reported on aggressive cytoreductive surgery in a group of 40 consecutive patients with stage III and IV ovarian cancer in which 87% were successfully cytoreduced to less than 2 cm before starting cisplatin, doxorubicin, and cyclophosphamide chemotherapy; however, only 30% of the patients achieved complete remission following chemotherapy despite the high rate of optimal cytoreduction. Moreover, while the estimated 3-year survival was 62%, the 3-year progression-free survival turned out to be only 29%, indicating that only a minority of patients would be cured even with successful cytoreductive surgery and cisplatin-based chemotherapy.

Since, in most nontertiary centers, a significant number of patients will not undergo cytoreductive surgery, Lawton et al (1989) evaluated the role of cytoreductive cisplatin-based combination chemotherapy followed by secondary cytoreductive surgery. Patients were treated with induction chemotherapy with reoperation at a median interval of 12.7 weeks. Of the 28 women who underwent reoperation, 16 (57%) had no macroscopic residual disease, 5 (18%) had less than 1 cm residual disease, 4 (14%) had less than 2 cm residual disease, and 3 (11%) had more extensive residual disease. However, as the authors point out, other factors may have been at work: "What proportion of our patient population was truly inoperable, as opposed to inoperable because of lesser surgical skills or diligence, is unknown. Indeed, the fact that omentectomy and/or hysterectomy was the most common procedure undertaken at the time of intervention surgery suggests that, in at least a proportion of our patients, optimal debulking surgery might have been performed at primary laparotomy."

Lawton's group did not evaluate the effect on survival of cytoreductive combination chemotherapy followed by secondary cytoreductive surgery. However, Neijt et al (1984) conducted a similar study in 47 patients on the effect of cytoreductive cisplatin-based chemotherapy for "unresectable" tumors followed by early secondary cytoreductive surgery. Although secondary cytoreductive surgery was successful in 63% of these patients, so that only residual masses of less than 1 cm remained, survival was not improved compared with survival among patients in whom secondary cytoreductive surgery was unsuccessful. Even when secondary surgical cytoreduction was successful, the survival rate was inferior to rates among those successfully cytoreduced at the time of initial diagnosis.

Clearly, optimal cytoreductive surgery is possible initially in most patients treated at tertiary medical centers. However, despite optimal surgery and cisplatin-based chemotherapy, the proportion of patients who will be cured will remain low, and secondary cytoreductive surgery following cytoreductive chemotherapy offers little benefit.

## SINGLE-AGENT CHEMOTHERAPY

Almost four decades ago, Seligman et al (1952) reported the first successful use of chemotherapy for palliation of advanced ovarian cancer, using the alkylating agent 2-chloro-2-hydroxydiethyl sulfide (hemisulfur) to control ascites in seven of 10 patients. Over the next 30 years, chemotherapy with alkylating agents, primarily phenylalanine mustard (melphalan), superseded radiation therapy as the most common adjuvant to surgery. It proved to be curative in a small percentage of patients with advanced disease and, when combined with other chemotherapeutic agents, resulted in higher response rates than when used alone.

Samuels et al (1962) reported "objective" responses to single-agent melphalan in six of seven women with advanced ovarian cancer treated at M.D. Anderson Hospital and Tumor Institute (MDAH) between 1956 and 1960. By 1963, these researchers had treated 93 patients with advanced ovarian adenocarcinoma with melphalan and reported a partial response (50% or more reduction in tumor size) in 51 (54.8%) (Burns et al, 1963).

At about the same time as the effectiveness of melphalan for palliation in advanced ovarian cancer was being reported, researchers were reporting encouraging results using three other alkylating agents. Masterson and Nelson (1965) reported a response rate of 50% in 280 patients treated with chlorambucil. In a study by Wallach and colleagues (1965), the response rate to treatment with triethylene triphosphoramide (thio-TEPA) in 144 patients was 64%, while Decker et al (1967) reported a response rate of 37% to cyclophosphamide.

The realization that alkylating agent therapy may be curative came in a 1966 report from MDAH, in which Rutledge and Burns reported that 13 patients treated with melphalan "had such unusually good responses that laparotomy was performed even to determine if an inoperable tumor had become removable or to evaluate the need for additional therapy. In each of the 13 patients, no tumor was found and chemotherapy was discontinued." Melphalan was discontinued in the 13 patients, and only two had recurrence at the time of the report. This report indicated the apparent cure of nonresectable malignancy by chemotherapy and, until recently, established melphalan as the treatment of choice for women with stage III and IV ovarian cancer. Their series was updated through the end of 1969, when they reported a 47% response rate to melphalan among 494 patients with advanced ovarian cancer (Smith and Rutledge, 1970) and a 5-year survival rate of 9% (Smith et al, 1972).

Melphalan replaced whole abdominal radiation for advanced ovarian cancer at most centers in 1975, following the MDAH report of a randomized clinical trial comparing melphalan with whole abdominal radiation. Although the survival rates reported for these two modalities were not significantly different, the morbidity associated with whole abdominal radiation was significantly greater than that for melphalan, leading many oncologists to abandon whole abdominal radiation based on this single report (Smith et al, 1975).

Single-agent melphalan was "replaced" by combination chemotherapy at most institutions following a National Cancer Institute report of a randomized clinical trial comparing melphalan to hexa-CAF (hexamethylmelamine, cyclophosphamide, methotrexate, and 5-fluorouracil). Young et al (1978) documented an overall response rate of 75% (30/40) and a complete response rate of 33% for hexa-CAF compared with rates of 54% and 16%, respectively, for melphalan alone.

Therefore, beginning in 1952, state-of-the-art adjuvant treatment for ovarian cancer progressed from single-agent alkylating agent chemotherapy for palliation of advanced disease to the demonstration that this chemotherapy could be curative in a small percentage of cases and the subsequent use of melphalan alone to replace whole abdominal radiation as the adjuvant treatment of choice, and finally to combination chemotherapy replacing the use of a single alkylating agent.

In 1976, single-agent chemotherapy continued to evolve with the seminal observation by Wiltshaw and Kroner that one of four patients responded to cisplatin as second-line chemotherapy after failing to respond to alkylating agent chemotherapy. By the 1980s, cisplatin-based chemotherapy had become one of the most widely used forms of adjuvant treatment for advanced ovarian cancer.

Other agents currently in use as adjuvant therapy for advanced ovarian cancer include doxorubicin, hexamethylmelamine, 5-fluorouracil, methotrexate, ifosfamide, prednimustin, taxol, carboplatin, mitomycin C, iproplatin, etoposide (VP16-213), mitoxantrone, hormones, and biologicals.

***Cisplatin*** Cisplatin (cis-diamminedichloroplatinum II) is a heavy metal that crosslinks strands of DNA in much the same way as the alkylating agents. Larger doses of cisplatin administered more frequently result in a statistically significant increase in objective response and median survival rates (Levin and Hryniuk, 1987).

The major dose-limiting toxicities of cisplatin are neurotoxicity and nephrotoxicity. Nephrotoxicity can usually be avoided by intense hydration. Litterst (1981) prevented renal toxicity in experimental animals by infusing cisplatin in 4% sodium chloride. Ozols et al (1985) reported the lack of significant nephrotoxicity using high-dose cisplatin (200 mg/m$^2$ over 5 days) in hyertonic saline in 19 patients with refractory ovarian cancer, 17 of whom did not respond to low-dose cisplatin; six (32%) responded. Systemic sodium thiosulfate reportedly helps prevent the nephrotoxicity seen with high-dose cisplatin (Pfeifle et al, 1985). Although cumulative dose-related peripheral sensory neuropathy now most often prohibits the continued use of cisplatin,

this problem may be alleviated somewhat by administering S-2, 3-aminopropylamino-ethylphosporothioic acid (WR-2721) with cisplatin, which has been reported to decrease the incidence of neuropathy significantly (Mollman et al, 1988).

***Doxorubicin (Adriamycin)*** Doxorubicin, an antitumor antibiotic, prevents DNA-dependent RNA synthesis (DiMarco et al, 1971). In 1975, DePalo et al reported that four of six patients responded to doxorubicin after failure to respond to melphalan, suggesting that non-alkylating agents could be used in sequence or in combination with standard alkylating agents. In the most recent report of long-term survival among patients treated with doxorubicin and melphalan, the Swedish Cooperative Ovarian Cancer Study Group reported on 148 patients with suboptimal stage III (palpable residual disease exceeding 10 cm after surgery) and stage IV disease who were randomized to melphalan alone or combined with doxorubicin. The authors reported statistically significant increases in response rate, median duration of response, median survival, complete response, and disease-free survival at 5 years (13.7% vs 4%) for the combination—an excellent 5-year survival rate for such large tumors (Trope, 1987).

***Hexamethylmelamine*** This drug, which has not been approved by the Food and Drug Administration (FDA), is structurally similar to the alkylating agent triethylenemelamine. Hexamethylmelamine is a substituted melamine derived from cyanuric chloride (Kiser et al, 1951). Wharton et al (1979) and Smith and Rutledge (1975) reported response rates of 31.8% and 46%, respectively, using hexamethylmelamine as first-line therapy in advanced ovarian cancer. Foster and coauthors (1986) reviewed all the trials using hexamethylmelamine in ovarian cancer and concluded that *"the questions regarding the role of hexamethylmelamine in the treatment of ovarian cancer remain unanswered."* However, Edmonson and colleagues (1988) and Bruckner and coauthors (1987) suggest that the addition of hexamethylmelamine to standard cisplatin-based combination chemotherapy improves long-term survival over cisplatin regimens without hexamethylmelamine.

***5-Fluorouracil*** The antimetabolite 5-fluorouracil (5-FU) is a fluorinated pyrimidine that inhibits the formation of thymidine. In a trial of 100 patients with advanced ovarian cancer randomized to hexamethylmelamine, 5-FU, or melphalan as first-line therapy, Smith and Rutledge (1975) reported response rates of 17% to 5-FU, 30% to melphalan, and 46% to hexamethylmelamine.

***Methotrexate*** Methotrexate, a folic acid antagonist, blocks the synthesis of thymidine and therefore DNA synthesis. Low-dose methotrexate has demonstrated minimal activity in advanced ovarian cancer (Greenspan and Bruckner, 1975). In addition, the use of high-dose methotrexate with citrovorum rescue factor was not associated with significant responses, with rates of 18% (Barlow and Piver, 1976) and 13% (Parker, 1979) reported.

**Ifosfamide** This alkylating agent is structurally related to cyclophosphamide. Although ifosfamide is active in the treatment of advanced ovarian cancer, there is no evidence that it is superior to other single alkylating agents (Yazigi et al, 1984). Hemorrhagic cystitis was originally the limiting factor precluding the use of ifosfamide, until the development of systemic thioluroprotector which prevents hemorrhagic cystitis. Ifosfamide was found to be effective as second-line therapy in a GOG study, which reported a 22% response rate among 37 patients previously treated with cisplatin (Sutton et al, 1989*a*).

**Prednimustin** Prednimustin, not yet approved by the FDA, is a chemical ester of prednisolone and chlorambucil. Leonard et al (1989) reported a pathologically confirmed response rate to the combination of hexamethylmelamine, 5-FU, cisplatin, and prednimustin, indicating that this compound shows significant activity.

**Taxol** A non-FDA approved drug, taxol is derived from a diterpene plant product isolated from the western yew *Taxus brevifolia*. The mechanism of action is antimicrotubule of the mitotic spindle, somewhat similar to that of vincristine and vinblastine. Of 40 evaluable patients receiving taxol as salvage therapy, 12 patients (30%) responded for periods lasting from 3 to 15 months, indicating significant activity for this agent (McGuire et al, 1989).

**Carboplatin** Carboplatin (cis-diammine-1,1-cyclobutane-dicaroxyl-platinum II), a second generation platinum analogue, is associated with significantly less neurotoxicity and nephrotoxicity than cisplatin. However, carboplatin causes significantly more myelosuppression and may therefore compromise optimal dosing when combined with other myelosuppressive agents. Moreover, in a carefully conducted study by Sleijfer et al (1989), carboplatin caused considerable loss of renal function. Adams et al (1989) conducted a randomized trial comparing cisplatin and carboplatin as first-line single-agent chemotherapy and found no significant difference in rates of response to these two platinum analogues, which appear to be cross-resistant. Third-generation platinum complexes, which lack cross-resistance with cisplatin, have recently been synthesized (Bitha et al, 1989).

**Mitomycin-C** Mitomycin-C is an antitumor antibiotic with a mechanism of action similar to that of alkylating agents. A 23% response rate has been reported in recurrent ovarian cancer (Creech et al, 1985).

**Iproplatin** Iproplatin (cis-dichloro-trans-dihydroxy-bis-isopropylamime platinum [CHIP]), a platinum analogue, is significantly less nephrotoxic than cisplatin and has been shown to be active in patients with ovarian cancer. Sessa (1986) reported a 27% (17/64) response rate in patients previously treated with cisplatin. In a randomized trial of cisplatin, carboplatin, and CHIP, each used in combination with cyclophosphamide, there were no significant differences in response, duration of response, or survival (Anderson et al, 1988).

**Etoposide (VP16-213)** Etoposide is a synthetic conjugate of podophyllotoxin that causes metaphase arrest and prevents cells from entering mitosis. Etoposide shows minimal activity when given as a single agent in advanced ovarian cancer, with the GOG reporting a response rate of only 8% among 24 previously treated patients (Slayton et al, 1979). In spite of this finding and the reported lack of in vitro synergy between etoposide and cisplatin (Tsai et al, 1989), the combination of these two drugs given intravenously and intraperitoneally is being evaluated in patients with advanced ovarian cancer (Reichman et al, 1989).

**Mitoxantrone** Mitoxantrone, an anthracenedione derivative, demonstrated only minimal activity in one study—with a response rate of 3% in 37 patients—when used as second-line chemotherapy (Coleman et al, 1989). However, Lawton et al (1986) reported a response rate of 25% in 40 evaluable patients with advanced ovarian cancer, only four of whom had not been treated previously. Because of its significant lack of vesicant activity and high level of tissue binding, mitoxantrone continues to be evaluated intraperitoneally in advanced ovarian cancer (Alberts et al, 1988*b*).

**Progestational Agents** Second-line hormonal therapy with a number of agents (17-alpha-hydroxyprogesterone-17-N-caproate, 17-alpha-hydroxyl-19-19 norprogesterone-17-N-caproate, 17-alpha-hydroxyl-6-methylprogesterone acetate, 6-dehydro-6-17-alpha-dimethylprogesterone, and megestrol acetate) has been reported in advanced ovarian cancer. Thigpen (1985) documented a response rate of only 12% in 176 patients treated with one of these progestational agents.

**Tamoxifen** This antiestrogen has been used for patients with refractory ovarian cancer. In the largest series on tamoxifen to date, Beecham et al (1988) observed a complete response rate of 9.5% (10/105) and a partial response rate of 7.6% (8/105) in patients with advanced ovarian cancer. However, Osborne et al (1988), after reporting disease progression in 98% of 51 patients treated with tamoxifen as second-line therapy, concluded that "evidence of substantial activity of tamoxifen in ovarian cancer has previously been overstated and . . . the true activity of this treatment is minimal."

**Gonadotropin-Releasing Hormone Analogue (Leuprolide Acetate)** Bruckner and Motwani (1989) reported therapeutic responses to this form of hormonal therapy in five patients with advanced ovarian cancer. Four of these patients had not responded to intensive chemotherapy, which included alkylating agents, cisplatin, and doxorubicin. Kavanagh et al (1989) reported a response rate of 17% in 18 ovarian cancer patients treated with leuprolide acetate as salvage therapy. When Parmar et al (1988) evaluated the gonadotropin-releasing hormone agonist D-Trp-6-LH-RH (decapeptyl), the overall response rate was 15% in 41 patients.

**Alpha- and Gamma-Interferons** Abdulhay et al (1984) evaluated treatment with the biologic response modifier alpha-interferon and reported a response rate of 19%

in 21 patients. Welander et al (1986) reported a response rate of 29% in 14 patients treated with gamma-interferon.

***Interleukin-2 (IL-2)*** Although IL-2 is active in renal cell cancer and melanoma, no responses to this agent were noted among nine women with ovarian epithelial cancer (Lotze et al, 1979, 1986; Chapman et al, 1988).

***Monoclonal Antibodies*** Monoclonal antibodies are thought to be potentially useful when coupled with a toxic material. Immunoconjugates have been formed by coupling monoclonal antibodies to radioisotopes, toxins, and cytotoxic drugs. Stewart et al (1989) reported 28 patients treated with $^{131}$I conjugated to HMFG-1, HMFG-2, or HI7E2 with an objective response rate of only 18%. Epenetos et al (1987) administered $^{131}$I-labeled monoclonal antibodies intraperitoneally to 15 patients with small-volume disease and reported a response rate of 56% (9).

## FIRST- AND SECOND-LINE CHEMOTHERAPY FOR STAGE III AND IV OVARIAN ADENOCARCINOMA

### First-Line Cisplatin-Based Combination Chemotherapy

Experiments by Rosenberg et al (1965) to evaluate bacterial replication in electrical fields demonstrated that the electric current between platinum and electrodes prevented the growth of *Escherichia coli* and that the platinum salt, not the electrical current, was responsible for this growth inhibition. In 1972, the first phase I clinical trials were initiated in the United States using cis-diamminedichloroplatinum II (cisplatin)—the most active platinum compound tested. At the same time, the National Institutes of Health of the United States supplied cisplatin to Wiltshaw and Carr (1974) of the United Kingdom for the first clinical trials in advanced ovarian cancer. These authors reported responses in seven (28%) of the first 25 patients treated between January, 1972, and March, 1973, all of whom had recurrent ovarian cancer after previous chemotherapy. This initial observation was updated in 1976 by Wiltshaw and Kroner who reported that nine (26.5%) of 34 patients with advanced ovarian cancer responded to cisplatin as second-line chemotherapy.

Based on the report by Wiltshaw and Kroner (1976) on the effectiveness of cisplatin as second-line chemotherapy and the 80% response rate to doxorubicin and cyclophosphamide reported by Lloyd et al (1976), researchers at the University of Indiana evaluated the three-drug combination of cisplatin, doxorubicin (Adriamycin) and cyclophosphamide (PAC) as first-line chemotherapy in advanced stage III and IV ovarian cancer. They reported a complete response rate of 37% in 35 evaluable patients and an overall response rate of 68.5% (Ehrlich et al, 1979). In 1983, this series was updated to a total of 56 patients and the response rate increased to 82% (Ehrlich et al, 1983). Hainsworth added hexamethylmelamine to the PAC regimen in 1988

and reported a response rate of 96% in 55 patients with advanced ovarian cancer.

Because so few other drugs were active against ovarian cancer, some researchers began evaluating the individual components of the PAC regimen (e.g., adding doxorubicin and/or cyclophosphamide to cisplatin), while others evaluated the addition of hexamethylmelamine to the PAC combination. In two studies in Italy comparing cisplatin and cyclophosphamide (PC) to PAC no significant increase in survival or progression-free survival was noted for either of the two treatments (Sessa, 1986; Conte et al, 1986). In both studies, most patients had suboptimal residual disease (> 2 cm) prior to receiving chemotherapy. The Danish Ovarian Cancer Group also found no difference in median survival between PC (21 months) and PAC (26 months) in a prospective, randomized clinical trial of 267 patients with stage III and IV ovarian cancer (Bertelsen et al, 1987). In another study comparing PC and PAC that included only stage III patients with less than or equal to 1 cm residual disease, Omura et al (1989) reported no significant difference in progression-free survival with PC (median-22.7 months) or PAC (median-24.6 months).

Each of these four studies concluded that adding doxorubicin to PC did not increase survival or progression-free survival for patients with advanced ovarian cancer. Based on these and other studies, PC became the standard therapy.

The same conclusion was reached in studies comparing PC to PAC plus hexamethylmelamine. Results of a clinical trial conducted in The Netherlands showed no difference in overall response, complete response, and survival rates in patients treated with PC and those treated with PAC plus hexamethylmelamine (Neijt et al, 1987). In a similar study, Edmonson and colleagues (1985) evaluated PC and PAC plus hexamethylmelamine and reported no difference between the two regimens in terms of responses, progression-free survival, or overall survival rates.

In a randomized clinical trial of 531 patients with advanced ovarian cancer treated with cisplatin alone (P), PC, or PAC, Italian researchers reported complete surgical response rates of 26% for PAC and 21% for PC and P, and no difference in survival or disease-free survival rates among the three arms, indicating that the addition of doxorubicin and/or cyclophosphamide to cisplatin may not increase the potential cure rate in this disease (Gruppo Interegionale Cooperativo Oncologico Ginecologia, 1987).

The exceptionally high response rates reported for PAC (82%) and PAC plus hexamethylmelamine (96%) are probably two to three times higher than the most accurate response rates reported for melphalan in the three clinical trials conducted by the GOG. Of the 193 patients in those studies, 16% showed complete responses and 17% showed partial responses, for an overall response rate of 33% (Thigpen et al, 1987). Given the high response rates to cisplatin-based chemotherapy (82 to 96%) compared with melphalan (33%) plus the value of debulking surgery demonstrated by Griffiths et al (1979), it was predicted almost a priori that the 5-year survival and disease-free survival rates would be significantly higher than, for example, the 9% survival rate reported by Smith et al (1972) in 494 patients with stage III disease treated with melphalan before the advent of aggressive debulking surgery. In that report, none of the patients who failed to respond to melphalan survived for 5 years compared with 16% of those who responded.

In the 1988 Hainsworth study of PAC plus hexamethylmelamine, in which 36% of the patients had optimal residual disease prior to chemotherapy, the 5-year progression-free survival rate was only 18% (10). The authors did not include three patients who survived for 45, 75, and 77 months and died of intercurrent disease without evidence of recurrent cancer, giving an overall 5-year survival rate of approximately 23% (13) (Table 14-6). Sutton et al (1989c) updated the 1983 study by Ehrlich of 56 patients in which only 30% of the patients were optimally debulked and the total cumulative dose of cisplatin was only 300 mg/m$^2$; they reported a 5-year survival rate of 23% (13) and the 5-year progression-free survival rate of 18%. This is the only study of cisplatin-based chemotherapy with a 10-year followup, and 9% of the patients are alive and 7% are alive with no evidence of disease.

At the National Cancer Institute, Louie et al (1986) used cisplatin, cyclophosphamide, hexamethylmelamine, and 5-fluorouracil (CHEX-UP) in a study of 62 patients, 24% of whom were optimally debulked, and reported a 5-year survival rate of 15% but only an 8% 5-year disease-free survival rate. In 1988, Piver reported a study of 40 patients with advanced ovarian cancer stages III and IV, a high percentage (87%) of whom were optimally debulked and were to receive a total of 820 mg/m$^2$ of cisplatin over a 12-month period. The protocol consisted of weekly induction cisplatin (P) followed by monthly PAC. The 5-year survival rate was 20% (8), but the 5-year disease-free survival rate was only 12.5% (5) (Piver, 1990).

In the reports by Hainsworth et al (1988), Sutton et al (1989c) and Louie et al (1986) of patients with limited residual disease prior to chemotherapy, survival was improved significantly. In the Hainsworth study, the median survival was 72 months compared with only 13 months for patients with extensive residual disease (p < 0.001). Sutton's group (1989c) reported similar results from a study in which patients with limited resid-

ual disease had statistically significant (p < 0.02) improved median progression-free survival and survival intervals (33.3 and 44.5 months, respectively) compared with patients who had suboptimal residual disease (16.4 and 22.5 months, respectively). Louie and associates reported an improved median survival of 23.8 months for a subset of patients with less than 2 cm residual disease compared with 15 months for those with more than 2 cm residual disease.

Thus, debulking surgery to limit residual disease to optimal levels prolongs survival compared with survival in patients with suboptimal residual disease. In 11 prospective studies using melphalan or PAC as first-line chemotherapy for stage III and IV ovarian cancer, the median survival with PAC (25 months) was significantly higher than with melphalan (14 months) (Levin and Hryniuk, 1987). However, it appears that debulking surgery and cisplatin-based chemotherapy will not result in more patients with advanced ovarian cancer being cured.

## Carboplatin

In response to the dose-limiting nephrotoxicity and neurotoxicity associated with cisplatin, second- and third-generation platinum compounds such as carboplatin have been developed. Carboplatin is significantly less neurotoxic, nephrotoxic and emetogenic than cisplatin; however, this compound is associated with severe thrombocytopenia. Because of its lack of nephrotoxicity, carboplatin can be administered on an outpatient basis without pre- or posthydration.

Results of a recent multicenter, randomized clinical trial comparing carboplatin (400 mg/m$^2$) and cisplatin (100 mg/m$^2$) in 173 previously untreated patients with stage III and IV advanced ovarian cancer demonstrated that these two compounds were of almost equal potential. The overall pathologic response and complete pathologic response rates were 57.3% and 26.8%, respectively, for carboplatin and 71.6% and 24.7% for cisplatin. With only a short followup, there was no statistically significant difference between the two therapies in terms of survival and progression-free survival (Mangioni et al, 1989). However, the authors cautioned that, because the significant myelosuppression associated with carboplatin required de-escalation of doses,

---

TABLE 14-6  Five-Year Survival With Cisplatin-Based Chemotherapy in Stage III and IV Ovarian Cancer

| Authors: | Sutton et al (1989c) | Louie et al (1986) | Hainsworth et al (1988) | Piver et al (1988b, 1990) |
|---|---|---|---|---|
| Regimen | PAC | CHEX-UP | H-PAC | P-PAC |
| Patients | 56 | 62 | 55 | 40 |
| Optimal residual disease | 30.0%* | 24.0%† | 36.0%† | 87.0%† |
| 5-year survival | 23.0% (13) | 15.0% (9) | 23.0% (13) | 20.0% (8) |
| 5-year progression free survival | 18.0% (10) | 8.0% (5) | 18.0% (10) 23.0% (13)‡ | 12.5% (5) |

\* = < 3 cm stage III
† = < 2 cm
‡ = three additional patients survived 45, 77, and 75 months, respectively, but died of intercurrent diseases with no evidence of recurrent ovarian cancer.
CHEX-UP = cisplatin, cytoxan, cyclophosphamide, hexamethylmelamine, and 5-fluorouracil; PAC = cisplatin, Adriamycin (doxorubicin), and cyclophosphamide; H-PAC = PAC plus hexamethylmelamine; P-PAC = PAC preceded by cisplatin (P).

carboplatin has the potential to adversely affect end results and decrease long-term progression-free survival and survival rates.

In a study of 103 previously untreated women with stage III and IV ovarian cancer who were randomized to either cyclophosphamide (1 g/m$^2$) plus cisplatin (60 mg/m$^2$) or carboplatin (150 mg/m$^2$) plus cyclophosphamide (1 g), progression-free survival was superior for the patients treated with cisplatin and cyclophosphamide (p = 0.005) (Edmonson et al, 1989). Owing to the clear superiority of this regimen, the clinical trial was aborted, and patients were encouraged to cross over to therapy with cisplatin and cyclophosphamide. Two other recent studies with short followup periods—one comparing carboplatin, doxorubicin, and cyclophosphamide with cisplatin, doxorubicin, and cyclophosphamide (ten Bokkel Huinink et al, 1988) and the other comparing carboplatin plus cyclophosphamide with cyclophosphamide plus cisplatin (Alberts et al, 1989)—demonstrated no difference in response rates.

According to McGuire and Abeloff (1989), "Carboplatin is clearly an important new drug in the armamentarium for epithelial ovarian cancer. Whether it will totally supplant cisplatin or serve as an alternative to cisplatin in specific patient populations requires longer followup of current studies."

Future clinical trials of carboplatin will add colony-stimulating factor to overcome the severe myelosuppression, and carboplatin may ultimately replace cisplatin as first-line chemotherapy in this disease.

## Second-Line Chemotherapy

For patients who respond to cisplatin but then suffer recurrence, the rate of response to retreatment with cisplatin-based chemotherapy is high. Gershenson et al (1989) reported a 100% overall response rate (nine complete and nine partial responses) in 18 patients who had responded to initial cisplatin-based chemotherapy and were retreated with the same after recurrence.

In a phase II clinical trial following progression of disease despite cisplatin combination chemotherapy, Alberts et al (1989a) reported a 40% response rate among 25 evaluable patients who received mitomycin-C and 5-FU as second-line chemotherapy. Similarly, Mulder et al (1989) reported six complete responses (five pathologically confirmed) in 11 patients with persistent ovarian cancer treated with high-dose cyclophosphamide and etoposide followed by autologous bone marrow transplantation. Of note, only patients with less than or equal to 2 cm residual disease responded.

Redman et al (1989) used epidoxorubicin and mitomycin-C in 33 evaluable patients, 32 of whom had previously received cisplatin, and reported complete or partial responses in 10 (30%). Sutton et al (1989a) used ifosfamide to treat 46 patients with advanced ovarian cancer whose disease was refractory or recurrent after cisplatin-containing combination chemotherapy; three (7%) had a complete response and 5 (13%) had a partial response. In 40 evaluable patients, McGuire et al (1989) used taxol as second-line chemotherapy and reported that 12 (30%) responded after progression of disease on cisplatin. Rosen et al (1987) treated 20

evaluable patients with hexamethylmelamine as second-line chemotherapy after they failed to respond to cisplatin-based multiple-agent chemotherapy; five objective responses were reported (four complete, one partial).

No long-term survival has been reported in any of the studies using non-cisplatin-based chemotherapy as second-line treatment, and most responses have been of short duration.

## Intraperitoneal Chemotherapy

Initially, intraperitoneal chemotherapy was used to control malignant ascites. Although there were some dramatic responses, they lasted only a short time. With the development of successful systemic chemotherapy, this modality was abandoned. However, in the early 1980s, researchers began reevaluating a possible role for intraperitoneal administration of cytotoxic agents, based on the rationale that cytotoxic agents with low solubility and high molecular weight clear the peritoneal cavity slowly compared with clearance from the systemic circulation. The low systemic clearance allows the use of higher doses of drugs intraperitoneally than could be given safely systemically.

With the discovery that cisplatin—the most active agent against ovarian cancer—could be administered intraperitoneally at significantly higher doses, using intravenous sodium thiosulfate to protect against nephrotoxicity, researchers were encouraged to apply this modality to patients who did not respond to intravenous cisplatin. Agents that have now been evaluated for safety, pharmacokinetic advantage, and possible effectiveness in ovarian carcinoma when used intraperitoneally include cisplatin, carboplatin, 5-FU, doxorubicin, mitoxantrone, melphalan, mitomycin-C, methotrexate, cytarabine, and etoposide (Markman et al, 1989).

In a prospective study of 31 patients who had previously responded to treatment with first-line intravenous cisplatin, Piver et al (1988c) reported a 26% (8) surgically documented response rate to second-line intraperitoneal cisplatin-based chemotherapy. The responders had stage III ovarian cancer with small residual disease (primarily ≤ 5 mm). Reichman et al (1989) treated 57 evaluable patients with intravenous cisplatin and intraperitoneal etoposide and reported a surgically documented response rate of 40%, with most responders having residual disease of less than 5 mm. Howell et al (1987b) reported on three sequential phase I/II clinical trials of intraperitoneal chemotherapy conducted between 1981 and 1985 that used cisplatin in combination with cytarabine, cytarabine and doxorubicin, or cytarabine and bleomycin. Of the 90 patients who had not responded to previous chemotherapy, 84% had been treated with cisplatin-based chemotherapy. Although response rates were not reported, the median survival for patients with less than 2 cm of residual disease was more than 4 years compared with only 8 months for those patients with more than 2 cm of residual disease. For those patients with small-volume disease (< 2 cm), the 4-year survival rate was 74%.

In retrospect, cisplatin plus cytarabine, bleomycin, and etoposide is probably not the ideal drug combination to use intraperitoneally for ovarian cancer. For example, it is not known whether cytarabine acts synergistically with cisplatin (Howell and Jill, 1985) or whether the low dose of bleomycin (2 units/m$^2$) is effective, since it is not pharmacologic; also, etoposide does not act synergistically with cisplatin (Tsai et al, 1989). Finally, the effect of intraperitoneal chemotherapy on long-term survival has not been established.

## SECOND-LOOK LAPAROTOMY

The concept of a second-look laparotomy to evaluate the status of a patient's cancer was described by Wagensteen et al in 1951 for patients with colon carcinoma. At that time, there was no effective adjuvant treatment, and second-look laparotomy was performed to determine whether colon cancer was present and, if so, whether to repeat resection to prolong survival.

When effective alkylating agent chemotherapy for ovarian cancer was developed in the 1960s (primarily using melphalan), second-look laparotomy was performed to confirm that patients considered clinically to be in complete remission as a result of chemotherapy were disease-free before treatment was discontinued. In the 1970s, when acute nonlymphocytic leukemia was reported to be associated with prolonged treatment with alkylating agent chemotherapy (Reimer et al, 1977), second-look laparotomy to document disease-free status became a preventive measure, and discontinuing treatment became a priority. By the 1980s, cisplatin-based chemotherapy had replaced alkylating agent chemotherapy, but discontinuing the treatment continued to be a priority owing to the significant neurotoxicity and nephrotoxicity associated with this regimen. Second-look laparotomy was performed to monitor disease status and indicate when to discontinue chemotherapy.

Unfortunately, with the more recent reports of a minimum recurrence rate of 50% after negative second-look laparotomy, even after successful treatment with cisplatin-based chemotherapy, this procedure is no longer considered a valuable indicator of when chemotherapy can be discontinued with minimal risk of recurrence. Focus has now shifted to the use of intraperitoneal chromic phosphate ($^{32}$P) (Varia et al, 1988) and whole abdominal radiation (Fuks et al, 1988) to prevent recurrence in patients with negative results on second-look laparotomy. Debate continues regarding the role of secondary cytoreductive surgery in improving survival when tumor is discovered on second-look laparotomy.

By definition, second-look laparotomy is designed to determine whether cancer is still present in patients treated with surgery followed by adjuvant treatment (primarily chemotherapy) who have no clinical or radiologic evidence of disease; it is not applicable to patients undergoing reoperation for persistent disease.

Findings at second-look laparotomy have been defined as follows:

*Negative*—Multiple biopsy samples and peritoneal cytologic washings contain no evidence of malignancy.

*Macroscopically Positive*—Visible disease is documented histologically.

*Microscopically Positive*—No visible disease, but one of the multiple biopsy or peritoneal samples contains evidence of malignancy.

The technique used for second-look laparotomy is similar to that of an initial staging laparotomy, with inspection and/or biopsy of the right leaf of the diaphragm, resection of any residual omentum, peritoneal washing cytology, paraaortic lymphadenectomy, and pelvic lymphadenectomy on the side of the tumor. All previous sites of known residual tumor from the initial surgery as well as all suspicious areas (usually white and granular), including adhesions, which frequently contain small clusters of tumor cells, should be biopsied.

In patients who respond to chemotherapy, there is a significant correlation between the mean percentage of positive biopsies at second-look laparotomy and the sites of known residual cancer after the initial surgery (Phibbs et al, 1983). However, Phibbs found no instance of disease at new sites when sites of previous residual cancer were disease-free.

The renewed controversy over the usefulness of second-look laparotomy is apparent when one considers the following questions raised by Young (1987a):

*Is the procedure required to definitely establish disease recurrence?* CT and/or ultrasound scans of the abdomen and pelvis are of minimal value in detecting occult residual disease at second-look laparotomy. Clarke-Pearson and colleagues (1986) reported that CT scans detected only 7% of tumor nodules less than or equal to 1 cm and only 37% of tumors greater than 1 cm. Murolo et al (1989) reported on 129 patients with stage III and IV ovarian cancer treated with six cycles of cisplatin or carboplatin chemotherapy prior to second-look laparotomy. Of the 94 patients with negative ultrasound scans, only 53 (56%) had no residual disease at second-look laparotomy.

Laparoscopy is a less invasive procedure, but it does not allow total visualization of the pelvis and abdomen and allows no visualization of the retroperitoneal lymph nodes. Piver et al (1980) reported a false-negative rate of 20% for second-look laparoscopy when second-look laparotomy was performed immediately after laparoscopic findings were deemed negative.

Although elevated levels of CA 125 prior to second-look laparotomy are highly predictive of disease, the converse is not true. Jacobs and Bast (1989) reported that 96% (234/243) of patients with elevated CA 125 levels prior to second-look laparotomy had disease. However, of the 336 patients with normal CA 125 levels prior to second-look laparotomy, 156 (46%) had disease. Thus, the overall accuracy of CA 125 in predicting the presence or absence of disease was 67% (390/579).

*Does the procedure either affect or define prognosis?* Most series report similar findings at second-look laparotomy: 40% of the patients have macroscopic disease, 20% have microscopic disease, and 40% have no evidence of disease.

Bertelsen et al (1988) reported on 267 patients with

stage III and IV ovarian cancer treated with cisplatin and cyclophosphamide. On second-look laparotomy in 157 of the patients, 45% had macroscopic residual, 15% had microscopic residual, and 40% had no residual disease. The 3-year survival rate for patients with no residual disease was 74%, 24% for those with microscopic residual disease, 28% for those with less than or equal to 1 cm residual disease, and 17% for those with greater than 1 cm residual disease. Moreover, the results of second-look laparotomy altered prognosis; in 29% of the patients found to have macroscopic residual disease, the tumor was completely resected, and the 3-year survival rate improved to 45%.

Similarly, Lippman et al (1988) reported that patients undergoing optimal resection (less than 2 cm residual mass) at second-look laparotomy had significantly longer survival than those with suboptimal resection ($p < 0.001$) (Fig. 14-4). Recently, Hoskins et al (1989) reported a 5-year survival rate of 62% for patients found to have microscopic disease at second-look laparotomy and a rate of 51% for those whose residual disease was rendered microscopic by cytoreductive surgery at the time of laparotomy. In contrast, for patients left with residual disease, whether less than or greater than 2 cm, the 5-year survival rate was less than 10% ($p = 0.013$).

Lippman (1988) reported that only stages I and II versus stages III and IV ($p = 0.002$) and optimal residual disease ($< 2$ cm) after initial surgery were significantly associated with a negative second-look laparotomy ($p < 0.001$). The 3-year actuarial survival rate was 80.7% for patients with no evidence of disease at second-look laparotomy, 49.1% for those with less than 2 cm residual disease, and 29.1% for those with greater than 2 cm residual disease. Patients undergoing optimal resection to less than 2 cm had a significantly better survival rate than those with greater than 2 cm residual disease ($p < 0.001$).

In the only prospective, randomized trial on the effect of second-look laparotomy on prognosis, Luesley and coauthors (1988) reported a contrary opinion. They treated 146 patients with five courses of cisplatin. Patients were then randomized to second-look laparotomy followed by either chlorambucil or whole abdominal radiation or to chlorambucil with no second-look laparotomy. Over a median followup of 46 months (range = 21 to 51), there was no difference in survival among the three groups. However, several caveats should be applied when one is interpreting these results. First, only 28% (46) of the 146 patients underwent optimal debulking at the time of the initial surgery. In addition, there is no evidence that chlorambucil is an effective consolidating agent after first-line cisplatin in ovarian cancer. Finally, most researchers now agree that whole abdominal radiation consolidation "does not enhance cure in stage III ovarian cancer" (Fuks et al, 1988).

*Does the procedure alter the selection of subsequent therapy?* As pointed out by Fuks, none of the patients with gross residual disease at second-look laparotomy survived 5 years when treated by whole abdominal radiation. The survival rate for patients whose residual disease is completely cytoreduced at second-look lapa-

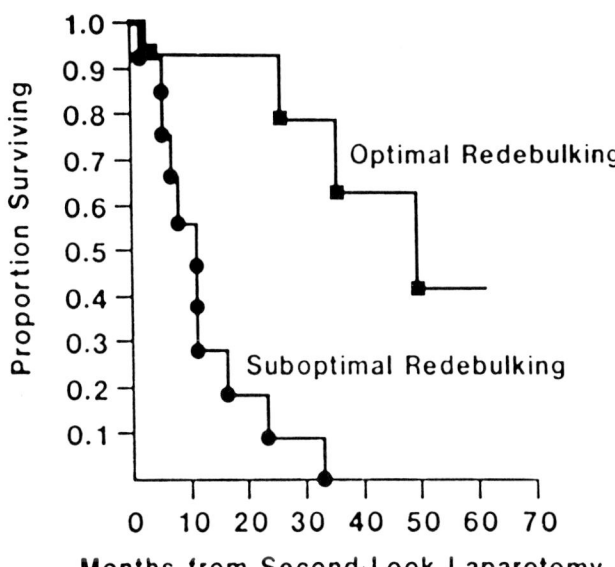

**FIGURE 14-4** Cumulative actuarial survival rates for 27 patients with ovarian cancer who underwent secondary cytoreductive operation for bulky disease ($> 2$ cm). The survival curves comparing 14 patients whose residual tumors had a maximum diameter of $< 2$ cm with 13 patients whose residual tumors were $> 2$ cm differed significantly. ($p = 0.001$). (From Lippman SM, Alberts DS, Slymen DJ, et al: Second-look laparotomy in epithelial ovarian carcinoma. Prognostic factors associated with survival duration. *Cancer* 61:2571, 1988.)

rotomy lies between that reported for patients with residual disease partly resected and that for patients with no residual disease. Of significance, seven of 14 patients with stage III disease and no microscopic residual disease at second-look laparotomy who were treated with whole abdominal radiation died. With this report, second-look laparotomy appears to have a negative effect on the selection of postoperative radiation.

However, one subset of patients with residual disease on second-look laparotomy might be helped by intraperitoneal cisplatin-based chemotherapy. Piver et al (1988c) reported that of 15 patients with stage III ovarian cancer initially who had residual disease (primarily less than or equal to 5 mm) on second-look laparotomy and who had responded to first-line intravenous cisplatin, 8 (53%) responded to second-line intraperitoneal chemotherapy, as documented on third-look laparotomy.

Moreover, in a nonrandomized, retrospective analysis, Varia et al (1988) reported a 4-year survival rate of 89% after second-look laparotomy in patients with no evidence of disease on laparotomy who were treated with intraperitoneal $^{32}$P compared with a rate of 67% for those who did not receive $^{32}$P. Corresponding survival rates were 59% for those treated with $^{32}$P versus 22% for those not treated with $^{32}$P for minimal residual disease ($< 2$ cm) at second-look laparotomy. In a small, similar study, Spencer et al (1989) reported no recurrences among 14 patients treated with $^{32}$P after a negative second-look laparotomy; however, disease recurred in four of 17 patients who were not treated with $^{32}$P ($p = 0.076$).

If these findings can be substantiated by other investigators, perhaps the findings at second-look laparotomy might allow for the effective use of intraperitoneal chemotherapy or $^{32}P$.

*Does the altered therapy change overall survival and survival for a definable and significant subset of patients?* At this time, it appears that survival rates will be improved for those patients who respond to intraperitoneal chemotherapy (Piver et al, 1988c; Howell et al, 1987b). However, longer followup is required. Moreover, patients who are candidates for intraperitoneal chemotherapy (primarily those with ≤ 5 mm residual disease) account for only 15 to 20% of those who come to second-look laparotomy. Furthermore, since 50% of patients with no evidence of disease at second-look laparotomy will have a recurrence, prospective trials are needed, such as the ongoing trial of $^{32}P$. Also, patients who undergo second-look laparotomy with cytoreduction to optimal disease (< 2 cm) seem to have an increased survival compared with those in whom cytoreductive surgery is not successful (Bertelsen et al, 1988; Lippman et al, 1988).

## BORDERLINE OVARIAN TUMORS

About 10 to 15% of all common epithelial ovarian tumors are classified as borderline. They are characterized by an unusual degree of epithelial cell stratification, increased mitotic activity, nuclear abnormalities, atypical cells, and the absence of stromal invasion. Because of the high cure rate associated with these tumors and the lack of histologic evidence of invasion, FIGO has proposed that this intermediate group of ovarian tumors be classified as a separate entity designated "carcinomas of low malignant potential." Similarly, the WHO has labeled this category of tumors "borderline ovarian malignancies."

Borderline ovarian tumors can be serous, mucinous, endometrioid, or clear cell. Of clinical importance is that about 25% of borderline tumors occur in patients under age 40 compared with less than 10% for invasive common epithelial tumors. Also important for younger patients who wish to preserve fertility is the fact that 25 to 40% of serous borderline tumors are bilateral at initial presentation in contrast to only 8% of mucinous borderline tumors.

Borderline serous ovarian carcinomas can be readily distinguished from the more invasive serous tumors by their lack of stromal invasion. However, interpreting stromal invasion in mucinous tumors can be difficult. The confusion about what constitutes borderline mucinous tumors versus invasive mucinous adenocarcinomas led Hart and Norris (1973) to define their own criterion based on the height of the atypical mucinous cells lining the glandular cyst: three layers or less would be borderline and four layers or more would be invasive. Subsequently, Hart (1977) added the presence of cribriform pattern of this criterion for invasive mucinous tumors. Many pathologists use the Hart and Norris

criteria for mucinous tumors rather than the FIGO or WHO definitions.

A discussion of the histology of borderline tumors is complicated because FIGO and WHO stress that the diagnosis be made on the primary ovary, regardless of the histopathology of any extraovarian metastasis. This contravenes the general pathologic principle of grading a neoplasm from the worst area. Thus, if there are invasive peritoneal implants from a primary borderline ovarian tumor, this tumor is still classified as borderline even though in reality these implants behave like invasive cancer. This was pointed out in a recent study by Bell (1988) of 56 borderline serous tumors associated with peritoneal implants and a followup of 4 or more years or until death. Of the 50 patients with noninvasive implants, 94% had no progression of disease, whereas only 17% of the six patients with invasive implants showed no progression.

Five-year actuarial survival rates for stage I borderline tumors range from 90 to 100%. Julian and Woodruff (1978), Katzenstein et al (1978), Minyi and Lijuan (1980), Genadry et al (1981), Barnhill et al (1985) each reported survival rates of 100%, while Hart and Norris (1973) reported 98%, Russell and Merkur (1979) 97%, Kolstad et al (1977) 90%, Chaitin et al (1985) 90%, and Aure et al (1971) 96% for stage IA and 94% for stage IB. Bjorkholm et al (1982, 1985) reported rates of 97% for stage IA, 98% for stage IB, and 94% for stage IC.

Of concern are the 20-year actuarial survival rates of 78% for stage IA and 86% for stage IB borderline tumors reported by Aure et al (1971). The results of Aure's study indicate that 14 to 22% of patients with stage I borderline ovarian tumors will die of their disease, if followed for a considerable period of time. If confirmed by other investigators, this report would indeed change the management of borderline ovarian tumors because conservative therapy (unilateral salpingo-oophorectomy or ovarian cystectomy) would be inappropriate for disease associated with a mortality rate between 14 and 22%, even at 20 years.

Five-year survival rates for stage II borderline ovarian tumors range from 96% (Minyi and Lijuan, 1980), 95% (Genadry et al, 1981), 93% (Julian and Woodruff, 1978) and 92% (Bjorkholm, 1982, 1985) to 66% (Kjorstad and Albeller, 1983) and 60% (Katzenstein et al, 1978). Still, these rates are considerably higher than the 20 to 40% 5-year survival rates for stage II invasive ovarian cancer. Also important are the significantly higher 5-year survival rates reported by some authors for stage III borderline ovarian carcinomas. Genadry reported a 5-year survival rate of 96%, Minyi and Lijuan (1980) 92%, and Bjorkholm 68%. Russell and Merkur (1979) reported only a 31% 5-year survival rate for stage III borderline ovarian carcinoma; however, some of their cases may have been invasive rather than borderline (Scully, 1982).

The first report of systematic surgical staging in stage I borderline tumors was reported by Yazigi in 1988. Two of 25 patients (8%) had malignant peritoneal cytology, none of 20 patients had metastasis to the omentum, none of 11 patients had metastasis to the diaphragm, none of 11 had peritoneal metastasis, three of 13 patients (23%) had pelvic lymph node metastasis, and one of 12 patients (8%) had aortic lymph node metastasis. Therefore, when one is considering conservative surgery (i.e., unilateral salpingo-oophorectomy or ovarian cystectomy) in a young patient with a borderline tumor, surgical staging would be of assistance.

The survival rate for patients with stage I borderline tumors without adjuvant therapy is important in formulating a treatment plan (e.g., the use of postoperative adjuvant therapy). Katzenstein et al (1978) reported a survival rate of 100% for 27 patients with stage IA and IB serous borderline tumors, 19 of whom received no treatment other than surgery.

In a study using more conservative surgery than salpingo-oophorectomy to treat patients with ovarian serous tumors of borderline malignancy, Lim-Tan et al (1988) treated 35 patients initially with unilateral cystectomy, with preservation of the remaining normal-appearing ovarian tissue; bilateral cystectomy; or unilateral cystectomy with contralateral oophorectomy or salpingo-oophorectomy, depending on the stage of disease. Nineteen patients with stage IA tumors were treated by unilateral cystectomy; of the nine who had no further treatment, all were alive with no clinical evidence of disease 3 to 14.2 years later. Four of these patients underwent ipsilateral oophorectomy or salpingo-oophorectomy 6 weeks to one year after the initial cystectomy, and all were clinically disease-free 5.8 to 11.5 years later. The remaining six patients in this group underwent hysterectomy and bilateral salpingo-oophorectomy 3 weeks to 3.5 years after cystectomy. Tumor was subsequently detected in two of these patients, one in the ipsilateral ovarian remnant and contralateral ovary 5 months after cystectomy, and the other in the contralateral ovary 2.5 years after cystectomy. However, all 19 stage IA patients are alive with no evidence of disease.

Therefore, Lim-Tan et al (1988) believe that ovarian cystectomy can be carried out in a young woman who wants to preserve fertility and who is willing to undergo careful and prolonged followup examination, if there is no tumor at the resection margin of the cyst. For all other patients with stage I borderline tumors, a unilateral salpingo-oophorectomy should be performed in those who desire to remain fertile, and total abdominal hysterectomy and bilateral salpingo-oophorectomy, with surgical staging, should be carried out in all others. If there is no evidence of metastasis, no further treatment is needed.

In a large series of stage II and III borderline tumors, Gershenson and Silva (1990) reported that six of 82 patients (7.3%) with stage II, III, or IV borderline ovarian tumors died of progressive ovarian cancer. Five- and 10-year survival rates of 95% were reported for 22 patients with benign peritoneal implants; 97% and 94%, respectively, for the 37 patients with noninvasive peritoneal implants; and 92% for 13 patients with invasive peritoneal implants.

In the largest single study (20 patients) on the use of systemic chemotherapy for metastatic borderline tumors, Gershenson and Silva reported complete and partial response rates of 40% each and no response in 20% among patients with macroscopic residual cancer after surgery determined by second-look laparotomy. These results indicate that borderline tumors are indeed sensitive to systemic chemotherapy.

## DYSGERMINOMA

This is the most common type of germ cell tumor, occurring twice as often as endodermal sinus tumors. Morphologically and ultrastructurally they are consistent with primordial germ cells and, in fact, arise from undifferentiated primordial germ cells. These tumors are the female homologue of the seminoma of the testes.

Dysgerminomas account for only 1 to 2% of all ovarian tumors and 3 to 5% of all ovarian malignancies. Fifteen to 20% occur during pregnancy or immediately post partum, only 2 to 5% of all other ovarian tumors are associated with pregnancy. Dysgerminomas constitute 25 to 30% of all ovarian cancers that coexist with pregnancy, yet the reason for this association is not known.

This type of tumor may contain syncytial giant cells that produce histochemically detectable human chorionic gonadotropin (HCG) (Ueda et al, 1972). On occasion, this may result in precocious puberty. In rare cases, women with dysgerminoma admixed with gonadoblastoma may be virilized due to hormonal stimulation by the surrounding stroma. Dysgerminomas have been reported to be associated with testicular feminization, Turner's syndrome, and the 46X,Y karyotype, each of which manifests genital abnormalities caused by the primary disease and not by the associated dysgerminoma. In contrast, sexual development is normal in almost all other patients with this tumor.

Dysgerminomas are distinguished from all other ovarian malignancies by their propensity for paraaortic lymph node metastasis in the absence of peritoneal metastasis and from all other ovarian germ cell tumors by a significant incidence of bilateral ovarian involvement and the high curability of metastasis by radiation therapy. Retroperitoneal spread is to the paraaortic nodes at approximately the second lumbar vertebra, just below the left renal vessels, and to the right of the third lumbar vertebra paraaortic nodes.

Although there is no specific marker for dysgerminomas, lactic dehydrogenase (LDH), a glycolytic enzyme present in many malignancies and other tissues in the body, is elevated in many cases. Serum LDH1 and LDH2 are the fractions characteristically elevated. Moreover, elevated levels of HCG or positive pregnancy tests have been reported in patients with pure dysgerminomas.

Treatment decisions are complicated by the frequent bilateral ovarian involvement in the absence of obvious metastasis, particularly in young patients who plan to bear children. Asadourian and Taylor (1969) and DePalo et al (1982) each have reported a 14% incidence of bilateral involvement in stage I disease. In the study by Asadourian and Taylor of 21 patients with clinical stage IA tumors (unilateral involvement) in whom both ovaries were removed, four (19%) were found to have occult microscopic involvement of the normal-appearing ovary. Even with bilateral ovarian involvement, however, the uterus can be preserved for future childbearing by means of in vitro fertilization.

The 1981 report by Gordon et al, which evaluated survival among patients with dysgerminoma in relation to histology, is useful because of the large size of the series and the fact that the authors reviewed the slides and separated pure dysgerminomas from mixed tumors. Such separation is important because of the low survival rate reported for the latter. In 1950, Mueller et al had reported a 5-year survival rate of 27% for dysgerminomas, but this low rate might be explained in part by the fact that this and many other early reports actually included dysgerminomas admixed with the more aggressive embryonal carcinoma, endodermal sinus tumor, or ovarian choriocarcinoma.

Gordon et al (1981) reported on 158 cases from the Ovarian Tumor Registry and the Oncology Service of the Johns Hopkins Hospital. Of the pure dysgerminomas in 136 patients, 78% were stage I (107), 10% were stage II (13), 5% were stage III (7), 0.7% were stage IV (1), and 6% were unclassified (8). There were no deaths among 72 patients with stage IA pure dysgerminomas measuring 10 cm or less, and only one death occurred among the patients with tumors measuring 15 cm or larger. These results were not statistically significant. However, among these 72 conservatively treated patients, (unilateral salpingo-oophorectomy without postoperative radiation), 12 (17%) recurred; among the 10 patients who were followed for at least 5 years after recurrence, there were four (6%) deaths (Table 14-7). The 5- and 10-year survival rates were 94% and 92%, respectively, for the patients with stage IA pure dysgerminomas treated conservatively in this series (Table 14-8).

Conservative treatment (unilateral salpingo-oophorectomy without postoperative radiation) is associated with a 6% mortality rate and a 17% recurrence rate in the earliest stage pure dysgerminoma, a highly radiocurable tumor. This raises serious questions about the validity of such treatment. The fact that conservative surgery may be problematic in stage IA dysgerminoma

is highlighted in a recent report from the Mayo Clinic by Buskirk et al (1987), in which 35% (5/14) of the patients with stage IA disease suffered a recurrence following treatment by unilateral salpingo-oophorectomy. Moreover, the relapse-free survival rate for stage IA was only 67% at 4 years.

Of significance is the fact that among the stage IA patients treated by pelvic radiation or no radiation, 38% relapsed in the paraaortic lymph nodes, again emphasizing the high propensity for paraaortic nodal metastasis in presumed localized dysgerminoma. Based on these findings, the authors recommended that stage IA patients who want to preserve future fertility receive 2,000 cGy to the ipsilateral common iliac and paraaortic nodes as adjuvant therapy to unilateral salpingo-oophorectomy. DePalo and colleagues affirmed this recommendation in a 1987 report of 12 patients with stage IA disease treated by unilateral salpingo-oophorectomy and radiation therapy to the ipsilateral hemipelvis and paraaortic lymph nodes, while shielding the contralateral ovary. Over a median followup of 77 months, there have been no relapses and no deaths.

Buskirk et al (1987) reported that in four of eight patients with clinical macroscopic paraaortic lymph node metastasis, tumor recurred in the mediastinal and supraclavicular areas after abdominal radiation therapy alone. Therefore, they recommended that patients with known paraaortic metastasis receive whole abdominal and paraaortic lymph node radiation and additional radiation treatment to the mediastinum and supraclavicular lymph nodes. The value of this recommendation is documented in a recent report by DePalo et al (1987). Among 10 patients with retroperitoneal paraaortic lymph node metastasis treated by pelvic, paraaortic, mediastinal, and supraclavicular radiation, there have been only three relapses and one death, with a median followup of 67 months (range = 24 to 96).

Although not reported in any large series, adjuvant therapy is probably not required in patients with stage IA dysgerminoma in whom biopsy results of the contralateral ovary show no evidence of germ cell tumor and in whom complete surgical staging (including evaluation of the diaphragm, omentum, ipsilateral pelvic nodes, paraaortic nodes, and peritoneal washings) is negative. In addition, the relapse rate would most likely be minor.

TABLE 14-7 Survival in Pure Ovarian Dysgerminoma (Stage IA) by Treatment

|  | Cases | Deaths | Survival(%) |
|---|---|---|---|
| Unilateral adnexectomy | 72 | 5* | 67 (94.4) |
| All other therapies | 14 | 3 | 11 (78.5) |
| TOTAL | 86 | 8 | 78 (90.6) |

Numbers in parentheses are actuarial survival rates.
* Includes one death without disease at autopsy.
*Source:* Gordon A, Lipton D, Woodruff JD: Dysgerminoma: A review of 158 cases from the Emil Novak Ovarian Tumor Registry. *Obstet Gynecol* 58:497, 1981.

TABLE 14-8 5-Year Survival for Pure Ovarian Dysgerminoma

| Stage | Cases | Deaths | Survival (%) |
|---|---|---|---|
| I | 94 | 12* | 82 (89.1) |
| II | 11 | 4 | 7 (63.6) |
| III | 7 | 3 | 4 (57.2) |
| IV | 1 | 1 | 0 (0) |
| V-k | 3 | 1 | 2 (66.7) |
| TOTAL | 116 | 21 | 95 (82.6) |

Numbers in parentheses are actuarial survival rates.
* Includes one death without disease at autopsy.
*Source:* Gordon A, Lipton D, Woodruff JD: Dysgerminoma: A review of 158 cases from the Emil Novak Ovarian Tumor Registry. *Obstet Gynecol* 58:497, 1981.

Future clinical trials may demonstrate that adjuvant chemotherapy could replace adjuvant radiation therapy as the treatment of choice. Early data supporting this contention come from Creasman et al (1979), who reported on the use of combination chemotherapy—methotrexate, actinomycin-D, and cyclophosphamide—following surgery in five patients with stage IA dysgerminoma. At the time of this report, all five patients were alive with no evidence of disease 3 to 36 months following diagnosis.

However, Gershenson et al (1986c) used cisplatin, bleomycin, and etoposide to treat two patients with metastatic dysgerminoma of the ovary, and both achieved complete remission, as documented by second-look laparotomy. Recently, Williams et al (1989) reported sustained, disease-free survival in seven of eight patients (88%) with metastatic dysgerminoma treated with cisplatin-based chemotherapy.

These two reports of a nearly 100% response rate to cisplatin-based chemotherapy in advanced dysgerminoma suggest that the effectiveness of this regimen may be equal to that of adjuvant radiation therapy in stage IA disease.

## ENDODERMAL SINUS TUMOR OF THE OVARY

Endodermal sinus tumor is the second most common malignant germ cell tumor of the ovary. In three large series, the median age has been reported to be 8 years (range = 1 to 45 years), and two-thirds of the patients were less than 20 years of age at diagnosis (Gallion et al, 1979); 19 years (range = 7 to 37) (Gershenson et al, 1983) and 19 years (range = 1 to 45) (Kurman and Norris, 1976b). Like immature teratomas of the ovary, endodermal sinus tumors are almost always unilateral. In a report by Kurman and Norris (1976b), six of the 71 tumors were bilateral, and all these were associated with extensive peritoneal metastasis.

Prior to 1976, embryonal carcinoma, a rare germ cell tumor, was often confused with endodermal sinus tumor of the ovary. However, in 1976, Kurman and Norris (1976a) described 15 cases of the ovarian germ cell tumor now referred to as embryonal carcinoma, separating them histologically, immunohistochemically, and clinically from the more common endodermal sinus tumor.

Embryonal carcinomas of the ovary and adult testes resemble each other, while endodermal sinus tumor of the ovary is similar in appearance to that of the infantile testes. These two types of tumors also differ in terms of age of occurrence, incidence, hormonal activity, and survival.

Using special histochemical techniques (immunoperoxidase), Kurman and Norris (1976a) were able to demonstrate alpha-fetoprotein (AFP) and beta human chorionic gonadotropin (HCG) in the tumor tissues of embryonal carcinoma, but only AFP in endodermal sinus tumor. Both tumors had elevated AFP levels. Because of the HCG activity in embryonal carcinoma, patients often have hormonal manifestations as well as positive pregnancy tests. All the patients with embryonal carcinoma reported by Kurman and Norris (1976a) had positive pregnancy tests and histochemical evidence of HCG in the tumor tissues. In contrast to the median age of 19 years (range = 1 to 45) reported by Kurman and Norris (1976b) for endodermal sinus tumors, the median age for embryonal carcinoma was 15 years (range = 4 to 28). Moreover, 60% of their patients with embryonal carcinoma patients had hormonal manifestations consisting of precocious puberty in premenarchal girls, abnormal vaginal bleeding in postmenarchal women, and a positive pregnancy test. In contrast, the patients with endodermal sinus tumor had negative pregnancy tests (Table 14-9). Of the 71 patients with endodermal sinus tumors, five had a benign cystic teratoma in the opposite ovary and 10 had an ipsilateral benign teratoma.

Until the recent discovery that adjuvant combination chemotherapy was effective in endodermal sinus tumors, the prognosis for these patients was extremely poor, even when the tumor was clinically confined to the ovary at initial diagnosis. Evidence for this was reported in the 1970s by Jimerson and Woodruff (1977) and Kurman and Norris (1976b). In these studies, only 9% (2/22) and 19% (5/27), respectively, of the patients with stage I endodermal sinus tumor of the ovary survived after treatment with surgery alone.

In stark contrast to these bleak survival rates for the earliest stage of this disease are reports of improved rates after adjuvant chemotherapy regimens—vincristine, actinomycin-D, and cyclophosphamide (VAC) and cisplatin, vinblastine, and bleomycin (PVB). In the 1985 update of the experience at M.D. Anderson Hospital and Tumor Institute by Gershenson et al, 94% (15/16) of the patients with stage I disease treated with VAC sustained long-term remission; 30% (3/10) of those with advanced disease treated with VAC also sustained long-term remission. In a not so salutary study, however, Slayton et al (1985), reporting for the GOG, found

**TABLE 14-9** Comparison of Characteristics Between Endodermal Sinus Tumor and Embryonal Carcinoma

| Characteristics | Endodermal Sinus Tumor | Embryonal Carcinoma |
|---|---|---|
| Median age | 19 years | 15 years |
| % Malignant ovarian germ cell tumors | 22% | 5% |
| Precocious puberty | — | + |
| Abnormal menstruation | — | + |
| Pregnancy test | — | + |
| Serum AFP | + | + |
| Tumor AFP | + | + |
| Tumor HCG | — | + |

Kurman RJ, Norris HJ: Embryonal carcinoma of the ovary. A clinicopathologic entity distinct from endodermal sinus tumor resembling embryonal carcinoma of the adult testis. *Cancer* 38:2420, 1976a; Kurman RJ, Norris HJ: Endodermal sinus tumor of the ovary. A clinical and pathologic analysis of 71 cases. *Cancer* 38:2404, 1976b.
AFP = alpha-fetoprotein; HCG = human chorionic gonadotropin.

that of 15 patients with stage IA disease treated with VAC chemotherapy, 47% failed to achieve remission; of the seven patients with stage IC disease treated with VAC, four (57%) did not respond to treatment. Thus, the total failure rate was 50% in stage I disease. Of the six patients with stage III and IV disease treated with VAC, only two sustained long-term remission without recurrence.

While VAC chemotherapy was being evaluated in germ cell tumors of the ovary, researchers were reporting excellent survival rates using PVB in patients with nonseminomatous germ cell tumors of the testes. By 1989, Williams et al, reporting for the GOG, used PVB in patients with stage II, III, IV, or recurrent endodermal sinus tumor of the ovary, all of whom had residual, unresected disease. Of the 29 patients evaluated, 55% (16) were disease-free. This appears to be somewhat higher than the earlier results of Gershenson et al (1983) and Slayton et al (1985), in which 31% (5/16) of the patients with advanced endodermal sinus tumor treated with VAC chemotherapy achieved remission. Although these numbers are too small for comparison, PVB appears to be superior to VAC in advanced endodermal sinus tumor of the ovary.

The use of adjuvant therapy for endodermal sinus tumor of the ovary is controversial. Gershenson et al (1985) reported a 94% sustained remission rate with VAC chemotherapy, while Slayton (1985) reported only a 50% sustained remission with the same therapy. The controversy settles not only on the percentage of long-term remissions reported by Gershenson but also on the significantly higher morbidity associated with PVB compared with VAC.

Only small series have been reported involving the adjuvant treatment of stage I endodermal sinus tumors with PVB. However, as seen in Table 14-10, the long-term remission rate with adjuvant PVB in 18 patients with stage I disease is 100% (Lokey et al, 1981; Wiltshaw et al, 1982; Carlson et al, 1983b); Gershenson et al, 1983; Vriesendorp et al, 1984; Davis et al, 1984; Taylor et al, 1985; Malone et al, 1986; and Sessa et al, 1987). Therefore, notwithstanding the excellent report of Gershenson using adjuvant VAC chemotherapy in

patients with stage I endodermal sinus tumor and its increased morbidity, PVB appears to be the treatment of choice.

It is not known, however, whether there is a need for adjuvant chemotherapy in patients with surgical stage I who have no evidence of metastasis outside the ovary and in whom AFP levels return to normal within a reasonable time after the tumor is resected. Only future prospective clinical trials can resolve this question.

To date, there are no large reports on salvage therapy for relapse after PVB for endodermal sinus tumor of the ovary. However, Williams et al (1989) reported sustained remissions in patients who crossed over to VAC chemotherapy after the disease had progressed during PVB therapy. Furthermore, they reported on seven patients treated with cisplatin and etoposide as second-line therapy, three of whom are progression-free; and 12 patients treated with VAC as second-line therapy, five of whom are progression-free.

Finally, Loehrer et al (1988) used cisplatin and ifosfamide with either vinblastine or etoposide as third-line therapy in testicular germ cell tumors after previous cisplatin chemotherapy. They reported durable, complete remissions in a significant number of patients. Therefore, cisplatin and etoposide, VAC, or cisplatin, ifosfamide, plus vinblastine or etoposide, would appear to be reasonable salvage therapy after PVB.

The use of second-look laparotomy in endodermal sinus tumors is also controversial. However, Curtin et al (1989) reported on the first two patients who had normalized AFP levels but who had persistent cancer at second-look laparotomy, indicating the value of second-look laparotomy if salvage therapy is available. However, the controversy on the value of second-look laparotomy continues because only one of the 15 patients with endodermal sinus tumor, reported by Gershenson in 1986a, who had undergone a second-look laparotomy had persistent disease; however, this was the only patient with an elevated AFP level prior to second-look laparotomy. The patient was subsequently treated with PVB and continued to have no evidence of disease 67 months after second-look laparotomy.

| TABLE 14-10  Results of Cisplatin, Vinblastine, and Bleomycin Therapy in Stage I Pure Endodermal Sinus Tumor ||| |
|---|---|---|
| Author | Patients | No. NED |
| Lokey et al (1981) | 2 | 2 |
| Wiltshaw et al (1982) | 4 | 4 |
| Carlson et al (1983) | 1 | 1 |
| Gershenson et al (1983) | 1 | 1 |
| Vriesendorp et al (1984) | 1 | 1 |
| Davis et al (1984) | 3 | 3 |
| Taylor et al (1985) | 1 | 1 |
| Malone et al (1986) | 1 | 1 |
| Sessa et al (1987) | 4 | 4 |
| Number with NED | 18 | 18 |
| | (100%) | |

NED = No evidence of disease.

## IMMATURE TERATOMAS

Immature teratomas are the third most frequent germ cell ovarian tumors, ranked behind dysgerminomas and endodermal sinus tumors. They account for about 15% of all germ cell tumors and 1% of all teratomas. Incidence peaks in the second decade, with a median age of 19 (range = 1 to 47) reported by Norris et al (1976), 19 reported by Gallion et al (1983), and 17 (range = 6 to 40) reported by Gershenson et al (1986b). This young median age is an important factor in treatment decisions.

Also important in this age group is the fact that immature teratomas are almost universally unilateral. None of the 58 cases reported by Norris et al (1976) and only three of 350 (0.8%) cases reported by Yanai-Inbar and Scully (1987) were bilateral. In the latter series, a mature teratoma (dermoid cyst) was present in the contralateral ovary of 10% of the patients.

Immature teratomas had been thought to be hormonally inert, with no serum or tissue markers. However, Perrone et al (1987) detected AFP by immunohistochemical reaction in three patients with immature teratoma, two of whom had elevated serum AFP levels. Recently, Gershenson (1986*b*) detected increased AFP levels in five of 16 (31%) patients with immature teratoma; none of the 16 had elevated levels of HCG.

Two important discoveries have improved our understanding of immature teratomas and have led to significant improvements in survival rates. The first report related the grade of these tumors—i.e., the amount of immature tissue present—to survival and the need for adjuvant treatment. The second report demonstrated that combination chemotherapy can result in long-term survival and actual cure.

Thurnbeck and Scully (1960) reported a grading system for ovarian teratomas based on the amount of immature tissue within the tumor (Table 14-11): Grade 0 consisted of mature tissue only, with no malignant potential; grade 1 contained small amounts of immature tissue, frequently immature neuroepithelium or cartilage with rare mitosis; grade 2 contained a moderate amount of immature elements; and grade 3 contained large amounts of immature (or embryonal) tissues with numerous mitoses. The lack of malignant potential in grade 0 ovarian teratomas was demonstrated in a report of 15 such patients by Woodruff and coauthors (1968). Fourteen patients were alive and well and one was lost to followup; none developed recurrent disease.

Norris and coauthors (1976) demonstrated the clear relation between grade and ultimate survival using the Thurnbeck and Scully grading system modified to take into consideration the amount of neural tissue within the tumor. Of their 40 patients with grade 1 disease, 85% (34) were treated by unilateral salpingo-oophorectomy alone. Thirteen (93%) of the 14 stage I, grade 1 patients were disease-free and the one patient with recurrence was salvaged with further surgery. For the 20 patients with grade 2 tumors and the six with grade 3 tumors, 55% and 33%, respectively, survived with no evidence of disease. Of the patients with metastasis (stages II and III) whose tissue was available for grading, all patients with grade 0 tumors were alive with no evidence of disease for more than 7 years, in contrast to less than 50% of the patients with grade 1 and grade 2 tumors.

Since the tumor grade is most important in deciding

on therapy and in gauging prognosis, one block of tissue should be examined for every centimeter of tumor. If the peritoneal implants are grade 0, no further treatment is required (Robboy and Scully, 1970).

Therefore, patients with stage 1, grade 0 teratoma who want to retain childbearing capacity require only salpingo-oophorectomy. Since bilaterality occurs in less than 1% of cases, unilateral salpingo-oophorectomy followed by chemotherapy and preservation of fertility is the treatment of choice for stage 1, grade 1, 2, or 3 patients and may also be appropriate for patients with advanced disease (stages II and III, grades 1, 2, or 3). Lee (1989*b*) reported the first successful pregnancy following conservative surgery (unilateral salpingo-oophorectomy) and combination chemotherapy in a patient with advanced (stage III) immature teratoma.

To date, the most effective adjuvant chemotherapy for immature teratomas appears to be vincristine, actinomycin-D, and cyclophosphamide (VAC) (Table 14-12). In 1986, Gershenson reported on the effectiveness of adjuvant VAC chemotherapy in the largest series from a single institution, conducted at M.D. Anderson (Table 14-13). Sustained remissions were achieved in 91% (10) of the 11 stage I patients treated with adjuvant VAC compared with 9% of 11 stage I patients treated by surgery alone. Moreover, long-term remission was 80% in 10 stage II and III patients with adjuvant VAC. The role of second-look laparotomy for patients with immature teratoma is unclear because in all 22 patients who underwent second-look laparotomies after chemotherapy the findings were negative.

In 1985, the GOG reported on the use of VAC chemotherapy in immature teratomas (Slayton 1985). All 15 stage IA patients—seven grade 3, seven grade 2, and one grade 1—achieved sustained remissions without recurrence. However, in a smaller subset of stage III pa-

---

**TABLE 14-11   Grading of Ovarian Teratomas**

| | |
|---|---|
| Grade 0 | All tissues mature; no mitotic activity |
| Grade 1 | Minor foci of embryonal tissue; rare mitosis |
| Grade 2 | Moderate quantities of embryonal tissue; moderate mitotic activity |
| Grade 3 | Large quantities of embryonal tissue |

*Source:* Thurlbeck WM, Scully RE: Solid teratoma of the ovary—A clinicopathological analysis of nine cases. *Cancer* 13:804, 1960.

---

**TABLE 14-12   Treatment Regimens for Immature Teratomas**

| Therapy | Dosage Schedule |
|---|---|
| PVB* | |
|   Cisplatin | 20 mg/m² intravenously daily for 5 days |
|   Vinblastine† | 12 mg/m², intravenous push day 1 |
|   Bleomycin‡ | 20 units/m², intravenous push weekly |
| VAC§ | |
|   Vincristine | 1.5 mg/m² (maximum, 2.0 mg; intravenous push, days 1 and 15 |
|   Actinomycin-D | 350 μg/m², intravenous push, days 1 to 5 |
|   Cyclophosphamide | 150 mg/m², intravenous push, days 1 to 5 |

\* Three to four courses given at 3-week intervals.
† Patients with previous radiotherapy received 9 mg/m²
‡ Maximum dose = 30 units; 10 units/m² for children age 13 and under
§ Six courses given at 4-week intervals
PVB = cisplatin, vinblastine, and bleomycin
VAC = vincristine, actinomycin-D, and cyclophosphamide
*Source:* Williams SD, Blessing JA, Moore DH, et al: Cisplatin, vinblastine and bleomycin in advanced and recurrent ovarian germ-cell tumors. *Ann Intern Med* 111:22, 1989.

TABLE 14-13 Sustained Remission* by Postoperative Treatment and Stage (N = 41)

| Treatment | Stage | | | | |
|---|---|---|---|---|---|
| | I | II | III | IV | Total |
| None (surgery alone) | 1/11 | 0 | 0/5 | 0 | 1/16 |
| Radiotherapy + chemotherapy | 0/1 | 0 | 0 | 0/1 | 0/2 |
| VAC | 10/11 | 2/3 | 6/7 | 0 | 18/21 |
| AcFuCy | 1/1 | 0 | 0 | 0 | 1/1 |
| Doxorubicin + cyclophosphamide | 0 | 0/1 | 0 | 0 | 0/1 |
| Total | 12/24 | 2/4 | 6/12 | 0/1 | 20/41 |

\* Sustained remission = no evidence of recurrent disease.
VAC = vincristine, actinomycin-D, cyclophosphamide; AcFuCy = actinomycin-D, 5-fluorouracil, cyclophosphamide.
*Source:* Gershenson DM, DelJunco G, Silva EG, et al: Immature teratoma of the ovary. *Obstet Gynecol* 68:624, 1986*b*.

tients or those with recurrent immature teratoma treated with the VAC regimen, only five (55%) remained disease-free.

More recently, in a GOG study by Williams and colleagues (1989), 26 patients with immature teratoma—stages II, III, and IV—were treated with a regimen consisting of cisplatin, vinblastine, and bleomycin (PVB) (Table 14-14). Response rates were not reported; however, 14 of the 26 (56%) were disease-free.

Although the numbers of patients with advanced disease treated with VAC (9) and PVB (26) in the GOG reports were small, the sustained disease-free recurrence rates were identical. Fatal and nonfatal pulmonary fibrosis from bleomycin is usually dose-related or occurs in patients who have previously undergone chest irradiation; however, either of these complications can occur in the absence of such predisposing factors (Trump et al, 1988; Dee et al, 1987). Therefore, PVB as adjuvant chemotherapy in stage I immature teratoma patients would appear to be contraindicated, especially given the sustained remission rates of 100% and 91% reported by Slayton et al (1985) and Gershenson (1986*b*), respectively, using the VAC regimen.

However, based on a recent report by Williams et al (1987), the GOG plans to study the effectiveness of bleomycin in combination with etoposide and cisplatin as adjuvant chemotherapy in early-stage immature teratomas. In this study, when vinblastine was replaced by etoposide to treat testicular germ cell tumors, there was no loss of efficacy and the peripheral neuropathy often

caused by vinblastine was precluded. However, the use of bleomycin in an adjuvant setting remains problematic because of the possibility of fatal pulmonary fibrosis. Whether VAC or PVB is more effective for advanced immature teratomas is still unsettled. Conceptually, cisplatin and etoposide without bleomycin may be the treatment of choice for advanced disease.

Rarely, a mature cystic teratoma (dermoid cyst) may contain a malignant element. Squamous cell carcinoma is the most common, followed by adenocarcinoma, undifferentiated carcinoma, carcinoid, malignant melanoma, and thyroid tissue. In a recent literature review, Kashimura et al (1989) reported on 2,176 mature cystic teratomas. Fifty-two (2.4%) had a malignancy, and 42 (1.9%) were squamous cell carcinoma. To date, no effective therapy has been reported.

## OVARIAN CHORIOCARCINOMA

Ovarian choriocarcinoma consists of an admixture of syncytiotrophoblasts and cytotrophoblasts, similar to uterine choriocarcinoma. This tumor may be a primary cancer resulting from an ovarian pregnancy (gestational) or may not be associated with an ovarian pregnancy (nongestational). In either case, HCG levels are elevated. Gestational ovarian choriocarcinoma is extremely rare, and to date only isolated cases have been reported. For an ovarian choriocarcinoma to be gestational, it must be presumed to follow an ovarian pregnancy, and there must be proof that there was no prior uterine choriocarcinoma. Nongestational ovarian choriocarcinoma is more common and is usually associated with other germ cell tumors—dysgerminoma, endodermal sinus tumor, pure embryonal carcinoma, and immature teratoma—as part of a mixed germ cell tumor.

Since ovarian choriocarcinomas are almost always unilateral, surgical treatment is similar to that for other germ cell tumors, with the exception of dysgerminoma, which is often bilateral. Only scattered reports describe the effectiveness of chemotherapy in this disease. Gerbie and coauthors (1975) treated four patients who had pure ovarian choriocarcinoma with MAC (methotrexate, actinomycin-D, and chlorambucil) chemotherapy. Three patients survived with no evidence of disease and one died of malignancy. However, of the three patients with ovarian choriocarcinoma mixed with other germ

TABLE 14-14 Disease-Free Survival in Stage II, III, IV, and Recurrent Germ-Cell Tumors of the Ovary After Treatment With Cisplatin, Vinblastine, and Bleomycin

| Cell Type | Total Disease-Free (%) |
|---|---|
| Endodermal sinus tumor | 16/29 (55) |
| Embryonal carcinoma | 1/4 (25) |
| Mixed germ cell tumor | 14/27 (52) |
| Immature teratoma | 14/26 (54) |
| Choriocarcinoma | 2/3 (67) |
| Dysgerminoma | 7/8 (88) |

*Source:* Williams SD, Blessing JA, Moore DH, et al: Cisplatin, vinblastine and bleomycin in advanced or recurrent ovarian germ-cell tumors. *Ann Intern Med* 111:22, 1989.

cell elements, only one survived and two died of the disease. In contrast, Wider and coauthors (1969) demonstrated complete responses to MAC chemotherapy in three of four cases of nongestational ovarian choriocarcinoma admixed with other germ cell elements. Williams et al (1989) reported disease-free survival in two of three patients with metastatic pure ovarian choriocarcinoma treated with cisplatin, vinblastine, and bleomycin (PVB).

Since ovarian choriocarcinoma is rarely bilateral and is associated with HCG, a specific tumor marker, conservative unilateral salpingo-oophorectomy allows fertility to be preserved in young patients. Adjuvant MAC chemotherapy is repeated until two consecutive normal HCG titers are achieved. Patients with metastatic choriocarcinoma could be treated with the best therapy for metastatic uterine choriocarcinoma, which includes at least methotrexate, actinomycin-D, and etoposide (VP16-213), although there are no reports on the use of these agents in ovarian choriocarcinoma.

## MIXED GERM CELL TUMORS

By definition, a mixed germ cell tumor of the ovary contains at least two malignant germ cell elements. Kurman and Norris (1976c) reported on 30 cases of mixed germ cell ovarian tumors, which represented 8% of the germ cell ovarian tumors seen at the Armed Forces Institute of Pathology, ranking fourth in incidence behind dysgerminoma (150), pure endodermal sinus tumor (71), malignant teratoma (50), mixed germ cell tumor (30) and pure embryonal carcinoma (12).

Histologically, dysgerminoma, the most common malignant element, was present in 70% of the 30 cases, followed by immature teratoma (53%), ovarian choriocarcinoma (20%), and pure embryonal carcinoma (16%). Endodermal sinus tumor and dysgerminoma constituted the most common combination of malignant elements present, accounting for one-third of the mixed germ cell tumors studied.

Gershenson and colleagues (1984) reported on 42 cases of mixed germ cell tumor of the ovary—19% of all malignant germ cell tumors seen at the M.D. Anderson Hospital and Tumor Institute. Dysgerminoma was the most common malignant element present (69%), followed by immature teratoma (62%), endodermal sinus tumor (60%), pure embryonal carcinoma (24%), and choriocarcinoma (10%). Again, dysgerminoma and endodermal sinus tumor was the most common combination of malignant elements seen. In both studies, the median age was 16, with age ranges of 5 to 33 in the Kurman and Norris study and 6 to 31 in the study by Gershenson et al. Depending on the cell types in the mixed germ cell tumors, serum levels of HCG, AFP, and LDH may be elevated.

Except for mixed germ cell tumors admixed with dysgerminoma, virtually all these tumors are unilateral. Therefore, in young patients, unilateral salpingo-oophorectomy and adjuvant chemotherapy would be appropriate treatment. If dysgerminoma is one of the elements, the probability of microscopic involvement of the contralateral ovary is about 20%, so this ovary should be biopsied.

In the study by Kurman and Norris, conducted prior to the modern era of surgical staging and the use of combination chemotherapy to treat patients with stage I mixed germ cell tumors, only 25% (3/12) of their patients survived when more than one-third of the tumor consisted of endodermal sinus tumor, a grade 3 immature teratoma, or ovarian choriocarcinoma. This compares to 100% (6/6) survival for those patients with tumors containing embryonal carcinoma, dysgerminoma or grade 1 or 2 immature teratoma.

Thus, the need for effective adjuvant chemotherapy, even for stage I mixed germ cell tumors, is clear. Slayton et al (1985), of the GOG, reported that five (83%) of six patients treated with adjuvant VAC chemotherapy for stage I mixed germ cell tumors had a long progression-free survival. In an update of their 1984 series, Gershenson and colleagues (1985) reported sustained remissions in 75% (9/12) of the stage I patients treated with adjuvant VAC chemotherapy. To date, there are only anecdotal case reports on the use of adjuvant cisplatin-based chemotherapy for patients with stage I mixed germ cell tumors. Moreover, there are no data to indicate definitively whether patients who are completely surgically staged and found to have surgical stage I mixed germ cell tumors even need adjuvant chemotherapy.

For metastatic mixed germ cell tumors, Slayton et al (1985) reported a failure rate of 100% in nine patients with stage II, stage III, or recurrent mixed germ cell tumor of the ovary treated with VAC chemotherapy. However, Gershenson et al (1985) reported that three (33%) of nine patients treated with VAC chemotherapy for stage III or IV tumors survived. Williams et al (1989) reported a 52% disease-free survival rate (14/27) (see Table 14-14) using PVB chemotherapy in a much larger series of patients with stage II, III, IV, or recurrent mixed germ cell tumors for the GOG.

Specific chemotherapy regimens for mixed germ cell tumors are less precise than for most ovarian tumors owing primarily to the combination of malignant elements present within the tumor. Conceptually, patients with mixed germ cell tumors that consist of more than one-third ovarian choriocarcinoma should receive methotrexate and actinomycin-D or MAC (methotrexate, actinomycin-D and chlorambucil) chemotherapy as part of their treatment. PVB or VAC chemotherapy would be used for patients with mixed germ cell tumors that consist of more than one-third endodermal sinus tumor, embryonal carcinoma, or immature teratoma.

## SEX CORD–STROMAL TUMORS

Sex cord–stromal tumors contain granulosa cells, theca cells, fibroblasts, and Sertoli and Leydig cells, either alone or in combination. The granulosa and Sertoli cells are thought to be derived from the sex cord of the embryonic gonad, whereas the other cells are derived from the stroma or its specialized derivatives, the Leydig and theca cells.

There are four major categories of sex cord–stromal tumors: (1) granulosa–stromal cell tumors composed of ovarian cell types, (2) Sertoli—stromal cell tumors containing cells of testicular type, (3) gynandroblastoma with cells characteristic of ovarian and testicular types, and (4) sex cord tumors with annular tubules (Table 14-15).

## Granulosa–Stromal Cell Tumors

Granulosa–stromal cell tumors contain granulosa cells, theca cells, and fibroblasts, alone or in combination. Kurman and coauthors (1979) demonstrated that granulosa cells produce estradiol, progesterone, and testosterone, and 75% of these tumors are endocrinologically active—feminizing (estrogenic) or virilizing (androgenic). These tumors cause postmenopausal bleeding and menometrorrhagia.

In addition, their increased estrogen production is reflected in endometrial changes. Cystic hyperplasia is the most common, with adenomatous hyperplasia occurring less often and endometrial adenocarcinoma present in fewer than 5% of cases (Stenwig et al, 1979). Virilizing symptoms—hirsutism, oligomenorrhea, or amenorrhea—occur in about 3% of patients.

Four tumor markers have been described for following patients with granulosa–stromal cell tumors. The most recent, *inhibin*, a peptide hormone produced by the granulosa cells, appears to be the most specific (Lappohn et al, 1989). Inhibin levels correlate with the size of residual tumor and response to therapy. Low levels of *follicular stimulating hormone* (FSH) also correlate well with elevated inhibin levels, but the rates of specificity and sensitivity of serum FSH were considered too

low. *Follicle regulatory hormone* (FRP) levels were elevated in 79% of 19 patients, and in all patients FRP levels paralleled the clinical course, including prediction of disease status at second-look laparotomy (Montz et al, 1989). Lomax and colleagues (1977) were the first to report markedly elevated levels of serum progesterone for metastatic disease. These levels returned to normal after a complete response to chemotherapy. Serum *estradiol* levels were reported to correlate with response to the treatment, but most often these levels are too low to be clinically useful.

There are two categories of granulosa–stromal cell tumors: granulosa cell tumors and tumors of the theca-fibroma group.

***Granulosa Cell Tumors*** Mistaking undifferentiated ovarian carcinomas for granulosa cell tumors is a frequent error in diagnosis that has significant therapeutic implications. Granulosa cell tumors are composed of granulosa cells either alone or combined with cells arising from the theca interna and externa. Previously, granulosa cell tumors and those with theca cell elements were considered together as granulosa–theca cell tumors for purposes of therapy, since the prognosis depends entirely on the granulosa cells and not on the presence or absence of theca cells. Although theca cells may be present with granulosa cell tumors, the term granulosa cell tumor is now accepted for tumors containing both cell types. These tumors are of two types—adult and juvenile.

***Adult granulosa cell tumors*** Adult granulosa cell tumors account for 5 to 10% of malignant ovarian tumors, 1 to 2% of all ovarian tumors, and 95% of all granulosa cell tumors. The median age of women with these tumors is between 45 and 55 years, with only 5% occurring in prepubertal girls.

Most adult granulosa cell tumors are stage IA at the initial operation and less than 5% are bilateral. Using rigid histologic criteria for diagnosing these tumors (i.e., nuclear grooves [characteristic of sex cord–stromal tumors in general], absence of ducts or mucin [as seen in ovarian adenocarcinoma], or acinar structures [as seen in ovarian carcinoids]), Norris and Taylor (1968) at the Armed Forces Institute of Pathology reported the best survival rates to date, with 97% and 93% of patients surviving 5 and 10 years, respectively. These excellent results included all patients with stages I, II, and III, but most patients had stage IA disease. The authors noted that long-term followup was necessary, since many deaths from this disease occur after 5 years and may occur as late as 20 to 30 years after the initial operation.

The malignant potential of adult granulosa cell tumors cannot be determined by the usual morphologic criteria because of the frequent absence of such findings as anaplasia, cellular atypia, abnormal or frequent mitosis, and hyperchromatic nuclei. Conservative unilateral salpingo-oophorectomy in younger patients desiring to retain future fertility, would be the treatment of choice, since about 95% of these tumors are unilateral at the initial operation; the 5- and 10-year actuarial survival rates have been reported to be 97% and 93%, respectively; and there is no documentation of effective

TABLE 14-15 Classification of Sex Cord–Stromal Tumors

Granulosa–stromal cell tumor
  Granulosa cell tumor
    Adult type
    Juvenile type
  Tumors in the thecoma-fibroma group
    Thecoma
      Typical
      Luteinized
    Fibroma-fibrosarcoma
      Fibroma
      Cellular fibroma
      Fibrosarcoma
    Stromal tumor with minor sex cord elements
    Sclerosing stromal tumor
    Unclassified
Sertoli–stromal cell tumors
  Sertoli cell tumor
  Leydig cell tumor
  Sertoli–Leydig cell tumors
    Well-differentiated
    Of intermediate differentiation
    Poorly differentiated
    With heterologous elements
Gynandroblastoma
Sex cord tumor with annular tubules
Unclassified

adjuvant therapy. For patients who do not wish to remain fertile, hysterectomy and bilateral salpingo-oophorectomy should be performed.

Whole abdominal radiation has not been successful in patients with metastatic disease. Of nine patients with optimal residual disease (≤ 2 cm), only one survived (Schwartz and Smith, 1976). There have been isolated reports of the use of cisplatin and doxorubicin with or without cyclophosphamide in metastatic adult granulosa cell tumors. Of the 10 reported cases, five patients had complete remissions, three had partial remissions, and two did not respond to therapy (Jacobs and Bast, 1989; Gershenson et al, 1987; Kaye and Davies, 1986; Camlibel and Caputo, 1983). PVB was used in two recent large series: Colombo et al (1986) reported six complete responses and three partial responses among 11 patients, while similarly, Pecorelli et al (1988) reported six complete responses and five partial responses among 13 patients.

### Juvenile granulosa cell tumors

Scully (1977) described a distinctive form of granulosa cell tumors, which he termed juvenile, 97% of which occur during the first three decades of life (Young et al, 1984a). These tumors account for about 5% of granulosa cell tumors. Juvenile granulosa cell tumors are associated with a common form of isosexual pseudoprecocity, occurring in 80% of cases. They are bilateral in only 2% of cases, and less than 2% have spread beyond the ovary at the time of the initial diagnosis.

Because of the low incidence of bilaterality and malignant potential, unilateral salpingo-oophorectomy in young patients and total abdominal hysterectomy and bilateral salpingo-oophorectomy in those who do not desire future fertility is the recommended treatment. For those with metastatic juvenile granulosa cell tumors, radiation therapy or chemotherapy has met with limited success (Flament et al, 1988).

## Tumors of the Thecoma-Fibroma Group

### Thecomas

Thecomas are divided into typical and luteinized forms, the latter containing thecoma or fibroma cells and steroid-type cells (Zhang et al, 1982). Most patients are postmenopausal. Postmenopausal bleeding has been reported to occur in 60%, and endometrial cancer has been found in 20% of patients with thecoma (Bjorkholm and Silfversward, 1980). In a large series of luteinized thecomas, 50% were estrogenic and 39% were nonfunctional, but 11% were androgenic (Zhang et al, 1982). Like granulosa cell tumors, only 3% are bilateral, and it is unclear whether there has ever been a malignant thecoma. The cases reported were probably low-grade fibrosarcomas.

### Fibroma-fibrosarcoma

Most fibromatous ovarian tumors are cellular fibromas, which are benign and only rarely exhibit mitosis. The median age of incidence is about 50 years. Fibromatous tumors are only infrequently associated with Meigs' syndrome (Meigs, 1954) or Gorlin's syndrome (basal cell nevus syndrome) (Raggio,

1983). Occasionally, fibromatous tumors show increased mitosis, and these are designated fibrosarcomas. Fibrosarcomas are characterized by hypercellularity, a high mitotic rate, and marked nuclear pleomorphism.

Pratt and Scully (1981) analyzed 17 cases of fibromatous ovarian tumors in an attempt to separate cellular fibromas from fibrosarcomas. Of the 11 cellular fibromas, two did recur, but all 11 patients were alive and well from 33 months to 13 years. Of the six patients with fibrosarcomas, all had an aggressive course, and four of the six died within 2 months to 4 years after initial diagnosis.

### Sclerosing Ovarian Stromal Tumors

Sclerosing ovarian stromal tumors are a rare, distinct subtype of sex cord–stromal tumors, 80% of which occur in the second and third decades. These tumors were originally described by Chalvardjian and Scully (1973) and were so named because of their characteristic feature—cellular areas undergoing collagenous sclerosis. These tumors are unilateral and benign. Unlike thecomas, they are rarely associated with estrogen production, although there have been sporadic reports of estrogen and androgen production.

## Sertoli–Stromal Cell Tumors (Androblastomas)

Sertoli–stromal cell tumors of the ovary are sex cord–stromal tumors that contain Sertoli cells, Leydig cells, and fibroblasts, either alone or in combination. These tumors represent 0.5% of all ovarian tumors and are the most commonly virilizing. They occur primarily in the second and third decades, at a median age of 25 years (Young and Scully, 1985). Virilization is noted in about 33%, 60% are inert, and only a small percentage are feminizing. Less than 2% are bilateral and have spread beyond the ovary at initial diagnosis.

### Sertoli Cell Tumors

Pure Sertoli ovarian tumors are of gonadal stromal origin and are composed entirely of Sertoli cells. These tumors account for about 4% of Sertoli–stromal cell tumors. Pure Sertoli cell tumors are more often associated with estrogenic manifestations followed by virilization. Tavassoli and Norris (1980) reported 28 cases of pure Sertoli cell ovarian tumors from the Armed Forces Institute of Pathology. Although all 28 cases were stage IA with no evidence of metastasis at the initial operation, two patients suffered a recurrence, one in the pelvis and one in the peritoneal cavity.

To date, all pure Sertoli cell ovarian tumors have been unilateral. Treatment should consist of unilateral salpingo-oophorectomy in younger patients who desire future fertility and hysterectomy and bilateral salpingo-oophorectomy in all other patients.

### Leydig Cell Tumors

Stromal–Leydig cell ovarian tumors are rare, virilizing tumors that occur in the ovarian stroma. These tumors consist of Leydig cells in a nodular formation and contain characteristic Reinke crystalloids. Sex cord–stromal elements, such as Sertoli or granulosa cells, are not present. In addition to the characteristics of Leydig cells, spindle-shaped stromal cells are present that are distinct from the stromal luteomas. All reported cases of Leydig cell tumors have occurred in perimenopausal women, and all these were benign. Treatment is similar to that described for Sertoli cell tumors.

***Sertoli–Leydig Cell Tumors*** In 1931, Meyer et al reported 26 cases of what was referred to as arrhenoblastoma. In 1958, Morris and Scully suggested that the term Sertoli–Leydig cell tumors be used in place of arrhenoblastoma to avoid the connotation that all arrhenoblastomas or androblastomas were masculinizing. However, the WHO histologic classification of ovarian tumors still uses both designations to describe these tumors.

Sertoli–Leydig cell tumors are divided into four categories. The most common tumors are the well-differentiated Pick's adenomas, consisting of hollow tubules separated by Leydig cells. Intermediate differentiated tumors contain more primitive Sertoli–Leydig cells arranged similarly to those of the sex cord of the embryonal testes. Poorly differentiated sarcomatoid tumors consist of cells resembling spindle-cell sarcomas. The fourth category is Sertoli–Leydig cell tumors with heterologous elements containing argentaffin cells, cartilage, skeletal muscle, and mucus-secreting epithelium. All four categories have well-differentiated Leydig cells identical to those seen in the male testes. Fourteen cases have been reported with elevated serum AFP (Motoyama et al, 1989).

The prognosis for these tumors relates to the stage and degree of differentiation. Most deaths occur among patients with poorly differentiated tumors. Because these tumors are almost always unilateral, the treatment of choice is unilateral salpingo-oophorectomy in the young patient with stage I disease. In all other women, total abdominal hysterectomy and bilateral salpingo-oophorectomy should be performed. To date, no therapy has been reported to be effective in metastatic disease.

### Gynandroblastoma

Gynandroblastomas of the ovary are rare sex cord–stromal ovarian tumors that contain both ovarian-type cells (granulosa stromal cells) and testicular-type cells (Sertoli or Leydig cells). These tumors may be associated with feminizing or virilizing symptoms. Since the original description by Meyer in 1931, there have been only occasional reports on the incidence of gynandroblastoma, and reports of death from the disease are even more rare. The malignant potential and treatment are generally similar to those of granulosa cell tumors.

### Sex Cord Tumors With Annular Tubules

In 1970, Scully described a distinct subtype of ovarian stromal tumor characterized by simple and complex ring-shaped tubules having patterns between granulosa cell tumors and Sertoli cell tumors and resembling a gonadoblastoma without the germ cell components

(Scully, 1970b). Sex cord tumors with annular tubules may contain Sertoli cells, granulosa cells, Leydig cells, theca cells, or fibroblasts, alone or in combination, and are often associated with Peutz-Jeghers syndrome. Of the reported cases, 50% have been accompanied by symptoms suggestive of hyperestrogenism, including menstrual dysfunction, postmenopausal bleeding, or sexual precocity. About 40% of these tumors are thought to produce estrogens, and about 20% have a malignant course (Young et al, 1982).

## LIPID CELL TUMORS

Lipid or lipoid cell tumors occur within the ovarian stroma and consist of large, round, polygonal cells with a vacuolated, lipid-rich cytoplasm. Hayes and Scully (1987) have suggested that the designation lipid or lipoid cell tumors be replaced by the term "steroid cell tumors, not otherwise specified." Microscopically, these tumors resemble adrenal cortical, hilar, Leydig, or lutein cells. Since hilar, adrenal cortical, and luteinized ovarian stromal cells are cytologically similar and many contain little or no lipid, the term lipid cell tumor may be inaccurate, and separation of these tumors into a specific category is often impossible. Roughly 30% are clinically malignant. Of the 63 tumors reported by Hayes and Scully, 50% were androgenic, 6% estrogenic, and 38% nonfunctional, and 6% of the patients had Cushing's syndrome.

Taylor and Norris (1967) reported virilization in 77% of their 30 patients with unilateral lipid cell tumors. Of the 22 patients available for followup, 18 had apparent clinical stage IA disease and four had disease outside the ovary. All tumors containing crystalloids of Reinke proved to be benign in character on followup. Three (17%) of the 18 patients with apparent stage IA disease died with lipid cell tumor, as did three of the four patients with extraovarian involvement.

Ireland and Woodruff (1976) reported 22 cases of lipid cell ovarian tumors from the Emil Novak Ovarian Tumor Registry. All 18 patients available for followup had stage IA disease, and there was only one (5%) tumor-related death.

## HILAR CELL TUMORS

Hilar cells are normally present in the ovarian hilus but may be located in any part of the ovary. Of the 22 cases of hilar cell tumor reported by Ireland and Woodruff (1976), patients' ages ranged from 11 to 75 years, 80% being age 40 and older. Significant virilization was associated with 75% of these tumors. Almost all these tumors are unilateral, and most authors consider them to be benign. No tumor-related deaths were reported.

## OVARIAN SARCOMAS

Ovarian sarcomas account for only 1% of all ovarian malignancies and occur primarily in postmenopausal women of low parity at a median age of approximately 59 years. These tumors grow rapidly, and most patients present with abdominal masses at the initial examination. The result is that most of these patients die within 2 years of diagnosis, since 80% have metastasis beyond the pelvis at the initial examination and, to date, there is no effective therapy to control this spread.

Ovarian sarcomas may consist of only sarcomatous elements or as one component along with other malignant elements. For clinical purposes, these tumors can be grouped into four categories—pure sarcomas, mixed homologous müllerian sarcomas (carcinosarcoma), mixed heterologous müllerian sarcomas (mixed mesodermal sarcomas), and other ovarian sarcomas. Pure sarcomas contain a single recognizable element, whereas mixed sarcomas contain two or more elements.

Classification remains disorganized, with many terms, such as mixed mesodermal sarcoma, malignant mixed mesodermal tumors, and carcinosarcoma, often used to refer to the same disease. Malignant mixed mesodermal tumors were originally described as carcinosarcomas to designate neoplasms with intermingling carcinomatous and sarcomatous elements. As used today, however, the term mixed mesodermal sarcomas refers to neoplasms in which the sarcomatous elements contain heterologous (foreign) tissues to the ovary, such as striated muscle, cartilage, bone, or fat. In contrast, the term carcinosarcoma has been used when the tumor contains sarcoma derived from tissue normally present in the ovary (homologous). However, many reports group carcinosarcoma and heterologous mixed mesodermal sarcomas as a single entity.

### Mixed Mesodermal Sarcoma

Carlson et al (1983*a*) reported on 12 cases of mixed mesodermal sarcoma of the ovary treated with whole abdominal radiation and vincristine, actinomycin-D, and cyclophosphamide (VAC) chemotherapy. Four of the 12 patients had complete tumor control; however, only one patient was currently alive. One patient died at 55 months of an unrelated cause, but with no evidence of malignancy at autopsy, and two died during therapy, again with no evidence of tumor at autopsy.

In 1984, Morrow and colleagues reported on 30 ovarian sarcomas, 15 carcinosarcomas, and 15 mixed mesodermal sarcomas. Four patients were alive and well at 6, 11, 22, and 32 months, respectively. In a protocol somewhat similar to that reported by Carlson et al, patients were treated with VAC chemotherapy and whole abdominal radiation, with VAC and pelvic radiation, or with VAC chemotherapy alone. Of the four patients treated with VAC and whole abdominal radiation, only one was alive with no evidence of disease. The same was true for those patients treated with VAC and pelvic radiation. All four patients treated with VAC alone died. Lele et al (1980) used various chemotherapy combinations to achieve a 12% response rate in 24 patients with mixed mesodermal tumors of the ovary, including two complete responses—one with VAC and one with 5-FU, actinomycin-D, and cyclophosphamide. These attempts at improving survival for ovarian sar-

comas with VAC chemotherapy with or without radiation were made before the discovery of newer agents such as doxorubicin, cisplatin, and ifosfamide.

Subsequently, doxorubicin was evaluated in patients with ovarian sarcomas. In 1986, Morrow reported only one partial remission among 10 evaluable patients in a study for the GOG. In 1987, Wheelock reported on six patients treated with cisplatin, doxorubicin, and cyclophosphamide (PAC) chemotherapy, five of whom died within less than 15 months. In contrast, Anderson et al (1989) reported on 10 patients with stage III and IV mixed mesodermal tumors of the ovary treated with PAC, cisplatin and cyclophosphamide, or with cisplatin and doxorubicin. Among the six patients with measurable disease, there were four complete and two partial responses.

### Adenosarcoma and Endometrioid Stromal Sarcoma

Clement and Scully (1977) described the first two cases of ovarian adenosarcoma as low-grade sarcomas associated with local pelvic recurrence and long-term survival. Kao and Norris (1978) reported 11 additional cases of adenosarcoma of the ovary and in the adnexal region. All of the five lowest grade tumors were confined to the ovary and did not recur after surgical excision, whereas two of the three intermediate-grade tumors extended beyond the ovary but were arrested by combination chemotherapy.

Before 1984, when Young and colleagues reported on 23 cases of endometrioid stromal sarcoma of the ovary, only nine cases of this rare tumor had been reported (Young et al, 1984*b*). The authors emphasized that these low-grade tumors had an indolent clinical course and should be separated from other ovarian sarcomas. They also recommended progesterone therapy in metastatic low-grade endometrioid stromal sarcoma.

### Fibrosarcomas

Most fibromatous ovarian tumors are benign and have only rare mitosis. Occasionally, there are fibromatous tissues with increased mitosis, which are designated fibrosarcomas. They are characterized by hypercellularity, high mitotic rate and marked nuclear pleomorphism. Pratt and Scully (1981) analyzed 17 cases of fibromatous ovarian tumors in an attempt to separate cellular fibromas from fibrosarcomas. Of the 11 cellular fibromas, two did recur, but all 11 were alive and well from 33 months to 13 years. Of the six fibrosarcomas, all pursued an aggressive course and four of the six patients were dead two months to four years after initial operation.

## REFERENCES

Abdulhay G, DiSaia P, Creasman W, et al: Human lymphoblastoid interferon in the treatment of advanced epithelial ovarian malignancies: A Gynecologic Oncology Group study. *ASCO Abstracts* No C-652, 1984, p 167.

Adams M, Kerby IJ, Rocker I, et al: A comparison of the toxicity and efficacy of cisplatin and carboplatin in advanced ovarian cancer. *Acta Oncol* 28:57, 1989.

Aguirre P, Scully RE: Malignant neuroectodermal tumor of the ovary. A distinctive form of monodermal teratoma. A report of five cases. *Am J Surg Pathol* 6:283, 1982.

Alberts DS, Garcia-Kendall D, Surwit EA: Phase II of mitomycin-C plus 5-FU in the treatment of drug-refractory ovarian cancer. *Semin Oncol* 15:22, 1988a.

Alberts DS, Green S, Hannigan E, et al: Improved efficacy of carboplatin/cyclophosphamide versus cisplatin/cyclophosphamide: Preliminary report of a phase III randomized trial in stages III-IV suboptimal ovarian cancer. *Proc ASCO* 8(588):151, 1989.

Alberts DS, Surwit EA, Peng YM, et al: Phase I clinical and pharmacokinetic study of mitoxantrone given to patients by intraperitoneal administration. *Cancer Res* 48:5874, 1988b.

Anderson H, Wagstaff J, Crowther D, et al: Comparative toxicity of cisplatin, carboplatin (CBDCA), and iproplatin (CHIP) in combination with cyclophosphamide in patients with advanced epithelial ovarian cancer. *Eur J Cancer Clin Oncol* 24:1471, 1988.

Anderson WA, Young DE, Peters WA, et al: Platinum-based combination chemotherapy for malignant mixed mesodermal tumors of the ovary. *Gynecol Oncol* 32:319, 1989.

Asadourian LA, Taylor HB: Dysgerminoma. An analysis of 105 cases. *Obstet Gynecol* 33:370, 1969.

Aure JC, Hoeg K, Kolstad P: Clinical and histologic studies of ovarian carcinoma: Longterm follow-up of 990 cases. *Obstet Gynecol* 37:1, 1971.

Bagley CM, Young RC, Canellos GP: Treatment of ovarian carcinoma: Possibilities for progress. *N Engl J Med* 287:856, 1972.

Barlow JJ, Piver MS: Methotrexate with citrovorum factor rescue alone and in combination with cyclophosphamide in ovarian cancer. *Cancer Treat Rep* 60:527, 1976.

Barlow JJ, DiCioccio RA, Dillard PH, et al: Frequency of an allele for low activity of alpha-L-fucosidase in sera: Possible increase in epithelial ovarian cancer patients. *J Natl Cancer Inst* 67:1005, 1981.

Barnhill D, Heller P, Brzozwski P, et al: Epithelial ovarian carcinoma of low malignant potential. *Obstet Gynecol* 65:53, 1985.

Bast RC, Klug TL, St. John E, et al: A radioimmunoassay using a monoclonal antibody to monitor the course of epithelial ovarian cancer. *N Engl J Med* 309:883, 1983.

Beecham JB, Blessing J, Creasman W, et al: Tamoxifen responsiveness, hormone receptors and tumor grade: Prospective study of 105 advanced ovarian cancer patients. *Gynecol Oncol* 29:136, 1988.

Bell DA, Weinstock MA, Scully RE: Peritoneal implants of ovarian serous borderline tumors: Histologic features and prognosis. *Cancer* 62:2212, 1988.

Berlin NI, VanScott EJ, Clendenning WE, et al: Basal cell nevus syndrome: Combined clinical staff conference at the National Institutes of Health. *Ann Intern Med* 64:403, 1966.

Bertelsen K, Hansen MK, Pedersen PH, et al: The prognostic and therapeutic value of second-look laparotomy in advanced ovarian cancer. *Br J Obstet Gynecol* 95:1231, 1988.

Bertelsen K, Jakobsen A, Andersen JE, et al: A randomized study of cyclophosphamide and cis-platinum with or without doxorubicin in advanced ovarian carcinoma. *Gynecol Oncol* 28:161, 1987.

Bitha P, Carvajal SG, Citarella RY, et al: A new family of water-soluble, third generation antitumor platinum complexes. *J Med Chem* 32:2063, 1989.

Bjorkholm E: Blood group distribution in women with ovarian cancer. *Int J Epidemiol* 13:15, 1984.

Bjorkholm E: *Personal communication*, 1985.

Bjorkholm E, Silfversward C: Theca cell tumors. Clinical features and prognosis. *Acta Radiol Oncol Radiat Phys Biol* 19:241, 1980.

Bjorkholm E, Pettersson F, Einhorn N, et al: Long-term follow-up and prognostic factors in ovarian carcinoma: The Radiumhemmet Series 1958-1973. *Acta Radiol Oncol* 21:413, 1982.

Boltz EM, Kefford RF, Leary JA, et al: Amplification of c-ras-Ki oncogene in human ovarian tumors. *Int J Cancer* 43:428, 1989.

Bourne T, Campbell S, Steer C, et al: Transvaginal colour flow imaging: A possible new screening technique for ovarian cancer. *Br Med J* 299:1367, 1989.

Bruckner HW, Motwani BT: Treatment of advanced refractory ovarian carcinoma with a gonadotropin-releasing hormone analogue. *Am J Obstet Gynecol* 161:1216, 1989.

Bruckner HW, Cohen CJ, Feuer E, et al: Long term follow-up in stage III and IV ovarian cancer. Controlled clinical trials utilizing cisplatin, doxorubicin, cyclophosphamide and hexamethylmelamine. *Proc ASCO* 6:121, 1987.

Buchsbaum HJ, Brady MF, Delgado G, et al: Surgical staging of carcinoma of the ovaries. *Surg Gynecol Obstet* 169:226, 1989.

Burns BC, Rutledge F, Gallagher HS: Phenylalanine mustard in the palliative management of carcinoma of the ovary. *Obstet Gynecol* 22:30, 1963.

Buskirk SJ, Schray MF, Malkasian GD, et al: Ovarian dysgerminoma: A retrospective analysis of results of treatment, sites of treatment failure and radiosensitivity. *Mayo Clin Proc* 62:1149, 1987.

Camlibel FT, Caputo TA: Chemotherapy for granulosa cell tumors. *Am J Obstet Gynecol* 145:763, 1983.

The Cancer and Steroid Hormone Study of the Centers for Disease Control and the National Institute of Child Health and Human Development: The reduction in risk of ovarian cancer associated with oral-contraceptive use. *N Engl J Med* 316:650, 1987.

Carlson JA Jr, Edwards C, Wharton JT, et al: Mixed mesodermal sarcoma of the ovary. Treatment with combination radiation therapy and chemotherapy. *Cancer* 52:1473, 1983a.

Carlson RW, Sikie BI, Turbow MM, et al: Combination cisplatin, vinblastine, and bleomycin chemotherapy (PVB) for malignant germ-cell tumors of the ovary. *J Clin Oncol* 1:645, 1983b.

Carmio-Pereira J, Cost FO, Henrigues E, et al: Advanced ovarian carcinoma: A prospective and randomized clinical trial of cyclophosphamide versus combination cytotoxic chemotherapy (hexaCAF). *Cancer* 48:1947, 1981.

Chaitin BA, Gershenson DM, Evans HL: Mucinous tumors of the ovary: A clinicopathologic study of 70 cases. *Cancer* 55:1958, 1985.

Chalvardjian A, Scully RE: Sclerosing stromal tumors of the ovary. *Cancer* 31:664, 1973.

Chapman PB, Kolitz JE, Hakes TB, et al: A phase I trial of intraperitoneal recombinant interleukin-2 in patients with ovarian carcinoma. *Invest New Drugs* 6:179, 1988.

Chatal JF, Fumoleau P, Saccavini JC, et al: Immunoscintigraphy of recurrences of gynecologic carcinomas. *J Nucl Med* 28:1807, 1987.

Chiara S, Conte PF, Bruzzone M, et al: Cisplatin and cyclophosphamide in early epithelial ovarian carcinoma. *Chemotherapia* 6:380, 1987.

Clarke DGC, Hilaris B, Roussis C, et al: The role of radiation therapy (including isotopes) in the treatment of cancer of the ovary. Results of 614 patients treated at Memorial Hospital in New York, New York. In Ariel IM (ed) *Progress in Clinical Cancer*, Vol 5. New York, Grune and Stratton, 1973, pp 227-235.

Clarke-Pearson DL, Bandy LC, Dudzinski M, et al: Computed tomography in evaluation of patients with ovarian carcinoma in complete clinical remission. *JAMA* 255:627, 1986.

Clement FB, Scully RE: Extrauterine mesodermal (müllerian) adenosarcoma. A clinical pathologic analysis of five cases. *Am Soc Clin Pathol* 59:276, 1977.

Coleman R, Clarke J, Gore M, et al: A phase II study of mitroxantrone in advanced carcinoma of the ovary. *Cancer Chemother Pharmacol* 24:200, 1989.

Colombo N, Sessa C, Landoni F, et al: Cisplatin, vinblastine and bleomycin combination chemotherapy in metastatic granulosa cell tumor of the ovary. *Obstet Gynecol* 67:265, 1986.

Conte PF, Bruzzone M, Chiara S, et al: A randomized trial comparing cisplatin plus cyclophosphamide versus cisplatin, doxorubicin and cyclophosphamide in advanced ovarian cancer. *J Clin Oncol* 4:965, 1986.

Council of Scientific Affairs: Magnetic resonance imaging of the abdomen and pelvis. *JAMA* 261:420, 1989.

Cramer DW, Welch WR: Determinants of ovarian cancer risk. II. Inferences regarding pathogenesis. *J Natl Cancer Inst* 71:717, 1983.

Cramer DW, Roth LM, Ulbright TM, et al: Evaluation of reproducibility of the World Health Organization classification of common ovarian cancers. *Arch Pathol Lab Med* 111:819, 1987.

Cramer DW, Welch WR, Cassells S, et al: Mumps, menarche, menopause and ovarian cancer. *Am J Obstet Gynecol* 147:1, 1983.

Cramer DW, Welch WR, Hutchison GB, et al: Dietary animal fat in relation to ovarian cancer risk. *Obstet Gynecol* 63:833, 1984.

Cramer DW, Welch WR, Scully RE, et al: Ovarian cancer and talc. A case-control study. *Cancer* 50:372, 1982.

Cramer DW, Willett WC, Bell DA, et al: Galactose consumption and metabolism in relation to the risk of ovarian cancer. *Lancet* 2:66, 1989.

Creasman WT, Fetter BF, Hammond CB, et al: Germ cell malignancies of the ovary. *Obstet Gynecol* 53:226, 1979.

Creech RH, Shah MK, Catalano RB, et al: Phase II study of low-dose mitomycin in patients with ovarian cancer previously treated with chemotherapy. *Cancer Treat Rep* 69:1271, 1985.

Currie JL, Bagne F, Harris C, et al: Radioactive chromic phosphate suspension: Studies on distribution, drug absorption, and effective therapeutic radiation in phantoms, dogs and patients. *Gynecol Oncol* 12:193, 1981.

Curtin JP, Rubin SC, Hoskins WJ, et al: Second look laparotomy in endodermal sinus tumor: A report of two patients with normal levels of alpha-fetoprotein and residual tumor at reexploration. *Obstet Gynecol* 73:893, 1989.

Davis HM, Zurawski VR, Bast RC, et al: Characterization of the CA 125 antigen associated with human epithelial ovarian carcinomas. *Cancer Res* 46:6143, 1986.

Davis TE, Loprinzi CL, Buchler DA: Combination chemotherapy with cisplatin, vinblastine and bleomycin for endodermal sinus tumor of the ovary. *Gynecol Oncol* 19:46, 1984.

Decker DG, Fleming TR, Malkasian GD, et al: Cyclophosphamide plus cisplatinum in combination. Treatment program for stage III or IV ovarian carcinoma. *Obstet Gynecol* 60:481, 1982.

Decker DG, Mussey E, Malkasian GD, et al: Adjuvant therapy for advanced ovarian malignancy. *Am J Obstet Gynecol* 97:171, 1967.

Dee GJ, Austin JK, Mutter DL: Bleomycin-associated pulmonary fibrosis: Rapidly fatal progression without chest radiotherapy. *J Surg Oncol* 35:135, 1987.

Dembo AJ: Abdominopelvic radiotherapy in ovarian cancer. Ten-year experience. *Cancer* 55:2285, 1985.

Dembo AJ, Bush RS, Beale HA, et al: A randomized clinical trial of moving strip versus open field whole abdominal radiation in patients with invasive epithelial cancer of the ovary. *Proc Am Soc Clin Oncol* 2:146, 1983.

DePalo GM, DeLena M, DiRe F, et al: Melphalan versus Adriamycin in the treatment of advanced carcinoma of the ovary. *Surg Gynecol Obstet* 141:899, 1975.

DePalo G, Lattuada A, Kenda H, et al: Germ cell tumors of the ovary: The experience of the National Cancer Institute of Milan. I. Dysgerminoma. *Int J Radiat Oncol Biol Phys* 13:853, 1987.

DePalo G, Pilotti S, Kenda R, et al: Natural history of dysgerminoma. *Am J Obstet Gynecol* 143:799, 1982.

Dickersin DR, Klein IW, Scully RE: Small cell carcinoma of the ovary with hypercalcemia. Report of 11 cases. *Cancer* 49:188, 1982.

DiMarco A, Zunino F, Silverstrini R, et al: Interaction of some daunomycin derivatives with deoxyribonucleic acid and their biological activity. *Biochem Pharmacol* 20:1323, 1971.

Dozois RR, Kempers RD, Dahlin DC, et al: Ovarian tumors associated with the Peutz-Jeghers syndrome. *Ann Surg* 172:233, 1970.

Edmonson JH, McCormack GW, Fleming TR, et al: Comparison of cyclophosphamide plus cisplatin versus hexamethylmelamine, cyclophosphamide, doxorubicin and cisplatin in combination as initial chemotherapy for stage III and IV ovarian carcinomas. *Cancer Treat Rep* 69:1243, 1985.

Edmonson JH, McCormack GW, Wieand HS, et al: Cyclophosphamide/cisplatin versus cyclophosphamide/carboplatin in stage III and IV ovarian carcinoma, a comparison of equally myelosuppressive regimens. *J Natl Cancer Inst* 81:1500, 1989.

Edmonson JH, Wieand HS, McCormack GW: Letters: Role of hexamethylmelamine in the treatment of ovarian cancer. Where is the needle in the haystack? *J Natl Cancer Inst* 80:1172, 1988.

Edwards C, Herson J, Gershenson DM, et al: A prospective randomized clinical trial of melphalan and cis-platinum versus hexamethylmelamine, Adriamycin and cyclophosphamide in advanced ovarian cancer. *Gynecol Oncol* 15:261, 1983.

Egli GE, Newton M: The transport of carbon particles in the human female reproductive tract. *Fertil Steril* 12:151, 1961.

Ehrlich CE, Einhorn LH, Stehman FB, et al: Treatment of advanced epithelial ovarian cancer using cisplatin, Adriamycin and Cytoxan. The Indiana University experience. *Clin Obstet Gynecol* 10:325, 1983.

Ehrlich CE, Einhorn LH, Williams SD, et al: Chemotherapy for stage III-IV epithelial ovarian cancer with cis-dichlorodiammineplatinum

(II), Adriamycin and cyclophosphamide: A preliminary report. *Cancer Treat Rep* 63:281, 1979.

Epenetos AA, Carr D, Johnson PM, et al: Antibody guided radiolocalization of tumors in patients with testicular or ovarian cancer using two radioiodinated monoclonal antibodies to placental alkaline phosphatase. *Br J Radiol* 59:117, 1986.

Epenetos AA, Munro AJ, Stewart S, et al: Antibiotic-guided irradiation of advanced ovarian cancer with intraperitoneal administered radiolabeled monoclonal antibodies. *J Clin Oncol* 5:1890, 1987.

Fanning J, Foon KA: Immunotherapy of gynecologic malignancies. *Semin Surg Oncol* 6:364-368, 1990.

Fathala MR: Incessant ovulation: A factor in ovarian neoplasia. *Lancet* 2:163, 1971.

Flament GV, Caillaud JM, and Demeocq FF: Juvenile granulosa cell tumor of the ovary in children. A clinical study of 15 cases. *J Clin Oncol* 6:990, 1988.

Fletcher WGH: Clinical dose-response curves of human malignant epithelial tumors. *Br J Radiol* 46:1, 1973.

Flynt TR, Gallup DG: The postmenopausal palpable ovary syndrome. A 14 year review. *Milit Med* 146:666, 1981.

Foster BJ, Clagett-Carr K, Marsoni S, et al: Role of hexamethylmelamine in the treatment of ovarian cancer. Where is the needle in the haystack? *Cancer Treat Rep* 70:1003, 1986.

Fuks Z: The role of radiation therapy in the management of ovarian carcinoma. *Israel J Med Sci* 13:815, 1977.

Fuks Z, Rizel S, Biran S: Chemotherapeutic and surgical induction of pathological complete remission and whole abdominal irradiation for consolidation does not enhance the cure of stage III ovarian carcinoma. *J Clin Oncol* 6:509, 1988.

Gallion HH, van Nagell JR Jr, Donaldson ES, et al: Immature teratoma of the ovary. *Am J Obstet Gynecol* 146:361, 1983.

Gallion HH, van Nagell JR Jr, Donaldson ES, et al: Adjuvant oral alkylating chemotherapy in patients with stage I epithelial ovarian cancer. *Cancer* 63:1070, 1989.

Gallion HH, van Nagell JR Jr, Powell DF, et al: Therapy of endodermal sinus tumor of the ovary. *Am J Obstet Gynecol* 135:447, 1979.

Gardner WU: Hormonal imbalances in tumorigenesis. *Cancer Res* 8:397, 1948.

Genadry R, Poliakoff S, Rotmensch J, et al: Primary, papillary peritoneal neoplasia. *Obstet Gynecol* 58:730, 1981.

Gerbie MV, Brewer JI, Tamimi H: Primary choriocarcinoma of the ovary. *Obstet Gynecol* 46:720, 1975.

Gershenson DM, Silva EG: Serous ovarian tumors of low malignant potential with peritoneal implants. *Cancer* 65:578, 1990.

Gershenson DM, Copeland LJ, DelJunco G, et al: Second look laparotomy in the management of malignant germ cell tumors of the ovary. *Obstet Gynecol* 67:789, 1986a.

Gershenson DM, Copeland LJ, Kavanagh JJ, et al: Treatment of malignant nondysgerminomatous germ cell tumors of the ovary with vincristine, dactinomycin and cyclophosphamide. *Cancer* 56:2756, 1985.

Gershenson DM, Copeland LJ, Kavanagh JJ, et al: Treatment of metastatic stromal tumors of the ovary with cisplatin, doxorubicin and cyclophosphamide. *Obstet Gynecol* 70:765, 1987.

Gershenson DM, DelJunco G, Copeland L, et al: Mixed germ cell tumors of the ovary. *Obstet Gynecol* 64:200, 1984.

Gershenson DM, DelJunco G, Herson J, et al: Endodermal sinus tumor of the ovary: The M.D. Anderson experience. *Obstet Gynecol* 61:194, 1983.

Gershenson DM, DelJunco G, Silva EG, et al: Immature teratoma of the ovary. *Obstet Gynecol* 68:624, 1986b.

Gershenson DM, Kavanagh JJ, Copeland LJ, et al: Re-treatment of patients with recurrent epithelial ovarian cancer with cisplatin-based chemotherapy. *Obstet Gynecol* 73:798, 1989.

Gershenson DM, Wharton JT, Kline RC, et al: Chemotherapeutic complete remission in patients with metastatic ovarian dysgerminoma. *Cancer* 56:2594, 1986.

Goldie JH, Coldman AJ: A mathematical model for relating the drug sensitivity of tumors to their spontaneous mutation rate. *Cancer Treat Rep* 63:1727, 1979.

Goldstein SR, Subramanyam B, Snyder JR, et al: The postmenopausal cystic adnexal mass. The potential role of ultrasound conservative management. *Obstet Gynecol* 73:8, 1989.

Gordon A, Lipton D, Woodruff JD: Dysgerminoma: A review of 158 cases from the Emil Novak Ovarian Tumor Registry. *Obstet Gynecol* 58:497, 1981.

Granowska M, Britton KE, Shepherd JH, et al: A prospective study of ¹²³I labeled monoclonal antibody imaging in ovarian cancer. *J Clin Oncol* 4:730, 1986.

Greenspan EM, Bruckner HW: Comparison of regression induction with triethylenethiophosphoramide or methotrexate in bulky stage III ovarian carcinoma. *Natl Cancer Inst Monograph* 42:173, 1975.

Griffiths CT, Fuller AF: Intensive surgical and chemotherapeutic management of advanced ovarian cancer. *Surg Clin N Amer* 58:131, 1978.

Griffiths CT, Parker LM, Fuller AF Jr: Role of cytoreductive surgical treatment in the management of advanced ovarian cancer. *Cancer Treat Rep* 63:235, 1979.

Gruppo Interegionale Cooperativo Oncologico Ginecologia: Randomized comparison of cisplatin with cyclophosphamide/cisplatin and with cyclophosphamide/doxorubicin/cisplatin in advanced ovarian cancer. *Lancet* 2:353, 1987.

Hacker NF, Berek JS, Lagasse LD, et al: Primary cytoreductive surgery for epithelial ovarian cancer. *Obstet Gynecol* 61:413, 1983.

Hainsworth JD, Grosh WW, Burnett LS, et al: Advanced ovarian cancer: Long-term results of treatment with intensive cisplatin-based chemotherapy of brief duration. *Ann Intern Med* 108:165, 1988.

Hanisch FG, Uhlenbruck G, Dienst C, et al: CA 125 and CA19-9; two cancer-associated sialylsaccharide antigens on a mucus glycoprotein from human milk. *Eur J Biochem* 149:323, 1985.

Hart WR: Ovarian epithelial tumors of borderline malignancy (carcinoma of low malignant potential). *Human Pathol* 8:541, 1977.

Hart WR, Norris HJ: Borderline and ovarian malignant mucinous tumors of the ovary. *Cancer* 31:1031, 1973.

Hayes MC, Scully RE: Ovarian steroid cell tumors (not otherwise specified). A clinicopathologic analysis of 63 cases. *Am J Surg Pathol* 11:835, 1987.

Henderson WJ, Hamilton TC, Griffith K: Talc in normal and malignant ovarian tissue. *Lancet* 1:499, 1979.

Hester LL, White L: Radioactive colloidal chromic phosphate in the treatment of ovarian malignancies. *Am J Obstet Gynecol* 103:911, 1969.

Hoover R, Gray LA, Fraumeni JF: Stilbestrol and the risk of ovarian cancer. *Lancet* 2:533, 1977.

Hoskins WJ, Rubin SC, Dulaney E, et al: Influence of secondary cytoreduction at the time of second-look laparotomy on the survival of patients with epithelial ovarian carcinoma. *Gynecol Oncol* 34:365, 1989.

Howell SB, Jill S: Lack of synergy between cisplatin and cytarabine against ovarian carcinoma in vitro. *Cancer Treat Rep* 70:409, 1985.

Howell SB, Schiefer M, Andrews PA, et al: The pharmacology of intraperitoneally administered bleomycin. *J Clin Oncol* 5:2009, 1987a.

Howell SB, Zimm S, Markman M, et al: Long-term survival of advanced refractory ovarian carcinoma patients with small-volume disease treated with intraperitoneal chemotherapy. *J Clin Oncol* 5:1607, 1987b.

International Federation of Gynecology and Obstetrics: Changes in definitions of clinical staging for carcinoma of the cervix and ovary. *Am J Obstet Gynecol* 156:246, 1987.

Ireland K, Woodruff JD: Review: Masculinizing ovarian tumors. *Obstet Gynecol Surv* 31:2, 1976.

Ishikura H, Scully RE: Hepatoid carcinoma of the ovary. A report of five cases of newly diagnosed tumor. *Cancer* 60:2775, 1987.

Jacobs A, Deppe G, Cohen CJ: Combination chemotherapy of ovarian granulosa cell tumor with cisplatinum and doxorubicin. *Gynecol Oncol* 14:294, 1989.

Jacobs I, Bast RC: The CA 125 tumor-associated antigen: A review of the literature. *Human Reprod* 4:1, 1989.

Jacobs I, Bridges J, Reynolds C: Multimodal approach of screening for ovarian cancer. *Lancet* 1:268, 1988.

Jimerson GK, Woodruff JD: Ovarian extraembryonal teratoma. II. Endodermal sinus tumor mixed with other germ cell tumors. *Am J Obstet Gynecol* 127:302, 1977.

Julian CG, Woodruff JD: The biologic behavior of low grade papillary serous carcinoma of the ovary. *Obstet Gynecol* 40:860, 1978.

Kabawat SE, Bast RC, Welch WR, et al: Immunopathologic characterization of a monoclonal antibody that recognized common sur-

face antigens of human ovarian tumors of serous, endometrioid and clear cell types. *Am J Clin Pathol* 79:98, 1983.

Kao GF, Norris HJ: Benign and low-grade variants of mixed mesodermal tumor (adenosarcoma) of the ovary and adnexal region. *Cancer* 42:1314, 1978.

Kashimura M, Shinohra M, Hirakawa T, et al: Clinical pathologic study of squamous cell carcinoma of the ovary. *Gynecol Oncol* 34:75, 1989.

Katzenstein ALA, Mazur MT, Mortan TE, et al: Proliferative serous tumors of the ovary. Histologic features and prognosis. *Am J Surg Pathol* 2:339, 1978.

Kavanagh JJ, Roberts W, Townsend P, et al: Leuprolide acetate in the treatment of refractory or persistent ovarian cancer. *J Clin Oncol* 7:115, 1989.

Kaye SB, Davies E: Cyclophosphamide, Adriamycin and cisplatinum for the treatment of advanced granulosa cell tumors using serum estradiol as a tumor marker. *Gynecol Oncol* 24:261, 1986.

Kaiser DW, Thurston JT, Dudley JR, et al: Cyanuric chloride derivatives. II. Substituted melamines. *J Am Chem Soc* 73:2984, 1951.

Kjorstad KE, Albeller V: Carcinoma of the ovary borderline lesions and their therapy. In Bender HG and Beck L (eds): *Carcinoma of the Ovary. Cancer Campaign, Vol. 7.* Stuttgart, Gustav Fischer Verlag, 1983, pp 131-135.

Klaassen D, Starreveld A, Shelly W, et al: External beam pelvic radiotherapy plus intraperitoneal radioactive chromic phosphate in early stage ovarian cancer. A toxic combination. *Int J Radiat Oncol Biol Phys* 11:1801, 1985.

Klemi PJ, Joensuu H, Maenpaa J, et al: Influence of cellular DNA content on survival in ovarian carcinoma. *Obstet Gynecol* 74:200, 1989.

Kolstad P, Davy M, Hoeg K: Individualized treatment of ovarian cancer. *Am J Obstet Gynecol* 128:617, 1977.

Kurman RJ, Norris HJ: Embryonal carcinoma of the ovary. A clinicopathologic entity distinct from endodermal sinus tumor resembling embryonal carcinoma of the adult testis. *Cancer* 38:2420, 1976a.

Kurman RJ, Norris HJ: Endodermal sinus tumor of the ovary. A clinical and pathologic analysis of 71 cases. *Cancer* 38:2404, 1976b.

Kurman RJ, Norris HJ: Malignant mixed germ cell tumors of the ovary. A clinical and pathologic analysis of 30 cases. *Obstet Gynecol* 48:579, 1976c.

Kurman RJ, Goebelemann U, Taylor CR: Steroid localization in granulosa-theca tumors of the ovary. *Cancer* 43:2377, 1979.

Kvale G, Heuch I, Nilssen S, et al: Reproductive factors and risk of ovarian cancer: A prospective study. *Int J Cancer* 42:246, 1989.

Lappohn RE, Burger HG, Bouma J, et al: Inhibin as a marker for granulosa cell tumors. *N Engl J Med* 321:790, 1989.

Lavin PT, Knapp RC, Malkasian G, et al: CA 125 for the monitoring of ovarian carcinoma during primary therapy. *Obstet Gynecol* 69:223, 1987.

Lawton F, Blackledge G, Chetiyawardana A, et al: A phase II study of mitoxantrone in epithelial ovarian cancer. *Proc ASCO* 5(436):112, 1986.

Lawton FG, Redman CW, Luesley DM, et al: Neoadjuvant (cytoreductive) chemotherapy combined with intervention debulking surgery in advanced, unresected epithelial ovarian cancer. *Obstet Gynecol* 73:61, 1989.

Lee JH, Kavanagh JJ, Wharton JT, et al: Allele loss at the c-Ha-ras1 locus in human ovarian cancer. *Cancer Res* 49:1222, 1989a.

Lee RB, Kelly J, Elg SA, et al: Pregnancy following conservative surgery and adjunctive chemotherapy for stage III immature teratoma of the ovary. *Obstet Gynecol* 73:853, 1989b.

Leiberman AJ, Kruse B, McSweeney MB: Transvaginal sonography: Comparison with transabdominal sonography in the diagnosis of pelvic masses. *Am J Radiol* 151:8, 1988.

Leichner PK, Bash SA, Back SC, et al: Effects of injection volume on the tissue dose, dose rate and therapeutic potential of intraperitoneal ³²P. *Radiology* 1401:193, 1981.

Lele SB, Piver MS, Barlow JJ: Chemotherapy in the management of mixed mesodermal tumors of the ovary. *Gynecol Oncol* 10:298, 1980.

Leonard RC, Smart GE, Livingstone JRB, et al: Randomized trial comparing prednimustine combination chemotherapy for advanced ovarian carcinoma. *Cancer Chemother Pharmacol* 23:105, 1989.

Levin L, Hryniuk WM: Dose intensity analysis of chemotherapy regimens in ovarian carcinoma. *J Clin Oncol* 5:756, 1987.

Liang AP, Levenson AG, Layde PM, et al: Risk of breast, uterine corpus and ovarian cancer in women receiving medroxyprogesterone injections. *JAMA* 249:2909, 1983.

Lim-Tan SK, Cajigas AG, Scully RE: Ovarian cystectomy for serous borderline tumors. A follow-up study of 35 cases. *Obstet Gynecol* 5:775, 1988.

Lippman SM, Alberts DS, Slymen DJ, et al: Second-look laparotomy in epithelial ovarian carcinoma. Prognostic factors associated with survival duration. *Cancer* 61:2571, 1988.

Litterst CL: Alterations in the toxicity of cis-dichlorodiammineplatinum (II) and tissue localization of platinum as a function of NaCl concentration in the vehicle of administration. *Toxicol Appl Pharmacol* 61:99, 1981.

Lloyd RE, Jones SE, Solomon SE, et al: Combination chemotherapy with Adriamycin (NSC-123127) and cyclophosphamide (NSC-26271) for solid tumors. A phase II trial. *Cancer Treat Rep* 60:77, 1976.

Loehrer PJ, Lauer R, Roth BJ, et al: Salvage therapy in recurrent germ cell cancer: Ifosfamide, cisplatin plus either vinblastine or etoposide. *Ann Intern Med* 109:540, 1988.

Lokey JL, Baker JJ, Price NA, et al: Cisplatin, vinblastine and bleomycin for endodermal sinus tumor of the ovary. *Ann Intern Med* 94:56, 1981.

Lomax CW, May HV, Panko WB, et al: Progesterone production by an ovarian granulosa cell carcinoma. *Obstet Gynecol* 50:339S, 1977.

Longo DL, Young RC: Cosmetic talc and ovarian cancer. *Lancet* 2:349, 1979.

Lotze MT, Chang AE, Seipp CA, et al: High-dose recombinant interleukin-2 in the treatment of patients with disseminated cancer. *JAMA* 256:3117, 1986.

Lotze MT, Custer MC, Rosenberg SA: Intraperitoneal administration of interleukin-2 in patients with cancer. *Arch Surg* 121:1373, 1979.

Louie KG, Ozols RF, Meyers CE, et al: Long term results of cisplatin containing combination chemotherapy regimens in the treatment of advanced ovarian carcinoma. *J Clin Oncol* 4:1579, 1986.

Luesley D, Blackledge G, Kelly K, et al: Failure of second-look laparotomy to influence survival in epithelial ovarian cancer. *Lancet* 2:599, 1988.

Lynch HT, Guinis MA, Albert S: Familial association of carcinoma of the breast and ovary. *Surg Gynecol Obstet* 138:717, 1974.

Lynch HT, Schuelke GS, Wells IC, et al: Hereditary ovarian carcinoma: Biomarker studies. *Cancer* 55:410, 1985.

MacBeth FR, MacDonald H, Williams CJ: Total abdominal and pelvic radiotherapy in the management of early stage ovarian carcinoma. *Int J Radiat Oncol Biol Phys* 15:353, 1988.

Malone JM, Gershenson DM, Creasy RK, et al: Endodermal sinus tumor of the ovary associated with pregnancy. *Obstet Gynecol* 68:86S, 1986.

Mangioni C, Bolis G, Pecorelli S, et al: Randomized trial in advanced ovarian cancer comparing cisplatin and carboplatin. *J Natl Cancer Inst* 81:1464, 1989.

Mann WJ, Patsner B, Cohen H, et al: Preoperative serum CA 125 levels in patients with surgical stage I invasive ovarian adenocarcinoma. *J Natl Cancer Inst* 80:208, 1988.

Mansi L, Panz N, Lastoria S: Diagnosis of ovarian cancer with radiolabeled monoclonal antibodies: Our experience using [131]I-B72.3. *Nucl Med Biol* 16:127, 1987.

Markman M, Hakes T, Reichman B, et al: Intraperitoneal therapy in the management of ovarian carcinoma. *Yale J Biol Med* 62:393, 1989.

Masterson JG, Nelson JH Jr: The role of chemotherapy in the treatment of gynecologic malignancy. *Am J Obstet Gynecol* 93:1102, 1965.

McGowan L, Parent L, Lednar W, et al: The woman at risk for developing ovarian cancer. *Gynecol Oncol* 7:325, 1979.

McGuire WP, Abeloff MD: Carboplatin substitution for cisplatin in the treatment of ovarian cancer—A word of caution. *J Natl Cancer Inst* 81:1438, 1989.

McGuire WP, Rowinsky EK, Rosenshein NB, et al: Taxol: A unique antineoplastic agent with significant activity in advanced epithelial neoplasms. *Ann Intern Med* 111:273, 1989.

Meigs JV: Fibroma of the ovary with ascites and hydrothorax. Meigs' syndrome. *Am J Obstet Gynecol* 67:962, 1954.

Mettlin C, Piver MS: A case controlled study of milk drinking and ovarian cancer risk. *Am J Epidemiol* 132:871-876, 1990.

Meyer R: Pathology of some special ovarian tumors and their relation to sex characteristics. *Am J Obstet Gynecol* 22:697, 1931.

Minyi T, Lijuan L: The characteristics of ovarian serous tumors of borderline malignancy. *Chinese Med J* 93:459, 1980.

Mitchell DG, Mintz MC, Spritzer CE, et al: Adnexal masses: MR imaging observations at 1.5T with US and CT correlation. *Radiol* 162:319, 1987.

Moebus V, Kreineberg R, Crombach G, et al: Evaluation of CA 125 as a prognostic and predictive factor in ovarian cancer. *J Tumor Marker Oncol* 3(2):251-258, 1988.

Mollman JE, Glover DJ, Hogan WM, et al: Cisplatin neuropathy. Risk factors, prognosis and protection by WR-2721. *Cancer* 61:2192, 1988.

Montz FJ, Rodgers KE, DiZerega GS, et al: Follicle regulatory protein (FRP): A new tumor marker for granulosa cell tumors. *Soc Gynecol Oncol Abst* 1989, No 101.

Morris JM, Scully RE: *Endocrine Pathology of the Ovary*. St. Louis, The CV Mosby Co, 1958, p 89.

Morrow CP, Bundy BN, Hoffman J, et al: Adriamycin chemotherapy for malignant mixed mesodermal tumor of the ovary. *Am J Clin Oncol* 9:24, 1986.

Morrow CP, d'Ablaing G, Brady LW, et al: A clinical and pathologic study of 30 cases of malignant mixed müllerian epithelial and mesenchymal ovarian tumors. Gynecologic Oncology Group study. *Gynecol Oncol* 18:278, 1984.

Motoyama T, Watanabe H, Gotoh A, et al: Ovarian Sertoli–Leydig cell tumor with elevated serum alpha fetoprotein. *Cancer* 63:2047, 1989.

Mueller CW, Tompkins P, Lapp WA: Dysgerminoma of the ovary: Analysis of 427 cases. *Am J Obstet Gynecol* 60:153, 1950.

Mulder POM, Willemse PHB, Aalders JG, et al: High-dose chemotherapy with autologous bone marrow transplantation in patients with refractory ovarian cancer. *Eur J Cancer Clin Oncol* 25:645, 1989.

Murolo C, Costantini G, Foglia T, et al: Ultrasound examination in ovarian cancer patients: A comparison with second look laparotomy. *J Ultrasound Med* 8:441, 1989.

Neijt JP, ten Bokkel Huinink WW, van der Burg ME, et al: Randomized trial comparing two combination chemotherapy regimens (CHAP-5 vs CP) in advanced ovarian carcinoma. *J Clin Oncol* 5:1157, 1987.

Neijt JP, van der Burg ME, Vriesendorp R, et al: Randomized trial comparing two combination chemotherapy regimens (Hexa-CAF vs CHAP-5) in advanced ovarian carcinoma. *Lancet* 2:594, 1984.

Norris HJ, Taylor HB: Prognosis of granulosa-theca tumors of the ovary. *Cancer* 21:255, 1968.

Norris HJ, Zerkin HJ, Benson WL: Immature (malignant) teratoma of the ovary. *Cancer* 37:2359, 1976.

Omura GA, Bundy BN, Berek JS, et al: Randomized trial of cyclophosphamide plus cisplatin with or without doxorubicin in ovarian carcinoma. A Gynecologic Oncology Group study. *J Clin Oncol* 7:457, 1989.

Osborne RJ, Malik ST, Slevin ML, et al: Tamoxifen in refractory ovarian cancer: The use of a loading dose schedule. *Br J Cancer* 57:115, 1988.

Ozols RF, Ostchega Y, Myers CE, et al: High dose cisplatin in hypertonic saline in refractory ovarian cancer. *J Clin Oncol* 3:1246, 1985.

Parker LM, Griffiths CT, Yankee RA, et al: High dose methotrexate with leucovorin rescue in ovarian cancer. Phase II study. *Cancer Treat Rep* 63:275, 1979.

Parmar H, Phillips RH, Rustin G, et al: Therapy of advanced ovarian cancer with D-Trp-6-LH-RH (decapeptyl) microcapsules. *Biomed Pharmacother* 42:531, 1988.

Pecorelli S, Wagener P, Bonazzi C, et al: Cisplatin, vinblastine, and bleomycin combination chemotherapy in recurrent or advanced granulosa cell tumor of the ovary. An EORTC Gynecologic Cancer Cooperative Group study. *Proc ASCO* 7:147, 1988.

Perrone T, Steeper TA, Dehner LP: Alpha-fetoprotein localization in pure ovarian teratoma. An immunohistochemical study of 12 cases. *Am J Clin Pathol* 88:713, 1987.

Pfeifle CE, Howell SB, Felthouse RD, et al: High dose cisplatin with sodium thiosulfate protection. *J Clin Oncol* 3:237, 1985.

Phibbs GD, Smith JP, Stanhope CR: Analysis of sites of persistent cancer at "second-look" laparotomy in patients with ovarian cancer. *Am J Obstet Gynecol* 147:611, 1983.

Piver MS: Radioactive colloids in the treatment of stage IA ovarian cancer. *Obstet Gynecol* 40:42, 1972.

Piver MS: Personal communication, 1989.

Piver MS, Baker TR, and Driscoll DL: Lack of substantial five year disease-free survival by primary aggressive surgery and cisplatin-based chemotherapy or by salvage intraperitoneal cisplatin-based chemotherapy. *Eur J Gynecol Oncol* 11:243-250, 1990.

Piver MS, Baker TR: The potential for optimal ($\leq$ 2 cm) cytoreductive surgery in advanced carcinoma at a tertiary medical center: A prospective study. *Gynecol Oncol* 24:1, 1986.

Piver MS, Barlow JJ, Lele SB: Incidence of subclinical metastasis in stage I and II ovarian carcinoma. *Obstet Gynecol* 52:100, 1978.

Piver MS, Barlow JJ, Lele SB, et al: Intraperitoneal chromic phosphate in peritoneoscopically confirmed stage I ovarian adenocarcinoma. *Am J Obstet Gynecol* 144:8, 1982.

Piver MS, Lele SB, Bakshi S, et al: Five and ten year estimated survival and disease-free rates after intraperitoneal chromic phosphate: Stage I ovarian adenocarcinoma. *Am J Clin Oncol* 11:515, 1988a.

Piver MS, Lele SB, Barlow JJ, et al: Second-look laparoscopy prior to proposed second-look laparotomy. *Obstet Gynecol* 55:571, 1980.

Piver MS, Lele SB, Marchetti DL, et al: The impact of aggressive debulking surgery and cisplatin-based chemotherapy on progression-free survival in stage III and IV ovarian carcinoma. *J Clin Oncol* 6:983, 1988b.

Piver MS, Lele SB, Marchetti DL, et al: Surgically documented response to intraperitoneal cisplatin, cytarabine and bleomycin after intravenous cisplatin-based chemotherapy in advanced ovarian adenocarcinoma. *J Clin Oncol* 6:1679, 1988c.

Piver MS, Malfetano J, Baker TR, et al: Adjuvant cisplatin based chemotherapy for stage I ovarian adenocarcinoma. A preliminary report. *Gynecol Oncol* 35:69, 1989.

Piver MS, Mettlin CJ, Tsukada Y, et al: Familial Ovarian Cancer Registry. *Obstet Gynecol* 64:195, 1984.

Pratt J, Scully RE: Cellular fibromas and fibrosarcomas of the ovary. Comparative clinical pathologic analysis of 17 cases. *Cancer* 47:2663, 1981.

Pratt J, Bhan AK, Dickersin JR, et al: Hepatoid yolk sac tumor of the ovary (endodermal sinus tumor with hepatoid differentiation). A light microscopical, ultrastructural and immunohistochemical study of seven cases. *Cancer* 50:2344, 1982.

Raggio M, Kaplan AL, Harberg JF: Recurrent ovarian fibromas with basal cell nevus syndrome (Gorlin's syndrome). *Obstet Gynecol* 61:95S, 1983.

Redman C, Lawton F, Stuart N, et al: Phase II study of combination 4′-epidoxorubicin and mitomycin-C in recurrent epithelial ovarian cancer. *Cancer Chemother Pharmacol* 23:51, 1989.

Reeves RD, Drake TS, O'Brien WF: Ultrasonographic versus clinical evaluation of pelvic mass. *Obstet Gynecol* 55:551, 1980.

Reichman B, Markman M, Hakes T, et al: Intraperitoneal cisplatin and etoposide in the treatment of refractory/recurrent ovarian carcinoma. *J Clin Oncol* 7:1327, 1989.

Reimer RI, Hoover R, Fraumeni JF, et al: Acute leukemia after alkylating agent therapy of ovarian cancer. *N Engl J Med* 297:177, 1977.

Robboy SJ, Scully RE: Ovarian teratoma with glial implants on the peritoneum. An analysis of 12 cases. *Human Pathol* 1:643, 1970.

Robey SS, Silva EG, Gershenson DH, et al: Transitional cell carcinoma in high-grade high-stage ovarian carcinoma. *Cancer* 63:839, 1989.

Rose DP, Boyar AP, Wynder EL: International comparisons of mortality rates for cancer of the breast, ovary, prostate and colon and per capita food consumption. *Cancer* 58:2363, 1986.

Rosen GF, Lurain JR, Newton M: Hexamethylmelamine in ovarian cancer after failure to cisplatin-based multiple-agent chemotherapy. *Gynecol Oncol* 27:173, 1987.

Rosenberg B, VanCamp L, Krigas T: Inhibition of cell division in *Escherichia coli* by electrolysis products from a platinum electrode. *Nature* 205:698, 1965.

Rulin MC, Preston AL: Adnexal masses in postmenopausal women. *Obstet Gynecol* 70:578, 1987.

Russell P, Merkur H: Proliferating ovarian epithelial tumors: A clinico-pathological analysis of 144 cases. *Austral NZ J Obstet Gynecol* 19:45, 1979.

Rutledge F, Burns BC: Chemotherapy for advanced ovarian cancer. *Am J Obstet Gynecol* 96:761, 1966.

Samuels ML, Howe CD, MacDonald EJ: *Alkylating Agents in the Treatment of Patients With Advanced Cancer of the Ovary, Carcinoma of the Uterine Cervix, Endometrium and Ovary*. Chicago. Yearbook Medical Publishers, 1962, p 329.

Schwartz PE, Smith JP: Treatment of ovarian stromal tumors. *Am J Obstet Gynecol* 125:402, 1976.

Scully RE: Common epithelial tumors of borderline malignancies (carcinomas of low malignant potential). *Bull de Cancer (Paris)* 69:228, 1982.

Scully RE: Ovarian tumors. *Am J Pathol* 87:686, 1977.

Scully RE: Recent progress in ovarian cancer. *Human Pathol* 1:73, 1970a.

Scully RE: Sex cord tumor with annular tubules. A distinctive ovarian tumor of the Peutz-Jeghers syndrome. *Cancer* 25:1107, 1970b.

Seligman AM, Rutenburg AM, Persky L, et al: Effect of 2-chloro-2′-hydroxydiethyl sulfide (hemisulfur mustard) on carcinomatosis with ascites. *Cancer* 5:354, 1952.

Senekjian EK, Weiser PA, Talerman A, et al: Vinblastine, cisplatin, cyclophosphamide, bleomycin, doxorubicin, and etoposide in the treatment of small cell carcinoma of the ovary. *Cancer* 64:1183, 1989.

Serov SF, Scully RE, Sobin LH: *Histological typing of ovarian tumors. International Classification of Tumors #9*. World Health Organization, Geneva, 1973.

Sessa C: European studies with cisplatin and cisplatin analogs in advanced ovarian cancer. *Eur J Cancer Clin Oncol* 22:1271, 1986a.

Sessa C, Bonazzi C, Landoni F, et al: Cisplatin, vinblastine and bleomycin combination chemotherapy in endodermal sinus tumor of the ovary. *Obstet Gynecol* 70:220, 1987.

Sessa C, Cavalli F, Kaye S, et al: Phase II study of iproplatin (CHIP) in advanced epithelial ovarian carcinoma. *Proc ASCO* 5(479):123, 1986.

Sevelda P, Dittrich C, Salzer H: Prognostic value of the rupture of the capsule in stage I epithelial ovarian carcinoma. *Gynecol Oncol* 35:321, 1989.

Silverburg E: Cancer statistics 1989. *Ca-A Cancer Journal for Clinicians*. Vol 39, No 1, Jan/Feb, 1989.

Skipper HL, Schabel FN, Lloyd HH: Experimental therapeutic and kinetic selection overgrowth of specifically and permanently drug resistant tumor cells. *Semin Hematol* 15:207, 1978.

Slayton RE, Creasman WT, Petty W, et al: Phase II trial of VP16-213 in the treatment of advanced squamous cell carcinoma of the cervix and adenocarcinoma of the ovary: A Gynecologic Oncology Group study. *Cancer Treat Rep* 63:2089, 1979.

Slayton RE, Park RC, Silverberg SG, et al: Vincristine, dactinomycin and cyclophosphamide in the treatment of malignant germ cell tumors of the ovary. A Gynecologic Oncology Group Study (A final report). *Cancer* 56:243, 1985.

Sleijfer DT, Smit EF, Meijer S, et al: Acute and cumulative effects of carboplatin on renal function. *Br J Cancer* 60:116, 1989.

Smith JP, Rutledge FN: Chemotherapy in the treatment of cancer of the ovary. *Am J Obstet Gynecol* 107:691, 1970.

Smith JP, Rutledge FN: Random study of hexamethylmelamine, 5-fluorouracil and melphalan in the treatment of advanced carcinoma of the ovary. *Natl Cancer Inst Monograph* 42:169, 1975.

Smith JP, Rutledge FN, Delclos L: Results of chemotherapy as adjunct to surgery in patients with localized ovarian cancer. *Semin Oncol* 2:277, 1975.

Smith JP, Rutledge FN, Wharton JT: Chemotherapy of ovarian cancer. New approaches. *Cancer* 30:1565, 1972.

Spencer TR, Marks RD, Fenn JO, et al: Intraperitoneal P-32 after negative second-look laparotomy in ovarian carcinoma. *Cancer* 63:2434, 1989.

Steiner M, Rubinov R, Borovik R, et al: Multimodal approach (surgery, chemotherapy and radiotherapy) in the treatment of advanced ovarian carcinoma. *Cancer* 55:2748, 1985.

Stenwig JT, Hazelkamp JT, Beecham JB: Granulosa cell tumors of the ovary: Clinical pathological study of 118 cases with long term follow-up. *Gynecol Oncol* 7:136, 1979.

Stewart JSW, Hird V, Sullivan M, et al: Intraperitoneal radioimmunotherapy for ovarian cancer. *Br J Obstet Gynecol* 96:529, 1989.

Sutton GP, Blessing JA, Homesley D, et al: Phase II trial of ifosfamide and mesna in advanced ovarian carcinoma: A Gynecologic Oncology Group Study. *J Clin Oncol* 7:1672, 1989a.

Sutton GP, Blessing JA, Photopulos G, et al: Phase II experience with ifosfamide/mesna in gynecologic malignancies: Preliminary report of Gynecologic Oncology Group studies. *Semin Oncol* 16:68, 1989b.

Sutton GP, Stehman FB, Einhorn LH, et al: Ten-year follow-up of patients receiving cisplatin, doxorubicin, and cyclophosphamide chemotherapy for advanced epithelial ovarian carcinoma. *J Clin Oncol* 7:223, 1989c.

Tavassoli FA, Norris HG: Sertoli tumors of the ovary. A clinical study of 28 cases with ultrastructural observations. *Cancer* 46:2281, 1980.

Taylor HB, Norris HJ: Lipid cell tumor of the ovary. *Cancer* 29:1953, 1967.

Taylor MH, Depetrillo AD, Turner R: Vinblastine, bleomycin and cisplatin in malignant germ cell tumors of the ovary. *Cancer* 56:1341, 1985.

Teilum G: Endodermal sinus tumors of the ovary and testes. Comparative morphogenesis of the so-called mesonephroma ovarii (chiller) and extraembryonic (yolk sac-allantoid) structures of the rat placenta. *Cancer* 12:1092, 1959.

ten Bokkel Huinink WW, vanderBurg ME, vanOsertom AT, et al: Carboplatin in combination therapy for ovarian cancer. *Cancer Treat Rev* 15:999, 1988.

Thigpen T: Single agent chemotherapy in the management of ovarian carcinoma. In: Alberts D, Surwit E (eds): *Ovarian Cancer*. Boston, Martinus Nijhoff, 1985, pp 115-146.

Thigpen T, et al: Chemotherapy for advanced or recurrent gynecologic cancers. *Cancer* 60:2104, 1987.

Thurnbeck WM, Scully RE: Solid teratoma of the ovary—A clinicopathological analysis of nine cases. *Cancer* 13:804, 1960.

Troche V, Hernandez E: Neoplasia arising in dysgenetic gonads. *Obstet Gynecol Surv* 41:74, 1986.

Trope C: Melphalan with or without doxorubicin in advanced ovarian cancer. *Obstet Gynecol* 70:582, 1987.

Trump DL, Bartel E, Pozniak M: Nodular pneumonitis after chemotherapy for germ cell tumors. *Ann Intern Med* 109:431, 1988.

Tsai CM, Gazdar AF, Venzon DJ, et al: Lack of in vitro synergy between etoposide and cis-diamminedichloroplatinum (II). *Cancer Res* 49:2390, 1989.

Ueda G, Hamanaka N, Hayakawa K, et al: Clinical histochemical and biochemical studies of an ovarian dysgerminoma with trophoblasts and Leydig cells. *Am J Obstet Gynecol* 114:748, 1972.

van't Veer LJ, Hermens R, vandenBerg-Bakker, et al: Ras oncogene activation in human ovarian cancer. *Oncogene* 2:157, 1988.

Vardi JR, Tadros GH, Foemmel R, et al: Plasma lipid-associated sialic acid and serum CA 125 as indicators of disease status with advanced ovarian cancer. *Obstet Gynecol* 74:379, 1989.

Varia M, Rosenman J, Venkatraman S, et al: Intraperitoneal chromic phosphate therapy after second look laparotomy for ovarian cancer. *Cancer* 61:919, 1988.

Vogl SE, Pagano M, Kaplan BH, et al: Cisplatin based combination chemotherapy for advanced ovarian cancer. *Cancer* 51:2024, 1983.

Vriesendorp R, Aalders JG, Sleifer DT, et al: Treatment of malignant germ cell tumors of the ovary with cisplatin, vinblastine and bleomycin (PVB). *Cancer Treat Rep* 68:779, 1984.

Wagensteen OH, Lewis FJ, Tongen LA: The second look in cancer surgery. *Lancet* 71:303, 1951.

Wallach RC, Kabakow B, Blinick G, et al: Thiotepa chemotherapy for ovarian carcinoma: Influence of remission and toxicity on survival. *Obstet Gynecol* 25:475, 1965.

Welander C, Homesley H, Levin E, et al: Phase II trial of the efficacy of human recombinant interferon gamma in recurrent ovarian adenocarcinomas. *Proc ASCO* Vol 5, p 221, No 863, 1986.

Wharton JT, Edwards CL, Rutledge FN: Long-term survival after chemotherapy for advanced epithelial ovarian carcinoma. *Am J Obstet Gynecol* 148:997, 1984.

Wharton JT, Rutledge FN, Smith JP, et al: Hexamethylmelamine: An evaluation of its role in the treatment of ovarian cancer. *Am J Obstet Gynecol* 133:833, 1979.

Wheelock J, Hancock K, Smith K: Cisplatin, doxorubicin and cyclophosphamide (PAC) in the treatment of mixed mesodermal tumor of the ovary. *Cancer Treat Rep* 71:1275, 1987.

Whittemore AS, Wu ML, Paffenbarger RS, et al: Personal and environmental characteristics related to epithelial ovarian cancer II. Exposures to talcum powder, tobacco, alcohol and coffee. *Am J Epidemiol* 128:1228, 1988.

Whittemore AS, Wu ML, Paffenbarger RS, et al: Epithelial ovarian cancer and the ability to conceive. *Cancer Res* 49:4047, 1989.

Wider JA, Marshall JR, Bardin CW, et al: Sustained remissions after chemotherapy for a primary ovarian cancer containing choriocarcinoma. *N Engl J Med* 280:1439, 1969.

Williams CJ, Mead GM, Macbeth FR, et al: Cisplatin combination chemotherapy versus chlorambucil in advanced ovarian carcinoma: Mature results of a randomized trial. *J Clin Oncol* 3:1455, 1985.

Williams SD, Blessing JA, Moore DH, et al: Cisplatin, vinblastine and bleomycin in advanced or recurrent ovarian germ-cell tumors. *Ann Intern Med* 111:22, 1989.

Williams SD, Brich R, Einhorn LH, et al: Treatment of disseminated germ-cell tumors with cisplatin, bleomycin and either vinblastine or etoposide. *N Engl J Med* 316:1435, 1987.

Wils J, vanGuens H: Chemotherapy consisting of cisplatin, doxorubicin and cyclophosphamide as an adjunct to surgery in stage IC-III epithelial ovarian carcinoma. *Am J Clin Oncol* 12:251, 1989.

Wiltshaw E, Carr B: Cis-platinum (II) diamminedichloride. Clinical experience of the Royal Marsden Hospitals and Institutes of Cancer Research, London. *Recent Results in Cancer Research* 48:178, 1974.

Wiltshaw E, Kroner T: Phase II study of cis-dichlorodiammineplatinum (II) (NSC-119875) in advanced adenocarcinoma of the ovary. *Cancer Treat Rep* 60:55, 1976.

Wiltshaw E, Stuart-Harris R, Barker GH, et al: Chemotherapy of endodermal sinus tumor (yolk sac tumor) of the ovary. Preliminary communication. *J Royal Soc Med* 75:888, 1982.

Woodruff JD, Protos P, Peterson WF: Ovarian teratomas. Relationship of histologic and oncogenic factors for prognosis. *Am J Obstet Gynecol* 102:702, 1968.

Wu ML, Whittemore AS, Paffenbarger RS, et al: Personal and environmental characteristics related to epithelial ovarian cancer. *Am J Epidemiol* 128:1216, 1988.

Yanai-Inbar I, Scully RE: Relation to ovarian dermoid cysts and immature teratomas: An analysis of 350 cases of immature teratoma and 10 cases of dermoid cyst with microscopic foci of immature tissue. *Int J Gynecol Pathol* 6:203, 1987.

Yancik R, Gloeckler L, Yates JW: Ovarian cancer in the elderly: An analysis of Surveillance, Epidemiology and End Results program data. *Am J Obstet Gynecol* 154:639, 1986.

Yazigi R, Sandstad J, Munoz AK: The primary staging in ovarian tumors of low malignant potential. *Gynecol Oncol* 31:402, 1988.

Yazigi R, Wild R, Madrid J, et al: Ifosfamide treatment of advanced ovarian cancer. *Obstet Gynecol* 63:163, 1984.

Young RC: A second look at second-look laparotomy. *J Clin Oncol* 9:1311, 1987a.

Young RC: Initial therapy for early ovarian carcinoma. *Cancer* 60:2042, 1987b.

Young RC: Personal communication, 1989.

Young RC, Chabner BA, Hubbard SP, et al: Advanced ovarian adenocarcinoma. A prospective clinical trial of melphalan (L-PAM) versus combination chemotherapy. *N Engl J Med* 299:1261, 1978.

Young RC, Decker DG, Wharton JT, et al: Staging laparotomy in early ovarian cancer. *JAMA* 250:3072, 1983.

Young RH, Scully RE: Ovarian tumors of probable wolffian origin. A report of eleven cases. *Am J Surg Pathol* 7:125, 1983.

Young RH, Scully RE: Ovarian Sertoli–Leydig cell tumors. A clinicopathological analysis of 207 cases. *Am J Surg Pathol* 9:543, 1985.

Young RH, Scully RE: Oxyphilic cell carcinoma of the ovary. *Am J Surg Pathol* 11:661, 1987.

Young RH, Dickersin GR, Scully RE: Juvenile granulosa cell tumor of the ovary. A clinicopathological analysis of 125 cases. *Am J Surg Pathol* 8:575, 1984a.

Young RH, Pratt J, Scully RE: Endometrioid stromal sarcomas of the ovary. A clinicopathologic analysis of 23 cases. *Cancer* 53:1143, 1984b.

Young RH, Welch WR, Dickersin GR, et al: Ovarian sex cord tumors with annular tubules. Review of 74 cases including 27 with Peutz-Jeghers syndrome and four with adenoma malignum of the cervix. *Cancer* 50:1384, 1982.

Zhang J, Young RH, Arseneau J, et al: Ovarian stromal tumors containing lutein or Leydig cells (luteinized thecomas and stromal

Leydig cell tumors): A clinical pathologic analysis of 50 cases. *Int J Gynecol Pathol* 1:270, 1982.

Zhou DJ, Gonzalez-Cadavid N, Ahuja H, et al: A unique pattern of proto-oncogene abnormalities in ovarian adenocarcinoma. *Cancer* 62:1573, 1988.

# *Chapter 15* | Cancer of the Vulva

*George W. Morley*

During the past 20 to 25 years, significant advances have been made in the diagnosis and management of vulvar malignancy. Prior to that time, residents training in obstetrics and gynecology were taught that (1) total vulvectomy was the preferred treatment for preinvasive disease, (2) radical vulvectomy with groin and pelvic lymphadenectomy was the treatment of choice for invasive disease, and (3) palliative vulvectomy was the treatment for incurable disease. Over the last several years, characteristics of this disease have changed, since patients have sought medical attention much earlier and physicians have become increasingly aware of the malignant potential of various vulvar lesions and the consequences of progressive disease. These lesions are now recognized at an earlier stage, and appropriate diagnosis and treatment have brought about a significant increase in the 5-year survival rates.

## INCIDENCE, PREVALENCE, AND EPIDEMIOLOGY

Carcinoma of the vulva accounts for approximately 5% of all gynecologic cancers treated in the United States today and is the fourth most common cancer of the female genital tract. The incidence of carcinoma in situ of the vulva is 0.7 per 100,000 women, and that of invasive carcinoma is 1.9 per 100,000. Its preinvasive stage appears to be on the rise, particularly among those of reproductive age, with approximately 75% of these lesions occurring in the premenopausal period. These younger patients tend to have multifocal lesions (Friedrich et al, 1980; Wilkinson et al, 1981; Cagler et al, 1982; Bernstein et al, 1983). Invasive disease, on the other hand, is predominantly a disease of elderly women, with the incidence being highest in the seventh decade of life. Over 75% of these patients have unifocal disease. Since these neoplasms occurring on the vulva differ significantly from those involving other skin surfaces of the body, the casual approach should be avoided.

Among those afflicted with this disease, the ratio of whites to blacks is about 3:1 (Friedrich et al, 1980).

The incidence of double primary tumors is approximately 10%; the other lesion usually involves the genital organs, the most common being the cervix (Choo, 1980; Green et al, 1958). Parity does not seem to play a role in the development of preinvasive or invasive carcinoma of the vulva, since studies suggest that both nulliparous and parous patients are susceptible to the same etiologic factors.

## ETIOLOGY AND ASSOCIATED DISEASES

Whereas the exact etiology of preinvasive and invasive lesions of the vulva is still unknown, certain etiologic factors are suspect, including venereal lesions of the vulva, nylon undergarments, tight wearing apparel, perineal deodorants, chemicals, broadened sexual activities, and trauma of all varieties. One predisposing factor related specifically to the vulvar tissues may be the environmental state of this area, which is frequently moist and warm and thus possibly gives rise to an unusual epithelial response to these external factors.

Malignant lesions of the vulva are frequently associated with some type of chronic vulvar abnormality, sometimes referred to as *chronic vulvar dystrophy* (Jeffcoate, 1966)—an all-inclusive term used by clinicians evaluating these patients. Even though some have been critical of this broad term (Charles, 1972), it is thought by most authorities to be a satisfactory clinical description, since a more specific diagnosis cannot be entertained without microscopic interpretation by the pathologist. Approximately 50% of all invasive carcinomas of the vulva rise in an area of chronic vulvar dystrophy; however, only 2 to 4% of the patients who have some type of chronic vulvar disease will ultimately experience a malignancy in this area.

Condylomatous lesions have recently been reported to be associated with atypical features of the epithelium, and 20 to 25% of the patients with preinvasive carcinomas of the vulva have existing or have had preexisting condyloma acuminatum (Woodruff, 1976; Crum et al, 1982). Those patients who have been treated for condyloma acuminatum over an extended period of time are considered at risk for the development of some type of malignant disease.

Furthermore, it has been reported that there is a 33% incidence of another primary lesion coexisting or having previously existed along with the preinvasive carcinoma of the vulva, and most of these malignancies involve other genital organs (Abell and Gosling, 1961). This suggests a common underlying causal factor. Lichen sclerosus et atrophicus has frequently been reported either antecedent to or concurrent with carcinoma of the vulva, although this finding has been challenged by some (Hart et al, 1975). Herpes vulvitis, syphilis, and other granulomatous lesions have all been identified as diseases associated with carcinoma of the vulva.

Immunosuppressed patients present a specific problem (Seski et al, 1978). For example, a significant increase in vulvar disease has been noted in patients undergoing long-term treatment with corticoids in the management of rheumatoid arthritis, systemic lupus erythematosus, and the like, and in patients receiving chemotherapy for treatment of an underlying malignant neoplasm. Diabetes mellitus and hypertension are seen in over 25% of the patients with invasive disease of the vulva. The cause–effect relationship has not yet been established, however, since these conditions may be directly related to the aging process itself.

## CLINICAL FEATURES AND HISTOLOGIC CHARACTERISTICS

Clinically, the preinvasive lesion presents as a flattened, slightly raised, reddened or whitish patch on the vulva and is often hyperkeratotic. It can be either discrete or coalescent and unifocal or multicentric in its location and origin. On occasion, these lesions are hyperpigmented. The multifocal lesion is seen much more commonly in the preinvasive state, and approximately 30 to 40% of these patients are asymptomatic (Friedrich et al, 1980; Kaplan et al, 1981). However, the most common complaint is uncontrollable pruritus of the vulva.

Preinvasive diseases of the vulva are divided into three groups: (1) carcinoma of the vulva in situ (simplex); (2) Bowen's disease of the vulva, and (3) Paget's disease of the vulva. The simplex lesion of the vulva is usually seen in the older age group, and its preinvasive stage is usually of short duration before the lesion invades the underlying structures. Bowen's disease of the vulva, on the other hand, occurs in younger patients with a median age of 43. It has a long preinvasive phase; however, if it is not therapeutically controlled, it has the potential to become an infiltrative lesion. Paget's disease of the vulva is seen in older women with a median age of 67. Grossly, this lesion appears as a soft, velvety, red, and thickened abnormality that tends to spread horizontally within the epidermis.

The invasive lesion of the vulva is primarily an exaggeration of the preinvasive disease in that it is more indurated, raised, nodular, and irregular. These lesions are more commonly ulcerated and unifocal. Patients frequently complain about the presence of a lump, bleeding, or pain; however, pruritus is still the most common complaint for all lesions of the vulva, being reported by over 50% of the patients.

The histologic features seen in the simplex type of carcinoma in situ are not particularly characteristic, but the degree of atypia is less marked and the lesion tends to be located in the basilar region. This lesion is the usual precursor for the commonest type of invasive carcinoma of the vulva, i.e., a well-differentiated, keratinizing squamous cell lesion that is present in over 85% of the patients with invasive disease.

The important histologic changes seen in Bowen's disease of the vulva involve the epithelial surfaces and the epidermis (Fig. 15-1). The characteristic feature is the "corps ronds," which are large cells containing clear, vacuolated cytoplasm and hyperchromatic nuclei. There appears to be a doubly-contoured halo around these nuclei (Abell and Gosling, 1961).

The microscopic features in extramammary Paget's disease consist of numerous large, pale, vacuolated cells with large vesicular nuclei and prominent nucleoli within the dermis (Fig. 15-2). Characteristically, these are parabasal in location and are frequently seen in the rete ridges where glandular formation is common. Mucicarmine- or alcian blue-stained sections reveal the presence of mucopolysaccharides in many of these cells (Parmley et al, 1975; Lee et al, 1975). Paget's cells may be differentiated along either squamous or secretory lines.

## DIAGNOSIS

Since the diagnosing physician is the physician of record, a high index of suspicion is required and the techniques for recognizing these lesions should be reviewed. In the past, there appeared to be a 1-year delay in diagnosis in over 30 to 35% of the cases reviewed. Commonly, these lesions would be treated with topical creams and antibiotic ointments. However, the incidence of diagnostic delay due to patient procrastination has decreased significantly since modesty and embar-

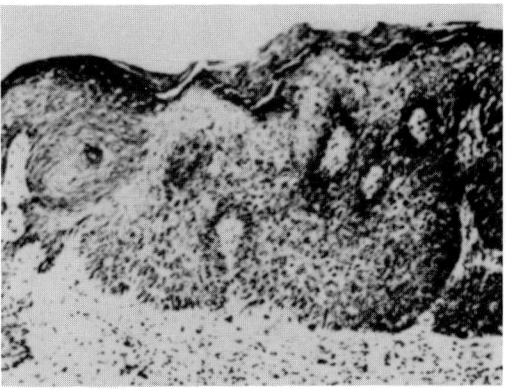

**FIGURE 15-1** Histologic features of Bowen's disease of the vulva. The corps ronds are large cells containing clear, vacuolated cytoplasm and hyperchromatic nuclei.

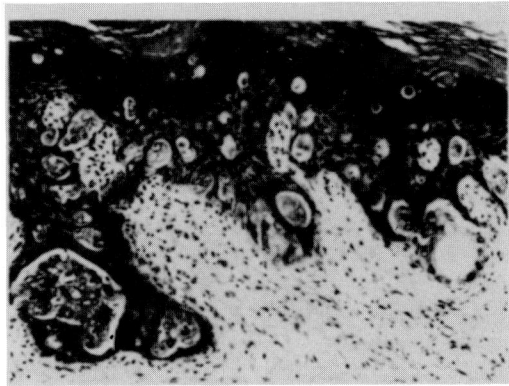

FIGURE 15-2 Histologic features of Paget's disease of the vulva. Note the characteristic large, pale, vacuolated cells with large vesicular nuclei located primarily in the parabasal layer.

rassment about seeking medical advice have lessened considerably, and delay on the part of physicians has declined markedly as a result of education in a variety of ways.

In performing the pelvic examination, one must inspect all vulvar tissues, including the perineal body, the perianal region, and the clitoral and periclitoral areas. On occasion, pubic hair growth will interfere with good visualization of this area, so that one must guard against superficial inspection of this region. All areas that appear chronically irritated should be thoroughly analyzed. A break in the continuity of the skin may be seen with the naked eye; however, a hand magnifying glass is a satisfactory aid in the clinical evaluation if one

desires a more detailed analysis of a suspected area. Colposcopy itself is thought to have limited value in the evaluation of the vulvar lesions.

Once the abnormality has been detected, a 1% toluidine blue nuclear stain may be applied to the vulva as an aid in localizing areas that are most suspect (Collins, 1966). From 3 to 5 minutes later, the area is "washed" with a 1 to 2% solution of acetic acid. Tissues that retain the dark blue color are biopsied. Most gynecologists, however, think this nuclear staining is of marginal value, since it cannot differentiate between benign and malignant disease and there is a consequent high incidence of false-positive and false-negative reporting.

After inspection, the vulvar tissue is palpated to determine the presence or absence of swelling or induration, and the lymph node–bearing region of the groin is evaluated at this time. A complete pelvic examination is performed and a Papanicolaou smear should be prepared for cytologic examination, since associated disease may coexist.

Often, when less suspect lesions are encountered, the attending physician will suggest a trial of creams, salves, or lotions in an effort to control the symptomatology, which is assumed to be caused by benign disease. This approach is probably unwise without biopsy confirmation; however, should it be chosen, it is mandatory that the patient be reexamined in 3 to 4 weeks. If a marked remission in the signs and symptoms has not taken place, a biopsy is required at that time.

Before treatment can be instituted, the diagnosis must be confirmed histologically by means of biopsies of the suspected lesions, either incisional biopsy of the ad-

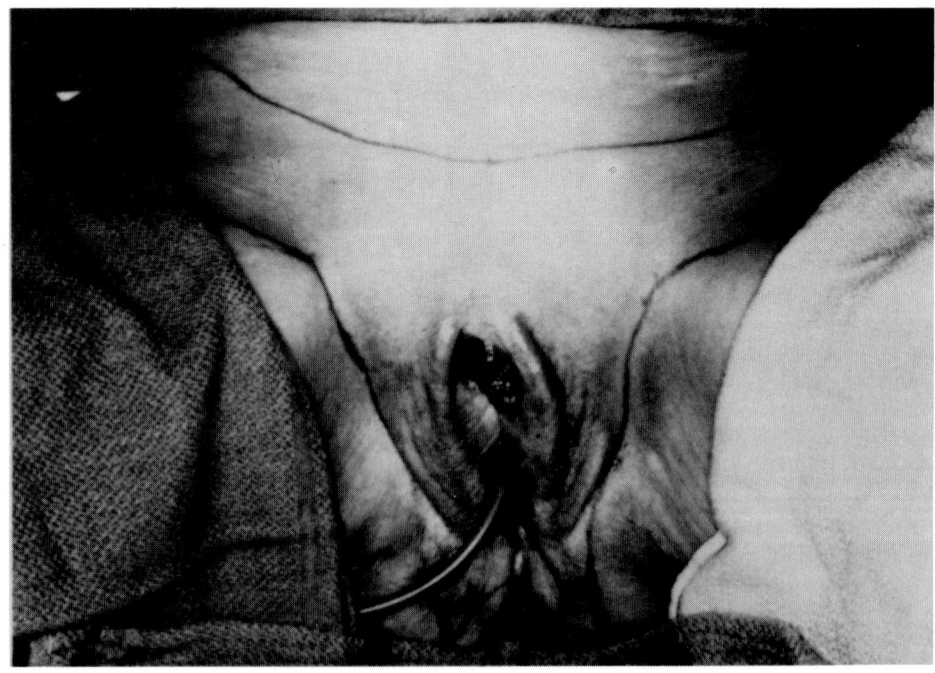

FIGURE 15-3 The trapezoid or butterfly incision is utilized in an en bloc radical vulvectomy and bilateral groin lymph node dissection and pelvic node exploration when indicated.

vancing edge or excisional biopsy of the lesion. There are a number of ways to obtain biopsy specimens of lesions of the vulva, all of which can be performed as outpatient procedures under local anesthesia with 1% lidocaine. A Keyes disposable dermatologic punch biopsy instrument can be used most satisfactorily for sampling purposes (Fig. 15-3). The pathologist is provided with a bit of tissue 4 to 6 mm in diameter and of appropriate depth for tissue analysis. Once the specimens have been taken, hemostasis can be satisfactorily accomplished using a 1% solution of ferric subsulfate (Monsel's solution) or other hemostatic agents of choice. Other biopsy instruments and techniques can be used for this purpose, depending on personal preferences.

Lastly, ever since lymphangiography was first described in 1952 (Kinmonth, 1952), it has been used in an attempt to define further the limits and extent of a variety of pelvic malignancies. Its overall accuracy in predicting the presence or absence of regional lymph node metastasis in vulvar malignancies has been reported to be 75 to 85% (Abitbol et al, 1965; Comas et al, 1969). Because this "predictability index" appears to be more accurate than that reported by others (Green et al, 1958; Way and Benedet, 1973; Morley, 1976) using clinical assessment of the regional lymph node–bearing tissue, lymphangiography is not recommended as a routine diagnostic aid in these patients.

## STAGING AND CLASSIFICATION

Prior to 1970, a number of authors proposed protocols for staging vulvar cancer based on the clinical evaluation of the extent of the disease; however, these reports were not only somewhat limited in scope but were also in direct conflict with one another (Taussig, 1940; McKelvey, 1970; Franklin, 1972). Correlation of results then became an impossible task.

During the past two decades, more attention has been focused on uniformity of clinical staging and reporting. In January 1971, the system of clinical staging of vulvar carcinoma that had just been approved by the International Federation of Obstetrics and Gynecology (FIGO) became effective. In spite of the inherent limitations of any classification system, it is important that all therapeutic results be reported in terms of these common denominators. This FIGO classification is used in reporting results in this chapter; however, in 1989 a new *surgical* staging was introduced as the current FIGO classification (Table 15-1). It is too early to evaluate the impact of this new classification on reported results; however, preliminary reports suggest an improved accuracy in the staging of carcinoma of the vulva.

## TREATMENT
### Preinvasive Carcinoma of the Vulva

Treatment of intraepithelial carcinoma of the vulva varies significantly depending primarily on the location and extent of the disease. These lesions can be treated surgically in a variety of ways: (1) wide local excision, (2) partial or hemivulvectomy, (3) subtotal or total vulvectomy, and (4) "skinning" vulvectomy. Cryosurgery has had only limited use and has been replaced by laser therapy in popularity.

***Surgical Therapy*** *Wide local excision* with 1-cm margins is an acceptable form of treatment for solitary preinvasive lesions of the vulva, and this more conservative approach preserves vulvar integrity and function. These solitary lesions occur more commonly now than had been previously recognized (Woodruff, 1976; Iversen et al, 1981; Bernstein et al, 1983), and they can be ideally managed in this way, especially in the younger patient. Every consideration should be given to obtaining a cosmetic result that is free from both deformity and sexual dysfunction without jeopardizing the primary goal—to cure the patient. Obviously, close followup observation is warranted in these patients.

If a lesion more broadly involves the vulvar tissues but not the skin over the clitoris, a *subtotal vulvectomy* with preservation of the clitoral tissues can be performed. This is an ideal approach for this type of patient.

Currently, a *skinning vulvectomy* with or without the application of a split-thickness skin graft to the operative site is the treatment of choice when surgical excision is the method of management in diffuse preinvasive disease (Rutledge et al, 1968; Hall, 1979; DiSaia and Rich, 1981; Kaplan et al, 1981). This approach provides satisfactory control of the disease, minimizes disfigurement of the area, and preserves the body of the clitoris for normal sexual response. The skin of the vulvar tissues can be readily separated from the underlying dermis with only a minimal amount of bleeding. Once all of the epidermis has been removed and hemostasis has been obtained by electrocoagulation, a decision must be made concerning whether or not a vulvoplasty using a split-thickness skin graft is indicated. The majority of these wounds can be closed primarily, with only minimal gaping of the vaginal introitus, but this depends on the lateral extent of the excision. Grafting is being used less often now than previously, since primary closure yields satisfactory cosmetic and functional results. One should not hesitate, however, to cover the denuded area with a split-thickness skin graft taken from the lateral buttock or posterior thigh region if coverage of the operative site seems to require this approach.

A Brown mechanical dermatome with a thickness setting of 0.018 inch is commonly used to obtain an appropriate skin graft. Several slitlike ("pie-crust") incisions are made in the donor skin graft to allow for drainage and stretching of the skin over the recipient area. Absolute hemostasis is a sine qua non in order to allow for maximum "take" of the graft. The edges of the graft are then secured to the lateral border of the recipient site with either continuous or interrupted absorbable suture material or by skin staples. An immobilizing stent is placed over the newly positioned skin graft and secured in the usual fashion. Dressings are

TABLE 15-1 FIGO Staging for Carcinoma of the Vulva

| | | |
|---|---|---|
| **Stage 0** | | |
| Tis | Carcinoma in situ intraepithelial carcinoma | |
| **Stage I** | | |
| T1 N0 M0 | Tumor confined to the vulva and/or perineum—2 cm or less in greatest dimension, nodes are not palpable | |
| **Stage II** | | |
| T2 N0 M0 | Tumor confined to the vulva and/or perineum—more than 2 cm in greatest dimension, nodes are not palpable | |
| **Stage III** | | |
| T3 N0 M0 | Tumor of any size with . . . | |
| T3 N1 M0 | 1) Adjacent spread to the lower urethra and/or the vagina, or the anus, and/or . . . | |
| T1 N1 M0 | 2) Unilateral regional lymph node metastasis | |
| T2 N1 M0 | | |
| **Stage IVA** | | |
| T1 N2 M0 | Tumor invades any of the following: | |
| T2 N2 M0 | Upper urethra, bladder mucosa, rectal mucosa, pelvic bone, and/or bilateral regional node metastasis | |
| T3 N2 M0 | | |
| T4 any N M0 | | |
| **Stage IVB** | | |
| Any T | Any distant metastasis including | |
| Any N, M1 | pelvic lymph nodes | |

**Rules for Clinical Staging**
The rules for staging are similar to those for carcinoma of the cervix.

**TNM Classification of Carcinoma of the Vulva (FIGO)**

*T* Primary tumor
    Tis Preinvasive carcinoma (carcinoma in situ)
    T1 Tumor confined to the vulva and/or perineum—$\leq$ 2 cm in greatest dimension
    T2 Tumor confined to the vulva and/or perineum—> 2 cm in greatest dimension
    T3 Tumor of any size with adjacent spread to the urethra and/or vagina and/or to the anus
    T4 Tumor of any size infiltrating the bladder mucosa and/or the rectal mucosa, including the upper part of the urethral mucosa and/or fixed to the bone

*N* Regional lymph nodes
    N0 No lymph node metastasis
    N1 Unilateral regional lymph node metastasis
    N2 Bilateral regional lymph node metastasis

*M* Distant metastasis
    M0 No clinical metastasis
    M1 Distant metastasis (including pelvic lymph node metastasis)

International Federation of Gynecology and Obstetrics. Annual report on the results of treatment in gynecological cancer. *Int J Gynecol Obstet* 28: 189-190, 1989

removed on the fifth postoperative day, and the patient is discharged from the hospital a day or two later. Again, close followup observation of these patients is mandatory.

***Laser Therapy*** More recently, *carbon dioxide laser vaporization therapy*, often guided by colposcopy (Caglar et al, 1982; Ferenczy, 1982), has become increasingly popular in the treatment of these lesions if the depth of vaporization does not exceed 3 mm. If the lesion can be seen, it can be eradicated in this manner; however, the patient must be highly motivated, since this mode of therapy causes significant irritation and discomfort that persists for approximately 4 weeks. The end result, however, is cosmetically excellent, and scar formation is minimal. Opposition to this form of therapy focuses on the fact that the pathologist is not given the opportunity to assess the status of the margins of the lesion and invasion cannot be ruled in or out, since there is no surgical specimen available for analysis. Furthermore, inhalation of the vaporized particles may be a health hazard to the operator and assisting personnel.

By comparison, the *medical management* of intraepithelial disease has been much more limited but deserves comment. Topical 5-fluorouracil (1% Efudex), applied once daily for approximately 6 weeks, is a simple, nonsurgical approach to the treatment of carcinoma in situ of the vulva (Krupp and Bohm, 1978; Lifshitz and Roberts, 1980; Carson et al, 1976). This mode of

therapy inhibits DNA production and brings about denudation of the epithelium. Again, these patients must be highly motivated, since the secondary inflammatory response is both irritating and painful. Short-term followup of these patients suggests a 75% response rate; however, long-term investigation is required, since a number of gynecologists feel that this method of treatment is not of particular value. Topical bleomycin, because of its known activity against squamous neoplasias, has had a trial; however, a reportedly poor response rate suggests that this form of therapy should not be used in the treatment of intraepithelial disease (Roberts et al, 1980). The use of interferon is still investigational.

Topical immunotherapy of vulvar carcinoma with dinitrochlorobenzene (DNCB) has been limited to the treatment of recurrent intraepithelial disease once the lesion has failed to respond to more conventional topical chemotherapy (Weintraub and Lagasse, 1973; Foster and Woodruff, 1981). This delayed induced hypersensitivity reaction is a nonspecific inflammatory response to the topical treatment which causes denudation of the epithelium with desquamation. If a lesion is sensitive to this initial challenge, the DNCB cream is applied topically each day for 1 to 2 weeks as indicated.

All the conservative approaches to the management of preinvasive carcinoma of the vulva are limited by a certain incidence of recurrence. Various reports suggest a 10 to 30% recurrence rate utilizing any of these therapeutic modalities (DiSaia and Rich, 1981; Benedet and Murphy, 1982); therefore, close followup evaluation is mandatory irrespective of the treatment used for these lesions. The incidence of recurrence is significant even in the presence of "negative margins" when the surgical specimen is reviewed by the pathologist. This observation may very well coincide with the currently popular causative factor, i.e., the human papillomavirus. It is well known that a number of these virus types exhibit a significant latency period between periods of activity.

***Extramammary Paget's Disease of the Vulva*** Although extramammary Paget's disease of the vulva is usually a preinvasive lesion, its management is different from that previously described for other preinvasive vulvar growths. Characteristically, this lesion grows horizontally within the epidermis, and the extent of the intraepidermal disease is often greater than that seen on inspection of the surface lesion. Furthermore, this lesion lies very close to the dermis, and its rete pegs tend to push into the dermis without actually penetrating it.

In view of these characteristic features, a patient with Paget's disease of the vulva should be treated not with a skinning vulvectomy but rather with a more traditional type of vulvectomy that includes the epidermis and underlying dermis. The dissection extends down to Colles' fascia of the vulva, which is the perineal extension of Scarpa's fascia from the abdominal wall. This type of dissection allows for a more adequate pathologic evaluation of the underlying tissue, since approximately one-third of all patients with extramammary Paget's disease of the vulva have invasive adenocarcinoma of the underlying apocrine gland structures (Boehm and Morris, 1971; Parmley et al, 1975; Hart and Millman, 1977). Should an invasive process be encountered, a more radical procedure is indicated, including a groin lymph node dissection. In addition, one must search for a second primary malignancy elsewhere, since this interrelationship also occurs in approximately 33% of these patients (Fenn et al, 1971; Breen et al, 1973; Creasman et al, 1975; Twombly, 1953). Associated malignancies of the cervix as well as mucinous carcinoma of the colon, bladder, gallbladder, and breast have been reported (Friedrich et al, 1975). On occasion, a skin graft will be required to cover the surgical defect satisfactorily. One must also remember that Paget's disease has a significant propensity to recur. Therefore, this area—including the site of the graft, if one is used—must be checked periodically for this complication (Beecham, 1976).

## Microinvasive Carcinoma of the Vulva

Although there is no universally accepted definition of microinvasive carcinoma of the vulva, an increasing number of early superficial lesions are being detected now that patients are more aware of alterations in the vulvar tissues. This enhanced patient awareness has been fortuitous, since it is now well recognized that these earlier lesions can be treated less radically with excellent results. A review of the literature indicates that a variety of therapeutic approaches have been proposed,

ranging from total vulvectomy alone to radical vulvectomy with bilateral groin lymphadenectomy (Wharton et al, 1974; DiPaola et al, 1975; Parker et al, 1975; DiSaia et al, 1979; Buscema et al, 1981; Chu et al, 1982). More recently, Hoffman et al (1983) reviewed 90 cases of Stage I squamous cell carcinoma of the vulva either treated with primary groin lymph node dissection or followed for 5 years. These authors assessed the size of the lesion, depth of invasion, histologic grade, confluence of the invasive tongues, and lymphovascular involvement as factors in determining the biologic propensity for lymph node metastases in these patients (Table 15-2). Confluence, depth of invasion, and lymphovascular involvement were all directly related to the risk of regional lymph node metastasis. Confluent carcinoma was defined as tongues of carcinoma extending into the dermis and joining with each other to form a large mass of carcinoma filling a 1-mm or greater stromal field. All of these lesions exhibiting nodal spread were of the confluent type; however, aproximately 50% of those showing confluence did not involve the lymph nodes. No patient was found to have nodal spread of disease in the absence of tumor confluence. Depth of stromal invasion was also useful in defining those patients more likely to have nodal metastases. The likelihood of nodal metastases increases significantly beyond the 3-mm threshold. The size of the lesion correlated closely with the depth of invasion and the chance of nodal spread. Although lymphovascular invasion was not a common feature observed in this study, it was seen in four of these patients, three of whom had regional lymph node involvement.

In 1979, DiSaia introduced the concept of utilizing superficial inguinal nodes as "sentinel nodes" in treatment planning for these early lesions. Using similar criteria, he noted that in 18 patients studied, there was no evidence of metastatic disease involving the superficial femoral nodes.

More recently, even though FIGO endorsement is lacking, the Internationl Society for the Study of Vulvar Disease has endorsed the definition of microinvasive carcinoma of the vulva as a solitary lesion, 2 cm or less in diameter, with a depth of invasion of 1 mm or less into the underlying stroma. Currently, the standardized measurement of the depth of invasion is from the dermal-epidermal junction (basement membrane) of the most superficial dermal papilla to the deepest point of invasion of the tumor. Based on a review of the litera-

---

TABLE 15-2 Microinvasive Carcinoma of the Vulva
(University of Michigan Series)

Depth of invasion versus nodal metastases/no. of patients

| | |
|---|---|
| ≤ 2 mm | 0/19 |
| ≤ 3 mm | 2/17 |
| ≤ 4 mm | 5/8 |
| ≤ 5 mm | 3/7 |

Confluence versus nodal metastases/no. of patients

| | |
|---|---|
| Confluent | 17/42 |
| Not confluent | 0/31 |

TABLE 15-3  Definition of Microinvasive Carcinoma of the Vulva from the International Society for the Study of Vulvar Disease

1. Lesion 2 cm or less in diameter.
2. Stromal invasion of 1 mm or less.*
3. Designated as Stage Ia lesion.

* Measured from the dermal-epidermal junction (basement membrane) of the most superficial dermal papilla to the deepest point of invasion.

ture as well as on personal communications, this definition has been generally accepted as Stage Ia disease (Table 15-3). These microinvasive lesions can be treated by wide local excision or by some type of vulvectomy, as dictated by the clinical situation. Regional groin lymph node dissection is not required. It must be remembered that the final staging is based on the microscopic assessment only *after* the entire lesion has been excised.

## Invasive Disease

Ever since Taussig reported on the treatment of invasive carcinoma of the vulva in 1940, the standard operation for the management of this disease has been radical vulvectomy and bilateral regional lymphadenectomy. Many American and European gynecologic surgeons felt for several years that the regional lymphadenectomy should include not only a routine groin lymph node dissection but also a pelvic lymphadenectomy (Green et al, 1958; Collins et al, 1973; Way, 1948; Boutselis, 1972). Over the past 20 years, these lesions of the vulva have been detected earlier and therefore have been considerably smaller than those seen so commonly during

the first half of this century. Currently, over 50% of the invasive lesions are classified as Stage I disease at the time of the initial diagnosis. Thus, by definition, the primary lesion is 2 cm or less in diameter, with no clinical evidence of regional lymph node involvement. For this reason, the results have been gratifying, since 40 years ago the 5-year survival rate was reported to be as low as 10 to 15% (Folsome, 1940; Way, 1940). Today, an overall 70 to 80% 5-year survival rate should be expected when appropriate radical surgery is instituted, irrespective of stage (Morley, 1976; Green, 1978; Iversen et al, 1981; Hopkins et al, 1991).

At the present time, the treatment of choice for invasive squamous cell carcinoma of the vulva is radical vulvectomy and bilateral groin lymphadenectomy, which is often expressed either as a femoral and inguinal or a superficial and deep groin lymph node dissection. Bilateral pelvic lymphadenectomy is no longer considered a routine part of this procedure, as will be noted later.

### *Radical Vulvectomy and Bilateral Groin Lymphadenectomy*
At operation, the patient is placed in the "ski position" so that the lower abdominal and perineal regions can be dissected without repositioning the patient. A two-team approach to groin dissections reduces the operating time considerably.

The technique for a radical vulvectomy and regional lymphadenectomy begins with the choice of incision. Although a variety of incisions have been described, the two most frequently used today are (1) the trapezoid or butterfly incision (Arbitol, 1973; Morley, 1976) (Fig. 15-4) and (2) the "three-in-one" incision utilizing separate incisions for the radical vulvectomy and the two groin lymph node dissections (Hacker et al, 1981). Both

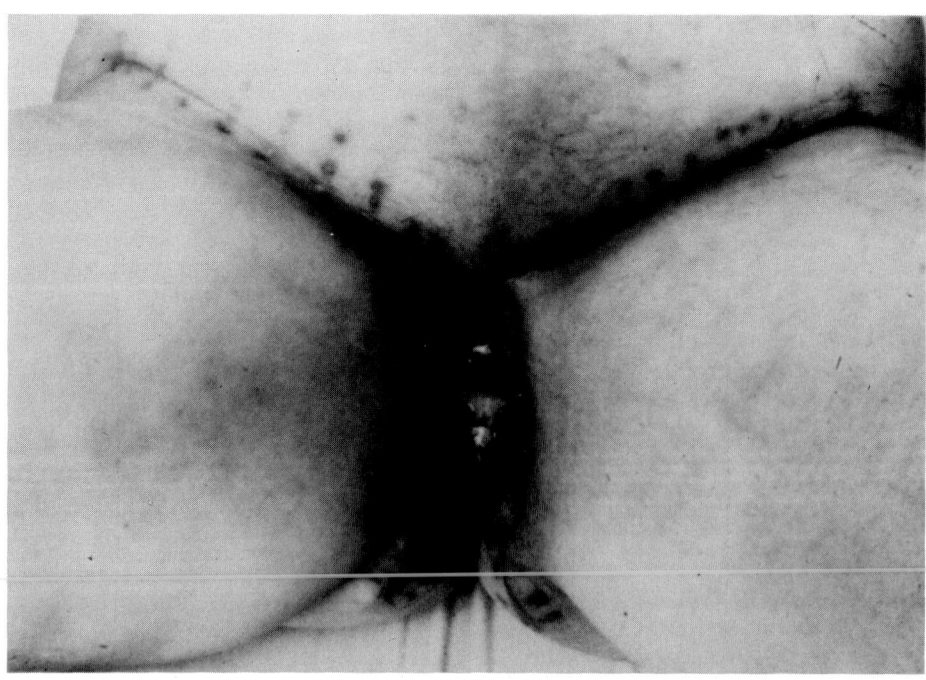

FIGURE 15-4  Wound healing is complete in about 2 months. A linear scar results from healing by wound contracture.

incisions are considered equally satisfactory, since survival rates are not altered in any way in either case. In general, the incision of choice is directly related to the extent of disease to be resected. The latter incision is now used more frequently since the lesions seen currently are smaller in size and many of the tumors do not involve the clitoral or paraclitoral areas.

Irrespective of which incision is chosen for the procedure, the *bilateral groin lymphadenectomy* consists of either an en bloc full-thickness dissection or an undermining dissection in each groin region. The full-thickness dissection, however, is designed to maintain circulation in the retained flaps.

In performing this operation an in-depth knowledge of the anatomic structures in the vulva and groin region is required. The groin lymph nodes are divided into two compartments—superficial and deep—and they are separated primarily by the fascia lata and the femoral sheath. In the classic description of this dissection, all of the groin lymph node–bearing tissue is resected by an en bloc dissection that mobilizes overlying fat from the underlying fascia lata. The lymph nodes in the superficial groin compartment lie alongside the major veins draining this area, including the saphenous, the external pudendal, the superficial circumflex iliac, and the superficial inferior epigastric vessels. During the dissection, a 6- to 7-cm segment of the saphenous vein is frequently excised; however, many gynecologic oncologists are convinced that this is not necessary and suggest that it may add to the dependent edema so commonly seen during the postoperative period in these patients. If a portion of the saphenous vein is to be resected, it is started just prior to its junction with the femoral vein. A transfixing suture ligature is used for the ligation. Caution must be exercised to avoid too much traction on this junction, which would create a tentlike effect of the femoral vein. The resected portion varies in length.

The superficial groin dissection can be simplified by lifting the fibroadipose tissue off the underlying fascia lata in the following manner: a medial incision at the top of the labiocrural line is carried down onto the fascia lata overlying the adductor longus muscle. By blunt dissection, the fibroadipose tissue is separated from the fascia lata medially to laterally and anterior to the femoral sheath overlying the femoral triangle. This anterior block of tissue contains the superficial inguinal lymph node–bearing tissue and the greater saphenous vein. Elevation of this tissue allows for easier dissection of the area, since the femoral vessels lie posterior to the fascia lata.

The fascia lata does not have to be routinely removed, as had been recommended by some in the past (Charles, 1972), unless it is directly involved; nor does the femoral nerve have to be exposed (deValera, 1968), since not only does it lie outside the femoral sheath, but there are no lymph nodes in this area.

The lymphatic vessels from the superficial groin lymph nodes then drain into the deep groin lymph node compartment in the region of the fossa ovalis. As the classic dissection progresses from lateral to medial, the femoral sheath overlying the femoral artery and vein is exposed and incised over these vessels. This sheath is opened through its full length from the base of the fossa ovalis downward to where the sartorius muscle laterally and the adductor muscle medially come together to form the apex of the femoral triangle. The deep groin lymph nodes lying medial and parallel to the femoral vein are then removed en bloc throughout the length of the femoral triangle. There are approximately six to eight lymph nodes in the deep compartment; the uppermost one is the gland of Cloquet or Rosenmuller's node, which is located just within the femoral canal. If appropriate traction is applied, this node can be included in this en bloc dissection. This part of the dissection is then completed and the femoral sheath is closed over the femoral artery and vein.

If the femoral sheath has been excised, the femoral vessels must be covered to avoid erosion and secondary hemorrhage caused by wound infection or other conditions. The sartorius muscle is then divided at its lateral insertion into the inguinal ligament, transposed medially, and attached to the medial portion of the inguinal ligament. This protects the vessels against direct exposure to infection and provides a protective cushion for this area.

Lastly, with regard to the groin lymph node dissection, the superficial groin lymph nodes, in draining into the deep groin lymph nodes, appear to drain primarily into the gland of Cloquet. If this is true, and if it is agreed that the gland of Cloquet lies in the fossa ovalis in the region of the inguinal canal, this sentinel node can be excised along with the en bloc dissection without any disruption of the femoral sheath in most cases. The more dependent or distal groin lymph nodes lying underneath the femoral sheath are probably involved only when the gland of Cloquet is positive for metastatic disease, and then only by paradoxical drainage.

As stated earlier, the lesions seen today are smaller than those seen previously, so that the degree of radical pelvic surgery can be modified yet equal control of disease can be achieved. One must remember that tumor spread from the primary site to the regional lymph nodes is by embolization and not by permeation or direct extension unless the lesion is very large. Therefore, radical resection of the non-lymph-node-bearing tissue seems unnecessary. This is why the three-in-one skin incision may become increasingly popular in the future.

For the *radical vulvectomy* portion of the procedure, the boundaries of the dissection should be defined. These are as follows: The lateral incision is a continuation of the groin incisions along the labiocrural crease laterally down into the region of the buttocks. This is then connected to a crescent-like incision anterior to the anal verge. If one chooses to use the three-in-one incision, the radical vulvectomy part of the procedure is essentially an elliptical incision involving similar boundaries, but with the anterior part of the incision beginning high over the symphysis pubis and extending laterally toward the labiocrural line.

The medial incision begins anterior to the external urethral meatus and continues posteriorly just inside the hymenal ring in a circumferential fashion; however, the outline of the dissection must be modified depending on the location and extent of the disease. This inner margin of resection leaves only the urethral and vaginal orifices intact. All the tissue superficial to the inferior fascia of the urogenital diaphragm is excised as an en bloc dissection. This inferior fascia is a direct extension into the vulvar region from the rectus abdominus fascia anteriorly and from the fascia lata laterally. These are all in the same fascial plane and are in contact with each other at the symphysis pubis and rami; thus, the plane of dissection can be established in this way. Adequate margins must be the number one priority.

This en bloc dissection can be facilitated by "bivalving" the upper portion of the vulvar specimen once the anterior dissection off the symphysis pubis has been completed. The ischiocavernosus and bulbocavernosus muscles, as well as the vestibular bulb, are excised as part of the specimen. The major blood supply to the vulva is through the clitoral vessels anteriorly and the pudendal vessels located posterolaterally in the fatty tissue and thought to be located at about 4 and 8 o'clock, respectively. Additional care must be taken in dissecting the perineal body free from the underlying rectal wall. Once the specimen is removed, the bleeding can be easily controlled. Most often the vulvar wound can be closed primarily, utilizing a layer closure, with the levator muscles being approximated in the midline posteriorly. Occasionally, the area over the symphysis remains open; however, this defect fills in quite readily with granulation tissue and ultimately forms a linear scar. A skin graft to the area is not required. All the wounds are closed in a preferential manner with or without the use of a variety of drains.

***Pelvic Lymph Node Dissection*** If there is an indication for a pelvic lymph node dissection, this procedure is performed after the groin lymph node dissection via an extraperitoneal approach. A linear incision is made through the aponeurosis of the external oblique muscle above and parallel to the inguinal ligament. This incision extends from the external inguinal ring to the anterior iliac spine. The oblique muscles are then divided the full length of the incision, using a finger dissection to separate the muscles from the underlying peritoneum and transversalis fascia. After the deep inferior epigastric vessels are doubly ligated and divided, the peritoneum can be mobilized and reflected medially and superiorly. This then exposes the regional lymph node chain up to and beyond the bifurcation of the iliac vessels. The ureter remains attached to the undersurface of the peritoneum and is also reflected medially.

The pelvic lymph nodes are then removed with both sharp and blunt dissection, with care taken to preserve the genitofemoral nerve overlying the iliopsoas muscle and the obturator nerve traversing the obturator space. This dissection includes the external iliac, internal iliac, common iliac (if indicated), and obturator lymph nodes. It must be remembered that the lowest group of the external iliac chain just above the inguinal ligament is always involved before the deeper ones. Once all these lymph node–bearing tissues are excised the peritoneum is repositioned and the opened inguinal ligament area

is reapproximated. Attachment to the lacunar ligament may be necessary to prevent the later development of a femoral hernia.

## REGIONAL LYMPH NODE ASSESSMENT

As stated previously, many gynecologic oncologists in the past considered a pelvic lymph node dissection to be a routine part of the radical surgical treatment for invasive carcinoma of the vulva. Currently, this concept has been modified by most authorities (Way, 1960; Green, 1978), and the pelvic lymph node dissection is no longer carried out routinely, thus allowing careful individualization of treatment. In patients in whom pelvic lymph node dissection was indicated, the frequency of pelvic lymph node involvement ranged from 17 to 26% (Franklin et al, 1971; Morley, 1976), and among those with positive pelvic lymph nodes, the 5-year survival rate was around 4 to 7%. External radiation to the pelvis is an optional form of therapy for these patients. The Gynecologic Oncology Group reported on a comparison of postoperative pelvic irradiation with a retroperitoneal lymphadenectomy when groin lymph nodes were positive (Homesley et al, 1986). In 114 patients, there was a 68% 2-year survival among those patients treated with irradiation versus 54% in the pelvic lymphadenectomy group.

*What then are the criteria for pelvic lymphadenectomy?* Given that pelvic lymph node dissection is no longer a part of routine treatment, the criteria for this procedure in the recent past have been (1) positive groin lymph nodes, (2) carcinoma of the clitoris, (3) carcinoma of the Bartholin gland, (4) melanoma of the vulva, and (5) urethral or vaginal extension of the malignancy. More recently, these criteria have been further modified, since a review of the literature has, except for a few isolated instances, divulged no reports of pelvic lymph node involvement without ipsilateral groin lymph node involvement in patients with carcinoma confined to the vulva; there have been essentially no instances of pelvic lymph node involvement without groin lymph node involvement in patients with carcinoma of the clitoris or carcinoma of the Bartholin gland. Parry-Jones reported in 1960 that he was unable to demonstrate drainage of the clitoral tissue in adults to other than the groin lymph node region, thus discounting any direct drainage into the pelvic lymph node area. In the older literature (Way, 1951; Franklin et al, 1971; Collins et al, 1963), it is stated that the chance of pelvic lymph node involvement without groin lymph node metastases is less than 3%. Currently, then, criteria for pelvic lymphadenectomy in the treatment of carcinoma of the vulva do not exist unless an individualized indication or preference exists. Retroperitoneal pelvic lymph node *exploration* may be an optional approach, since the external iliac nodes are more likely to be involved before any of the other pelvic nodes. This exploration can be easily performed by palpation, with the examining finger inserted into the pelvis through an enlarged femoral ring area. As noted later, melanoma of the vulva is no longer considered an indication for routine pelvic lymphadenectomy.

In spite of the common misbelief that there is bilateral lymphatic drainage of one-sided vulvar lesions, one must recall from a study of the lymphatic drainage of the vulva, that there are no interlacing or anastomotic connections between the two sides of the labia except in the midline in the region of the clitoris, the posterior fourchette, and the perineal body. Lymphatic drainage of unilateral lesions is based upon the prevailing path of least resistance, so that drainage is into the ipsilateral groin lymph node area. Paradoxical or retrograde drainage into the contralateral lymph nodes occurs only when the drainage on the ipsilateral side is obstructed by neoplasm.

In view of these observations, one might suggest unilateral groin lymph node dissection for unilateral disease not involving midline tissues when the lymph nodes from the ipsilateral groin lymph node dissection are negative for metastases (Morris, 1977; Iversen et al, 1981). In the future, a unilateral or hemiradical vulvectomy may also be the treatment of choice for the unilaterally oriented primary lesion.

## RESULTS OF TREATMENT

From a collected series (all references in this chapter), 1,292 patients were treated with radical vulvectomy and regional lymphadenectomy during the period 1926 to 1978 (Table 15-4). The overall 5-year survival rate for this group of patients (when reported) for all stages of carcinoma of the vulva was approximately 66.6%. When this treatment was chosen for patients with Stage I (T1 N0 M0) disease, the overall 5-year survival rate was approximately 87%.

It is well known that one of the most significant prognostic factors in evaluating patients with invasive carcinoma of the vulva is the presence or absence of regional lymph node involvement. It has been stated that almost irrespective of how large the primary lesion is, the prognosis will be quite favorable if the regional lymph nodes are negative. In this same series, the overall 5-year survival rate for all stages of carcinoma without regional lymph node involvement was 81.2%. For those with regional lymph node involvement, the 5-year survival rate was 41.7%. Similarly, when only Stage I disease was analyzed, patients without lymph node in-

volvement had a 92.6% 5-year survival, while those with lymph node involvement had about a 50% 5-year survival, although the reports on this issue are limited. These are all absolute survival figures. When one expands these figures to include more current observations, it is comforting to know that the results in the absence of positive regional lymph nodes continue to be favorable and that survival rates still decrease about 50% stage for stage when regional lymph nodes are involved.

The number of lymph nodes involved and unilateral versus bilateral involvement were not reported frequently enough to allow us to draw any conclusions. Lymph node metastasis did correlate directly with stage of disease, size of lesion, and depth of invasion. From this review, it is estimated that for all stages of disease combined, the incidence of regional lymph node metastasis was 40% and for Stage I disease, 12%.

Occasionally, an even more radical surgical approach to the treatment of carcinoma of the vulva is indicated, depending on the size and location of the primary tumor. A number of investigators have reported a 50 to 70% 5-year survival rate in this small group of patients who underwent some type of pelvic exenteration (Thornton et al, 1973; Kaplan and Kaufman, 1975; Morley, 1976; Cavanagh and Shepherd, 1982). The prognosis is much improved if the lesion is geographically located in such a way that only an anterior or posterior pelvic exenteration is required and the 5-year survival rate approximates 80%. If a total pelvic exenteration is necessary because of anterior and posterior involvement, the lesion is considered to be far advanced and a poorer prognosis must be anticipated.

Recently, radiation therapy for advanced vulvar malignancies has been utilized and the results presented have been promising (Morley et al, 1989).

## POSTOPERATIVE COURSE AND COMPLICATIONS

Once the immediate postoperative and postanesthetic period has passed, patients undergoing this type of surgery usually have a progressively satisfactory course. Most surgeons caring for these patients require that they

TABLE 15-4  Radical Vulvectomy and Groin Lymphadenectomy for Carcinoma of the Vulva—All Stages

| Reference | No. of Patients | Survival Rates (%) | | |
|---|---|---|---|---|
| | | Overall | Negative Nodes | Positive Nodes |
| Morley (1976) | 229 | 66.8 | 83.8 | 37.5 |
| Iversen et al (1981) | 76 | 79 | | 52 |
| Green (1958) | 69 | 61 | 86 | 47 |
| Way (1960) | 81 | 49 | 77 | 42 |
| Krupp (1973) | 100 | | 81 | 42 |
| Figge and Gaudenz (1974) | 50 | 62 | | 42 |
| | | (Absolute = 58) | | |
| Hacker et al (1981) | 100 | 86 | | 70 |

remain strictly confined to bed for 48 to 72 hours, assuming a modified semi-Fowler's position so that the wounds are free of tension and somewhat immobilized. During this period of time, "log-rolling" is permitted to improve circulation. Once this period has passed, the patient is allowed to be up and about with very few limitations, and the in-dwelling catheter is removed after about 5 days.

Whereas wound breakdown is common among these patients, the separations are not significant in most instances, and usually patients are discharged from the hospital in 14 to 21 days. One wonders about the adequacy of the procedure if some degree of wound separation does not occur.

Complications related to the radical surgery used in the treatment of invasive carcinoma of the vulva are classified into two groups: immediate and delayed (Table 15-5). Parenthetically, it must be stated that these patients are all subject to complications unrelated to the procedure itself; however, in spite of the fact these patients are often quite elderly, these complications occur very infrequently.

## Immediate Complications

The most common complication encountered in the postoperative period involves the wound itself, with some degree of wound infection and secondary wound disruption occurring in approximately 40 to 50% of the cases (Figge and Gaudenz, 1974; Morley, 1976; Green, 1978). Often disruption is more an annoyance than a significant complication, and it is treated conservatively using the physician's favorite remedies. On occasion, these wounds are left open at the time of surgery and are allowed to heal secondarily. Once separation has occurred, patients are treated with frequent dressing changes, sitz baths, whirlpool therapy, and debridement if required. A number of topical agents such as zinc oxide, honey, and Elase have been tried in an effort to accelerate healing (Cavanagh et al, 1970; Sedlacke et al, 1976). Shortly after wound disruption has taken place and the infection has cleared, islands of granulation tissue begin to appear. Once this "proud flesh" covers the entire exposed wound, the patient is instructed about self-care of the wound and is then prepared for discharge from the hospital. A visiting nurse may call on these patients two or three times a week for a short period of time.

It is not uncommon for these patients to develop a low-grade fever during the postoperative period, since sepsis secondary to the wound infection or to urinary tract infection is a frequent but not serious postoperative complication. Usually these infections can be controlled if the appropriate therapeutic precautions are taken. Osteitis pubis, on the other hand, is a serious complication, although extremely rare, and may occur if one has been too aggressive in surgically dissecting the tissue attached to the periosteum covering the symphysis pubis. Reports of isolated cases indicate that this is a significant complication in these elderly patients.

Hemorrhage as a complication occurs infrequently, either as a result of the surgery and wound infection or secondary to the frequent use of prophylactic anticoagulants. It must be remembered that these patients are often elderly and frequently self-administer other anticoagulants such as salicylates for control of pain caused by a variety of conditions. Therefore, these patients must be observed closely during the postoperative period, since hemorrhage, for whatever reason, can occur during the first 10 to 14 days after surgery. Although a frightening experience for the patient, hemorrhage can usually be controlled in a straightforward manner.

Thromboembolic disease, on the other hand, occurs with some frequency, since these patients are often elderly and usually immobilized for 2 to 3 days after surgery. Although the increased use of prophylactic anticoagulant therapy in these patients has reduced the incidence of thrombophlebitis significantly, its indiscriminate use might, again, cause bleeding at the operative site. Pulmonary embolization itself is rarely reported as a complication of this procedure.

An overall postoperative surgical and hospital mortality of 1 to 4% seems reasonable when one realizes that some of these patients are in the ninth decade of life (Rutledge and Sinclair, 1968; Figge and Gaudenz, 1974; Morley, 1976). If one were to report more recent experience, this rate would be even further reduced.

Not infrequently, a lymphocyst appears in the groin in the region of the femoral triangle. This complication occurs in approximately 10% of the cases and can be prevented by careful ligation of the lymphatic vessels at the time of surgical dissection. Should a lymphocyst appear, it can be treated by periodic needle aspiration of the cyst fluid followed by local compression to the area. Seldom is surgical intervention required.

## Late Complications

Delayed complications related to this procedure primarily involve the vaginal introitus, urinary tract system, and lower extremities. Introital stenosis of the vagina secondary to scar formation may cause dyspareunia, local fissuring, or a feeling of inelasticity and numbness in the area. This abnormality can be easily corrected by means of relaxing incisions of the introitus, which often can be performed under local anesthesia as an outpatient procedure. Mobilization and advancement of the posterior vaginal mucosa to cover the denuded perineal body at the time of surgery is recommended if the radical dissection in this area causes one to anticipate this type of complication.

**TABLE 15-5** Complications Related to Radical Vulvectomy and Regional Lymphadenectomy

| Immediate | Delayed |
| --- | --- |
| Wound infection | Introital stenosis |
| Wound disruption | Hyperkeratosis |
| Sepsis | Pevic relaxation |
| Hemorrhage | Stress urinary incontinence |
| Thromboembolic disease | Micturition misdirection |
| Lymphocyst | Chronic leg edema |

Pelvic relaxation with the development of a cystocele and/or rectocele secondary to introital gaping is encountered in approximately 20% of the cases. This relaxation may be more apparent than real, since the vulvar tissues that previously covered this area have been surgically removed; however, it must be realized that the vulvar tissues themselves may have provided anatomic support to the vaginal walls. If these lesions become symptomatic, appropriate surgical measures can be prescribed. On occasion, patients will report symptoms of stress urinary incontinence that may or may not be related to the previous radical pelvic surgery. In either case, these patients can be treated satisfactorily with some type of suprapubic urethropexy.

In the future, the gynecologic surgeon should pay more attention to the position of the external urethral meatus at the conclusion of the operation, since these patients complain of an embarrassing misdirection of the urinary stream during micturition, and they frequently must attach a plastic deflector to their excretory receptacle. Hooding of the urethra may also cause urinary splatter. This complication can be prevented at the time of surgery by repositioning the external urethral meatus through a stab wound approximately 1 to 2 cm up the anterior vaginal wall. Again, this should be performed only when this complication is anticipated. Stenosis of the external urethral meatus does occur on rare occasions and, if not corrected, can cause serious urinary retention. An external urethral meatotomy is the treatment of choice for this complication.

Probably the most annoying late complication is significant swelling of the lower extremities. As a preventive measure, elastic stockings at least up to the knees should be worn for the first 6 months after surgery in the hope of minimizing chronic obstructive lymphangitis with secondary chronic lymphedema of the lower extremity. Again, as stated before, preservation of the saphenous vein at the time of groin lymph node dissection may help significantly to reduce this complication at no therapeutic expense to the patient.

## OTHER TREATMENT MODALITIES

The role of radiation therapy in the primary treatment of invasive carcinoma of the vulva is probably limited, since the results have not been favorable and the vulvar tissues respond poorly to this type of exposure. There does, however, appear to be an indication for its use in far advanced lesions, and this is being evaluated (Latourette et al, 1972; Boronow et al, 1987). Currently, the relative merits of pelvic irradiation versus pelvic lymphadenectomy in those patients demonstrating metastasis to the groin lymph nodes are being studied by a number of investigators (Daly and Million, 1974; Morley, 1976). Those recommending pelvic irradiation support the concept of treating the external disease with radical vulvectomy and groin lymph node dissection and treating the internal disease with pelvic irradiation.

A number of investigators are reporting on the relative value of preoperative irradiation in the management of some invasive carcinomas of the vulva, especially when the lesion is unusually large or strategically located (Boronow, 1973, 1982; Acosta et al, 1978; Jafari and Magalotti, 1981). These results are too preliminary to allow any final conclusions to be drawn at this time. However, with improved radiotherapeutic methods and techniques appearing on the clinical horizon, this may be the method of the future under certain circumstances. Boronow et al (1987) have reported a 75% 5-year survival rate for the combined treatment of primary cases of vulvar cancer.

The experience with chemotherapy in the treatment of advanced or recurrent carcinoma of the vulva has been disappointing. Various single chemotherapeutic agents and a variety of combinations have been tried. However, one must await the reports of the ongoing studies being carried out by various collaborators (Deppe et al, 1977; Iversen, 1982).

## REHABILITATION

The long-term rehabilitation of these patients is an extremely important part of the followup care and observation. Most often, they are able to return to full activity and lead active and rewarding lives. Sexual intercourse, when desired, is certainly permissible, and in most cases patients are able to participate satisfactorily, since the caliber and depth of the vagina are seldom altered. On occasion, a stricture of the introitus is encountered, but this can be remedied easily, as indicated previously.

From a cosmetic point of view, there is a significant alteration in the appearance of the perineum—a change that can threaten the patient's body image and self-esteem. The patient must continue to be mindful of the importance of this treatment, which was required to control this potentially fatal disease (Fig. 15-4). Fortunately, most of these women are in the older age group, and this anatomic alteration does not seem to threaten their emotional and sexual stability as much as it would in younger patients.

Although many plastic procedures have been attempted, vulvoplasties have not been particularly successful to date. At the present time, myocutaneous gracilis flaps are being evaluated in patients who desire this type of rehabilitation (Dinner et al, 1979; Wheeless et al, 1979). Silastic implants similar to those used in augmentation mammoplasties have been mentioned. The classic Z-plasty approach to the management of extensive vulvar defects has also been recommended (Julian et al, 1971; Rankin and Pinkney, 1973). It is my opinion that none of the reconstructive procedures should be performed at the time of the primary surgery, but rather should be deferred until later, when they may prove to be necessary. If sexual function is satisfactory and only local appearance is of concern, the patient should probably receive sexual counseling rather than undergo surgical correction of the postoperative disfigurement.

## UNUSUAL MALIGNANCIES OF THE VULVA

*Verrucous carcinoma of the vulva,* with its distinctive clinical and pathologic features, is a variant of an epi-

**304** | UNIT II Sites

dermoid carcinoma. It is a locally aggressive, nonmeta-static, warty, fungating tumor that gradually increases in size and pushes into, rather than invades, the underlying structures. There is often an active inflammatory response in the surrounding stroma (Isaacs, 1976). Fewer than 50 cases have been reported in the literature to date.

Microscopically, these lesions show an outward growth of the papillary processes composed of well-differentiated squamous cell carcinoma covered with parakeratosis and keratin. The cells are large and contain eosinophilic cytoplasm with marked nuclear atypism, loss of polarity, and few mitotic figures (Foye et al, 1969; Selim and Lankerani, 1979). Despite their aggressive clinical appearance, these tumors tend to grow slowly and invade locally, and rarely spread to regional lymph nodes. Distant metastases are also quite uncommon (Japaze et al, 1982). At present, once this verrucous variety of invasive carcinoma of the vulva is diagnosed, wide surgical excision appears to be the treatment of choice. However, since lymph node metastasis has been reported infrequently, one should consider regional lymph node dissection in the larger and recurrent lesions.

Whereas over 90% of malignancies involving the vulva are of the epidermoid type, a significant number of nonsquamous cell carcinomas involve the vulvar tissues (Table 15-6). *Primary carcinoma of the Bartholin gland* accounts for approximately 5% of all vulvar cancers, and over 200 cases have been reported in the world literature (Dodson et al, 1978; Leuchter et al, 1982). The Bartholin gland duct is lined by squamous epithelium that becomes transitional as it approaches the adenomatous part of the gland. Only about 50% of Bartholin gland tumors are of the nonepidermoid type, since the other half of these lesions involve the duct itself. Based on a review of the literature, radical vulvectomy and bilateral groin lymphadenectomy are recommended as the treatment of choice for all histologic types of Bartholin gland carcinoma (Chamlian et al, 1972; Leuchter et al, 1982). Again, pelvic lymph node dissection is not necessary unless there is groin lymph node involvement. Unfortunately, these lesions are clinically misdiagnosed as a Bartholin cyst or Bartholin abscess in more than half of the patients at the time of

initial inspection (Chamlian et al, 1972). Increased physician awareness and frequent biopsy of suspected lesions, especially in the elderly patient, are in order. The overall 5-year survival rate approximates 70% for this small group of patients; this rate is significantly below that reported for all carcinomas of the vulva and is probably directly related to the delay in diagnosis. For unexplained reasons, the left Bartholin gland is involved more frequently than the right.

*Basal cell carcinoma* is rarely encountered on the female external genitalia. This lesion is a locally invasive, nonmetastatic tumor that usually involves the labium majus (Cruz-Jimenez and Abell, 1975; Breen et al, 1975). Wide local excision is generally recommended as the treatment of choice, since these lesions uniformly respond satisfactorily to this form of treatment (Palladino et al, 1969).

Approximately 500 cases of *melanoma of the vulva* have been reported in the literature to date, and the overall 5-year survival rate—irrespective of the therapeutic modality used—approximates 50% (Yackel et al, 1970; Morrow and Rutledge, 1972; Chung et al, 1975; Karlen et al, 1975; Podratz et al, 1982; Jaramillo et al, 1985; Rose et al, 1988). Nowhere in the field of gynecologic oncology is the term "vagaries of neoplasia" more applicable than in the evaluation of the responses to treatment of vulvar melanomas. Although there have been a number of satisfactory responses to wide local excision, there have also been a number of failures after the radical surgical procedures. This lesion most often affects the labia minora or the clitoris. Until recently, the treatment of choice has been radical vulvectomy and bilateral groin and pelvic lymphadenectomy (Yackel et al, 1970; Morrow and Rutledge, 1972; Fenn and Abell, 1973).

It is hoped that as histologic types become better understood and the depth of invasion can be more accurately identified, the scientific approach to the treatment of this unusually aggressive disease will improve. The lentigo maligna type, which involves just the epidermis, has the best prognosis and requires less radical surgery. The nodular type of melanoma has the worst prognosis, and this is directly related to its potential for vertical growth. The superficial spreading type fits between these two extremes. It is well known that melanoma is spread via the lymphatic and hematogenous routes, with the lungs and brain being quickly involved once it becomes blood-borne. The prognosis is extremely guarded when lymph node metastasis is found.

The FIGO classification for staging carcinoma of the vulva does not appear to be applicable to these melanomas; therefore, another method should be used in determining the preferred type of treatment for these patients (Table 15-7). A number of consultants recommend wide local excision for Clark Level I and II disease (Clark et al, 1969) or a Breslow (1970) depth of invasion of less than 1.5 mm unless palpable regional lymph nodes are encountered. Some state that no patient with invasive melanoma of the vulva 1 mm or less below the granular layer of the vulvar skin has succumbed to the disease (Chung et al, 1975). Radical vulvectomy with groin and pelvic lymphadenectomy (if groin nodes are

---

TABLE 15-6 Nonsquamous Cell Malignancies of the Vulva

Carcinoma of the Bartholin gland
Malignant melanoma of the vulva
Basal cell carcinoma of the vulva
Adenocystic basal cell carcinoma of the vulva
Adenoid squamous carcinoma of the vulva
Sarcomas of the vulva
  Leiomyosarcoma
  Neurogenous sarcoma
  Rhabdomyosarcoma
  Other sarcomas
Other malignancies
  Primary—hydradenocarcinoma
  Secondary—breast, etc.

---

**TABLE 15-7**  Classification of Melanomas of the Vulva

| Clark Levels | Chung's Modification |
|---|---|
| I  Intraepithelial | Intraepithelial |
| II  Extension into papillary dermis | < 1-mm invasion into dermis or lamina propria |
| III  Filling dermal papillae | 1- to 2-mm invasion into subepithelial tissue |
| IV  Invasion of collagen in reticular dermis | > 2-mm invasion into fibrous or fibromuscular tissue |
| V  Extension into subcutaneous fat | Extension into subcutaneous fat |

Breslow's Depth of Invasion
I  ≤ 0.75 mm from skin surface
II  0.76-1.4 mm from skin surface
III  ≥ 1.5 mm from skin surface

---

positive) are recommended as the treatment of choice for Level III, IV, and V disease or if the depth of invasion is 1.5 mm or greater. A prospective randomized study of therapeutic trials in patients with vulvar melanoma is imperative to confirm currently recommended treatment programs.

The role of chemotherapy and/or immunotherapy in the treatment of melanoma of the vulva is an ongoing study and will be reported in the future by other investigators.

*Adenoid cystic carcinoma* of the vulva is an exceedingly rare tumor that causes unrelenting pain, since the neoplasm characteristically involves the perineural and neural tissues (Abell, 1963; Dodson et al, 1978). This lesion is uniformly treated with radical vulvectomy and groin lymph node dissection; however, it is prone to local recurrence and metastasis, even though its course is often protracted and insidious. *Adenoid squamous cell carcinoma*, on the other hand, which is often attributed to solar damage, is treated in the same way as the usual variety of squamous cell carcinoma of the vulva and the survival rates are not statistically different (Lasser and Morris, 1974).

*Sarcomas of the vulva* constitute a rare and perplexing group of malignant neoplasms that are infrequently reported in the literature (DiSaia et al, 1971; Piver et al, 1972; Davos and Abell, 1976; Gallup et al, 1976). Leiomyosarcoma appears to be the most frequently encountered sarcoma in this small group of patients. From a review of over 35 cases (DiSaia et al, 1971; Tavassoli et al, 1979), wide local excision is recommended as the initial treatment of choice, with a 5-year survival rate approximating 100%. Locally recurring lesions are similarly treated. Rhabdomyosarcoma, on the other hand, is an aggressive, rapidly growing tumor that requires aggressive surgical and medical management as the only hope for improving the 5-year survival (Piver et al, 1973). Neurogenous sarcomas, embryonal sarcomas, epithelioid sarcomas, hemangiopericytomas, dermatofibrosarcomas, and others have all been reported to involve the vulvar tissues. Although too few cases are available for significant analysis of the response to treatment, radical surgery is probably the treatment of choice for these lesions. Size of the tumor, extent of infiltration, and degree of mitotic activity obviously must play important roles in the final decision regarding the therapeutic approach.

## SUMMARY

Malignant lesions of the vulva, especially in the preinvasive stage, appear to be increasing in frequency. This is thought by some to be directly related to the use of a variety of synthetic undergarments and to the changes in sexual activity; however, more scientific studies are required before such a cause–effect relationship can be accepted. Whatever the cause, if these lesions of the vulva are diagnosed in the preinvasive or early invasive stage without regional lymph node involvement, the prognosis is quite favorable and the 5-year survival rates are well over 90%. Treatment of these preinvasive and invasive lesions of the vulva is primarily surgical. Other therapeutic modalities are used only when the disease is resistant to surgical therapy, when the lesion has extended to the regional lymph nodes, or when systemic involvement has been identified. Occasionally, surgery is contraindicated for medical reasons.

Guidelines and prognostic factors for the future include the following:

1. Surgical staging of disease will increase its accuracy and the accuracy of prognostications.
2. Five-year survival rates for all stages of disease will drop about 50% if groin lymph nodes are positive.
3. In unilateral labial lesions, no contralateral lymph node assessment is indicated if the ipsilateral groin nodes are negative.
4. If groin nodes are negative, pelvic lymph node treatment is not indicated.
5. The overall incidence of positive groin lymph nodes is approximately 35%.

Again, given early diagnosis and early instituation of appropriate therapy, malignancy of the vulva is a curable disease in the great majority of cases.

## REFERENCES

Abell MR: Adenocystic basal cell carcinoma of the vestibular glands of the vulva. *Am J Obstet Gynecol* 86:470-482, 1963.

Abell MR, Gosling JR: Intra-epithelial and infiltrative carcinoma of the vulva: Bowen's type. *Cancer* 14:318, 1961.

Abitbol MM: Carcinoma of the vulva: Improvements in the surgical approach. *Am J Obstet Gynecol* 117:483, 1973.

Abitbol MM, Meng C-H, Romney SL: Anatomic and therapeutic aids of lymphangiography in pelvic malignancy. *Am J Obstet Gynecol* 93:95, 1965.

Acosta AA, Given FT, Frazier AB, Cordoba RB, Luminari A: Preoperative radiation therapy in the management of squamous cell carcinoma of the vulva: Preliminary report. *Am J Obstet Gynecol* 132:198, 1978.

Barnhill DR, Hoskins WJ, Metz P: The use of rhomboid flap after partial vulvectomy. *Obstet Gynecol* 62:444-447, 1983.

Beecham CT: Paget's disease of the vulva: Recurrence in skin grafts. *Obstet Gynecol* 47(Suppl):55s, 1976.

Benedet JL, Murphy KJ: Squamous carcinoma in situ of the vulva. *Gynecol Oncol* 14:213-219, 1982.

Bernstein SG, Kovaks BR, Townsend DE, Morrow CP: Vulvar carcinoma in situ. *Obstet Gynecol* 61:304, 1983.

Boehm F, Morris JM: Paget's disease and apocrine gland carcinoma of the vulva. *Obstet Gynecol* 38:185, 1971.

Boronow RC: Therapeutic alternative to primary exenteration for advanced vulvo-vaginal cancer. *Gynecol Oncol* 1:223-225, 1973.

Boronow RC: Combined therapy as an alternative to exenteration for locally advanced vulvo-vaginal cancer. *Cancer* 46:6, 1982.

Boronow RC, Hickman BT, Reagan MT, Smith RA, Steadham RE: Combined therapy as an alternative to exenteration for locally advanced vulvovaginal cancer. II. Results, complications, and dosimetric and surgical considerations. *Am J Clin Oncol* 10:171-181, 1987.

Boutselis JG: Radical vulvectomy for invasive squamous cell carcinoma of the vulva. *Obstet Gynecol* 39:827, 1972.

Breen JL, Neubecker RD, Greenwald E, Gregori KA: Basal cell carcinoma of the vulva. *Obstet Gynecol* 46:122, 1975.

Breen JL, Smith CI, Gregori KA: Extramammary Paget's disease. *Clin Obstet Gynecol* 21:1107, 1973.

Breslow A: Thickness, cross-sectional areas, and depth of invasion in the prognosis of cutaneous melanoma. *Ann Surg* 172:902-908, 1970.

Buscema J, Stern JL, Woodruff JD: Early invasive carcinoma of the vulva. *Am J Obstet Gynecol* 140:563-569, 1981.

Caglar H, Tamer S, Hreshchyshyn MM: Vulvar intraepithelial neoplasia. *Obstet Gynecol* 60:346, 1982.

Carson TE, Hopkins WJ, Wurzel JF: Topical 5-fluorouracil in the treatment of carcinoma in situ of the vulva. *Obstet Gynecol* 47(Suppl):59s, 1976.

Cavanagh D, Beazley J, Ostapowicz F: Radical operations for carcinoma of the vulva. *J Obstet Gynaecol Br Commonw* 77:1037-1040, 1970.

Cavanagh D, Shepherd JH: The place of pelvic exenteration in the primary management of advanced carcinoma of the vulva. *Gynecol Oncol* 13:318-322, 1982.

Chamlian DL, Taylor HB: Primary carcinoma of the Bartholin gland: A report of 24 patients. *Obstet Gynecol* 46:122, 1975.

Charles HA: Carcinoma of the vulva. *Br Med J* 1:397-402, 1972.

Choo CY: Double primary epidermoid carcinoma of the vulva and cervix. *Gynecol Oncol* 9:324-333, 1980.

Chu J, Tamini KH, Ek M, Figge DC: Stage I vulvar cancer: Criteria for micro-invasion. *Obstet Gynecol* 59:176, 1982.

Chung AF, Woodruff JW, Lewis JL Jr: Malignant melanoma of the vulva: A report of 44 cases. *Obstet Gynecol* 45:638, 1975.

Clark WH Jr, From L, Bernardino EA, Mihm MC: The histogenesis and biologic behavior of primary human malignant melanomas of the skin. *Cancer Res* 29:705-727, 1969.

Classification and staging of malignant tumors in the female pelvis. *Acta Obstet Gynecol Scand* 50:7, 1971.

Collins CG: A clinical stain for use in selecting biopsy sites in patients with vulvar diseases. *Obstet Gynecol* 28:158, 1966.

Collins CG, Collins JH, Barclay DL, Nelson EW: Cancer involving the vulva. *Am J Obstet Gynecol* 87:762, 1963.

Comas MR, Morris CH, Averette HE: Lymphography and vulvar carcinoma. *Obstet Gynecol* 33:177, 1969.

Creasman WT, Gallagher S, Rutledge F: Paget's disease of the vulva. *Gynecol Oncol* 3:133-148, 1975.

Crum CP, Fu YS, Levine RU, Richart RM, Townsend DE, Fenoglio CM: Intra-epithelial squamous lesions of the vulva: Biologic and histologic criteria for the distinction of condylomas from the vulvar intra-epithelial neoplasia. *Am J Obstet Gynecol* 144:77, 1982.

Cruz-Jimenez PR, Abell MR: Cutaneous basal cell carcinoma of the vulva. *Cancer* 36:1860, 1975.

Daly JW, Million RR: Radical vulvectomy combined with elective node irradiation for TxNo squamous cell carcinoma of the vulva. *Cancer* 32:161-165, 1974.

Davos I, Abell MR: Soft tissue sarcomas of the vulva. *Gynecol Oncol* 4:70-86, 1976.

Dean RE, Taylor ES, Weisbrod DM, Martin JW: The treatment of premalignant and malignant lesions of the vulva. *Am J Obstet Gynecol* 119:59, 1974.

Deppe G, Bruckner HW, Cohen CJ: Adriamycin treatment for advanced vulvar carcinoma. *Obstet Gynecol* 50(Suppl):13s, 1977.

deValera E: Radical vulvectomy. *Am J Obstet Gynecol* 101:78-83, 1968.

Dinner MI, Peters CR, Martinbeau PW, Bolsky RL: A perineal reconstruction following extensive radical vulvectomy. *Gynecol Oncol* 8:78-83, 1979.

DiPaola GR, Gomez-Rueda N, Arrighi L: Relevance of micro-invasion in carcinoma of the vulva. *Obstet Gynecol* 45:647-649, 1975.

DiSaia PJ, Creasman WT, Rich WM: An alternative approach to early cancer of the vulva. *Am J Obstet Gynecol* 133:825-830, 1979.

Di Saia PJ, Rich WM: Surgical approach to multi-focal carcinoma in situ of the vulva. *Am J Obstet Gynecol* 140:136-145, 1981.

DiSaia PJ, Rutledge F, Smith JP: Sarcoma of the vulva: Report of 12 patients. *Obstet Gynecol* 38:180, 1971.

Dodson MG, O'Leary JA, Orfei E: Adenoid cystic carcinoma of the vulva. *Obstet Gynecol* 51(Suppl):26s, 1978.

Donaldson ES, Powell DE, Hanson MB, van Nagell JR Jr: Prognostic parameters in invasive vulvar cancer. *Gynecol Oncol* 11:184-190, 1981.

Fenn ME, Abell MR: Melanomas of the vulva and vagina. *Obstet Gynecol* 41:902, 1973.

Fenn ME, Morley GW, Abell MR: Paget's disease of the vulva. *Obstet Gynecol* 38:660, 1971.

Ferenczy A: Using lasers to treat condylomas and VIN. *Contemp Obstet Gynecol* 20:57, 1982.

Figge CD, Gaudenz R: Invasive carcinoma of the vulva. *Am J Obstet Gynecol* 119:382, 1974.

Folsome GE: Benign and malignant tumors of the vulva. *JAMA* 114:1499, 1940.

Foster DC, Woodruff JD: The use of dinitrochlorobenzene in the treatment of vulvar carcinoma in situ. *Gynecol Oncol* 11:330-339, 1981.

Foye G, Marsh MR, Minkowitz S: Verrucous carcinoma of the vulva. *Obstet Gynecol* 43:484, 1969.

Franklin EW III: Clinical staging of carcinoma of the vulva. *Am J Obstet Gynecol* 40:277, 1972.

Franklin EW III, Rutledge FD: Prognostic factors in epidermoid carcinoma of the vulva. *Obstet Gynecol* 37:892, 1971.

Friedrich EG Jr, Wilkinson EJ, Fu YS: Carcinoma in situ of the vulva: Continuing challenge. *Am J Obstet Gynecol* 136:830, 1980.

Friedrich EG Jr, Wilkinson EJ, Steingraeber PH, Lewis JD: Paget's disease of the vulva and carcinoma of the breast. *Obstet Gynecol* 46:130, 1975.

Gallup DG, Abell MR, Morley GW: Epithelioid sarcoma of the vulva. *Obstet Gynecol* 48(Suppl):14s, 1976.

Green TH Jr: Carcinoma of the vulva: A reassessment. *Obstet Gynecol* 52:462, 1978.

Green TH Jr, Ulfelder H, Meigs JV: Epidermoid carcinoma of the vulva: An analysis of 238 cases. Parts I and II. *Am J Obstet Gynecol* 73:834 and 848, 1958.

Hacker NF, Leuchter RS, Berek JS, Castaldo TW, Lagasse LD: Radical vulvectomy and bilateral groin lymphadenectomy through separate groin incisions. *Obstet Gynecol* 58:574, 1981.

Hall DJ, Goplerud DR, Dunn LJ: A new technique for vulvar skin grafting. *Obstet Gynecol* 54:343, 1979.

Hart WR, Millman RB: Progression of intra-epithelial Paget's disease of the vulva in invasive carcinoma. *Cancer* 40:2333-2337, 1977.

Hart WR, Morris HJ, Helwig EB: Relation of lichen sclerosus et atrophicus of the vulva to development of carcinoma. *Obstet Gynecol* 45:369, 1975.

Hoffman JS, Kumar NB, Morley GW: Microinvasive squamous carcinoma of the vulva: Search for a definition. *Obstet Gynecol* 61:615-681, 1983.

Homesley HD, Bundy BN, Sedlis A, Adcock L: Radiation therapy versus pelvic node resection for carcinoma of the vulva with positive groin nodes. *Obstet Gynecol* 68:733-740, 1986.

Hopkins MP, Reid GC, Vettrano I, Morley GW: Squamous cell carcinoma of the vulva: Prognostic factors influencing survival. *Gynecol Oncol* 43:113-117, 1991.

Isaacs HJ: Verrucous carcinoma of the female genital tract. *Gynecol Oncol* 4:259-269, 1976.

Iversen T: Irradiation and bleomycin in the treatment of inoperable vulvar carcinoma. *Acta Obstet Gynecol Scand* 61:195- 197, 1982.

Iversen T, Abeler V, Aalders J: Individualized treatment of Stage I carcinoma of the vulva. *Obstet Gynecol* 57:85, 1981.

Jafari K, Cartnick EN: Microinvasive carcinoma of the vulva. *Am J Obstet Gynecol* 125:274, 1976.

Jafari K, Magalotti M: Radiation therapy in carcinoma of the vulva. *Cancer* 47:686-692, 1981.

Japaze H, Dinh TV, Woodruff JD: Verrucous carcinoma of the vulva: Study of 24 cases. *Obstet Gynecol* 60:462, 1982.

Jaramillo BA, Ganjei P, Averette HE, Sevin B-U, Lovecchio JL: Malignant melanoma of the vulva. *Obstet Gynecol* 66:398-401, 1985.

Jeffcoate TNA: Chronic vulval dystrophies. *Am J Obstet Gynecol* 95:61, 1966.

Julian CG, Callison J, Woodruff JD: Plastic management of extensive vulvar defects. *Obstet Gynecol* 38:193, 1971.

Kaplan AL, Kaufman RH: The management of advanced carcinoma of the vulva. *Gynecol Oncol* 3:220, 1975.

Kaplan AL, Kaufman RH, Birken RA, Simkin S: Intra-epithelial carcinoma of the vulva with extension to the anal canal. *Obstet Gynecol* 58:368-371, 1981.

Karlen JR, Piver S, Barlow JJ: Melanoma of the vulva. *Obstet Gynecol* 45:181, 1975.

Kinmouth JB: Lymphangiography in man: Method of outlining lymphatic trunks at operation. *Clin Sci* 2:13, 1952.

Krupp PI, Bohm IW: 5-Fluorouracil topical treatment on in situ vulvar cancer: A preliminary report. *Obstet Gynecol* 51:702, 1978.

Krupp PJ, Lee FY, Batson HWK, Allen PM, Collins JH: Carcinoma of the vulva. *Gynecol Oncol* 1:345-362, 1973.

Lasser AM, Morris JM: Adenoid squamous cell carcinoma of the vulva. *Cancer* 33:224, 1974.

Latourette HB: Radiation therapy in carcinoma of the vulva: A review of 53 patients. *Cancer* 30:997-1000, 1972.

Lee SC, Roth LM, Ehrlich C, Hall JM: Extra-mammary Paget's of the vulva. *Gynecol Oncol* 3:133-148, 1977.

Leuchter RS, Hacker NF, Voet RL, Berek JS, Townsend DE, Lagasse LD: Primary carcinoma of the Bartholin gland: A report of 14 cases and a review of the literature. *Obstet Gynecol* 60:361, 1982.

Lifshitz S, Roberts JA: Treatment of carcinoma in situ of the vulva with topical 5-fluorouracil. *Obstet Gynecol* 56:242, 1980.

McKelvey JL: Carcinoma of the vulva: Classifications, treatment and results. *Proc Natl Cancer Conf* 6:361-364, 1970.

Morley GW: Infiltrative carcinoma of the vulva: Results of surgical treatment. *Am J Obstet Gynecol* 124:874, 1976.

Morley GW: Cancer of the vulva: A review. *Cancer* 48:597-601, 1981.

Morley GW, Hopkin MP, Lindenauer SM, Roberts JA: Pelvic exenteration, University of Michigan: 100 patients at 5 years. *Obstet Gynecol* 74:6, 934-943, Dec. 1989.

Morris JM: A formula for selective lymphadenectomy: Its application to cancer of the vulva. *Obstet Gynecol* 50:152, 1977.

Morrow CP, Rutledge FN: Melanoma of the vulva. *Obstet Gynecol* 39:745-752, 1972.

Palladino VS, Duffy JL, Bures GJ: Basal cell carcinoma of the vulva. *Cancer* 24:460, 1969.

Parker RT, Duncan I, Rampone J, Creasman W: Operative management of early invasive epidermoid carcinoma of the vulva. *Am J Obstet Gynecol* 123:349, 1975.

Parmley HT, Woodruff JD, Julian CG: Invasive vulvar Paget's disease. *Obstet Gynecol* 46:341, 1975.

Parry-Jones E: Lymphatics of the vulva. *Br J Obstet Gynaecol* 67:919, 1960.

Piver MS, Barlow JJ, Wang JJ, Shah NK: Combined radical surgery, radiation therapy and chemotherapy in infants with vulvo-vaginal and embryonal rhabdomyosarcoma. *Obstet Gynecol* 42:522, 1973.

Piver MS, Tsukada Y, Barlow J: Epithelioid sarcoma of the vulva. *Obstet Gynecol* 40:839, 1972.

Podratz KC, Gaffey TA, Symmonds RE, Johansen KL, O'Brien PC: Melanoma of the vulva: An update. *Gynecol Oncol* 16:153-168, 1983.

Rankin RP Jr: The use of Z-plasty in gynecologic operations. *Am J Obstet Gynecol* 117:231, 1973.

Roberts JA, Watring WG, Lagasse LD: Treatment of vulvar intra-epithelial neoplasia with local bleomycin. *Cancer Clin Trials* 3:351-354, 1980.

Rose PG, Piver S, Tsukada Y, Lau T: Conservative therapy for melanoma of the vulva. *Am J Obstet Gynecol* 159:52-55, 1988.

Rutledge F, Sinclair M: Treatment of intraepithelial carcinoma of the vulva by skin excision and graft. *Am J Obstet Gynecol* 102:806, 1968.

Sedlacek TB, Mangan CE, Giuntoli RL, Mikuta JJ: Zinc sulfate: An adjunct to wound healing in patients undergoing radical vulvectomy. *Gynecol Oncol* 4:324-327, 1976.

Selim MA, Lankerani MR: Verrucous carcinoma of the vulva. *J Reprod Med* 22:93, 1979.

Seski JC, Reinhalter ER, Silva J Jr: Abnormalities of lymphocyte transformations in women with intraepithelial carcinoma of the vulva. *Obstet Gynecol* 52:332-336, 1978.

Taussig FJ: Cancer of the vulva: An analysis of 155 cases. *Am J Obstet Gynecol* 40:764, 1940.

Taussig FJ: Carcinoma of the vulva. *Am J Obstet Gynecol* 40:277, 1972.

Tavassoli FA, Norris HJ: Smooth muscle tumors of the vulva. *Obstet Gynecol* 53:213, 1979.

Thornton WN Jr, Flanagan WC Jr: Pelvic exenteration in the treatment of advanced malignancy of the vulva. *Am J Obstet Gynecol* 117:774, 1973.

Trelford JD, Silverton JS: Successful plastic procedures of the perineum. *Gynecol Oncol* 7:239-247, 1979.

Twombly GH: The technique of radical vulvectomy for carcinoma of the vulva. *Cancer* 6:516-530, 1953.

Way S: The anatomy of the lymphatic drainage of the vulva and its influence on the radical operation for carcinoma. *Ann R Coll Surg Engl* 3:187, 1948.

Way S: *Malignant Disease of the Female Genital Tract*. London, Churchill Livingstone, 1951, pp 46-47.

Way S: Carcinoma of the vulva. *Am J Obstet Gynecol* 79:692, 1960.

Way S, Benedet JL: Involvement of inguinal lymph nodes in carcinoma of the vulva. *Gynecol Oncol* 1:119-122, 1973.

Weintraub I, Lagasse LD: Reversibility of vulvar atypia by DNCB-induced delayed hypersensitivity. *Obstet Gynecol* 41:195, 1973.

Wharton JT, Gallagher S, Rutledge FD: Microinvasive carcinoma of the vulva. *Am J Obstet Gynecol* 118:159, 1974.

Wheeless CR Jr, McGibbon B, Dorsey JH, Maxwell GP: Gracilis myocutaneous flap in reconstruction of the vulva and female perineum. *Obstet Gynecol* 54:97, 1979.

Wilkinson EJ, Friedrich EG, Eduard G, Fu YS: Multicentric nature of vulvar carcinoma in situ. *Obstet Gynecol* 58:69, 1981.

Woodruff JD: Vulvar atypia and carcinoma in situ. *J Reprod Med* 17:155, 1976.

Yackel DB, Symmonds RE, Kempers RD: Melanoma of the vulva. *Obstet Gynecol* 35:625, 1970.

# Chapter 16 | Cancer of the Vagina and Fallopian Tube

*Edward Podczaski    Arthur L. Herbst*

## CANCER OF THE VAGINA

The majority of vaginal malignancies are metastatic (Gompel and Silverberg, 1985) and may be the first manifestation of an occult neoplasm arising, in many cases, from an endometrial or cervical carcinoma. From 12 to 14% of endometrial carcinomas metastasize to the vagina, presumably by retrograde spread through submucosal lymphatics (Way, 1951). Less commonly, vaginal metastases are from tumors of the ovary, rectum, and kidney (Bergman, 1966; Nerdrum, 1966). Choriocarcinoma can also present as hemorrhagic mulberry-like lesions in the vagina (MacRae, 1951).

Primary vaginal cancer is uncommon and represents approximately 1 to 3% of all female genital tract malignancies. Vaginal cancers comprise a heterogenous group of tumors, with endodermal sinus tumors and embryonal rhabdomyosarcomas (sarcoma botryoides) predominating in infancy; clear cell carcinomas in adolescence and young adulthood; and squamous cell carcinomas (the most common variety), adenocarcinomas, melanomas, and sarcomas in later adult life. By definition, these malignant neoplasms arise in the vagina and do not involve the external os of the cervix superiorly or the vulva inferiorly; the former tumors are classified as cervical and the latter as vulvar. Vaginal cancers are staged according to criteria set forth by the International Federation of Gynecology and Obstetrics (FIGO) (Table 16-1).

### Diagnosis and Treatment

Regardless of tumor histology, the majority of affected patients present with abnormal vaginal bleeding or discharge. Anterior vaginal tumors occasionally produce urinary tract symptoms, whereas cancers of the posterior wall may produce constipation, tenesmus, or pain on defecation. From 10 to 20% of patients with vaginal carcinomas can be asymptomatic at the time of diagnosis (Pride et al, 1979; Gallup et al, 1987; Sulak et al, 1988). Such tumors are usually detected as gross lesions or when the cytology is found to be abnormal at the time of a routine visit.

It is a paradox that cancers of the vagina arise in a clinically accessible site yet are often not diagnosed until late in the course of the disease. Delay in the diagnosis of these cancers frequently occurs, in part because of their rarity, as well as because of a lack of recognition that the abnormal symptoms may be due to malignancy. In approximately 20% of patients, there is a delay of over 7 months from the onset of symptoms to the initiation of therapy (Herbst et al, 1970). In general, the length of time the patient has been symptomatic is related to the size of the tumor and its spread; patients with longstanding symptoms usually have larger tumors that are more difficult to treat.

A definitive diagnosis can usually be made by biopsy of a visible or palpable lesion. Occasionally, an abnormal cytology report leads to a careful pelvic examination that will reveal a primary vaginal malignancy. In the course of the examination, the vaginal speculum should be carefully rotated so as not to obscure a small lesion.

Treatment of vaginal cancer is predicated on the location and size of the lesion, the pertinent lymphatic drainage, and the regional anatomy. Effective therapy is complicated by the proximity of these lesions to the bladder, ureters, and rectum. As a basis for the origin and treatment of invasive vaginal neoplasms, we will initially consider the anatomy and embryology of the vagina and its related structures.

### Vaginal Anatomy and Embryology

The vagina is a fibromuscular tube that forms the distal portion of the female reproductive tract. Its anterior surface is anatomically related to the bladder base and urethra. The lower three-fourths of the posterior wall is in contact with the rectum, while the upper one-fourth is separated from the rectosigmoid by the pouch of Douglas. At the superior end of the vagina, the cervix projects through the anterior vaginal wall creating a circular sulcus that entirely surrounds the cervix, thereby forming the vaginal fornices (Fig. 16-1).

The vaginal wall consists of three layers: the muscularis, the mucosa, and the adventitia. On gross examination, the mucosal membrane has numerous folds or rugae separated by transverse folds. This mucosal surface is lined by a stratified, nonkeratinizing squamous epithelium. The vaginal mucosa contains no glands and is lubricated by transudation across the mucosa as well as by secretions from the cervix (Weiss and Greep, 1977). Under the influence of estrogens, the vaginal mucosa thickens due to proliferation and maturation of epithelial cells. The muscularis of the vagina is composed of two poorly defined muscle layers, an inner circular layer and an external layer of longitudinal smooth muscle fibers. It encircles a highly vascular submucosa that contains a venous plexus and loose connective tissue. The adventitia lies outside the muscularis and consists of blood vessels, lymphatics, and connective tissues that anchor the vagina to neighboring structures (Goss, 1973).

The paired vaginal arteries arise from the adjacent

| TABLE 16-1 | FIGO System Used for Staging Vaginal Cancers |
|---|---|
| Stage 0 | Carcinoma in situ. |
| Stage I | Carcinoma is limited to the vaginal wall. |
| Stage II | Carcinoma has involved subvaginal tissue but has not extended to the pelvic wall. |
| Stage III | Carcinoma has extended to the pelvic wall. |
| Stage IV | Carcinoma has extended beyond the true pelvis or has involved the mucosa of the bladder or rectum. (Bullous edema as such does not consign a patient to Stage IV.) |
| Stage IVa | Adjacent organs are involved (bladder, rectum). |
| Stage IVb | Distant organs are involved. |

*Source: American Joint Committee on Cancer: Manual for Staging of Cancer, 3rd ed. Philadelphia, JB Lippincott Co, 1988, p 170.*

internal iliac arteries, or uterine vessels. The vaginal arteries lie lateral to the vagina and anastomose with the uterine, inferior vesical, and middle rectal arteries. The longitudinal anterior and posterior azygos arteries develop from lateral anastomotic branches that join in the midline (Fig. 16-2). Branches of the internal pudendal artery supply the distal vagina. The vaginal venous plexus communicates with the vesical, hemorrhoidal, and uterine plexus and eventually drains into the hypogastric vein.

Vaginal lymphatics form a meshed net in the mucosal membrane and anastomose with lymphatic vessels in the muscularis (Plentl and Friedman, 1971). The lymphatics of the upper vagina communicate with those of the cervix and drain into the pelvic nodes. The posterior vaginal wall is defined by lymphatics that anastomose with the rectal lymphatic system; lymph from the posterior vagina is channeled to the deep pelvic nodes, such as the inferior gluteal, sacral, and rectal nodes. The anterior wall is drained by lymphatics that drain to the nodes of the lateral pelvic walls. The lymphatics of the distal one-third of the vagina drain to both inguinal and pelvic nodes (Fig. 16-3).

Although the developmental origin of the vagina in humans has been investigated for over 100 years, it still remains controversial. As early as 1927, Bloomfield and Frazier pointed out that the descriptions of vaginal development could be divided into three main groups, depending on the structures believed to participate in vaginal embryogenesis. Three origins of the vagina have been proposed: (1) the epithelium derived from the Müllerian ducts, (2) epithelium derived from both Müllerian and Wolffian ducts, and (3) the urogenital sinus. Vaginal embryogenesis is a complex process, since three epithelial layers interact over a limited area. Probably mediated by biochemical factors, these tissue interactions cannot be accurately deciphered by conventional histologic techniques, and these difficulties have precluded a definitive understanding of vaginal development.

The occurrence of lower genital tract anomalies and clear cell carcinomas in women exposed to diethylstilbestrol (DES) in utero stimulated further interest in determining the developmental origin of the vagina. As frequently happens, pertinent details about the sequential development of the vagina have come to light as a result of the recognition of congenital anomalies and experimentation with animal models.

Current findings now support the opinion that both the urogenital sinus and the Müllerian ducts participate in vaginal development (Ulfelder and Robboy, 1976). At 4 weeks of development, the Müllerian (paramesonephric) duct system begins as an invagination of the coelomic epithelium in the urogenital fold just lateral to the cranial end of the mesonephric ducts (Prins et al, 1976). The paired Müllerian ducts extend caudally, fuse in the midline, and reach the urogenital sinus by 7 weeks of gestational age. The septum formed by the fusion of the Müllerian ducts disappears, forming a single cavity, the uterovaginal canal.

The simple columnar epithelium of the vagina is transformed into a stratified epithelium of polygonal cells. The vaginal plate arises at the urogenital sinus and exhibits progressive cephalad growth into the uterovaginal canal, thereby obliterating the vaginal lumen. The vaginal plate then cavitates, leaving behind the stratified squamous epithelium of the vagina (Prins et al, 1976; Forsberg and Kalland, 1981). In women, in utero exposure to DES results in hormonally mediated persistence of Müllerian glandular epithelium (adenosis) within the vagina. Evidence from experimental animal studies suggests that the vaginal stroma can direct the differentiation of the vaginal epithelium toward squamous or glandular (adenosis) tissue (Cuhna and Fujii, 1981).

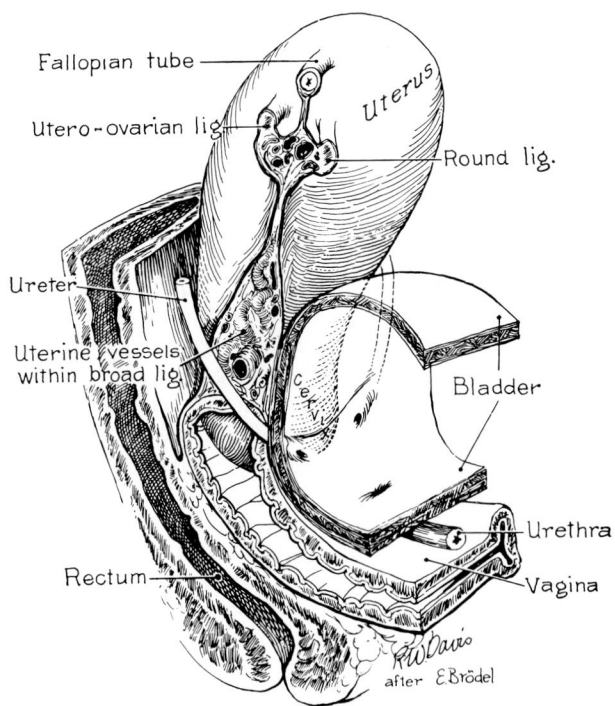

FIGURE 16-1 The Anatomic relationships among the vagina, bladder, ureters, and rectum. (From Pritchard, JA, MacDonald PC: *Williams Obstetrics,* 15th ed. New York, Appleton-Century-Crofts, 1976, p 24.)

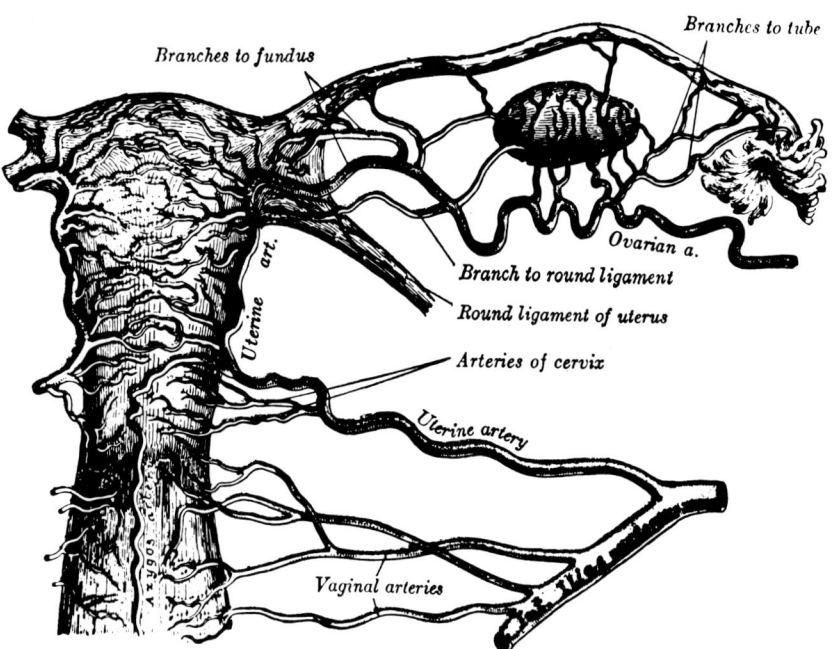

Branches to tube

Branches to fundus

Ovarian a.

Branch to round ligament

Round ligament of uterus

Uterine art.

Arteries of cervix

Uterine artery

Vaginal arteries

FIGURE 16-2 Arterial blood supply of the vagina. (From Goss CM [ed]: *Gray's Anatomy*, 29th ed. Philadelphia, Lea and Febiger, 1973, p 645.)

## Squamous Cell Carcinomas

Squamous cell carcinomas are the most common of vaginal malignancies and account for about 90% of primary vaginal malignancies (Perez et al, 1973; Rubin et al, 1985; Herbst, 1992). The patient's age at diagnosis ranges from 25 to 98, and the incidence peaks between the fifth and seventh decades of life. Over 75% of these lesions occur after age 50 (Rubin et al, 1985; Gallup et al, 1987). Although potential predisposing factors have been extensively investigated, factors such as reproductive and marital history, menstrual patterns, and local irritants have not been correlated with tumor occurrence.

***Diagnosis*** The most common site for a squamous cell carcinoma is the upper third of the vagina. According to Plentl and Friedman (1971), 51% of carcinomas arise from the upper vagina, 19% from the middle third, and 30% from the distal third. Fifty-seven percent of the tumors originate from the posterior wall, 27% from the anterior wall, and 16% from the lateral wall.

Tumor size may range from an occult lesion (< 1 cm2 ) to a large mass measuring 8 by 10 cm (Pride et al, 1979). Grossly, these tumors may be polypoid, fungating masses or indurated, ulcerative plaques. On microscopic examination, the carcinoma consists of malignant squamous cells infiltrating from vaginal epithelium and extending beneath the submucosa (Fig. 16-4). Cords of malignant cells advance into the submucosa and are usually surrounded by inflammatory cells. Initially, local extension is into the submucosa, with later spread into the paracolpos and parametria. Squamous cell carcinomas are usually moderately differentiated and nonkeratinizing (Perez et al, 1974). The degree of histologic differentiation, based on the amount of keratinization and the number of squamous

pearls, does not constitute a sound basis for assessing prognosis (Perez et al, 1974; Pride et al, 1979; Peters et al, 1985b).

One major prognostic factor is the stage of the tumor at the time of diagnosis. Tumor stage is assessed by an examination under anesthesia, cystoscopy, proctoscopy, and radiologic studies. In addition, the pretherapy evaluation usually includes a barium enema and an intravenous pyelogram. Vaginal carcinomas are staged according to the FIGO criteria (see Table 16-1). When Pride et al (1979) reviewed 338 patients, they found a typical distribution of stage: 91 patients (27%) had Stage I tumors, 156 (46%) had Stage II, and 91 (27%) had Stage III or IV disease.

***Treatment*** Therapy must be individualized with regard to tumor location, volume, and depth of invasion (Pride et al, 1979). Both operation and irradiation therapy have been effective, considering the limits imposed by the proximity to the bladder and rectum and the risk of fistula formation from these organs to the vagina. Most patients with invasive carcinomas have been managed with a combination of external-beam therapy plus intracavitary or interstitial radiation sources (Perez et al, 1974; Peters et al, 1985b). Large Stage I lesions (greatest tumor diameter exceeding 2 cm) and nearly all Stage II to IV tumors are treated with external-beam therapy initially in order to reduce the size of the primary tumor mass, thereby rendering intravaginal therapy more effective (Pride et al, 1979).

Patients with Stage I disease are treated with a variety of methods depending on the extent and thickness of the lesion (Perez et al, 1977). Superficial tumors may be treated with an intracavitary insertion alone. If the lesion is thicker, a single-plane interstitial implant can be used along with the intracavitary cylinder. The addition

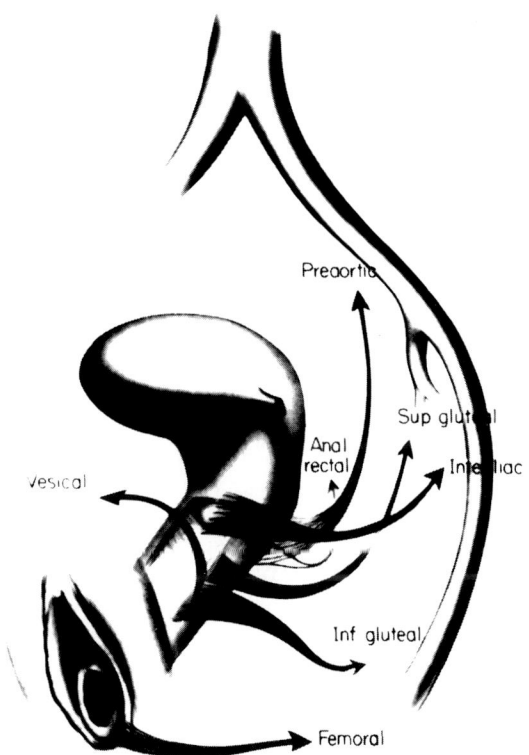

FIGURE 16-3 Lymphatic drainage of the vagina. (From Plentl AA, Friedman EA: *Lymphatic System of the Female Genitalia. The Morphologic Basis of Oncologic Diagnosis and Therapy.* Philadelphia, WB Saunders Co, 1971, p 55.)

of interstitial radiotherapy to the vaginal cylinder increases the depth dose without delivering excessive radiation to the vaginal mucosa. Larger tumors are treated with 4,000 to 5,000 cGy over 4 to 5 weeks using superor megavoltage equipment, followed by intracavitary and/or interstitial radiotherapy with a total tumor dose of approximately 7500 cGy. Carcinomas of the upper third of the vagina are treated technically as if the lesion

involved the cervix, which usually requires use of a tandem (if the uterus is present) and ovoids to provide the appropriate dosimetry. If the distal vagina is involved, the pelvic port should include the inguinal areas (Perez et al, 1974), since spread of the tumor would be similar to that of vulvar carcinoma. Kucera and Vavra (1991), in a series of 934 patients treated with irradiation, noted results were best for low-stage tumors, those in the upper one-third of the vagina and if the tumor was well differentiated.

Surgical intervention is useful for smaller tumors of the upper third of the vagina as well as for lesions that appear after previous radiotherapy; it is also used as an adjunct to radiation therapy for more advanced lesions and to treat tumors that do not respond to irradiation (Rutledge, 1967; Herbst et al, 1970). Surgically resectable tumors of the upper third of the vagina can be treated with radical hysterectomy, partial vaginectomy, and pelvic lymphadenectomy. In general, posterior wall tumors in the upper vagina present fewer treatment problems than do those in the distal vagina or on the anterior wall, which are located more closely to the rectum and bladder. Patients with central recurrences or persistence of tumor after radiotherapy are candidates for exenterative surgery.

Five-year survival rates appear to be related to tumor area, diameter, and clinical stage, decreasing with increasing tumor size and advanced clinical stage. Among 338 cases described in six published reviews, Pride et al (1979) found an overall 5-year survival rate of 44%; by stage, these rates were 74% for Stage I tumors, 45% for Stage II, and 16% for Stage III. The high proportion of tumors of advanced stage as well as the treatment problems imposed by the proximity of the bladder and rectum, probably accounts for the low 5-year salvage rate of 44%.

Treatment failures resulted from lack of local disease control as well as distant metastases. The frequency of local radiation failures and distant metastases increases with advanced-stage tumors. Perez and coworkers (1988) documented distant metastases in 16% of Stage

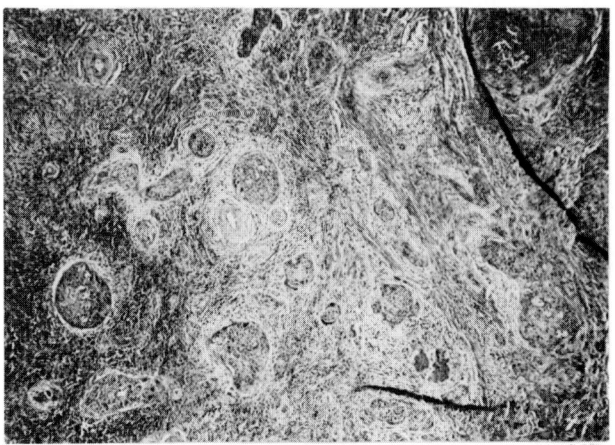

FIGURE 16-4 (*A*) Surgical specimen of exophytic squamous cell carcinoma of the upper vagina. (*B*) Photomicrograph of primary squamous cell carcinoma of the vagina; nests of malignant squamous cells infiltrate the underlying stroma. (Courtesy of Dr. Elizabeth Alenghat, Department of Pathology, The University of Chicago Hospitals and Clinics.)

I, 46% of Stage IIb, 62% of Stage III, and 50% of Stage IV disease. In advanced tumor stages, local or pelvic failures are likely associated with nonhomogeneous distribution of the radiation dose and the presence of hypoxic, less radiosensitive subpopulations of tumor cells (Perez et al, 1977).

## Carcinoma in Situ

Benedet and Sanders (1984) reviewed 136 cases of carcinoma in situ of the vagina collected over a 30-year interval. The patients ranged in age from 17 to 77, with a mean of age of 55 years. Eighty-five percent of the patients presented with an abnormal Pap smear. Colposcopy is useful for determining the extent of the lesion and selecting a biopsy site. White epithelium with punctation was the most frequent colposcopic pattern seen in the patients reviewed by Benedet and Sanders (1984). Definitive diagnosis is always established by biopsy. Microscopically, vaginal dysplasias demonstrate the same characteristics as those found in intraepithelial neoplasia of the cervix. These neoplastic alterations are limited to the squamous epithelium and include the presence of abnormal mitoses, nuclear pleomorphism, and loss of cellular polarity (Fig. 16-5).

Vaginal carcinoma in situ most commonly involves the upper third of the vagina and may demonstrate a unifocal or multifocal distribution. Eighty-three percent of the patients described by Benedet and Sanders (1984) had lesions confined to the upper third of the vagina. Fifty patients (37%) had multifocal lesions, as defined by pathologic findings or colposcopic impressions. Lenehan et al (1986) described similar findings; 88% of their patients had disease located in the upper third of the vagina, and 29 of 59 patients (49%) had multifocal disease.

The natural history of intraepithelial neoplasia of the vagina has been less well studied than that in the cervix. Although dysplastic changes appear slow to advance, progression to invasive disease has been documented (Hummer et al, 1970; Lenehan et al, 1986). However, the factors influencing the transition from in situ to invasive vaginal carcinoma and the time required are unknown.

The close association of vaginal carcinoma in situ with squamous neoplasia of the lower genital tract is well established. Of 25 patients reviewed by Gallup and Morley (1975), only five were without a history of prior genital tract dysplasia or invasive carcinoma. Of the 136 patients with vaginal carcinoma in situ reviewed by Benedet and Sanders (1984), there were 24 (18%) patients with invasive carcinomas of the cervix or vulva and 72 (53%) patients with dysplasia of the cervix or vulva.

Jimerson and Merrill (1976) described eight patients with severe dysplasia or carcinoma in situ of the vagina following hysterectomy; in all eight, the lesion was confined to the vaginal apex. This observation led to the conclusion that incomplete removal of the dysplastic vagina at the time of hysterectomy was a common factor in vaginal cuff dysplasia. Colposcopy or the application of Lugol's solution prior to hysterectomy to outline the abnormal epithelium will decrease the risk of this complication.

Because of uncertainty regarding the biologic behavior of vaginal dysplasias, the wide age range of the patients, and the frequently multifocal nature of this disease, it is difficult to formulate a single therapeutic approach. Since the disease is preinvasive and limited to the epithelial layer, optimal therapy should result in minimal damage to the normal vaginal mucosa. Available methods of treatment include excisional biopsy, partial/total vaginectomy with or without skin grafting, topical 5-fluorouracil (Ballon et al, 1979), laser vaporization (Capen et al, 1982), and local radiation (Benedet and Sanders, 1984), with radiation being the least frequently utilized of these modalities.

To ensure satisfactory sexual function after treatment of vaginal dysplasia, local ablative techniques have become popular. Although considerable success has been reported with carbon dioxide laser therapy (Jobson and Homesley, 1983), some researchers have noted a failure rate of approximately 50% (Woodman et al, 1984; Lenehan et al, 1986). Failures of local treatment may result from incomplete therapy or difficulties in colposcopic assessment. Krebs (1989) reported that topical 5-fluorouracil was as effective as laser therapy and eradicated 81% of vaginal intraepithelial neoplasia.

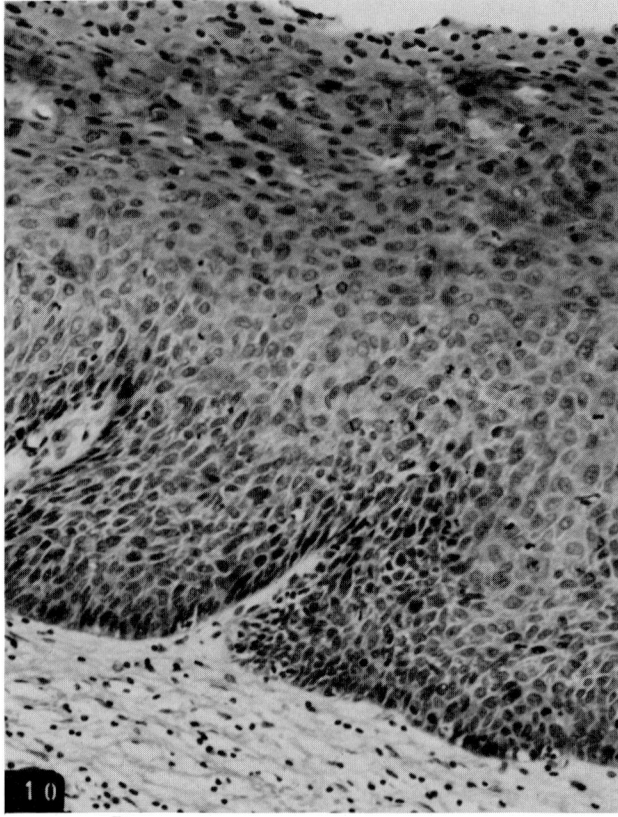

**FIGURE 16-5** Vaginal intraepithelial neoplasia showing nuclear pleomorphism, loss of cellular polarity, and abnormal mitoses. The process is limited to the squamous epithelium. (Courtesy of Dr. Elizabeth Alenghat, Department of Pathology, The University of Chicago Hospitals and Clinics.)

## Verrucous Carcinoma

Verrucous carcinoma is an extremely uncommon variant of squamous cell carcinoma with distinctive clinical and pathologic features (Isaacs, 1976). The tumor presents as a warty, fungating, grayish-pink to white mass that gradually increases in size and pushes into rather than invades contiguous structures. Grossly, it may be confused with condyloma acuminatum. The characteristic histologic pattern is a densely keratinized layer covering large papillary fronds and a well-circumscribed, deep margin comprising rows of bulbous, well-oriented rete ridges (Fig. 16-6).

When a verrucous carcinoma is diagnosed, wide surgical excision apparently yields the best results; inadequate excision leads to recurrence. Radiotherapy of such lesions is not recommended, since there have been case reports of rapid, radiation-induced transformation to a more malignant neoplasm (Gallousis, 1972).

## Adenocarcinoma

Approximately 10% of primary vaginal malignancies are adenocarcinomas (Rubin et al, 1985). Whenever this diagnosis is considered, it is necessary to rule out metastatic lesions from the bowel, uterus, or ovary. The

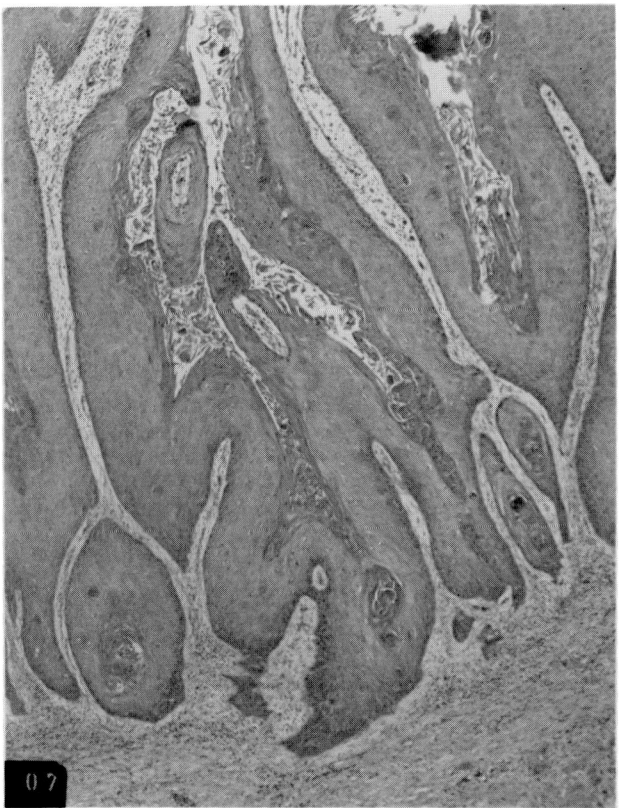

**FIGURE 16-6** Microscopic appearance of a verrucous carcinoma. The characteristic pattern is that of a densely keratinized layer covering large papillary fronds. The tumor appears to push into rather than invade the stroma. (Courtesy of Dr. Elizabeth Alenghat, Department of Pathology, The University of Chicago Hospitals and Clinics.)

most common variety is the clear cell adenocarcinoma, which can occur spontaneously as well as in women exposed to diethylstilbestrol (DES) in utero.

### *DES Exposure and Clear Cell Adenocarcinomas of the Vagina*

In 1970, Herbst and Scully reported seven cases of vaginal adenocarcinoma occurring in women 15 to 22 years of age. Six of the tumors were clear cell carcinomas and one was an endometrioid carcinoma. In a subsequent study these tumors were associated with maternal ingestion of DES which was prescribed to prevent abortion or prematurity (Herbst et al, 1971). The Registry for Research on Hormonal Transplacental Carcinogenesis was established in 1971 to centralize data on the natural history, pathology, and epidemiology of these cancers occurring in females born after 1940, whether or not there was a history of maternal medication. As of February, 1992, the Registry had accessioned 580 cases of clear cell carcinoma of the vagina and cervix. In utero exposure to synthetic estrogens has been documented in approximately 60% of the women with available maternal histories. In an additional 12%, the mothers had been treated with another hormone or with an unidentified medication. In 24% there was no apparent maternal hormone usage. The youngest DES-exposed patient to develop clear cell adenocarcinoma was 7 years of age at the time of diagnosis and in 1992 the oldest patient was 42 years (Herbst, 1992).

The risk of clear cell adenocarcinomas developing in DES-exposed women from birth through age 34 is one in 1,000 (Melnick et al, 1987). The greatest number of DES-exposed patients with these tumors were born in the United States between 1950 and 1952, the period when DES was apparently most frequently prescribed in pregnancy. Factors related to the risk for clear cell adenocarcinoma in DES-exposed women were evaluated in a case-control study by Herbst et al, (1986). Time of exposure to DES during pregnancy (prior to the 12th week of gestation) was found to be a critical risk factor.

Figure 16-7 summarizes the incidence of clear cell adenocarcinomas in DES-exposed females according to the age at diagnosis. Clear cell adenocarcinoma was virtually nonexistent before age 15; a sharp rise in the incidence rate began at age 15, with an irregular plateau from ages 17 to 22. The median age at diagnosis was 19 years. Thereafter, the incidence gradually decreases, although the shape of the curve beyond age 25 is uncertain at this time owing to the limited number of observations (Melnick et al, 1987).

Two types of cells have been identified in the glands of adenosis—the mucinous cell resembling endocervical epithelium and the tuboendometrial cell simulating fallopian tube epithelium or proliferative endometrium. Robboy and coworkers (1982) blocked and serially sectioned 20 specimens of uterus and vagina removed because of a clear cell carcinoma of the cervix or vagina. In 18 of 20 cases, tuboendometrial cells were intimately related to the tumor, either surrounding it or abutting

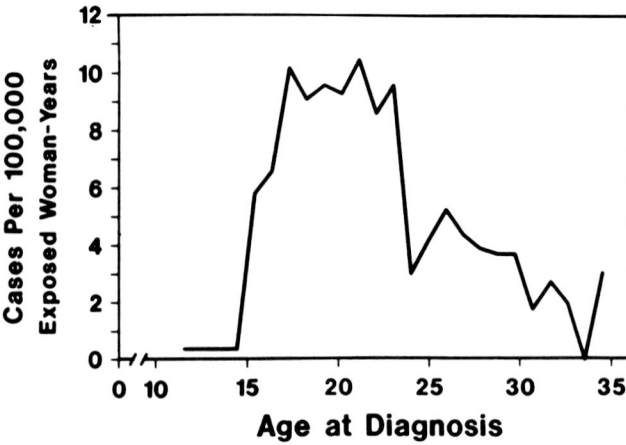

FIGURE 16-7  Incidence of clear cell adenocarcinomas by age at diagnosis among white females in the United States. (From Melnick S, et al: Rates and risks of diethylstilbestrol-related clear-cell adenocarcinoma of the vagina and cervix. An update. *N Engl J Med* 316:514-516, 1987. Reprinted with permission from the *New England Journal of Medicine*.)

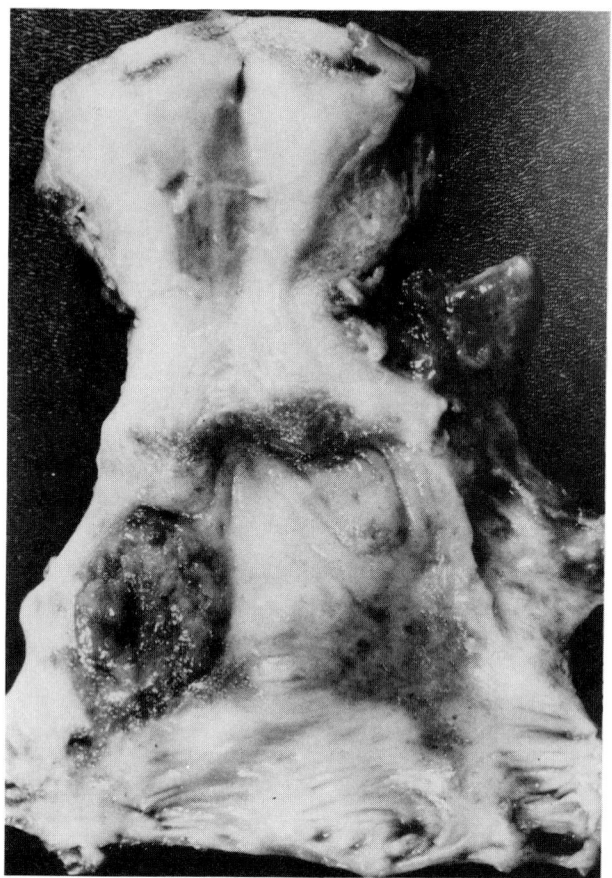

FIGURE 16-8  Clear cell adenocarcinoma of the anterior vaginal wall. (From Herbst AL, Scully RE: Adenocarcinoma of the vagina in adolescence. A report of 7 cases including 6 clear-cell carcinomas [so-called mesonephromas]. *Cancer* 25:745-757, 1970.)

its inferior border. In six of the vaginal carcinomas, the adenosis surrounding the tumor was entirely of the tuboendometrial type.

The topographic relationships in this study strongly suggested that clear cell carcinomas are associated with tuboendometrial rather than mucinous epithelium. The tumor arises in regions where the concentration of tuboendometrial epithelium is greatest. Furthermore, in most specimens, foci of atypical tuboendometrial epithelium (a possible transition from adenosis to carcinoma) were noted immediately adjacent to the tumor. These observations have led to the hypothesis that patients exposed to DES prior to the 18th week of gestation have a larger volume of adenosis (and resulting tuboendometrial epithelium), which may provide a large substrate for later development of a carcinoma.

***Pathology and Histology***  Grossly, clear cell adenocarcinomas are usually exophytic, polypoid masses and may contain areas of necrosis; they may appear as indurated or ulcerative plaques (Fig. 16-8). Tumors confined to the vaginal lamina propria have also rarely been reported. These adenocarcinomas have no particular colposcopic features and are diagnosed by means of careful inspection and palpation. The smallest vaginal tumor accessioned into the registry was 0.2 cm in its greatest diameter (Chambers et al, 1978); the largest measured 8 × 10 cm.

Three histologic patterns of clear cell carcinomas are observed—tubulocystic, solid, and papillary—either alone or in combination (Fig. 16-9). The most frequent, the tubulocystic pattern, is characterized by tubules and cysts lined by hobnail cells. The solid pattern consists of sheets of tumor cells with clear cytoplasm. The least frequent, papillary, has numerous papillae within cysts or tubules.

Vaginal clear cell carcinomas are staged according to the FIGO criteria (see Table 16-1). Of 315 vaginal clear cell adenocarcinomas analyzed in the registry (Table 16-2), 234 (74%) were classified as stage I while the remaining 81 (26%) were stage II lesions.

***Treatment***  Therapy of clear cell adenocarcinomas parallels that used for squamous malignancies of the cervix and vagina, taking into consideration the very young age of patients undergoing treatment as well as tumor size and location. Table 16-2 summarizes the therapeutic modality utilized in 315 cases of vaginal clear cell tumors. Stage I and small Stage II tumors have frequently been treated with radical hysterectomy, partial or complete vaginectomy, and replacement of the vagina by a split-thickness graft along with pelvic lymphadenectomy. Full pelvic irradiation was the most commonly used therapeutic modality for Stage II disease and large tumors.

In order to preserve fertility, some patients have undergone local resection of tumor and local radiotherapy utilizing an implant or transvaginal cone to treat the primary tumor bed and adjacent pelvic tissues (Wharton et al, 1975). Since metastases to regional nodes can occur with small vaginal tumors, retroperitoneal node dissections are performed prior to initiation of radiotherapy.

Senekjian et al (1987) reviewed 219 cases of stage I

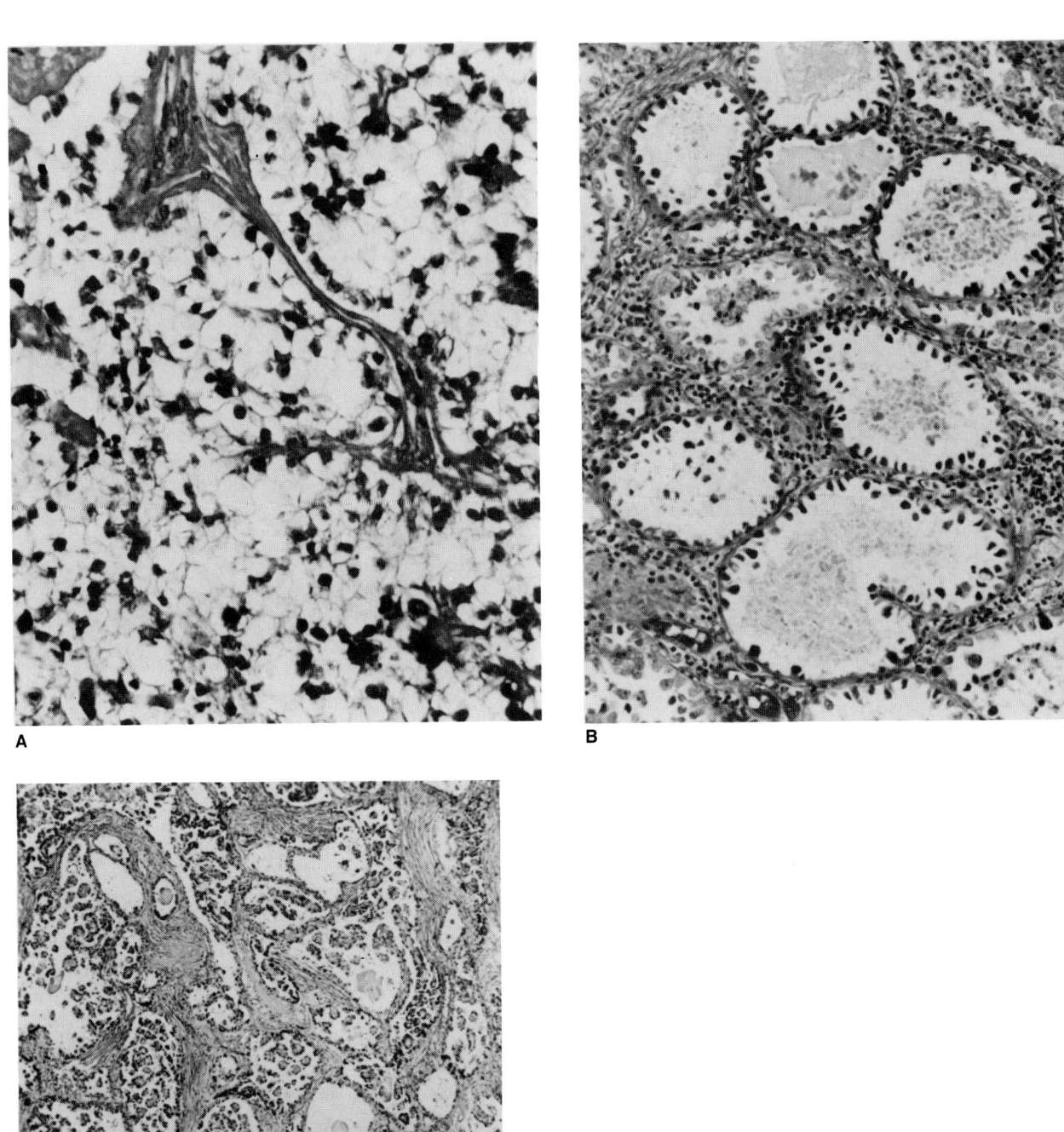

FIGURE 16-9 Histologic patterns of clear cell adenocarcinomas: solid pattern (*A*), tubulocystic type (*B*), and papillary pattern (*C*). (From Robboy SJ, et al: Female genital tract changes related to prenatal diethylstilbestrol exposure. In Blaustein A (ed): *Pathology of the Female Genital Tract*, 2nd ed. New York, Springer-Verlag, 1982, pp 99-118; and Scully RE, et al: Vaginal and cervical abnormalities, including clear-cell adenocarcinoma, related to prenatal exposure to stilbestrol. *Ann Clin Lab Sci* 4:222-233, 1974.)

TABLE 16-2 Therapeutic Modality Used in Treatment of Vaginal Clear Cell Carcinomas

|  | Stage I | Stage II |
|---|---|---|
| Surgery |  |  |
| Radical hysterectomy and vaginec- tomy | 127 | 14 |
| Modified radical hysterectomy and vaginectomy | 3 | 0 |
| Simple hysterectomy and vaginectomy | 2 | 0 |
| Local excision/vaginectomy | 27 | 2 |
| Exenteration | 1 | 7 |
| Other | 2 | 0 |
| Total | 162 | 23 |
| Radiation |  |  |
| Intracavitary/interstitial implant only | 3 | 1 |
| External-beam only | 2 | 0 |
| External-beam and intracavitary/inter- stitial implant | 23 | 28 |
| Total | 28 | 29 |
| Chemotherapy | 0 | 1 |
| Surgery and radiation | 40 | 23 |
| Surgery and chemotherapy | 2 | 0 |
| Radiation and chemotherapy | 0 | 2 |
| Surgery, radiation, and chemotherapy | 1 | 2 |
| Other/unknown | 1 | 1 |

*Source: Data from the Registry for Research on Hormonal Transplacental Carcinogenesis, 5841 South Maryland Avenue, Chicago, Illinois 60637.*

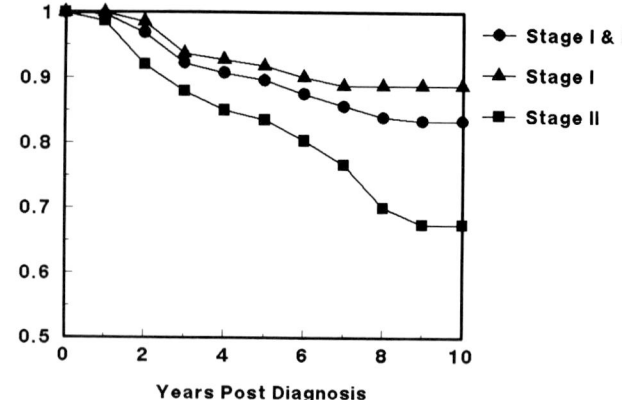

**Proportion Surviving**

FIGURE 16-10 Survival of patients with Stage I and II vaginal clear cell adenocarcinomas as calculated by life-table methods.

vaginal clear cell adenocarcinomas, of which 176 had conventional therapy and 43 patients underwent local therapy. They noted that the survival of patients with small vaginal tumors treated by local excision and then irradiation is comparable to those with conventional extensive therapy. The clinical and pathologic characteristics of the two groups were similar. Treatment consisted of vaginectomy in nine cases, local excision alone in 17 cases, and local irradiation (with or without local excision) in 17 cases. Disease recurred in nine of the 26 patients (35%) treated with vaginectomy or local excision alone. However, in the subgroup of patients treated with local irradiation, the rate of recurrence was similar to that seen with conventional therapy. The authors concluded that selected patients with Stage I vaginal tumors who wish to retain their reproductive potential can be treated by a combination of wide local excision, retroperitoneal node dissection, and staging laparotomy followed by local radiotherapy. The best candidates are those with tumors less than 2 cm in diameter, a predominant tubulocystic pattern, and a depth of invasion less than 3 cm.

Overall 5-year survival rates, regardless of the mode of therapy, were 92% among patients with Stage I tumors and 84% among those with Stage II disease. Survival for patients with Stage I and II disease, (as calculated by life-table methods) is summarized in Figure 16-10.

It has been noted that the age of the patient at the time of diagnosis correlates with patient survival. Patients 15 years of age or younger have had a shorter survival than those 19 years of age or older. This age correlation was found to be related to differences in the behavior of the tumor in terms of its predominant histologic pattern. The best survival rates were associated with the tubulocystic pattern, which is the predominant pattern in patients older than 19 years of age (Herbst et al, 1979*a*).

Clear cell adenocarcinomas demonstrate local spread as well as metastases via blood vessels and lymphatics. Approximately 17% of Stage I vaginal carcinomas have been reported to have nodal metastases (Herbst et al, 1979*b*; Scully and Welch, 1981). Persistent or recurrent disease has been noted in over 25% of registry cases. The proportion of patients with Stage I and II disease who suffered recurrence (as calculated by life-table methods) is summarized in Figure 16-11. Most recurrences are detected within 3 years of primary therapy; but isolated recurrences of clear cell adenocarcinoma have occurred as long as 20 years after initial therapy. Furthermore, approximately one-third of recurrences are detected at distant sites, such as the lungs or supraclavicular nodes (Robboy et al, 1974).

Depending upon the location of the tumor recurrence, therapy has consisted of additional radical sur-

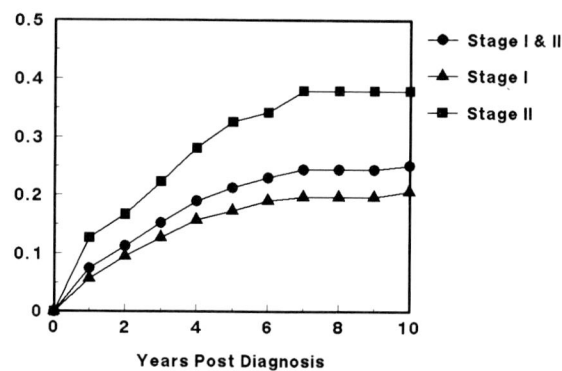

**Proportion Recurring**

Figure 16-11 Proportion of patients with Stage I and II vaginal clear cell adenocarcinomas who developed recurrent disease as calculated by life-table methods.

gery or extensive radiation in localized pelvic disease and systemic chemotherapy in cases of metastatic disease. Multiple agent cytotoxic chemotherapy is usually prescribed. Cisplatin 75 to 100 mg/M$^2$ with 3 to 5 days of continuous infusion, and 5-FU, 1 gm/M$^2$ every 3 to 4 weeks, are currently recommended. Unfortunately, no single agent or combination of chemotherapeutic agents has been found to be an effective therapy for these recurrences. Radiation therapy has also been used for solitary metastases, in which case the site of recurrence as well as the area of lymphatic drainage is often treated. In patients with pulmonary metastases, palliative therapy has consisted of actinomycin D and whole-lung irradiation (1,800 cGy). Results of cytotoxic chemotherapy (single-agent or combination) or hormonal therapy (progestins) for systemic disease have been disappointing.

Although the majority of patients with clear cell adenocarcinomas are diagnosed at the time of initial presentation, 19 patients have been reported to develop clear cell adenocarcinomas during follow-up after in utero DES exposure (Registry, unpublished). Sander et al (1986) analyzed data available from 10 patients with vaginal adenosis in whom clear cell adenocarcinoma developed during subsequent observation. These patients were described as having "metachronous" cancers and were compared with the much larger group of patients who initially presented with clear cell adenocarcinomas and associated adenosis (the "synchronous group"). Patients developed carcinomas during followup (the metachronous group) were uniformly asymptomatic; 50% had a negative Pap smear. All had Stage I disease and none had metastases. Six of the 10 patients had lesions on the posterior vaginal wall. In contrast, the synchronous group, who initially presented with clear cell adenocarcinomas, often had lesions arising from the anterior vaginal wall. Eighty percent were symptomatic, and approximately 17% had lymph node metastases.

Carlson et al (1989) described the eleventh patient with a "metachronous" cancer after 8 years of careful followup preceding the diagnosis of a clear cell adenocarcinoma. In contrast to the cases analyzed by Sander et al (1986), the patient had Stage II disease arising from the anterior vaginal wall, which was treated with definitive radiotherapy. Such observations emphasize the necessity of careful, regular examinations in women with a history of DES exposure. The majority of such malignancies have been small and were discovered only through systematic palpation, inspection, and cytologic examination.

### Incidence of Dysplasia in DES-Exposed Women

The existence of an extensive transformation zone in the DES-exposed female has prompted some to hypothesize that DES-exposed progeny are at higher risk for squamous cell neoplasia (Stafl and Mattingly, 1974). Presumably, this larger transformation zone would increase the risk of exposure of the immature metaplastic epithelium to a potential carcinogen.

Whether patients with in utero DES-exposure are at increased risk for dysplasia remains an unanswered question. Data from a case-control study by Robboy et al (1981) did not demonstrate such an increased risk; however, in a subsequent publication, these investigators reported an incidence rate for dysplasia and carcinoma in situ among DES-exposed offspring that was significantly higher than that in non–DES-exposed, matched subjects (Robboy et al, 1984). The DES-exposed patients also had increased rates of genital herpes compared with the matched subjects (11.8% vs. 6.3%). The latter study has been criticized because of the possibility that the higher incidence of dysplasia among the DES-exposed patients was related to the increased rate of genital viral infections and to ascertainment bias (Bornstein et al, 1988). DES-exposed women had larger areas of metaplasia and therefore were more likely to undergo biopsy. Richart (1986) has also questioned the later study by Robboy et al since it did not differentiate human papillomavirus–induced lesions from true dysplasias.

A common problem in the diagnosis of dysplasia in DES-exposed patients is the misidentification of immature metaplastic cells for dysplastic squamous cells (Robboy et al, 1978). When the ultrastructural features of lesions diagnosed as grade III cervical intraepithelial neoplasia (CIN III) in DES-exposed females were examined by Lawrence et al (1980), they found that the majority of the lesions were more compatible with lesser degrees of dysplasia or metaplasia. DNA microspectrophotometry has been used to differentiate dysplasia from immature squamous metaplasia, and it was found that mature or immature metaplasia was euploid, whereas moderate and severe dysplasias was aneuploid (Fu et al, 1978). Although microspectrophotometry is time-consuming and has been utilized primarily in research laboratories, the development of a computerized method of performing such an analysis should allow more widespread use of this technique (Wied et al, 1983).

### Vaginal Melanomas

Vaginal melanomas are rare. Approximately 3% of malignant melanomas involve the female genital tract (Ariel, 1981). As such, the frequency of malignant melanomas of the female genital tract is proportionate with its contribution to total body surface area. The majority of these genital tract lesions arise on the vulva (Ariel, 1981; Morrow and DiSaia, 1976). However, malignant melanomas account for 2.7% of vaginal malignancies, and more than 125 vaginal melanomas have been reported (Lee et al, 1984; Liu et al, 1987; Reid et al, 1989b).

Malignant melanomas of mucosal surfaces appear to arise from in situ melanocytes. Nigogosyan and coworkers (1964) systematically assessed the vaginal epithelium of 100 women examined at autopsy. Melanocytes were found in three cases. Benign melanosis has been reported in the vagina as well as in the cervix (Tsukada, 1976; Deppisch, 1983), and atypical melanocytic hyperplasia of the vagina has been documented (Bottles et al, 1984). Furthermore, Lee and coworkers (1984) have noted progression of preexisting vaginal melanosis into a malignant melanoma.

The age distribution for this neoplasm has ranged from 22 to 83 years, with an average age of 55 (Morrow and DiSaia, 1976). The majority of patients are postmenopausal and present with vaginal bleeding, discharge, or a mass. Tumor size may vary from 0.5 to 7.5 cm, with approximately 30% being 2 cm or less in diameter (Morrow and DiSaia, 1976). The appearance of the tumor is variable: it may present as a small nodule, a flat plaque, or a fungating polypoid mass (Fig. 16-12). Usually, the tumor is blue-black or black-brown in appearance. The majority of these tumors develop in the distal third of the vagina, commonly on the anterior wall.

Malignant melanoma is a neoplasm of melanin-producing cells (Fig. 16-13). Histologically, these tumors are similar to malignant melanoma elsewhere in the body and should fulfill the following criteria: intra- and extracellular melanin; junctional activity; extreme cellular pleomorphism; large, hyperchromatic, atypical nuclei; and, in early tumors, a bandlike inflammatory cell infiltrate beneath the lesion (Laufe and Bernstein, 1971).

Vaginal melanomas have a poor prognosis, with 5-year survival rates of approximately 21% (Chung et al, 1980). This grim prognosis may be related to the invasiveness of these tumors and the resultant depth of penetration at the time of diagnosis. Chung and co-workers (1980) evaluated 19 cases of vaginal melanoma using a method previously described for vulvar melanomas (Chung et al, 1975). Positive nodes were found only with lesions penetrating the subepithelial tissues 1 mm or more.

In a more recent retrospective review, Reid et al (1989*b*) analyzed 15 patients with vaginal melanomas. All tumors were of the nodular type and 66% involved the distal third of the vagina. The cumulative 5-year survival was 17.4%. Tumor thickness (6 mm or less)

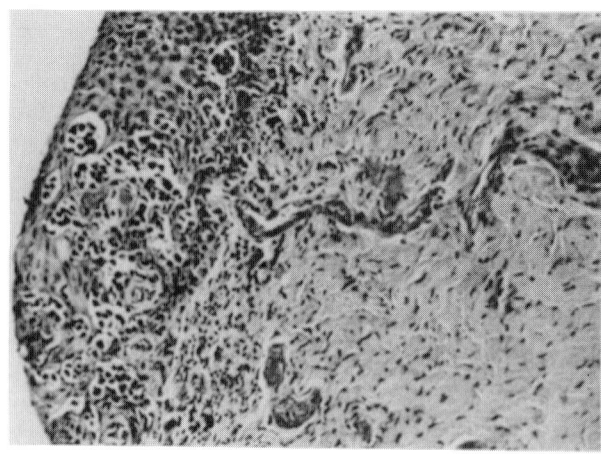

FIGURE 16-13 Nests of melanoma cells at the dermal-epidermal junction and within the epidermis. (From Laufe LE, Bernstein ED: Primary malignant melanoma of the vagina. *Obstet Gynecol* 37:148-154, 1971. Reprinted with permission from The American College of Obstetricians and Gynecologists.)

significantly affected the disease-free interval, whereas tumor size (less than 3 cm) was a major factor in patient survival.

Although the optimal treatment of this uncommon disease is unclear, most cases diagnosed since 1960 have been treated with radical surgery. By extrapolation from the experience with vulvar melanomas (Podratz et al, 1983), a wide local excision with a 2- to 3-cm margin is worthy of consideration if technically feasible. In the past, malignant melanoma was felt to be radioresistant (Collantes et al, 1967). Of eight patients treated primarily with irradiation, only one showed evidence of local control (Chung et al, 1980). More recently, Borazjani et al (1990) noted improved survival for patients whose tumors had less than six mitoses per 10 high power field. Subtotal vaginectomy at any level is also therapeutically undesirable; microscopically, there can be multiple foci of melanoma within the vagina even with a small primary lesion (Ehrmann et al, 1962). Consequently, most tumors are now managed by extended radical procedures, with the location and extent of the tumor determining whether anterior, posterior, or total exenteration is performed (Morrow and DiSaia, 1976; Ariel, 1981).

## Vaginal Sarcomas

Peters and coworkers (1985) reviewed 68 cases of sarcoma of the adult vagina reported up until 1985. Analysis of those lesions limited to one vaginal wall and/or one of the three vaginal segments indicated that these tumors arise with approximately equal frequency throughout the vagina. Sarcomas of the adult vagina histologically resemble those arising within the uterus. The most common histologic type was *leiomyosarcoma*, which accounted for 68% of the reported cases. Tavassoli and Norris (1979) studied the clinical and pathologic features of 60 vaginal smooth muscle tumors in order to determine the pathologic characteristics that

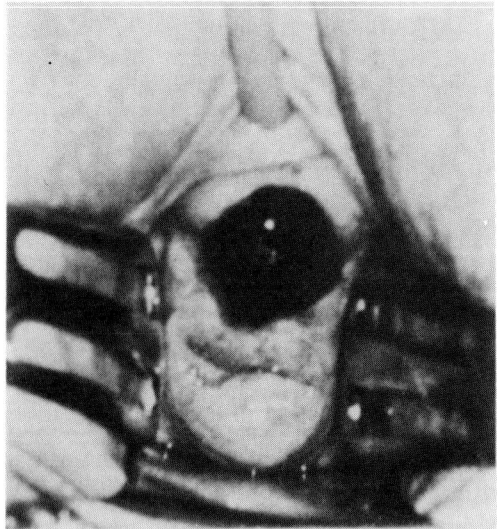

FIGURE 16-12 A melanoma arising from the distal anterior vaginal wall. (From Laufe LE, Bernstein ED: Primary malignant melanoma of the vagina. *Obstet Gynecol* 37:148-154, 1971. Reprinted with permission from The American College of Obstetricians and Gynecologists.)

best define leiomyosarcoma. A neoplasm with moderate to marked atypia and five or more mitotic figures per 10 high-power fields was felt to merit this designation.

Because of the rarity of these lesions, the optimal approach to treatment is not clear, but treatments now utilized are similar to those for other sarcomas of the female genital tract. Surgical resection is the therapy of choice and may necessitate radical surgery for complete excision (Reid et al, 1989*a*). Although combination chemotherapy has dramatically improved the results of therapy in pediatric sarcomas, its role in the treatment of adult vaginal sarcomas remains undefined. Radiation therapy may be beneficial; however, no cures have been reported with its use (Peters et al, 1985*a*).

## Embryonal Rhabdomyosarcomas (Sarcoma Botryoides)

The highly malignant rhabdomyosarcoma of the vagina, sarcoma botryoides, has a peak incidence between the first and second years of life. The average age at onset of symptoms was 27.5 months in a Mayo Clinic series and 38.8 months in 58 cases in the literature reviewed by Hilgers et al (1970). Between 85 and 90% of cases occurred in girls less than 5 years of age, with approximately two-thirds of these lesions appearing during the first 2 years of life (Fig. 16-14); in two cases the tumor was noted at birth. Rarely does it occur in a young child over 8 years of age. In approximately 80% of the cases, the presenting complaint was a vaginal mass and/or bleeding. The tumor seems to appear initially in the form of small papillae or nodules arising from hypertrophic vaginal rugae (Hilgers et al, 1970); with further growth, pedunculated or sessile polypoid masses appear that resemble a bunch of grapes (Fig. 16-15). The proliferation of tissue can extend beneath the vaginal epithelium as well as into the lumen. Microscopically, the tumor is identified by the presence of rhabdomyoblasts (strap cells) that contain cross-striations (Fig. 16-16). In addition, infiltration of tumor beneath the vaginal epithelium results in a distinct subepithelial dense zone, the cambium layer (Fig. 16-17).

Hilgers (1975) reviewed the literature on pelvic ex-

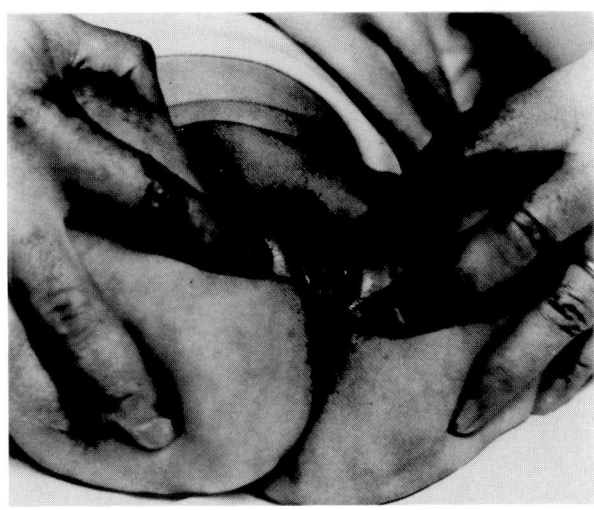

**FIGURE 16-15** Gross appearance of sarcoma botryoides, a polypoid tumor that resembles a bunch of grapes. (From Hilgers RD, et al: Embryonal rhabdomyosarcoma (botryoid type) of the vagina. A clinicopathologic review. *Am J Obstet Gynecol* 107:484-502, 1970.)

enteration in 21 cases of embryonal rhabdomyosarcoma. This form of treatment was found to be a relatively ineffective means of curing patients with tumor that extended beyond the limits of the vagina. Piver, Barlow, and coworkers (1973) reported three infants with vulvovaginal rhabdomyosarcomas successfully treated with radical surgery and postoperative radiotherapy and combination chemotherapy. The three infants treated at 10 to 15 months of age, continue to be free of disease at 14 to 16.5 years after treatment was completed (Piver and Rose, 1988).

The addition of chemotherapy and radiotherapy to surgery greatly increases the survival of patients with

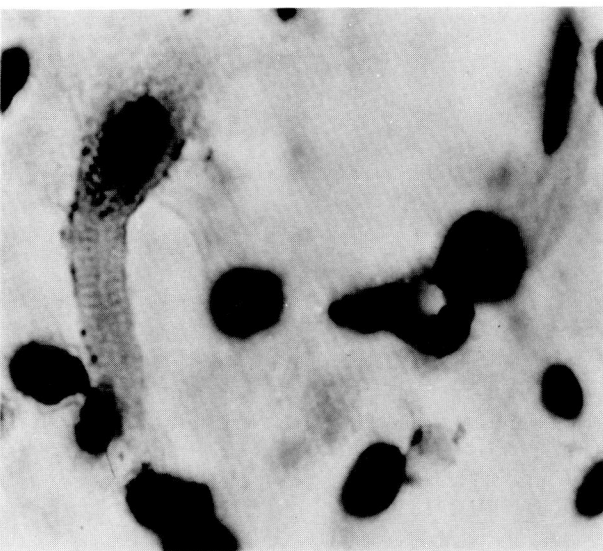

**FIGURE 16-16** Rhabdomyoblast cells of sarcoma botryoides. (From Hilgers RD, et al: Embryonal rhabdomyosarcoma (botryoid type) of the vagina. A clinicopathologic review. *Am J Obstet Gynecol* 107:484-502, 1970.)

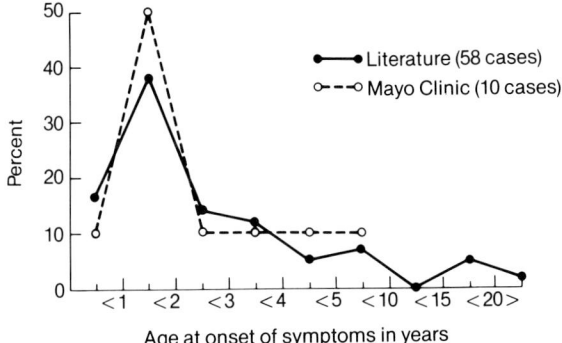

**FIGURE 16-14** Age distribution of patients with vaginal rhabdomyosarcomas at onset of symptoms. (From Hilgers RD, et al: Embryonal rhabdomyosarcoma (botryoid type) of the vagina. A clinicopathologic review. *Am J Obstet Gynecol* 107:484-502, 1970.)

rhabdomyosarcoma. Dewhurst (1980) reported six patients also treated by a combined approach. Three patients received chemotherapy (vincristine, cyclophosphamide, and actinomycin D) and radiation with or without extended hysterectomy. All three were free of disease 1.5 to 3 years after therapy.

The Intergroup Rhabdomyosarcoma Study used a multimodality approach to patients with vaginal tumors (Hays et al, 1985). Patients underwent chemotherapy (vincristine and actinomycin D with or without cyclophosphamide and doxorubicin), irradiation, and/or surgery. Mean patient age was 1.8 years. There was only one tumor-related death among 24 evaluable patients. Only two of the 24 patients underwent exenterative surgery. Eighteen of the 24 patients had gross residual tumor after conservative surgery or biopsy only. With the advent of effective chemotherapy, pelvic exenteration—at one time the recommended treatment for embryonal rhabdomyosarcoma of the vagina—is rarely necessary.

A rare benign polyp that may resemble sarcoma botryoides has been reported in pregnant females, adult women, and infants (Norris and Taylor, 1966; Miettinen et al, 1983; Mitchell et al, 1987). These polyps are termed *pseudosarcoma botryoides*; microscopically, they contain large, atypical mesenchymal cells or giant cells but no rhabdomyoblasts. Furthermore, the closely packed subepithelial mesenchymal layer—the cambium of sarcoma botryoides—is absent in these benign tumors (Fig. 16-18). They are adequately treated by local excision.

Sarcoma botryoides almost always occurs in children under the age of 8, and the physician should hesitate before making the diagnosis of an embryonal rhabdomyosarcoma in an adult.

### Endodermal Sinus Tumor

The endodermal sinus (yolk sac) tumor is a rare germ cell malignancy that is usually found in the ovary (Fig. 16-19). These neoplasms are also known to occur in extragonadal sites, presumably resulting when germ cells become misplaced during their migration to the urogenital ridge. They have also been documented in the pineal gland, retroperitoneum, stomach, liver, and sacrococcygeal region as well as in the infant vagina (Teilum, 1971).

Young and Scully (1984) described nine cases of endodermal sinus tumor of the vagina and reviewed 32 cases previously reported in the literature. All the tumors have occurred in children age 2 years or younger. Patients who presented with vaginal bleeding or discharge have had polypoid or sessile tumors. With the use of immunohistochemical techniques, it has been possible to demonstrate alpha-fetoprotein (AFP) in some endodermal sinus tumors of the vagina (Norgaard-Pedersen et al, 1979; Dewhurst and Ferreira, 1981). Furthermore, serum AFP levels correlated with the clinical course in one of the patients reported (Norgaard-Pedersen et al, 1979). This tumor marker appears to be useful as a guide to diagnosis and for monitoring the patient's response to treatment.

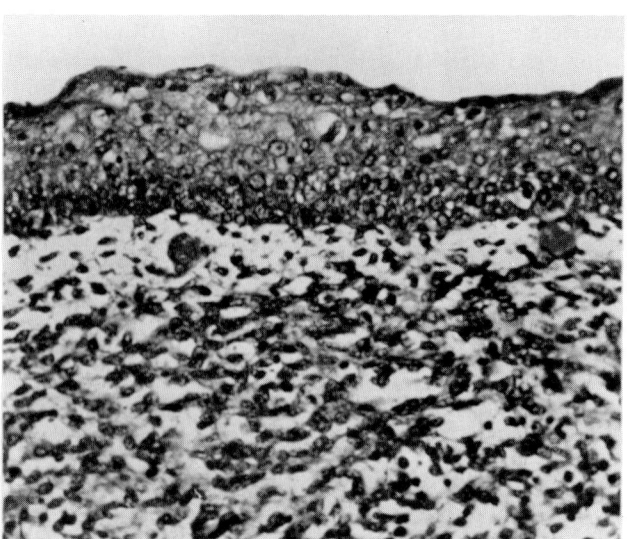

FIGURE 16-17  The cambium layer of sarcoma botryoides beneath the epithelium. (From Hilgers RD, et al: Embryonal rhabdomyosarcoma (botryoid type) of the vagina. A clinicopathologic review. *Am J Obstet Gynecol* 107:484-502, 1970.)

The introduction of effective chemotherapeutic agents has significantly changed the treatment and prognosis of patients with this tumor. Six of the nine patients reported by Young and Scully (1984) underwent surgery and chemotherapy initially (vincristine, actinomycin-D, and cyclophosphamide)(VAC), with radiation therapy in two cases. All six children were alive and free of disease from 2 to 9 years postoperatively. Of the 32 patients previously reported, 18 died of disease despite the frequent use of radical surgery; only 10 were free of disease from 4 months to 7 years postoperatively. Copeland et al (1985) treated six patients with endodermal sinus tumors of the vagina and cervix. Five patients were treated with excisional surgery and all received chemotherapy (usually vincristine, actinomycin D, and cyclosphosphamide)(VAC). Four of the six patients were disease-free from 2 to 23 years after treatment. Recently, Collins et al (1989) noted tumor regression in a 5-month-old patient after VAC therapy alone.

## CANCER OF THE FALLOPIAN TUBE

Primary fallopian tube carcinoma is the least common of the female genital tract malignancies. Its relative frequency varies from 0.3 to 1.1% of all gynecologic cancers; to date, approximately 1,400 cases have been reported in the world literature (Sedlis, 1978; Hershey et al, 1981; Eddy et al, 1984b; McMurray et al, 1986; Podratz et al, 1986; Pfeiffer et al, 1989; Rose et al, 1990). Using data from the National Cancer Institute's Surveillance, Epidemiology, and End-Results (SEER) Program, Rosenblatt and colleagues estimated an average annual incidence of 3.6 tubal cancers per million women per year, a rate which did not substantially change from 1977 to 1984. Since no single individual or institution has treated a large number of affected

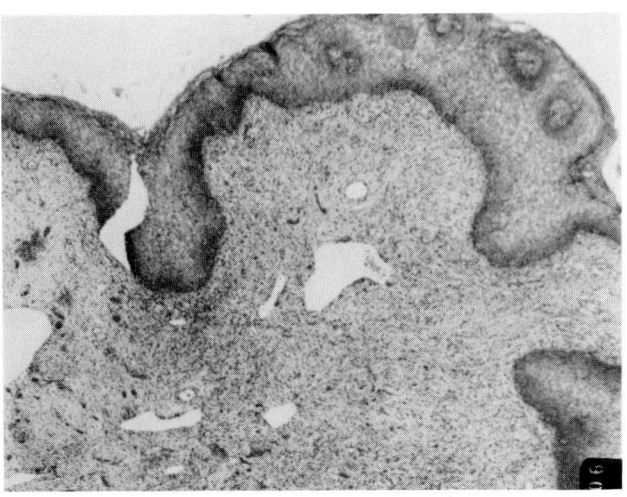

A

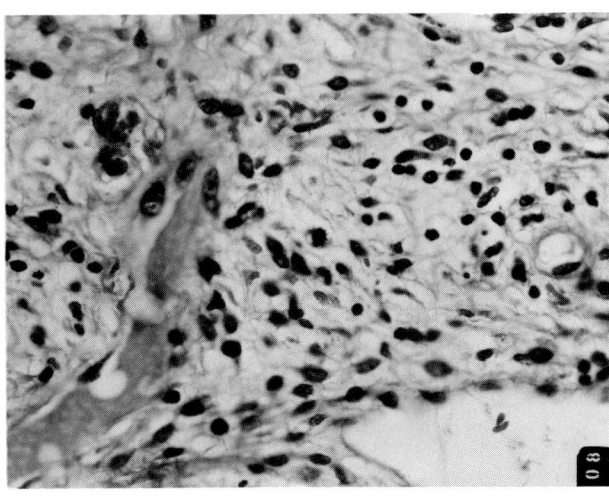

B

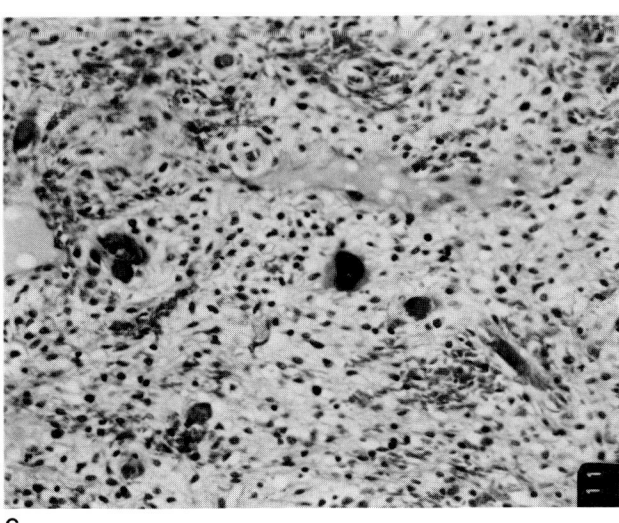

C

FIGURE 16-18 Microscopic appearance of a pseudosarcoma botryoides. (*A*) An intact epithelium overlying an edematous stroma. Note the absence of a cambium layer. (*B and C*) An edematous stroma with areas of giant cells. No rhabdomyoblasts (strap cells) are evident in these photographs. (Courtesy of Dr. Elizabeth Alenghat, Department of Pathology, The University of Chicago Hospitals and Clinics.)

patients, most reports have reviewed collections of diverse cases, often variously treated. In 1945, Mitchell and Mohler compiled 449 cases in a comprehensive review; Sedlis (1961) collected an additional 232 cases over the next decade.

Approximately 85% of fallopian tube malignancies are metastatic from other sites (Plentl and Friedman, 1971), frequently arising from the ovary, endometrium, or gastrointestinal tract. Usually transperitoneal spread results in serosal metastases, whereas lymphatic dissemination from the primary sites may involve the muscularis or mucosa. In some patients, carcinoma of the fallopian tube may be part of a multifocal upper genital tract malignancy. Of 64 tubal cancers reported by Rose and colleagues (1990), 24 were felt to be part of such a multifocal process.

Hu and co-workers (1950) proposed the following criteria for a primary tubal carcinoma:

1. Grossly, the main tumor is in the tube.
2. Microscopically, the mucosa should be mainly involved and should show a papillary pattern.
3. If the tubal wall is involved, the transition between benign and malignant tubal epithelium should be demonstrable.

Affected patients have been reported to range in age from 18 to 80 years, with the peak incidence between the ages of 50 and 60 (Sedlis, 1961; Hanton et al, 1966). Approximately 9% of the affected patients were below age 40 (Sedlis, 1961). Data from the SEER Program indicated that the rates of tubal cancer increased sharply with age, reached a peak at ages 60 to 64, and leveled off at age 65 and beyond (Rosenblatt et al, 1989).

As with other carcinomas, the etiology of primary tubal malignancies remains obscure. Many authors have associated chronic salpingitis with tubal carcinomas (Jones, 1965). Such an association may explain the high incidence of low parity seen in women with tubal carcinomas. Over 50% of patients reviewed by Sedlis (1961) and 27% of the patients reviewed by Hu et al (1950) were nulliparous. However, pelvic inflammatory disease is a common diagnosis, while tubal carcinomas are uncommonly rare.

## Symptoms

The clinical detection of fallopian tube carcinoma presents a challenge. Carcinoma of the oviduct, like epithelial malignancies of the ovary, is often asymptomatic.

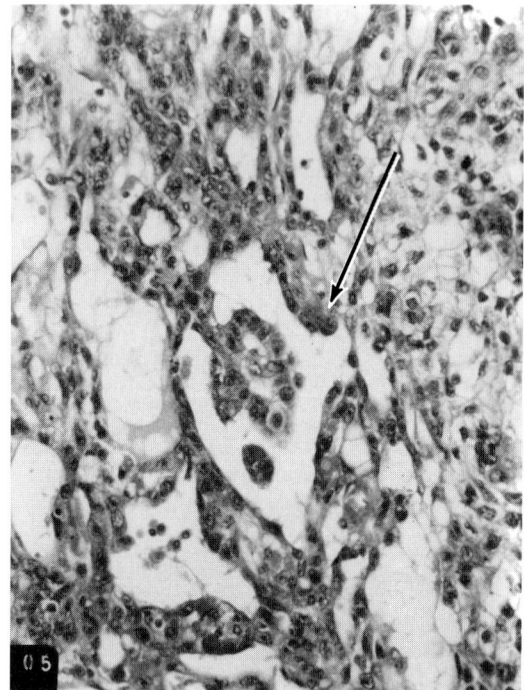

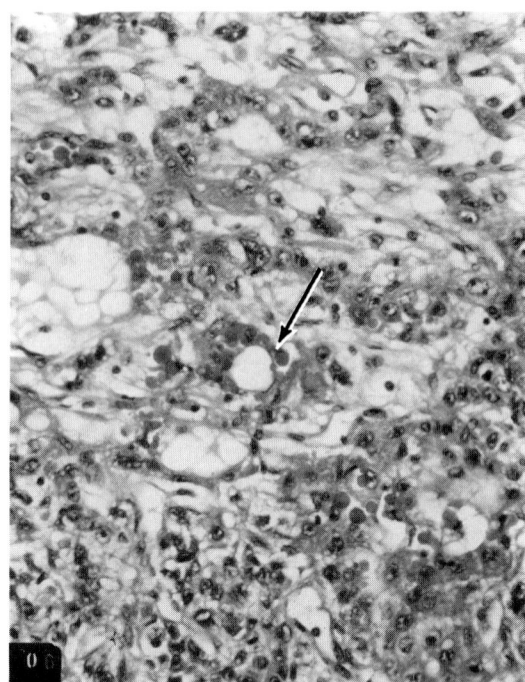

**FIGURE 16-19** Microscopic appearance of an endodermal sinus tumor. (*A*) The glomeruloid body is indicated by an arrow. (*B*) Hyaline globules are indicated by an arrow. (Courtesy of Dr. Elizabeth Alenghat, Department of Pathology, The University of Chicago Hospitals and Clinics.)

The disease is uncommon and has a subtle clinical presentation. Of 780 cases reviewed by Jones (1965), only 10 were correctly diagnosed preoperatively. The accuracy of preoperative diagnosis improved little over the next 20 years. According to a recent review (Eddy et al, 1984*b*), the correct preoperative diagnosis was made in only 2 of 71 patients with tubal carcinomas. In eight patients (12%) the diagnosis of a tubal carcinoma was incidental, discovered on pathologic examination, and unrecognized at the time of laparotomy.

Vaginal bleeding or discharge is the most commonly reported symptom and is seen in over 50% of affected patients (Sedlis, 1978). The next most frequent presenting complaint is pelvic or lower abdominal pain. A pelvic or adnexal mass has been detected in approximately 60% of patients with fallopian tube carcinoma (Sedlis, 1978; Eddy et al, 1984*b*). The classic triad (hydrops tubae profluens) consisting of pelvic pain, a pelvic mass, and vaginal discharge is observed in less than 15% of cases (Sedlis, 1978; Kinzel, 1976; Hanton et al, 1966).

Cervicovaginal cytology may be positive in patients with tubal carcinoma and may offer the first clue to an underlying malignancy. However, routine cytologic smears are generally ineffective as a screening test for fallopian tube carcinoma. Approximately 10% of the patients reported by Yoonessi (1979) had Pap smears suggestive of or positive for adenocarcinoma.

## Pathology

Grossly, the tumor may vary from several millimeters to 13 cm in diameter (Hanton et al, 1966). In most cases, the middle or distal portion of the tube is involved and forms a tubular, distended structure resembling a hydrosalpinx (Fig. 16-20). The fimbriated end is closed in about half the cases (Novak and Woodruff, 1979). The lumen of the tube may be filled with papillary or solid tumor that is grey to pink in color, with areas of necrosis and hemorrhage.

The tumor arises in the right and left tubes with approximately equal frequency; the incidence of bilateral tubal carcinoma ranges from 13 to 26% in large series (Hanton et al, 1966; Sedlis, 1978; Yoonessi, 1979). Although some workers have felt that bilateral tumors result from multifocal neoplasia, others have found bilateral tumors in advanced disease (Schiller and Silverberg, 1971).

Primary tubal malignancies are usually adenocarcinomas with papillary to medullary (solid) growth patterns (Fig. 16-21). Tumor grade varies from well-differentiated papillary neoplasms (Grade 1) to tumors with predominantly solid features (Grade 3). Although Hu et al (1950) and Momtazee and Kempson (1968) reported a worse prognosis with undifferentiated tumors, Hayden and Potter (1960) found no correlation between tumor grade and prognosis. More recently, Boutselis and Thompson (1971), and Podratz et al (1986) were unable to relate degree of tumor differentiation and survival. The mixture and gradations of tumor growth patterns frequently precluded a histologic assessment of tumor grade (Hanton et al, 1966).

## Staging

The FIGO staging for gynecologic malignancies does not include an official classification for tubal carcinoma. However, most individuals use a modification of the

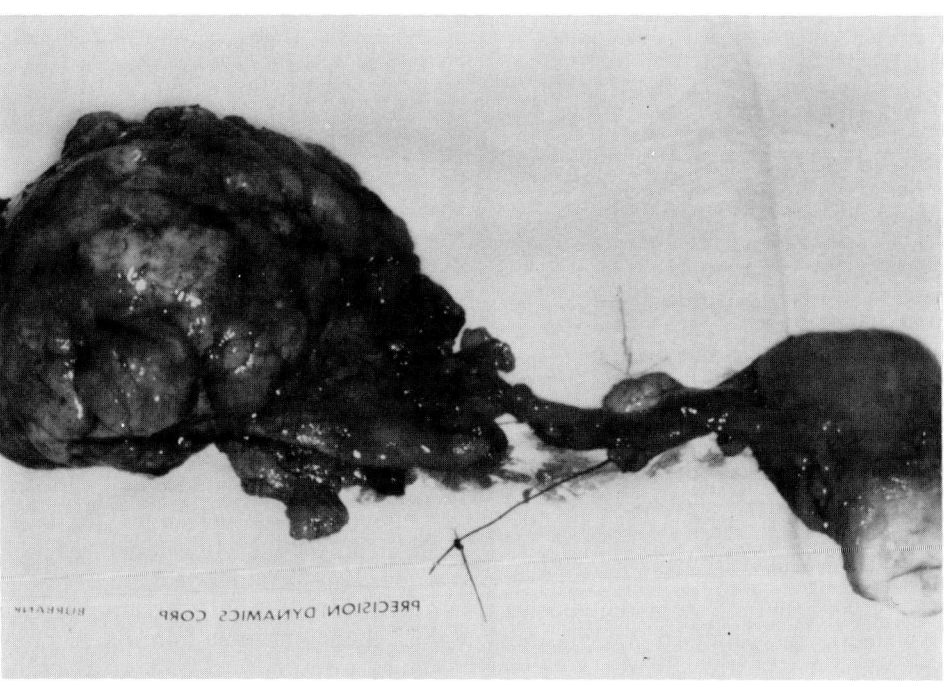

**FIGURE 16-20** External appearance of a large, tubal adenocarcinoma. Ipsilateral ovary was grossly normal. (Courtesy of Dr. John B. Wheelock, Department of Obstetrics and Gynecology, Keesler United States Air Force Medical Center, Biloxi, Mississippi.)

FIGO ovarian staging protocol to evaluate tubal malignancies. Dodson et al (1970) have proposed such a system (Table 16-3), which has been used in a number of retrospective studies.

A different concept was introduced by Schiller and Silverberg (1971), who proposed a staging classification similar to Dukes' system for colon carcinomas (Table 16-4). This scheme was predicated on the assumption that the fallopian tube is a hollow viscus with a muscular wall (similar to the colon) and, therefore, that the mechanics of tumor penetration and spread would differ from those of epithelial tumors of the ovary. A similar concept had been described earlier by Erez et al (1967).

## Natural History

As tubal carcinomas enlarge, the tumor may penetrate through the serosa or spill malignant cells out of the open, fimbriated end, contaminating the peritoneum. As with ovarian epithelial carcinomas, transcoelomic spread is a major factor in treatment failures (Denham and Maclennan, 1984). Sedlis (1961) found metastases in 29% of 232 patients with fallopian tube carcinoma, the most frequent site being the peritoneum.

Tubal carcinomas can also spread by lymphatic dissemination. The tubes are permeated by a rich lymphatic network within the mesosalpinx. Invariably, ef-

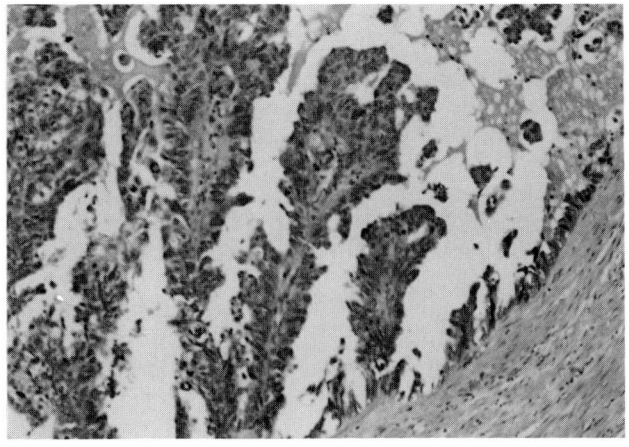

A

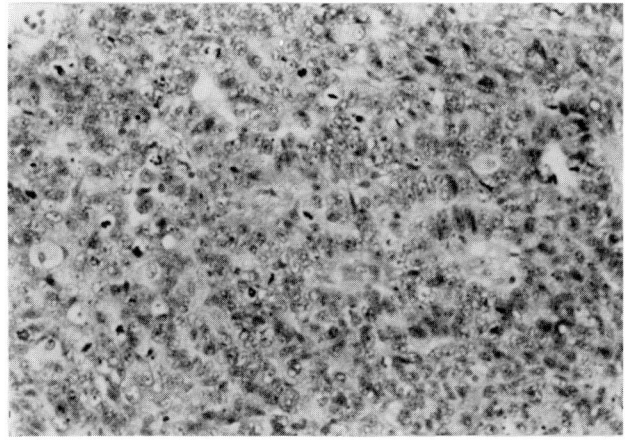

B

**FIGURE 16-21** (*A*) Microscopic appearance of a well-differentiated papillary adenocarcinoma of the fallopian tube. (Courtesy of Dr. Elizabeth Alenghat, Department of Pathology, The University of Chicago Hospitals and Clinics.) (*B*) Microscopic appearance of a poorly differentiated tubal carcinoma with a predominantly solid growth pattern. (Courtesy of Dr. Paul Kaminski, Department of Obstetrics and Gynecology, Milton S. Hershey Medical Center, Pennsylvania State University.)

TABLE 16-3   Clinical and Operative Staging for Fallopian Tube Carcinoma as Proposed by Dodson et al (1970)

| | |
|---|---|
| Stage I | Growth limited to the tube. |
| Stage Ia | Growth limited to one tube; no ascites. |
| Stage Ib | Growth limited to both tubes; no ascites. |
| Stage Ic | Growth limited to one or both tubes; ascites present with malignant cells in fluid. |
| Stage II | Growth involving one or both tubes with pelvic extension. |
| Stage IIa | Extension and/or metastases to the uterus or ovary. |
| Stage IIb | Extension to other pelvic tissues. |
| Stage III | Growth involving one or both tubes with widespread intraperitoneal metastases (the omentum, bowel, and its mesentery). |
| Stage IV | Growth involving one or both tubes with distant metastases outside the peritoneal cavity. |

TABLE 16-4   Clinical and Operative Staging of Fallopian Tube Carcinoma as Proposed by Schiller and Silverberg (1971)

| | |
|---|---|
| Stage 0 | Carcinoma in situ (limited to the tubal mucosa). |
| Stage I | Tumor extending into the submucosa and/or muscularis but not penetrating to the serosal surface of the tube. |
| Stage II | Tumor extending to the serosa of the fallopian tube. |
| Stage III | Direct extension of tumor to the ovary and/or endometrium. |
| Stage IV | Extension of tumor beyond the reproductive organs ( e.g., other pelvic organs, abdominal viscera, peritoneal implants). |

ferent lymphatics accompany the infundibulopelvic ligament and terminate in the paraaortic lymph node chain. Frequently, some lymphatics follow a pelvic course in the broad ligament and terminate at the interiliac lymph nodes. Tamimi and Figge (1981) demonstrated paraaortic lymph node metastases in five of 15 patients. The paraaortic nodes were the only sites of metastases in two patients, indicating that paraaortic lymph node involvement can be an early feature in the spread of disease. Inguinal node metastases have also been documented from fallopian tube carcinoma (Yoonessi, 1979; Tamimi and Figge, 1981). In these cases, neoplastic cells may be carried in a retrograde fashion toward the uterine fundus. Lymphatic efferents from the corpus follow the round ligament and terminate outside the pelvis in the femoral nodes (Plentl and Friedman, 1971).

## Treatment

Total abdominal hysterectomy with bilateral salpingo-oophorectomy is the essential step in the operative management of fallopian tube carcinoma. However, the staging of tubal carcinoma is based on the findings at laparotomy and requires an adequate intraoperative assessment. Ideally, omentectomy, evaluation of the paraaortic lymph nodes, and peritoneal cytologic examination should be an integral part of the surgical staging of fallopian tube carcinoma.

The optimal treatment of this disease is still undefined, but further therapy should be considered when the disease has extended beyond the tubal serosa. Radiation directed solely at the pelvis is inadequate insofar as the disease has the potential for intraperitoneal dissemination (McMurray et al, 1986). Further treatment with radiotherapy or chemotherapy should be considered once effective staging and primary surgery have been performed. The role of radical surgery in achieving optimal tumor debulking, with chemotherapy as an adjunctive therapeutic modality, requires further evaluation. However, some workers have demonstrated a sur-

vival advantage for patients who have minimal residual disease after the initial surgery (Eddy et al, 1984b; Podratz et al, 1986). More recently, Barakat et al (1991) reported an 83% five-year survival in platinum-treated patients with stages II, III, and IV disease who had no gross residual disease following surgery. In their platinum-treated patients with gross residual disease, the five-year survival was only 29%.

Second-look laparotomy has been used in the evaluation of patients with tubal carcinomas who achieved a complete response to initial surgery and adjunctive chemotherapy and/or radiation therapy. Rose and colleagues reviewed the experience with second-look laparotomy in tubal cancer. Of 45 second-look procedures reported since 1980, 31 were negative. However, 8 of the 31 patients (26%) with a "negative" second-look have subsequently demonstrated recurrent disease.

Serial CA 125 determinations may effectively assess disease activity in patients with tubal cancers. CA 125 has been immunohistochemically demonstrated in normal tubal epithelium, as well as in carcinomas (Neunteufel and Breitenecker, 1989). Furthermore, elevated serum CA 125 levels have been documented in patients with tubal cancers (Niloff et al, 1984; Kol et al, 1990).

## Radiotherapy

The role of adjunctive radiotherapy in the management of tubal carcinoma is unclear. Schray and coworkers (1987) administered postoperative radiotherapy to 34 patients with tubal cancer. Fifteen of the patients (44%) survived disease-free until intercurrent death or to a median followup of 70 months. Intraperitoneal radioactive isotopes (gold-198, phosphorus-32) have been used in patients with no gross residual disease after surgery (Benedet et al, 1977). Radioactive isotopes have the potential for controlling microscopic disease in individuals with intraperitoneal dissemination. Unfortunately, experience with this form of therapy is too limited to allow any conclusions about its efficacy.

## Chemotherapy

Using a regimen of cisplatin (50 mg/m$^2$ of body surface area), doxorubicin (37.5 mg/m$^2$ of body surface area), and progestins with or without cyclophosphamide, Deppe and coworkers (1980) reported surgically proven complete remissions in two patients with advanced fallopian tube carcinoma. Both patients began chemotherapy with bulky residual disease and had negative second-look laparotomies after 10 to 13 cycles of treatment. Chemotherapy was administered every 3 weeks, and no severe drug-related toxicity occurred in either patient.

Peters et al (1989) identified 46 patients with measurable disease who received chemotherapy for advanced or recurrent carcinoma of the fallopian tube. The response rate was 9% with single-agent therapy, 29% with multiagent therapy without cisplatin, and 81% with cisplatin-containing regimens. Subsequent reports have also corroborated the activity of cisplatin-based combination chemotherapy in fallopian tube cancers (Morris et al, 1990; Barakat et al, 1991).

## Survival and Prognosis

The stage or extent of disease at diagnosis appears to be the most important factor in determining the prognosis of fallopian tube carcinoma. Patients with tubal carcinoma that has not extended to the tubal serosa appear to have the best chance for long-term survival (Schiller and Silverberg, 1971). Ten of 11 patients with tumor limited to the tubal mucosa survived for 5 years as compared with 7 of 13 patients in whom the tumor had penetrated the submucosa or muscularis. Furthermore, patients with disease extending beyond the pelvis but confined to the peritoneal cavity (Stage III) do not fare as well as patients with disease confined to the fallopian tube (Stage I) or pelvis (Stage II) (Eddy et al, 1984*b*).

## Sarcomas of the Fallopian Tube

This is a very rare pathologic diagnosis. The majority of these tumors are of the mixed Müllerian type. The stromal component may contain tissues that are homologous or heterologous to the Müllerian duct system. So far 26 cases of mixed Müllerian tumors of the fallopian tube have been reported in the literature (Hanjani et al, 1980; Deppe et al, 1984; Muntz et al, 1989; Seraj et al, 1990; van Dijk et al, 1990).

Patients have ranged in age from 14 to 76 years, with most tumors occurring in the fifth and sixth decades of life. Clinically, these tumors are similar to tubal carcinomas in presentation. Usually the patient is asymptomatic until the tumor has reached considerable size.

The recommended treatment is surgery followed by radiation therapy or chemotherapy. Some patients with advanced disease have shown clinical responses to vincristine, actinomycin D, and cyclophosphamide chemotherapy or regimens containing cisplatin (Hanjani et al, 1980; Deppe et al, 1984). Prognosis is poor, with most patients surviving for less than 2 years, although long-term survival has been seen when the tumor is confined to the tube at the time of surgery.

## REFERENCES

Ariel IM: Malignant melanoma of the female genital system: A report of 48 patients and review of the literature. *J Surg Oncol* 16:371-383, 1981.

Ballon SC, Roberts JA, Lagasse LD: Topical 5-fluorouracil in the treatment of intraepithelial neoplasia of the vagina. *Obstet Gynecol* 54:163-166, 1979.

Barakat RR, Rubin SC, Saigo PE, et al: Cisplatin-based combination chemotherapy in carcinoma of the fallopian tube. *Gynecol Oncol* 42:156-160, 1991.

Benedet JL, White GW, Fairey RN, Boyes DA: Adenocarcinoma of the fallopian tube. Experience with 41 patients. *Obstet Gynecol* 50:654-657, 1977.

Benedet JL, Sanders BH: Carcinoma in situ of the vagina. *Am J Obstet Gynecol* 148:695-700, 1984.

Bergman F: Carcinoma of the ovary. A clinicopathological study of 86 autopsied cases with special reference to mode of spread. *Acta Obstet Gynecol Scand* 45:211-231, 1966.

Bloomfield A, Frazier JE: The development of the lower end of the vagina. *J Anat* 62:9-32, 1927.

Borazjani G, Prem KA, Okagaki T, et al: Primary malignant melanoma of the vagina: A clinicopathologic analysis of 10 cases. *Gynecol Oncol* 37:264, 1990.

Bornstein J, Adam E, Adler-Storthz K, Kaufman RH: Development of cervical and vaginal squamous cell neoplasia as a late consequence of in utero exposure to diethylstilbestrol. *Obstet Gynecol Surv* 43:15-21, 1988.

Bottles K, Lacey CG, Miller TR: Atypical melanocytic hyperplasia of the vagina. *Gynecol Oncol* 19:226-230, 1984.

Boutselis JG, Thompson JN: Clinical aspects of primary carcinoma of the fallopian tube: A clinical study of 14 cases. *Am J Obstet Gynecol* 111:98-101, 1971.

Capen CV, Masterson BJ, Magrina JF, Calkins JW: Laser therapy of vaginal intraepithelial neoplasia. *Am J Obstet Gynecol* 142:973-976, 1982.

Carlson JA, Morgan M, Boothby R, Rubin M: Stage II papillary clear cell adenocarcinoma of the vagina during observation in a diethylstilbestrol-exposed daughter. *Gynecol Oncol* 32:86-87, 1989.

Chambers J, Rogers LW, Julian CG: Minute clear cell carcinoma of vagina with early metastasis to pelvic lymph nodes. *Am J Obstet Gynecol* 131:223-225, 1978.

Chung AF, Casey MJ, Flannery JT, et al: Malignant melanoma of the vagina—report of 19 cases. *Obstet Gynecol* 55:720-727, 1980.

Chung AF, Woodruff JM, Lewis JL Jr: Malignant melanoma of the vulva. A report of 44 cases. *Obstet Gynecol* 45:638-646, 1975.

Collantes TM, Pratt JH, Dockerty MB: Primary malignant melanoma of the vagina. *Obstet Gynecol* 29:508-514, 1967.

Collins HS, Burke TW, Heller PB, et al: Endodermal sinus tumor of the infant vagina treated exclusively by chemotherapy. *Obstet Gynecol* 73:507, 1989.

Copeland LJ, Sneige N, Ordonez NG, et al: Endodermal sinus tumor of the vagina and cervix. *Cancer* 55:2558-2565, 1985.

Cunha GR, Fujii H: Stromal-parenchymal interactions in normal and abnormal development of the genital tract. In Herbst AL, Bern HA (eds): *Developmental Effects of Diethylstilbestrol (DES) in Pregnancy*. New York, Thieme-Stratton, 1981, pp 179-193.

Denham JW, Maclennan KA: The management of primary carcinoma of the fallopian tube. Experience of 40 cases. *Cancer* 53:166-172, 1984.

Deppe G, Bruckner HW, Cohen CJ: Combination chemotherapy for advanced carcinoma of the fallopian tube. *Obstet Gynecol* 56:530-532, 1980.

Deppe G, Zbella E, Friberg J, Thomas W: Combination chemotherapy for mixed Müllerian tumor of the fallopian tube. *Cancer* 54:1517-1520, 1984.

Deppisch LM: Cervical melanosis. *Obstet Gynecol* 62:525-526, 1983.

Dewhurst J: *Practical Pediatric and Adolescent Gynecology*. New York, Marcel Dekker, 1980.

Dewhurst J, Ferreira HP: An endodermal sinus tumour of the vagina in an infant with seven year survival. *Br J Obstet Gynecol* 88:859-862, 1981.

Dodson MG, Ford JH, Averette HE: Clinical aspects of fallopian tube carcinoma. *Obstet Gynecol* 36:935-939, 1970.

Eddy GL, Copeland LJ, Gershenson DM: Second-look laparotomy in fallopian tube carcinoma. *Gynecol Oncol* 19:182-186, 1984*a*.

Eddy GL, Copeland LJ, Gershenson DM, et al: Fallopian tube carcinoma. *Obstet Gynecol* 64:546-552, 1984*b*.

Ehrmann RL, Younge PA, Lerch VL: The exfoliative cytology and histogenesis of an early primary malignant melanoma of the vagina. *Acta Cytol* 6:245-254, 1962.

Erez S, Kaplan AL, Wall JA: Clinical staging of carcinoma of the uterine tube. *Obstet Gynecol* 30:547-550, 1967.

Forsberg JG, Kalland T: Embryology of the genital tract in humans and in rodents. In Herbst AL, Bern HA (eds): *Developmental Effects of Diethylstilbestrol (DES) in Pregnancy*. New York, Thieme-Stratton, 1981, pp 4-25.

Fu Y, Robboy SJ, Prat J: Nuclear DNA study of vaginal and cervical squamous cell abnormalities in DES exposed progeny. *Obstet Gynecol* 52:129-137, 1978.

Gallousis S: Verrucous carcinoma. Report of three vulvar cases and review of the literature. *Obstet Gynecol* 40:502-507, 1972.

Gallup DG, Morley GW: Carcinoma in situ of the vagina. A study and review. *Obstet Gynecol* 46:334-340, 1975.

Gallup DG, Talledo OE, Shah KJ, Hayes C: Invasive squamous cell carcinoma of the vagina: A 14-year study. *Obstet Gynecol* 69:782-785, 1987.

Gompel C, Silverberg SG: *Pathology in Gynecology and Obstetrics*. Philadelphia, JB Lippincott Co, 1985.

Goss CM (ed): *Gray's Anatomy*, 29th ed. Philadelphia, Lea and Febiger, 1973.

Hanjani P, Petersen RO, Bonnell SA: Malignant mixed Müllerian tumor of the fallopian tube. Report of a case and review of literature. *Gynecol Oncol* 9:381-393, 1980.

Hanton EM, Malkasian GD, Dahlin DC, Pratt JH: Primary carcinoma of the fallopian tube. *Am J Obstet Gynecol* 94:832-839, 1966.

Hayden GE, Potter EL: Primary carcinoma of the fallopian tube with report of 12 new cases. *Am J Obstet Gynecol* 79:24-31, 1960.

Hays DM, Shimada H, Raney RB, et al: Sarcomas of the vagina and uterus: The Intergroup Rhabdomyosarcoma Study. *J Pediat Surg* 20:718-724, 1985.

Herbst AL: Problems of Prenatal DES Exposure. In Herbst AL, Mishell DR, Stenchever MA, and Droegemueller W (eds): *Comprehensive Gynecology* (2nd ed.) St. Louis, Mosby Yearbook, 1992, Chap. 14.

Herbst AL, Scully RE: Adenocarcinoma of the vagina in adolescence. A report of 7 cases including 6 clear-cell carcinomas (so-called mesonephromas). *Cancer* 25:745-757, 1970.

Herbst AL, Anderson S, Hubby MM, et al: Risk factors for the development of diethylstilbestrol-associated clear cell adenocarcinoma: A case-control study. *Am J Obstet Gynecol* 154:814-822, 1986.

Herbst AL, Cole P, Norusis MJ, et al: Epidemiological aspects and factors related to survival in 384 registry cases of clear cell adenocarcinoma of the vagina and cervix. *Am J Obstet Gynecol* 135:876-886, 1979*a*.

Herbst AL, Green TH, Ulfelder H: Primary carcinoma of the vagina. An analysis of 68 cases. *Am J Obstet Gynecol* 106:210-218, 1970.

Herbst AL, Norusis MJ, Rosenow PJ, et al: An analysis of 346 cases of clear cell adenocarcinoma of the vagina and cervix with emphasis on recurrence and survival. *Gynecol Oncol* 7:111-122, 1979*b*.

Herbst AL, Ulfelder H, Poskanzer DC: Adenocarcinoma of the vagina. Association of maternal stilbestrol therapy with tumor appearance in young women. *N Engl J Med* 284:878-881, 1971.

Hershey DW, Fennell RH, Major FJ: Primary carcinoma of the fallopian tube. *Obstet Gynecol* 57:367-370, 1981.

Hilgers RD: Pelvic exenteration for vaginal embryonal rhabdomyosarcoma. A review. *Obstet Gynecol* 45:175-180, 1975.

Hilgers RD, Malkasian GD, Soule EH: Embryonal rhabdomyosarcoma (botryoid type) of the vagina. A clinicopathologic review. *Am J Obstet Gyencol* 107:484-502, 1970.

Hu CY, Taymor ML, Hertig AT: Primary carcinoma of the fallopian tube. *Am J Obstet Gynecol* 59:58-67, 1950.

Hummer WK, Mussey E, Decker DG, Dockerty MB: Carcinoma in situ of the vagina. *Am J Obstet Gynecol* 108:1109-1116, 1970.

Isaacs JH: Verrucous carcinoma of the female genital tract. *Gynecol Oncol* 4:259-269, 1976.

Jimerson GK, Merrill JA: Cancer and dysplasia of the post-hysterectomy vaginal cuff. *Gynecol Oncol* 4:328-334, 1976.

Jobson VW, Homesley HD: Treatment of vaginal intraepithelial neoplasia with the carbon dioxide laser. *Obstet Gynecol* 62:90-93, 1983.

Jones OV: Primary carcinoma of the uterine tube. *Obstet Gynecol* 26:122-129, 1965.

Kinzel GE: Primary carcinoma of the fallopian tube. *Am J Obstet Gynecol* 125:816-820, 1976.

Kol S, Gal D, Friedman M, Paldi E: Preoperative diagnosis of fallopian tube carcinoma by transvaginal sonography and CA-125. *Gynecol Oncol* 37:129-131, 1990.

Krebs HB: Treatment of vaginal intraepithelial neoplasia with laser and topical 5-fluorouracil. *Obstet Gynecol* 73:657-660, 1989.

Kucera H, Vavra N: Radiation management of primary carcinoma of the vagina: Clinical and histopathological variables associated with survival. *Gynecol Oncol* 40:12, 1991.

Laufe LE, Berstein ED: Primary malignant melanoma of the vagina. *Obstet Gynecol* 37:148-154, 1971.

Lawrence WD, Shingleton HM, Gore H, Soong SJ: Ultrastructural and morphometric study of diethylstilbestrol-associated lesions diagnosed as cervical intraepithelial neoplasia III. *Can Res* 40:1558-1567, 1980.

Lee RB, Buttoni L, Dhru K, Tamimi H: Malignant melanoma of the vagina: A case report of progression from preexisting melanosis. *Gynecol Oncol* 19:238-245, 1984.

Lenehan PM, Meffe F, Lickrish GM: Vaginal intra-epithelial neoplasia: Biologic aspects and management. *Obstet Gynecol* 68:333-337, 1986.

Liu L, Hou Y, Li: Primary malignant melanoma of the vagina: A report of seven cases. *Obstet Gynecol* 70:569-572, 1987.

MacRae DJ: Chorionepithelioma occurring during pregnancy. *J Obstet Gynaecol Br Emp* 58:373-380, 1951.

McMurray EH, Jacobs AJ, Perez CA, et al: Carcinoma of the fallopian tube. Management and sites of failure. *Cancer* 58:2070-2075, 1986.

Melnick S, Cole P, Anderson D, Herbst A: Rates and risks of diethylstilbestrol-related clear-cell adenocarcinoma of the vagina and cervix. An update. *N Engl J Med* 316:514-516, 1987.

Miettinen M, Wahlstrom T, Vesterinen E, Saksela E: Vaginal polyps with pseudosarcomatous features. A clinicopathologic study of seven cases. *Cancer* 51:1,148-1,151, 1983.

Mitchell RM, Mohler RW: Primary carcinoma of the fallopian tube. *Am J Obstet Gynecol* 50:283-292, 1945.

Mitchell M, Talerman A, Sholl JS, et al: Pseudosarcoma botryoides in pregnancy: Report of a case with ultrastructural observations. *Obstet Gynecol* 70:522-526, 1987.

Momtazee S, Kempson RL: Primary adenocarcinoma of the fallopian tube. *Obstet Gynecol* 32:649-656, 1968.

Morrow CP, DiSaia PJ: Malignant melanoma of the female genitalia: A clinical analysis. *Obstet Gynecol Surv* 31:233-271, 1976.

Muntz HG, Rutgers JL, Terraza HM, Fuller AL: Carcinosarcomas and mixed Müllerian tumors of the fallopian tube. *Gynecol Oncol* 34:109-115, 1989.

Nerdrum TA: Vaginal metastases of hypernephroma. *Acta Obstet Gynecol Scand* 45:515-524, 1966.

Neunteufel W, Breitenecker G: Tissue expression of CA-125 in benign and malignant lesions of the ovary and fallopian tube: A comparison with CA 19-9 and CEA. *Gynecol Oncol* 32:297-302, 1989.

Nigogosyan G, De La Pava S, Pickren JW: Melanoblasts in vaginal mucosa. Origin for primary malignant melanoma. *Cancer* 17:912-913, 1964.

Niloff JM, Klug TL, Schaetzl E, et al: Elevation of serum CA 125 in carcinomas of the fallopian tube, endometrium, and endocervix. *Am J Obstet Gynecol* 148:1057-1058, 1984.

Norgaard-Pedersen B, Lundborg CJ, Laursen AM, Hagerstrand I: infantile vaginal tumor with alpha-fetoprotein synthesis. *Acta Path Microbiol Scand* 87A:223-226, 1979.

Norris HJ, Taylor HB: Polyps of the vagina: A benign lesion resembling sarcoma botryoides. *Cancer* 19:227-232, 1966.

Novak ER, Woodruff JD: *Novak's Gynecologic and Obstetric Pathology With Clinical and Endocrine Relations*. Philadelphia, WB Saunders Co, 1979.

Perez CA, Arneson AN, Dehner LP, Galakatos A: Radiation therapy in carcinoma of the vagina. *Obstet Gynecol* 44:862-872, 1974.

Perez CA, Arneson AN, Galakatos A, Samanth HK: Malignant tumors of the vagina. *Cancer* 31:36-44, 1973.

Perez CA, Camel HM, Galakatos AE, et al: Definitive irradiation in carcinoma of the vagina: Long-term evaluation of results. *Int J Radiat Oncol Biol Phys* 15:1283-1290, 1988.

Perez CA, Korba A, Sharma S: Dosimetric considerations in irradiation of carcinoma of the vagina. *Int J Radiat Oncol Biol Phys* 2:639-649, 1977.

Peters WA, Andersen WA, Hopkins MP: Results of chemotherapy in advanced carcinoma of the fallopian tube. *Cancer* 63:836-838, 1989.

Peters WA, Kumar NB, Andersen WA, Morley GW: Primary sarcoma of the adult vagina: A clinicopathologic study. *Obstet Gynecol* 65:699-704, 1985a.

Peters WA, Kumar NB, Morley GW: Carcinoma of the vagina. Factors influencing treatment outcome. *Cancer* 55:892-897, 1985b.

Pfeiffer P, Mogensen H, Amtrup F, Honore E: Primary carcinoma of the fallopian tube. A retrospective study of patients reported to the Danish Cancer Registry in a five-year period. *Acta Oncologica* 28:7-11, 1989.

Piver MS, Rose PG: Long-term follow-up and complications of infants with vulvovaginal embryonal rhabdomyosarcoma treated with surgery, radiation therapy, and chemotherapy. *Obstet Gynecol* 71:435-437, 1988.

Piver MS, Barlow JJ, Wang JJ, Shah NK: Combined radical surgery, radiation therapy and chemotherapy in infants with vulvovaginal embryonal rhabdomyosarcoma. *Obstet Gynecol* 42:522-526, 1973.

Plentl AA, Friedman EA: *Lymphatic System of the Female Genitalia. The Morphologic Basis of Oncologic Diagnosis and Therapy.* Philadelphia, WB Saunders Co, 1971.

Podratz KC, Gaffey TA, Symmonds RE, et al: Melanoma of the vulva: An update. *Gynecol Oncol* 16:153-168, 1983.

Podratz KC, Podczaski ES, Gaffey TA, et al: Primary carcinoma of the fallopian tube. *Am J Obstet Gynecol* 154:1319-1326, 1986.

Pride GL, Schultz AE, Chuprevich TW, Buchler DA: Primary invasive squamous carcinoma of the vagina. *Obstet Gynecol* 53:218-225, 1979.

Prins RP, Morrow CP, Townsend DE, DiSaia PJ: Vaginal embryogenesis, estrogens, and adenosis. *Obstet Gynecol* 48:246- 250, 1976.

Pritchard JA, MacDonald PC: *Williams Obstetrics,* 15th ed. New York, Appleton-Century-Crofts, 1976.

Reid GC, Morley GW, Schmidt RW, Hopkins MP: The role of pelvic exenteration for sarcomatous malignancies. *Obstet Gynecol* 74:80-84, 1989a.

Reid GC, Schmidt RW, Roberts JA, et al: Primary melanoma of the vagina: A clinicopathologic analysis. *Obstet Gynecol* 74:190-199, 1989b.

Richart RM: The incidence of cervical and vaginal dysplasia after exposure to DES. *JAMA* 255:36-37, 1986.

Robboy SJ, Herbst AL, Scully RE: Clear-cell adenocarcinoma of the vagina and cervix in young females: Analysis of 37 tumors that persisted or recurred after primary therapy. *Cancer* 34:606-614, 1974.

Robboy SJ, Keh PC, Nickerson RJ, et al: Squamous cell dysplasia and carcinoma in situ of the cervix and vagina after prenatal exposure to diethylstilbestrol. *Obstet Gynecol* 51:528-535, 1978.

Robboy SJ, Noller KL, O'Brien P, et al: Increased incidence of cervical and vaginal dysplasia in 3,980 diethylstilbestrol-exposed young women. *JAMA* 252:2979-2983, 1984.

Robboy SJ, Szyfelbein WM, Goellner JR, et al: Dysplasia and cytologic findings in 4,589 young women enrolled in Diethylstilbestrol-Adenosis (DESAD) Project. *Am J Obstet Gynecol* 140:579-586, 1981.

Robboy SJ, Welch WR, Young RH, et al: Topographic relation of cervical ectropion and vaginal adenosis to clear cell adenocarcinoma. *Obstet Gynecol* 60:546-551, 1982.

Rose PG, Piver MS, Tsukada Y: Fallopian tube cancer. The Roswell Park experience. *Cancer* 66:2661-2667, 1990.

Rosenblatt KA, Weiss NS, Schwartz SM: Incidence of malignant fallopian tube tumors. *Gynecol Oncol* 35:236-239, 1989.

Rubin SC, Young J, Mikuta JJ: Squamous carcinoma of the vagina: Treatment, complications and long-term follow-up. *Gynecol Oncol* 20:346-353, 1985.

Rutledge FN: Cancer of the vagina. *Am J Obstet Gynecol* 97:635-655, 1967.

Sander R, Nuss RC, Rhatigan RM: Diethylstilbestrol-associated vaginal adenosis followed by clear cell adenocarcinoma. *Int J Gynecol Pathol* 5:362-370, 1986.

Schiller HM, Silverberg SG: Staging and prognosis in primary carcinoma of the fallopian tube. *Cancer* 28:389-395, 1971.

Schray MF, Podratz KC, Malkasian GD: Fallopian tube cancer: The role of radiation therapy. *Radiother Oncol* 10:267-275, 1987.

Scully RE, Welch WR: Pathology of the female genital tract after prenatal exposure to diethylstilbestrol. In Herbst AL, Bern HA (eds): *Developmental Effects of Diethylstilbestrol (DES) in Pregnancy.* New York, Thieme-Stratton, 1981, pp 26-45.

Sedlis A: Primary carcinoma of the fallopian tube. *Obstet Gynecol Surv* 16:209-226, 1961.

Sedlis A: Carcinoma of the fallopian tube. *Surg Clin North Am* 58:121-129, 1978.

Senekjian EK, Frey KW, Anderson D, Herbst AL: Local therapy in Stage I clear cell adenocarcinoma of the vagina. *Cancer* 60:1319-1324, 1987.

Seraj IM, King A, Chase D: Malignant mixed Müllerian tumor of the oviduct. *Gynecol Oncol* 37:296-301, 1990.

Stafl A, Mattingly RF: Vaginal adenosis: A precancerous lesion? *Am J Obstet Gynecol* 120:666-677, 1974.

Sulak P, Barnhill D, Heller P, et al: Nonsquamous cancer of the vagina. *Gynecol Oncol* 29:309-320, 1988.

Tamimi HK, Figge DC: Adenocarcinoma of the uterine tube: Potential for lymph node metastases. *Am J Obstet Gynecol* 141:132-137, 1981.

Tavassoli FA, Norris HJ: Smooth muscle tumors of the vagina. *Obstet Gynecol* 53:689-693, 1979.

Teilum G: *Special Tumors of Ovary and Testis and Related Extragonadal Lesions. Comparative Pathology and Histologic Identification.* Philadelphia, JB Lippincott Co, 1971.

Tsukada Y: Benign melanosis of the vagina and cervix. *Am J Obstet Gynecol* 124:211-212, 1976.

Ulfelder H, Robboy SJ: The embryologic development of the human vagina. *Am J Obstet Gynecol* 126:769-776, 1976.

van Dijk CM, Kooijman CD, van Lindert ACM: Malignant mixed Müllerian tumor of the fallopian tube. *Histopathology* 16:300-302, 1990.

Way S: Vaginal metastases of carcinoma of the body of the uterus. *J Obstet Gynaecol Br Emp* 58:558-572, 1951.

Weiss L, Greep RO: *Histology.* New York, McGraw-Hill, 1977.

Wharton JT, Rutledge FN, Gallagher HS, Fletcher G: Treatment of clear cell adenocarcinoma in young females. *Obstet Gynecol* 45:365-368, 1975.

Wied GL, Bartels PH, Dytch HE, Bibbo M: Rapid DNA evaluation in clinical diagnosis. *Acta Cytol* 27:33-37, 1983.

Woodman CBJ, Jordan JA, Wade-Evans T: The management of vaginal intraepithelial neoplasia after hysterectomy. *Br J Obstet Gynecol* 91:707-711, 1984.

Yoonessi M: Carcinoma of the fallopian tube. *Obstet Gynecol Surv* 34:257-270, 1979.

Young RH, Scully RE: Endodermal sinus tumor of the vagina: A report of nine cases and review of the literature. *Gynecol Oncol* 18:380-392, 1984.

# Chapter 17

# Management of Molar Pregnancy and Gestational Trophoblastic Tumors

*Ross S. Berkowitz*    *Donald P. Goldstein*

*Gestational trophoblastic diseases* (GTD) comprise a spectrum of interrelated conditions, including molar pregnancy, invasive mole, placental-site trophoblastic tumors, and choriocarcinomas that have varying propensities for invasion and metastasis. *Gestational trophoblastic tumors* (GTT) are uncommon solid tumors that are highly curable even with widespread dissemination (Bagshawe, 1976; Goldstein and Berkowitz, 1982). While GTT most commonly occur after a molar gestation, they may follow any pregnancy.

Important advances have been made in the detection, management, and monitoring of patients with molar pregnancy and GTT. In this chapter, we will review these advances and discuss basic principles of treatment based upon our clinical experience at the New England Trophoblastic Disease Center (NETDC).

## MOLAR PREGNANCY

### Pathologic and Chromosomal Features

Hydatidiform mole may be categorized as either complete or partial based on gross morphology, histopathology, and karyotype (Table 17-1).

*Complete hydatidiform moles* have no identifiable embryonic or fetal tissues, and the chorionic villi show generalized swelling and diffuse trophoblastic hyperplasia. Usually complete moles have a 46,XX karyotype, and all molar chromosomes have a paternal origin (Kajii and Ohama, 1977). They appear to arise from a defective ovum that has been fertilized by a haploid sperm, which then duplicates its own chromosomes (Yamashita et al, 1979). About 10% of complete moles have a 46,XY chromosomal pattern (Pattillo et al, 1981), and the molar chromosomes are also entirely of paternal origin.

The influence of the parental genome on embryonic development has been studied in a mouse model of nuclear transplantation (Surani et al, 1986). When the entire murine genome is paternally derived, like a complete mole, embryonic development is limited but trophoblastic growth is exuberant. In contrast, when the entire murine genome is maternally derived, embryonic development is more advanced and trophoblastic growth is scanty. The development of molar pregnancy in humans, therefore, seems to be analogous to this model.

*Partial hydatidiform moles* are characterized by the following histopathologic features: (1) chorionic villi of varying sizes with focal swelling and focal trophoblastic hyperplasia, (2) villous scalloping and stromal trophoblastic inclusions, and (3) identifiable fetal or embryonic tissues (Szulman and Surti, 1978a). Usually, partial moles have a triploid karyotype, which results from fertilization of an apparently normal ovum by two sperm (Szulman and Surti, 1978b). When fetuses are identified with partial moles, they generally exhibit the stigmata of triploidy, including growth retardation, hydrocephalus, microphthalmos and syndactyly of the hands and feet (Doshi et al, 1983). While some partial moles may have a diploid karyotype, it is difficult to distinguish a diploid partial mole from a twin gestation with a complete mole.

### Complete Molar Pregnancy: Presenting Signs and Symptoms

*Vaginal Bleeding* Vaginal bleeding is the most common presenting sign in patients with complete mole, occurring in 97% of our patients (Berkowitz and Goldstein, 1981). The endometrial cavity may be expanded by large volumes of blood, and "prune juice"–like fluid may leak into the vagina as the intrauterine clots undergo oxidation and liquefaction.

*Excessive Uterine Size* The endometrial cavity may also be expanded by both the proliferation of chorionic tissue and retained clots. In general, excessive uterine size—i.e., when the uterus is larger than would be expected based on gestational age—is associated with markedly elevated human chorionic gonadotropin (hCG) values because the expansion is due in part to hyperplastic trophoblastic tissue. While excessive uterine enlargement is considered one of the classic signs of complete mole, half our patients lack this clinical finding.

*Preeclampsia* Preeclamptic toxemia is diagnosed in 27% of our patients with complete mole, so that the possibility of a complete molar pregnancy should be considered whenever toxemia develops early in pregnancy. Although preeclampsia is often associated with hypertension and hyperreflexia, eclamptic convulsions rarely occur. Toxemia develops almost exclusively in patients with excessive uterine enlargement and markedly elevated hCG levels. Curry et al (1975) also reported that 81% of their patients with molar pregnancy and toxemia had an enlarged uterus.

**TABLE 17-1** Complete versus Partial Molar Pregnancy:
Histopathologic and Chromosomal Features

|  | Complete Mole | Partial Mole |
|---|---|---|
| Fetal or embryonic tissue | Absent | Present |
| Hydatidiform swelling of chorionic villi | Diffuse | Focal |
| Trophoblastic hyperplasia | Diffuse | Focal |
| Scalloping of chorionic villi | Absent | Present |
| Trophoblastic stromal inclusions | Absent | Present |
| Karyotype | 46,XX (mainly); 46,XY | Triploid (mainly); diploid |

chest usually reveals diffuse rales, and a chest roentgenogram may demonstrate bilateral diffuse pulmonary infiltrates. Fortunately, respiratory distress generally resolves within 72 hours with cardiovascular and respiratory support.

Respiratory insufficiency usually occurs in patients with a markedly enlarged uterus. Twiggs et al (1979) reported pulmonary complications in 12 (27%) of 44 patients with a molar pregnancy 16 weeks in size or larger.

Hankins et al (1987) detected only a minimal number of trophoblastic cells in the pulmonary arterial blood of six women undergoing evacuation of large molar pregnancies. None of these women experienced significant pulmonary compromise or hemodynamic instability, and these authors speculated that respiratory insufficiency in patients with mole may be due in part to the cardiopulmonary changes induced by preeclampsia, anemia, hyperthyroidism, and vigorous transfusion therapy.

***Hyperemesis Gravidarum*** Hyperemesis requiring antiemetic and/or intravenous therapy was noted in 26% of our patients with complete mole. Infrequently, a severe electrolyte imbalance may ensue, requiring parenteral fluids. Although the etiology is still unclear, hyperemesis occurs primarily in patients with an excessively enlarged uterus and markedly elevated hCG values. Masson et al (1985) reported high serum hCG levels during the first trimester in women with nausea and vomiting.

***Hyperthyroidism*** Hyperthyroidism was diagnosed in 7% of our patients with complete mole. These patients may present with tachycardia, warm skin, and tremor, and the diagnosis can be confirmed by detecting elevated serum levels of free thyroxine ($T_4$) and triiodothyronine ($T_3$). If hyperthyroidism is suspected, beta-adrenergic blockers should be administered prior to evacuation, since anesthesia or surgery may precipitate thyroid storm and thus lead to hyperthermia, convulsions, atrial fibrillation, or cardiovascular collapse. Pretreatment with beta-adrenergic blockers may prevent or rapidly reverse many of these metabolic and cardiovascular complications.

Some investigators have suggested that hCG is the thyroid stimulator in patients with molar pregnancy (Nisula and Taliadouros, 1980), since positive correlations between serum hCG and serum total $T_4$ or total $T_3$ concentrations have been observed in some but not all studies. However, we performed thyroid function tests in 47 patients with complete mole and observed no significant correlation between serum hCG levels and free $T_4$ or $T_3$ index values (Amir et al, 1984). Therefore, the thyrotropic factor in molar pregnancy has not been clearly identified.

***Trophoblastic Embolization*** Acute respiratory distress develops in 2% of patients with complete mole, presumably owing to trophoblastic embolization to the pulmonary vasculature (Kohorn, 1987). After molar evacuation, patients may experience tachypnea and tachycardia in the recovery room. Auscultation of the

***Theca Lutein Ovarian Cysts*** Prominent theca lutein ovarian cysts (greater than 6 cm in diameter) develop in about half our patients with complete mole (Berkowitz and Goldstein, 1981). These cysts contain amber or serosanguineous fluid and are usually bilateral and multilocular. Ovarian enlargement is seen almost exclusively in patients with markedly elevated hCG values. The formation of theca lutein cysts may also be related to increased serum levels of prolactin (Osathanondh et al, 1986). While theca lutein cysts are usually detected at presentation, they may also enlarge significantly after molar evacuation. The mean time for spontaneous regression of these cysts is 8 weeks, as reported by Montz et al (1987). These investigators observed that only three of 99 patients suffered acute surgical complications (torsion or rupture). If patients have marked symptoms of pelvic pressure, theca lutein cysts may be aspirated percutaneously under ultrasound guidance or laparoscopically (Berkowitz et al, 1980).

## Partial Molar Pregnancy: Presenting Signs and Symptoms

Patients with partial molar pregnancy usually do not show the clinical features characteristic of complete mole. In general, they present with the signs and symptoms of missed or incomplete abortion. When 81 patients with partial mole were followed at the NETDC between January, 1979, and August, 1984, excessive uterine enlargement and preeclampsia were detected in only three and two patients, respectively (Berkowitz et al, 1985). Szulman and Surti (1982) also reported that only nine (11%) of their 81 patients with partial mole had excessively enlarged uteri. In addition, none of our patients had prominent theca lutein ovarian cysts, hyperthyroidism, or hyperemesis. Preevacuation hCG values were measured in 30 patients and exceeded 100,000 mIU/ml in only two (7%). The diagnosis of partial mole may be considered only after histologic review of curettage specimens.

## Ultrasonographic Diagnosis

**Complete Mole** Ultrasonography is both sensitive and reliable in detecting a complete molar pregnancy. Because of marked diffuse swelling of the chorionic villi, complete mole produces a characteristic vesicular sonographic pattern. If the pregnancy is normal, the gestational sac and fetal heart beat should be identifiable after the 6th week of gestation. However, it may be difficult to distinguish an early mole from degenerating chorionic tissues, since molar chorionic villi in the first trimester may be too small to be visualized on ultrasound. Measuring hCG at the time of ultrasound may help in the diagnosis of complete mole.

**Partial Mole** Ultrasonography may also contribute to the diagnosis of partial molar pregnancy. Sixty-one of our patients with partial mole who were clinically thought to have a missed or an incomplete abortion underwent preevacuation ultrasound (Berkowitz et al, 1985). In 16 patients (26.2%), ultrasound suggested molar disease because of cystic spaces in the placenta.

Recently, we conducted a study to determine whether sonographic criteria could be established to diagnose reliably the presence of partial mole prior to evacuation (Fine et al, 1989). Two criteria were found to be significantly associated with this diagnosis: (1) cystic changes in the placenta and (2) a ratio of transverse-to-anteroposterior gestational sac dimension greater than 1.5. When both criteria were met, the frequency of partial mole was 87%. Sonographic features can therefore be helpful in differentiating partial mole from other cases of missed or incomplete abortion.

## Serum Levels of hCG and Its Free Subunits in Complete and Partial Mole

Monoclonal antibodies have recently been developed that enable sensitive and specific measurement of hCG and its free subunits, alpha- and beta-hCG. While complete moles have higher levels of percent-free beta-hCG, partial moles have higher levels of percent-free alpha-hCG (Berkowitz et al, 1989). Trophoblastic cells in complete and partial mole differ significantly in the manner in which they secrete the free subunits of hCG. The levels of percent-free beta-hCG may reflect trophoblastic differentiation and hyperplasia, since they increase progressively from normal pregnancy after 5 weeks' gestation (mean = 0.4%), to partial mole (mean = 1.0%), to complete mole (mean = 2.4%), to gestational choriocarcinoma (mean = 9.2%) (Ozturk et al, 1988; Berkowitz et al, 1989). Thus, trophoblastic cells secrete greater amounts of free beta-hCG as cellular atypia and proliferation increase.

## Natural History of Complete and Partial Molar Pregnancy

The potential for complete hydatidiform moles to exhibit local invasion or metastasis is well known. Following molar evacuation, uterine invasion and metastasis occur in 15% and 4% of these patients, respectively (Berkowitz and Goldstein, 1986).

We reviewed 858 patients with complete mole to identify factors that might predispose to postmolar tumor. At the time of presentation, 41% of the patients had the following signs of marked trophoblastic growth: hCG level greater than 100,000 mIU/ml, uterine size large for gestational age, and theca lutein cysts larger than 6 cm in diameter. After molar evacuation, 31% showed uterine invasion and 8.8% were found to have metastases. The risk for persistent tumor was considerably lower among patients who did not present with signs of marked trophoblastic proliferation. Following evacuation, only 3.4% of these women showed invasion, and metastases were noted in 0.6%. Therefore, patients with complete moles who have markedly elevated hCG values and excessive uterine enlargement are at increased risk for postmolar tumor, while those without an enlarged uterus, theca lutein cysts, or high hCG levels are categorized as being at low-risk.

Risk for postmolar GTT also appears to be increased in women older than 40 years of age. Tow (1966) reported that 37% of such women developed persistent tumor. Complete moles in older women are more frequently aneuploid, and this may be related to the increased potential for local invasion and metastasis.

Between January, 1979, and January, 1989, 16 (6.6%) of 240 patients with partial mole followed at the NETDC were found to have persistent GTT (Rice et al, 1990). Nonmetastatic tumor developed in all 16 patients. Prior to molar evacuation, 15 were thought clinically to have a missed abortion. Only one patient presented with an excessively enlarged uterus and theca lutein ovarian cysts and was believed to have molar disease. No patient presented with toxemia, hyperemesis, or hyperthyroidism. None of the evacuated partial molar tissues showed marked trophoblastic hyperplasia. Those patients with partial mole who developed persistent tumor had no clinical or pathologic features that distinguished them from other patients with partial mole.

The reported risk for persistent tumor after partial mole has ranged from 0 to 11% (Berkowitz et al, 1988) (Table 17-2). Of 597 patients with partial mole studied at nine centers, 22 (3.7%) developed persistent GTT after uterine evacuation. In general, patients with persistent tumor following partial mole have nonmetastatic disease. However, both Stone and Bagshawe (1976) and Wong and Ma (1984) have each reported metastases in two patients following partial mole.

## Treatment of Molar Pregnancy

After a molar pregnancy has been diagnosed, the patient is carefully evaluated for possible medical complications, including preeclampsia, electrolyte imbalance, hyperthyroidism, and anemia. Once the patient has been stabilized, a decision must be made regarding the most appropriate method of evacuation based on reproductive preferences.

If the patient no longer desires to maintain fertility, *hysterectomy* may be performed, and prominent theca lutein ovarian cysts may be aspirated at the time of surgery. Although hysterectomy eliminates the risks of

TABLE 17-2 Persistent Tumor After Partial Molar Pregnancy

| Series | Patients (No.) | Persistent Tumor (No.) |
|---|---|---|
| Stone and Bagshawe, 1976 | 194 | 5* |
| Vassilakos et al, 1977 | 56 | 0 |
| Czernobilsky et al, 1982 | 25 | 1 |
| Lawler et al, 1982 | 15 | 0 |
| Szulman and Surti, 1982 | 49 | 2 |
| Wong and Ma, 1984 | 35 | 4* |
| Berkowitz et al, 1985 | 81 | 8 |
| Ohama et al, 1986 | 56 | 0 |
| Bolis et al, 1988a | 86 | 2 |
| Total | 597 | 22 (3.7%) |

* Two patients in each study had metastases.

local invasion, it does not prevent metastasis, so that gonadotropin followup is still mandatory.

In patients who desire to preserve fertility, *suction curettage* is the preferred method of evacuation, regardless of uterine size (Berkowitz et al, 1987). As the cervix is being dilated, the passage of retained blood may result in brisk blood loss. Shortly after suction evacuation begins, uterine bleeding can generally be well controlled, and the uterus rapidly regresses in size. If the uterus is larger than 14 weeks in size, the surgeon should place one hand on top of the fundus and should massage the uterus to stimulate uterine contraction. During evacuation, a pitocin intravenous drip can also be employed to stimulate myometrial contraction. When suction evacuation is thought to be complete, sharp curettage should be performed to remove any residual molar tissue. Curettings from both suction and sharp curettage should then be submitted separately for pathologic review.

**Prophylactic Chemotherapy** Although the use of chemoprophylaxis at the time of molar evacuation remains controversial (Goldstein, 1974), several investigators have reported that such treatment reduces the risk for postmolar tumor.

Between July, 1965, and June, 1979, at the NETDC, 247 patients with complete mole received actinomycin D prophylactically at the time of evacuation. Uterine invasion subsequently occurred in only 10 (4%) patients, and no patient showed evidence of metastases. Furthermore, all 10 of these patients later achieved remission after only one additional course of chemotherapy.

In an important randomized, prospective trial in patients with complete mole, chemoprophylaxis reduced the incidence of postmolar tumor from 47% to 14% in these patients with high-risk mole (Kim et al, 1986). However, such treatment did not significantly influence the frequency of tumor in patients with low-risk mole (6% with vs. 8% without chemoprophylaxis).

Recently, we reviewed our experience with adminis-

tering prophylactic actinomycin-D to patients with high-risk complete mole (Berkowitz et al, 1987). Only 10 (11%) of 93 patients so treated developed postmolar tumor. Chemoprophylaxis was more commonly unsuccessful in patients whose preevacuation hCG values were markedly elevated. Prophylactic chemotherapy may be of benefit in patients with high-risk complete moles, particularly when hormonal followup is unavailable or unreliable.

**Hormonal Followup** After molar evacuation, all patients must be followed by means of hCG measurements to ensure remission. Measurements should be obtained weekly until hCG values are normal for 3 weeks and then monthly until they are normal for 6 months.

Patients are advised to use reliable contraception during the entire interval of followup. Because of the risk for uterine perforation and bleeding, intrauterine devices should not be inserted until normal levels of hCG are achieved. If the patient does not desire surgical sterilization, she must decide whether to use oral contraceptives or barrier methods.

Although the incidence of postmolar tumor has been reported to be increased in patients who used oral contraceptives (Stone et al, 1976), data from the NETDC, the University of Southern California, and the Gynecologic Oncology Group do not support this finding (Berkowitz et al, 1981b; Morrow et al, 1985; Curry et al, 1989). The contraceptive method also did not influence the mean hCG regression time. We therefore believe that oral contraceptives may be safely prescribed after molar evacuation.

## GESTATIONAL TROPHOBLASTIC TUMORS

After a molar pregnancy, persistent GTT may have the histologic features of either molar tissue or choriocarcinoma, whereas after a nonmolar gestation, they may have the features of only choriocarcinoma. Gestational choriocarcinoma does not contain chorionic villous structures but is composed of sheets of both cytotrophoblasts and syncytiotrophoblasts.

*Placental-site trophoblastic tumor* (PSTT), an uncommon variant of choriocarcinoma, is composed almost entirely of mononuclear intermediate trophoblasts and does not contain chorionic villi (Finkler et al, 1988). Because PSTT secrete only small amounts of hCG, the tumor burden may become quite large before hCG levels are detectable.

### Natural History

**Nonmetastatic Disease** Locally invasive GTT develops in 15% of patients after complete mole and infrequently after other pregnancies (Berkowitz and Goldstein, 1981). Trophoblastic tumor may perforate the myometrium, producing intraperitoneal bleeding, or may erode into uterine vessels, causing vaginal hemorrhage. In addition, bulky necrotic tumor may serve as a nidus for uterine sepsis.

| TABLE 17-3 | Staging of Gestational Trophoblastic Tumors |
|---|---|
| Stage I | Confined to uterine corpus |
| Stage II | Metastases to pelvis and vagina |
| Stage III | Metastases to lung |
| Stage IV | Distant metastases |

**Metastatic Disease** Metastatic GTT occurs in 4% of patients after complete mole and infrequently after other gestations. Most often, metastases are associated with choriocarcinoma, which has a propensity for early vascular invasion with widespread dissemination. The most common metastatic sites are the lung (80%), vagina (30%), brain (10%), and liver (10%). Cerebral and hepatic metastases are uncommon unless the lungs and/or vagina are involved concurrently. Because trophoblastic tumors are perfused by fragile vessels, metastases are often hemorrhagic, and patients may present with associated signs and symptoms such as hemoptysis or acute neurologic deficits.

## Staging System

The International Federation of Gynecology and Obstetrics (FIGO) has begun to report data on GTT using an anatomic staging system (Table 17-3). *Stage I* includes all patients with tumor confined to the uterus. *Stage II* comprises all patients with tumor outside the uterus but localized to the vagina and/or pelvis. *Stage III* includes all patients with pulmonary metastases with or without uterine, vaginal, or pelvic involvement. *Stage IV* patients have far-advanced disease in which the brain, liver, kidneys, or gastrointestinal tract are involved. These patients are in the highest risk category because they are most likely to be resistant to chemotherapy. In general, Stage IV tumors are choriocarcinoma and commonly follow a nonmolar pregnancy.

It is also helpful to employ prognostic factors to predict the likelihood of drug resistance and to assist in the selection of optimal chemotherapy. The World Health Organization has published a *prognostic scoring system*, based on one developed by Bagshawe (1976), that reliably predicts the potential for chemotherapy resistance (Table 17-4). When the prognostic score is 8 or greater, the patient is considered to be at high risk and will require intensive combination chemotherapy to attain remission. In general, patients with Stage I disease have a low-risk score and patients with Stage IV disease have a high-risk score. Therefore, the distinction between low and high risk applies primarily to Stage II or III GTT.

## Diagnostic Evaluation

Optimal management of GTT requires a thorough evaluation of the extent of the disease. All patients with persistent tumor should undergo careful assessment that includes a complete history and physical examination; hCG levels; and hepatic, thyroid, and renal function tests. The metastatic workup should include a chest roentgenogram, ultrasonography of the abdomen and pelvis, head computed tomography (CT) and in some cases selective angiography of abdominal and pelvic structures.

CT of the head has facilitated the early diagnosis of asymptomatic cerebral lesions (Athanassiou et al, 1983). In patients with choriocarcinoma and/or metastases, hCG levels in cerebrospinal fluid (CSF) should be measured to detect cerebral tumor. Bagshawe and Harland (1976) have reported that a plasma:CSF-hCG ratio less than 60 strongly suggests central nervous system involvement by GTT. However, because rapid changes in plasma hCG levels may not be promptly reflected in the CSF, a single plasma:CSF hCG ratio may be misleading (Berkowitz et al, 1981c).

## Management

**Stage I GTT** Tables 17-5 and 17-6 review the NETDC protocol for the management of Stage I disease as well as the results of therapy. The selection of treatment is

| TABLE 17-4 | Scoring System Based on Prognostic Factors to Predict Resistance to Chemotherapy | | | |
|---|---|---|---|---|
| | Score* | | | |
| Prognostic Factors | 0 | 1 | 2 | 4 |
| Age (yr) | $\leq 39$ | $> 39$ | | |
| Antecedent pregnancy | Hydatidiform mole | Abortion | Term | |
| Interval† | 4 | 4 to 6 | 7 to 12 | $> 12$ |
| hCG (IU/liter) | $< 10^3$ | $10^3$ to $10^4$ | $10^4$ to $10^5$ | $> 10^5$ |
| ABO groups (female × male) | | 0 × A | | B |
| | | A x O | AB | |
| Largest tumor, including uterine tumor | | 3 to 5 cm | 5 cm | |
| Site of metastases | | Spleen | GI tract | Brain |
| Number of metastases identified | | 1 to 4 | 4 to 8 | $> 8$ |
| Prior chemotherapy | | | Single drug | Two or more drugs |

* The total score for a patient is obtained by adding the individual scores for each prognostic factor: $\leq 4$ = low risk, 5 to 7 = moderate risk, $\geq 8$ = high risk.
† Interval = time (months) between end of antecedent pregnancy and start of chemotherapy.
*Source: Gestational Trophoblastic Diseases.* Report of a WHO Scientific Group, Technical Report Series 692, World Health Organization, Geneva, 1983, p 51.

TABLE 17-5   NETDC Treatment Protocol for Stage I GTT

*Initial Therapy:*
Single-agent chemotherapy OR
Hysterectomy with adjunctive chemotherapy

*Resistant Tumors:*
Combination chemotherapy
Hysterectomy with adjunctive chemotherapy
Local uterine resection
Pelvic infusion

*Followup:*
hCG—Weekly until normal × 3
     Monthly until normal × 12
Contraception—12 consecutive months of normal hCG levels

NETDC = New England Trophoblastic Disease Center.

based primarily on the patient's desire to preserve fertility.

If the patient no longer wishes to remain fertile, hysterectomy with adjuvant single-agent chemotherapy may be performed as primary treatment. Adjuvant chemotherapy is administered for three reasons: (1) to reduce the likelihood of disseminating viable tumor at surgery, (2) to maintain a cytotoxic level of the drug in case viable tumor is disseminated at surgery, and (3) to treat occult metastases. Occult pulmonary metastases may be detected by CT in about 40% of patients with presumed nonmetastatic disease (Mutch et al, 1986). Chemotherapy may be safely administered at the time of hysterectomy without increasing operative morbidity. At the NETDC, 28 patients were treated with primary hysterectomy and adjuvant chemotherapy, and all achieved complete remission with no additional therapy.

Nonmetastatic PSTT should be treated with hysterectomy because of its poor response to chemotherapy. Because PSTT is generally resistant to chemotherapy, there are few if any long-term survivors with metastases despite intensive multimodal therapy. Patients with PSTT showing five or more mitoses/10 high-power fields are at particular risk for metastases and a fatal outcome (Lathrop et al, 1988).

Single-agent chemotherapy is the preferred treatment in patients with Stage I disease who desire to retain fertility. Primary single-agent chemotherapy induced complete remission in 347 (93.0%) of 373 patients with Stage I GTT. The remaining 21 resistant patients later achieved remission with either combination chemotherapy or surgical intervention. If the patient is resistant to chemotherapy and wants to preserve fertility, local uterine resection may be considered. When local resection is planned, ultrasound and/or arteriography may identify the site of resistant tumor (Berkowitz et al, 1983).

***Stage II and III GTT*** The NETDC protocol for the management of Stage II and III disease as well as the results of treatment are outlined in Tables 17-7 to 17-9. While patients at low risk are managed initially with single-agent chemotherapy, those at high risk are treated with primary combination chemotherapy.

Between July, 1965, and December, 1990, 26 patients with Stage II disease were managed at the NETDC and all attained remission. Single-agent chemotherapy induced complete remission in 16 (88.9%) of 18 low-risk patients. In contrast, only 2 of 8 high-risk patients achieved remission with single-agent treatment.

Vaginal metastases may bleed profusely because they may be highly vascular and friable. Bleeding may be controlled by packing the vagina or performing local excision. One or two courses of chemotherapy may lead to marked tumor regression and reduced vascularity. Infrequently, angiographic embolization of the hypogastric arteries may be necessary to control vaginal hemorrhage.

Between July, 1965, and December, 1990, 121 patients with Stage III tumors were treated at the NETDC, and 120 (99.7%) attained complete remission. Single-agent chemotherapy induced complete remission in 67

TABLE 17-6   Results of Therapy in Stage I GTT (Confined to Uterine Corpus)—NETDC (July, 1965, to December, 1990)

| Remission Therapy | No. of Patients (%) | No. of Remissions (%) |
|---|---|---|
| *Initial Therapy:* | 380 (94.8%) | |
| Sequential MTX/Act D | | 347 (91.3%) |
| Hysterectomy | | 28 (7.4%) |
| MAC | | 3 (0.8%) |
| EMA | | 2 (0.5%) |
| *Resistant Tumors:* | 21 (5.2%) | |
| MAC | | 10 (47.6%) |
| EMA | | 6 (28.6%) |
| Hysterectomy | | 2 (9.5%) |
| Local uterine resection | | 2 (9.5%) |
| Pelvic infusion | | 1 (4.8%) |
| TOTALS | 401 | 401 (100%) |

NETDC = New England Trophoblastic Disease Center; MTX = methotrexate; Act-D = actinomycin-D; MAC = methotrexate, actinomycin-D, cyclophosphamide; EMA = etoposide, methotrexate, actinomycin-D.

TABLE 17-7   NETDC Treatment Protocol for Stages II and III GTT

*Low Risk\*:*
Initial therapy
    Single-agent chemotherapy
Resistant tumors
    Combination chemotherapy
*High risk\*:*
Initial therapy
    Combination chemotherapy
Resistant tumors
    Second-line combination chemotherapy
*Followup:*
hCG
    Weekly until normal × 3
    Monthly until normal × 12
Contraception
    12 consecutive months of normal hCG levels

NETDC = New England Trophoblastic Disease Center.
\* Local resection optional.

TABLE 17-8 Results of Therapy in Stage II GTT (Metastases to Pelvis and Vagina)—NETDC (July, 1965, to December, 1990)

| Remission Therapy | No. of Patients | No. of Remissions(%) |
|---|---|---|
| *Low Risk:* | 18 (69.2%) | |
| Initial therapy | | |
|    Sequential MTX/Act-D | | 16 (88.9%) |
| Resistant tumors | | |
|    MAC | | 2 (11.1%) |
| *High Risk:* | 8 (31.8%) | |
| Initial therapy | | |
|    Sequential MTX/Act-D | | 2 (25.0%) |
|    MAC | | 4 (50.0%) |
| Resistant tumors | | |
|    MAC | | 1 (12.5%) |
|    CHAMOCA | | 1 (12.5%) |
| TOTALS | 26 | 26 (100%) |

NETDC = New England Trophoblastic Disease Center; MTX = methotrexate; Act-D = actinomycin-D; MAC = methotrexate, actinomycin-D, cyclophosphamide; CHAMOCA = Bagshawe multiagent regimen.

(84.8%) of 79 patients with low-risk disease and in 13 (31.0%) of 42 patients with high-risk disease. All patients who were resistant to single-agent treatment later achieved remission with combination chemotherapy.

Thoracotomy has a limited role in the management of Stage III disease and should be performed if the diagnosis is seriously in doubt. Furthermore, if a patient has a persistent viable pulmonary nodule despite intensive chemotherapy, pulmonary resection may be performed. However, an extensive metastatic workup should be carried out to exclude other sites of persistent disease. It is important to emphasize that fibrotic nodules may persist indefinitely on chest roentgenogram even after complete remission is confirmed by hCG measurements.

Hysterectomy may be required in patients with metastases to control uterine hemorrhage or sepsis. In patients with bulky uterine tumor, hysterectomy may reduce the tumor burden and thereby limit the need for chemotherapy.

***Stage IV GTT*** Tables 17-10 and 17-11 outline the NETDC protocol for managing Stage IV disease as well as the results of therapy. These patients are at high risk for rapidly progressive disease despite intensive therapy.

All patients with Stage IV disease should be treated with intensive combination chemotherapy and the selective use of radiation therapy and surgery (Surwit and Hammond, 1980). Before 1975, only 6 (30%) of 20 patients with Stage IV tumors attained complete remission. However, after 1975, 14 (77.8%) of 18 patients with Stage IV disease achieved remission. This dramatic improvement in survival resulted from intensive multimodal therapy.

The management of hepatic disease is particularly problematic and challenging. If a patient is resistant to systemic chemotherapy, hepatic arterial infusion of chemotherapy may induce complete remission in selected cases. Hepatic resection may also be necessary to control bleeding or to excise resistant disease.

If cerebral metastases are detected, whole-brain irradiation is promptly instituted at our Center. Concurrent administration of chemotherapy and brain irradiation may reduce the risk of spontaneous cerebral bleeding (Weed and Hammond, 1980). Brain irradiation may be both hemostatic and tumoricidal. Yordan et al (1987) reported deaths due to cerebral involvement in 11 (44%) of 25 patients treated with chemotherapy alone, but no deaths occurred in 18 patients treated with both brain irradiation and chemotherapy.

In contrast, Athanassiou et al (1983) and Rustin et al (1989) reported excellent remission rates in patients with cerebral metastases who were treated with chemotherapy alone. Eighty percent of their patients with cerebral tumor achieved remission with intensive combination chemotherapy that included intravenous and

TABLE 17-9 Results of Therapy in Stage III GTT (Metastases to Lung)—NETDC (July, 1965, to December, 1990)

| Remission Therapy | No. of Patients | No. of Remissions (%) |
|---|---|---|
| *Low Risk:* | 79 (65.3%) | |
| Initial therapy | | |
|    Sequential MTX/Act-D | | 67 (84.8%) |
| Resistant tumors | | |
|    MAC | | 12 (15.2%) |
| *High Risk:* | 42 (34.7%) | |
| Initial therapy | | |
|    Sequential MTX/Act-D | | 13 (31.0%) |
|    MAC | | 12 (28.6%) |
|    EMA | | 9 (21.4%) |
| Resistant tumors | | |
|    MAC | | 2 (4.8%) |
|    CHAMOCA | | 1 (2.4%) |
|    5-FU-Adria | | 1 (2.4%) |
|    VPB | | 2 (4.8%) |
|    EMA | | 1 (2.4%) |
| TOTALS | 121 | 120 (99.7%) |

NETDC = New England Trophoblastic Disease Center; MTX = methotrexate; Act-D = actinomycin-D; MAC = methotrexate, actinomycin-D, cyclophosphamide; CHAMOCA = Bagshawe multiagent regimen; 5-FU-Adria = 5-fluorouracil, Adriamycin (doxorubicin); VPB = vinblastine, cisplatin, bleomycin; EMA = etoposide, methotrexate, actinomycin-D.

TABLE 17-10 NETDC Treatment Protocol for Stage IV GTT

*Initial Therapy:*
Combination chemotherapy
Brain metastases—Whole-head irradiation (3,000 rads), craniotomy to manage complications
Liver metastases—Resection to manage complications
*Resistant Tumors\*:*
Second-line combination chemotherapy
*Followup:*
hCG—Weekly until normal × 3
  Monthly until normal × 24
Contraception—24 consecutive months of normal hCG levels

NETDC = New England Trophoblastic Disease Center.
\* Local resection optional.

TABLE 17-11  Results of Therapy in Stage IV GTT (Distant Metastases)—NETDC (July, 1965, to December, 1990)

| Remission Therapy* | No. of Remissions (%) |
| --- | --- |
| *Before 1975* | 6/20 (30%) |
| Initial therapy | |
|   Sequential MTX/Act-D | 5 |
| Resistant tumors | |
|   MAC | 1 |
| *After 1975* | 14/18 (77.8%) |
| Initial therapy | |
|   Sequential MTX/Act-D | 2 |
|   MAC | 2 |
| Resistant tumors | |
|   High-dose MTX/Act-D | 4 |
|   MAC | 1 |
|   CHAMOCA | 1 |
|   VPB | 1 |
|   EMA | 3 |

* Radiation therapy and surgery utilized when indicated. MTX = methotrexate; Act-D = actinomycin-D; MAC = methotrexate, actinomycin-D, cyclophosphamide; CHAMOCA = Bagshawe multiagent regimen; VPB = vinblastine, cisplatinum, bleomycin; EMA = etoposide, methotrexate, actinomycin-D.

intrathecal methotrexate. Therefore, excellent cure rates can be attained in patients with cerebral metastases using chemotherapy alone.

Craniotomy should be performed to manage life-threatening complications and thereby provide the opportunity for chemotherapy to induce remission. Craniotomy may be required to provide acute decompression or to control bleeding. Infrequently, cerebral tumor that is resistant to chemotherapy may be amenable to resection. Fortunately, patients with cerebral metastases who attain remission usually have no residual neurologic deficits.

## Followup

All patients with Stages I, II, and III GTT should be followed with weekly hCG measurements until values are normal for 3 weeks and then monthly until values are normal for 12 months. Patients are advised to use contraception during the entire interval of monitoring. For patients with Stage IV disease, hCG should be measured weekly until normal for 3 weeks and then monthly until values are normal for 24 months. These patients require prolonged followup because they are at increased risk for late recurrence.

## CHEMOTHERAPY

### Single-Agent Chemotherapy

**Selection of Agent**  Single-agent chemotherapy with either actinomycin-D (Act-D) or methotrexate (MTX) has achieved comparable and excellent cure rates in both nonmetastatic and metastatic GTT (Osathanondh et al, 1975). An optimal regimen should maximize the remission rate while minimizing morbidity.

Methotrexate with folinic acid rescue (MTX-FA) has been the preferred single-agent protocol at the NETDC

since 1974 (Berkowitz et al, 1986). Between September, 1974, and September, 1984, 185 patients with GTT were treated with primary MTX-FA at the NETDC. Complete remission was attained in 162 (87.6%) patients, and 132 (81.5%) of these patients required only one course of MTX-FA to achieve remission. MTX-FA induced remission in 147 (90.2%) of 163 patients with Stage I disease and in 15 (68.2%) of 22 patients with low-risk Stage II and III tumors. Resistance to MTX-FA was more common in patients with choriocarcinoma, metastases, and pretreatment hCG levels greater than 50,000 mIU/ml. Following MTX-FA, thrombocytopenia, granulocytopenia, and hepatotoxicity occurred in only 3 (1.6%), 11 (5.9%), and 26 (14.1%) patients, respectively. No patient required platelet transfusions or developed sepsis due to myelosuppression, and no patient experienced marked nausea or alopecia. Not only does MTX-FA achieve an excellent remission rate with minimal toxicity, but it also effectively limits chemotherapy exposure (Berkowitz et al, 1981*a*).

**Administration**  hCG levels are measured weekly after each course of chemotherapy, and the hCG regression curve serves as the primary basis for determining the need for further treatment. After the first treatment, further chemotherapy is withheld as long as the hCG level is falling progressively. Additional single-agent chemotherapy is not administered at any predetermined or fixed time interval. A second course of chemotherapy is administered under the following conditions: (1) when the hCG level plateaus for more than 3 consecutive weeks or rises again, and (2) when the hCG level does not decline by one log within 18 days after the initial treatment has been completed.

If a second course of MTX-FA is necessary, the dosage of MTX is unchanged if the patient's response to the first treatment was adequate. An adequate response is defined as a decline in the hCG level by one log following a course of chemotherapy. When the response to the first treatment is inadequate, the dosage of MTX is increased 2 mg/kg in four divided doses. If the response to two courses of MTX-FA is inadequate, the patient is considered to be resistant to MTX, and Act D is promptly substituted.

### Combination Chemotherapy

Modified triple therapy with MTX-FA, Act D, and cyclophosphamide had been the preferred combination drug regimen at the NETDC (Berkowitz et al, 1984). Ten (71.4%) of 14 patients with high-risk metastatic GTT achieved remission with modified triple therapy. However, triple therapy is inadequate as an initial treatment in patients with metastases whose prognostic score indicates that they are at high risk (score ≥ 8) (DuBeshter et al, 1987). Triple therapy induced remission in only 5 (45%) of 11 patients with a high-risk score. Curry et al (1989) and Gordon et al (1989) also observed that triple therapy achieved remission in only 5 (62%) of 8 patients and 11 (46%) of 24 patients, respectively, with metastatic GTT and a high-risk score.

Etoposide (VP-16) has proved to be a highly effective antitumor agent in GTT. Primary oral etoposide induced complete remission in 56 (93.3%) of 60 patients with nonmetastatic and low-risk metastatic GTT (Wong et al, 1986). Bagshawe (1984) reported an 83% remission rate in patients with a high-risk score using a new combination regimen that includes etoposide, MTX, Act D, cyclophosphamide, and vincristine (EMA-CO) which may currently be the preferred treatment for metastatic GTT and a high-risk score. Bolis et al (1988b) also reported that primary treatment with EMA-CO induced complete sustained remission in 76% of patients with metastatic GTT and a high-risk score. Most likely, the optimal combination drug regimen will include MTX, Act D, and etoposide and perhaps other agents, administered in the most dose-intensive manner (Surwit, 1987).

Patients who require combination chemotherapy must be treated intensively to achieve remission. We administer combination chemotherapy as frequently as toxicity permits until the patient attains 3 weekly normal hCG values. After normal hCG levels are achieved, additional chemotherapy is administered to reduce the risk of relapse.

## SUBSEQUENT PREGNANCIES

### Pregnancies After Hydatidiform Mole

Patients with complete molar pregnancies can anticipate normal reproduction in the future (Berkowitz et al, 1991). Patients with complete moles, treated at the NETDC, had 1,162 subsequent pregnancies between June, 1965, and December, 1989. These gestations resulted in 803 (69.1%) full-term live births, 84 (7.2%) premature deliveries, 9 (0.8%) ectopic pregnancies, and 6 (0.5%) stillbirths (Table 17-12). First-trimester spontaneous abortion occurred in 190 (16.4%) pregnancies, and major and minor congenital malformations were detected in only 35 (3.9%) of 893 infants. Primary cesarean section was performed in only 49 (17.0%) of

288 full-term and premature births between January, 1979, and December, 1989.

Limited data are available concerning the subsequent pregnancy experience in patients with partial mole (Berkowitz et al, 1991). Between June, 1965, and December, 1989, patients with partial mole at the NETDC had 107 later pregnancies that resulted in 79 (73.9%) term live births, 1 (0.9%) stillbirth, 2 (1.8%) moles, and 1 (0.9%) premature delivery. First-trimester spontaneous abortion occurred in 16 (14.9%) pregnancies, and major or minor congenital anomalies were detected in only two (2.5%) infants. The preliminary information regarding subsequent conceptions after partial mole is therefore reassuring.

When a patient has had a molar pregnancy, she is at increased risk for molar disease in a later conception. Fifteen of our patients have had at least two documented molar gestations (Rice et al, 1989). The risk of molar disease in a later conception is about 1%. Patients may have an initial complete or partial mole and then in a later pregnancy develop the other type of molar disease. Importantly, four of our patients have had a normal subsequent term gestation after two prior molar pregnancies.

Therefore, to confirm normal development, we recommend ultrasonography during the first trimester of any later pregnancy. Furthermore, the placenta or chorionic tissues from later pregnancies should undergo pathologic review, and hCG levels should be measured 6 weeks after the completion of any future pregnancy to exclude occult trophoblastic disease.

## After GTT

Patients with GTT who are successfully managed with chemotherapy can also expect normal reproduction in the future (Walden and Bagshawe, 1976; Berkowitz et al, 1991). Between June, 1965, and December, 1989, patients who received chemotherapy at the NETDC for GTT had 385 subsequent pregnancies. These later ges-

| TABLE 17-12 Subsequent Pregnancies in Patients with Complete Mole—NETDC (June, 1965 to December, 1989) | |
|---|---|
| Outcome | Number (%) |
| Term delivery | 803 (69.1%) |
| Stillbirth | 6 (0.5%) |
| Premature delivery | 84 (7.2%) |
| Spontaneous abortion | |
|   1st trimester | 190 (16.4%) |
|   2nd trimester | 18 (1.5%) |
| Therapeutic abortion | 37 (3.2%) |
| Ectopic pregnancy | 9 (0.8%) |
| Repeat molar pregnancy | 15 (1.3%) |
| Total no. of pregnancies | 1,162 |
| | No./deliveries (%): |
| Congenital malformations | 35/893 (3.9%) |
| Primary cesarean section | 49/288 (17.0%)* |
| * January, 1979, to December, 1989. | |

| TABLE 17-13 Subsequent Pregnancies in Patients With Gestational Trophoblastic Tumors—NETDC (June, 1965, to December, 1989) | |
|---|---|
| Outcome | Number (%) |
| Term delivery | 275 (71.4%) |
| Stillbirth | 6 (1.5%) |
| Premature delivery | 14 (3.6%) |
| Spontaneous abortion | |
|   1st trimester | 58 (15.1%) |
|   2nd trimester | 7 (1.9%) |
| Therapeutic abortion | 20 (5.2%) |
| Ectopic pregnancy | 4 (1.0%) |
| Repeat molar pregnancy | 1 (0.3%) |
| Total no. of pregnancies | 385 |
| | No./deliveries (%): |
| Congenital malformations | 6/295 (2.0%) |
| Primary cesarean section | 28/189 (14.8%)* |
| * January, 1979, to December, 1989. | |

tations resulted in 275 (71.4%) full-term live births, 14 (3.6%) premature deliveries, 4 (1.0%) ectopic pregnancies, and 6 (1.5%) stillbirths (Table 17-13). First-trimester spontaneous abortion occurred in 58 (15.1%) pregnancies, and major and minor congenital malformations were diagnosed in only 6 (2.0%) of 295 infants. It is particularly reassuring that the frequency of congenital anomalies has not increased since chemotherapy can be teratogenic. Primary cesarean section was performed in only 28 (14.8%) of 189 later full-term and premature deliveries between January, 1979, and December, 1989. Risk for obstetric complications does not appear to be increased in subsequent pregnancies.

Song et al (1988) performed cytogenetic studies on the peripheral lymphocytes from 94 children from later pregnancies and reported no increase in chromosomal aberrations. The growth and development of these children were also evaluated through adolescence and proved to be normal.

## SUMMARY

Since the introduction of chemotherapy in 1956, dramatic advances have taken place in the management of GTT. It is hoped that further improvement in our understanding and treatment of this disease will be fostered by the development and acceptance of a uniform terminology and staging system, which will permit rational comparison and sharing of data among different institutions. An International Society for the Study of Trophoblastic Disease has been established to promote understanding of GTT through a free exchange of ideas and experience. Cooperative studies are now needed to allow critical evaluation of current therapies and the development of new treatment regimens.

## REFERENCES

Amir SM, Osathanondh R, Berkowitz RS, Goldstein DP: Human chorionic gonadotropin and thyroid function in patients with hydatidiform mole. *Am J Obstet Gynecol* 150:723-728, 1984.
Athanassiou A, Begent RHJ, Newlands ES, Parker D, Rustin GJS, Bagshawe KD: Central nervous system metastasis of choriocarcinoma: 23 years experience at the Charing Cross Hospital. *Cancer* 52:1728-1735, 1983.
Bagshawe KD: Risks and prognostic factors in trophoblastic neoplasia. *Cancer* 38:1373-1385, 1976.
Bagshawe KD: Treatment of high-risk choriocarcinoma. *J Reprod Med* 29:813-820, 1984.
Bagshawe KD, Harland S: Immunodiagnosis and monitoring of gonadotropin-producing metastases in the central nervous system. *Cancer* 38:112-118, 1976.
Berkowitz RS, Goldstein DP: Pathogenesis of gestational trophoblastic neoplasms. *Pathobiol Ann* 11:391-411, 1981a.
Berkowitz RS, Goldstein DP: Management of molar pregnancy and gestational trophoblastic tumors. In Knapp RC, Berkowitz RS (eds): *Gynecologic Oncology*. New York, Macmillan, 1986, pp 425-443.
Berkowitz RS, Birnholz J, Goldstein DP, Bernstein MR: Pelvic ultrasonography and the management of gestational trophoblastic disease. *Gynecol Oncol* 15:403-412, 1983.
Berkowitz RS, Goldstein DP, Bernstein MR: Laparoscopy in the management of gestational trophoblastic neoplasms. *J Reprod Med* 24:261-264, 1980.

Berkowitz RS, Goldstein DP, Bernstein MR: Modified triple chemotherapy in the management of high-risk metastatic gestational trophoblastic tumors. *Gynecol Oncol* 19:173-181, 1984.
Berkowitz RS, Goldstein DP, Bernstein MR: Natural history of partial molar pregnancy. *Obstet Gynecol* 66:677-681, 1985.
Berkowitz RS, Goldstein DP, Bernstein MR: Ten years experience with methotrexate and folinic acid as primary therapy for gestational trophoblastic disease. *Gynecol Oncol* 23:111-118, 1986.
Berkowitz RS, Goldstein DP, Bernstein MR: Partial molar pregnancy: A separate entity. *Contemp Ob/Gyn* 31:99-102, 1988.
Berkowitz RS, Goldstein DP, Bernstein MR: Reproductive experience after complete and partial molar pregnancy and gestational trophoblastic tumors. *J Reprod Med* 36:3-8, 1991.
Berkowitz RS, Goldstein DP, DuBeshter B, Bernstein MR: Management of complete molar pregnancy. *J Reprod Med* 32:634-639, 1987.
Berkowitz RS, Goldstein DP, Jones MA, Marean AR, Bernstein MR: Methotrexate with citrovorum factor rescue—Reduced chemotherapy toxicity in the management of gestational trophoblastic neoplasms. *Cancer* 45:423-426, 1981a.
Berkowitz RS, Goldstein DP, Marean AR, Bernstein MR: Oral contraceptives and postmolar trophoblastic disease. *Obstet Gynecol* 58:474-478, 1981b.
Berkowitz RS, Osathanondh R, Goldstein DP, Martin PM, Mallampati SR, Datta S: Cerebrospinal fluid human chorionic gonadotropin levels in normal pregnancy and choriocarcinoma. *Surg Gynecol Obstet* 153:687-689, 1981c.
Berkowitz RS, Ozturk M, Goldstein DP, Bernstein MR, Hill L, Wands JR: Human chorionic gonadotropin and free subunits' serum levels in patients with partial and complete hydatidiform moles. *Obstet Gynecol* 74:212-216, 1989.
Bolis G, Belloni C, Bonazzi C, Mangili G, Presti M, Zanaboni F, Mangioni C: Analysis of 309 cases after hydatidiform mole: Different follow-up program according to biologic behavior. *Tumori* 74:93-96, 1988a.
Bolis G, Bonazzi C, Landoni F, Mangili G, Vergadoro F, Zanaboni F, Mangioni C: EMA/CO regimen in high-risk gestational trophoblastic tumor (GTT). *Gynecol Oncol* 31:439-444, 1988b.
Czernobilsky B, Barash A, Lancet M: Partial moles: A clinicopathologic study of 25 cases. *Obstet Gynecol* 59:75, 1982.
Curry SL, Blessing JA, DiSaia PJ, Soper JT, Twiggs LB: A prospective randomized comparison of methotrexate, dactinomycin and chlorambucil versus methotrexate, dactinomycin, cyclophosphamide, doxorubicin, melphalan, hydroxyurea and vincristine in "poor prognosis" metastatic gestational trophoblastic disease: A Gynecologic Oncology Group study. *Obstet Gynecol* 73:357-362, 1989.
Curry SL, Hammond CB, Tyrey L, Creasman WT, Parker RT: Hydatidiform mole—Diagnosis, management and long-term follow-up of 347 patients. *Am J Obstet Gynecol* 45:1-8, 1975.
Curry SL, Schlaerth JB, Kohorn EI, Boyce JB, Gore H, Twiggs LB, Blessing JA: Hormonal contraception and trophoblastic sequelae after hydatidiform mole (A Gynecologic Oncology Group study). *Am J Obstet Gynecol* 160:805-811, 1989.
Doshi N, Surti U, Szulman AE: Morphologic anomalies in triploid liveborn fetuses. *Hum Pathol* 14:716-723, 1983.
DuBeshter B, Berkowitz RS, Goldstein DP, Cramer DW, Bernstein MR: Metastatic gestational trophoblastic disease: Experience at the New England Trophoblastic Disease Center, 1965-1985. *Obstet Gynecol* 69:390-395, 1987.
Fine C, Bundy AL, Berkowitz RS, Boswell SB, Berezin AF, Doubilet PM: Sonographic diagnosis of partial hydatidiform mole. *Obstet Gynecol* 73:414-418, 1989.
Finkler NJ, Berkowitz RS, Driscoll SG, Goldstein DP, Bernstein MR: Clinical experience with placental site trophoblastic tumors at the New England Trophoblastic Disease Center. *Obstet Gynecol* 71:854-857, 1988.
Goldstein DP: Prevention of gestational trophoblastic disease by use of actinomycin-D in molar pregnancies. *Obstet Gynecol* 43:475-479, 1974.
Goldstein DP, Berkowitz RS: *Gestational Trophoblastic Neoplasms—Clinical Principles of Diagnosis and Management*. Philadelphia, WB Saunders Co, 1982, 301 pp.
Gordon AN, Gershenson DM, Copeland LJ, Stringer CA, Morris M, Wharton JT: High-risk metastatic gestational trophoblastic disease:

Further stratification into clinical entities. *Gynecol Oncol* 34:54-56, 1989.

Hankins G, Wendel GD, Snyder RR, Cunningham FG: Trophoblastic embolization during molar evacuation—Central hemodynamic observations. *Obstet Gynecol* 69:368-372, 1987.

Kajii T, Ohama K: Androgenetic origin of hydatidiform mole. *Nature* 268:633-634, 1977.

Kim DS, Moon H, Kim KT, Moon YJ, Hwang YY: Effects of prophylactic chemotherapy for persistent trophoblastic disease in patients with complete hydatidiform mole. *Obstet Gynecol* 67:690-694, 1986.

Kohorn EI: Clinical management and the neoplastic sequelae of trophoblastic embolization associated with hydatidiform mole. *Obstet Gynecol Surv* 42:484-488, 1987.

Lathrop JC, Lauchlan S, Nayak R, Ambler M: Clinical characteristics of placental site trophoblastic tumor (PSTT). *Gynecol Oncol* 31:32-42, 1988.

Lawler S, Fisher RA, Pickthall U, et al: Genetic studies on hydatidiform moles. I. The origin of partial moles. *Cancer Genet Cytogenet* 5:309, 1982.

Masson GM, Anthony F, Chau E: Serum chorionic gonadotrophin (hCG), schwangersschaftsprotein 1 (SP1), progesterone and oestradiol levels in patients with nausea and vomiting in early pregnancy. *Br J Obstet Gynaecol* 92:211-215, 1985.

Montz FJ, Schlaerth JB, Morrow CP: Natural history of theca lutein cysts. *Gynecol Oncol* 26:414, 1987.

Morrow P, Nakamura R, Schlaerth J, Gaddis O, Eddy G: The influence of oral contraceptives on the postmolar human chorionic regression curve. *Am J Obstet Gynecol* 151:906-914, 1985.

Mutch DG, Soper JT, Baker ME, Bandy LC, Cox EB, Clarke-Pearson DL, Hammond CB: Role of computed axial tomography of the chest in staging patients with nonmetastatic gestational trophoblastic disease. *Obstet Gynecol* 68:348-352, 1986.

Nisula BC, Taliadouros GS: Thyroid function in gestational trophoblastic neoplasia—Evidence that the thyrotropic activity of chorionic gonadotropin mediates the thyrotoxicosis of choriocarcinoma. *Am J Obstet Gynecol* 138:77-85, 1980.

Ohama K, Ueda K, Okamoto E, et al: Cytogenetic and clinicopathologic studies of hydatidiform moles. *Obstet Gynecol* 68:259, 1986.

Osathanondh R, Berkowitz RS, deCholnoky C, Smith BS, Goldstein DP, Tyson JE: Hormonal measurements in patients with theca lutein cysts and gestational trophoblastic disease. *J Reprod Med* 31:179-182, 1986.

Osathanondh R, Goldstein DP, Pastorfide GB: Actinomycin D as the primary agent for gestational trophoblastic disease. *Cancer* 36:863-866, 1975.

Ozturk M, Berkowitz R, Goldstein D, Bellet D, Wands JR: Differential production of human chorionic gonadotropin and free subunits in gestational trophoblastic disease. *Am J Obstet Gynecol* 158:193-198, 1988.

Pattillo RA, Sasaki S, Katayama KP, Roesler M, Mattingly RF: Genesis of 46,XY hydatidiform mole. *Am J Obstet Gynecol* 141:104-105, 1981.

Rice LW, Berkowitz RS, Lage JM, Goldstein DP, Bernstein MR: Persistent gestational trophoblastic tumor after partial hydatidiform mole. *Gynecol Oncol* 36:358-362, 1990.

Rice LW, Lage JM, Berkowitz RS, Goldstein DP, Bernstein MR: Repetitive complete and partial hydatidiform mole. *Obstet Gynecol* 74:217-219, 1989.

Rustin GJS, Newlands ES, Begert RHJ, Dent J, Bagshawe KD: Weekly alternating etoposide, methotrexate, actinomycin D/vincristine and cyclophosphamide chemotherapy for the treatment of CNS metastases of choriocarcinoma. *J Clin Oncol* 7:900-903, 1989.

Song H-Z, Wu P-C, Wang Y, Yang XY, Dong SY: Pregnancy outcomes after successful chemotherapy for choriocarcinoma and invasive mole: Long-term follow-up. *Am J Obstet Gynecol* 158:538-545, 1988.

Stone M, Bagshawe KD: Hydatidiform mole: Two entities. *Lancet* 1:535, 1976.

Stone M, Dent J, Kardana A, Bagshawe KD: Relationship of oral contraception to development of trophoblastic tumour after evacuation of a hydatidiform mole. *Br J Obstet Gynaecol* 83:913-916, 1976.

Surani MAH, Barton SC, Norris ML: Nuclear transplantation in the mouse: Heritable differences between parental genomes after activation of the embryonic genome. *Cell* 45:127-136, 1986.

Surwit EA: Management of high-risk gestational trophoblastic disease. *J Reprod Med* 32:657-662, 1987.

Surwit EA, Hammond CB: Treatment of metastatic trophoblastic disease with poor prognosis. *Obstet Gynecol* 55:565-570, 1980.

Szulman AE, Surti U: The syndromes of hydatidiform mole. I. Cytogenetic and morphologic correlations. *Am J Obstet Gynecol* 131:665-771, 1978a.

Szulman AE, Surti U: The syndromes of hydatidiform mole. II. Morphologic evolution of the complete and partial mole. *Am J Obstet Gynecol* 132:20-27, 1978b.

Szulman AE, Surti U: The clinicopathologic profile of the partial hydatidiform mole. *Obstet Gynecol* 59:597-602, 1982.

Tow WSH: The influence of the primary treatment of hydatidiform mole on its subsequent course. *J Obstet Gynaecol Br Commonw* 73:545-552, 1966.

Twiggs LB, Morrow CP, Schlaerth JB: Acute pulmonary complications of molar pregnancy. *Am J Obstet Gynecol* 135:189-194, 1979.

Vassilakos P, Riotton G, Kajii T: Hydatidiform mole: Two entities. *Am J Obstet Gynecol* 127:167, 1977.

Walden PAM, Bagshawe KD: Reproductive performance of women successfully treated for gestational trophoblastic tumors. *Am J Obstet Gynecol* 125:1108-1114, 1976.

Weed JC Jr, Hammond CB: Cerebral metastatic choriocarcinoma: Intensive therapy and prognosis. *Obstet Gynecol* 55:89-94, 1980.

Wong LC, Ma HK: The syndrome of partial mole. *Arch Gynecol* 234:161, 1984.

Wong LC, Choo YC, Ma HK: Primary oral etoposide therapy in gestational trophoblastic disease: An update. *Cancer* 58:14-17, 1986.

Yamashita K, Wake N, Araki T, Ichinoe K, Makoto K: Human lymphocyte antigen expression in hydatidiform mole: Androgenesis following fertilization by a haploid sperm. *Am J Obstet Gynecol* 135:597-600, 1979.

Yordan EL Jr, Schlaerth J, Gaddis O, Morrow CP: Radiation therapy in the management of gestational choriocarcinoma metastatic to the central nervous system. *Obstet Gynecol* 69:627-630, 1987.

# UNIT III | Management of Complications of Disease and Treatment

# Chapter 18 | Urinary Tract Involvement in Gynecologic Cancer

### Gary P. Kearney    Sabah S. Tumeh

Often, in dealing with cancers of the female reproductive system, the gynecologic oncologist in effect confronts genitourinary diseases, so profound are the implications of these tumors for the urinary tract. Therefore, an approach to these cancers must include not only a command of current gynecologic techniques but also an appreciation of the recent advances in urologic surgery.

## TYPES OF URINARY TRACT INVOLVEMENT

### Cervical Cancer

Usually, the spread of cervical carcinoma first distorts the base of the bladder and later involves the lower ureters. In patients with direct extension into the ureters, the adventitial layer is involved first, followed by encroachment on the muscularis and, occasionally, the mucosa. As the disease progresses into the lumen of the ureter, obstruction ensues.

Ureteral obstruction can also result from compression of the ureters by adjacent tumor-filled lymphatics. Lymphogenous spread of cervical carcinoma usually occurs in an orderly fashion, after the base of the broad ligaments and parametrium have become involved. The paracervical, internal iliac, obturator, external iliac, and sacral nodes are involved first, followed by the aorta, mediastinal, and supraclavicular nodes.

In carcinoma of the cervix, death most often results from uremia secondary to ureteral obstruction. Obstruction occurs most frequently where the ureter passes through the cardinal ligament, 3 to 6 cm from the ureterovesical junction. This area is at particular risk for both tumor extension and radiation damage (Bugbee, 1934; Drexler and Howes, 1934; Rhamy and Stander, 1961 and 1962).

### Uterine Carcinoma and Sarcoma

*Carcinoma of the endometrium* grows slowly, and approximately three-fourths of women have localized disease at the time of diagnosis. However, 10% of patients with clinical Stage I disease and 36% with Stage II disease will be found to have pelvic lymph node metastases on histologic study (Morrow et al, 1973). The mechanisms of spread include extension to the endocervix and invasion into the myometrium, with subsequent lymphatic involvement.

The paths of lymphatic extension reflect the segment of the uterus involved by the carcinoma. Lesions of the fundus may be drained by lymphatics that join with lymphatic vessels from the fallopian tube, drain into the ovarian plexus, and follow the ovarian vessels to the aortic lymph nodes. The lower segment of the corpus and the cervix drain to the pelvic lymph nodes. If the endocervix is involved, contiguous spread into the endopelvic fascia may result in tumor extension to the pelvic sidewalls through the cardinal ligaments. The tumor can also extend to the pelvic sidewalls along the base of the broad ligaments. If there is obstructive retrograde lymphatic flow, periurethral metastases may result.

Endometrial carcinoma is associated with a lower incidence of urinary tract involvement compared with carcinoma of the cervix. Bladder involvement is rare, occurring most often in the context of a poorly differentiated tumor that invades the myometrium and extends through the lower anterior uterine wall into the bladder (Buchsbaum and Schmidt, 1978). Ureteral obstruction occurs somewhat more frequently as a consequence of pelvic node involvement.

The hematogenous route is most important in the spread of *leiomyosarcoma*, with metastases most often involving the lungs and liver. Leiomyosarcomas also frequently extend into the broad ligaments, but lymphatic spread is less common. Resection may be difficult, and the disease usually recurs quickly; few patients survive longer than 1 year.

Local involvement is of greater significance in *endometrial stromal sarcoma*. This tumor infrequently invades the myometrium and may compress or directly involve the bladder, urethra, or ureters.

### Ovarian Cancer

Cancer of the ovary can either compress the bladder superiorly, giving rise to urinary frequency and urgency if the tumor is posterior to the uterus in the cul-de-sac, or displace the uterus and bladder anteriorly, with consequent ureteral compression. Such compression may be due to pressure of the tumor against the lateral pelvic walls or at the pelvic inlet or extension to pelvic and paraaortic lymph nodes (Mitty, 1980; Walsh et al, 1981). Ureteral obstruction occurs in 40 to 80% of large ovarian neoplasms. In one patient with an ovarian mass, oliguria developed in association with elevated intraabdominal pressure. Operative decompression of the abdomen reversed the oliguric state (Celoria et al, 1987).

### Vulvar Cancer

Vulvar cancer is usually slow-growing and superficial, with spread to the groin and pelvic nodes. Treatment most often involves radical vulvectomy and bilateral groin resection. With untreated longstanding disease, however, fungating, ulcerative extension to the urethra, bladder, vagina, or rectum may take place. In these patients, partial or total exenteration may increase survival somewhat. Urinary incontinence can occur after radical vulvectomy unless urethral plication is carried out prophylactically.

# DIAGNOSTIC ASSESSMENT OF THE URINARY TRACT

In patients with gynecologic neoplasms, preoperative assessment of the urinary tract is important, since it not only determines whether the urinary tract is involved in the cancer but can also evaluate renal function and define any congenital urinary tract anomalies before surgery is undertaken.

Routine followup of these patients also demands that the status of the urinary tract be assessed. Symptoms of ureteral obstruction occurring after treatment should prompt immediate studies; this is particularly true in cervical carcinoma, since ureteral obstruction is one of the few objective signs of recurrent disease.

## Excretory Urography

Excretory urography remains the most important technique for assessing the urinary tract in patients with gynecologic neoplasms, since it can provide detailed morphologic and functional information. In many cases, findings on excretory urography lead to a change in staging. In one series, 16 of 86 patients (21%) shown by excretory urography to have ureteral obstruction had no palpable evidence of lateral parametrial or pelvic wall tumor (Van Nagell et al, 1975).

Spataro (1988) has reported that new, low-osmolality contrast agents provide significantly higher urinary iodine concentrations than do conventional, high-osmolality ionic contrast media. The low-osmolality agents also produce better quality excretory urograms, are better tolerated, and cause fewer side effects and serious adverse reactions. In one of the earlier prospective studies comparing these two types of media, Katayama et al (1988) used ionic contrast media in 168,363 patients. In those given the low-osmolality agents, the overall incidence of adverse reactions (of all types) was 3%; severe reactions occurred in 0.04% and very severe reactions in 0.004%. These rates were 13%, 0.22% and 0.04%, respectively, in the group given the high-osmolality agents. These data imply that to prevent a severe reaction, nonionic contrast medium should be used in patients with a history of a previous reaction.

In contrast, Lasser et al (1987) reported a smaller drop in the incidence of such reactions in 6,763 patients randomized to receive low doses of corticosteroids prior to injection of the contrast agent. The incidence of all types of reactions was 6% among the patients pretreated with steroids compared with 9% among those

not so treated. Severe reactions occurred in 0.20% and 0.52% of these two groups, respectively.

Urographic results can also alert the physician to possible treatment complications. As Lang et al (1973) have noted, the urographic demonstration of encasement of the parametrial segment of the ureter by tumor is an indication that the ureter is at particular risk for obstruction following surgery or radiation therapy.

Followup urographic studies have also been shown to be an accurate means of both monitoring urinary tract abnormalities and assessing their significance. In 20 of 126 patients with irradiated cervical carcinoma, ureteral obstruction devoted or progressed after treatment; in 16 patients this represented recurrence of the disease, and of these, 14 (87.5 per cent) died within 6 months to 4.5 years. In contrast, six patients with mild urographic changes ascribed to radiation effect on the bladder mucosa were all alive 6 months to 6 years following treatment. Of seven patients who demonstrated urographic improvement after radiation therapy, two (28.6 per cent) died during the followup period. Among the 99 patients without urographic changes there were 10 deaths (10.1 per cent) (Ruponen et al, 1974).

## Computed Tomography

Computed tomography (CT) is a useful, noninvasive method for assessing gynecologic cancers, since it can provide morphologic information. In cervical cancer, CT allows staging with an accuracy greater than 70% (Stanley and Lee, 1980). It can also be of value in assessing possible recurrence. CT detected correctly local recurrent cervical disease in 85% of patients in a study by Heron et al (1988). Six equivocal, two false-positive, and two false-negative CT results were due either to difficulty in differentiating recurrent disease from changes related to radiotherapy or to the failure of CT to detect small areas of local recurrence in 39 of 70 patients examined. CT studies are also valuable in assessing pelvic sidewall extension and detecting metastases in clinically inaccessible areas as well as in showing hydronephrosis and indicating the site of ureteral obstruction (Fig. 18-1). CT can also be employed to document urine extravasation and to define its extent (Mitty, 1980).

The most important disadvantage of CT is its inability to differentiate recurrent tumor from radiation fibrosis, but only in a small percentage of patients (Walsh et al, 1981). This was a particular problem with hydronephrosis; two of the four false-negative or equivocal findings represented cases of hydronephrosis ascribed to recurrent disease rather than to radiation fibrosis. In patients who have not previously undergone radiation treatment, CT findings should be less ambiguous.

## Ultrasonography

Ultrasonography is useful in evaluating tumor extension through the central pelvis and for detecting hydronephrosis due to extension or treatment (Samuels and

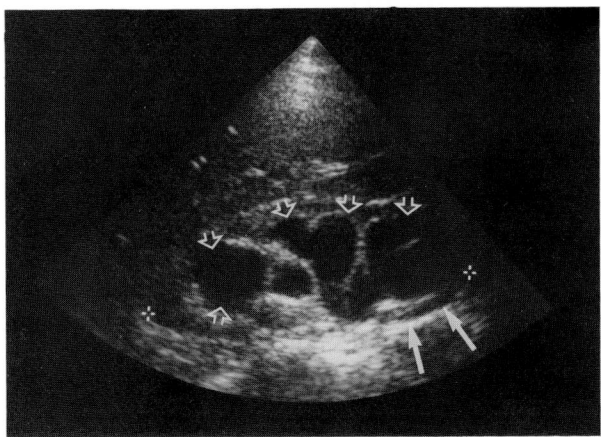

A

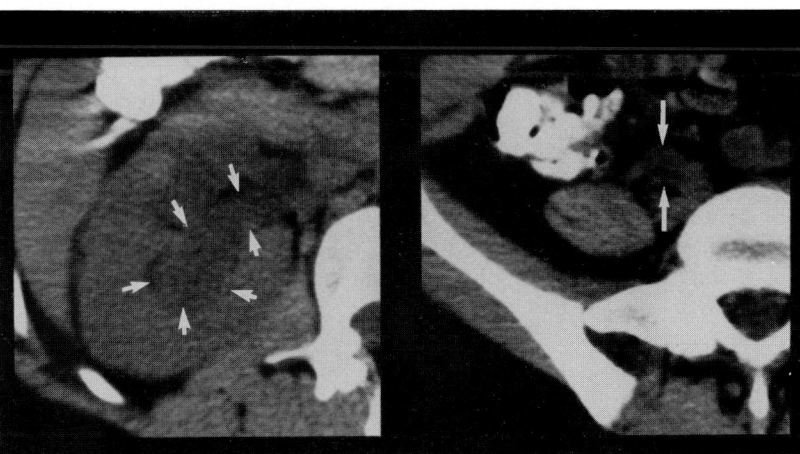

B

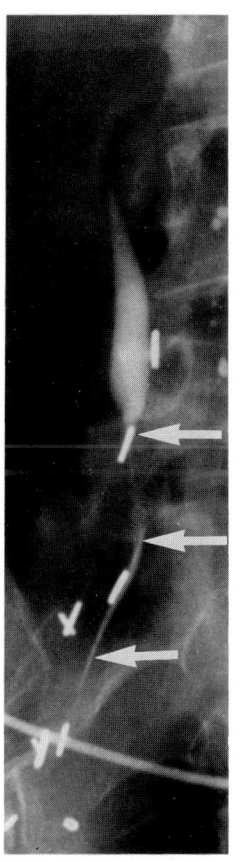

D

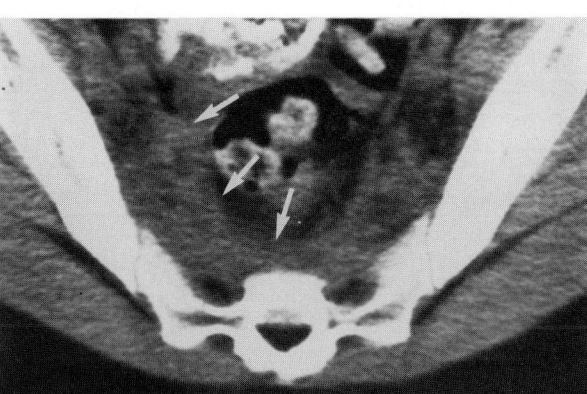

C

FIGURE 18-1 Following hysterectomy and radiotherapy for carcinoma of the cervix, this patient presented with diminished renal function.

(*A*) Longitudinal sonogram of right kidney showing marked dilatation of the collecting system (open arrows) and proximal ureter (solid arrows). The rest of the ureter cannot be seen because gas in the overlying bowel prevented the ultrasound beam from reaching posterior structures, in this case the ureter. Although ultrasonography detected the hydronephrosis, it did not indicate the level of obstruction, which is generally more accurately depicted by CT.

(*B*) CT scans, obtained without intravenous contrast enhancement, through the right kidney (*left panel*) and midabdomen (*right panel*) reveal dilatation of the collecting system (small arrows) and middle of the right ureter (large arrows).

(*C*) CT scan through the pelvis revealing marked thickening of the presacral soft tissues on the right due to radiation fibrosis. The fibrotic mass encased the right ureter, causing obstruction.

(*D*) Antegrade pyeloureterogram showing narrowing of the proximal few centimeters of the right ureter (arrows).

Silver, 1978; Walsh et al, 1980). Although sonography cannot provide the precision and detail afforded by CT, sonography is a noninvasive tool that is particularly well suited for serial evaluations, since it involves neither ionizing radiation nor the injection of contrast media, as is required for urography.

Nevertheless, ultrasonography has some weaknesses. First, it does not penetrate air and may therefore miss significant lesions located behind air-filled loops of bowel. Second, obese patients pose a special problem, particularly when an evaluation of the peritoneum is needed. Third, ultrasound is extremely sensitive (at a rate approaching 100%) in detecting high-grade hydronephrosis. Of course, this is only achieved at the expense of a low specificity—i.e., too many patients with minimal separation of fat in the renal sinus will be diagnosed as having grade 1 hydronephrosis. If Doppler ultrasound is applied in such cases, it will suggest an arterial or venous cause for this central fat separation in about 40% of cases (Scola et al, 1989). Furthermore, sonography provides no information regarding the function of a hydronephrotic kidney, which may have to be evaluated by either excretory urography or nuclear scintigraphy. Finally, because of the subtlety of minimal separation of renal sinus fat, ultrasound may fail to detect early obstruction. Depending on the clinical situation, further evaluation of the patient using invasive techniques such as retrograde pyelography may then be necessary.

## Magnetic Resonance Imaging (MRI)

MRI is rapidly evolving into a useful imaging modality in the staging and followup of gynecologic tumors. Although the spatial resolution of MRI is inferior to that of CT, its superior contrast resolution as well as its ability to display images in the sagittal, coronal, and transaxial projections make it a better choice in this clinical setting. For example, MRI can differentiate endometrium from myometrium, allowing one to assess the depth of myometrial invasion by endometrial carcinoma (Hricak et al, 1986). It has also proved to be of value in excluding invasion of the rectum, bladder, and pelvic sidewalls by carcinoma of the uterine cervix (Togashi et al, 1986, Hricak et al, 1988). MRI does have two main advantages. First, it can be used to estimate tumor size fairly accurately and may thus be of help in selecting a particular mode of therapy. Second, it has been used successfully to differentiate fibrotic tissue from residual or recurrent tumor (Ebner et al, 1988). However, it should be noted that different tissues may have similar MR signals, which precludes tissue characterization; for example, current MRI techniques are not able to differentiate endometrial carcinoma from hyperplasia or blood clots (Hricak et al, 1986). Furthermore, MRI offers no advantage over CT in evaluating lymph node involvement by gynecologic tumors; both techniques use a size criterion to estimate the likelihood of such involvement.

## Cystoscopy

While excretory urography is important in all stages of cervical carcinoma, cystoscopy should be performed for staging purposes only in patients with clinical Stage III and IV tumors. This technique is not indicated in patients with endometrial carcinoma, since this lesion rarely involves the bladder (Van Nagell et al, 1975)

Cystoscopy can show bladder distortion or displacement by a mass; a finding of bullous edema also suggests the presence of adjacent tumor. When lesions are visualized directly, biopsy permits a precise diagnosis to be made. Cystoscopy is useful after radiation therapy if urinary symptoms have developed; direct inspection of the tissues can disclose, for example, infection, telangiectatic vessels, or fistulas.

Cystometry may be indicated if there are symptoms of urgency or frequency, and the assessment of bladder capacity and sphincter function can provide valuable information in cases of incontinence. Morphologic de-

tail and the presence of vesicoureteral reflux can be determined from cystograms.

In patients with bladder injury or known tumor involvement of the bladder, cystoscopy is best performed under general or regional anesthesia, since it is poorly tolerated under local anesthesia in such patients. However, urodynamic bladder studies must be performed under local anesthesia.

## Retrograde and Antegrade Pyelography

*Retrograde pyelography* can provide detailed information regarding ureteral obstruction that may not be obtainable by excretory urography. Retrograde studies should, however, be undertaken with extreme caution. Contrast injection beyond a high-grade obstruction can lead to sepsis and pyonephrosis that may require placement of a retrograde catheter to decompress the collecting system. If decompression is unsuccessful, surgical intervention will be necessary, usually a percutaneous nephrostomy under local anesthesia. Because of the potential for serious complications, retrograde pyelography should never be performed unless the information to be derived is absolutely essential to diagnosis. In a patient with ureteral obstruction and a nonfunctioning kidney who is doing well clinically, retrograde studies are rarely indicated; they should be carried out only if urinary diversion is contemplated.

If the patient has a nonfunctioning kidney without sepsis and it is absolutely essential to define the anatomy, an *antegrade pyelogram* using a small-gauge spinal needle is employed because there is less risk of infection in an obstructed collecting system.

If sepsis is suspected in the context of a nonfunctioning kidney, the urine in the renal pelvis on the impaired side should be aspirated, and culture and Gram stains should be carried out to rule out an infected hydronephrosis (pyonephrosis).

## THE KIDNEYS

### Injury

Studies by Goldberg (1972) showed that radiation treatment in 28 patients with Stage II or III carcinoma of the cervix was followed by a change in the rate of creatinine clearance. Although the change was relatively small, it was statistically significant, suggesting that radiation therapy may be associated with a reduction in the glomerular filtration rate and thus might prolong the action of drugs that are normally cleared by this mechanism. It was conjectured that this finding might represent a hormonal effect rather than stem from direct damage to the kidney.

Combined surgical and radiation treatment may result in a high incidence of renal damage. Of 72 patients with Stage I or II cervical carcinoma treated with radical hysterectomy and postoperative radiotherapy, only 17 showed no alterations in renal function after treatment. In 37 cases there were changes in creatinine clearance, reflecting glomerular damage, while 24 showed abnormal concentration and dilution, suggesting a lesion in the tubulointerstitial tract. Results of both concentration and dilution tests were abnormal in only 10% of the patients (Marziale 1979).

## Diagnosis

Before surgical or radiation theory is begun, baseline kidney function should be assessed, with determinations repeated frequently during treatment and throughout the followup period.

## Management

Steckel et al (1974) have studied the possibility of protecting the normal kidney from radiation damage during treatment for disseminated ovarian carcinoma by inducing hypoxia through intraarterial infusions of epinephrine. After such treatment, 2 of 25 patients had no evidence of nephropathy on either side, while 3 showed nephropathy on the side that had not been protected. In one case in which the patient had multiple renal arteries on both sides, epinephrine infusion into the dominant renal artery on one side succeeded in protecting only 60 to 70% of the kidney, as estimated by the normal perfusion areas. At autopsy it was found that radiation nephropathy had affected the segment of the kidney that had not been protected during treatment.

## THE URETERS

### Injury

***Obstruction by Tumor*** Ureteral obstruction is the most common urinary tract complication of gynecologic cancers. It occurs with particular frequency in cervical carcinoma and, as has been noted, is the cause of death in most fatal cases.

Between 1951 and 1981, 2,016 new patients with invasive carcinoma of the cervix (Stages I to IV) were seen at the Louisiana State University Medical Center (Bahrassa and Ampil, 1987). Ureteral obstruction developed in 137 cases of early-stage disease (12%) after treatment of the malignancy was completed and in 18% of those with advanced cervical carcinoma. Ninety-four (69%) of these patients died, and autopsy results were available in 28 cases. The rate of biopsy-proven recurrent or persistent carcinoma in patients with post-treatment obstruction was 40% for those with early-stage disease and 66% for those with disease in an advanced stage.

Because of the serious implications of urinary tract obstruction in cervical carcinoma, it has been recommended that tumors in patients with evidence of obstruction be classified as Stage IIIb in the International Federation of Obstetrics and Gynecology (FIGO) system. Luciani et al (1987) investigated the usefulness of aspiration biopsy cytology under fluoroscopic guidance in establishing the true nature of ureteral stenosis in 15 patients with known primary malignancy previously

treated with surgery, radiotherapy, or chemotherapy. The sites of the primary tumors were the cervix (6), bladder (2), prostate (2), uterine corpus (2), pancreas (1), stomach (1), and rectum (1). Thirteen patients had metastatic ureteral involvement. Since there were no false-positive or false-negative cytologic findings, the rate of diagnostic accuracy was 100%. The results of this study and a review of the literature indicate that aspiration biopsy cytology offers an accurate, minimally invasive way to diagnose the ureteral strictures that often complicate cancer and obviates more aggressive diagnostic procedures such as exploratory laparotomy.

The management of malignant ureteral obstruction (MUO) has undergone major changes with the availability of percutaneous drainage techniques and new ureteral stents for endoscopic insertion (Zadra et al, 1987). Obstruction almost always occurs in the distal ureter; in one series, it was found to be at or near the ureterovesical junction in 96 per cent of cases in which the site of obstruction could be localized (Van Nagell et al, 1975). Obstruction in the proximal portion of the ureter without distal involvement is rare, most likely because ureteral lymphatics drain segmentally into regional nodes, and there are no continuous longitudinal channels in the ureteral wall or periureteral sheath (Miller and Spear, 1973). In some cases, however, the tumor may metastasize to lymphatics outside the pelvis before extensive intrapelvic involvement becomes evident (Parente, 1960; Cherry et al, 1953). This may result in ureteral obstruction if the proximal ureter is involved (Perch, 1971; Anderson, 1973; Miller and Spear, 1973).

Ureteral obstruction after treatment of cervical carcinoma is usually a sign of recurrent tumor. In patients with recurrent disease, ureteral involvement often signals the presence of unresectable tumor and consequently a poor prognosis.

***Obstruction After Surgery*** Transient ureteral obstruction after surgery most likely reflects a combination of postoperative edema, infection, and impaired lymph flow. Chronic ureteral obstruction can result from devascularization of distal ureters, since this segment of the ureter also receives much of its blood supply from the hypogastric vessels. Ureteral obstruction can also result from the inadvertent inclusion of the ureter in a bulk ligature introduced to stem bleeding from the uterine artery or vein (Wesolowski, 1969). This possibility underscores the need for precise visualization of bleeding vessels.

Between July, 1980, and September, 1987, 3,185 major gynecologic operations were performed in a residency program (Mann et al, 1988). Ureteral injury occurred in 17 cases, 14 (0.04%) of which were accidental.

***Radiation Stricture*** Radiation has been shown to evoke a sequence of histologic changes in the ureter. In the *acute stage*, which occurs during or shortly after irradiation, there is hyperemia and edema; microvascular injury; epithelial cell degeneration; endothelial degeneration, necrosis, and proliferation; and subendothelial and medial vascular fibrosis. In this stage, muscle may degenerate because of vascular insufficiency and may be replaced by fibrous tissue. The *subacute stage* is marked by continuing epithelial degeneration and vascular damage and by the infiltration of inflammatory cells. In the *chronic stage* there is slow progression of an endarteritis obliterans, which in turn leads to increasing epithelial and muscular atrophy. Lost muscle continues to be replaced by fibrous tissue, which may contract. This last stage usually begins 6 months after treatment and may still be evident 10 or more years later (Cosbie, 1941).

In general, however, ureters are resistant to radiation injury. Over a 27-year period (1959 to 1986), 10 of 328 patients (3%) treated with curative intent using primary radiation therapy for carcinoma of the cervix developed obstructive ureteropathy due to fibrosis (Parliament et al, 1989). The mean age of these patients was 45 years, and the median time to obstruction was 26 months. In eight cases, the obstruction was unilateral and involved the parametrial portion of the ureter in at least five cases. No predisposing risk factor was found to be associated with the development of obstructive ureteropathy. After corrective surgery, renal function remained normal in eight patients, and hydronephrosis resolved in four.

In a series of 100 asymptomatic women who had been treated 5 years previously with radiation, evidence of ureteral injury was found on examination in only 4, while 5 patients showed improvement on excretory urograms compared with pretreatment studies (Underwood et al, 1977). While stricture may result simply from the effects of radiation on the ureteral wall, especially if errors are made in radiotherapy, in many instances other factors are probably also involved. It has been suggested that the tumor itself may result in a permanent desmoplastic response in the ureter or that ureteral fibrosis may follow necrosis of tumor invading the ureteral wall or sheath (Alfert and Gillenwater, 1972). Pelvic infection (Widholm and Mattsson, 1972) or surgical manipulation of an irradiated ureter (Alfert and Gillenwater, 1972) may also cause a subclinical ureteral injury to proceed to frank stricture.

Ureteral obstruction develops and, in many cases, resolves sooner after surgery than after radiation therapy (Mallik, 1960). In a study of patients with carcinoma of the cervix who were treated either surgically or with radiation, it was also noted that urinary tract infections occurred in the surgically treated group during the immediate postoperative period, whereas they developed an average of 14.5 months after treatment in patients who had received radiation therapy (Mickal et al, 1972). The combination of surgery and radiation therapy constitutes a particularly high risk for the development of stricture (Shingleton et al, 1969) and other urinary tract complications (Mikuta et al, 1977; Rotman et al, 1979).

The overall incidence of urinary and bowel complications has been reported to be as high as 20% among patients undergoing radiation therapy for cancer of the cervix (Chau et al, 1962; Lang et al, 1973). However, in the vast majority of these patients whose exposure to the radiation dose was carefully controlled, radiation

injury occurred in 1 to 3% (Gray and Kottmeier, 1957; Kottmeier and Gray, 1961).

A comprehensive survey was carried out at the Yale Medical Center of 964 consecutive patients who received interstitial and/or external beam radiation therapy for malignant disease of the pelvis between 1963 and 1968 (Dean and Lytton, 1978). These patients received daily doses of 200 rads, i.e., a total of more than 6,000 rads over a 6-week period. Among the 964 patients studied, there were 203 urologic problems—an incidence of 21%. Pure radiation injury alone was seen in 2.5% of these patients; the remainder had evidence of recurrent or persistent tumor. Of the total group, 493 were treated for gynecologic malignancy, 240 for genitourinary malignancy, 172 for bowel malignancy, and 59 for other tumors. Gross hematuria was found in only five patients, and this occurred late in all instances; three of these patients had tumor instances; three of these patients had tumor invading the bladder and the remaining two had received a total dose exceeding 7,000 rads.

Obstruction of the ureter occurred in 35 cases; only 1 of these cases could be associated with the effects of radiation alone, and this occurred after 44 months. Recurrent cancer was associated with obstruction in the remaining 34 cases. Eleven patients developed fistulas, half of which occurred early and half late; nine of these patients had been treated for carcinoma of the cervix. Nine of the 11 had received more than 6,000 rads, and 5 of the 9 had tumor in the fistula. There appeared to be no prevalence of associated conditions such as diabetes, anemia, or previous urinary tract difficulties in this group of patients. Thus, it appears that when the urinary tract does undergo radiation injury, gynecologic malignancy is generally associated with recurrent and/or persistent tumor rather than with the effects of radiation alone, although excessive radiation itself can result in complications in a small percentage of patients.

*Fistula*  The tissue trauma and disruption of the blood supply associated with hysterectomy or radiation therapy can lead to ureterovaginal or vesicovaginal fistulas. Ureterovaginal fistulas, which are more common, were reported in some studies to occur after approximately 10 per cent of radical hysterectomies (Morton, 1947; Douglas and Birnbaum, 1954; Brunschwig and Frick, 1956), but more recent studies show a far lower incidence. Patients with cancers of more advanced stage (Calame and Nelson, 1967) and those who have had previous radiation therapy or postoperative urinary infection are at greater risk for fistula formation.

## Diagnosis

*Intraoperative Injury*  While unrecognized operative ureteral injury can result in kidney damage or fistula formation, these complications can be avoided in most cases with immediate repair. However, ureteral injuries are recognized intraoperatively in only about 30% of cases (Mattingly and Borkowf, 1978). This rate of detection could be greatly improved if care were taken to assess the continuity of the urinary tract intraoperatively whenever injury may have occurred. By intravenously injecting half of a standard ampule of indigo carmine or methylene blue, one can identify the side of the leak and outline the ureter. (If the patient has hypertension, indigo carmine should not be used because it has been known to induce hypertensive crises.)

***Obstruction or Stricture*** A classic symptom of ureteral obstruction or stricture is a dull, constant ache in the lower lumbar region or groin that may be referred to the flank, lower abdomen, thigh, or leg. If there is an associated urinary tract infection, systemic symptoms, including anorexia, malaise, chills, and fever, may be found. Ureteral obstruction does not, however, invariably give rise to symptoms. Richie et al (1979) reported on a series of 82 patients with ureteral obstruction secondary to metastatic disease, 35 of whom had carcinoma of the cervix. They noted that fewer than 55% of the group as a whole complained of urinary tract symptoms.

In patients with known gynecologic malignancy who experience the characteristic pain or symptoms of a urinary tract infection, ureteral obstruction must be ruled out. Urinalysis and urine culture should be carried out as a first step, after which a limited intravenous pyelographic study or renal ultrasonography should be performed.

***Fistula*** The presence of a ureterovaginal fistula following radiation therapy or radical hysterectomy is signaled by spontaneous drainage of urine from the vagina, usually associated with ureteral obstruction. Staining of a vaginal tampon after the intravenous injection of indigo carimine or methylene blue will confirm the presence of a urovaginal fistula. One can determine which ureter is involved by means of excretory urography; occasionally, such fistulas are bilateral (Fig. 18-2) (Ignatoff and Graham, 1974).

## Management

***Intraoperative Injuries*** Limited in situ ureteral repairs should be reserved for patients with no history of previous radiation therapy, crushing injury, or devascularization of the ureter. When there has been a simple suture ligature of a ureter in such patients, deligation and placement of an inlying ureteral stent is frequently all that is necessary. If the ureter has been transected, formal repair by ureteroureterostomy and/or ureteral reimplantation is necessary. If the ureteral division is low in the pelvis, ureteral reimplantation is the safest approach, since achieving a urine-tight closure by ureteroureterostomy can be technically difficult. If there is loss of adequate ureteral length, a tension-free anastomosis can be fashioned by using a Boari bladder flap. In this procedure, a flap is separated from the bladder and sutured to form a tube, bridging the gap between the bladder and ureter. This technique can also be combined with nephropexy, or mobilization of the kidney, in order to bring the kidney a few centimeters closer to the bladder. Transureteroureterostomy should be reserved for patients in whom the bladder has received

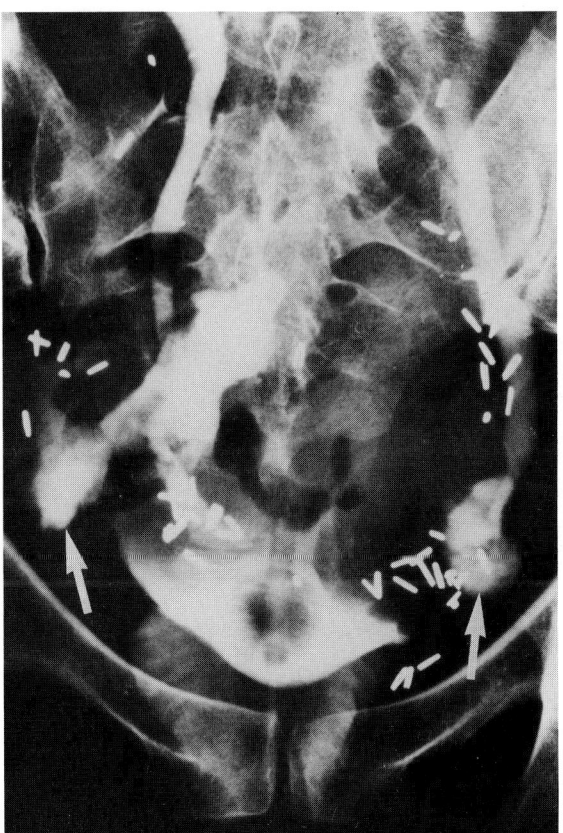

FIGURE 18-2 IV intravenous pyelogram demonstrating bilateral ureterovaginal fistulas after radical hysterectomy treated successfully with bilateral percutaneous nephrostomy and antegrade passage of double-J stents.

high-dose radiation, those with pelvic fixation, and those in whom tissue healing cannot be anticipated.

***Obstruction or Stricture*** Ureteral stricture may be treated by introducing an internal ureteral stent via a cystoscope (Fig. 18-3) (Pellman et al, 1977; Kearney et al, 1979). If this fails to relieve the obstruction, a number of techniques may be employed, including ureteroneocystostomy with or without a flap, transureteroureterostomy, or creation of a urinary conduit (usually with the colon). The procedure of choice depends on the findings at exploration: the site of obstruction, the length of damaged ureter, the vascularity of the ureter proximal to the affected segment, the technical ease with which the ureter and bladder may be mobilized, and the condition of the bladder wall.

***Fistula*** Management of fistula depends on the patient's condition. In the absence of flank pain or fever, the patient should be watched for approximately 3 weeks, since instrumentation sooner after radical hysterectomy can result in failure and possibly enlargement of the fistula (Calame and Nelson, 1967). Prentiss and Mullenix (1951) have summarized our contention that when ureteral injuries are accompanied by ureterovaginal fistulas, it is most important to preserve function until healing takes place. In many cases, such a course will

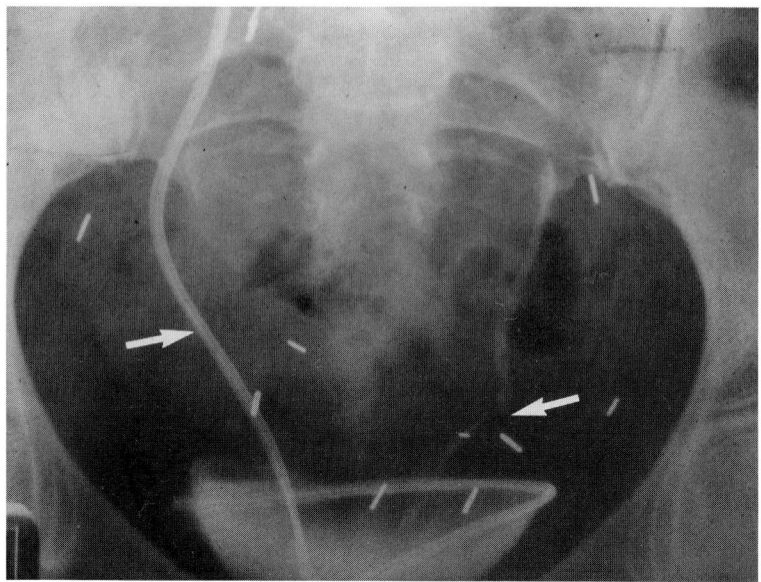

FIGURE 18-3 Endoscopic placement of a right ureteral stent for ureteral obstruction and fistula after radical hysterectomy for cervical carcinoma (left arrow). A left ureterovaginal fistula has healed spontaneously (right arrow).

permit spontaneous healing of the fistula. Treatment of ureterovaginal fistula resembles that carried out for ureteral stricture. In a study by Maillet et al (1987), 40 patients with urinary fistulas were treated with interventional radiology. Antegrade percutaneous catheterization of the ureter and fistula bypass enabled ureteral stenting in 36 patients (90%); 28 (70%) were treated successfully. In five of the 40 patients (12.5%), nephrectomy was required after failure of the percutaneous technique.

## THE BLADDER

### Injury

*Invasion* In gynecologic cancers, extension to the bladder occurs less frequently and at a later clinical stage of disease than does ureteral obstruction. Bladder involvement is most often found with carcinoma of the cervix and, according to the FIGO staging scheme, would require that such cases be classified as Stage IV disease.

Extension of cervical carcinoma to the bladder in the absence of distant metastases does not preclude a good outcome. A retrospective study of 53 such patients treated at the M.D. Anderson Hospital by radiation or exenteration revealed a 30% 5-year survival rate, with exenteration providing no therapeutic advantage over radiation (Million et al, 1972).

*Intraoperative Injuries* Direct bladder injury usually occurs on the posterior bladder wall, above and between the ureteral orifices, where the vaginal cuff is sutured.

During radical (Wertheim) hysterectomy, the bladder is also at risk for neurologic injury. In simple hysterectomies, complete disruption of bladder innervation may be avoided, since accessory nerves to the bladder are preserved near the ureterovesical junction. Radical hysterectomy, on the other hand, involves extensive dissection of the pelvic sidewalls and the distal portion of the ureter. This can result in severe functional injury, since the hypogastric web that passes from the pelvic side-

walls to the bladder—the uterine, vesical, and vaginal arteries—constitutes the bladder's major parasympathetic nerve supply.

Complications secondary to Wertheim hysterectomy can, however, persist for years after the operation. In one study, followup over 5 to 15 years after radical hysterectomy revealed that 27 of 46 patients (59%) had urinary tract symptoms (Fraser, 1966). The most common symptoms were urgency, stress incontinence, diminished or total absence of bladder sensation, and the need to strain in order to commence micturition. Nineteen patients (42%) had abnormally high residual urine volumes, eight (17%) had urinary tract infections, and six showed radiologic evidence of chronic pyelonephritis.

*Ulceration* The pathogenesis of irradiation bladder ulcers has been outlined by Masterson and Rutledge (1967). In the bladder, radiation first results in mucosal erythema and edema that later progress to petechial hemorrhage and then telangiectasia. Subsequent submucosal edema and fibrosis result in urgency and diminished bladder capacity and a diagnosis of radiation cystitis. Acute and chronic cystitis, with or without pyelonephritis, may occur if there is a secondary infection. If submucosal vascular obliterations are extensive, mucosal ulceration may result; if the ulceration deeply penetrates the submucosa, segments of vessel walls may slough into the bladder lumen, producing hematuria. The fibrosis, when marked, may be palpable vaginally as thickening at the base of the bladder. If fibrosis is widespread, vascular alterations may involve the blood supply to the rectum and paravaginal tissues, and the entire pelvis may become rigid and fixed.

In one series, the types of symptoms were found to vary according to the time interval from the beginning of radiation treatment to the onset of symptoms (Masterson and Rutledge, 1967). When the ulcers developed within a few months of irradiation, dysuria, nocturia, frequency, and urgency were the most common symptoms, whereas gross hematuria was usually found in addition to the irritative symptoms when ulcers developed a year after treatment.

These radiation ulcers are usually single, occur in the supratrigonal area, and range from a few millimeters to 4 cm in size. On cystoscopic examination, sharp ulcer margins can often be seen, with surrounding submucosal edema, telangiectasia, and petechial hemorrhage. In some cases, biopsy may be necessary to determine the nature of the lesion. Repeated biopsies should be avoided, however, since they provide limited additional information and can lead to fistula formation. Occasionally, it may be impossible to distinguish radiation necrosis from tumor even by histologic examination (Barber and Brunschwig, 1970; Cowan, 1975; Duncan et al, 1977).

**Fistula** Vesicovaginal fistulas may develop after surgical or radiation treatment, especially in the wake of high-dose irradiation. Invasion by tumor also predisposes to the development of fistulas, since tumor necrosis after irradiation can result in a tissue deficit. In the series by Lang et al (1973), four of the six patients in whom fistulas developed after conventional radiotherapy had Stage IV disease. Although advanced disease increases the likelihood of fistula formation after irradiation, this complication is not inevitable; in 53 patients with Stage IV carcinoma of the cervix and bladder invasion treated by irradiation or exenteration, vesicovaginal fistulas developed during treatment in only 2 (Million et al, 1972).

**Functional Disturbances** Radical surgery in gynecologic malignancy can have a profound effect on bladder and urethral function. It is well known that patients undergoing radical hysterectomy have difficulty voiding for several weeks after surgery, and frequently catheters are left in place until the patient is completely ambulatory. In addition, urinary incontinence is not an infrequent sequela to radical vulvectomy. Many gynecologic surgeons will perform urethropexy prophylactically at the time of radical vulvectomy to prevent this complication.

Nordling and Meyhoff (1979) performed urodynamic investigations in four patients undergoing radical hysterectomy and found significant detrusor areflexia (hypotonic bladder). All of these patients had normal urethral and anal sphincter functions.

It is essential to maintain Foley catheter drainage for a period of time after radical surgery until the patient is completely ambulatory and pain-free because of the high residual urine volumes observed in many of these patients. As a practical measure, recatheterization is not carried out unless the patient is experiencing abdominal discomfort associated with a distended bladder and/or the voiding pattern is unsatisfactory, since it is anticipated that residual volumes may exceed several hundred milliliters for a period of time. Prophylactic antibiotics are administered to these patients because of the known high residual urine volume and the propensity for urinary tract infection. Nordling et al (1981) studied seven patients known to have bladder denervation and sensitivity to carbachol after radical hysterectomy, and they compared the results with those in normal women. After

radical hysterectomy, urethral sensitivity to sympathetic nervous system transmitters was increased when there were signs and symptoms of damage to the pelvic nerves supplying the bladder.

It is well known that patients who have undergone extensive radiation therapy have had a high incidence of irritative bladder symptoms such as urgency, frequency, and discomfort on voiding, most of which can be managed effectively with antispasmodics. The vast majority of these patients were being treated for gynecologic tumors, and a considerable number had genitourinary tumors and other malignant tumors of the pelvis. The prevalence of chronic bladder symptoms 5 to 11 years after radiotherapy for cervical carcinoma was investigated by Parkin et al (1987) by means of a postal questionnaire. Of the 66 replies (68%), only 29 (44%) of the patients were asymptomatic; 17 (26%) had severe symptoms, the most common being urgency and urge incontinence (45%) and significant frequency and nocturia (35%); voiding problems were less common. Thus, bladder dysfunction is a common long-term complication of radiotherapy for cervical carcinoma.

## Diagnosis

**Intraoperative Injuries** The detection of any direct bladder injury during operative treatment is extremely important. With preoperative placement of a three-way catheter, the bladder can be filled with sterile normal saline containing indigo carmine or methylene blue dye during the operative procedure; in this way, any unrecognized leak will become evident (Fig. 18-4). Cystography should also be performed prior to removal of the catheter to confirm the absence of bladder leakage.

**Ulceration** Irritative bladder symptoms should prompt an evaluation to determine their cause, for example, infection, recurrent tumor, or radiation therapy. Cultures usually resolve the question of infection. Cystoscopy must be carried out to rule out direct invasion by tumor. Bladder biopsies may be needed to rule out tumors; however, biopsy is fraught with hazard in the setting of previous radiation therapy because the bladder does not heal well.

**Vesicovaginal Fistulas** In a study by Kursh et al (1988), most of the patients who developed vesicovaginal fistulas had suffered severe postoperative abdominal pain, distention or paralytic ileus, or both. Hematuria and symptoms of bladder irritability were also noted, and prolonged postoperative fever and increased white blood cell counts were common.

The presence of a vesicovaginal fistula, which is also suggested by drainage of urine through the vagina, can be confirmed by dye cystography with insertion of a vaginal tampon to demonstrate staining. The fistula is usually located above and between the ureteral orifices. Excretory urography may show a characteristic double-contrast appearance (Fig. 18-5), but the upper tract is generally normal unless there is an associated uretero-vaginal fistula; definition of both lower ureteral segments is essential to rule out this possibility. Cystoscopy

UROLOGIC DRAINAGE SYSTEM

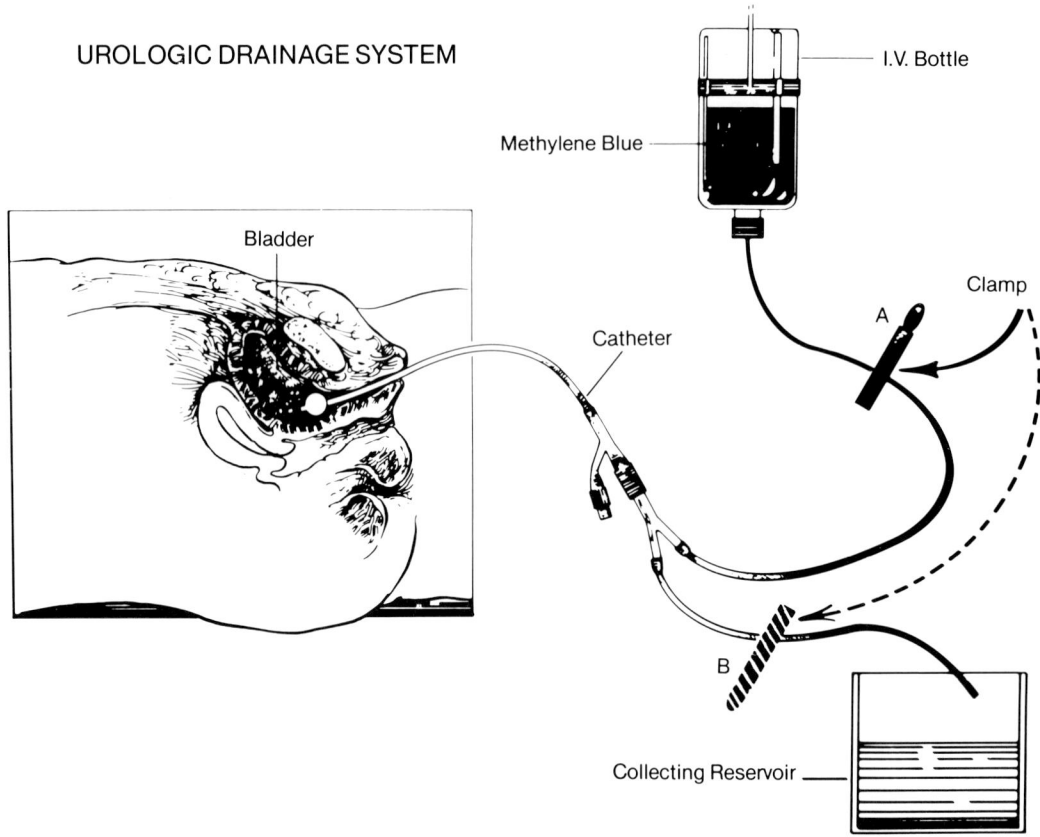

**FIGURE 18-4** Use of three-way catheter bladder irrigation to rule out vesicovaginal fistula.

can be used to confirm the presence of the fistula as well as to determine its size and appearance. Biopsy of the vaginal apex and margins of the fistula is necessary to rule out recurrent tumor.

## Management

**Invasion** If the bladder is involved by tumor, segmental resection may provide an alternative to cystectomy. In this procedure, the bladder is opened anteriorly where it is free from tumor. Use of electrocoagulation will reduce bleeding substantially. The involved segment of the bladder is excised, including wide margins. If the tumor extends to the trigone in the vicinity of the ureteral orifice, either double-J stents or feeding tubes can be placed, depending on the size of the ureter. One must also visualize the ureter as it passes into the pelvis so as not to damage this structure.

Once the involved area is excised, the bladder is repaired in the usual fashion with a layered closure. The bladder is then filled with saline that contains indigo carmine or methylene blue dye in order to assess its integrity. Adequate drainage is of the utmost importance, especially since the pelvic peritoneum is frequently removed as part of a radical procedure. Drainage should include suction, if necessary, to prevent intraperitoneal spillage of urine. Postoperatively, the pelvis should be kept in a dependent position.

The drain should be left in the bladder as long as there is any evidence of leak on gravity cystography. A drainage film is also recommended prior to removal in more difficult cases. If the pelvis has been irradiated, it may be necessary to send the patient home on catheter drainage for several weeks to ensure adequate healing of the bladder.

**Intraoperative Injuries** In patients who have undergone previous radiation therapy, bladder injuries may be complicated by poor tissue healing and, possibly, a persistent vesicocutaneous fistula. In the absence of previous radiation therapy, most such injuries can be treated easily with layered bladder closure (without tension), extraperitoneal drainage, and Foley catheter and/or suprapubic catheter drainage. The use of omentoplasty to bring a new blood supply to potentially devascularized tissue is a useful adjunct to the standard closure technique.

**Ulceration** If the patient experiences urgency, frequency, and dysuria, antispasmodics should be given initially. If this measure fails, one has few options. If bleeding is a problem, application of diluted silver nitrate solutions or ethyl alcohol (or, rarely, dilute formalin) can be tried, but this may further compromise bladder function. If there are irritative bladder symptoms or if bleeding cannot be controlled, hydrostatic dilatation with a Helm-

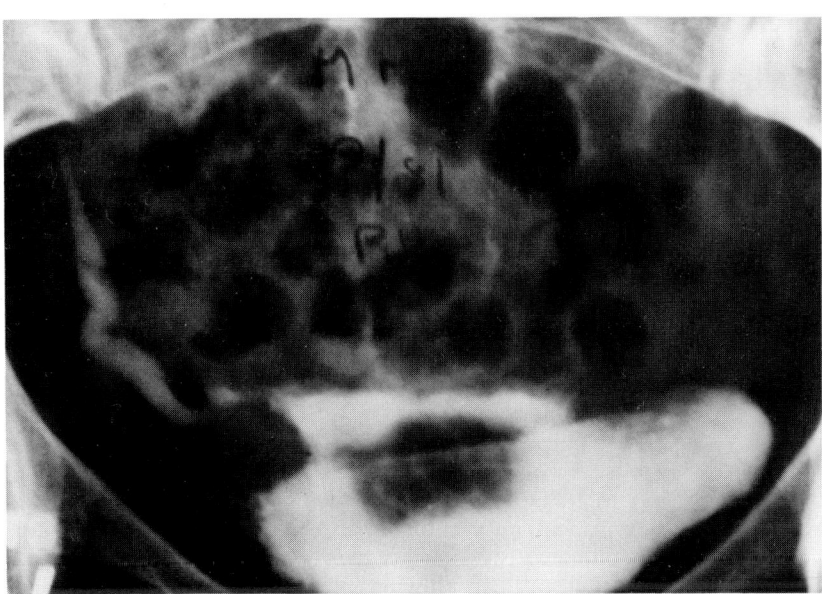

FIGURE 18-5 Vesicovaginal fistula. The double contour on cystography shows vaginal apex.

stein balloon can be tried; although this will stop the bleeding, the long-term result is seldom satisfactory. Some form of supravesical diversion will probably then be necessary.

One can temporize by placing a suprapubic tube if the patient is bleeding massively; however, urinary tract diversion without a cystectomy will generally solve the major problem. Again, diversion is frequently necessary in this setting of radiation, and some form of diversion should be carried out above the radiated field.

Local fulguration of visible bleeding lesions of the bladder may be possible, but often the bleeding is diffuse and not amenable to local therapy. In patients who have persistent, intractable irritative bladder symptoms and/ or hematuria with clots that are not controlled by local measures, urinary diversion followed by instillation of 10% formalin in the defunctionalized bladder may be necessary. Although treatment using the Helmstein intravesical balloon technique has met with some success in Europe, it has not been widely employed or accepted in the United States. Ligation of internal iliac vessels has proved ineffective.

Conservative treatment consisting of sedatives to control urgency and frequency, and antibiotics for supervening infection as well as for avoiding prolonged catheter drainage, should be tried before any operative intervention (Masterson and Rutledge, 1967). If surgery is necessary, the most limited procedure is indicated. A study of 77 patients with severe radiation necrosis has shown that those treated with conservative operation did better and required fewer surgical procedures than did those in whom radical cystectomy or pelvic exenteration was carried out (Barber and Brunschwig, 1970).

***Fistula*** A vesicovaginal fistula without recurrent tumor in patients who have not undergone radiation therapy is generally repaired 3 to 6 months after surgery, since premature closure frequently results in surgical failure. Spontaneous closure can occur if the fistula is small; therefore, in selected cases, watchful waiting for up to 6 months is warranted. The patient and family must be constantly reassured during the period before repair can be attempted. A variety of techniques, including the use of tampons and rubber pants or an intravaginal menstrual tasset cup connected to a leg bag, may keep the patient more comfortable during the waiting period. In three women with large, incurable urinary tract fistulas, palliation was achieved by occluding the distal ureters with isobutyl-2-cyanoacrylate (Bucrylate) and creating a permanent bilateral percutaneous nephrostomy (Stern et al, 1987).

While the vaginal approach can be used if the fistula is low and small, most large and/or complicated vesicovaginal fistulas are best approached suprapubically (O'Conor et al, 1973). Separation of the fistula from the bladder wall by wide mobilization, division of all adhesions, and excision of devascularized tissue is essential. Additional layers of tissue must be interposed and the fistula must be closed to achieve surgical success. The use of peritoneum, omentum (Kiricuta and Goldstein, 1972), gracilis muscle (Öbrink and Bunne, 1978), or the labial fat pad (Keettel et al, 1978) is an important adjunct in irradiated cases. Nonabsorbable suture can be utilized for the vagina, but chromic catgut or polyglycolate sutures should be used for the bladder. If the fistula is near the ureteral tunnel, kinking and compromise of the ureter during the repair as well as postoperative ureteral obstruction due to edema can be avoided by placing temporary splinting catheters in the ureters (O'Conor, 1980). During the healing process, urethral catheter drainage is generally the preferred method of urinary diversion.

Hedlund and Lindstedt (1987) treated 45 patients with urovaginal fistulas due to operative gynecologic procedures and radiotherapy. Fistulas were vesicovaginal and urethrovaginal in 36, ureterovaginal in six, and rectovesicovaginal in three. Reconstruction was performed in 40 patients, mainly via a transvesical approach. Twenty-four of 26 patients not treated with irradiation experienced primary healing, with no failures noted. Of the 14 patients treated with irradiation, nine showed primary healing, and treatment was unsuccessful in three.

# TECHNIQUES OF UROLOGIC MANAGEMENT

## Percutaneous Nephrostomy

Percutaneous ultrasound-guided nephrostomies were found to be useful in 21 patients with ureteral occlusion or lesions secondary to advanced gynecologic malignancies in a study by Pedersen and Juul (1988). One perinephric hematoma and one perinephric abscess (4%) occurred during primary percutaneous nephrostomy diversion of 53 renal units performed by Soper et al (1988). Out of 34 patients, one death (3%) occurred as a result of sepsis related to the nephrostomy. This technique produced immediate and reliable urinary diversion without the morbidity and mortality associated with operative techniques and should be considered as a means of relieving ureteral obstruction (a) in patients with untreated cervical carcinoma who may thus derive prolonged palliation or cure, (b) as a temporizing method of urinary diversion in patients with complications related to previous urinary conduits, and (c) in patients with benign or chemotherapy-sensitive pelvic malignancies that are causing ureteral obstruction. In patients with recurrent carcinoma of the cervix, use of this approach should be individualized according to the expected duration of functional palliation.

An evaluation by Culkin et al (1987) of percutaneous nephrostomy drainage for palliation of metastatic ureteral obstruction in 27 patients revealed an increase in survival with decreased morbidity over a followup of 3 to 25 months. Mean survival for all patients (n = 19) was 6.6 months, with eight patients still alive as of this writing. Perioperative mortality was 11.1% (3/27), and postoperative complications consisted of hemorrhage requiring transfusion in 29.6% (8/27), gastrointestinal bleeding in 3.7% (1/27), and dislodged nephrostomy tube in 44.4% (12/27) of patients studied. Percutaneous nephrostomy drainage causes less morbidity than with open surgical procedures, and length of survival depends mainly on the histology of the primary tumor in patients with metastatic ureteral obstruction.

Percutaneous nephrostomy is a rapid and relatively safe form of short- or long-term management for urinary obstruction irrespective of the underlying cause. Probably the most common indication for this procedure in gynecology is urinary tract obstruction secondary to pelvic malignancy. This technique can be used to temporize renal function, to allow palliative therapy, and to assess the residual functional capacity of the obstructed kidney (Hedegaard and Wallace, 1987).

## Internal Urinary Drainage (Inlying Ureteral Stents)

Use of the inlying ureteral stent has greatly improved the quality of life of the patient with gynecologic malignancy. The inlying stent is helpful in patients undergoing urinary diversion with total pelvic exenteration as well as in those who suffer damage to the ureter during gynecologic surgery.

Spurlock et al (1987) reported on a patient with calyceal rupture and perirenal urinoma formation secondary to distal ureteral obstruction by cervical carcinoma. Preoperative diagnosis was established using CT and renal scanning. The urinoma resolved after surgical placement of a ureteral stent. In 1988, Thomas described a technique that has proved successful for stenting tortuous and dilated ureters using a combination of an open-ended catheter and a markedly floppy Bentson guidewire to negotiate the ureteral curves.

Because of substantial technologic improvements over the past 10 years, it is now also possible to bypass ureteral obstruction or fistulas by means of self-contained internal urinary stents. These stents can be inserted using transluminal percutaneous techniques if cystoscopic insertion fails (Smith et al, 1978; Smith et al, 1979; Gunther et al, 1980).

The technique of stent placement has evolved over the last 15 years (Singh et al, 1979). In 1967, Zimskind reported the use of open-end silicone tubes to bypass areas of obstruction and fistula. Three years later, Marmar was the first to recognize the importance of closing one end of the tube to allow insertion of a splint within the catheter, and multiple sideholes were introduced to improve drainage. In 1973, Orikasa et al used an additional segment of catheter as a "pusher" to hold the ureteral stent in place as the splint was withdrawn. The first significant improvement over these silicone catheters was achieved by Gibbons, who developed a silicone catheter with a distal flange to prevent its upward migration, a spiral wire for rigidity, and soft flanges to prevent expulsion (Gibbons et al, 1974, 1976).

These early catheters presented several problems. They were difficult to insert, requiring ureteral dilation. Despite the distal flange, retraction did occur, necessitating the addition of a small silicone tail to allow retrieval. Because of these drawbacks, better techniques were sought, and in 1978 Hepperlen described a J-shaped catheter that could be inserted utilizing the Seldinger approach (Seldinger, 1953; Hepperlen et al, 1978). The technique employed arterial catheters that were widely available and effectively suspended the catheter from the kidney. The catheter could be straightened using a wire stylette passed to the kidney cystoscopically through a previously placed, open No. 6 French whistle-tipped catheter.

When it was discovered that this catheter, too, could migrate upward into the renal pelvis, Finney (1978) fashioned a stent that had curves at both ends (Camach et al, 1979; Mardis et al, 1979). These *double-J ureteral stents* will be discussed in detail, since they can be used to solve most of the problems incurred during placement of inlying ureteral stents both endoscopically and at open surgery. In some cases, these more ideal catheters cannot be utilized for technical reasons; Kearney et al (1979) have outlined a technique whereby most standard ureteral catheters can be fashioned into ureteral stents to avoid the high cost of maintaining a stock of custom-made products.

Insertion of percutaneous indwelling ureteral stents was performed or attempted by Skriver et al (1987) in 10 patients with ureteral obstruction or postoperative urinary extravasation. All patients had previously undergone unsuccessful attempts at endoscopic retrograde stent placement. The percutaneous double-J stent was inserted properly in eight patients (73%) and was functionally successful in seven (64%).

Complications associated with ureteral stents include irritative bladder symptoms to the extent of trigonal erosion and compression (usually occurring with hard catheters without a J tip), upward migration (emphasizing the importance of adequate length to prevent retraction), and downward migration (principally seen with catheters without an upward J tip). Crystalloid encrustation can occur over time with any ureteral stent; however, internal crystalline obstruction within the tubing does not usually prevent the flow of urine around the catheter, so that stones rarely form in the patient with gynecologic malignancy. Microscopic hematuria and pyuria cannot be avoided, but urinary infection, including pyelonephritis, can be prevented with prophylactic antibiotics. Sterile reflux due to the stent will occur, but this presents no problems. With ureteral obstruction and/or fistula, operative palliative diversion is associated with a high operative mortality, thus making internal drainage particularly attractive.

Before diversion is carried out, the issue of quality of life should be addressed. Grabstald and McPhee (1973) have described a useful life as one in which the patient has minimal pain and few complications, possesses full mental faculties, and is able to return home for at least 2 months to participate in family life.

The ideal stent can be described as one that is (1) made of silicone (since this is softer than polyethylene, is flexible, and resists encrustation better than other materials); (2) radiopaque for easy radiologic identification; (3) of uniform diameter, without barbs that would impede passage; (4) able to pass easily in either direction during surgery as well as at cystoscopy; and (5) not likely to migrate in either direction. In addition, it should be able to withstand sterilization in the autoclave. Silicone elastomers and many plastics should not be sterilized in solutions, which are absorbed to a significant degree by these materials. Two cases of fractured polyethylene double-pigtail ureteral catheters in patients with pelvic cancer were reported by Welch et al (1985), emphasizing the need for timely replacement of stents (within 4 to 6 months). Keeping a record of all patients with stents to allow for timely recall is therefore advisable.

The double-J ureteral catheter best fulfills these criteria (Fig. 18-6). The J hooks are on either end of the stent and are angled in opposite directions so that the proximal J can hook into the lower calyx or renal pelvis while the distal J curves outward into the bladder. This

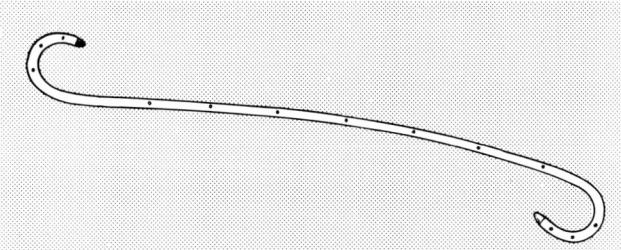

**FIGURE 18-6** Double-J ureteral stent produced by the Medical Engineering Corporation, Washington, D.C.

design prevents the distal J tip from impinging directly on the bladder mucosa and thus reduces the discomfort. The stent, produced by the Medical Engineering Corporation in Washington, D.C., is supplied in several sizes (Nos. 6, 7, and 8.5 French) and lengths (16, 26, 28, and 30 cm). The lengths listed refer to the straight portion of the stent and do not include the hooked ends. Drainage holes are located at 1-cm intervals, and the device bears standard markings at 5-cm increments for accuracy in passage.

The stent is supplied with both ends closed, but the distal end is clipped for endoscopic insertion, and the stylette wire is passed the full length to straighten the two J's. In addition, a separate pusher catheter is threaded over the stylette and inserted against the open end of the stent during retrograde catheterization (Fig. 18-7). The stylette and pusher catheter are removed by withdrawing the stylette while holding the ureteral stent in place with the pusher. During an open operation, this catheter can be passed easily through a ureterotomy or transvesically, as indicated, in which case no pusher catheter is needed. The stylette is inserted through the drainage holes to straighten the appropriate length of the ureteral stent and is passed manually through the open ureter. When the wire is withdrawn, the J will reform, thus preventing migration of the device.

If, for example, injury has occurred to the lower ureter, it is important to have the bladder filled with saline containing indigo carmine or methylene blue dye and to measure the length of ureter to the bladder with either a separate ureteral catheter or a feeding tube prior to insertion of the stent. Passing the stent into the bladder while the filled bladder is compressed manually will demonstrate free reflux of dye-stained urine into the open proximal ureter, indicating successful passage of the stent into the bladder. Failure to pass the catheter far enough may result in incorrect placement of the ureteral stent, i.e., above the ureterovesical junction, and open exploration may be necessary to retrieve it. In the case of a divided ureter, the opposite stent would be passed into the renal pelvis. The stent is later removed endoscopically as an outpatient procedure using foreign body forceps or a stylette with a small hook formed at its end. This is done easily under local anesthesia (Finney, 1978).

Inlying ureteral stents are less likely to result in infection than are stents that exit through the flank to provide external drainage. The inlying stent can be left in place for prolonged periods, and patients are usually

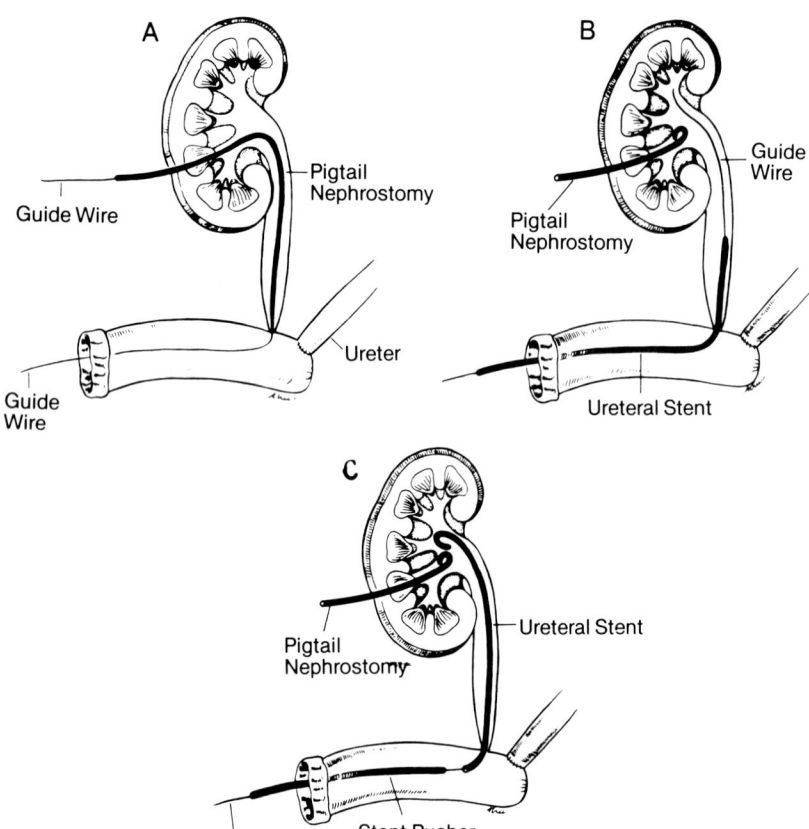

FIGURE 18-7 Placement of ureteral stent. *A*; The guidewire is advanced through the ureteral stenosis and ileal conduit. *B*, The stent is advanced proximal to the stenosis. The guidewire has been withdrawn from the pigtail nephrostomy and repositioned in the renal pelvis. *C*, The ureteral stent is now properly positioned with the proximal end in the renal pelvis and the distal end in the ileal conduit. (From Fowler JE, Jr, Raife MJ, and Sennott RI: A method for placement of a ureteral stent following supravesical intestinal diversion. *J Urol* 124:547, 1980, by permission of The Williams and Wilkins Company.)

unaware of its presence. Routinely, in a complicated case, we may leave these catheters in for several weeks to allow healing, and care must be taken to record that a stent has been placed so that it will not be left in inadvertently.

Occasionally, the ureteral catheter may retract above the ureteral junction. Retrieval can usually be carried out in a simple manner utilizing fine alligator grasping forceps under fluoroscopic control or by direct ureteroscopic maneuvers.

When endoscopic placement of a ureteral stent is not possible, an antegrade guide wire is passed beyond the obstruction and/or fistula into the bladder after percutaneous nephrostomy, the end of the wire is grasped cystoscopically, and a ureteral stent is placed either antegrade or retrograde, again obviating operative intervention (Smith et al, 1979).

Lang et al (1979) described the percutaneous antegrade introduction of ureteral stents in five patients (two with ureterovaginal fistulas, two with ureterocutaneous fistulas, and one with ureteral stricture). In all cases, stenting was followed by healing or resolution of the lesions, although in one patient with ureterovaginal fistula and in one with ureterocutaneous fistula, there was subsequent cicatricial ureteral stricture requiring further treatment.

Double stents have been routinely used in patients undergoing urinary diversion, especially with transverse colon and ileal conduits. The Medical Engineering Corporation has produced a diversionary stent 95 cm in length that has holes for the first 8 cm and can be brought through the kidney and out through the stoma;

however, we have found the short, 24-cm catheter more effective for the transverse colon conduit, fixing it with absorbable sutures to the stoma and placing it in the renal pelvis. In high-risk patients undergoing urinary diversion, especially those who have received previous radiation therapy, this additional safety measure can help avoid the catastrophic complication of leakage from the ureterocolic anastomosis.

With the earlier types of stents, the complication rate was significant. Today, there is virtually no contraindication to the use of stents. Their routine use in urologic procedures is increasing for all types of malignancies involving the genitourinary tract in both men and women. Principal gynecologic applications are in patients with carcinoma of the cervix, endometrium, or ovary or with genitourinary involvement from colonic metastases. Stents may be employed in ureteral injuries, including ureterovaginal and ureterocutaneous fistulas, and for postoperative drainage in patients undergoing ureterointestinal conduit placement, ureteroureteral anastomosis, ureteral neocystostomy, and ureterolysis. These devices can also be used for temporary drainage in case of urinary sepsis or uremia.

## Urinary Diversion

Since many of these patients have other disabilities, management of the urinary tract must be integrated with other aspects of patient care. The introduction of the colonic conduit and, more recently, the continent types of urinary diversion reflect the continued search for an ideal method (Hampel et al, 1986).

Urinary diversion may be performed as part of a pelvic exenterative procedure to treat recurrent or extensive disease, or it may be performed alone, either for palliation or for treatment of urinary tract complications. In pelvic exenteration, radical hysterectomy and lymphadenectomy are combined with removal of the bladder (anterior exenteration), rectosigmoid (posterior exenteraton), or both (total exenteration). Exenteration is not carried out as a palliative procedure; if tumor is discovered in the paraaortic lymph nodes or abdominal viscera or adherent to the pelvic sidewalls, the procedure must be discontinued.

Although exenteration is occasionally performed for severe complications of therapy, diversion without exenteration is more common in such cases, which may include patients with extensive bladder scarring after radiation. Most of these patients have undergone extensive pelvic irradiation or are candidates for future pelvic irradiation. This must be borne in mind when one is selecting the appropriate type of urinary diversion at the time of exenterative surgery.

In a study by Krause et al (1987), urologic surgery was required because of complications related to radiotherapy for gynecologic cancer in 17 patients. Four had recurrent malignant disease, and 13 had no evidence of cancer. The median interval to onset of the urologic complications was 18 months (range = 0 to 144 months). Ileal substitution was performed because of bilateral ureteral obstruction in two cases, and transureteroureterostomy was used to treat unilateral obstruction in one case. Fourteen patients who underwent urinary diversion developed vesicovaginal fistulas; the procedures included cutaneous ureterostomy and ligation of the contralateral ureter in six cases, cutaneous ureterostomy and transureteroureterostomy in three, and ileal conduit diversion in five. The diversion procedure should be selected based on the patient's fitness, her status with regard to recurrence of malignancy, and the distribution of function between the two kidneys.

Historically, the Bricker operation, which has been used since 1955, has been the standard procedure. Excellent long-term studies have now been carried out to determine the complications of this type of urinary diversion (Jaffee and Bricker, 1950; Jaffee et al, 1968; Schmidt et al, 1973).

Fallon et al (1979) have reported on 43 patients who underwent pelvic exenteration for gynecologic malignancy between 1965 and 1976 with a minimum of 2 years of followup. Thirty-four patients had been treated previously with radiation, in most cases 3,000 rads of external radiation plus one or two radium implants. Another nine patients had received no radiation therapy before undergoing surgery. The operations were performed by a team of gynecologic and urologic surgeons, with the latter performing the urinary diversions. Of the 43 cases, 24 had total and 19 had anterior exenterations. Urinary diversion included 33 ileal conduits and 8 colon conduits with 2 cutaneous ureterostomies. The ureterocolic anastomoses were not stented and were effected with 4-0 chromic catgut sutures. No antireflux tunnels were created.

Six patients experienced significant early urologic complications, three of whom had undergone ileal conduit diversion and three colonic diversion. All three patients with colonic diversion developed ureteroileal fistulas, two of which resolved spontaneously with observation and one of which required unilateral nephrostomy. Among those patients with ileal conduits, a ureteroileal anastomotic fistula occurred in one, a conduit-vaginal fistula occurred in the second, and conduit ischemia developed in the third; in the last patient, a new urinary conduit had to be created, and the patient died during the postoperative period. The patient with the ureterocolic anastomotic leak had bilateral nephrostomies and died in the postoperative period as well (Fallon et al, 1979).

We have reviewed some of the common problems associated with urinary diversion. In exenteration, the main problem with ileal conduit or low sigmoid conduit diversion or the use of cecum is that this tissue falls within the irradiated field, so that the probability that stricture or fistula will develop at the anastomotic site is greater. The transverse colon is uniquely suited for the gynecologic patient because both the bowel segment utilized and the anastomosis between the ureter and the colon are above the irradiated field. The incidence of stomal stenosis is lower with the transverse colon, and this type of bowel can be used in either an isoperistalic or a reverse peristaltic mode. Antirefluxing intestinal anastomoses can be performed to reduce the possibility of pyelonephritis in the young patient with a high likelihood of cure, although in the vast majority of gynecologic patients this is unnecessary.

We prefer to use the transverse colon rather than the sigmoid colon, since the sigmoid colon may still lie within the irradiated field, and while the advantage of eliminating a bowel anastomosis is attractive, this approach will generally convert a dry-end sigmoid colostomy to a wet proximal colostomy.

The versatility and other advantages of the transverse colon conduit for urinary diversion have been described and implemented in 50 patients (Schmidt and Buchsbaum, 1986). The transverse colon segment is indicated for primary supravesical diversion as well as for salvage of problems related to ileal conduits *especially after radiation therapy.*

Fifty-five patients with advanced carcinoma of the cervix and vesicovaginal fistula were managed with urinary diversion using the transverse colon as a conduit in a surgical technique described by Kisner and Kesner (1987). This form of urinary diversion is recommended for such patients. The review by Orr et al (1982) of 119 pelvic exenterations performed between 1969 and 1981 illustrates our approach to the management of this problem. Of the 115 who had a concurrent supravesical urinary diversion, 56 had an anterior exenteration and 59 had total exenteration. An ileal segment was used in 97 patients and a transverse colon conduit in 16; two sigmoid conduits were utilized. In 85 patients, intestinal anastomoses were constructed using gastrointestinal staplers, resulting in a significantly shortened mean operating time. Ureteral stents were used routinely. In all patients, closure of the pelvic defect was attempted using peritoneal flaps, omental grafts, or a sigmoid lid to prevent late bowel obstruction.

There were no significant gastrointestinal complications. Clinical pyelonephritis developed in 24 patients (20.9%); no difference was noted between the transverse colon and ileal conduit groups. Among the patients with ileal conduits, 10.3% experienced a urinary leak or fistula despite use of the ureteral stent. There were no urinary fistulas or leaks in the small number of patients who received the transverse colon conduit. Of those patients with urinary fistula, six underwent a second operative procedure, and three of these patients died (50%). This result reflects the general experience that reoperation is associated with a high mortality rate in patients who have undergone urinary diversion complicated by fistula. Those patients who did well and were treated conservatively with spontaneous healing of the fistula generally fared much better. The reported incidence of urinary leak or fistula after urinary diversion for exenteration ranges between 5 and 22%, depending on the type of intestinal conduit, the nature of the surgery, and whether ureteral stents are used (Symmons et al, 1948; Barber and Brunschwig, 1966; Schoenberg and Makuta, 1973; Schmidt et al, 1976; Rutledge et al, 1977; Schlesinger et al, 1979).

Currently, for all patients undergoing urinary diversion, a transverse colon conduit is considered the procedure of choice if there is a history or possibility of radiation therapy (Fig. 18-8) (Schmidt et al, 1975). A gastrointestinal stapler (GIA or TA-55) [see Chapter 19] is used in all procedures. We have had no problems with this approach using the double-J ureteral stent in all patients. The anastomosis is created over the stent, which is anchored to the stoma with nonabsorbable suture. If the viability of the ureter is in question at the time of anastomosis, the stent should be left in for a prolonged period of time (i.e., in excess of 2 to 3 weeks), with a drain placed at the butt end of the loop. Routinely, in patients in whom the ureter is considered to be of good quality, a drain associated with the pelvic portion of the procedure is utilized. In this manner, if a leak develops later, the fistula will drain as a cutaneous fistula. A drainage tract can be easily reestablished, with the expectation of spontaneous closure.

If spontaneous closure does not occur, percutaneous nephrostomy is performed with vacuum suction of the conduit. When a gastrointestinal stapler has been used,

it has been our practice to remove the staples from the butt end of the loop and close this area in a conventional two-layer fashion, with chromic sutures for the inner layer and Lembert nonabsorbable sutures for the outer layer. It has been stated that if the stapler alone is used, stones do occur; however, these tend to be small and to pass spontaneously, and are of little clinical significance unless an augmentation procedure is planned. Our technique of creating a transverse colon conduit is similar to that described by Schmidt et al (1975).

The patient undergoes extensive mechanical cleansing with a mild laxative, liquid diet, and enemas, followed by an oral antimicrobial agent with neomycin and erythromycin base immediately prior to surgery. High-dose intravenous aminoglycosides are given immediately preoperatively. A long midline incision is used to facilitate the exenterative procedure. The conduit may be created either before or after the pelvic portion of the procedure. If creation of the conduit precedes exenteration, the stoma should not be created until afterward to prevent traction on the ureterocolic anastomosis. Virtually the entire length of transverse colon is utilized, since dramatic shortening of the conduit can occur after division [Fig. 18-9]. Great care should be taken not to place traction on the splenocolic ligament, since the splenic capsule tears easily. Blood supplied from the middle colic artery is easily noted, generally without the need for transillumination of the mesocolon. The greater omentum is dissected away from the superior surface of the transverse colon, and mesenteric vessels are ligated with fine suture. Bowel continuity is reestablished with the GIA and TA-55, with the conduit inferior to the bowel anastomosis.

Over a small kidney basin, the proximal and blind end of the divided conduit is opened, and the intestinal contents are irrigated with neomycin solution until the effluent is clear. A decision is then made as to which end of the conduit will be the stomal end. In general, we have found that placing the conduit in reverse peristaltic fashion provides the best mobility. The butt end of the loop

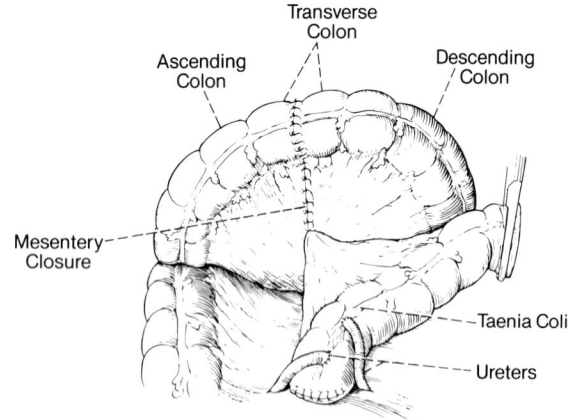

FIGURE 18-8 Completed urinary conduit using the transverse colon with placement of ureterocolic anastomoses in the taenia coli.

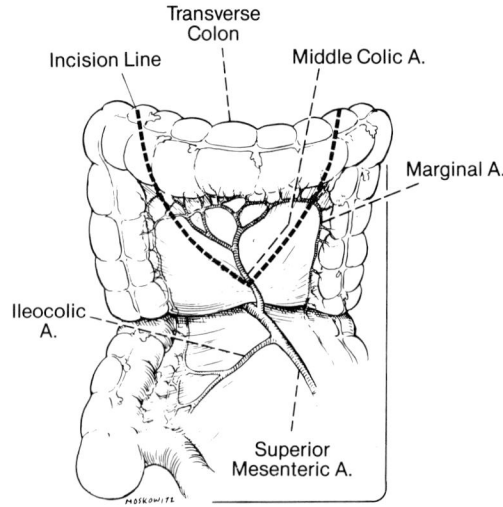

FIGURE 18-9 Segment of transverse colon used for a urinary conduit. Note that the line of incision in the mesentery requires most of the transverse colon. The blood supply to the urinary conduit is based on the middle colic artery.

is then closed with loosely running chromic suture that is pulled tight after the bowel clamp has been removed. A second layer of interrupted 4-0 silk Lembert sutures with a carefully placed corner stitch completes the anastomosis.

The ureters have been previously dissected proximally, in the retroperitoneal space to the level of the renal pelvis, and brought anteriorly through small stab wounds adjacent to the proximal portion of the colon conduit. Great care is taken to achieve a gentle curve without kinking of the right ureter anterior to the duodenum or of the left ureter anterior to the great vessels. The operator then creates the ureterocolic anastomoses in end-to-end fashion without attempting an antireflux procedure on the taenia; these anastomoses are performed over an 8.5 double-J ureteral stent. Absorbable interrupted 4-0 chromic catgut or polyglycolate sutures are used with all knots on the outside.

No attempt is made to reperitonealize the anastomosis or suture the butt end of the loop to the parietal peritoneum. Stomal position is established at a later time, after a decision has been made as to whether the pelvic colon should be divided as well. In general, a right upper quadrant stoma through the rectus muscle is utilized. A full-thickness core of abdominal wall, fascia, rectus muscle, and posterior peritoneum is removed. The seromuscular portion of the conduit is sutured to the anterior abdominal fascia at four quadrants. Lastly, subcuticular skin is approximated to the distal end of the conduit with absorbable 2-0 chromic catgut suture.

Wound closure is performed in a routine fashion using internal retention sutures of 1-0 proline with near-far, far-near sutures without external retention sutures. A temporary urostomy appliance is utilized for the first 5 days. Drainage of the urinary conduit is carried out only in specific high-risk circumstances in addition to the routine drains associated with cystectomy or exenteration. We believe that early serious urinary complications can be avoided by instituting routine ureteral stent drainage.

## Palliative Diversion

Palliative urinary diversion as performed in patients with advanced pelvic malignancy has virtually no place in the treatment of patients with gynecologic malignancy. Meyer et al (1980) reviewed their experience with 90 patients with pelvic malignancy and bilateral ureteral obstruction treated with *open surgical nephrostomy*. Eighty-three patients underwent bilateral nephrostomies, three had unilateral skin ureterostomies, and three had ileal loop diversions. Forty-four patients had carcinoma of the cervix, 19 had carcinoma of the bladder, and 12 had colonic tumors. The median survival for these 90 patients was 3.3 months, with a mean survival of 8.5 months. Forty-two per cent (38 of 90) did not leave the hospital after urinary diversion. The younger population (27 to 49 years) had a significantly shorter survival time, with a median survival of 2 months.

In 1979, Holden et al addressed the issue of the value of palliative urinary diversion in nephrostomies in 218 consecutive uremic patients. This report described six patients who died as a direct result of the nephrostomy

complications—a significant immediate postoperative mortality. They reviewed the outcome of diversions performed in unselected patients between 1955 and 1974. Their series included 94 men and 124 women; carcinoma of the cervix was the most common diagnosis (70 patients). Unilateral nephrostomies were performed in 167 patients. Twelve patients had minor complications (e.g., catheters falling out or urinary infection). Major life-threatening complications occurred in 99 patients (45%). Patient survival was broken down by stage: stage A patients had localized disease confined to the organ of origin, stage B patients had local extension or regional nodal metastasis, and stage C patients had disseminated disease. Among the stage A patients, 88% were alive 2 years after nephrostomy. In contrast, 32 and 49% of patients in stages B and C, respectively, died within 2 months.

Based on this and other studies, palliative urinary diversion, if carried out in selected patients, can clearly result in a useful life with minimal pain and few complications (Brin et al, 1975). In addition, diversion should be carried out only in patients in whom further therapy holds promise for survival with advanced disease or in those who have diseases with an unpredictable natural history.

At present, open nephrostomy is probably rarely indicated. There are many newer techniques in which inlying ureteral stents can be placed under local anesthesia, obviating the morbidity of an operative procedure.

In patients whom this approach is not possible, percutaneous nephrostomy offers an alternative means of palliative diversion in patients with short-term survival. Irrespective of the underlying cause, it is a less morbid procedure than open surgical procedures under anesthesia. The main determinant of length of survival is the histology of the primary tumor in patients with metastatic ureteral obstruction. Percutaneous nephrostomy should be considered for relief of ureteral obstruction in patients with untreated cervical carcinoma who may enjoy prolonged palliation or cure, in patients with complications of previous urinary conduits as a temporizing method of urinary diversion, and in patients with benign or chemotherapy-sensitive pelvic malignancies causing ureteral obstruction.

Percutaneous nephrostomy, if carried out on a temporary basis, can gradually be converted to an adequate permanent nephrostomy with the use of fascial dilators and progressively larger catheters.

*Cutaneous ureterostomy* is uniquely suited for supravesical urinary diversion in patients whose short-term life expectancy is limited but satisfactory, especially the high-risk patient with a solitary functioning kidney. This technique has the significant advantage of providing an extraperitoneal supravesical urinary diversion without requiring a colonic anastomosis. The stoma is brought out through the anterior abdominal wall and can be easily cared for. Unlike conduit diversion, this operation does not require prolonged bowel preparation and is effective, particularly in high-risk patients with poor nutrition.

The kidney is mobilized through a transverse extraperitoneal incision from within Gerota's fascia. The lower pole of the kidney is rotated anteriorly, and a formal nephropexy to the anterior abdominal musculature is carried out. The ureter is brought out in a straight line from the renal pelvis to the anterior abdominal wall via a small incision made through the rectus muscle and anterior rectus fascia. A small horseshoe incision is made in the skin, the spatulated ureter is stented with an inlying 8.5 double-J ureteral stent, and the skin-to-ureteral anastomosis is then created. If two functioning renal units exist, one may consider the options of contralateral nephrectomy and/or angiographic infarction. When two renal units are needed in cases of marginal renal function, it is recommended that one kidney at a time be diverted, with measurements of total renal function. If the creatinine clearance is greater than 22 ml/min/m$^2$, the contralateral kidney can be sacrificed if the patient has a limited life expectancy (Harrison, 1982).

Over a 21-year period (1963 to 1984), 46 patients underwent permanent urinary diversion using cutaneous ureterostomy (MacGregor et al, 1987). In 37 patients, this method of diversion was employed for palliation in pelvic malignancies. In 70%, diversion was carried out secondary to ureteral obstruction, while in the others it was performed to relieve lower urinary tract symptoms or because of failure of an alternative form of diversion. Although cutaneous ureterostomy is no longer indicated as a primary form of palliative diversion, it may be used as an alternative to open nephrostomy tube placement or intestinal conduit should other, more conservative forms of management fail.

Schutten et al (1987) treated 24 patients who had a malignant pelvic mass with a diverting cutaneous ureterostomy. Necrosis developed in four cases (17%), and one patient (4%) required surgical correction to relieve stenosis. The remaining patients had a well-functioning ureterocutaneostomy until death, which occurred on average 174 days later.

In patients with ureteral obstruction due to tumor and/or fibrosis whose nonobstructed kidney is functionally impaired, *transureteroureterostomy* may be a valuable option for renal preservation if the bladder has been irradiated (Hendren and Hensle, 1980; Hodges et al, 1980). Infection, calculous disease, retroperitoneal fibrosis, and tuberculosis are contraindications to this procedure. Frozen sections of the ureter used for the anastomosis should be examined to ensure normal anatomy and rule out cancer. The ureter should cross above the inferior mesenteric artery, and the anastomosis should be tension free. One should not mobilize the recipient ureter in such a way that angulation would result.

# REFERENCES

Alfert HJ, Gillenwater JY: The consequences of ureteral irradiation with special reference to subsequent ureteral injury. *J Urol* 107:369, 1972.

Anderson CB: Recurrent carcinoma of cervix: Cause of proximal bilateral ureteral obstruction. *Urology* 2:454, 1973.

Bahrassa F, Ampil F: Posttreatment ureteral obstruction in invasive carcinoma of uterine cervix. *Int J Radiat Oncol Biol Phys* 13:23, 1987.

Barber HRK, Brunschwig A: Urinary tract fistulas following pelvic exenteration. *Obstet Gynecol* 28:754, 1966.

Barber HRK, Brunschwig A: Definitive treatment of radiation necrosis: 5-year results in 77 patients. *Obstet Gynecol* 35:344, 1970.

Brin EN, Schiff J Jr, Weiss RN: Palliative urinary diversion for pelvic malignancy. *J Urol* 113:619, 1975.

Brunschwig A, Frick HC: Urinary tract fistulas following radical surgery treatment of carcinoma of the cervix (exclusive of exenterations). *Am J Obstet Gynecol* 72:479, 1956.

Buchsbaum HJ, Schmidt JD: *Gynecologic and Obstetric Urology.* Philadelphia, WB Saunders, 1978, p 363.

Bugbee HG: Ureteral occlusion following radium implantation into the cervix. *J Urol* 32:439, 1934.

Calame RJ, Nelson JH Jr: Ureterovaginal fistula as a complication of radical pelvic surgery. *Arch Surg* 94:876, 1967.

Camach MF, Pereiris R, Carrion H, Bondhus M, Politano VA: Double end pig-tail ureteral stent: Useful modification of a single ended ureteral stent. *Urology* 13:516, 1979.

Celoria G, Steingrub J, Dawson JA, Teres D: Oliguria from high intra-abdominal pressure secondary to ovarian mass. *Crit Care Med* 15:78, 1987.

Chau TM, Fletcher GH, Rutledge FN, Dodge DG Jr: Complications in high-dose whole pelvis radiation in female pelvic cancer. *Am J Roentgenol* 87:22, 1962.

Cherry CP, Glücksmann A, Dearing R, Ways S: Observations on lymph node involvement in carcinoma of the cervix. *J Obstet Gynaecol Br Commonw* 60:368, 1953.

Cosbie WG: The complications of irradiation treatment of carcinoma of the cervix. *Am J Obstet Gynecol* 42:1003, 1941.

Cowan PN: False cytodiagnosis of bladder malignancy due to previous radiotherapy. *Br J Urol* 47:405, 1975.

Culkin DJ, Wheeler JJ, Marsans RE, Nam SI, Canning JR: Percutaneous nephrostomy for palliation of metastatic ureteral obstruction. *Urology* 30(3):229, 1987.

Dean RJ, Lytton B: Urological complications of pelvic radiation. *J Urol* 119:64, 1978.

Douglas RG, Birnbaum SF: Urological complications following radiological and surgical treatment of carcinoma of the cervix. *South Med J* 47:559, 1954.

Duncan RE, Bennett DW, Evans AT, et al: Radiation-induced bladder tumors. *J Urol* 118:43, 1977.

Drexler LS, Howes WE: Ureteral obstruction in carcinoma of the cervix. *Am J Obstet Gynecol* 28:197, 1934.

Ebner F, Kressel HY, Mintz MC, Carlson JA, Cohen EK, Schiebler M, Gefter W, Axel L: Tumor recurrence vs. fibrosis in the female pelvis: Differentiation with MR at 1.5.T. *Radiology* 166:333, 1988.

Fallon B, Loening S, Hawtrey CE, Lifshitz SG, Buchsbaum HJ: Urologic complications of pelvic exenteration for gynecologic malignancy. *J Urol* 122:159, 1979.

Finney RP: Experience with new double-J ureteral catheter stent. *J Urol* 120:678, 1978.

Fraser AC: The late effects of Wertheim's hysterectomy on the urinary tract. *J Obstet Gynaecol Br Commonw* 73:1002, 1966.

Gibbons RP, Correa RJ Jr, Cummings KB, Mason JT: Experience with inlying ureteral stent catheters. *J Urol* 115:222, 1976.

Gibbons RP, Mason JT, Correa RJ Jr: Experience with indwelling silicone rubber ureteral stents. *J Urol* 111:594, 1974.

Goldberg DM: Changes in intestinal and renal function after pelvic irradiation: Correlation of clinical and experimental observations. *Clin Radiol* 23:225, 1972.

Grabstald H, McPhee M: Nephrostomy and the cancer patient. *South Med J* 66:217, 1973.

Gray MJ, Kottmeier HL: Rectal and bladder injuries following radium therapy for carcinoma of the cervix at the Radiumhemmet. *Am J Obstet Gynecol* 74:1294, 1957.

Gunther R, Altwein JE, Alken P: Internal urinary diversion by percutaneous ureteral splint. *Br J Urol* 52:165, 1980.

Hampel N, Bodner DR, Persky L: Ileal and jejunal conduit urinary diversion. *Urol Clin North Am* 13(2): 207, 1986.

Harrison JH: Personal communication, 1982.

Hedegaard CK, Wallace D: Percutaneous nephrostomy: Current indications and potential uses in obstetrics and gynecology. Literature review and report of a case. *Obstet Gynecol Surv* 42:671, 1987.

Hedlund H, Lindstedt E: Urovaginal fistulas: 20 years of experience with 45 cases. *J Urol* 137:926, 1987.

Hendren WH, Hensle TW: Transureteroureterostomy: Experience with 75 cases. *J Urol* 123:826, 1980.

Hepperlen TW, Mardis HK, Kammandel H: Self-retained internal ureteral stents: A new approach. *J Urol* 119:731, 1978.

Heron CW, Husband JE, Williams MP, Dobbs HJ, Cosgrove DO: The value of CT in the diagnosis of recurrent carcinoma of the cervix. *Clin Radiol* 39:496, 1988.

Hodges CV, Barry JM, Fuchs EF, Pearse HD, Tank ES: Transureter-oureterostomy: 25-year experience with 100 patients. *J Urol* 123:834, 1980.

Holden S, McPhee M, Grabstald H: The rationale of urinary diversion in cancer patients. *J Urol* 121:19, 1979.

Hricak H, Lacey CG, Sandles SG, Chang YC, Winkler ML, Stern JL: Invasive cervical carcinoma: Comparison of MR imaging and surgical findings. *Radiology* 166:623, 1988.

Hricak H, Stern JL, Fisher MR, Shapeero LG, Winkler ML, Lacey CG: Endometrial carcinoma staging by MR imaging. *Radiology* 160:431, 1986.

Ignatoff JM, Graham JB: Bilateral ureterovaginal fistula. *Urology* 4:585, 1974.

Jaffee BM, Bricker EM: Bladder substitution after pelvic evisceration. *Surg Clin North Am* 30:1511, 1950.

Jaffee BM, Bricker EM, Butcher HR Jr: Surgical complication of ileal segment diversion. *Ann Surg* 167:367, 1968.

Katayama H, Kozuta T, Takashima T, Matsuura K, Yamaguchi K: Adverse reactions to contrast media: High-osmolality vs. low-osmolality media (Abstract). *Radiology* 169:421, 1988.

Kearney GP, Mahoney EM, Brown HP: Useful technique for long-term urinary drainage by inlying ureteral stent. *Urology* 14:126, 1979.

Keettel WC, Sehring FG, de Prosse CA, Scott JR: Surgical management of urethrovaginal and vesicovaginal fistulas. *Am J Obstet Gynecol* 131:425, 1978.

Kiricuta I, Goldstein AMB: The repair of extensive vesicovaginal fistulas with pedicled omentum: A review of 27 cases. *J Urol* 108:724, 1972.

Kisner CD, Kesner KM: Use of the transverse colon conduit for vesicovaginal fistula in late-stage carcinoma of the cervix. *Br J Urol* 59:234, 1987.

Kottmeier HL, Gray MJ: Rectal and bladder injuries in relation to high radiation dosage in carcinoma of the cervix: A five-year followup. *Am J Obstet Gynecol* 82:74, 1961.

Krause S, Hald T, Steven K: Surgery for urologic complications following radiotherapy for gynecologic cancer. *Scand J Urol Nephrol* 21:115, 1987.

Kursh ED, Morse RM, Resnick MI, Persky L: Prevention of the development of a vesicovaginal fistula. *Surg Gynecol Obstet* 166:409, 1988.

Lang EK, Wood M, Brown R, Pirkle TN, Johnson B, Right JR, Chance HL, Trichel DE, St. Barton DC: Complications within the urinary tract related to treatment of carcinoma of the cervix. *South Med J* 66:228, 1973.

Lang EK, Lanasa JA, Garrett J, Stripling J, Palomar J: The management of urinary fistulas and strictures with percutaneous ureteral stent catheters. *J Urol* 122:736, 1979.

Lasser EC, Berry CC, Talner LB, Santini LC, Lang EK, Gerber FH, Stolberg HO: Pretreatment with corticosteroids to alleviate reactions to intravenous contrast media. *N Engl J Med* 317:845, 1987.

Luciani L, Scappini P, Pusiol T, Piscioli F: The role of aspiration cytology in the management of ureteral obstruction in patients with known cancer. *Cancer* 59:1936, 1987.

MacGregor PS, Montie JE, Straffon RA: Cutaneous ureterostomy as palliative diversion in adults with malignancy. *Urology* 30:31, 1987.

Maillet PJ, Pelle FD, Leriche A, Leclercq R, Demiaux C: Fistulas of the upper urinary tract: Percutaneous management. *J Urol* 138:1382, 1987.

Mallik MD: A study of the ureters following Wertheim's hysterectomy. *J Obstet Gynaecol Br Emp* 67:556, 1960.

Mann WJ, Arato M, Patsner B, Stone ML: Ureteral injuries in an obstetrics and gynecology training program: Etiology and management. *Obstet Gynecol* 72:82, 1988.

Mardis HK, Hepperlen TW, Kammandel H: Double pig-tail ureteral stent. *Urology* 14:23, 1979.

Marmar JL: The management of ureteral obstruction with silicone rubber splint catheters. *J Urol* 104:386, 1970.

Marziale P: Renal function after Wertheim-Meigs operation for cervical cancer. *Gynecol Oncol* 8:27, 1979.

Masterson BJ, Rutledge F: Irradiation ulcer of the urinary bladder. *Obstet Gynecol* 30:23, 1967.

Mattingly RF, Borkowf HI: Acute operative injury to the lower urinary tract. *Clin Obstet Gynaecol* 5:123, 1978.

Meyer JE, Yatsuhashi M, Green TH: Palliative urinary diversion in patients with advanced pelvic malignancies. *Cancer* 45:2968, 1980.

Mickal A, Torres JE, Schlosser JV: Complications of the therapy for carcinoma of the cervix. *Am J Obstet Gynecol* 112:556, 1972.

Mikuta JJ, Giuntoli RL, Rubin EL, et al: The "problem" radical hysterectomy. *Am J Obstet Gynecol* 128:119, 1977.

Miller WA, Spear JL: Periureteral and ureteral metastases from carcinoma of the cervix. *Radiology* 107:533, 1973.

Million RR, Rutledge F, Fletch GH: Stage IV carcinoma of the cervix with bladder invasion. *Am J Obstet Gynecol* 113:239, 1972.

Mitty H: CT for diagnosis and management of urinary extravasation. *Am J Radiol* 134:497, 1980.

Morley GW, Lindenauer SM, Cerny JC: Pelvic exenterative surgery in recurrent pelvic carcinoma. *Am J Obstet Gynecol* 109:1175, 1971.

Morrow CP, DiSaia PJ, Townsend DE: Current management of endometrial carcinoma. *Obstet Gynecol* 42:399, 1973.

Morton DG: Surgical treatment of cervical cancer; Wertheim operation; pelvic lymphadenectomy. *Am J Roentgenol* 57:685, 1947.

Nordling JH, Meyhoff HH: Dissociation of urethral and anal sphincter activity in neurogenic bladder dysfunction. *J Urol* 122:352, 1979.

Nordling JH, Meyhoff HH, Hald T, Gerstenberg T, Walter S, Christensen NJ: Urethral denervation supersensitivity to noradrenaline after radical hysterectomy. *Scand J Urol Nephrol* 15:21, 1981.

Öbrink A, Bunne G: Gracilis interposition in fistulas following radio-therapy for cervical cancer. *Urol Int* 33:370, 1978.

O'Conor VJ Jr: Review of experience with vesicovaginal fistula repair. *J Urol* 123:367, 1980.

O'Conor VJ Jr, Sokol JK, Bulkley GJ, Nanninga JB: Suprapubic closure of vesicovaginal fistula. *J Urol* 109:51, 1973.

Orikasa S, Tsuji I, Siba T, Ohashi N: New technique for transurethral insertion of silicone rubber into an obstructed ureter. *J Urol* 110:184, 1973.

Orr JW, Shingleton HM, Hatch KD, Taylor PT, Austin JM Jr, Partridge EE, Soong SJ: Urinary diversion in patients undergoing pelvic exenteration. *Am J Obstet Gynecol* 142:883, 1982.

Parente JT: Metastases in cancer of the cervix. *Am J Surg* 99:343, 1960.

Parkin DE, Davis JA, Symonds RP: Long-term bladder symptomatology following radiotherapy for cervical carcinoma. *Radiother Oncol* 9:195, 1987.

Parliament M, Genest P, Girard A, Gerig L, Prefontaine M: Obstructive ureteropathy following radiation therapy for carcinoma of the cervix. *Gynecol Oncol* 33:237, 1989.

Pedersen H, Juul N: Ultrasound-guided percutaneous nephrostomy in the treatment of advanced gynecologic malignancy. *Acta Obstet Gynaecol Scand* 67:199-201, 1988.

Pellman C, Sall S, Calanog A: The relief of ureteral obstruction by internal ureteral stent in patients with gynecologic malignancy. *Gynecol Oncol* 5:152, 1977.

Perch GA: Carcinoma of the cervix involving the upper urinary tract. *J Urol* 106:562, 1971.

Prentiss RJ, Mullenix RB: Management of ureteral injuries in pelvic surgery. *JAMA* 145:1244, 1951.

Rhamy RK, Stander RW: Postradiation ureteral stricture. *Surg Gynecol Obstet* 113:615, 1961.

Rhamy RK, Stander RW: Pyelographic analysis of radiation therapy in carcinoma of the cervix. *Am J Obstet Gynecol* 87:41, 1962.

Richie JP, Withers G, Ehrlich RM: Ureteral obstruction secondary to metastatic tumors. *Surg Gynecol Obstet* 148:355, 1979.

Rotman J, John MJ, Moon SH, Choi KN, Stowe SM, Abitol A, Herskovic T, Sall S: Limitations of adjunctive surgery in carcinoma of the cervix. *Int J Radiat Oncol Biol Phys* 5:327, 1979.

Ruponen S, Grönroos M, Mäkinen E, et al: Prognostic value of urography in irradiated cervical carcinoma. *Ann Chir Gynaecol Fenn* 63:127, 1974.

Rutledge FN, Smith JP, Wharton JT, O'Quinn EG: Pelvic exenteration: Analysis of 296 patients. *Am J Obstet Gynecol* 149:881, 1977.

Samuels BI, Silver TM: Diagnostic ultrasound in the evaluation of patients with gynecologic cancer. *Surg Clin North Am* 58(1):3, 1978.

Schlesinger RE, Ballon SC, Watring WG, Moore JG: Choice of intestinal segment for urinary conduit in surgical gynecological obstetrics. *Surg Gynecol Obstet* 148:445, 1979.

Schmidt JD, Buchsbaum HJ: Transverse colon conduit diversion. *Urol Clin North Am* 13(2):233, 1986.

Schmidt JD, Buchsbaum HJ, Jacoby EC: Transverse colon conduit for supravesical urinary tract diversion. *Urology* 8:542, 1976.

Schmidt JD, Hawtrey CE, Buchsbaum HJ: Transverse colon conduit: Preferred method of urinary diversion for radiation-treated pelvic malignancies. *J Urol* 113:308, 1975.

Schmidt JD, Hawtrey CE, Flocks RH, Coe DA: Complications, results and problems of ileal conduit diversion. *J Urol* 109:210, 1973.

Schoenberg W, Makuta JJ: Technique for preventing urinary fistulas following pelvic exenteration and ureteroileostomy. *J Urol* 110:294, 1973.

Schutten BT, Teilum D, Sondergaard O, Fischer AB: Cutaneous ureterostomy in cancer patients. *Scand J Urol Nephrol* 21:159, 1987.

Scola FH, Cronan JJ, Schepps B: Grade 1 hydronephrosis: Pulsed Doppler ultrasound evaluation. *Radiology* 171:519, 1989.

Seldinger SI: Catheter replacement of the needle in percutaneous arteriography: A new technique. *Acta Radiol* 39:360, 1953.

Shingleton HM, Fowler WC Jr, Pepper FD Jr, et al: Ureteral strictures following therapy for carcinoma of the cervix. *Cancer* 24:77, 1969.

Singh B, Kim H, Wax SH: Stent vs. nephrostomy: Is there a choice? *J Urol* 121:268, 1979.

Skriver EB, Miskowiak J, Mygind T: Percutaneous introduction of double-J ureteral stents. *Scand J Urol Nephrol* 21:47, 1987.

Smith AD, Lang PH, Renke DB, Miller RP: Extraction of ureteral calculi from patients with ileal loops: A new technique. *J Urol* 120:623, 1978.

Smith AD, Miller RP, Renke DB, Lang PH, Greeley EE: Insertion of the Gibbons ureteral stent using endourological techniques. *Urology* 14:330, 1979.

Soper JT, Blaszczyk TM, Oke E, Clarke PD, Creasman WT: Percutaneous nephrostomy in gynecologic oncology patients. *Am J Obstet Gynecol* 158:1126, 1988.

Spataro RF: New and old contrast agents: Pharmacology, tissue opacification, and excretory urography. *Urol Radiol* 10:2, 1988.

Spurlock JW, Burke TW, Dunn NP, Heller PB, Collins HS, Park RC: Calyceal rupture with perirenal urinoma in a patient with cervical carcinoma. *Obstet Gynecol* 70(3PT2):511, 1987.

Stanley RJ, Lee JKT: Value of CT in detection of lymphatic metastases from tumors of genitourinary tract origin (Abstract). *Radiologic Society of North America Annual Meeting*, 1980.

Steckel RJ, Collins JD, Snow HD, et al: Radiation protection of the normal kidney by selective arterial infusions. *Cancer* 34:1046, 1974.

Stern JL, Maroney TP, Lacey CG: Management of incurable urinary fistulas by percutaneous ureteral occlusion. *Obstet Gynecol* 70:958, 1987.

Swann RW, Rutledge FN: Urinary conduit in pelvic cancer patients: A report of 16 years' experience. *Am J Obstet Gynecol* 119:6, 1974.

Symmons RE, Pratt JH, Welsh JS: Exenteration operations: Experience with 118 patients. *Am J Obstet Gynecol* 101:66, 1948.

Thomas R: Catheterizing a tortuous ureter. *J Urol* 140:778, 1988.

Togashi K, Nishimura K, Itoh K, Fujisawa I, Asato R, Nakano Y, Itoh H, Torizuka K, Ozasa H, Mori T: Uterine cervical cancer: Assessment with high-field MR imaging. *Radiology* 160:431, 1986.

Underwood PB Jr, Lutz MH, Smoak DL: Ureteral injury following irradiation therapy for carcinoma of the cervix. *Obstet Gynecol* 49:663, 1977.

Van Nagell JR Jr, Sprague AD, Roddick JW: The effect of intravenous pyelography and cystoscopy on the staging of cervical cancer. *Gynecol Oncol* 3:87, 1975.

Walsh JW, Amendola MA, Hall DJ, Tisnado J, Goplerud DR: Recurrent carcinoma of the cervix: CT diagnosis. *Am J Radiol* 136:117, 1981.

Walsh JW, Brewer WH, Schneider V: Ultrasound diagnosis in diseases of the uterine corpus and cervix. *Semin Ultrasound* 1:30, 1980.

Welch RA, Malviya VK, Deppe G: Fractured ureteral catheters in gynecologic oncology. *Gynecol Oncol* 22:356, 1985.

Wesolowski S: Bilateral ureteral injuries in gynecology. *Br J Urol* 41:666, 1969.

Widholm O, Mattsson T: Urinary tract infections in association with radium therapy for gynecologic cancer. *Acta Obstet Gynaecol Scand* 51:247, 1972.

Zadra JA, Jewett MA, Keresteci AG, et al: Nonoperative urinary diversion for malignant ureteral obstruction. *Cancer* 60:1353, 1987.

Zimskind PE, Fetter TR, Wilkerson JL: Clinical use of the long-term indwelling silicone rubber ureteral splints inserted cystoscopically. *J Urol* 97:840, 1967.

# Chapter 19

# Gastrointestinal Operations in Gynecologic Oncology

*Neville F. Hacker*  *Jonathan S. Berek*
*Leo D. Lagasse*

In patients with gynecologic malignancies, the gastrointestinal tract may be involved because of local extension of disease from the cervix, vagina, or vulva or distant dissemination from ovarian cancer. In addition, bowel complications of therapy, particularly radiotherapy, may necessitate medical or surgical intervention. Therefore, a thorough understanding of the principles of gastrointestinal surgery is mandatory for the surgical management of these patients.

In some cases, such as bowel obstruction or fistula, the need for bowel surgery is known in advance, and appropriate planning can be carried out. More frequently, however, especially in the management of patients with ovarian cancer, the need for bowel surgery may not be apparent until the abdomen has been opened and explored. Therefore, when one is operating on patients with ovarian cancer, it is important to anticipate the possible need for bowel resection, initiate suitable preoperative bowel preparation, and assemble a surgical team capable of dealing with any eventuality. Clearly, it would be desirable for the operating surgeon to be both facile in gynecologic and gastrointestinal surgical techniques and well acquainted with the relevant disease processes.

## PREOPERATIVE INVESTIGATIONS

In women under 40 years of age with no symptoms or signs referable to the bowel, Hemoccult testing of the stool at the time of rectal examination is the only preoperative gastrointestinal investigation required. In older women, a barium enema or colonoscopy should be performed to exclude concurrent primary bowel cancer in patients with a pelvic mass. There is a known association between primary colonic cancer and cancer of the ovary (Lynch et al, 1981). Gastrointestinal malignancies, particularly of the colon, may also metastasize to ovaries. Such metastases may be solid but are more often predominantly cystic, may be very large, and may closely simulate primary ovarian cancer (Scully, 1979).

If the bowel is obstructed, erect and supine abdominal films will reveal dilated loops of bowel, usually with fluid levels evident in the erect films. Jejunum is characterized by valvulae conniventes, i.e., mucosal folds that are regularly spaced and resemble a concertina. These become much less prominent in the ileum. The colon, except for the cecum, shows haustral folds

and is situated more peripherally. Unlike the valvulae conniventes, haustral folds are spaced irregularly, and the indentations are not situated opposite one another.

The number of fluid levels in the erect film reflects the degree of obstruction and its site in the small bowel; the more distal the obstruction, the greater the number of fluid levels. High colonic obstruction may also demonstrate fluid levels in the small bowel because of incompetence of the ileocecal valve, whereas low colonic obstruction will usually reveal a markedly dilated cecum, without small bowel fluid levels.

The two major categories of diagnostic contrast agents currently used to opacify the lumen of the gastrointestinal tract are barium sulfate suspensions and the iodinated water-soluble materials such as Gastrografin. Barium sulfate suspensions allow better mucosal definition and are less irritating if aspirated into the tracheobronchial tree but are more irritating to the peritoneum. In the small bowel, barium suspensions remain liquid because of the large amount of retained fluid proximal to the obstruction. However, if a colonic obstruction is present, orally administered barium may become impacted due to the absorption of water by the colonic mucosa.

Because the water-soluble contrast media do not irritate the peritoneum, they are useful for examining patients with a suspected perforation. However, these agents are hyperosmolar, averaging approximately six times the osmolarity of normal serum—a characteristic that may lead to acute pulmonary edema if they are aspirated. Similarly, dilution of these agents by large volumes of fluid drawn into the bowel lumen limits their usefulness in the diagnosis of small bowel obstruction.

Based on the above properties of these contrast agents, the following recommendations may be made for the evaluation of intestinal obstruction (Ott and Gelfand, 1983). If the clinical history and plain abdominal films suggest colonic or distal small bowel obstruction, a barium enema should be performed initially. If colonic obstruction has been excluded, oral administration of barium sulfate is the preferred approach. Any suspicion of intrinsic bowel disease on barium enema would require colonoscopy for further preoperative evaluation.

For obstruction of the small bowel, we prefer initially to pass a long gastrointestinal tube, such as a Miller-Abbott or Cantor tube. These tubes are propelled by peristalsis, their onward progress being arrested at the site of obstruction. Not only do they frequently localize the site of obstruction, they also effectively decompress the small bowel preoperatively and protect the site of anastomosis postoperatively in the event of bowel resection. In addition, the presence of a long tube to differentiate proximal from distal small bowel is extremely helpful intraoperatively in patients with matted, inseparable loops of bowel when only surgical bypass is feasible. This is sometimes the case in obstruction due to advanced ovarian cancer or following whole-abdomen radiation. If necessary, barium sulfate may be injected through the tube to help localize the site or sites of obstruction.

## PREOPERATIVE BOWEL PREPARATION

Small bowel resection and reanastomosis should be safe, regardless of previous bowel preparation, provided there is no impairment of the blood supply to either segment and no advanced peritoneal sepsis. Colonic resection requires adequate preoperative bowel preparation to optimize healing and decrease the risk of anastomotic leakage. Schrock and colleagues (1973) reported that 98% of colon reanastomoses should heal without leakage if the bowel is adequately prepared; the segments are well vascularized; and there is no significant sepsis, previous irradiation, or carcinoma at the site of anastomosis.

Thorough bowel preparation should be undertaken for any patient known to require large bowel surgery and for any patient undergoing laparotomy for ovarian cancer. We prefer to use both a mechanical and an antibiotic bowel preparation, the details of which are presented in Table 19-1.

In a prospective, randomized, double-blind clinical study of 116 patients, Clarke and colleagues (1977) reported that directly related septic complications occurred in 43% of the placebo group but in only 9% of the group receiving neomycin and erythromycin base. The erythromycin-neomycin preparation produced a 4- to 5-log decrease in the concentration of both aerobes and anaerobes in the colonic lumen compared with the placebo group.

---

**TABLE 19-1  Bowel Preparation**

Preoperative day 3:
  Low-residue diet
  Colace, 1 capsule at 6 P.M.
Preoperative day 2:
  Clear liquid diet
  Magnesium citrate, 100 ml at 8 A.M.
  Tapwater enema at night × 2
Preoperative day 1:
  Clear-liquid diet
  Magnesium citrate, 100 ml at 8 A.M.
  Oral neomycin, 1 gm q4h × 4 doses
  Oral erythromycin base, 1 gm q4h × 4 doses
  Tapwater enemas until no solid stool at night
  Commence IV fluids at 8 A.M. to correct fluid and electrolyte imbalance caused by bowel cleansing

---

## POSTOPERATIVE CARE

Following small bowel resection under ideal circumstances, the patient should take nothing orally for at least 4 days. Although not mandatory, a nasogastric tube is desirable. After the passage of flatus, clear liquids may be commenced, followed 24 hours later by a low-residue diet if liquids are well tolerated. If the bowel has been previously irradiated, we prefer to protect the anastomosis with a long gastrointestinal tube that has been passed preoperatively or a Baker tube passed at the time of surgery. In irradiated patients, nothing should be given by mouth for at least 7 days to decrease the risk of anastomotic leak.

Following large bowel resection, the patient should take nothing orally for at least 6 days. Patients receiving intravenous fluids secrete more gastric juices than the intestinal tract is able to propel forward, so that nasogastric suction for the first 48 to 72 hours is desirable to prevent vomiting and aspiration.

If a long period of postoperative ileus is anticipated, we prefer to perform a gastrostomy, since prolonged nasogastric suction is distressing to the patient. Patients suitable for gastrostomy include those who have had previous abdominal radiation, and those who have a small bowel obstruction from ovarian cancer with significant residual disease on bowel serosa. Once flatus is passed, the gastrostomy tube can be clamped, and prior to removal of the tube, oral fluids can be given to see whether they are tolerated.

If colonic resection is planned or anticipated, we administer perioperative antibiotics, usually cefoxitin, 2 gm 2 hours preoperatively and 2 gm every 6 hours for two additional doses.

Should large bowel resection be performed in the absence of preoperative preparation, a 5-day course of broad-spectrum antibiotics, such as gentamicin and clindamycin, should be given.

## TECHNIQUES FOR BOWEL REANASTOMOSIS

Following resection of a segment of bowel and a wedge-shaped segment of mesentery, reanastomosis is usually performed by either an open two-layered or a closed one-layered end-to-end technique. Prior to reanastomosis, all fat must be cleared off the serosa for a distance of about 1 cm from the cut end.

### Open Two-Layered Anastomosis

This is the most common technique employed. With proximal and distal bowel ends approximated with crushing clamps, an outer posterior layer of interrupted 3-0 silk Lembert (seromuscular) sutures are placed. The crushing clamps (e.g., Kocher or Bainbridge) are then removed, and traumatized tissue is excised (Fig. 19-1).

An inner continuous full-thickness layer of 3-0 chromic catgut is used to complete the posterior part of the anastomosis. Two separate sutures are required.

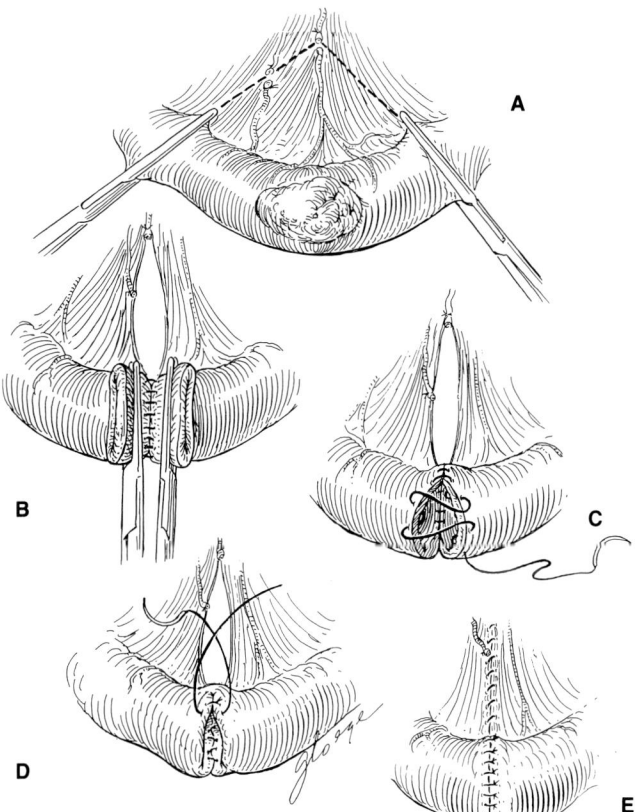

FIGURE 19-1   Hand-sewn end-to-end enteroenterostomy. (*A*) The tumor and bowel are resected along with the mesentery. (*B*) The posterior seromuscular layer is sutured. (*C*) The Connell stitch is placed. (*D*) The anterior seromuscular layer is placed. (*E*) Closure of the mesentery. (From Berek JS, Hacker NF [eds]: *Practical Gynecologic Oncology*. Baltimore, Williams and Wilkins, 1989, p 529.)

Each starts centrally and progresses laterally. When each corner is reached, the needle is brought from inside the bowel lumen out through the bowel wall. This continuous layer is then continued anteriorly as a Connell stitch to complete the inner layer of the anastomosis. The Connell stitch passes outside to inside, then inside to outside on each segment of bowel. The anterior part of the anastomosis is completed by placing interrupted 3-0 silk Lembert sutures, after which the defect in the mesentery is closed with interrupted silk or catgut. The patency of the lumen is tested by invaginating one wall of the intestine through the anastomosis with the tip of the index finger.

## Closed One-Layered Anastomosis

This technique was particularly common prior to the advent of thorough mechanical and antibiotic bowel preparation because it decreased the amount of possible peritoneal contamination with bowel organisms. With the bowel ends approximated with crushing clamps, a series of interrupted 3-0 silk Lembert sutures are placed anteriorly and left untied. The clamps are then rotated through 180 degrees to allow insertion of the posterior

Lembert sutures. With steady traction being applied to the anterior and posterior sutures, the clamps are removed. Each suture is tied while traction is maintained to keep the bowel lumens apposed. A final check is made for defects, and after patency of the lumen is confirmed by digital invagination, the mesentery is approximated.

## Side-to-Side Anastomosis

This is particularly useful when a bypass is being performed rather than a bowel resection, such as may be applicable for palliation of bowel obstruction in patients with inoperable ovarian cancer. This approach is best avoided in patients who have a better prognosis because of the problems with blind loop syndrome.

The segments of bowel to be anastomosed are approximated after atraumatic, linen-shod intestinal clamps have been applied more distally to prevent spillage of bowel contents. A row of interrupted 3-0 silk Lembert sutures are placed and tied, forming the posterior layer of the anastomosis. Incisions are then made into each lumen, about one-quarter inch from the suture line.

A full-thickness, continuous suture of 3-0 chromic catgut is inserted to complete the posterior layer and is continued anteriorly as a Connell suture. The anterior part of the anastomosis is completed with a series of interrupted 3-0 silk Lembert sutures.

## Surgical Stapling

During the past decade, sophisticated surgical stapling devices for bowel anastomosis have become available, and recent reports of their use in the management of gynecologic malignancies attest to their safety (Wheeless and Dorsey, 1981; Delgado, 1981). These devices facilitate anastomosis and thus allow better utilization of operating time, particularly in poor-risk patients. Stapled anastomoses are probably no better than sutured anastomoses under normal circumstances but are superior after low anterior resection of the colon, when poor exposure makes suturing technically more difficult.

Chassin (1980) retrospectively studied complications after 812 gastrointestinal procedures performed by the same group of surgeons using either the stapling devices or hand-sewn sutures. There was no statistically significant difference in the incidence of complications between the sutured and stapled groups (4.4 versus 4.1%).

The main disadvantage of the stapling devices is their increased cost. Provided the blood supply to the tissues is adequate and there is no tension on the anastomosis, the only contraindication to the use of staples is the presence of tissues that are too thick or too thin for the size of the staples. If the tissues are too thick, necrosis might occur, while if they are too thin, bleeding and anastomotic leakage are likely. The other problem with excessive use of stapling devices is that residents in training receive less exposure to the techniques of hand-sewn anastomoses.

**Stapling Instruments** Three stapling instruments are required for gastrointestinal operations.

**Thoracoabdominal Stapler (TA-30®, TA-55®, or TA-90®)*** The TA® stapler applies a double-staggered row of staples either 30, 55, or 90 mm long. Two sizes of staples are available with the TA® devices. The 3.5-mm staple is 3.5 mm in leg length and 4.0 mm across the base, while the 4.8-mm staple has a leg length of 4.8 mm and is also 4.0 mm across the base. After the jaws of the TA® device are optimally tightened, the degree of compression of tissues is approximately 1.5 mm using the 3.5-mm staple and 2.0 mm using the 4.8-mm staple. These devices close a lumen in an everting fashion.

**Gastrointestinal Anastomosis Stapler (GIA®)** This device applies two double-staggered rows of staples, while a knife, which is part of the instrument, divides the tissues between the two double rows. It inverts the tissue at the site of the anastomosis. Only one staple size is available, so no adjustment can be made for tissues of varying size. The GIA® compresses tissues to a thickness of approximately 1.75 mm.

**End-to-End Anastomosis Stapler (EEA®)** This is a most useful stapling device for the gynecologic oncologist because it facilitates the low colorectal anastomosis that is frequently needed after pelvic exenteration or extirpation of ovarian cancer from the pelvis. The device applies a double-staggered row of staples that approximates two tubular structures in inversion, while the knife cuts the tissue just inside the staple line. Only one staple size is available, which compresses the tissues to a thickness of approximately 2.0 mm. Four cartridge sizes are available in a disposable curved instrument, the respective diameters being 21, 25, 28, and 31 mm. Metal sizers are available to determine the diameter of the bowel lumen. The new premium CEEA device is easier to use, because the anvil disarticulates from the main instrument.

**Stapling Techniques** The three most common gastrointestinl procedures performed with the stapling devices in gynecologic oncology are the functional end-to-end anastomosis (small or large bowel), the side-to-side enteroenterostomy, and the low anterior resection with end-to-end anastomosis.

**Functional End-to-End Anastomosis (Fig. 19-2)** The bowel resection is performed by applying the GIA® stapler across the proximal and distal ends of the segment to be removed. This leaves both the proximal and distal bowel loops stapled closed. The antimesenteric corner of the staple line is excised from each loop, the antimesenteric borders are approximated, and one arm of the GIA® is then inserted into each bowel lumen. After the bowel ends are evenly aligned on the instrument, it is closed and fired. The GIA® is withdrawn, and the common opening is closed with one application of the TA-30® or TA-55® stapler. Prior to its removal, the edge of the instrument is used as a guide to excise redundant tissue.

*GIA®, TA®, EEA®, and PURSTRING™ are trademarks of United States Surgical Corporation.

**Side-to-Side Enteroenterostomy (Fig. 19-3)** The bowel segments to be anastomosed are approximated using traction sutures. After a small opening is made with a scalpel into the lumen of both bowel loops on the antimesenteric borders, one arm of the GIA® is inserted into each lumen. The bowel segments are evenly aligned on the instrument, which is then closed and fired. The GIA® is withdrawn and the common opening is closed with the TA-30® or TA-55® stapler.

**Low Anterior Resection with End-to-End Anastomosis (Fig. 19-4)** Following resection of the involved segment of rectosigmoid, the proximal segment is mobilized sufficiently to allow approximation of the two segments without tension. The PURSTRING™ instrument is used to place a PURSTRING™ suture around the proximal and distal ends of the lumen. The EEA® is introduced into the rectum and advanced to the site of anastomosis. The instrument is opened to allow the anvil to protrude from the rectum, and the anvil is passed into the proximal colon with the aid of Allis clamps, after which the two pursestring sutures are tied. The instrument is closed and fired. It is preferable to place a couple of Lembert sutures over the anterior staple line to protect it during removal of the instrument. With the newer CEEA instrument, the proximal colon may be prepared with the anvil and anvil shaft separated from the instrument. The anvil shaft is then engaged in the instrument shaft, prior to closure and firing. To remove the EEA®, the instrument is opened and gently rotated. To check the anastomosis, the pelvis should be filled with saline and air introduced into the rectum by means of a 50-ml bulb syringe passed through the anus. Any escape of bubbles indicates an imperfect anastomosis.

# TECHNIQUES FOR MINOR GASTROINTESTINAL PROCEDURES

In the management of gynecologic malignancies, a number of minor procedures are regularly performed, particularly in patients with ovarian cancer or complications of radiation therapy. Four common procedures—gastrostomy, ileostomy or jejunostomy, Baker-tube stitchless plication, and colostomy—are described below.

## Gastrostomy

In gynecologic oncology, a gastrostomy is usually performed when the need for prolonged postoperative decompression of the stomach is anticipated. This obviates the use of a nasogastric tube, which patients find irritating and uncomfortable. Two types of gastrostomies are applicable, as described below.

**Stamm Gastrostomy** This is the simplest type and the technique we most commonly use. A small incision is made at the midportion of the anterior wall of the stomach, and a Foley catheter, previously brought into the peritoneal cavity through a separate stab incision in

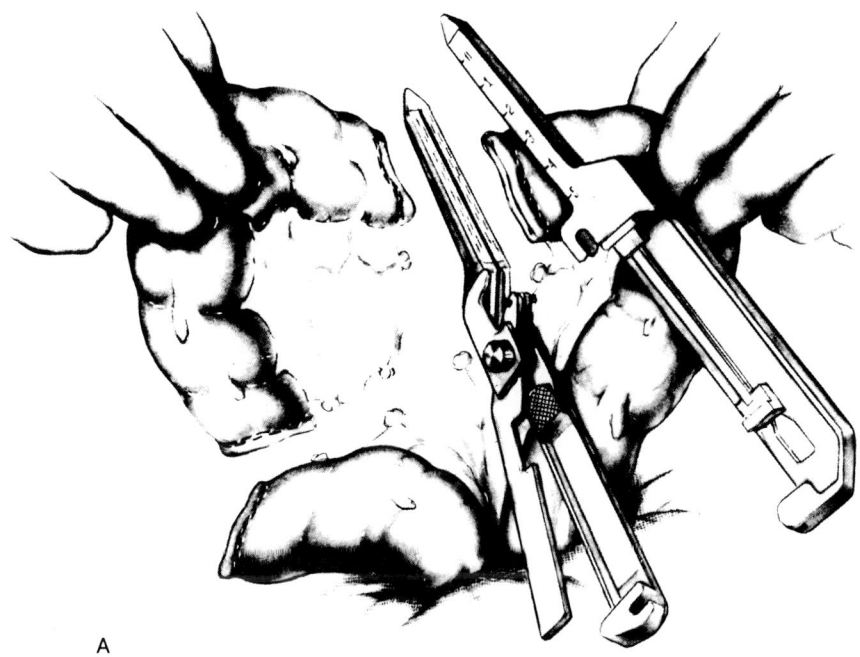

A

**FIGURE 19-2** (*A*) Bowel resection is performed with two applications of the GIA®. The GIA® is applied to the bowel in a scissor-like manner. The instrument is then closed and the staples are fired. A double-staggered staple line is placed on the specimen side and another on the patient side while the bowel between the two staple lines is resected by a knife in the GIA®. The GIA® is then reapplied and the specimen resected.

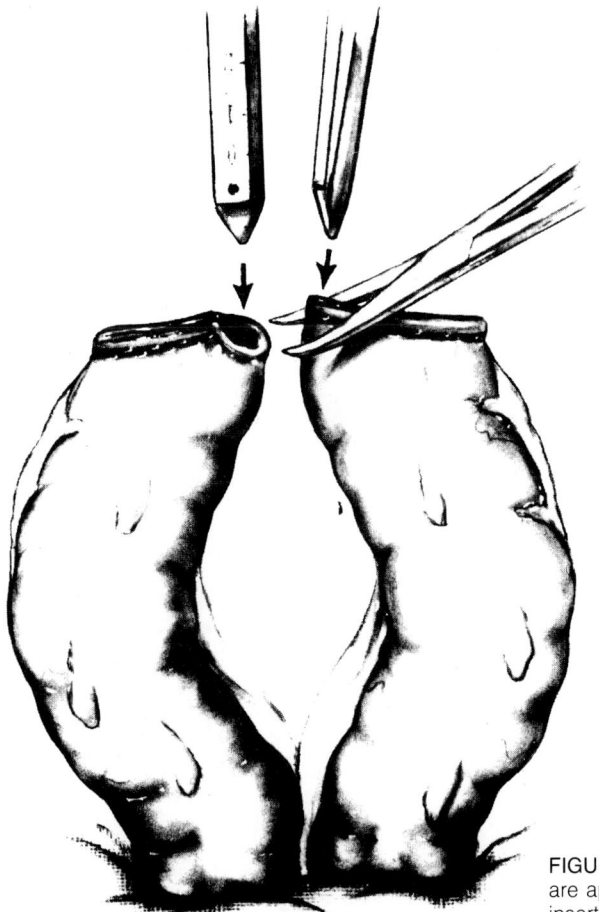

**FIGURE 19-2 (cont.)** (*B*) The antimesenteric borders of the bowel loops are approximated, the corners are resected, and one fork of the GIA® is inserted into each bowel lumen with the bowel ends evenly aligned. *(Continued on p. 366.)*

B

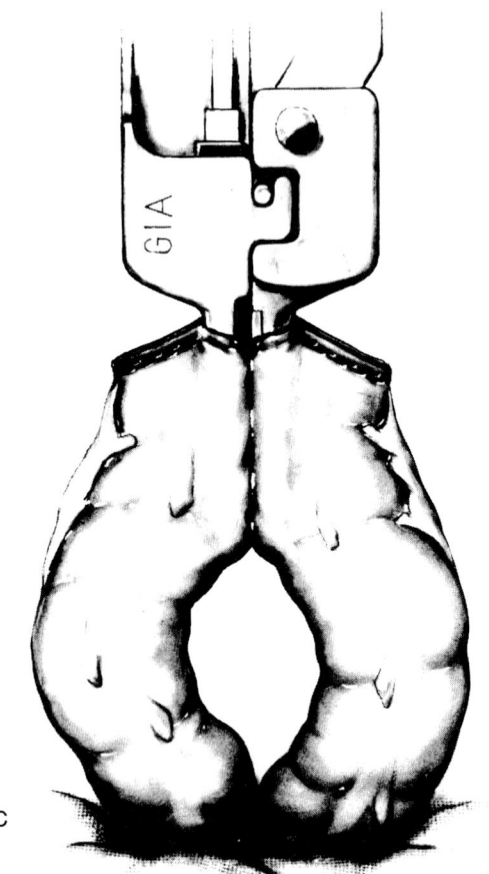

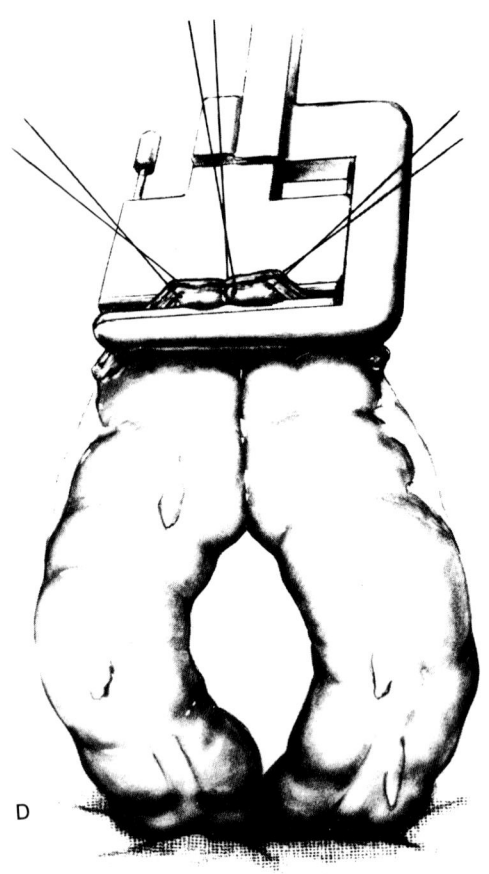

FIGURE 19-2  (continued)  (*C*) The instrument is closed and the staples are fired. As the two double-staggered staple lines are created to join the bowel walls, the knife assembly in the GIA® divides the bowel between the two lines, creating a stoma. After the GIA® forks are withdrawn, the anastomotic staple line should be inspected for adequate hemostasis. (*D*) The now common opening can then be closed with one application of the TA-30® or TA-55®. (Ravitch M, Steichen F (eds): *Principles and practice of surgical stapling.* Year Book Medical Publishers, 1987, p 10.)

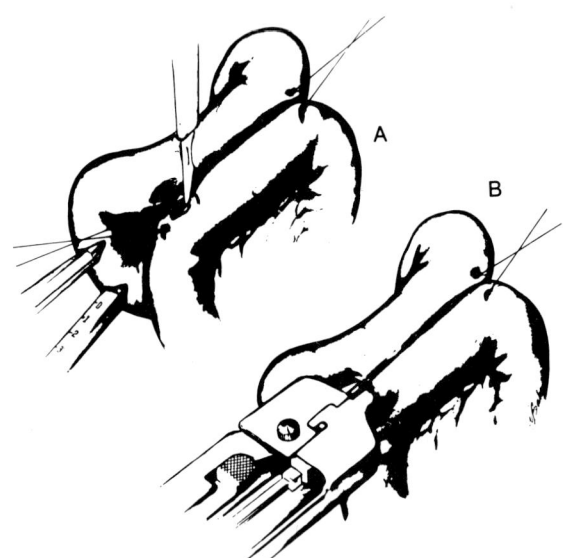

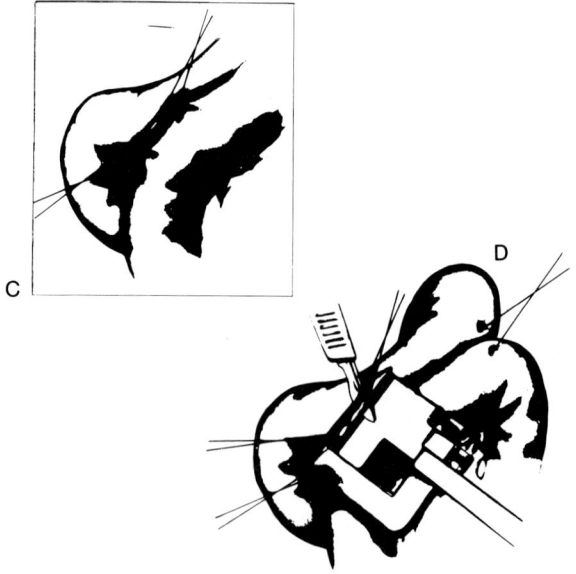

FIGURE 19-3  Enteroenterostomy performed using the GIA®. (*A*) The bowel segments are approximated side by side by means of traction sutures. A stab wound is made into the lumen of both bowel loops on the antimesenteric borders. (*B*) The forks of the GIA® are inserted fully of these openings to ensure maximal stomal size, and the tissue edges are evenly aligned. (*C*) Two double-staggered staple lines are placed so as to join the walls of the bowel while the knife assembly in the GIA® divides the bowel between these lines to create a stoma. (*D*) The anastomotic staple lines should be inspected for hemostasis before the now common stab wound is closed with the TA-55®. (Copyright © 1974, 1980, 1988 United States Surgical Corporation. All rights reserved. Reprinted with the Permission of United States Surgical Corporation.)

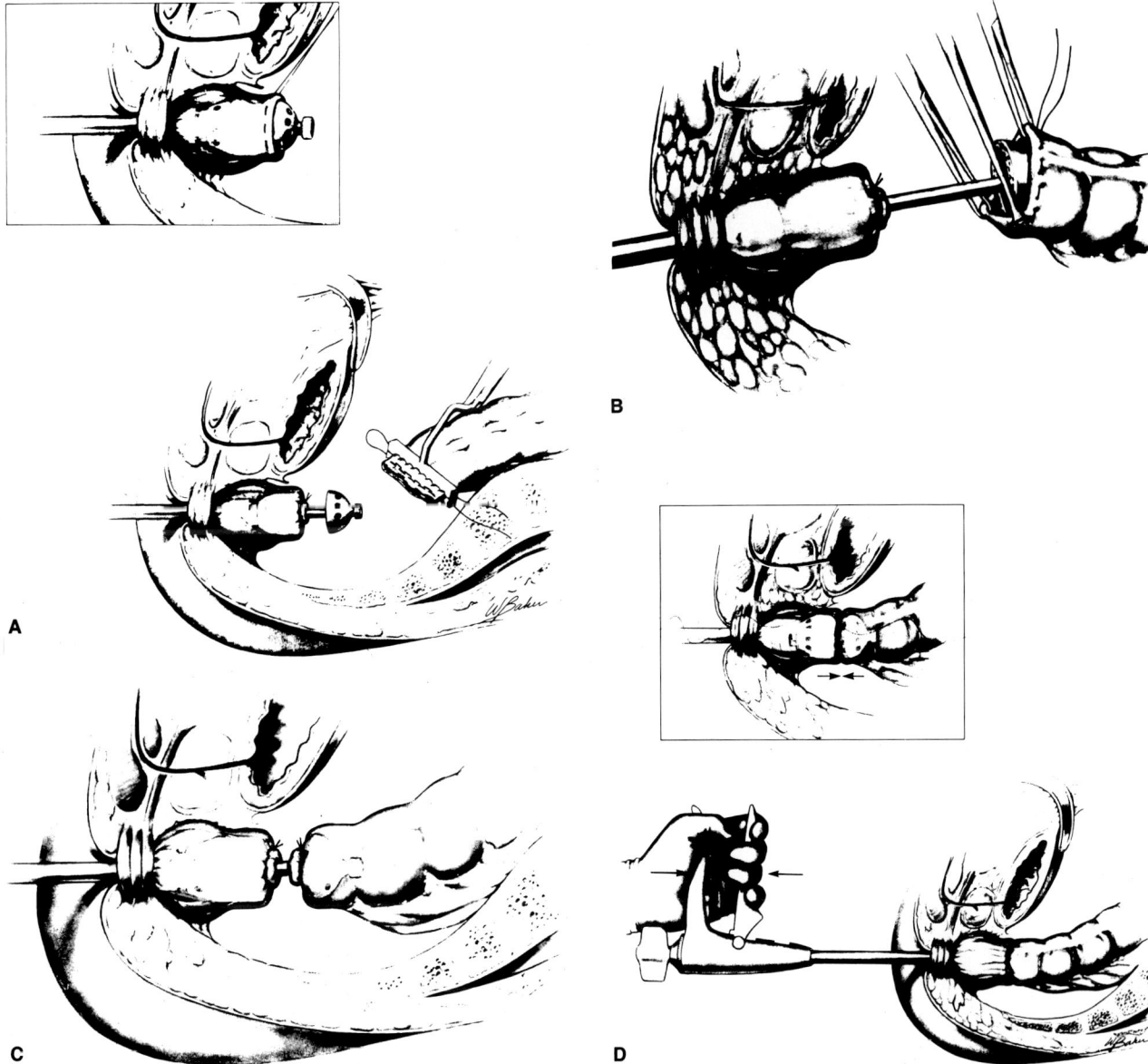

**FIGURE 19-4** When the EEA® is used to perform the anastomosis, the stapler is introduced into the anus and advanced to the level of the PURSTRING™ instrument. (*A*) When this instrument has been removed, the EEA® is opened to allow the anvil to protrude from the rectum, and the PURSTRING™ suture is tied. (*B*) The tissue edges are grasped with three Allis clamps placed equidistantly. As traction is applied on the clamps, the anvil portion of the EEA® is introduced into the proximal colon. (*C*) The Allis clamps are removed and the PURSTRING™ suture is tied. The tissue should be snug against the cartridge and anvil to prevent bunching or overlap as the tissue is approximated. (*D*) With all tissues incorporated within the loading unit, the EEA® is closed and the staples are fired. A circular double-staggered row of staples join the bowel, while a circular blade in the EEA® creates the stoma. (Copyright © 1974, 1980, 1988 United States Surgical Corporation. All rights reserved. Reprinted with the Permission of United States Surgical Corporation.)

the left upper quadrant of the abdomen, is introduced into the stomach. Two or three successive PURSTRING™ sutures of 3-0 chromic catgut are used to invert the stomach wall about the tube, and interrupted sutures of 3-0 black silk are used to approximate the serosa of the stomach to the peritoneum around the gastrostomy tube.

***Witzel Gastrostomy*** This procedure is similar to the Stamm gastrostomy except that after the first purse-string suture has been placed, the Foley catheter is laid along the serosal surface of the stomach and is buried within the stomach wall for a distance of about 1 inch

with either Lembert sutures or a continuous seromuscular suture. This technique produces a serosal tunnel for the tube before it exits from the abdomen, which may reduce the likelihood of leakage of gastric contents after the tube has been removed. With either technique, leakage is usually minimal and the artificial fistula will close within 2 or 3 days.

## Ileostomy or Jejunostomy

The site for the ileostomy should be selected to ensure that the appliance will not come into contact with the costal margin or the anterior superior iliac spine. A site in the right or left iliac fossa is usually suitable. A circular incision about 2 cm in diameter is made at the selected site, and the circle of skin is removed. The fat is then incised to expose the anterior rectus sheath, and a 2-cm longitudinal incision is made in the peritoneum. The opening in the abdominal wall is dilated to accept two fingers. Using Babcock clamps, the operator brings the end of the ileum or jejunum out through the opening and then sutures it to the skin edges using everting interrupted sutures of 3-0 chromic catgut. The cut edge of the mesentery is sutured to the paracolic peritoneum to obliterate a potential site of internal herniation.

## Baker-Tube Stitchless Plication

Placement of a Baker tube is particularly useful in patients with prior irradiation who are undergoing small bowel resection or lysis of multiple adhesions with serosal damage (Baker, 1968). The No 18 French Baker tube, 270 cm long with a 5-ml bag at its tip, is passed through either a jejunostomy or a gastrostomy of the Stamm type. We have routinely introduced the Baker tube through a jejunostomy and have encountered no postoperative problems, although this route is reported to be more commonly associated with persistent leakage or intestinal obstruction after the Baker tube has been removed (Chassin, 1980). After the tube is passed through a stab incision in the abdominal wall, it is introduced into the bowel and advanced by milking the balloon. Intermittent suction allows evacuation of gas and intestinal contents. When local factors make antegrade passage difficult, retrograde passage via a cecostomy may be used.

## Colostomy

Colostomies are usually performed in either the transverse or the sigmoid colon, since the colon in both regions possesses a mesentery that permits easier delivery of the bowel. If the colostomy is to be permanent, a terminal or end colostomy should be performed, and it should be placed as far distal as is compatible with the disease in order to permit the maximal amount of fluid absorption prior to evacuation of the stool. The surgical technique is similar to that for an ileostomy.

If temporary fecal diversion is required, a transverse colostomy is usually performed. The simplest technique is to bring a loop of transverse colon out through a separate transverse incision in the right upper quadrant just lateral to the rectus abdominis muscle after a segment of omentum has been removed. If the transverse colon is tensely distended because of distal obstruction, it is preferable to decompress it first by inserting a No 16 needle attached to low-pressure suction.

Traditionally, the loop is maintained by a glass or Silastic rod passed through a small opening in the transverse mesentery, and the loop is matured 48 hours later. However, the bulky nature of the loop colostomy and rod make it difficult to manage subsequently, and it is preferable to mature the colostomy immediately by making a 4-cm incision along the antimesenteric border

of the colon, preferably in a taenia. Any bowel contents are aspirated, the operative field is irrigated with 0.1% kanamycin solution, and the full thickness of the colon wall is sutured to the skin with interrupted 3-0 chromic catgut. Immediate fixation of bowel mucosa to skin eliminates serositis and edema of the bowel wall (Patey, 1951), and subcutaneous infection rarely occurs (Chassin, 1980). It is not necessary to transect the colon completely and construct a double-barreled colostomy in order to divert the fecal stream completely (Chassin 1980), since the longitudinal incision in the colon permits the posterior wall to prolapse, resulting in functionally separate distal and proximal stomas.

Another technique, which we are using increasingly, consists of transecting the transverse colon with the GIA®, suturing the distal end to the fascia, and leaving it buried subcutaneously. The proximal end may be left stapled until 48 hours postoperatively if the bowel has not been prepared preoperatively.

# BOWEL SURGERY IN OVARIAN CANCER

In the management of patients with ovarian cancer, bowel surgery may be required as part of the primary or secondary cytoreductive effort or to relieve bowel obstruction.

## Cytoreduction

In an analysis of sites of metastases in patients with Stage III ovarian cancer, Hacker and colleagues (1983) reported the colon to be involved in 68% of cases and the small bowel in 59% of cases. Frequently, the disease is confined to the serosa, and bowel resection can be avoided by meticulous dissection of the tumor mass from the noninvaded muscularis (Griffiths and Fuller, 1978). In fact, of patients having optimal cytoreductive operations, defined as involving a residual tumor mass 1.5 cm or less in its largest diameter, Hacker et al reported that bowel resection was required in only 16% of patients. For patients having secondary cytoreductive operations for ovarian cancer, Berek and colleagues (1983) reported that bowel resection was required in 53% of cases.

In patients with ovarian cancer and no evidence of impending bowel obstruction, bowel resection should be considered only if it will allow optimal cytoreduction. When performed under these circumstances, it does not add significantly to the operative morbidity (Hacker et al, 1983; Berek et al, 1983).

For all patients undergoing laparotomy for ovarian cancer, the bowel should be thoroughly prepared preoperatively in case colonic resection is required. If cul-de-sac disease is palpable on rectal examination, it is desirable to perform the operation with the patient in a modified lithotomy ("ski") position to facilitate primary reanastomosis with the EEA® should rectosigmoid resection be required. We no longer protect the rectosigmoid reanastomosis with a temporary colostomy unless the bowel is unprepared, the patient has received previous pelvic radiation, or there is active pelvic infection (Berek et al, 1984).

## Bowel Obstruction

Intestinal obstruction is a common outcome for patients with advanced ovarian cancer for whom conventional methods of treatment have failed. Obstruction is related partly to mechanical blockage and partly to motility problems caused by tumor involvement of the serosa and mesentery.

Only palliative treatment is available to these patients, and the decision to operate is often a difficult one and can be made only after discussion with the patient and her family. Castaldo and colleagues (1981) suggested that surgical relief of obstruction should be attempted if the projected life expectancy is at least 2 months. Krebs and Goplerud (1983) reported that patient age, nutritional status, tumor spread, presence of ascites, and type of previous therapy all correlated well with the prognosis. Bowel obstruction in the presence of rapidly accumulating ascites was associated with successful palliation in less than 20% of cases.

In four recent series, the operative mortality among 268 patients who underwent operations for bowel obstruction due to ovarian cancer was 14% (Table 19-2) and major complications were common. Prior radiation therapy and the need for multiple anastomoses increased the complication rate (Castaldo et al, 1981). Common complications included enterocutaneous fistulas, disruption of the suture line, sepsis, short bowel syndrome, gastrointestinal hemorrhage, and pulmonary embolism. Recurrent bowel obstruction may also occur. Increasing the use of pre- and postoperative hyperalimentation in these malnourished patients decreases the complication rate.

Conservative management should be tried initially, including intravenous fluids and passage of a long gastrointestinal tube. If the obstruction is not relieved within 4 or 5 days, surgery may be indicated after the above considerations have been taken into account.

Multiple sites of obstruction may be present. Tunca and colleagues (1981) reported small bowel obstruction in 52% of patients, colonic obstruction in 33%, and small and large bowel obstruction in 15%. Frequently there were multiple sites of small bowel obstruction. A Cantor tube introduced preoperatively or a Baker tube introduced at laparotomy will define sites of small

bowel obstruction, but a barium enema is an important preoperative step to ascertain possible sites of obstruction in the colon.

In this palliative situation, intestinal bypass rather than resection is usually appropriate, since it is usually less morbid than resection and median survival times for the two procedures are not significantly different (Tunca et al, 1981). Piver and colleagues (1982) reported that among patients undergoing intestinal bypass, side-to-side enterocolostomy was the most frequently performed procedure. Colostomy may be necessary when there is distal large bowel obstruction, and on occasion, ileostomy or jejunostomy may be required when the colon is completely encased in tumor.

In up to 18% of patients, no relief of obstruction can be provided because of extensive carcinomatosis. In this group, placement of a gastrostomy tube will facilitate terminal care. Because of the likelihood of continued poor bowel function postoperatively, consideration may be given to nutritional support using an elemental diet delivered through a needle-catheter jejunostomy (Ballon, 1982).

Median survival for patients undergoing surgery for intestinal obstruction from ovarian cancer has ranged from 2.5 months (Piver et al, 1982) to 7 months (Tunca et al, 1981), although Castaldo and colleagues (1981) reported that 4 of 23 patients (17%) survived for more than 12 months.

## BOWEL SURGERY IN PELVIC EXENTERATION

Pelvic exenteration is usually performed for centrally recurrent carcinoma of the cervix but may also be performed for primary or recurrent carcinoma of the uterine corpus, vagina, or vulva. Almost all patients will have had previous pelvic radiation. In an analysis of 296 patients undergoing pelvic exenteration, Rutledge and colleagues (1977) reported that 176 patients (59.5%) required total pelvic exenteration, 85 anterior exenteration (28.7%), and 35 (11.8%) posterior exenteration.

If the disease is in the upper vagina, it is usually possible to preserve the rectal sphincter without compromising the surgical margins. In such patients, rectal substitution performed at the time of pelvic exenteration can obviate permanent colostomy and improve the psychologic adjustment of these patients (Lagasse et al, 1973). Following resection of the rectosigmoid segment, the distal sigmoid must be adequately mobilized in order to reach the rectal stump without tension. This necessitates freeing the descending colon and splenic flexure from their lateral peritoneal attachments and mobilizing a wide cuff of sigmoid mesentery close to its base to preserve the blood supply provided by the marginal artery of Drummond. The anastomosis is made with the EEA®. Prior to insertion of the stapling device, the bowel should preferably be dilated to 3.2 cm, which is the outer diameter of the largest EEA® cartridge. Dilatation may be accomplished with the sizing instruments

TABLE 19-2  Operations for Bowel Obstruction in Ovarian Tumor

| Reference | No. of Cases | Operative Mortality | % Mortality |
|---|---|---|---|
| Castaldo et al (1981) | 25 | 3 | 12.0 |
| Piver et al (1982) | 49 | 9 | 18.4 |
| Krebs and Goplerud (1983) | 104 | 12 | 11.5 |
| Tunca et al (1981) | 90 | 13 | 14.4 |
| Totals | 268 | 37 | 13.8 |

supplied by the manufacturer. Chassin (1980) cautions that the use of EEA® cartridges smaller than 31 mm may produce a lumen too small for optimal function of the rectum. Wheeless and Dorsey (1981) reported that 10 patients (30%) who underwent low anastomosis with the EEA® stapler developed a mild degree of stricture at the anastomotic site. The stenosis was found on routine rectal examination and was managed by placing the patients on stool softeners for 3 to 4 months; in all cases, the stenosis gradually disappeared.

For all patients who have undergone previous pelvic radiation, the anastomosis should probably be protected with a temporary transverse or sigmoid colostomy. Schrock and colleagues (1973) reported disruption in 10% of low colorectal anastomoses, in spite of the fact that most of their patients had not received previous radiation therapy. Although disruption was not prevented by proximal decompression, use of the transverse colostomy did appear to prevent mortality due to leakage.

Four to 6 months after exenteration, the integrity of the anastomosis can be evaluated by instillation of a radiopaque contrast medium into the distal segment. Sphincter function is evaluated by instilling saline and then injecting air into the neorectum. The colostomy may be closed after a satisfactory sphincteric mechanism and a healed anastomosis have been demonstrated (Lagasse et al, 1973).

## SMALL BOWEL SURGERY AFTER RADIATION THERAPY

Significant intestinal injuries probably occur in about 5% of patients receiving 5,000 cGy or more to some portion of the abdomen (Morgenstern et al, 1977). In a review of 71 patients requiring surgical intervention for small bowel injury secondary to radiation therapy, Smith (1982) reported that the principal indication for operation was obstruction (62 patients). Four patients experienced perforation with peritonitis, four had enterovaginal fistulas, and one had an enterovesical fistula. In 48% of the patients, the injuries developed within 1 year after the completion of treatment and in 74% within 2 years.

Patients with small bowel obstruction should initially be treated conservatively with intravenous fluids and no oral intake. If there is vomiting despite the absence of oral intake, a long intestinal tube should be passed, and the patient should be started on central or peripheral hyperalimentation. If there has been more than 10% loss of body weight, central hyperalimentation for 7 to 10 days preoperatively, and again postoperatively, is indicated.

When operating on an irradiated bowel, the operator should perform as conservative a procedure as possible. Extensive lysis of adhesions should be avoided because serosal injuries heal poorly in these patients, and subsequent perforation and/or fistula formation is frequent (Morgenstern et al, 1977). Meticulous care must be taken to identify any serosal defects and repair them

with 3-0 black silk sutures. Extensive resection and multiple anastomoses should be avoided. Agglutinated loops of bowel should not be dissected out of the pelvis but should be bypassed with a side-to-side anastomosis of the small intestine to the ascending or transverse colon.

In a review of the world literature, Swan et al (1976) reported a 21% mortality among the resected group and a 10% mortality among the bypass group; anastomotic dehiscence occurred in 36% of the resected group but in only 6% of the bypass group. Smith (1982) reported a 33% postoperative mortality in the resected group and a 21% mortality in the bypass group. Most deaths in the resected group were the result of dehiscence of the anastomosis, while most deaths in the bypass group were due to medical complications.

Stapling devices may be used safely on irradiated bowel (Wheeless and Dorsey, 1981; Delgado, 1981), although we have noticed that in the first few months after irradiation, the bowel may be too edematous to accept the 3.5-mm staples available with the GIA® device.

Because of the need for prolonged postoperative nasogastric suction, it is desirable to replace the long gastrointestinal tube intraoperatively with a gastrostomy tube and a Baker tube. Postoperatively, suction should be continued until flatus is passed, which usually takes 10 to 14 days. Hyperalimentation should be continued until adequate oral intake is tolerated, and broad-spectrum antibiotic therapy that was begun 24 hours preoperatively should be continued for at least 5 days postoperatively.

### Management of Small Bowel Fistulas

In the practice of gynecologic oncology, small bowel fistulas are usually seen in patients who have had prior pelvic or abdominal irradiation. Many of these fistulas follow pelvic exenteration; Berman and colleagues (1976) reported an incidence of 13% among 101 patients who underwent this procedure.

Spontaneous closure often occurs if the patient is well nourished and there is no distal obstruction, so that conservative management consisting of nasogastric suction and hyperalimentation should be tried initially in nonirradiated patients. Somatostatin may be used to decrease gastrointestinal secretions and hasten closure. Great care must be taken to protect surrounding skin from the gastrointestinal contents; this is best achieved by treating the fistula as a stoma and applying an appropriate collecting bag. If obstruction is present, an operation will be required; this is common in enteroperineal fistulas after pelvic exenteration.

Berman and colleagues (1976) reported a 10-point plan (described below) for the surgical management of small bowel fistulas.

Preoperatively, the patient should undergo a Gastrografin upper gastrointestinal study to attempt to localize the site of the fistula. A Gastrografin enema should also be performed to exclude an associated large bowel fistula. A long intestinal tube should be passed to reduce drainage of small bowel contents, to decompress the bowel, and to help identify afferent loops of bowel at the time of surgery. Hyperalimentation, using 25% dextrose and 5% amino acids, should be delivered through a central line, provided that the patient is not febrile. Early surgical intervention should be planned after correction of anemia and acid-base and electrolyte abnormalities. The interval between fistula development and surgical intervention should be less than 14 days if possible. Prophylactic antibiotic coverage using an aminoglycoside or cephalosporin for the gram-negative aerobic bacteria and clindamycin, carbenicillin, or metronidazole (Flagyl) for the anaerobes should commence 24 hours preoperatively.

At laparotomy, the involved segment of bowel is isolated and transected proximally and distally (Fig. 19-5). One or both ends of the isolated bowel segment should be brought to the skin as mucous fistulas to prevent closed-loop obstruction. The proximal segment of small bowel should then be anastomosed to the distal segment or to the ascending or transverse colon. If the bowel wall is heavily irradiated and the vasculature impaired, the safety of the anastomosis may be increased by closing the transected bowel ends and using a side-to-side technique.

Postoperative care should be as previously described.

## LARGE BOWEL SURGERY AFTER RADIATION THERAPY

In a series of 72 patients with large bowel injuries secondary to radiation for cervical cancer reported by

ENTEROPERINEAL FISTULAE

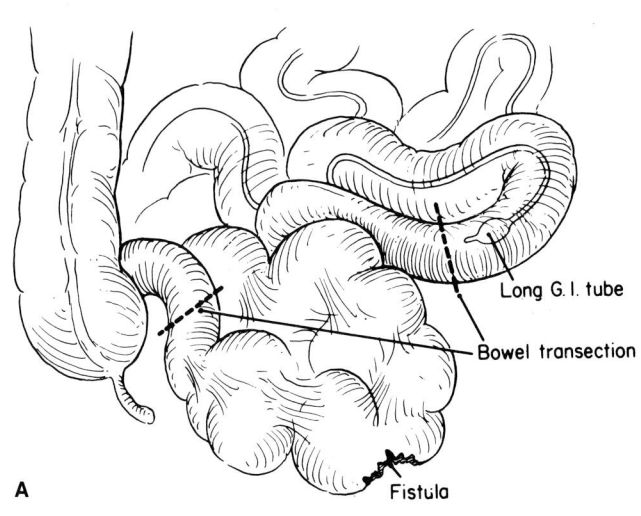

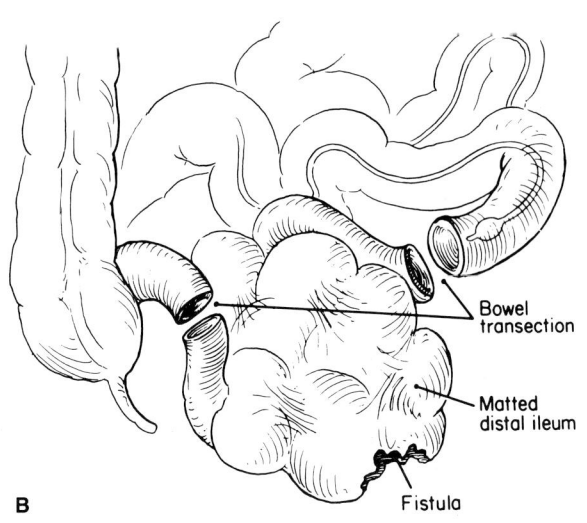

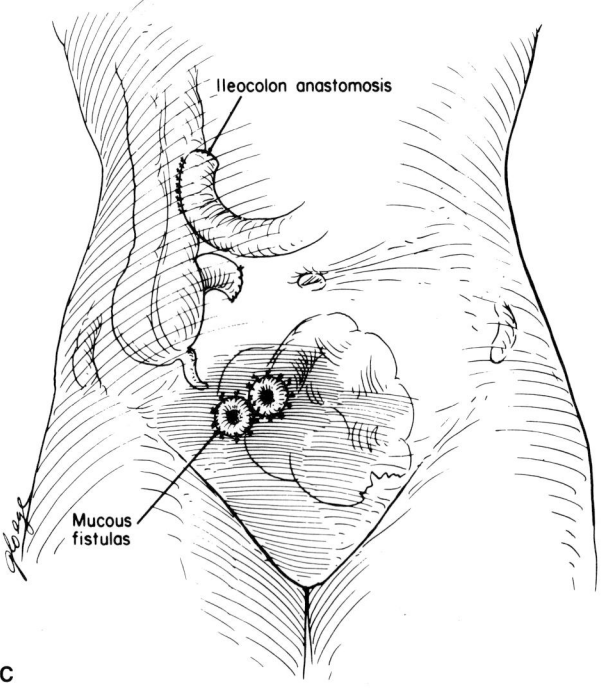

FIGURE 19-5   (*A*) Identification of loops of small bowel proximal to a fistula by locating small bowel tube. (*B*) Transection of bowel proximal and distal to the fistula. (*C*) Creation of an enterocolic anastomosis and mucous fistulas. (From Berman ML, et al: Enteroperineal fistulae following pelvic exenteration: A 10-point program of management. *Gynecol Oncol* 4:368, 1976.)

Smith et al (1969), 30 had rectovaginal fistulas, 18 had sigmoiditis, 17 had obstruction, 5 had perforation, and 2 had fistulas. In 18 of the 30 patients (60%) in whom rectovaginal fistulas developed, a vesicovaginal fistula also developed, and most had vaginal vault necrosis before the fistula appeared.

## Management of Radiation-Induced Rectovaginal Fistula

Because of the poor vascularity of the tissues, radiation-induced fistulas are very likely to recur after repair by any technique that does not introduce a new blood supply to the fistula site.

Once a rectovaginal fistula has developed, diversion of the fecal stream is mandatory. If the patient is elderly and in poor medical condition, or the fistula is so large that repair is unrealistic, an end sigmoid colostomy should be performed. However, if fistula repair is considered feasible, a temporary loop transverse or sigmoid colostomy is applicable. The fistula should be biopsied to rule out recurrent carcinoma. It is also important to document sphincter function and the absence of rectal stricture before attempting surgical repair.

Three or 4 months should elapse between colostomy formation and fistula repair to allow the inflammatory response in the surrounding tissues to subside, and adequate preparation of the distal bowel should be carried out preoperatively.

After the fistula site is exposed by utilizing a Schuchardt incision, the fibrotic margins of the fistula are excised until distinct layers of bowel and vagina can be separated. The bowel is widely mobilized from the vagina to allow closure without tension. This may require a laparotomy to facilitate the dissection. After adequate mobilization, the edges of the rectal mucosa are closed transversely with inverting 3-0 catgut sutures, and a second layer of sutures is placed in the submucosa.

At this point, a vascular pedicle should be used to reinforce the sutures lines. Omentum may be partly mobilized from the transverse colon or stomach and brought down into the pelvis. Alternatively, the bulbocavernosus fat pad or gracilis muscle may be used as pedicle grafts. Either one is mobilized on its vascular pedicle, delivered to the fistula site via a subcutaneous tunnel under the labial and vaginal mucosa, and sutured above the repaired fistula (Fig. 19-6). The vaginal mucosa is closed vertically over the pedicle, and the skin is closed over the site of the bulbocavernosus or gracilis muscle. The temporary colostomy is closed about 6 months later, after there is radiologic and endoscopic evidence of fistula closure.

White and colleagues (1982) reported 14 bulbocavernosus muscle grafts in 12 patients for closure of radiation-induced rectovaginal fistulas, with success in all but 1 patient. The fistulas varied in diameter from 1 to 4 cm and had an average diameter of 2 cm.

Bricker and Johnston (1979) described the use of proximal colon as a vascular pedicle graft to close the fistula (Fig. 19-7). By filleting the antimesenteric border of the colon, a similar technique can be used to treat rectal stricture, which is frequently associated with a radiation-induced rectovaginal fistula. The authors reported on five patients in whom complicated fistulas and strictures were successfully corrected, with restoration of normal rectal function.

If the fistula or stricture is not too low, resection of the involved bowel segment and primary reanastomosis using the EEA® stapler may be preferable.

## Management of Proctosigmoiditis

Severe rectal bleeding may result from radiation injury to the rectosigmoid, necessitating multiple blood transfusions. Conservative measures should be tried initially; however, if these fail, sigmoid colostomy to divert the fecal stream is frequently necessary.

In order to avoid colostomy in a patient with persistent bleeding from proctosigmoiditis, Leuchter and colleagues (1982) reported the successful use of the Nd:YAG laser attached to a fiberoptic endoscope. Four treatments over 6 months were required to control all bleeding points. General anesthesia was not necessary and no morbidity was encountered.

# MEDICAL MANAGEMENT OF GASTROINTESTINAL SYNDROMES

Operations on, or radiation to, the gastrointestinal tract may be associated with alterations in intestinal function, clinically manifested as the malabsorption syndrome. Three conditions that warrant special mention are short bowel syndrome, blind loop syndrome, and radiation enteritis. Before discussing these conditions, we will describe the normal mechanism of absorption.

Following digestion in the stomach and upper small intestine by gastric, pancreatic, and intestinal juices, nutrients are absorbed in varying degrees throughout the small and large intestines. The proximal small intestine is a major site for the absorption of iron, folic acid, calcium, water-soluble vitamins, and fat (monoglycerides and fatty acids). Sugars are absorbed in the proximal and mid-small bowel, while most amino acid absorption takes place in the middle of the small intestine and to some extent in the proximal and distal areas. The distal small bowel is the major absorptive area for bile salts and vitamin $B_{12}$. Water and electrolytes are absorbed mainly in the colon, particularly the cecum.

Clinically, malabsorption syndromes are manifested as diarrhea, weight loss, anemia, and passage of abnormal stools that are characteristically pale and greasy because of their increased fat content. Signs and symptoms of specific vitamin deficiencies such as glossitis, cheliosis, muscle tenderness, peripheral neuritis, and dermatitis from deficiencies of the B-complex vitamins also occur.

## Short Bowel Syndrome

Approximately 90 to 120 cm of small intestine are required for adequate absorption. Resection of ileum will impair the absorption of bile salts and vitamin $B_{12}$,

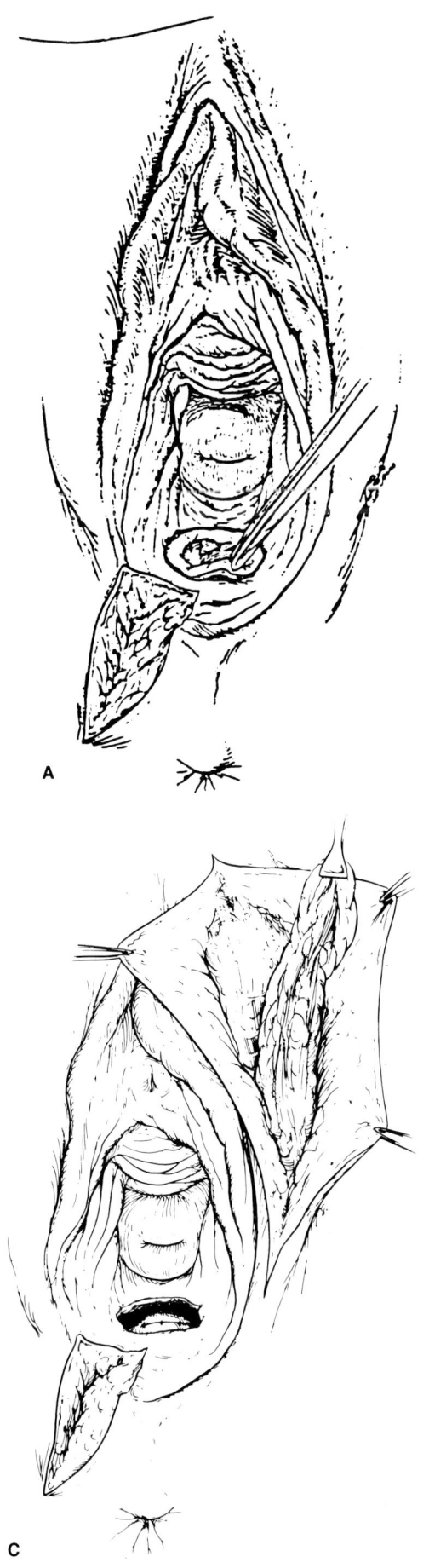

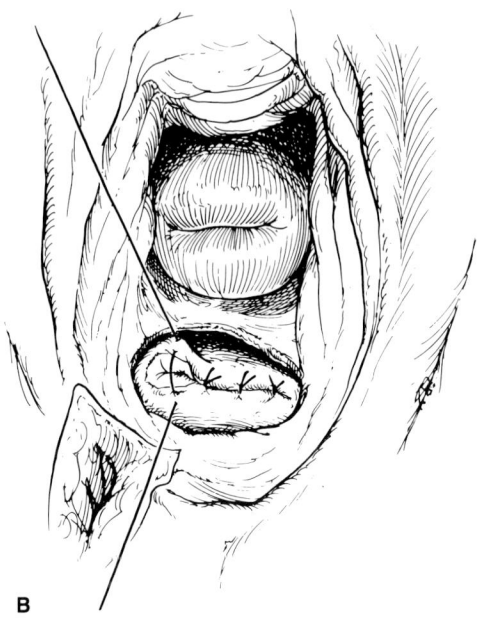

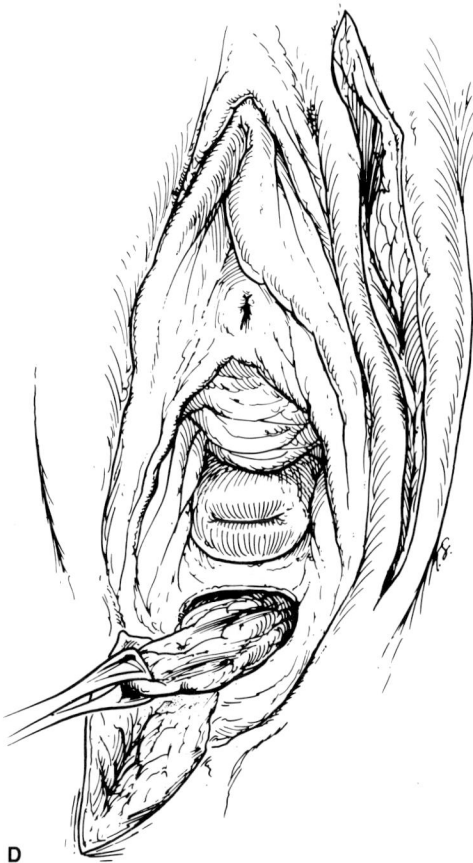

**FIGURE 19-6** Use of the bulbocavernosus muscle (Martius procedure) for repair of radiation-induced rectovaginal fistula. (*A* Schuhardt incision with the formation of vaginal collar. (*B*) Closure of the rectal layer with interrupted fine chromic catgut suture. (*C*) Mobilization of the left bulbocavernosus muscle and labial fat pad. (*D*) A pedicle graft is placed over the rectal closure. *(Continued on p. 374)*

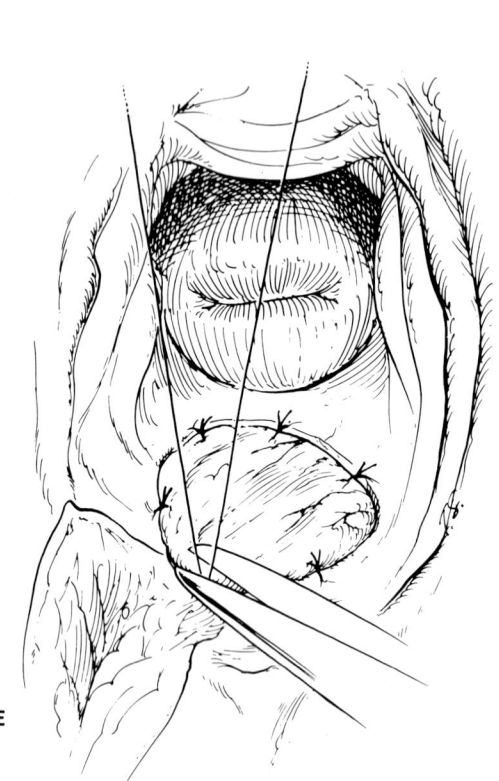

E

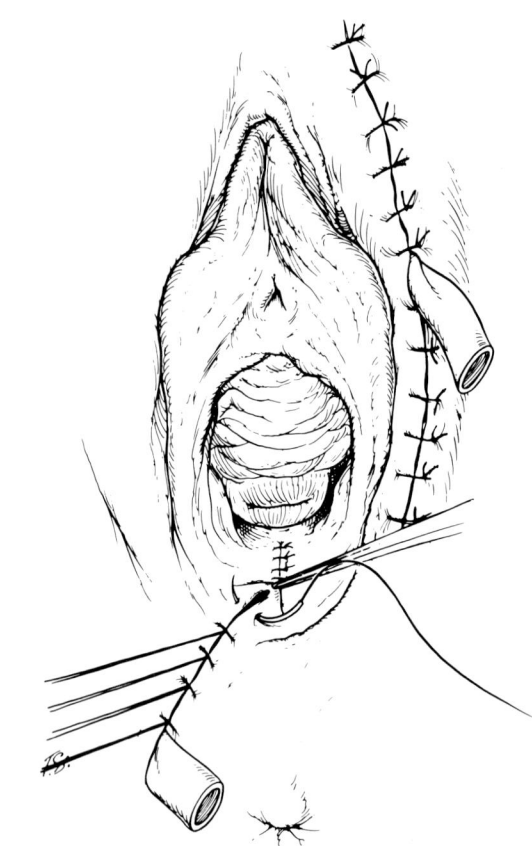

F

FIGURE 19-6 (continued) (E) The labial pad is sutured in place. (F) Closure of the vagina and labium major and Schuhardt incision. (From White AJ, et al: Use of the bulbocavernosus muscle (Martius procedure) for repair of radiation-induced rectovaginal fistulas. *Obstet Gynecol* 60:114, 1982, by permission from The American College of Obstetricians and Gynecologists.)

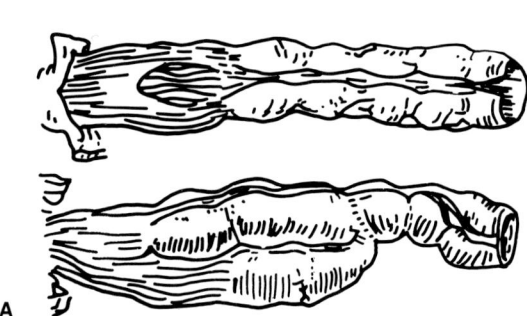

A

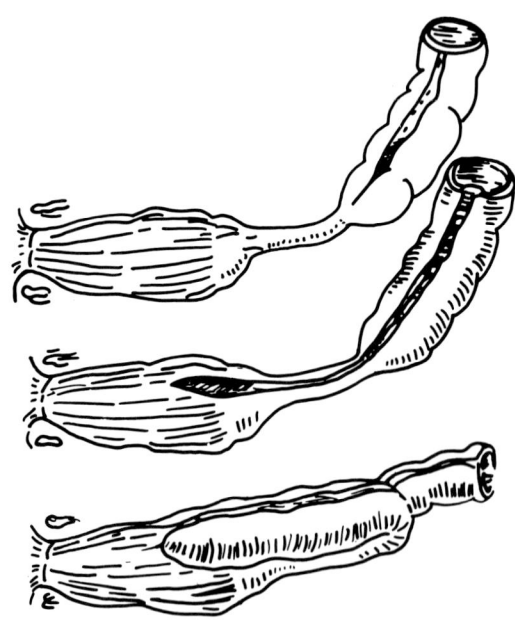

B

FIGURE 19-7 Repair of postirradiation rectovaginal fistula and stricture (A) The proximal end of the colon is anastomosed end-on to the fistula, and the bowel lumen can be increased by an antimesenteric slit to a fistulous defect of any size. (B) A long stricture can be opened by filleting the normal colon and strictured area and by folding the normal colon over to be sutured to the edges of the stricture. (From Bricker EM, Johnson WD: Repair of postirradiation-rectovaginal fistula and stricture. *Surg Gynecol Obstet*. 148:499, 1979. By permission of *Surgery, Gynecology & Obstetrics*.)

whereas jejunal resection will impair absorption of fat, calcium, and folic acid. Postoperatively, the remaining segment of intestine will show progressive improvement in absorptive capacity associated with dilatation and, to a lesser extent, lengthening, with associated hypertrophy and hyperplasia of the mural components (Scheflan et al, 1976).

Regardless of the segment resected, the diet should be high in protein, and frequent feeding (six times daily) is recommended. Calcium as well as vitamins A, D, and K and the B-complex vitamins should be given orally. If the distal ileum has been resected, parenteral vitamin $B_{12}$ will be required, while folic acid may be required for persistent megaloblastic anemia. Oral iron—or, if necessary, parenteral iron—may be required for iron deficiency anemia. Elemental diets may be useful. In addition to the usual drugs used to reduce hypermotility (Lomotil, codeine, paregoric), cholestyramine, which chelates bile salts, is often very helpful.

In severe cases, total parenteral nutrition may be indicated. An indwelling Hickman catheter is placed in the cephalic vein, and the patient is taught how to manage hyperalimentation at home. Although initially this may be required daily, with progressive hypertrophy of the residual mucosa, it is sometimes possible slowly to wean the patient off parenteral nutrition.

## Blind or Stagnant Loop Syndrome

A loop of intestine is "blind" when it has been removed from the mainstream of the intestinal tract but still retains a functional connection. Examples include a loop of terminal ileum that has been partially excluded by either a side-to-side or end-to-end ileotransverse colostomy or an obstructed loop of small intestine in the pelvis that has been bypassed by a side-to-side anastomosis.

Bacterial colony counts rarely exceed $10^4$/ml of jejunal fluid, the major mechanism limiting bacterial growth being normal peristalsis (Greenberg and Isselbacher, 1974). Stasis and overgrowth of bacteria take place in the blind loop, with subsequent extension of bacteria into the upper small intestine. Certain species of *Bacteroides* and coliforms are the most common offending organisms (Swan, 1974).

Bacterial overgrowth alters bile salt metabolism, which accounts for the steatorrhea. The bacteria (especially anaerobic gram-positive bacteria) may cause intraluminal deconjugation of bile salts, with production of free bile acids. Unconjugated bile acids may be absorbed in the proximal small bowel by nonionic diffusion. The overall decrease in bile salt concentration serves to impair intraluminal micelle formation and hence fat absorption. Impaired absorption of vitamin $B_{12}$ associated with the blind loop syndrome appears to be related to the uptake of vitamin by the bacteria (Scheflan et al, 1976).

Typical symptoms include malaise, weight loss, malodorous diarrhea, and abdominal pain (Swan, 1974). Diagnosis of malabsorption due to bacterial overgrowth in the small intestine is established by (1) increased fecal fat, usually in the range of 15 to 30 gm/24 hours; (2)

macrocytic, megaloblastic anemia; (3) impaired absorption of vitamin $B_{12}$ that is not corrected by intrinsic factor; and (4) colony counts greater than $10^5$/ml in cultures of duodenal or jejunal fluid. Absorption of D-xylose and findings on peroral small bowel biopsy may be normal.

Permanent cure of this syndrome would necessitate surgical correction of the blind loop. However, since this is not a practical consideration in gynecologic oncology patients with this syndrome, therapy should consist of intermittent courses of antimicrobial therapy.

## Radiation Enteritis

Persistent diarrhea and malabsorption may develop shortly after the completion of pelvic or abdominal radiotherapy, or there may be a latent period of several years before the onset of diarrhea. Steatorrhea ranging from 10 to 70 gm/day is common, but impaired absorption of calcium, iron, D-xylose, or vitamin $B_{12}$ is less common (Scheflan et al, 1976). Diarrhea and malabsorption may be refractory to all methods of treatment, including antibiotics, pancreatic enzymes, a gluten-free diet, adrenal corticosteroids, anticholinergic drugs, and opiates. Occasionally these patients require intermittent hospitalization and parenteral nutrition.

## ACKNOWLEDGMENT

The authors would like to thank Dr. Felicien M. Steichen and Dr. Mark M. Ravitch for allowing them to reprint several drawings from *Stapling Techniques: General Surgery,* second edition, published by the United States Surgical Corporation, Norwalk, Connecticut; and from Ravitch M, Steichen F (eds): *Principles and Practice of Surgical Stapling,* Year Book Medical Publishers, 1987, p 10.

## REFERENCES

Baker JW: Stitchless plication for recurring obstruction of the small bowel. *Am J Surg* 116:316, 1968.

Ballon SC: Early post-op nutrition with needle-catheter jejunostomy. *Contemp Obstet Gynecol* 19:181, 1982.

Berek JS, Hacker NF, Lagasse LD: Rectosigmoid colectomy and reanastomosis to facilitate resection of primary and recurrent gynecologic cancer. *Obstet Gynecol* 64:715, 1984.

Berek JS, Hacker NF, Lagasse LD, Nieberg RK, Elashoff RM: Survival of patients following secondary cytoreductive surgery in ovarian cancer. *Obstet Gynecol* 61:189, 1983.

Berman ML, Lagasse LD, Watring WG, Moore JG, Smith M: Enteroperineal fistulae following pelvic exenteration: A 10 point program of management. *Gynecol Oncol* 4:368, 1976.

Bricker EM, Johnston WD: Repair of postirradiation rectovaginal fistula and stricture. *Surg Gynecol Obstet* 148:499, 1979.

Castaldo TW, Petrilli ES, Ballon SC, *et al*: Intestinal operations in patients with ovarian carcinoma. *Am J Obstet Gynecol* 139:80, 1981.

Chassin JL: *Operative Strategy in General Surgery,* Vol 1. New York, Springer-Verlag, 1980.

Clarke JS, Condon RE, Bertlett JG, *et al*: Preoperative oral antibiotics reduce septic complications of colon operations. *Ann Surg* 186:251, 1977.

Delgado G: The automatic stapler versus the conventional gastrointestinal anastomosis in gynecologic malignancies. *Gynecol Oncol* 12:302, 1981.

Greenberg NJ, Isselbacher KJ: Disorders of absorption. In *Harrison's Principles of Internal Medicine*, 7th ed. New York, McGraw-Hill Book Co, 1974, p 1456.

Griffiths CT, Fuller AF: Intensive surgical and chemotherapeutic management of advanced ovarian cancer. *Surg Clin North Am* 58:131, 1978.

Hacker NF, Berek JS, Lagasse LD, Nieberg RK, Elashoff RM: Primary cytoreductive surgery for epithelial ovarian cancer. *Obstet Gynecol* 61:413, 1983.

Krebs HB, Goplerud DR: Surgical management of bowel obstruction in advanced ovarian carcinoma. *Obstet Gynecol* 61:237, 1983.

Lagasse LD, Berman ML, Watring WG, Ballon SC: The gynecologic oncology patient: Restoration of function and prevention of disability. In McGowan L (ed): *Gynecologic Oncology*. New York, Appleton-Century-Crofts, 1978, pp 398-400.

Lagasse LD, Johnson GH, Smith ML, *et al*: Use of sigmoid colon for rectal substitution following pelvic exenteration. *Am J Obstet Gynecol* 116:106, 1973.

Leuchter RS, Petrilli ES, Dwyer RM, Hacker NF, Castaldo TW, Lagasse LD: Nd:YAG laser therapy of rectosigmoid bleeding due to radiation injury. *Obstet Gynecol* 59:655, 1982.

Lynch HT, Lynch PM, Albano WA, et al: The cancer family syndrome: A status report. *Dis Colon Rectum* 24:311, 1981.

Morgenstern L, Thompson R, Friedman NB: The modern enigma of radiation enteropathy: Sequelae and solutions. *Am J Surg* 134:166, 1977.

Ott DJ, Gelfand DW: Gastrointestinal contrast agents. Indications, uses and risks. *JAMA* 249:2380, 1983.

Patey DH: Primary epithelial apposition in colostomy. *Proc R Soc Med* 44:423, 1951.

Piver MS, Barlow JJ, Lele SB, Frank A: Survival after ovarian cancer induced intestinal obstruction. *Gynecol Oncol* 13:44, 1982.

Rutledge FN, Smith JP, Wharton JT, O'Quinn AG: Pelvic exenteration: An analysis of 296 patients. *Am J Obstet Gynecol* 129:881, 1977.

Scheflan M, Galli SJ, Perrotto J, Fischer JE: Intestinal adaptation after extensive resection of the small intestine and prolonged administration of parenteral nutrition. *Surg Gynecol Obstet* 143:757, 1976.

Schrock TR, Deveney CW, Dunphy JE: Factors contributing to leakage of colonic anastomoses. *Ann Surg* 177:513, 1973.

Scully RE: *Tumors of the Ovary and Maldeveloped Gonads*. Washington DC, Armed Forces Institute of Pathology, 1979, p 337.

Smith JP: Complications related to the radiated gastrointestinal tract. In Delgado G, Smith JP (eds): *Management of Complications in Gynecologic Oncology*. New York, John Wiley and Sons, 1982, p 104.

Smith JP, Golden PE, Rutledge FN: The surgical management of intestinal injuries following irradiation for carcinoma of the cervix. In *Cancer of the Uterus and Ovary*. University of Texas, MD Anderson Hospital, and Tumor Institute of Houston, Chicago, Year Book Medical Publishers, 1969, p 241.

Swan RW: Stagnant loop syndrome resulting from small bowel irradiation injury and intestinal bypass. *Gynecol Oncol* 2:441, 1974.

Swan RW, Fowler WC Jr, Boronow RC: Surgical management of radiation injury to the small intestine. *Surg Gynecol Obstet* 143:325, 1976.

Tunca JC, Buchler DA, Mack EA, Ruzicka FF, Crowley JJ, Carr WF: The management of ovarian-cancer–caused bowel obstruction. *Gynecol Oncol* 12:186, 1981.

Wheeless CR, Dorsey JH: Use of the automatic surgical stapler for intestinal anastomosis associated with gynecologic malignancy. Review of 283 procedures. *Gynecol Oncol* 11:1, 1981.

White AJ, Buchsbaum HJ, Blythe JG, Lifshitz S: Use of the bulbocavernosus muscle (Martius procedure) for repair of radiation-induced rectovaginal fistulas. *Obstet Gynecol* 60:114, 1982.

# Chapter 20 | Cardiopulmonary Complications*

**Herbert B. Hechtman**    **Richard Welbourn**

**Gideon Goldman**

Cardiopulmonary complications are commonplace after major surgery. Anticipation and early recognition of these problems will minimize the morbidity and mortality associated with delayed or inappropriate therapy. In this chapter, we will review the common mechanisms underlying failure of the heart and lungs as well as the rationale for therapy. Our focus will be on the older woman requiring major surgery who might be at high risk because of preexistent heart or lung disease or because of complicating factors related to the primary gynecologic problem, such as inanition, ascites, or chemotherapy.

* This research was supported in part by The National Institutes of Health; The Brigham Surgical Group, Inc.; and The Trauma Research Foundation.

## IDENTIFICATION OF RISK FACTORS

Most risk factors are readily noted on history taking and physical examination. Seldom are invasive diagnostic tests and cardiopulmonary monitoring indicated in the healthy patient undergoing major surgery. However, the presence of certain signs and symptoms must on occasion prompt vigorous and extensive evaluation in order to minimize morbidity.

### Airways Disease

Resistance to air flow is common in patients with bronchitis and is usually due to a reduction in airways diameter because of excess secretions or constriction of bronchial smooth muscle. This results in an increase in the expiratory work of breathing, which in the extreme can lead to carbon dioxide retention and ventilatory failure. There is, however, a broad pathologic spectrum in chronic bronchitis. Some patients may simply complain of a productive cough, while others may wheeze.

Our concern is with the patient who has significant functional impairment. For example, active exhalation signifies major airways disease. Exhalation is normally a passive process that relies on the elasticity of the lungs. In severe bronchitis, active work may be required for exhalation, with recruitment of the accessory muscles of respiration. Unfortunately, compression of the thoracic cage during active exhalation must, of course, increase intrathoracic pressure. Pressure surrounding the airways may then exceed intrabronchial pressure, particularly in patients with emphysema, in whom lung elastic recoil is reduced. In order to maintain airway patency, such patients must exhale slowly to prevent major increases in intrathoracic pressure. Furthermore, they must purse their lips during exhalation. This form of self-employed positive end-expiratory pressure is used by patients with severe chronic lung disease to raise airways pressure and thereby prevent collapse of the bronchi. Such patients have minimal pulmonary reserves and are at extreme risk.

### Sputum Production

*Smoking* predisposes to chronic bronchitis and is associated with both increased mucous sputum production and a decreased ability of the cilia to clear secretions. This may lead to airway obstruction, with distal atelectasis and pneumonia. With bronchial irritants such as allergens or an upper respiratory infection, mucus plugging may also be present. Smoking increases the levels of carbon monoxide in blood, impairing delivery of oxygen to the tissues, and raises nicotine levels, which alters cardiovascular function. Although smoking cessation is thought to lead to maximal benefit within 8 weeks, carbon monoxide and nicotine levels fall by 24 hours and ciliary function and sputum production return to normal after 2 weeks (Ashburn and Stanley, 1988). Consumption of 20 cigarettes a day increases the risk for postoperative complications, but the presence of a productive cough is probably a better indication of risk (Jackson, 1988; Warner et al, 1984). A forced expiratory volume of less than 2 liters in one second ($FEV_1$) or an $FEV_1$-to-forced vital capacity (FVC) ratio below 0.75 is a reliable indicator of high risk (Manning, 1989). Thus, a history of smoking and auscultatory signs of retained secretions should be sought, and chest physiotherapy, antibiotics, and bronchodilators should be initiated, if necessary (Jackson, 1988).

### Lung Displacements

Three acute pulmonary problems may occur in the perioperative period. *Massive atelectasis* may be suspected on physical exam, but confirmation by chest x-ray is necessary. Repeated bronchoscopy may be needed to reexpand the lung. *Pleural effusions* may be malignant or nonmalignant, and large effusions should be tapped dry (Fig. 20-1). Occasionally, effusions may be due to improper placement of central lines, with infusion or bleeding into the chest. Treatment entails removal of the line and fluid evacuation. *Pneumothorax* secondary to lung lacerations because of a thoracentesis or subclavian vein catheterization is an extreme hazard to a patient who requires pressure breathing during general anesthesia. Procedures that expose patients to the risk of lung laceration should be avoided in the perioperative period. If subclavian catheterization must be done, a chest x-ray during exhalation is necessary to exclude a pneumothorax (Figure 20-2).

### Myocardial Infarction and Heart Failure

These are two common causes of postoperative morbidity and mortality. As with pulmonary disease, the preoperative history and physical examination are important in identifying underlying cardiac problems. Five prevalent risk factors have been correlated with postoperative cardiovascular complications: (1) prior myocardial infarction, (2) presence of congestive heart failure, (3) arrhythmias, (4) abnormalities on the electrocardiogram (such as bundle branch block), and (5) history of a previous cerebrovascular accident (Goldman et al, 1978). In the majority of cases, these risk factors can be detected by the initial screening history and physical exam. The two primary adjunctive diagnostic modalities available for evaluating potential cardiac problems are the electrocardiogram and the chest radiograph. Neither has much value as a routine screening test (Robbins and Mushlin, 1979), and they are not usually obtained in women under 30 years of age who are undergoing surgery and are in good health. (Rees et al, 1976).

*Myocardial Infarction* Patients undergoing surgery within 6 months of a myocardial infarction are particularly vulnerable to cardiac complications, the reinfarction rate being between 15 and 30%. Even a remote history of myocardial infarction still poses a threat of reinfarction in 3 to 6% of cases (Steen et al, 1978). Other factors associated with an increased risk of developing a postoperative coronary artery occlusion include (1) age above 70 years; (2) findings of dyspnea, orthopnea, or edema; (3) Grade ¾ mitral murmur; (4) more than five premature ventricular contractions per minute; and (5) a tortuous, calcified aorta on chest x-ray (Robbins and Mushlin, 1979). Stable angina is not a significant factor. The mortality after perioperative myocardial infarction is approximately 50%, with reports ranging from 35 to 70%.

Patients who have recently had a myocardial infarction demand careful perioperative management, including constant monitoring by means of electrocardiography and insertion of both intraarterial and pulmonary artery catheters. These catheters can also be used for volume infusions and in the treatment of hypo- or hypertension.

Patients with unstable angina usually require preoperative treatment with beta-adrenergic blocking agents and/or nitrates. These medications should be continued

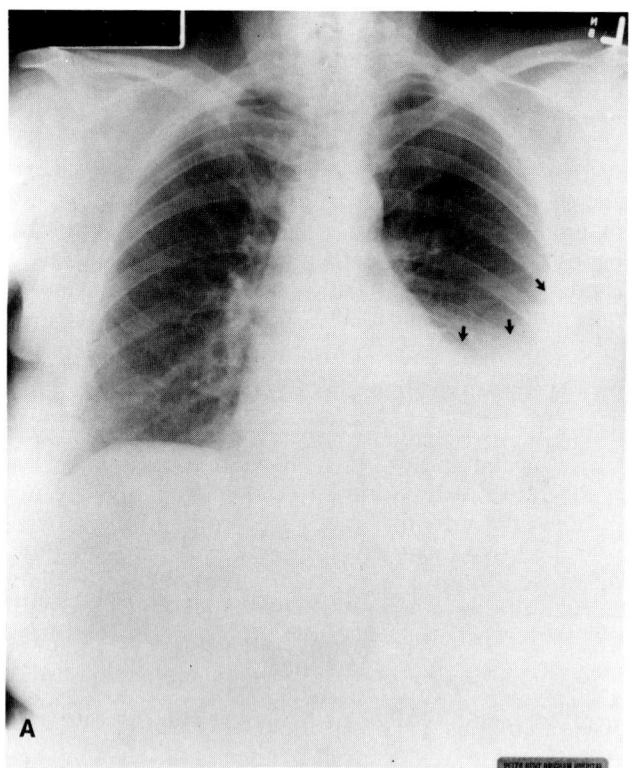 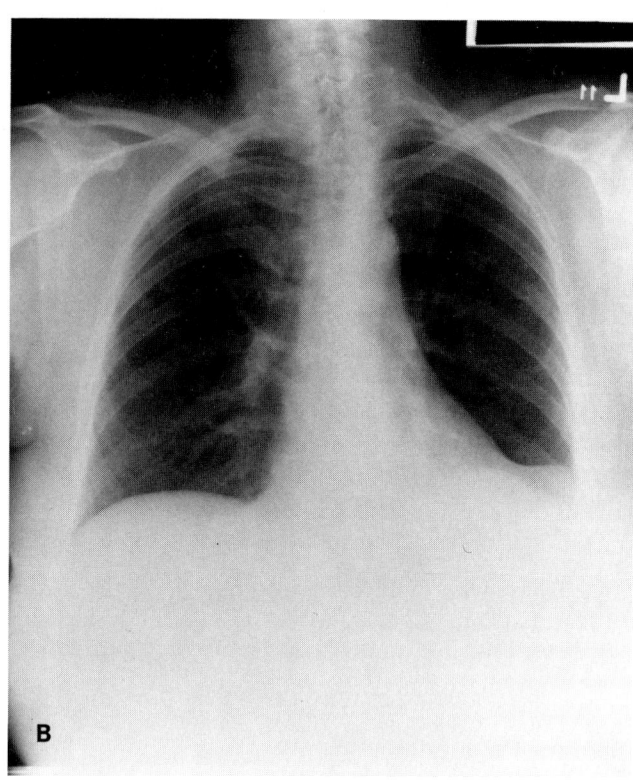

FIGURE 20-1 On this posterior-anterior chest x-ray, a large, homogeneous density can be seen at the left base. Proof that this is fluid was the observation on a lateral decubitus projection of a layering-out of the density (A). Following thoracocentesis, there was a marked decrease in the amount of fluid (B).

in oral form until the morning of surgery and then readministered as early as possible after surgery. Intravenous nitroglycerin has been shown to decrease the incidence of perioperative myocardial ischemia effectively in patients with angina (Fusciardi et al, 1980).

**Congestive Heart Failure** The presence of congestive heart failure secondary to ischemic, valvular, or hypertensive heart disease is associated with a higher incidence of postoperative complications. In addition, a history of or preoperative signs indicating pump failure will also increase the chances of subsequent problems. The postoperative development of cardiogenic pulmonary edema is associated with a mortality of over 50% (Goldman et al, 1978).

Patients with extreme ventricular enlargement on chest x-ray, congestive heart failure, or a history of previous episodes of failure should be treated preoperatively with digitalization, diuretics, and nitrates to reduce preload or afterload as indicated. Surgery should be postponed until the existing cardiovascular insufficiency has been reversed or at least stabilized. The prophylactic use of digitalis is not recommended for elderly patients or those with minimal left ventricular chamber enlargement (Hillis and Cohn, 1978).

**Valvular Heart Disease** Patients with significant valvular heart disease are at increased risk for congestive heart failure postoperatively. This patient population has been shown to have a mortality approaching 10% (Goldman et al, 1978) and should undergo perioperative monitoring with systemic as well as pulmonary artery catheters. Previous episodes of bacterial endocarditis require antibiotic prophylaxis, usually gentamicin and vancomycin. The use of antibiotics in patients with mitral valve prolapse is a matter of controversy, and most clinicians do not recommend prophylaxis in this setting.

### Hypertension

Approximately one-third of surgical patients present with a previous history of hypertension or are found to have elevated blood pressure preoperatively. Severe hypertension increases the risk of cardiovascular complications. A diastolic pressure greater than 110 torr should under most circumstances be a contraindication to surgery (Goldman and Caldera, 1979). It has been shown that patients with poorly controlled hypertension lack adequate autoregulation of the systemic vasculature and are susceptible to wide fluctuations in blood pressure during surgery. This magnifies the possible occurrence of hypertensive cardiovascular disease and is the primary reason for increased risk in these patients (Feigal and Blaisdell, 1979).

Surgery should be delayed until hypertension is adequately controlled. Initial treatment involves the use of diuretics, usually a thiazide. If the diastolic pressure remains unacceptably high, a second agent such as al-

venous procainamide is also a useful agent and can be substituted for lidocaine if initial therapy is ineffective.

Due to the lack of predictable markers, it is difficult to determine which patients are at increased risk for supraventricular tachyarrhythmias (Rogers et al, 1952). These arrhythmias are more apt to occur in the elderly population. In general, the prophylactic use of digitalis preoperatively is not recommended. If a supraventricular arrhythmia occurs perioperatively, the goal of treatment is to control the rate of ventricular response. Administration of digoxin or propranolol is effective in the majority of cases. Verapamil, a calcium channel blocker, is useful as an initial form of therapy (Arono et al, 1979).

## Systemic Factors

A variety of conditions may directly or indirectly influence cardiopulmonary function. For example, electrolyte imbalance can adversely affect cardiac contractility and induce arrhythmias. Age and obesity influence pulmonary function, as does ascites. For example, extreme obesity has been shown to correlate with operative mortality. After surgery for uterine neoplasms, mortality was 20% among women weighing over 300 pounds but was less than 2% among lighter women (Feigal and Blaisdell, 1979). Failure of other organ systems may have indirect, although important, effects on the lungs. Thus, the comatose or stuporous patient may aspirate gastric contents more easily and is much more vulnerable to ventilatory failure. Liver failure slows the rate of drug metabolism, so that vigilance is required when one is using drugs that depress cardiopulmonary function.

## Tumor-Related Factors

***Pulmonary Metastasis*** Discrete tumor nodules ordinarily do not produce much lung dysfunction (Fig. 20-3). In contrast, lymphangitic spread may lead to severe abnormalities in respiratory gas exchange (Fig. 20-4). This form of malignant growth occurs when small tumor emboli become trapped within the pulmonary microvasculature, grow into the interstitium, and invade lymphatics. The process may be extremely rapid, occurring over a matter of weeks. Lymphangitic spread can be suspected but not confirmed on chest x-ray. Often, transbronchial or open lung biopsy is needed for a definitive diagnosis, particularly when other, potentially reversible entities such as infection with *Pneumocystis carinii* may be present. A favorable therapeutic response in the presence of lymphangitic spread is so remote that cessation of vigorous therapy should be strongly considered if this diagnosis is confirmed.

***Thrombophlebitis*** Pelvic malignancy is often associated with deep venous phlebitis and pulmonary embolism. This is thought to be due to the release of proaggregatory factors from the tumor combined with the lesion's direct compressive effect on pelvic veins. The preventive use of heparin, 5,000 units subcutaneously every 12 hours starting preoperatively, must be weighed against

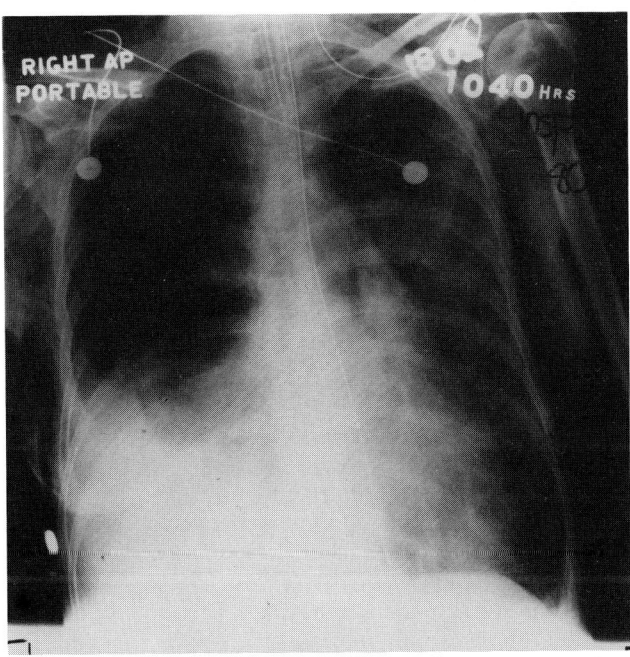

FIGURE 20-2 This 45-year-old woman was recuperating from severe sepsis and respiratory failure when a right-sided central venous feeding line was placed. Extensive mediastinal and left-sided subcutaneous emphysema had been present for more than 1 day and was thought to be related to the use of mechanical ventilation with positive end-expiratory pressure. Air was dissected from a ruptured small airway proximally into the mediastinum and subcutaneous tissues. On the right, there is a 30% pneumothorax and a significant amount of pleural fluid. This was considered to be a problem directly related to the central venous catheter, which was positioned on the right. Hyperalimentation fluid was obtained from the right pleural space by thoracocentesis.

phamethyldopa, propranolol, or clonidine should be added. Oral treatment should be continued until the morning of surgery; thereafter, the intravenous agents nitroprusside or nitroglycerin usually provide adequate blood pressure control. For problems related to excess volume loading, intravenous furosemide should constitute initial therapy. Subsequently, if diuresis is ineffective, a second agent such as alphamethyldopa, propranolol, or hydralazine may be desirable.

## Cardiac Arrhythmias

It is estimated that 5% of general surgical patients develop significant intraoperative or postoperative arrhythmias. (Goldman et al, 1978). Alterations in electrolyte balance secondary to diuretic use, hypoxia, hypercapnia, and certain general anesthetics combined with surgical stress predispose these individuals to conduction abnormalities. To prevent perioperative ventricular arrhythmias, prophylaxis with antiarrhythmic agents is indicated for patients with a recent ischemic episode or those with coronary artery disease complicated by complex ventricular ectopy (Goldman et al, 1977). Lidocaine is the agent of choice for both prophylaxis and therapy in ventricular tachyarrhythmias. An intravenous injection of 100 to 200 mg followed by an infusion of 1 to 4 mg/min is recommended. Intra-

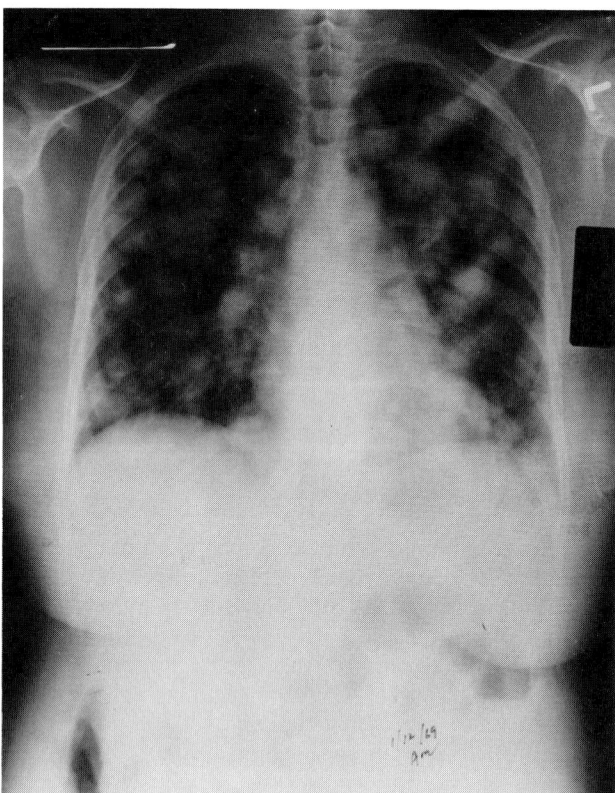

FIGURE 20-3 A 33-year-old woman presented with flulike symptoms and normal menstrual cycling. A lower abdominal mass could be palpated. The multiple metastatic nodules noted on the chest x-ray proved to be secondary to endometrial carcinoma.

the risk of bleeding from operative sites—a risk heightened by potential thrombocytopenia secondary to radiation and chemotherapy. A more satisfactory alternative would be the use of compression boots, which can be applied preoperatively from ankle to midthigh and can be removed once the patient becomes ambulatory.

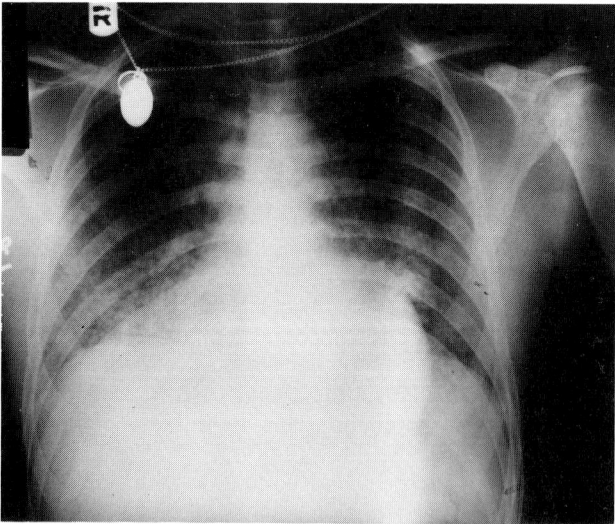

FIGURE 20-4 A diffuse interstitial process is present bilaterally and is consistent with lymphatic spread of cancer in a patient with known breast malignancy.

**Chemotherapy** Surgical procedures are frequently performed in women who have been or are currently being treated with chemotherapy. Several of these agents are known to cause cardiopulmonary dysfunction. For example, doxorubicin is toxic to the myocardium and can indirectly lead to respiratory failure via myocarditis and cardiac failure. On the other hand, radiotherapy directed to the diaphragms in patients with ovarian carcinoma is usually not given in sufficient doses to injure lung parenchyma or produce myocarditis.

Other chemotherapeutic agents can produce direct lung toxicity. For example, pulmonary fibrosis occasionally complicates administration of the alkylating agents busulfan and cyclophosphamide. The antimetabolite methotrexate has also been found to be associated with pulmonary infiltrates.

Bleomycin is the chemotherapeutic agent usually associated with adverse pulmonary effects. Frequently used in the treatment of recurrent or disseminated squamous cell carcinoma of the cervix, vagina, and vulva, this antibiotic is associated with a 3% incidence of fatal pneumonitis and pulmonary fibrosis (McCord and Fridovich, 1978). Excess collagen deposition is characteristic of this complication. The mechanism involved is unknown, as is a means for predicting which patients are vulnerable to pulmonary changes. The incidence of pulmonary fibrosis appears to be increased in elderly patients, especially when drug doses exceed 400 mg. Of equal and great importance is the fact that bleomycin sensitizes the lungs to oxygen, so that low inspired concentrations become potentially toxic. As a result, patients with a history of bleomycin administration are at high risk for developing acute respiratory failure (ARF) in the perioperative period (Gould et al, 1972).

## Sepsis

Patients with sepsis may become so ill that the typical responses to infection, i.e., fever and leukocytosis, are not consistently present. Often the secondary sequelae of bacteremia are the only clues available to the clinician. These are hypotension unexplained by volume loss or myocardial infarction, thrombocytopenia, leukopenia or leukocytosis, and multisystem organ failure. The clinical presentation of multisystem failure varies. Typically, patients become confused or stuporous. Pulmonary abnormalities are manifested by permeability edema with hypoxemia or ventilatory failure, along with high respiratory rates and carbon dioxide retention. Cardiac output tends to be normal, although resistant hypotension is frequent. Oliguria or nonoliguric renal failure with a rising creatinine level is common. Bilirubinemia is frequent, as are inconsistent elevations in other measurements of liver function. Superficial gastric ulcerations with guaiac-positive or frankly hemorrhagic nasogastric fluid may also be seen.

The initial manifestation of severe infection in approximately 40% of patients who are eventually proved to have sepsis is ARF. The corollary is also true that in surgical patients with severe sepsis—that is, with hypotension and bacteremia—ARF is likely to intervene. ARF evolving in this setting of sepsis is associated with a mortality of over 50% (Walker and Eiseman, 1975).

Death usually occurs late, 2 to 3 weeks after the onset of symptoms, when the patient succumbs to progressive multisystem organ failure.

Lung damage in sepsis is characterized by an increase in capillary permeability and a general extravasation of a protein-rich exudate throughout the pulmonary interstitium. Clinically, this appears as a diffuse, patchy infiltrate on chest x-ray in patients whose pulmonary arterial wedge pressure is in the normal range (Fig. 20-5). While gram-negative pathogens are most often implicated in sepsis, gram-positive organisms are equally capable of mediating the systemic sequelae of organ failure. Repeat blood cultures may be required to identify the causative agent. To be successful in treating septic ARF, one must identify the septic focus and organism(s).

### Clinical Problems Closely Associated with ARF

***Disseminated Intravascular Coagulation (DIC)*** This phenomenon is usually a manifestation of a significant underlying illness such as sepsis. However, DIC has also been noted to occur during uncomplicated major surgery (McLoughlin et al, 1979). This has been documented by declines in fibrinogen, plasminogen, and platelet counts as well as by the appearance of fibrin monomer, increased fibrinolytic activity, and fibrin degradation products. In the setting of major surgery, there have usually been no untoward cardiopulmonary effects despite the fact that indices of DIC are as marked as those noted in severe sepsis. Infrequently, bulky tumors, when manipulated, may release procoagulants that trigger DIC. In this setting, bleeding may be a problem, as may longer term effects, particularly acute tubular necrosis. Clinically, we conclude that DIC itself is not a common cause of ARF.

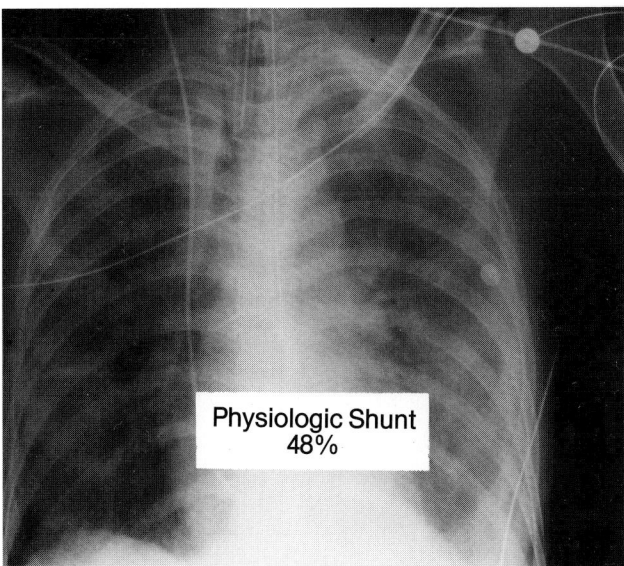

**FIGURE 20-5** This patient developed septicemia 5 days postoperatively, manifested initially by severe dyspnea and tachypnea. A chest x-ray showed a diffuse interstitial edema. Pulmonary arterial wedge pressure was 6 mm Hg, indicating permeability edema. Hypoxemia was severe.

***Pancreatitis*** The empiric relationship between severe pancreatitis and ARF is not disputed, although the mechanism is conjectural. The leading thesis is that pancreatic enzymes activate complement. In turn, the complement fragment C5a is released, which activates white blood cells. These cells aggregate and are then sequestered in the lungs, where they cause endothelial cell damage. The difficulty with these theories is the lack of correlation between hypoxemia and high amylase or lipase levels. Pancreatitis may also lead to pleural effusions via retroperitoneal lymphatics. Thoracentesis may document pancreatitis, since the pleural effusion is rich in amylase.

***Shock*** This ill-defined entity has been thought to be an important determinant of organ failure, hence the use of the term *shock lung* to describe ARF. However, in multiple clinical, primate, and dog studies, severe hemorrhagic hypotension has not been found to be causally related to the subsequent development of ARF.

***Blood Transfusion*** Stored blood contains microaggregates that are thought capable of inducing ARF. Once trapped in the lungs, the microaggregates may activate other cells such as platelets and leukocytes, which, in turn, can release vasoactive and vasotoxic agents. This reasoning has stimulated the use of fine mesh sieves to filter out microaggregates from blood prior to infusion. Unfortunately, the data linking blood transfusion to ARF are weak; there is little evidence to substantiate an association with respiratory failure even when massive quantities of blood are used, providing there are no transfusion reactions.

### Anesthesia

General inhalation and spinal anesthetic techniques are inherently safe and have similar complication rates. It is principally the duration of anesthesia that is a risk factor. Operations of longer than 3.5 hours are associated with an increased number of complications (Jackson, 1988). The choice of anesthetic technique is often based on secondary considerations. For example, spinal or epidural anesthesia should be favored in a patient who has had a recent pneumothorax. On the other hand, hypotension due to sepsis may be more difficult to manage under spinal anesthesia. Airway control with proper minute ventilation can be better assured using general anesthesia and may be of importance in patients who have only marginally compensated for their increased respiratory work in whom hypnotics, analgesics and a supine position during surgery may induce ventilatory failure.

### Intravascular Volume

Undetected fluid shifts may confuse volume assessments in seriously ill patients. Pulmonary and systemic microvascular permeability may be altered by drugs, radiation, tumor, or bacteria and result in protein leakage. Fluid may be sequestered as ascites, in the walls of the peritoneal cavity or bowel, or as pulmonary edema. The venous capacitance vessels may be inoperative and may fail to regulate the volume of venous return. Further, compliance of the ventricles and their contractility are often disordered. Because of these factors, the usual signs of volume status, pulse rate, blood pressure, jugular venous distention, and urine flow may be misleading.

Patients with borderline left ventricular function secondary to coronary or hypertensive heart disease are particularly sensitive to volume infusions. Small increases in preload, i.e., left ventricular end-diastolic fiber stretch or volume, can precipitate heart failure. This results in increased end-diastolic pressure or pulmonary arterial wedge pressure. These high left ventricular filling pressures are transmitted retrograde, elevating pulmonary capillary pressure and leading to pulmonary edema.

## PULMONARY COMPLICATIONS

### Atelectasis

Atelectasis is the most common postoperative respiratory complication, usually occurring on the first to third day after surgery (Fig. 20-6). The incidence of atelectasis is approximately 10% for lower abdominal operative procedures (Pierce and Robertson, 1977). Extending the incision into the upper abdomen increases the complication rate by a factor of 2. In addition to the location of the surgical incision, smoking, obesity, duration of anesthesia, and chronic obstructive lung disease are other risk factors that increase the incidence of atelectasis (Hechtman et al, 1980). The degree of lung collapse is variable. Minimal atelectasis may present as a subtle linear density on radiography. Collapse of a lung segment represents an extension of the same process and is usually readily apparent on chest x-ray. In the extreme, an entire lobe or lung may be collapsed, with shift of the mediastinum.

In the immediate postoperative period, the patient's ability to inspire deeply and exhale completely is significantly reduced. These two dynamic volumes make up the vital capacity (VC). The postoperative reduction in VC is more pronounced as the surgical incision is made higher in the abdomen. The fact that VC correlates with the ability to cough suggests a mechanism of atelectasis in patients with low VC. Failure to cough and clear secretions leads to airway obstructions and distal lung collapse as alveolar gas is absorbed.

High concentrations of inspired oxygen, in a range that can be delivered only by a mechanical ventilator and endotracheal tube, increase the risk of atelectasis. Open systems used to deliver oxygen seldom result in an inspired concentration greater than 50% and therefore pose a lesser risk. Unlike the case with nitrogen, in which there is no peripheral utilization by the body and the nitrogen tension of pulmonary artery blood equals that of systemic arterial blood, the transpulmonary uptake of oxygen is substantial. Flowing blood removes alveolar oxygen at a rapid rate. Failure to ventilate alveoli that are filled with 100% oxygen promptly leads to atelectasis. Within minutes the lung segment becomes airless and has an appearance like that of liver. The ventilation/perfusion ratio need not be zero to lead to atelectasis. In theory, low ratios such as 0.1 make the lung vulnerable to atelectasis, since the amount of oxygen removed by the blood exceeds alveolar filling via the airways.

The phenomenon of *absorption atelectasis* is probably the greatest hazard of breathing 100% oxygen. It is seen in any setting in which ventilation is limited. Patients at greatest risk are those with reduced functional residual capacity (FRC), which is the volume of air in the lungs at the end of a normal tidal ventilation.

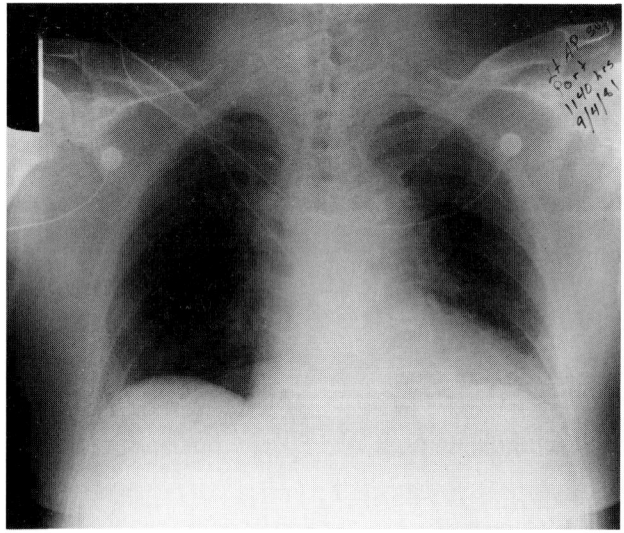

A

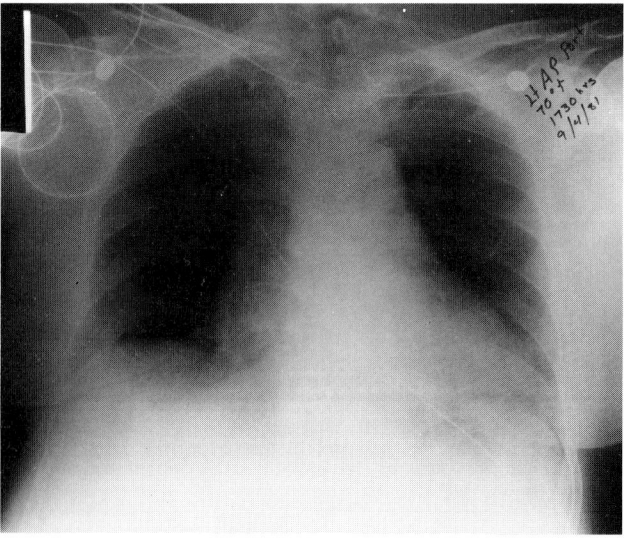

B

FIGURE 20-6  Several hours after extubation following a general anesthetic, stridor and cyanosis developed in this patient, and he was reintubated. An x-ray showed atelectasis, evidenced by marked shagginess of the left cardiac silhouette (*A*). Chest physiotherapy resolved these abnormalities in 5 hours (*B*).

Such patients include those suffering from acute ventilatory and respiratory failure.

In cases of prolonged atelectasis, failure to clear secretions allows local bacterial proliferation, resulting in pneumonia. Predictably, the incidence of pneumonia parallels that of atelectasis, since the same risk factors predispose to both. The incidence is about 5% following lower abdominal surgery and most often involves dependent lung segments.

## Aspiration

Perioperatively, patients are at increased risk for aspirating gastric contents. Endotracheal intubation and extubation are critical times when gastric secretions can reflux and enter the tracheobronchial tree. The majority of episodes involving aspiration are clinically silent, with relatively little gastric fluid contaminating the lungs. Postoperatively, cases of suspected atelectasis may actually be unrecognized aspiration. As many as 16% of patients have been shown to suffer occult aspiration after general anesthesia (Culver et al, 1951). Prolonged endotracheal intubation, even with the use of a high-volume, low-pressure cuff, is associated with a 20% aspiration rate (Spray et al, 1976).

The appearance of clinical signs after aspiration depends upon the amount and type of fluid aspirated. Gastric fluid with a pH below 3 is likely to cause severe damage due to protein denaturation of lung parenchyma. However, pancreatic and biliary secretions may also be noxious. Massive bilateral aspiration is associated with a mortality approximating 90%. The mortality for all clinically recognized cases of aspiration is high and probably reflects the fact that the debilitated patient who is older and more likely to have a significant underlying illness is most vulnerable to aspiration. Therapy for this problem is supportive; steroids appear to offer no benefit.

## Pulmonary Embolus

Over a century ago, Virchow described the classic triad of factors predisposing to thromboembolism: stasis of flow, vessel injury, and enhanced coagulability of the blood. Pulmonary embolism remains a frequent cause of respiratory failure (Fig. 20-7). Pelvic surgery in particular is associated with an increased incidence of embolism. As with aspiration, it is difficult to estimate the true incidence of the problem. Fifty per cent of episodes are without symptoms. Even large emboli may present simply with hypotension and no other signs. Conversely, symptomatic cases may frequently be misdiagnosed. Most occur between the third and sixth day following surgery. The vast majority of venous thrombi occur in the thighs and iliofemoral venous system.

## Oxygen Toxicity

Pulmonary oxygen toxicity is an important manifestation of oxygen overdosage observed in experimental animals. Its importance in humans is likely but difficult to document. Adverse effects on the lungs are related

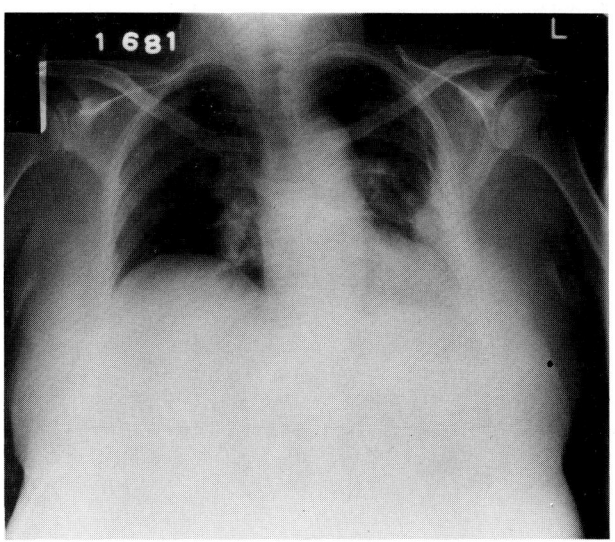

**FIGURE 20-7** This 61-year-old woman developed chest pain and shortness of breath on the 10th postoperative day. The chest film shows a wedge-shaped, pleura-based density in the left lower lobe. This radiographic density is consistent with a pulmonary infarct but is not specific. Other causes of such a density include pneumonia or atelectasis. Additional x-ray views confirmed the presence of a left pleural effusion, which is usually the earliest radiographic sign of infarction.

solely to the tension of inspired $O_2$. The injury is thought to be due to excess formation of superoxide anion and hydrogen peroxide (McCord and Fridovich, 1978). In addition, it is likely that relative insufficiency of the protective enzymes catalase and superoxide dismutase permit and probably magnify oxygen toxicity. These enzymes rapidly clear oxygen free radicals. Finally, in experimental hypoxia, the number of alveolar neutrophils has been correlated with a rise in levels of the chemoattractant leukotriene B4, an oxygenation product of arachidonic acid (Taniguchi et al, 1986).

Experimentally, the most significant noxious effect of oxygen is on endothelial and alveolar type I cells, while alveoar type II cells are seemingly resistant. Changes in cellular morphology have been observed within 48 hours of $O_2$ exposure in otherwise healthy lungs. Patients treated with the chemotherapeutic agent bleomycin are extremely sensitive to oxygen administration. Judicious use of perioperative $O_2$ is therefore essential in these patients, since any increase in oxygen tension may precipitate ARF (Goldner et al, 1978).

## Ventilatory and Respiratory Failure

***Inadequate Alveolar Ventilation*** Failure to generate sufficient alveolar ventilation to excrete carbon dioxide is a general definition of ventilatory failure. This may be due to mechanical displacement or compression of the lungs because of pleural air or fluid. Since these mechanical states are easily reversed, the diagnosis must be vigorously pursued. Even substantial volumes of fluid and air are easily missed on chest x-rays taken by the portable technique. Such films must be of reasonable quality, and patients should be positioned in as upright a posture as possible. Instability of the blood pressure may force one to obtain lateral decubitus films.

The usual setting of ventilatory failure is the postoperative patient who cannot be weaned from the mechanical ventilator. Certain factors, particularly age, chronic airways disease, ascites, and diminished mentation, increase the risk. Most of these patients are easily recognized preoperatively. Usually, we make no attempt to wean them from ventilatory support until the morning after surgery, when the majority of anesthetic drugs have been metabolized.

On occasion, ventilatory failure is not anticipated. In the early postoperative period, iatrogenic factors can precipitate ventilatory problems, particularly an excess use of narcotics in patients in whom the muscle-paralyzing drugs have still not cleared. One reason for delayed hepatic metabolism of these agents in prolonged surgical procedures may be related to hypothermia secondary to cold transfusions of blood and evaporational cooling. Thus, after 2 hours, a xiphoid-to-pubis midline incision combined with a 4-unit blood transfusion will result in an average decline in patient temperature to 34°C. Increasing the temperature of the operating room may be necessary, as well as anticipating the problem and using a blood warmer and a heating blanket under the patient.

Monitoring the sedated patient in the recovery room with regard to the adequacy of ventilation requires continuous assessment of vital signs. It is virtually impossible to estimate tidal volume or minute ventilation quantitatively by bedside inspection of chest-cage motion. Since most patients receive supplementary oxygen, the usual consequence of hypoventilation is not hypoxia but hypercarbia and respiratory acidosis. The cardiovascular response is hypertension and tachycardia; on occasion, the only respiratory manifestation may be tachypnea. Evaluation requires arterial blood gas analysis.

A variety of acute pulmonary and systemic problems can cause or aggravate ventilatory failure. Examples of pulmonary problems include pneumonia, acid aspiration, and ARF. Systemic illnesses such as cerebrovascular accidents may lead to major difficulties with muscle function and coordination of chest wall mechanics. A computed tomographic (CT) scan may be needed to differentiate stroke from electrolyte abnormalities or metabolic encephalopathies, all of which can decrease neural control mechanisms as well as directly induce weakness of the muscles of ventilation. Patients with hepatitis and renal failure or sepsis are also vulnerable to these metabolic effects on muscle function.

Ventilatory failure may be due to increased work requirements. The hypermetabolic patient with increased catabolism due to operative trauma or sepsis must excrete increased amounts of $CO_2$. The oral, nasogastric, or intravenous use of hyperalimentation, particularly carbohydrates, can force further $CO_2$ production. Therefore, nutritional support must be used judiciously, since hyperalimentation will not prevent or reverse muscle weakness and may indeed cause or perpetuate ventilatory failure by increasing the need for minute ventilation to excrete $CO_2$.

Ventilatory failure may be prolonged, lasting for weeks or even months. Underlying mechanisms beyond the initiating catastrophic illness, which has often been resolved, are unknown. Many patients appear alert and may even be taking food by mouth. However, their muscle coordination and reserves for doing ventilatory work are severely impaired, and respiratory control mechanisms may function abnormally. Attempts to wean frequently fail, that is, the respiratory rate increases and $CO_2$ is retained. Despite these multiple failures, however, weaning trials should be continued.

***Acid-Base Imbalance*** Arterial partial pressure of carbon dioxide ($PCO_2$) must be interpreted with respect to pH; the latter is the first part of the arterial blood gas report to be examined. For example, an acid pH and elevated $PCO_2$ strongly suggest a primary respiratory acidosis due to hypoventilation. Mixed acid-base defects are common. Thus, an elevated pH and $PCO_2$ are often seen during the liberal use of loop diuretics such as furosemide, which leads to excess excretion of $Cl^-$ and reabsorption of $HCO_3^-$. The resultant homeostatic response to this primary metabolic alkalosis in a spontaneously breathing patient is hypoventilation, $CO_2$ retention, and a compensatory respiratory acidosis. Calculation of the "base excess" may assist in deriving the net acid-base status in mixed defects. In this example, base excess may be used to quantitate the amount of intravenous $0.1 N$ HCl needed to correct a severe metabolic alkalosis.

***Hypoxemia*** Acute respiratory failure is a clinical state of severe hypoxemia requiring supplemental oxygen. The disorder is a manifestation of abnormalities in peripheral bronchoalveolar capillary units. Although many conditions result in hypoxemia, such as pulmonary compression or major airway obstruction, these are examples of ventilatory failure in which mechanical events are the cause of maldistribution of ventilation and in which mechanical therapy can usually resolve the gas exchange abnormality.

The ultimate cause of hypoxia in ventilatory or respiratory failure is perfusion of poorly ventilated or nonventilated lung segments. Diffusion barriers in ARF secondary to interstitial edema are of lesser significance. Airway obstructions due to mucus plugs or bronchospasm are important causes of decreased ventilation and hypoxia. Another common cause of reduced alveolar ventilation is critical airways closure. The *closing volume* at which critical closure occurs is defined as that lung volume at which there is collapse of peripheral airways. This occurs primarily in the dependent portions of the lungs. Smoking and age adversely affect the closing volume (Leblanc et al, 1970). Prior to the fifth decade of life in normal lungs, the FRC comfortably exceeds the closing volume for a person in the supine position. With advancing age, a rise in closing volume occurs, and the ratio of FRC to closing volume diminishes. Above age 50, the closing volume surpasses the FRC, permitting small-airway closure at the end of each expiration. Smoking accelerates the aging process of the lungs by approximately 10 years.

With increasing age and smoking history, airway closure may occur during normal tidal ventilation. Surgical patients have unique problems. The supine position elevates the diaphragm and leads to an average reduction in FRC of 20%. This is thought to be the explanation of the hypoxia of recumbency.

Other poorly understood events related to surgery tend to cause reductions in the FRC. Delayed falls in FRC on the first postoperative day are associated with incisions that extend into the upper abdomen. It is conjectured that the failure to cough adequately, sigh, and deep-breathe prevents surfactant either from being synthesized by alveoli or from working properly to reduce surface tension. Surfactant is a metastable phospholipid, the mechanical effects of which are in large part determined by physical factors such as its molecular thickness on the alveolar wall. Stretching alveoli and surfactant by periodic deep breathing makes surfactant more effective; surface tension is reduced and FRC increases. It is unlikely that the phenomenon of microatelectasis, which was often invoked to explain the hypoxia that followed many major surgical procedures, ever existed as a true pathologic state. In atelectasis the alveoli become gasless and alveolar walls become intimately approximated—a condition that is difficult to reverse. Hypoxia associated with a reduction in FRC following surgery is probably not microatelectasis, since it can be so easily corrected. More likely, the fall in FRC is due to a surfactant-related decline in compliance. Hypoxia may then result from critical closure. The lack of precision in this field is due to the difficulty in measuring surfactant in situ.

***Pneumonia and Systemic Sepsis*** The most common cause of ARF is infection, either a local pneumonia or systemic sepsis (Vito et al, 1974). The bacteriology is often complex, and identification of these infectious agents may be difficult. Unusual organisms may be found in patients who have been immunosuppressed. Even lung lavage with 10 to 20 ml of saline may yield misleading bacteriologic results. On occasion, transbronchial or open lung biopsy is needed, particularly to exclude the possibility of rare organisms such as *P. carinii*.

At least 50% of patients with ARF have radiologic evidence of pneumonia. However, the complacent acceptance of pneumonia as the principal site of major infection and cause of ARF may lead one to overlook life-threatening infradiaphragmatic infections. Common primary or secondary gynecologic problems that may cause ARF include ascending urinary tract infection, infected hematomas, abscesses of the pelvis, deep infections of the operative wound, occult injury to the ureters or rectum, and anastomotic leaks from enteroenterostomies. Nonbacterial events that may lead to ARF include bowel infarction secondary to radiation or volvulus and pancreatitis.

## MEDIATORS OF ARF

### Inflammation

Although infection is the most common cause of ARF, the general process leading to respiratory and multisystem organ failure is inflammation. Because there is an inappropriate systemic inflammatory response to localized injury or infection, several of the pulmonary manifestations of sepsis are believed to be secondary to circulating mediators such as interleukin 1 and tumor necrosis factor or to agents contained in polymorphonuclear leukocytes (PMN). Some of the same mediators may also be produced by the lungs themselves. It is thought that pharmacologic manipulations will be used to modify the activity of these inflammatory agents. Ultimately, it is hoped that we will be able to modify the generalized activation of inflammatory cells and thereby prevent their localization in the lungs. This generalized and unbridled inflammatory response seen in ARF may be self-destructive in a manner similar to autoimmune disease.

The lungs may uniquely cause leukocytes to become entrapped. It is likely that neutrophil and endothelial receptors are involved. For example, the complement system may lead to leukocyte entrapment in the lungs. Experimental work has shown that agents such as pancreatic enzymes and perhaps bacterial products stimulate the complement cascade, causing the generation of C5a. This complement fragment is a potent chemoattractant that will upregulate the adherence of leukocytes and lead to their sequestration and synthesis of arachidonic acid derivatives as well as oxygen free radicals. The intravascular clumps of white blood cells are then mechanically filtered by the pulmonary microvasculature. Here, neutrophils may release damaging proteases such as elastase.

### Bronchoconstriction

Platelets are involved early in the course of ARF. Within 1 hour of experimental embolization or acid aspiration in dogs, significant numbers of platelets are trapped in the lungs, where they release serotonin (5-hydroxytryptamine [5HT]). While the mechanism of platelet entrapment in embolization involves the interaction of thrombin in the clot with platelet surface receptors, the mechanism of platelet sequestration following acid aspiration and ARF is less clear. It is likely that the thrombocytopenia that characterizes severe sepsis in humans is at least partly related to the entrapment of platelets in the lungs.

Serotonin is a potent constrictor of smooth muscle. The platelet release reaction provides a high concentration of this amine in strategic locations in the lungs, which in turn is thought to induce pulmonary vascular and bronchial smooth muscle constriction. The former leads to pulmonary hypertension and the latter to regions of diminished ventilation. The fact that areas of reduced alveolar ventilation fail to elicit a prominent hypoxic pulmonary vascular constrictive response, so that perfusion is redirected away from these poorly ventilated regions, is an important cause of the severe hypoxia. However, the reason for incomplete activity of this normal homeostatic function is unknown.

A second cause of hypoxia is the fact that 5HT leads to a fall in FRC. Bronchial constriction induced by 5HT occurs in very small peripheral airways and has the effect of increasing airways resistance as well as decreasing compliance. The fall in compliance leads to a decrease in FRC and the problems of critical airway closure.

## Oxygenation Products of Arachidonic Acid and Lung Metabolism

Many potent vasoactive and bronchoactive spasminogens are produced by the lungs themselves, as well as by platelets and leukocytes. Oxygenation products of arachidonic acid may be processed by the enzymes lipoxygenase or cyclooxygenase to yield either leukotrienes (LT) or prostanoids (Fig. 20-8). The rate-limiting step for the arachidonic acid cascade is activation of the acylhydrolases in cells. These enzymes liberate arachidonic acid from membrane phospholipid. Cell receptors in control of these events are often similar from cell to cell. Certain hormones, however, are able selectively to stimulate specific cells whose unique enzyme composition determines the end product of arachidonic acid. Thus, cycyclooxygenase contained in most cells transforms arachidonic acid into endoperoxides. In endothelium the presence of the unique enzyme prostacyclin synthetase converts the endoperoxides to the vasodilator and antiaggregator prostacyclin. Angiotensin will selectively trigger this event. On the other hand, platelets and leukocytes contain thromboxane (Tx) synthetase and therefore produce as a final product thromboxane $A_2$ ($TxA_2$), a potent smooth muscle constrictor and proaggregator. Without an enzyme to transform the endoperoxides, they will spontaneously degrade to prostaglandins of the E and F series.

Products of arachidonic acid such as the leukotrienes (LTB4 and LTD4) and $TxA_2$ not only induce important

vasospastic and bronchospastic events (Ogletree and Brigham, 1982) but have other properties that make them central to the inflammatory process (Klausner et al, 1989b). For example, hydroxyeicosatetraenoic acid (HETE) and LTB4 are powerful chemoattractants and may be responsible for recruiting leukocytes to the lungs. The oxygenation products of arachidonic acid also include vasotoxic agents. Thus, LTC4 and LTD4 induce permeability edema, an action that may not be direct but may be mediated by superoxide anion or other free radicals. This vasotoxicity has been proved in the systemic circulation. The action of LT in the lungs still requires clarification.

Other metabolic activities of the lungs may eventually prove to be of significance for both pulmonary and systemic organ function. For example, degradation of the peptide angiotensin I to the active systemic vasoconstrictor angiotensin II occurs by means of a converting enzyme located on the surface of the pulmonary endothelium. The same enzyme degrades the vasodilator bradykinin to an inactive form. In addition to synthesizing the prostanoids $TxA_2$ and prostacyclin, the lungs actively degrade other vasoactive prostaglandins. Thus, over 90% of the prostaglandins $PGE_2$ and $PGF_2$ are inactivated in a single passage. Several amines are also cleared by the lungs. Up to 70% of excess plasma serotonin is removed by active transport in a single circuit. Selectivity in this process of clearance of amines is shown by the ability of the endothelium to remove norepinephrine but not epinephrine or dopamine. In theory, depressed or inappropriate metabolic functioning of the lungs may lead to local or systemic vasoactive and vasotoxic consequences.

## Pharmacologic Adjuncts in Therapy of ARF

During the first 1 to 2 days of ARF, platelet-derived 5HT is an important determinant of hypoxia. At this time, administration of a 5HT antagonist ketanserin can lead to reversal of a substantial portion of the physiologic shunt (Fig. 20-9) as well as a decrease in peak inspiratory pressure. After several days, 5HT no longer appears to be a significant determinant of hypoxia.

In the later stages of ARF, pulmonary edema due to increased permeability is likely to be an important cause of maldistributed ventilation and hypoxia. The mechanism of enhanced permeability is often leukocyte-related and may depend in part on products of arachidonic acid metabolism. Thus, in experimental ARF induced by acid aspiration, either cyclooxygenase or thromboxane synthetase inhibitors prevent leukocyte entrapment in the lungs and limit the volume of edema fluid and the rise in physiologic shunting. Inhibitors of LTC4, LTD4, and LTE4 also reduce the volume of edema fluid. These data illustrate the importance of archidonic acid metabolites in injury induced by leukocytes but should not be interpreted as excluding toxicity of other white blood cell agents such as the neutral proteases, that is, collagenase and elastase, as well as oxygen free radicals. The release of oxygen free radicals by neutrophils has been demonstrated in experimental studies of shock and ischemia (Klausner et al, 1989a). Antioxidants have proved ef-

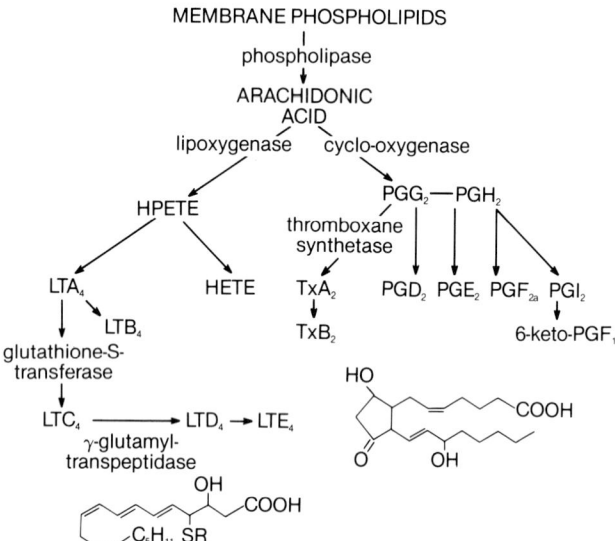

**FIGURE 20-8** Membrane-derived arachidonic acid is processed to a variety of cyclooxygenase derivatives, such as thromboxane $A_2$ and $PGI_2$. The end product depends upon the cell type. Leukotrienes (LT) C, D, and E are the prominent spasminogens that result from 5-lipoxygenase activity. *Bottom left:* General structure of LTs. *Bottom right:* Structure of $PGE_2$. HETE = hydroxyeicosatetraenoic acid; HPETE = hydroperoxyeicosatetraenoic acid. (From Hechtman H B et al: Prostaglandin and thromboxane mediation of cardiopulmonary failure. *Surg Clin NA* 63:265, 1983.)

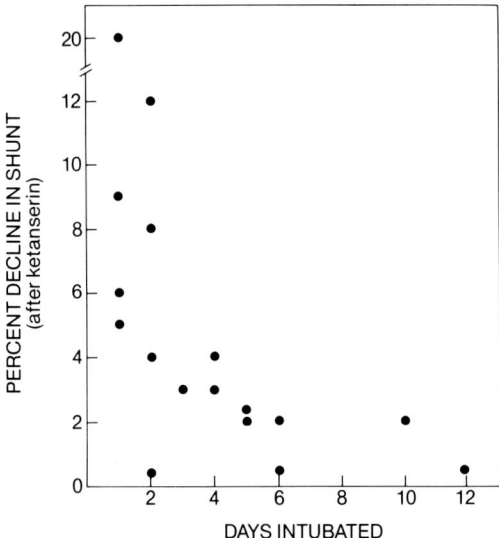

FIGURE 20-9 Early in the course of ARF, 5HT is an important determinant of $Q_S/Q_T$. Treatment with ketanserin is effective therapy.

fective in some forms of ARF (Klausner et al, 1989*a*) but not in others. Currently, experiments are focused on the use of monoclonal antibodies directed against leukocyte and/or endothelial adhesion receptors, and these antibodies have been shown experimentally to be effective in preventing organ failure (Simpson et al, 1988).

The therapeutic avenues that need to be explored continue to broaden. Our general objectives are to maintain the integrity of the inflammatory reaction. At the same time, we would like to limit and localize this homeostatic response and prevent the uncontrolled recruitment and generalized activation of all inflammatory mediators.

## PULMONARY EDEMA

The pulmonary edema noted in ARF is rich in protein and occurs at low pulmonary capillary pressures. These are the hallmarks of permeability edema and are in contrast to the high pressure or hydrostatic edema evident at pulmonary arterial wedge pressure (PAWP) values exceeding 20 to 25 mm Hg. Even though permeability edema occurs at relatively low hydrostatic pressures, the event is very pressure-sensitive. Any increase in PAWP will exacerbate permeability edema. Although this edema is initially distributed uniformly throughout the lung, after several days the gravitationally dependent regions of the lung will contain greater amounts of fluid.

Pharmacologic agents may be used to control permeability edema by lowering pulmonary perfusion pressure. Drugs such as nitroglycerin have been shown to be of value in experimental settings, but these smooth muscle vasodilators may be hazardous in patients with systemic hypotension. Ideally, the identification of possible vasospastic agent(s) that produce increases in pulmonary perfusion pressure may point to the use of

specific therapy to reduce pulmonary hypertension and thereby edema formation.

Several homeostatic mechanisms exist to minimize the functional importance of pulmonary edema. The first pertains to the uniform architecture of alveolar-capillary units. One side of the alveolar-capillary interface where bidirectional gas transfer occurs is thin; a thicker area of loose connective tissue containing a network of collagen fibers is present on the other side of the capillary. Initial accumulation of edema is limited to the area of thickened connective tissue, thus minimizing any deleterious effect on gas exchange. Second, the pulmonary lymphatics have a large reserve and can clear more than 20 times the amount of interstitial fluid normally removed from the lung (Uhley et al, 1961). This lymphatic reserve capacity takes several days to become functional. It is unique to the lungs and minimizes the accumulation of lung water. The final defense against edema is the fact that the ingress of interstitial fluid causes an increase in interstitial hydrostatic pressure and a decrease in oncotic pressure. These changes limit further edema formation. Pulmonary dysfunction occurs only when the capacity of these several mechanisms to protect lung function is overwhelmed, allowing alveolar flooding.

## ACUTE RESPIRATORY FAILURE

### Diagnosis

Dyspnea is a significant symptom and must be evaluated carefully using chest x-ray and arterial blood gas measurements. Other presenting signs of ARF are nonspecific. Tachypnea is common, with respiratory rates in the 30s; however, this is often noted in any serious illness. Not only is the respiratory rate increased but the minute ventilation is elevated. This drive to hypocarbia and increased pH is probably related to interstitial pulmonary edema and stimulation of local stretch receptors. Respiratory alkalosis is common and is a primary event, not a response to metabolic acidosis or to the hypoxia that is invariably present during room-air breathing in patients suffering from ARF. On occasion the stimulus to hyperventilation is extreme, and the arterial carbon dioxide pressure ($PaCO_2$) may be driven down to the 20s. This heightened work requirement may lead to fatigue and ventilatory failure. Excess sedation may also contribute to ventilatory failure and a rising $PaCO_2$.

Physical examination of the chest may help to evaluate the possibility of ventilatory failure due to atelectasis, effusion, or pneumothorax. Auscultatory examination of the patient with ARF or ventilatory failure is usually nonspecific. Wheezing and fine rales may or may not be present. Although the chest x-ray is important, negative findings must be interpreted with great caution. Most often the x-ray will be taken by the portable technique. Positioning of the patient is difficult, the view is anteroposterior, and the phase of the respiratory cycle is hard to control. Furthermore, the tachypneic patient will usually not be able to hold his or her breath for long periods of time and certainly not at total lung capacity. The absence of edema on the radiograph does not exclude ARF.

## Respiratory Gas Exchange

Arterial blood gases may indicate hypoxia—a finding consistent with ARF but not uniquely diagnostic. Typically, blood gases show a pattern of primary respiratory alkalosis with hypoxia. The fact that alveolar ventilation is normal or even excessive is shown by the low $PaCO_2$. The simultaneous presence of a low $PaCO_2$ and a low arterial oxygen pressure $(PaO_2)$ is common and relates to the ability of the body to regulate $CO_2$ excretion easily by changing minute ventilation. The converse is not true; increasing ventilation will not necessarily increase oxygen uptake. The following common clinical example may serve as an illustration; if the endotracheal tube is inadvertently positioned too low in the trachea, so that ventilation is delivered only to the right lung, blood that perfuses the left lung will neither pick up $O_2$ nor excrete $CO_2$. The initial systemic response will be a severe fall in $PaO_2$ and a moderate rise in $PaCO_2$. If the right lung is now hyperventilated, we can not only return $PaCO_2$ to a normal value but produce hypocarbia without much difficulty. This can be explained by the almost linear relationship of $CO_2$ excretion to ventilation. Oxygen uptake is different. Blood perfusing the right lung will be 100% oxygenated. Hyperventilation will add little more oxygen. Even 100% oxygen breathing will increase the oxygen content only modestly in relation to the amount of $O_2$ that can be dissolved in plasma.

The hypoxia of ARF is due to perfusion of poorly ventilated or nonventilated lung segments. In the example of the incorrectly positioned endotracheal tube, the entire left lung is perfused but not ventilated. In patients with ARF, hypoxia is due to perfusion of alveoli that are fluid-filled and airless or that are poorly ventilated or not at all ventilated because of airway closure.

The hypoxemia associated with pulmonary embolism is also due to perfusion of poorly ventilated alveoli, but the reason for this is obscure. Emboli lead to direct mechanical obstruction of the vasculature. Impairment of ventilation is indirect and due to secondary humoral or neurohumoral effects. Experimentally, it can be shown that platelets are trapped by emboli. Platelet 5HT is released and is responsible, at least in part, for bronchoalveolar obstruction in adjacent nonembolized lung segments. It is these perfused but poorly ventilated segments that cause hypoxia. Inhibitors of the bronchospasm induced by 5HT will completely reverse the hypoxemia of experimental embolism (Fig. 20-10).

## Edema and Lung Function

Pulmonary edema will cause abnormalities in respiratory gas exchange. However, the degree of hypoxia is not a good index of the volume of interstitial or intraalveolar fluid (Hechtman et al, 1973). This is due to the uneven distribution of interstitial fluid and to the fact

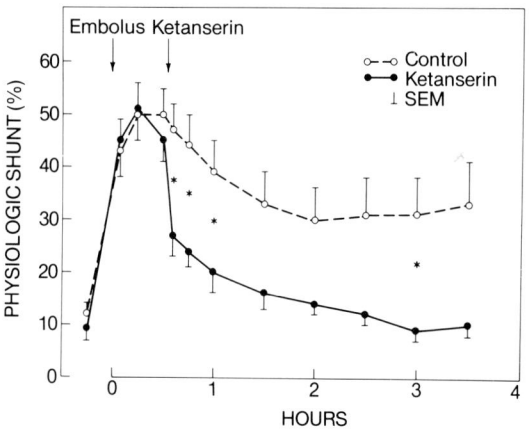

**FIGURE 20-10** After experimental pulmonary embolism, administration of IV ketanserin inhibits 5HT and reverses $Q_S/Q_T$. (From Huval W V et al: Therapeutic benefits of 5-hydroxytryptamine inhibition following pulmonary embolism. *Ann Surg* 197:220, 1983.)

that intraalveolar edema need not totally eliminate alveolar gas exchange. Alveolar fluid can be layered along the walls of the air sacs as the lungs expand and air enters the alveoli. As the FRC increases, alveoli that may have been completely fluid-filled now begin to participate in gas exchange, although there are undoubtedly limitations to diffusion. Large tidal volumes will improve oxygenation, since alveoli are more likely to contain gas at some phase of the ventilatory cycle.

The difficulty in quantitating lung edema is well recognized. Chest radiography by the portable technique is relatively insensitive to changes in lung water, due largely to the difficulty of holding air volumes constant. This variability in the air/fluid ratio confuses x-ray interpretation. Varying air volumes also account for the lack of correlation between blood gases and lung water. Changes in FRC and tidal volume directly affect oxygen exchange.

## Lung Compliance

Another functional defect that characterizes ARF is an increase in lung stiffness or a fall in compliance. This is measured as a rise in the peak inspiratory pressure at a constant tidal volume. Changes in inflow pressure may be substantial, although they are not primarily determined by lung edema but rather by agents that act on parenchymal smooth muscle. These spasminogens, such as 5HT, $TxA_2$, and LTD4, may act to reduce compliance independently of lung water.

The initial manifestation of ARF developing intraoperatively may be a rise in inspiratory pressure. For example, a transfusion reaction may activate white blood cells via complement and lead to their entrapment in the lungs. The metabolic consequence of this event may be the synthesis of $TxA_2$ and LT, with resultant sharp increases in peak inspiratory pressure to 30 or 40 cm $H_2O$. In normally compliant lungs, inspiratory pressure ranges between 10 and 15 cm $H_2O$ at high tidal volumes.

## Congestive Heart Failure

The presence of pulmonary edema should spark an investigation to determine whether this event is possibly related to either fluid overloading or primary ventricular failure. These patients' physiologic volume status can no longer be calculated from an intake and output record, nor can it be derived from a simple measure of body weight. This difficulty is due to the current use of crystalloid infusions that enter into equilibrium with a space far larger than the vascular volume. Certain clinical facts and their interpretation regarding volume status remain valid no matter what type of fluid is infused. Thus, volume overload should be suspected in the patient who is hypertensive and has a brisk diuresis or in the patient who has received rapid, large-volume infusions without loss.

In patients without sepsis, sinus tachycardia is an early sign of left ventricular failure. It is seldom of diagnostic use in patients with ARF because so many other factors may influence heart rate. Other findings on physical examination may be of more value in the diagnosis of congestive failure, such as the presence of a gallop rhythm or the observation that an important risk factor exists (e.g., acute hypertension or disturbances in cardiac rhythm). Tachyarrhythmias such as atrial flutter or atrial tachycardia may be triggered by left atrial stretch due to volume overload. An electrocardiogram (ECG) tracing is necessary to define the precise type of rhythm disturbance.

Other estimates of cardiac function include neck vein distention, which is a semiquantitative measure of central venous or right atrial pressure. Although central venous pressure may be used to assess right ventricular function, it is, at best, an unreliable guide to left ventricular function. The ECG is used to detect possible myocardial infarction, an important risk factor in the development of congestive heart failure and pulmonary edema. The portable chest x-ray has little to offer with regard to a direct evaluation of cardiac function. The anteroposterior projection, with the patient in a semi-sitting posture but not at a fixed distance from the x-ray source, does not provide sufficient information with which to judge either absolute cardiac dimensions or relative changes from day to day.

## Therapeutic Trial

A brief trial of therapy may be used in an attempt to confirm a presumptive diagnosis of high-pressure pulmonary edema and distinguish it from increased permeability edema. Thus, the effect of controlling tachyarrhythmias should be noted. If excess volume is considered to have induced respiratory failure, therapeutic steps to be considered are volume restriction and diuresis. The use of a positive inotropic agent such as dopamine or dobutamine may be attempted. If systemic pressure can be easily maintained and a diuresis established, therapy should be continued while the underlying cardiopulmonary problem is investigated. At any time, therapeutic failure or paradoxical results indicate the need for new, vigorous diagnostic procedures, including invasive catheterizations.

## INVASIVE DIAGNOSTIC PROCEDURES

### Arterial Blood Gas Analysis and Acid-Base Therapy

**pH and Paco$_2$** Precise evaluation of acid-base status and respiratory gas exchange can only be done by analysis of arterial blood using Clark and Severinghaus electrodes. Interpretation of these data should start with the pH, which will define whether the patient is acidotic or alkalotic. Next, the Paco$_2$ is examined to see whether it deviates from normal and, if so, whether this deviation can explain the pH abnormality. If the pH is paradoxically high or low relative to the Paco$_2$, a mixed respiratory and metabolic disorder exists. Commonly, patients manifest both a primary respiratory alkalosis and a primary metabolic alkalosis. In such a case, the blood pH is excessively high and is not fully explained by the moderate fall in Paco$_2$, e.g., a pH of 7.55 with a Paco$_2$ of 35 mm Hg. A precise estimate of the degree of metabolic alkalosis requires calculation of the *base excess*, which is the milliequivalent excess or deficit of acid after mathematical correction of the Paco$_2$ to 40 mm Hg. The base excess has some diagnostic importance but assumes real clinical value when therapy is being considered to adjust acid-base abnormalities using acid or base infusions.

Metabolic alkalosis may become severe. Usually it occurs secondary to removal of HCl by nasogastric suctioning; to the infusion of citrate anticoagulant with blood transfusions; or to the use of loop diuretics such as furosemide, which promotes renal retention of HCO$_3^-$ and loss of Cl$^-$. Treatment of a severe alkalosis, such as one in which the pH exceeds 7.55, is suggested to avert arrhythmias due to low plasma concentrations of K$^+$, Ca$^{2+}$, and Mg$^{2+}$. Furthermore, alkalosis will shift the hemoglobin-oxygen affinity state in such a way that offloading of O$_2$ in the peripheral tissues is impaired. This can be a significant problem, particularly in elderly patients with coronary artery disease whose myocardial oxygen delivery, which normally depends on flow regulation, is limited by arteriosclerosis.

Treatment of metabolic alkalosis depends on its severity. If the patient has the mechanical reserve capacity, she should be permitted to ventilate spontaneously to allow respiratory compensation. If the pH remains elevated, an infusion of 0.1 N HCl via a central venous line should be considered. A slower but useful approach is to administer the carbonic anhydrase inhibitor acetazolamide to force the secretion of an alkaline urine.

Underlying renal functional abnormalities due to ureteral obstruction or damage from cisplatin chemotherapy may set the stage for metabolic acidosis. This can be accentuated by acute tubule damage with oliguric or nonoliguric renal failure. Although causes of the metabolic defects may be multiple and difficult to determine, a general definition of the metabolic or respiratory nature of the problem should be straightforward.

***Oxygen Tension*** Oxygen tension is the last of the three measurements of arterial blood to be analyzed. During room-air breathing, $Pao_2$ should be above 75 mm Hg; lower values may be secondary to hypoventilation. This is easily documented if the $PaCO_2$ is elevated. If supplementary oxygen is being inhaled, the $Pao_2$ must be interpreted; accuracy in the estimate of the fraction of oxygen inspired ($F_iO_2$) is limited when patients are not intubated and use various types of nasal prongs or masks for delivery of oxygen. Under these circumstances, detailed assessment of the alveolar-arterial (A-a) or inspired arterial gradient is impossible. In contrast, the $F_iO_2$ may be accurately set to within 1% in intubated patients using most volume-cycled ventilators. Patients receiving oxygen in this setting thus have a predictable $F_iO_2$ and an interpretable oxygen gradient that can be used to monitor therapy. There are few practical advantages in a closer analysis of the defect in oxygen transport, such as calculating physiologic and/or anatomic shunting.

Maintenance of the $Pao_2$ above 60 mm Hg is a therapeutic goal. Initially, adjustments are made in the $F_iO_2$. Failure to raise the $Pao_2$ above 40 mm Hg usually calls for endotracheal intubation and mechanical ventilation. If $F_iO_2$ values above 70 to 80% are required in this setting, the danger of absorption atelectasis and oxygen toxicity becomes sufficiently great to warrant the introduction of other techniques, such as increased tidal volume or end-expiratory pressure.

Usually the $PaCO_2$ may be allowed to fall to 50 mm Hg without undue hazard to the patient. Hemoglobin remains 83% saturated at this partial pressure, and under most conditions, with the exception of significant coronary artery disease, it is hard to demonstrate adverse effects. However, potential risks increase if patients are maintained at a $Pao_2$ of 50 mm Hg, since oxygen reserves are severely limited. At this point on the oxygen-hemoglobin dissociation curve, small declines in $O_2$ tension lead to rapid declines in the percent saturation.

The fact that the per cent saturation of hemoglobin changes slowly as the $Pao_2$ rises above 50 mm Hg means that at this position of the dissociation curve, per cent saturation is insensitive to major changes in $Pao_2$. Thus, even though saturation is a simple spectrophotometric measure, it is of limited value in the patient population under discussion.

## Arterial Catheterization

Radial artery catheterization with a 20-gauge cannula should be routinely employed preoperatively in patients at risk for cardiopulmonary complications. A number of factors have already been described. Other risk factors include prolonged operative procedures and settings in which extubation will be delayed for 1 or more days. The incidence of clinically significant complications for radial artery catheters is less than 0.2% even though the rate of arterial thrombosis may be as high as 40%. Ischemic problems are avoided if patency of the ulnar artery is assured by means of the Allen test before insertion of the arterial line.

The arterial catheter is routinely used to sample blood for gas and pH analysis and to monitor arterial pressure. The monitoring feature is convenient and usually in accord with cuff pressures. However, in arteriosclerosis, significant errors in measurement may occur. This is particularly true in states of hypertension in which there may be overestimates of systolic pressure and underestimates of diastolic pressure by as much as 40 mm Hg. Mean arterial pressure remains valid. Thus, in the setting of hypertension, the intraarterial monitor should be validated using standard cuff technique. This is particularly true if there are clinical reasons for treating systolic hypertension, as in a patient with a systolic pressure exceeding 170 mm Hg in the immediate postoperative period. Before an antihypertensive such as nitroprusside is administered, the hypertension should be confirmed and the response to therapy monitored by cuff measurements as well as by arterial catheterization.

## Lung Scans and Angiography

Pulmonary embolism must be considered when hypoxemia develops in the postoperative period. Patients with malignancies are at increased risk for emboli at any time, particularly after surgery. This latter period is particularly difficult diagnostically, in part because of problems in transporting the patient to the diagnostic facility. Second, the high incidence of atelectasis and pneumonia noted on chest x-ray in postoperative and seriously ill patients reduces the accuracy of radionuclide scans. In regions of nonaerated or collapsed alveoli, the pulmonary hypoxic response leads to reduced blood flow. Abnormal radionuclide perfusion scans using iodinated macroaggregated albumin may therefore be interpreted as perfusion defects consistent with emboli. Ventilation scans using inert gas tracers such as xenon-133 help reduce the incidence of such false-positive reports.

Many seriously ill patients who become hypoxemic also have potential clotting disorders. Platelet counts and other clotting factors are often low, and bleeding sites, such as those occurring with superficial gastritis, are frequent. Thus, it is generally wise to confirm the diagnosis of embolism with a pulmonary angiogram. The high risk of clinical bleeding makes heparinization hazardous and prohibits the use of fibrinolytic agents. If anticoagulation presents unacceptable hazards, insertion of a vena caval filter is a reasonable alternative. This is usually done under local anesthesia via an internal jugular vein cutdown.

## Pulmonary Artery Catheterization

In 1970 Swan and Ganz described the flow-directed pulmonary artery catheter. The advantage of this device was that one could insert the catheter at the bedside and measure right- and left-sided cardiac filling pressures. The primary data derived with this catheter are central venous pressure (CVP) or right aterial pressure, pulmonary arterial pressure (PAP), and pulmonary arterial (capillary) wedge pressure (PAWP). PAWP provides an estimate of the filling pressure of the left ventricle in the same fashion as CVP estimates the filling pressure of the right ventricle. PAWP is obtained through inflation of a small balloon located near the tip of the catheter that occludes flow in a small pulmonary arterial branch. Since there is no kinetic energy loss, the tip of the catheter distal to the balloon senses pressure in the pulmonary veins or effectively in the left atrium. Because the catheter is soft and its frequency response is not high, systolic and diastolic pressure fluctuations tend to result in under- and overestimations of true values. Average pressures, however, should be accurate.

In patients whose pulse rate is slow, pulmonary arterial diastolic pressure should allow a good estimate of PAWP, providing that pulmonary vascular resistance is not increased. Soon after insertion of the pulmonary catheter, pulmonary end diastolic pressure and PAWP should be compared. If they are within 1 to 2 mm Hg of each other, pulmonary diastolic pressure may be used in lieu of PAWP should the balloon burst or the catheter no longer wedge—two common occurrences. On the other hand, if the pulse is slow, any difference between the pulmonary end-diastolic pressure and PAWP may serve as an estimate of pulmonary vascular resistances.

PAWP is normally 5 to 10 mm Hg—several mm Hg higher than CVP. Mean PAP is 10 to 15 mm Hg. The typical patient with ARF has a PAWP between 10 and 15 mm Hg, with a mean PAP of 20 to 25 mm Hg. Pulmonary embolism, on the other hand, leads to obstruction of the pulmonary vasculature, with pulmonary hypertension and a normal PAWP. In patients with large emboli or other causes of high pulmonary vascular resistance, severe pulmonary hypertension may develop. Even with a normal PAWP, such patients may transmit from the pulmonary artery to the pulmonary capillaries pressures sufficient to cause hydrostatic pulmonary edema. Pulmonary hypertension may also cause right ventricular dilatation, with a shift of the interventricular septum to the left. This will encroach on the left ventricle, acutely reducing its compliance and causing PAWP to rise. Thus, right ventricular failure may result in increases in PAWP as well as in CVP.

Classic teaching argues that end-diastolic pressure estimates the fiber stretch of ventricular muscle. Unfortunately, the relationship of ventricular pressure and volume—i.e., compliance—is unpredictable, as shown by studies in which PAWP does not correlate with volume measured by gated blood pool scans. Based on these findings, neither PAWP nor CVP can be taken as a certain index of ventricular function or as a criterion of functional vascular volume. On the other hand, the importance of a high PAWP in defining hydrostatic pulmonary edema remains valid.

The measurement of cardiac output (CO) by thermodilution is easily accomplished with the pulmonary artery catheter. Within 1 minute of the rapid injection of 10 ml of 5% dextrose in water into the CVP port, the distal thermistor bead located at the tip of the catheter records and electronically integrates the temperature-time curve, allowing immediate display of CO in liters per minute. Three injections should be carried out, and each measure of CO should agree within 0.5 liters/min. Dividing CO by body surface will yield the cardiac

index (CI). The normal CI value in women is 3.0 liters/min·m². Stress induced by sepsis, hemorrhage, or surgical trauma leads to variable increases in CI, particularly after therapy with fluid and blood. If the CI remains below 2.5 liters/min·m² despite resuscitative efforts, the prognosis is poor.

***Techniques of Pulmonary Artery Catheterization*** A catheter can be placed in the pulmonary artery using the medial antecubital vein or an external jugular, internal jugular, or subclavian vein. One disadvantage of the antecubital route is the high incidence of thrombophlebitis, which limits the catheter residence to short periods. In addition, axillary venospasm may make catheterization difficult. Cannulating the external jugular vein is at times impossible because of the angle between the external jugular vein and the subclavian vein. Furthermore, the difficulty in preventing catheter movement and the location of the catheter near the hairline increase the risk of sepsis. Also, it is difficult to maintain the sterility of internal jugular vein catheters because of their location. Despite these objections, the internal jugular vein has become the site of choice.

Another route used for cannulation of the superior vena cava is the subclavian vein. Outside the operating room, this location allows easy access to the central venous system with minimal complications. A contraindication to the use of the subclavian vein is a severe coagulopathy. Relative contraindications include significant emphysema, upper chest wall deformity, adjacent infection, or burns.

The patient should be placed supine in the Trendelenburg position to ensure positive pressure in the vein, allowing its distention. The patient's head should be turned slightly away from the side of catheterization. A small rolled towel placed longitudinally between the scapulae will allow the shoulders to fall back onto the bed. Patients are continuously monitored on ECG. Drugs such as procainamide must be available to treat arrhythmias. The area of cannulation should be cleansed with povidone-iodine soap. A fat-soluble agent such as acetone is applied to remove fatty oils and loose cutaneous scales.

Before insertion, the catheter balloon is tested for leaks, and all lumens are flushed to ensure their patency. The infraclavicular site for percutaneous needle puncture is around the midclavicular line. A needle 2 to 2.5 inches in length and 2.5 mm in diameter attached to a syringe is inserted beneath the clavicle in a horizontal plane, with its tip aimed at the posterior aspect of the sternal notch. The syringe is frequently aspirated until a free flow of blood is obtained. It is then disconnected and the catheter is introduced. The patient is asked to hold his or her breath while the needle is detached from the syringe to minimize the risk of air embolism. The needle is withdrawn and a 10-cm segment of catheter is left within the central venous system. If difficulty is encountered in advancing the catheter, both needle and catheter should be removed together. Withdrawal of the catheter, with the needle in place, may result in transection of the catheter and embolism of the distal segment.

Once the central vein is cannulated, a pressure transducer is connected to the pulmonary artery port, the balloon is inflated with 0.75 ml of air, and the catheter is slowly advanced into the right atrium and ventricle. Catheter location can be verified by the pressure trace. The catheter should not remain in the right ventricle for an unduly long period, since arrhythmias are most common in this location. The catheter is then advanced into the pulmonary artery and further along until the wedge pressure pattern is seen. Placement of the catheter in the wedge position may be confirmed using three criteria: (1) a manometric pressure tracing showing a waveform characteristic of that seen in the left atrium, (2) a pressure lower than the main PAP, and (3) withdrawn blood having a high oxygen tension similar to the $Pao_2$ in arterial blood. The balloon is then deflated and a pulmonary artery tracing confirmed. The average distance from insertion site to wedge position is 30 to 35 cm. The catheter is secured firmly with a suture, and the point of cannulation should be covered with povidone-iodine and a sterile gauze pad.

The two pressure ports of the pulmonary artery catheter are coupled to pressure transducers. In addition, both ports are slowly flushed with diluted heparinized saline at a rate of 3 to 4 ml/hr using a Millipore system. This will virtually assure line patency. Unless it is absolutely necessary, the CVP port should not be used for infusions. This prohibition is absolute for the pulmonary arterial port and includes the use of vasoactive drugs.

Chest x-rays are obtained after catheter insertion in order to assure proper positioning. The catheter tip is usually located in a right lower lobular artery and should not extend more than half the distance from the mediastinum to the chest wall. X-rays may detect unsuspected complications such as a pneumo- or hemothorax. Redressings and application of antibiotic ointment at 24-hour intervals are advised. Depending upon the type of adverse reaction, reported complication rates have varied from 1 to 21%. Most investigators report a 1 to 7% incidence of noninfectious mechanical problems. Common complications include pneumothorax, arterial puncture, hemomediastinum, hemothorax, hydromediastinum, hydrothorax, and multiple premature ventricular beats. Rare complications comprise brachial plexus or thoracic duct injury, air embolism, catheter embolism, arteriovenous fistula, endocarditis, venobronchial fistula, osteomyelitis of the clavicle, and even death. Any indwelling catheter can serve as a focus of infection. If the etiology of a postoperative fever cannot be readily determined, the pulmonary artery catheter must be removed and the tip cultured for bacteria and fungi.

### Treatment for Low-Flow States

Patients in a low-flow state require vigorous treatment. Our general focus is on improving oxygen transport, the principal determinants of which are arterial oxygen content and blood flow. Oxygen content, in turn, is a function of hemoglobin and oxygen tension. Surprisingly, the ideal hemoglobin or hematocrit (Hct) has not been defined. Retrospective data point to ideal Hct values in the low 30s. It is possible that the difficulty in defining the ideal Hct reflects the neutralizing effects of increased $O_2$ content with a rising Hct and the reduced microcirculatory flow as viscosity increases with the Hct change.

Minute ventilation should be set to minimize increases in airways pressure. This can be done by using assist/control settings as well as reducing tidal volume and end-expiratory pressure. Successful adjustments of the respirator should be tested by measuring cardiac outputs by thermodilution.

In hypovolemic patients, adjustments of the ventilator often accompany intravenous infusions designed to adjust the PAWP to between 10 and 12 mm Hg. This filling pressure range has been found to maximize CO in most patients with ARF (Hechtman, 1979).

Inotropic agents such as dopamine and dobutamine may be used if CO or urinary output is still not ideal. Ordinarily, digitalis preparations are avoided unless an arrhythmia is being treated, since these drugs cause frequent hazardous fluctuations in pH and potassium levels. The pulmonary artery catheter should be used frequently to validate the benefits of inotropic and volume therapy with regard to flow and filling pressures.

Other measurements obtained by means of the pulmonary artery catheter have less clinical value. Mixed venous blood gases and pH from pulmonary artery blood may be used to calculate the *physiologic shunt*. The physiologic shunt is without question the most sensitive assessment of oxygen uptake by the lungs, since it takes into account the variability in venous oxygen content, which can fluctuate because of changes in flow and systemic oxygen extraction. Unfortunately, the refined measurement of physiologic shunting seldom leads to changes in management.

Mixed venous oxygen tension ($P_vo_2$) reflects the oxygen reserve capacity, i.e., whether additional oxygen could have exited the capillary bed if needed. Normal $P_vo_2$ is between 35 and 45 mm Hg; lower oxygen tensions are hazardous, since they imply exhaustion of oxygen reserves and tissue hypoxia. This is usually a result of low flow, a clinical problem readily identified by measuring CO.

## RESPIRATORY MANAGEMENT

### Mechanical Ventilation

Severe pulmonary distress may require either temporary or long-term support of lung function. In addition to increasing inspired oxygen, the major means by which pulmonary function is maintained are by endotracheal intubation and mechanical ventilation.

Mechanical ventilatory support is required when there is a rapid fall in $Pao_2$ despite supplementary oxygen breathing. Thus, a fall in $Pao_2$ to 50 mm Hg despite oxygen delivered by face mask is an indication for intubation. A second indication is the presence of acute ventilatory failure, manifested by a high respiratory rate and respiratory fatigue. Concern for fatigue is increased in the elderly, stuporous, or obese patient whose $Paco_2$ is rising.

Often the indication for postoperative reintubation and ventilatory support is the presence of severe hypoxemia secondary to ARF. Occasionally, heightened respiratory work and fear of fatigue call for mechanical ventilatory support. Most often these problems of ventilatory insufficiency are noted during the period when extubation is being considered. At such times, patients who have been supported by mechanical ventilation for days to weeks seldom have difficulty with oxygenation; their problem is usually a limited energy reserve, manifested by a rising respiratory rate and rising $PaCO_2$ during the weaning attempt.

In the majority of patients with respiratory complications, adequate gas exchange is easily maintained by mechanical support. A tidal volume between 8 and 12 ml/kg with a rate of 12 to 15 cycles per minute will normally maintain the $PaCO_2$ between 38 and 42 mm Hg. The second goal of therapy is to ensure an adequate arterial $PO_2$. Initially, the ventilator is set to deliver an $F_iO_2$ at or below 50%. In most patients, this level of inspired oxygen will achieve a desired $PaO_2$ above 60 mm Hg. Arterial blood gases should be measured after a delay of 15 minutes to allow equilibration with the new $F_iO_2$. Should the $PaO_2$ still remain unacceptably low, sedatives or narcotics such as diazepam or morphine can augment oxygenation by enhancing patient compliance with the ventilatory cycle, thus discouraging active exhalation and maintaining an elevated FRC. If arterial oxygen tension remains low, positive end-expiratory pressure (PEEP) should be utilized. PEEP will increase the FRC and minimize the physiologic shunt (Hechtman et al, 1973). Levels of PEEP between 5 and 10 cm $H_2O$ are usually sufficient to improve oxygenation. An occasional patient with poor lung compliance may require a level of PEEP equal to or in excess of 15 cm $H_2O$. When levels greater than 10 cm $H_2O$ are employed, a pulmonary artery catheter should be inserted to monitor CO, since this amount of PEEP adversely affects venous return and CO. PEEP is most effective if exhalation is entirely passive. Thus, paralytic agents such as pancuronium bromide may be useful.

### Airway Control

In patients without ventilatory failure, particularly those with low blood flow and hypotension, hypoxia may best be treated using continuous positive airway pressure. With this form of ventilatory support, patients must breathe spontaneously. Endotracheal intubation can be achieved by the nasotracheal or orotracheal route. The latter airway is most commonly used but is not always the optimal means of management. Orotracheal tubes are generally poorly tolerated in awake patients. Furthermore, the frequency of laryngeal injury after nasotracheal intubation is approximately half that seen with an orotracheal tube. The principal reason for this is the smaller-sized tube used via the nasal route and the decreased tube curvature. In addition, the nasotracheal tube is more stable, thus reducing the potential for damage due to movement of the tube. Certain complications unique to nasal intubation include necrosis of the nose and septum as well as maxillary sinusitis.

Furthermore, airways resistance due to the smaller tube size may necessitate a large and perhaps unacceptable amount of respiratory work during weaning.

If, after 2 to 4 weeks of nasotracheal or orotracheal intubation, weaning from mechanical ventilation cannot be anticipated, a tracheostomy should be performed. The advantages of this are several. First, there is a significantly reduced dead space. In addition, access to the tracheobronchial tree facilitates pulmonary toilet. Tracheostomy tends to be tolerated better by the conscious patient because it is less likely to stimulate coughing and gagging. Finally, patients are able to swallow and eat more easily with a tracheostomy.

## TREATMENT OF SEPSIS

Reversal of the symptoms of cardiopulmonary failure is the first step in the treatment of sepsis. Vigorous diagnostic steps must then be taken to document the underlying problem. If the etiologic problem is sepsis, its source must be found. Clinical judgment must be keen, since improvement in organ function does not necessarily reflect reversal of sepsis. Thus, improvement in oxygenation may be due to exhaustion of a platelet source of 5HT and therefore abatement of bronchoconstriction. Furthermore, after several days, pulmonary lymphatic function may expand sufficiently to reverse edema. Decisions regarding surgical intervention to drain an abscess or to correct the conditions that led to sepsis should, of course, take into account the benefits and hazards. The argument that the patient is too ill to undergo surgery does not consider the critical question of mortality associated with sepsis complicated by ARF, which exceeds 50%.

## REFERENCES

Arono WS, Larder D, Plasceria G, Wong W, Karlsburg RP, Ferlinz J: Verapamil in atrial fibrillation and atrial flutter. *Clin Pharmacol Ther* 26:578-583, 1979.

Ashburn MA, Stanley TH: Anesthesiology update: The preanesthetic evaluation. *Comprehensive Ther* 14:27-32, 1988.

Beutler G, Milsark IW, Cerami AC: Passive immunization against cachectin/tumor necrosis factor protects mice from lethal effect of endotoxin. *Science* 229:869-871, 1985.

Culver GA, Makel HP, Beecher HK: Frequency of aspiration of gastric contents by lungs during anesthesia and surgery. *Ann Surg* 133:289-294, 1951.

Feigal DW, Blaisdell FW: The estimation of surgical risk. *Med Clin North Am* 63:1131-1143, 1979.

Fusciardi J, Dalox M, Cariat P, Harari A, Ducardonet P, Viars P: Prevention of myocardial ischemia by nitroglycerin in patients with severe coronary artery disease undergoing non-cardiac surgery. *Anesthesiology* 53:S80-S84, 1980.

Goldman L, Caldera DL: Risk of general anesthesia and elective operations in the hypertensive patient. *Anesthesiology* 50:285-292, 1979.

Goldman L, Caldera DL, Nussbaum SR, Southwick FS, Drogstad DJ, Murray B, Burke DJ, O'Malley TA, Goroll AH, Caplan CH, Nolan J, Carabello B, Slater EE: Multifactorial index of cardiac risk in non-cardiac surgical procedures. *N Engl J Med* 297:845-850, 1977.

Goldman L, Caldera DL, Southwick FS, Nussbaum SR, Murray B, O'Malley TA, Goroll AH, Caplan CH, Nolan J, Burke DS, Drogstad DJ, Carabello B, Slater EE: Cardiac risk factors and complications in non-cardiac surgery. *Medicine* 57:357-365, 1978.

Goldiner PL, Carlon GC, Cuitkovic E, Schwiezer O, Howland WS: Factors influencing postoperative morbidity and mortality in patients treated with bleomycin. *Br Med J* 1:1664-1667, 1978.

Gould VE, Tosco R, Wheelis RF: Oxygen pneumonitis in man: Ultrastructural observations on the development of alveolar lesions. *Lab Invest* 26:499-508, 1972.

Hechtman HB: Evaluation and general treatment procedures in critical illness. In Hechtman HB (ed): *Acute Respiratory Failure: Etiology and Treatment*. Boca Raton, Florida, CRC Press, 1979, pp 179-192.

Hechtman HB, Krausz MM, Utsunomiya T, Valeri CR: Preoperative assessment of the high risk surgical patient. *Surg Clin North Am* 60:1349-1358, 1980.

Hechtman HB, Weisel RD, Vito L, Ali J, Bergerc RL: Independence of pulmonary shunting and pulmonary edema. *Surgery* 74:300-306, 1973.

Hillis LD, Cohn PF: Non-cardiac surgery in patients with coronary artery disease. *Arch Intern Med* 138:972-975, 1978.

Jackson CV: Preoperative pulmonary evaluation. *Arch Intern Med* 148:2120-2127, 1988.

Klausner JM, Paterson IS, Kobzik L, Valeri CR, Shepro D, Hechtman HB: Oxygen-free radicals mediate ischemia-induced lung injury. *Surgery* 105:192-199, 1989a.

Klausner JM, Paterson IS, Kobzik L, Valeri CR, Shepro D, Hechtman HB: Thromboxane A$_2$ mediates increased pulmonary microvascular permeability following limb ischemia. *Circ Res* 64:1178-1189, 1989b.

Leblanc P, Ruff F, Milic-Emili J: Effect of gas and body position on "airway closure" in man. *J Appl Physiol* 28:448-451, 1970.

Manning FC: Preoperative evaluation in the elderly patient. *Am Fam Physician* 39:123-128, 1989.

McCord JM, Fridovich I: The biology and pathology of oxygen radicals. *Ann Intern Med* 89:122-127, 1978.

McLoughlin GA, Grindlinger GA, Manny J, Valeri CR, Lipinski B, Mannick JA, Hechtman HB: Intrapulmonary clotting and fibrinolysis during abdominal aortic aneurysm surgery. *Ann Surg* 190:623-630, 1979.

Ogletree ML, Brigham KL: Effect of cyclo-oxygenase inhibitors on pulmonary vascular response to endotoxin in unanesthetized sheep. *Prostaglandins, Leukotrienes, Med* 8:489-502, 1982.

Pierce AK, Robertson J: Pulmonary complications of general surgery. *Ann Rev Med* 28:211-217, 1977.

Rees NM, Roberts CJ, Bligh AS, Evans KT: Routine preoperative chest radiography in non-cardiopulmonary surgery. *Br Med J* 1:1333-1335, 1976.

Robbins JA, Muslin AI: Preoperative evaluation of the healthy patient. *Med Clin North Am* 63:1145-1156, 1979.

Rogers WR, Wrobleski F, LaDue JS: Supraventricular tachycardia complicating surgical procedures. *Circulation* 7:192-199, 1952.

Simpson PJ, Todd RF, Fantone JC, Mickelson JK, Griffin JG, Lucchesi BR: Reduction of canine myocardial infarction injury by a monoclonal antibody (Anti-Mol, Anti-CD18) that inhibits leukocyte adhesion. *J Clin Invest* 81:624-629, 1988.

Spray BS, Zuidema GD, Cameron JL: Aspiration pneumonia: Incidence of aspiration with endotracheal tubes. *Am J Surg* 131:701-703, 1976.

Steen PA, Tinker JH, Tarhan S: Myocardial reinfarction after anesthesia and surgery. *JAMA* 239:2566-2570, 1978.

Taniguchi H, Taki F, Takagi K, Satake T, Sugiyama S, Ozawa T: The role of leukotriene B$_4$ in the genesis of oxygen toxicity in the lung. *Am Rev Resp Dis* 133:805-808, 1986.

Uhley H, Leeds SE, Sampson JJ, Friedman M: Some observations of the role of the lymphocytes in experimental acute pulmonary edema. *Cancer Res* 9:288-291, 1961.

Vito L, Dennis RC, Weisel RD, Hechtman HB: Sepsis presenting as acute respiratory insufficiency. *Surg Gynecol Obstet* 138:896-900, 1974.

Walker L, Eiseman B: The changing pattern of posttraumatic respiratory distress syndrome. *Ann Surg* 182:693-697, 1975.

Warner MA, Divertie MB, Tinker JH: Preoperative cessation of smoking and pulmonary complications in coronary artery bypass patients. *Anesthesiology* 60:380-383, 1984.

# Chapter 21 | Infection in the Patient with Gynecologic Malignancy

### Ruth Tuomala

Infection may be encountered during all phases of diagnosis, evaluation, and management of gynecologic cancer. Although the impact of such infections varies somewhat depending on the type, location, and extent of the specific lesion and the treatment indicated, it is clear that infection is a major cause of morbidity and mortality among oncologic patients (Gurwith et al, 1978a; Inagaki et al, 1974; Davy, 1974; Bodey, 1975). Infection associated with diagnostic procedures and antitumor therapy as well as with the tumor itself results directly in morbidity, exposure to antimicrobial toxicity, additional surgical procedures, prolonged hospitalization, and higher costs (Mayo and Wenzel, 1982). Indirectly, the presence of infection may delay definitive tumor management and thus increase mortality (Kottmeier, 1964; Cho and Choi, 1979).

Much of the material presented in this chapter can be applied to oncologic patients in general; however, it is not meant to be an exhaustive discussion of infectious diseases in malignancy. Host factors and specific organisms that influence the incidence, presentation, and course of infection in patients with gynecologic malignancy will be presented as well as guidelines for the diagnosis, treatment, and prevention of such infections. In addition, there is a section on infection in the neutropenic patient.

## PATHOGENESIS OF INFECTION

All infections result from an interaction between the host and the infecting organism(s) or pathogen(s) (Fig. 21-1). If the host's defense mechanisms are functioning properly, they will protect against infection. Physical barriers, such as the skin and mucous membranes, as well as clearance mechanisms, such as respiratory tract cilia and cough reflex, are the first line of defense in preventing infective organisms from gaining access to the body. If these mechanisms fail, local and systemic humoral and cellular immunity plus phagocytic mechanisms come into play to keep invading organisms from multiplying, causing local infection, and disseminating throughout the body, with systemic effects. Whether or not the organisms cause infection depends not only on host defense mechanisms but also on the number of organisms present at a potential site of infection, interactions between these organisms, and the inherent pathogenicity or virulence of the organisms themselves.

In the cancer patient, susceptibility to infection and the host-organism interaction can be influenced by a number of factors. Any tumor, by virtue of its location, size, growth characteristics, and degree of metastatic spread, may alter the incidence of infection (Dionigi et al, 1980). Tumors may ulcerate into mucous membranes, skin, or other tissues colonized by potential pathogens, thus disrupting the physical barrier to invasion and exposing tumor surfaces to bacterial colonization. Tumor cell growth and surface characteristics may alter the number and types of colonizing organisms, potentially increasing the risk of infection (Pizzo and Schimpff, 1983). Rapidly growing tumors may undergo necrosis, promoting invasion of the tumor by colonizing organisms. Such tumor infection may remain

localized or may gain access to the bloodstream, sometimes through erosion of the tumor into blood vessels. Large tumors may obstruct clearance mechanisms that would normally prevent the multiplication of organisms, so that infection may develop behind the area of obstruction.

Tumors of the lower genital tract are in contact with organisms that normally colonize this area. Vulvar, vaginal, or invasive cervical tumors can disrupt the integrity of the local mucocutaneous barriers and allow these potential pathogens to enter the bloodstream and surrounding soft tissues. With rapid growth and necrosis, lower genital tract tumors may become infected and become a focus of dissemination during diagnostic and therapeutic manipulations. Uterine tumors, including gestational trophoblastic neoplasms (Lacey et al, 1976), can become infected if the lower genital tract flora gains access to the tumor through extension of the lesion to colonized surfaces or as a result of diagnostic and therapeutic procedures that inadvertently introduce bacteria to the tumor site.

All gynecologic tumors that extend into the parametrium or intraabdominal cavity can cause infection even if the tumor mass is not colonized or infected. For example, cervical or uterine tumor growth may lead to ureteral obstruction. This may be associated with urinary tract infection secondary to manipulations performed to relieve obstruction or with pyelonephritis and even perinephric abscess proximal to the obstruction. Any tumor mass that is contiguous with bowel, particularly cancer of the ovary, may erode into the bowel and lead to a localized intraabdominal abscess or to spillage of bowel flora into the peritoneal cavity, leading to acute peritonitis.

The diagnosis and treatment of cancer can also increase the risk of infection and alter its severity and prognosis by modifying host defense mechanisms and influencing the spectrum of causative organisms. All invasive diagnostic and therapeutic procedures, including surgery, are associated with the risk of infection. Vulvar, vaginal, and cervical biopsies may all lead to local infection. In addition, procedures such as cervical biopsy or conization and dilatation and curettage of the uterine cavity may spread local organisms to the upper genital tract and bloodstream. Major surgical procedures such as hysterectomy, radical hysterectomy, radical vulvectomy, and bowel resection all carry substantial risks of postoperative sepsis from pelvic, wound, and urinary tract sources.

Chemotherapy may alter host defenses in several ways, foremost of which are its myelosuppressive and immunosuppressive effects (Klainer and Beisel, 1969; Cone et al, 1981; Dionigi et al, 1980). Chemotherapeutic regimens may suppress bone marrow function and protein synthesis, and quantitative and qualitative defects in granulocytes and lymphocytes are common consequences. Defects both in complement synthesis and antibody formation and in cell-mediated immunity may ensue. At present, most of the chemotherapeutic agents used for gynecologic cancers are not associated with profound immunosuppression such as that seen with the remission-induction chemotherapy applied to retic-

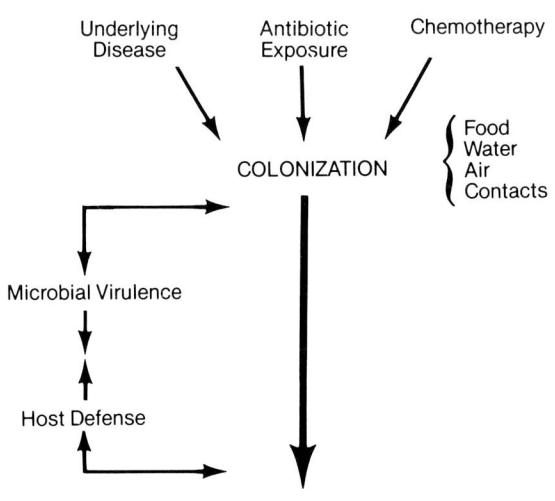

**Figure 21-1** Origin of infection in cancer patients: Exposure leads to colonization, which leads to infection. (From Pizzo PA, Schimpff SC: Strategies for the prevention of infection in the myelosuppressed or immunosuppressed cancer patient. *Cancer Treat Rep* 67:224, 1983.)

ulohematopoietic cancers or the total myelosuppression seen with bone marrow transplantation. However, as chemotherapeutic regimens for solid tumors have become more aggressive, this situation is changing. In fact, the effect of neutropenia on the risk of infection is already of concern to the gynecologic oncologist (Chambers and Schwartz, 1986). In addition, chemotherapy alters the effectiveness of the immune system even if severe neutropenia does not result (Bodey, 1986b).

Another toxic effect of chemotherapy is erosion of the mucocutaneous barrier. Systemic effects such as mucositis or gastrointestinal tract ulceration plus the direct toxic effects of local skin sloughing can lead to infection.

The early and delayed effects of radiation therapy may also be associated with infection. Local application of radium may be associated with pelvic infection or pyometra. External-beam therapy can cause radiation dermatitis, which may become superinfected and lead to more invasive cellulitis (Husseinzadeh et al, 1984). With extensive x-ray beam therapy, the bone marrow may be suppressed, leading to neutropenia. Both radiation therapy and chemotherapy may cause tumors to shrink; if such tumors are near the bowel, perforation and spillage of intestinal contents may occur (Bodey, 1975). More often, the delayed effects of radiation therapy can lead to gastrointestinal and genitourinary obstruction, strictures, perforation, and fistula formation and thereby to local and systemic infection. The long-lasting effect on irradiated tissue may be an increased risk for infection during later surgical procedures.

Instrumentation during any stage of care for the patient with cancer may increase the risk of infection. Many cases of infection are preceded within days by a procedure that has provided a pathway for invasion of bacteria. Indwelling bladder catheters used at the time of operative procedures or for supportive care can give rise to urinary tract infections and septicemia. With the use of intravenous lines and indwelling catheters perioperatively or for chemotherapy or supportive care, breaks in the skin barrier represent potential sites for organism invasion. Use of intraperitoneal catheters for administering chemotherapy may provide a route of access for infection or may lead to bowel erosion.

Nutritional deficits associated both with the malignancy itself and with various antitumor therapies are rarely a primary factor in increasing infection rates; rather, poor nutrition is an additive factor that influences the outcome of infection by interfering with delayed hypersensitivity and by retarding wound healing (Dionigi et al, 1980).

Finally, the organisms causing infection as well as the types of infections seen are affected by tumor therapy and management. Multiple hospitalizations, surgical procedures, exposure to antibiotics, and immunosuppression all serve to increase the risk of infection and influence the composition of microbial flora colonizing body surfaces. To some extent, alterations in the flora determine the organisms seen at the site of infections and thereby change the presentation and outcome of infections in patients with cancer.

# MICROBIOLOGIC CONSIDERATIONS

In general, infections in patients with solid tumors are *autoinfections*—i.e., they are caused by organisms that colonize various host surfaces—and 90% are bacterial in origin (Bodey, 1975; Cho and Choi, 1979). Although the endogenous flora in a patient with cancer may be exactly the same as that in a normal, healthy host, it is frequently altered during the course of the disease as a result of contact with organisms acquired largely from the hospital environment. Up to 50% of the infections that occur during the advanced stages of malignant disease are caused by such nosocomial bacteria.

Colonized surfaces that may give rise to infection include the skin, respiratory tract, gastrointestinal tract (including the pharynx and anorectal areas), and genital tract. Most significant and unique to the patient with gynecologic malignancy is the flora of the lower genital tract, which is polymicrobial and includes both aerobic and anaerobic organisms. Its exact composition varies among individuals and appears to be influenced by age, hormonal status, sexual experience, and possibly immune status. Cell type may also affect flora, possibly because of differences in the adherence of the bacteria to cell surfaces and in cell turnover (Mårdh and Weström, 1976). Although the vulva, vagina, and cervix are colonized with similar species of organisms, the exact types and quantities of organisms present in each of these areas may be distinct, representing "ecologic niches" for bacteria within the lower genital tract (Bartlett et al, 1978).

Lower genital tract flora has been studied in various patient populations (Bartlett et al, 1977; Linder et al, 1978; Larsen and Galask, 1980). On average, 4.7 to 6.7 mixed aerobic and anaerobic species per person were found, and the prevalence of some of these endogenous bacteria is presented in Table 21-1. Table 21-2, which lists all the bacterial species of the lower genital tract flora isolated during an investigation by Bartlett et al (1977), shows the diversity of organisms present in normal, asymptomatic women.

Results of surveys to determine the prevalence of

TABLE 21-1 Average Prevalence of Lower Genital Tract Flora

| Organism | Range (%) | Average (%) |
|---|---|---|
| *Lactobacillus* spp. | 10-97 | 75 |
| *Staphylococcus albus* | 5-75 | 50 |
| *Gardnerella vaginalis* | 8-40 | 30 |
| *Enterococcus* | 5-35 | 25 |
| *Streptococcus viridans* | 2-30 | 15 |
| Group B streptococcus | 5-20 | 12 |
| *Escherichia coli* | 3-24 | 10 |
| *Staphylococcus aureus* | 1-12 | 5 |
| *Peptococcus* | 8-64 | 30 |
| *Peptostreptococcus* | 10-30 | 20 |
| *Bacteroides* spp. | 5-35 | 20 |
| *B. fragilis* | 1-9 | 3 |
| *Fusobacterium* | 2-23 | 5 |

TABLE 21-2   Bacteria Isolated in Concentrations of $> 10^6$ cfu/gm in 52 Specimens of Vaginal Secretions from 22 Women

| Organism | No. of Women Harboring Organism (%)* | No. of Specimens Harboring Organism (%)* | Mean Concentration |
|---|---|---|---|
| Aerobes and facultative anaerobes | | | |
|   Gram-positive cocci | 18 (91) | 36 (69) | |
|     *Staphylococcus epidermidis* | 9 (41) | 29 (56) | 7.5‡ |
|     *Staphylococcus aureus* | 1 (5) | 1 (2) | 6.7 |
|     Streptococci | 13 (59) | 22 (42) | 6.8 |
|       α-Hemolytic | 3 (14) | 3 (6) | 6.6 |
|       Group B | 1 (5) | 1 (2) | 6.6 |
|       *Enterococcus* | 6 (27) | 8 (15) | 7.0 |
|       Nonhemolytic (not group A or D) | 8 (36) | 10 (19) | 6.8 |
|   *Lactobacillus* species | 11 (50) | 25 (48) | 8.7 |
|   *Corynebacterium* species | 7 (31) | 26 (50) | 7.2 |
|   *Escherichia coli* | 2 (9) | 2 (4) | 6.4 |
| Anaerobic bacteria | | | |
|   Cocci | 16 (73) | 38 (73) | |
|     *Peptococcus* | | | |
|       *prevotii* | 6 (27) | 11 (21) | 7.6 |
|       *morbillorum* | 3 (14) | 7 (13) | 9.9 |
|       *assacharolyticus* | 5 (23) | 6 (12) | 8.2 |
|       *magnus* | 5 (23) | 9 (17) | 8.1 |
|       *variabilis* | 5 (23) | 5 (10) | 8.9 |
|       *constellatus* | 1 (5) | 1 (2) | 9.7 |
|       *species* | 4 (18) | 4 (8) | 8.9 |
|       Total | 14 (64) | 34 (65) | 8.7 |
|     *Peptostreptococcus* | | | |
|       *anaerobius* | 3 (14) | 8 (15) | 8.3 |
|       *intermedius* | 3 (14) | 5 (10) | 7.8 |
|       *micros* | 2 (9) | 4 (8) | 10.1 |
|       *productus* | 1 (9) | 2 (6) | 8.3 |
|       Total | 5 (23) | 18 (35) | 8.3 |
|     Unidentified gram-positive cocci | 2 (9) | 4 (8) | 9.6 |
|     *Veillonetta* | 2 (9) | 2 (4) | 7.6 |
|     *Gaffkya anaerobia* | 1 (5) | 1 (2) | 8.1 |
|   Gram-positive bacila | 12 (55) | 36 (69) | |
|     *Lactobacillus* | | | |
|       *plantarum* | 4 (18) | 7 (13) | 7.9 |
|       *fermentum* | 3 (24) | 4 (8) | 9.7 |
|       *acidophilus* | 1 (5) | 5 (10) | 8.2 |
|       *minutus* | 2 (9) | 2 (4) | 8.7 |
|       *casei* | 1 (5) | 1 (2) | 9.0 |
|       *crispatis* | 1 (5) | 1 (2) | 7.9 |
|       *species* | 6 (27) | 7 (13) | 7.7 |
|     Total | 10 (45) | 24 (46) | 8.2 |
|     *Eubacterium* | | | |
|       *lentum* | 5 (23) | 10 (19) | 8.6 |
|       *limosum* | 1 (5) | 1 (2) | 9.8 |
|       *alactolyticum* | 2 (9) | 2 (4) | 8.1 |
|       *rectale* | 1 (5) | 1 (2) | 5.8 |
|       species | 2 (9) | 2 (4) | 7.7 |
|       Total | 8 (36) | 16 (31) | 8.4 |
|     Propionibacteria | 3 (14) | 4 (8) | 8.6 |
|     *Bifidobacterium breve* | 1 (5) | 1 (2) | 8.6 |
|     Unidentified non-spore forming | | | |
|       gram-positive bacilli | 4 (18) | 9 (17) | 8.7 |
|     *Clostridium* species§ | 4 (18) | 4 (4) | 8.2 |
|   Gram-negative bacilli | 9 (14) | 29 (56) | |
|     *Bacteroides* | | | |
|       *melaninogenicus* | 8 (36) | 17 (33) | 7.6 |
|       *fragilis* | 1 (5) | 6 (12) | 8.5 |
|       *oralis* | 4 (18) | 6 (12) | 8.1 |

*(Continued on next page.)*

TABLE 21-2  Bacteria Isolated in Concentrations of > $10^6$ cfu/gm in 52 Specimens of Vaginal Secretions from 22 Women *(continued)*

| Organism | No. of Women Harboring Organism (%)* | No. of Specimens Harboring Organism (%)* | Mean Concentration |
|---|---|---|---|
| *capillosis* | 1 (5) | 1 (2) | 9.5 |
| *ruminicola* | 1 (5) | 1 (2) | 8.0 |
| *pneumocintes* | 1 (5) | 1 (2) | 10.3 |
| species | 2 (14) | 15 (29) | 9.1 |
| Fusobacteria | 5 (23) | 7 (13) | 8.5 |

* Includes each specimen from 17 college students and one randomly selected specimen from each of the 5 volunteers who supplied multiple samples.
† A total of 52 specimens were examined.
‡ Mean concentration exressed as $\log_{10}$ cfu/gm.
§ Includes *Clostridium perfringens (one)*, *Cl. tertium* (one), *Cl. glycolicum* (one), and *Clostridium* species (one).
*Source:* Bartlett JG et al: Quantitative bacteriology of the vaginal flora. *J Infect Dis* 136:274, 1977.

specific organisms in the lower genital tract have been compared with cultures of infection sites. Bacterial species frequently found at sites of infection are classified as "potential pathogens"; other organisms that are part of the normal lower genital tract flora do not usually cause local or systemic infections and are considered to have "low pathogenic potential." Certain bacterial species, such as *Escherichia coli* and *Bacteroides fragilis*, appear to be underrepresented in the lower genital tract relative to the rate at which they are found to be pathogens at the site of infections (Larsen and Galask, 1980). Most likely this is due to their particular virulence or invasiveness. For example, the presence of a polysaccharide capsular antigen that helps to resist phagocytosis and opsonization while enhancing tissue invasiveness is one such virulence factor.

The pathogenic potential of the lower genital tract flora may also depend in part on interactions between bacteria. The number and types of organisms present and the relative proportion of potential pathogens at the site of infection may be important determinants of the incidence and severity of infection.

Although some investigators who surveyed populations of women with diverse gynecologic tumors could find no differences in the lower genital tract flora between women with and without malignancy (Blythe, 1978; Thadepalli et al, 1982), others have suggested that both qualitative and quantitative differences may in fact exist. Two studies of patients with invasive cervical carcinoma showed an apparent increase in the prevalence of potentially pathogenic bacteria in the cervix. In one, Mead (1978) found changes in the cervical flora similar to those previously described in immunosuppressed women, including a relative increase in the prevalence of *E. coli* and anaerobic species with a concomitant decrease in the prevalence of lactobacilli. In a study of cervical biopsy cultures performed at the Brigham and Women's Hospital, we found both quantitative and qualitative differences between women with malignancy and a control group of women with benign disease (Tuomala et al, 1983) (Tables 21-3 and 21-4). There was a marked shift toward anaerobic species and an increase in the average number of colony-forming units of bacteria per sample in the women with invasive cervical cancer. It is not clear whether these potential

differences in the lower genital tract flora are clinically significant, although the presence and quantity of specific potential pathogens in the endogenous flora may prove to be risk factors for infection at various stages in the diagnosis and therapy of cervical carcinoma.

The major aerobic pathogens of importance in the patient with gynecologic malignancy are the Enterobacteriaceae, including *E. coli* and *Klebsiella* species; *Pseudomonas* species; streptococci, including *Viridans* streptococci and enterococci; and *Staphylococcus aureus*. With the exception of *S. aureus*, these organisms are often found in combination with other aerobic or anaerobic organisms at the site of infection.

Although anaerobic bacteria may be the sole pathogens at an infection site, they are more often found as part of a polymicrobial infection. The most numerous anaerobic pathogens are the anaerobic gram-positive cocci, including anaerobic streptococci, peptococci, and peptostreptococci. Bacteroides species, including *fragilis*, *bivius*, and *melaninogenicus*, must be considered major anaerobic pathogens in wound and soft tissue infections; the prevalence of infections with *Clostridium perfringens* and other anaerobic bacteria, although considerable, is much lower.

In patients with malignancy, colonization by potential pathogens acquired from the hospital environment becomes an important factor over the course of the disease. Not surprisingly, tertiary centers and facilities caring for patients over the long term report a higher incidence of nosocomial infections (Young, 1981). Hospitalized patients may become colonized by organisms via air, water, food, and direct transmission from patient to patient by way of personnel or equipment (Kramer et al, 1982; Levine et al, 1974). Administration of an-

TABLE 21-3  Organisms Isolated per Sample

| | Cases (13) | Controls (11) |
|---|---|---|
| *Anaerobes* | 2.53 | 0 |
| Concentration | $10^{5.2}$ cfu/gm | |
| *Aerobes, facultative* | 1.46 | 0.45 |
| Concentration | $10^{4.6}$ cfu/gm | $10^{3.5}$ cfu/gm |

**TABLE 21-4** Organisms Recovered from Patients with Cervical Cancer

| Organism | Frequency of Isolation (%) | Mean Concen-tration* |
|---|---|---|
| Anaerobes | | |
| *Bacteroides* spp. | 8/13 (61.5) | 4.69 ± 1.29 |
| Anaerobic cocci | 7/13 (53.8) | 5.50 ± 1.39 |
| Gram-positive bacilli | 4/13 (30.8) | 5.13 ± 1.52 |
| *Clostridium* | 3/13 (23.1) | 5.13 ± 1.26 |
| Aerobes | | |
| Aerobic staphylococci | 6/13 (46.2) | 4.16 ± 0.81 |
| Aerobic streptococci | 6/13 (46.2) | 4.88 ± 0.42 |
| From controls | | |
| *Staphylococcus* spp. | 2/11 (18) | 3.78 ± 0.99 |
| *Candida albicans* | 1/11 (9) | 3.04 |
| *Corynebacterium* spp. | 1/11 (9) | 2.47 |
| α-Hemolytic streptococcus | 1/11 (9) | 4.30 |

* $Log_{10}$ cfu/gm of tissue. Same study group as in Table 21-3.

**TABLE 21-5** Causes of Fever in the Gynecologic Oncology Patient

*Postoperative*
  Early
    Pulmonary
    Wound infection (streptococcal)
    Peritonitis
  Early to intermediate
    Urinary tract infection
    Pelvic infection
      Pelvic cellulitis
      Vaginal cuff abscess
      Pelvic inflammatory disease
  Late
    Pelvic infection
    Pelvic abscess
    Intraabdominal abscess
    Wound infection
    Pelvic thrombophlebitis
*Nonoperative causes*
  Anesthesia-related
  Hepatitis
  Tumor-related
  Drug fever
  Intercurrent systemic infection
  Intravenous site infection

tibiotics as either prophylaxis or therapy fosters this recolonization and may also be partially responsible for promoting the survival of organisms with relatively greater resistance from among the normal flora. The virulence of acquired organisms is highly variable, although any opportunistic pathogen may cause infection if present in sufficient numbers in a susceptible host. Acquired flora of particular concern in oncologic patients includes *Pseudomonas aeruginosa*, *Serratia marcescens*, other Enterobacteriaceae, various fungi, and with the increasing use of indwelling venous catheters, skin flora including methicillin-resistant *S. aureus*, *S. epidermidis*, and *Corynebacterium*, and *Bacillus* species.

## FEVER AND INFECTION IN THE PATIENT WITH GYNECOLOGIC MALIGNANCY

When a patient with cancer presents with fever, a diagnosable infection is the cause in about two-thirds of the cases (Table 21-5). Infection may be defined by the presence of positive results on culture or may be clinically evident with or without positive cultures. The types of infection seen among gynecologic oncology patients vary according to the patient's general state of health, the types of organisms involved, whether there is recent or ongoing hospitalization, and whether or not recent surgery or immunocompromise are factors to be considered. Recently, morbidity due to infection specifically on gynecologic oncology services has been reviewed (Brooker et al, 1987; Chambers and Schwartz, 1986; Dvoretsky et al, 1988). These reviews suggest that such morbidity is similar in presentation to the previously well-described problems related to infection seen on general oncology services. Rates of infection are similar, with 11 to 18% of gynecologic oncology patients suffering a major infection during hospitalization for their primary diagnosis. At present, gynecologic patients probably have shorter hospital stays for infection and associated complications, reflecting the less pro-

found complications of neutropenia and immune suppression in this group as opposed to patients seen on general oncology services. However, specific diagnoses, risk factors for infection, prognostic factors, and problems encountered during evaluation and therapy are the same. The most common of these infections and the organisms most frequently associated with them will now be discussed in more detail.

### Bacteremia

On average, 25 to 50% of blood cultures drawn when the patient presents with fever will document bacteremia. The primary focus of infection giving rise to bacteremia may or may not be obvious; no single primary site of infection can be said to predispose to bacteremia disproportionately. Infections that present with high fever are most likely to produce positive cultures. In addition, invasive infection is more likely to result in bacteremia when the patient is neutropenic (EORTC, 1978).

The outcome of bacteremia depends upon the patient's underlying clinical condition including stage and presence of ongoing malignancy or other comorbid conditions (Talcott et al, 1988), the site of infection, the infecting organisms, and to some extent the adequacy and immediacy of therapy (Klastersky, 1988). Overall, half the patients with solid tumors who presented with infections that eventually proved fatal had bacteremia.

Four organisms account for the majority of isolates from oncologic patients with bacteremia: *E. coli*, *K. pneumoniae*, *P. aeruginosa*, and *S. aureus*. The exact proportions of these bacterial isolates vary with the patterns of infection in individual hospitals and on individual tumor services. Patterns of bacteremia for a group of patients with gynecologic malignancy have not been well defined. The previously mentioned recent reviews plus analysis of reviews from large oncology services suggest that generally the patterns of bacteremia are similar. However, bacteremia due to *P. aeruginosa* may be seen somewhat less frequently in gynecology patients, while polymicrobial bacteremias are seen proportionately more frequently (Elting et al, 1986). Polymicrobial bacteremias may involve more than one species of aerobic or anaerobic organism or both aerobic and anaerobic organisms being isolated from the bloodstream during an episode of sepsis. The prognosis with respect to both fatalities and recurrence of bacteremia once initial therapy has been completed tends to be the worst for gram-negative bacillemias and for polymicrobial bacteremias.

***Escherichia coli*** *E. coli* is a major contributor to bacteremias in patients with solid tumors. In 25% of cases in which *E. coli* is isolated from the bloodstream, the organisms may be found in combination with another gram-negative enteric bacillum or with anaerobic organisms. *E. coli* is a normal colonizer of both the lower genital tract and the gastrointestinal tract, so that breaks in the defense barriers of either of these systems may lead to invasive infection and bacteremia. In addition, *E. coli* is a frequent urinary tract pathogen, so that the urinary tract may be the source of bacteremia.

*E. coli* bacteremia presents as an acute episode characterized by shaking chills and high fevers. Ten to 30% of patients present with signs of systemic sepsis and septic shock, including hypotension, hypovolemia, changes in mental status, and multisystem failure. Two-thirds of the fatalities due to *E. coli* bacteremia occur within the first 24 hours (Grose et al, 1978; Bodey et al, 1986), probably owing to endotoxemia that causes a shocklike picture. *E. coli* may cause sepsis at any stage of malignancy. Strains resistant to common antimicrobial agents may be responsible for bacteremias that occur while the patient is taking antibiotics and for recurrent bacteremias after the completion of initial therapy for infections cause by coliforms or other gram-negative enteric bacilli (Grose et al, 1978).

***Klebsiella pneumoniae*** *K. pneumoniae* is a member of the Enterobacteriaceae. It is a normal colonizer of the lower genital tract and gastrointestinal tract but is less prevalent under healthy conditions than is *E. coli*. Its prevalence both as a colonizer and in the presence of invasive infection increases with exposure to antimicrobial agents. *Klebsiella* may enter the bloodstream through the gastrointestinal, genitourinary, or genital tract and occasionally through the respiratory tract.

The clinical presentation of *K. pneumoniae* sepsis is similar to that of *E. coli* bacteremia. *Klebsiella* infection may result in death 20 to 60% of the time—a wide variation that is perhaps related to the adequacy of initial antibiotic therapy. Along with *E. coli*, *Klebsiella* is one of the major organisms causing recurrent bacteremias after initial therapy, particularly therapy for other gram-negative bacillemias (Grose et al, 1978).

***Pseudomonas aeruginosa*** *P. aeruginosa* is seen as a cause of bacteremia less frequently in patients with solid tumors than in those with hematologic malignancies. *Pseudomonas* is not a frequent colonizer of the lower genital tract in most patient populations, and although it may be found in the gastrointestinal tract, it is not often isolated from gynecologic intraabdominal and postoperative infections. *Pseudomonas* is a frequent colonizer of the respiratory tract and is a major contributor to sepsis from this source. Infection of the local soft tissues in the anorectal area may also result in bacteremia. *P. aeruginosa* is frequently found in hospital environments, and patients with more advanced stages of disease or who have been hospitalized frequently tend more often to be colonized by this organism.

The clinical presentation of *Pseudomonas* bacteremia is similar to that of other gram-negative bacillemias. Thirty percent of these patients may present with characteristic indurated, ulcerated skin lesions with necrotic centers called ecthyma gangrenosum that are seen in the groin, axillary, and perianal areas. Bacteremia with *P. aeruginosa* may result in a disproportionately high number of fatalities (Armstrong et al, 1971). The bacteria are encapsulated and may be particularly virulent in patients with defective humoral immunity, especially defective opsonizing antibody. *Pseudomonas* septicemia also tends to occur in patients with neutropenia and in those with advanced disease, which may contribute to the high case-fatality ratio.

***Staphylococcus aureus*** The incidence of bacteremia caused by *S. aureus* is increasing for all types of malignancy. *S. aureus* is a common skin colonizer during all stages of malignant disease. Invasive infection and bacteremia are most often a direct result of an identifiable breach in the mucocutaneous barrier that allows this organism to enter the body (Carney et al, 1982a). Perhaps the major sources of skin breaks that lead to *S. aureus* bacteremia are invasive monitoring devices and indwelling lines such as intravenous catheters and long lines for central venous access. Staphyloccocal bacteremia presents as an acute, nonspecific illness, with no particular predilection for the immunocompromised host (Kilton et al, 1979; Carney et al, 1982a). It is somewhat more common in the bedridden patient with debilitating advanced disease. Although metastatic foci of infection occur occasionally, surprisingly few cases of staphylococcal endocarditis result from bacteremia. This experience has resulted in slightly less stringent criteria for the duration of treatment of patients with malignancy who have documented staphylococcal bacteremia (Carney et al, 1982b). There is a lower rate of mortality associated with *S. aureus* than with gram-negative septicemia (in the range of 4%), and the outcome of staphylococcal bacteremia depends more upon the host's underlying clinical condition than upon the initial focus of infection or the disease presentation. If *S. aureus* is suspected, initial antimicrobial therapy should include a penicillinase-resistant, semisynthetic penicillin or cephalosporin, and the foci of infection should be removed if possible. In services that are beginning to encounter strains of methicillin-resistant *S.*

*aureus*, initial coverage may need to include vancomycin (Rubin et al, 1988).

***Other Bacteria*** All types of aerobic streptococci may cause bacteremia in patients with malignancy. A very low but constant level of sepsis due to the enterococcus is found in patients with gynecologic malignancy in particular. Enterococcal septicemia may potentially occur after any invasive diagnostic or therapeutic gynecologic procedure, such as cervical conization or dilatation and curettage. In addition, enterococcal sepsis may be seen in postoperative patients, arising from intraabdominal or wound sepsis and, in particular, urinary tract infections.

*Streptococcus pneumoniae* is an uncommon cause of sepsis in patients with gynecologic malignancy. When it does occur, it is most often found in patients with preexisting lung disease or a history consistent with recent pulmonary compromise, such as prolonged anesthesia or aspiration. The pneumococcus is an encapsulated bacterium, and defects in humoral immunity, particularly those occurring after splenectomy, may predispose to pneumococcal septicemia and more severe disease (Chou et al, 1983). Pneumococcal bacteremia may present as a fulminating illness, with a mortality rate of up to 40 to 50%. Eighty percent of the time, presenting symptoms include those of an upper respiratory infection.

Anaerobic bacteremia does occur in patients with gynecologic malignancy, with anaerobes frequently contributing to a polymicrobial bacteremia along with aerobes. Anaerobic gram-positive cocci, *Bacteroides* species, and *Clostridia* are most often isolated from the blood in cases of postoperative infection or intraabdominal sepsis, either peritonitis or abscess formation.

*Bacteroides* bacteremia may be associated with tumors—either obstruction due to tumor or infection of the tumor tissue itself. Occasionally, bacteremia with *Bacteroides fragilis* may be the first sign of malignancy (Dionigi et al, 1980). *B. fragilis* bacteremia is characterized by high spiking fevers with repeated chills, obtundation, shock, and a high white blood cell count (Sinkovics and Smith, 1970), although occasionally the presentation may be milder. Death ensues 25 to 45% of the time, with the outcome dependent upon the patient's condition and to some extent the site of the primary infection. Bacteremia due to septic thrombophlebitis with septic embolization may be associated with a particularly bad prognosis.

*Clostridia perfringens* may be isolated in up to 4% of cases of sepsis in patients with uterine infections. When *Clostridia* is present at the site of a soft tissue infection, bacteremia may result in up to 90% of cases. The source of clostridial bacteremia may be the gastrointestinal or urinary tract or the tumors themselves. Up to 75% of patients with clostridial bacteremia present with fulminating sepsis with tachycardia, hypotension, oliguria, jaundice, and intravascular hemolysis. Exotoxins are responsible for the characteristic intravascular hemolysis and hemoglobinuria that contribute to the shock and renal failure associated with clostridial sepsis. Despite prompt initiation of antibiotic therapy and occasional use of antitoxin, death from *Clostridia* often occurs within 12 to 24 hours of the onset of bacteremia.

## Intraabdominal Infection

Intraabdominal sepsis arises more often in patients with gynecologic malignancy than in any other group of cancer patients, with the exception of those with bowel cancer. The possibility of intraabdominal sepsis has major implications for diagnosis and therapy in terms of both antibiotic selection and surgical intervention.

Intraabdominal infection may be a complication of diagnostic procedures, a postoperative complication, a delayed complication of radiation therapy (such as perforation or fistula formation), or a complication of chemotherapy (including instillation of drugs via an indwelling peritoneal catheter). In addition, the tumor itself may be the primary focus of sepsis in the absence of any invasive procedures. For example, in tumors that have been contaminated with lower genital tract flora, superinfection and abscess can develop. An intraabdominal tumor may also cause intestinal perforation, with spillage of bowel contents or localized abscess formation.

Two major types of intraabdominal sepsis are of concern: peritonitis and abscess formation. *Peritonitis* occurs when a bacterial load is presented acutely to the peritoneal cavity through a break in a mucocutaneous barrier, such as bowel or uterine perforation or spillage of organisms from the fallopian tubes in cases of upper genital tract infection. The resulting acute generalized peritoneal inflammation causes dramatic signs, with a high fever, diffuse pain, guarding, and abdominal rigidity. In addition to the consequences of bacteremia, the rapid and voluminous sequestration of intraabdominal fluid accompanying this acute peritoneal inflammation may cause dramatic and potentially fatal metabolic and cardiovascular alterations, with shocklike collapse. Occasionally, the onset of peritonitis is more insidious. With advanced malignancy or steroid therapy, intraabdominal sepsis may present with fever and few diagnostic clinical signs. If a patient with fever is at high risk for intraabdominal sepsis, needle aspiration of peritoneal fluid that reveals polymorphonuclear leukocytes and the presence of bacteria on Gram stain can be diagnostic.

The late effect of intraperitoneal leakage or spillage of bacterial flora is *abscess formation*, occurring 5 to 7 days later. Following diffuse peritonitis, localized abscess formation is commonly found in dependent portions of the peritoneal cavity, such as the subhepatic space, the cul-de-sac, and the paracolic gutters. The abscess may be diffuse or fairly well walled-off and confined to immediate areas of contamination in the pelvis, near the bowel, or within tumor tissue itself. Abscess formation less often results in bacteremia and is more likely to present as spiking fevers without a clinically obvious source.

Organisms that cause intraabdominal sepsis are found among the lower genital tract or gut flora, particularly that of the more heavily colonized large bowel.

Intraabdominal infection is most often polymicrobial, with mixed aerobic and anaerobic bacteria, and may cause either polymicrobial or single-organism bacteremia.

The pathophysiology of intraabdominal infection due to contamination of the peritoneal cavity by polymicrobial flora has been elucidated in an elaborate series of animal experiments using bacteriologic and antimicrobial probes. The initial peritonitis stage of intraabdominal sepsis is due to aerobic organisms, chiefly *E. coli*. If this bacteremia goes untreated, the mortality from *E. coli* peritonitis is high, while survivors of untreated peritonitis inevitably develop intraabdominal abscesses. Anaerobic organisms are always involved in abscess formation, and most require the presence of more invasive aerobes to be fully pathogenic. The exception to this is *B. fragilis*, which is capable of forming abscesses on its own. The presence of a capsular polysaccharide surface antigen that resists phagocytosis and opsonization is responsible for this particular pathogen's virulence. *B. fragilis* is found in intraabdominal abscesses approximately 60% of the time.

After intraabdominal spillage of polymicrobial flora, one must provide antimicrobial coverage for both gram-negative enteric bacilli and anaerobes, including *B. fragilis*, to prevent both the major morbidity and mortality associated with peritonitis and abscess formation. Such therapy should be instituted promptly whenever spontaneous intraabdominal sepsis is suspected or when the large bowel is inadvertently entered at the time of surgery. Whenever one suspects a pelvic abscess due to lower genital tract flora or infection of a tumor mass, multiorganism coverage must also be instituted and specific coverage for *B. fragilis* provided. Often, antimicrobial therapy for intraabdominal abscesses, infected tumor masses, and peritonitis with a large exudative reaction is not sufficient for cure. Unless the patient responds promptly to antibiotic therapy, surgical intervention to drain the peritoneum or abscess or to resect infected tissue is warranted; delay serves only to increase morbidity.

The placement and manipulation of intraperitoneal catheters are clearly associated with intraperitoneal infection. However, it appears that only a minority of these infections are related to actual bowel perforation with spillage of intraluminal contents. Rather, skin flora are commonly implicated, *Staphylococcus epidermidis* being the most frequent isolate in one series (Kaplan et al, 1985). In this same series, 35% of the patients eventually had intraperitoneal infection, as diagnosed by positive Gram stain. All these patients eventually needed antibiotic therapy, and in 26% the intraperitoneal catheter had to be removed to effect a cure.

One complication of intraabdominal infection is *septic pelvic thrombophlebitis*. Such localized intravascular infection of the major pelvic veins involves a heparinase-producing *B. fragilis*. The typical presentation includes hectic, spiking fevers that have no clear source and do not respond to antibiotics. The patient occasionally presents with respiratory symptoms due to septic embolization. Treatment consists of heparin therapy in addition to antibiotics. Sometimes ligation of the inferior vena cava and right ovarian vein above the level of the clot is required, particularly if the patient presents with multiple septic emboli.

## Postoperative Infections

Virtually all surgical procedures performed during diagnosis and therapy of gynecologic malignancy may result in localized postoperative infection. The risk of infection correlates most strongly with contamination of the operative site by potential pathogens. Although procedures that expose the upper genital tract, intraabdominal cavity, or skin wounds to lower genital tract flora may result in significant postoperative infection, those in which the operative site is contaminated by bowel flora lead to an even greater incidence of such infections.

Upper genital tract infections may complicate cervical biopsy and conization, dilatation and curettage to diagnose endometrial carcinoma or to treat gestational trophoblastic neoplasms, and even radiation therapy with intracavitary radium. The onset of such infections may be either acute or more insidious, with subacute signs. It is not clear whether colonization of the lower genital tract by any potential pathogen in particular will increase the risk of such iatrogenic pelvic infections. However, if appropriate, screening for sexually transmitted organisms (such as *Neisseria gonorrhoeae*) should be carried out, and the patient should be treated accordingly prior to such procedures. To date, there is no evidence that other prophylactic use of antimicrobials is warranted.

Cultures of the lower genital tract may not accurately reveal the organisms present at the site of upper genital tract infection. Therapy is based on the assumption that upper genital tract infections are polymicrobial, often of mixed (aerobic and anaerobic) etiology. In acute illness, aerobic organisms such as streptococci, coliforms, and occasionally *N. gonorrhoeae* are of particular concern, while anaerobes (including the *Bacteroides* species) are of concern, with more indolent infection and abscess formation. Unless the infection appears to be particularly mild, antibiotic therapy should be administered by the parenteral route.

After hysterectomy, the risk of infection ranges from 7 to 30% and may be even higher after radical hysterectomy. Morbidity after vaginal hysterectomy usually consists of pelvic infections, such as cuff cellulitis or pelvic abscess. After either simple or radical abdominal hysterectomy, there is risk for both pelvic and major abdominal wound infection. Causative organisms include the aerobic and anaerobic lower genital tract flora contaminating the operative site at the time of entry in the vagina. Abdominal wound infections may be due to skin colonizers such as *S. aureus* and streptococcal species but may also involve lower genital tract flora.

Posthysterectomy pelvic cellulitis presents as fever and lower pelvic pain, with an indurated and often exquisitely painful vaginal cuff 2 to 5 days after surgery. Although both aerobic and anaerobic organisms may contribute to this type of infection, the response to simple broad-spectrum therapy that does not include extensive coverage for *B. fragilis* is often prompt and gratifying. In cases of life-threatening illness or when there is a suggestion of early abscess formation, antimicrobial coverage for gram-negative enteric bacilli, streptococci, anaerobic cocci, *B. fragilis* must be provided. Drainage of the vaginal cuff can be a helpful adjunct to antibiotic therapy.

*Postoperative pelvic abscesses* of the vaginal cuff, of the pelvic floor and sidewalls, or at the site of intraabdominal blood collections tend to present more than 5 days after hysterectomy or other intraabdominal pelvic surgical procedures and may not become manifest until after the patient has been discharged from the hospital. The bacteriology and management are similar to those of spontaneous pelvic abscesses, described previously.

*Wound infection* may occur at the sites of skin incisions after abdominal surgical procedures or after either simple or radical vulvectomy. Patients who have undergone radiation therapy in addition to surgery are at particular risk for wound infection. Postoperative wound infections may present acutely with fever and marked incisional pain accompanying erythema, induration, warmth, and tenderness. When this occurs 24 to 48 hours after surgery, the group A beta-hemolytic streptococci are the most likely causative organisms. However, a less immediate onset with the same type of erythematous, indurated wound is more typical. Often a wound infection is the cause of a spiking, low-grade fever, but the source does not become obvious until a collection of pus is discovered through either spontaneous drainage or wound exploration.

*S. aureus* and other skin flora are frequently isolated from postoperative wound infections. After operation on the genital tract, mixed flora may also be found, and a Gram stain of material from an open skin wound or incisional collection can be helpful when one is choosing antimicrobial therapy prior to culture results. Because of their unique exposure to mixed aerobic/anaerobic pathogens at the time of surgery, patients with gynecologic malignancy are at risk for several distinct but uncommon types of "synergistic" wound infections at the site of abdominal or vulvar incisions. The clinical presentation in such infections reflects the invasion of tissue planes by both aerobic and anaerobic organisms. Aerobic organisms cause initial tissue infection and damage, while anaerobic organisms cause further tissue destruction in an atmosphere of decreased oxygen tension. In addition to operative exposure to polymicrobial flora, obesity, diabetes, debilitating disease, and previous radiation therapy are all risk factors for the development of synergistic infections (Meltzer, 1983).

Synergistic infections may progress rapidly, with tissue infection and necrosis spreading along fascial lines or through the subcutaneous tissue in a matter of hours, as in necrotizing fasciitis or cellulitis. In such cases, fever and signs of systemic sepsis are almost always present. Examination of skin and subcutaneous tissues will reveal areas of skin necrosis and underlying crepitation, and x-rays may reveal a subcutaneous gas pattern. Necrotizing synergistic infection must be distinguished from necrotizing wound infection due to *C. perfringens*. In other cases, sometimes referred to as "progressive synergistic bacterial gangrene," synergistic wound infections have an insidious onset and lack systemic signs, although local pain is often intense. By the time the characteristic skin changes become apparent, i.e., central necrosis with surrounding erythema of a violaceous hue, subcutaneous tissue necrosis may be far more advanced than the superficial appearance of the lesion would suggest.

The original description of synergistic wound infections by Meleney (1931) was of mixed aerobic staphylococci and microaerophilic streptococci. Since that time, combinations of *E. coli* and other gram-negative enterics or aerobic streptococci with anaerobic cocci and *Bacteroides* species have been reported (Daly et al, 1978; Meltzer, 1983). In cases of suspected synergistic wound infections, antibiotic therapy must provide broad-spectrum coverage for both aerobes and anaerobes, although antimicrobial therapy alone will rarely halt the progression of these infections. Most often, cure is achieved only after debridement of all affected tissues, with subsequent healing by secondary intention. In cases of rapidly progressive disease, prompt debridement may be lifesaving. Infected tissue undermines the skin and has been described as grey, stringy, and devitalized, with a purulent and malodorous or "dishwater" discharge. All such tissue must be totally resected, with the margins of resection extended to healthy-appearing, bleeding tissue. Fascial grafting with synthetic grafts may be necessary (Daly et al, 1978).

The risk of major pelvic or wound infection after simple hysterectomy, either vaginal or abdominal, is significantly reduced (but not eliminated) by perioperative antimicrobial prophylaxis. Although some studies suggest a benefit to prophylaxis for radical hysterectomy, efficacy has not been as clearly demonstrated for reducing major infection after radical hysterectomy, perhaps because the risk of infection tends to be greater with longer surgical procedures. If such prophylaxis is to be used to prevent infection after hysterectomy, it must be administered appropriately. Parenteral antibiotics should be given just prior to surgery and continued postoperatively for less than 24 hours; extending either preoperative or postoperative prophylaxis is of no benefit. Usually broad-spectrum, first generation antimicrobials such as cefazolin are employed; doxycycline has also been demonstrated to be effective. More expensive and toxic regimens that provide additional coverage for anaerobes and resistant gram-negative enteric bacilli do not appear to afford any additional benefit; furthermore, superinfection or infection due to resistant organisms is a potential danger.

By using properly functioning, active drains at the intraperitoneal operative site or subperitoneal vaginal cuff, one can prevent some instances of postoperative infection (Creasman et al, 1982; Swartz and Tanaree, 1975). It is not clear whether the use of drains is as effective as or enhances the efficacy of perioperative antimicrobial prophylaxis.

The incidence of infection after hysterectomy for cervical cancer may be influenced by the timing of previous cervical conization. For the past 20 years, results of reports of infections occurring after hysterectomy performed at varying intervals following conization have been conflicting (Williams, 1970; Elkins et al, 1982). Many investigators have shown that the risk is increased if simple hysterectomy is performed 48 hours to 3 weeks after cervical conization, presumably owing to the inflammatory changes and suppuration observed microscopically from 48 hours to 60 days after conization, both at the site of conization and extending to the parametrium (Wisborg, 1972; Orr et al, 1982; Osoba, 1958; Skaarup et al, 1971; Mikuta et al, 1977; Laubach and McGanity, 1965; DeCenzo et al, 1971; Doran and Shier, 1964). This led to the recommendation that hysterectomy should be either performed immediately after conization, with the decision for surgery based on a frozen section of the cervical specimen, or delayed for at least 6 weeks. However, more recent investigations suggest that the conization-hysterectomy interval is no longer an important consideration, since perioperative antimicrobial prophylaxis has sufficiently reduced the risk of posthysterectomy infection (Orr et al, 1982; Mann et al, 1981; Lerner et al, 1980; Forney et al, 1975). Others have noted that this interval is also probably unimportant in radical hysterectomy, since the parametrium is excised in this particular procedure (Webb and Symmonds, 1979). Since few pathology laboratories have a proven record of accuracy in interpreting cervical cone frozen sections, it seems reasonable to postpone either simple or radical hysterectomy until at least 3 weeks after conization, whenever possible.

When the large bowel is entered at laparotomy in patients with bowel obstruction or when unprepared bowel is inadvertently entered at the time of laparotomy, the risk of postoperative sepsis is so high that antibiotics are used therapeutically to prevent major sequelae (i.e., peritonitis and abscess formation). When bowel entry is anticipated as part of a planned surgical procedure, such as exenteration, the incidence of postoperative infection can be reduced through the use of antimicrobial prophylaxis. If there is no evidence of bowel dysfunction, the administration of oral nonabsorbable broad-spectrum antibiotics in addition to mechanical cleansing does reduce the incidence of major postoperative infections. A regimen such as 1 gm of oral erythromycin base and 1 gm of neomycin given three times during the afternoon and evening prior to surgery has been shown to be efficacious in this setting.

Parenteral perioperative prophylaxis with agents that provide anaerobic coverage, such as cefoxitin or metronidazole, also decreases operative site infection. There is no justification for using both oral and parenteral agents simultaneously. A reasonable approach to perioperative prophylaxis at the time of elective bowel surgery would be mechanical cleansing plus oral nonabsorbable antibiotics in patients with adequate bowel function; parenteral antibiotics would be reserved for those with bowel dysfunction or obstruction.

The efficacy of perioperative antibiotics to prevent wound infection after vulvectomy has not been clearly demonstrated. Incisions in the radical procedure are also at risk for breakdown due to necrosis. To reduce such wound complications, one can use separate incisions for vulvectomy and lymph node dissection and active drains

under skin and subcutaneous flaps (Byron et al, 1965; Hacker et al, 1981).

## Urinary Tract Infection

Urinary tract infection (UTI), the most common hospital-acquired infection, is a major source of sepsis and bacteremia in the gynecologic oncology patient. The most important risk factor in the etiology of these infections is the presence of an indwelling bladder catheter. These catheters are used routinely during the perioperative period in patients undergoing simple hysterectomy and other intraabdominal surgical procedures and, over a longer term, after radical hysterectomy and radical vulvectomy. Furthermore, indwelling catheters may be employed as part of long-term supportive care during advanced stages of disease.

The incidence of UTI (e.g., pyelonephritis secondary to ascending bacteria) correlates directly with the length of time the catheter is in place. Although meticulous catheter care and use of closed drainage systems may delay or lower the incidence of infection, such measures will not alter this correlation. Intermittent bladder irrigation with sterile or antibiotic-containing solutions has not convincingly demonstrated any decrease in the incidence of UTI in patients with indwelling bladder catheters (Savage et al, 1982). Oral or parenteral antimicrobial prophylaxis does not lower the incidence of catheter-related bacteriuria and probably promotes infections involving bacteria that are resistant to the prophylactic agents used (Bodey, 1975).

In addition to indwelling bladder catheters, ileal conduits and urinary tract obstruction secondary to tumor or fibrosis can be factors in increasing the incidence of upper UTI.

Although infection may remain localized to the lower urinary tract, bacteria may ascend to the upper tract, causing acute pyelonephritis. Upper UTI may occur more frequently in the setting of altered ureteral motility and bacteriuria secondary to obstruction; in neutropenic patients; and immediately after catheterization, cystoscopy, or other procedures that introduce an acute bacterial load to the urinary tract. Occasionally, kidneys may be seeded with organisms from bacteremia that originated at another focus.

Acute upper UTI does not typically lead to renal damage. However, in the presence of obstruction, renal parenchymal damage can lead to chronic pyelonephritis and papillary necrosis. Renal or perirenal abscess may also result from untreated infection.

Any upper UTI may be associated with an acute, febrile, painful presentation and bacteremia, but a more insidious presentation that consists of fever with developing flank or abdominal pain should raise the question of a perirenal or renal abscess.

Organisms that most often cause UTI in patients with gynecologic cancer include *E. coli*, *Proteus* species, *Klebsiella* species, enterococci, *P. aeruginosa*, and occasionally *Staphylococcus* species and fungi such as *Candida*. The enterococcus is a particularly common pathogen of the perioperative period. *Pseudomonas*, staphylococci, and *Candida* should be considered in patients with more advanced disease and multiple hospitalizations.

Asymptomatic bacteriuria in the presence of a catheter often will not be cured until the catheter is removed, and the patient should be treated with oral antibiotics to which the offending bacteria are sensitive. Upper UTI should be treated promptly with parenteral antibiotics. Initial therapy of a UTI in a patient with sepsis should be guided by the results of Gram staining of a drop of unspun urine. If bacteria are found, infection is likely, and morphologic characteristics can aid in identifying the infecting organism.

Certain clinical features at presentation should prompt further urinary tract testing. If there is no clear-cut etiology (e.g., recent urinary tract instrumentation, presence of an indwelling catheter), if the response to therapy is delayed, or if there is a possibility of obstruction based on either a history suggestive of tumor or an atypical presentation of a UTI with abdominal and back pain that is disproportionate to the usual symptoms associated with pyelonephritis, a more extensive evaluation is in order. Intravenous pyelography or ultrasonography or both should be performed to look for obstruction or immobility, which suggests a perirenal abscess. Both these problems will often require surgical management in conjunction with antibiotic therapy.

In general, mortality from UTI—even when the infection is associated with bacteremia—is lower than that associated with other soft tissue foci of infection and bacteremia. However, in many cases, death from UTI may be preventable. One recent study suggests that the presence of an indwelling bladder catheter should be considered a major risk factor for death among hospitalized patients (Platt et al, 1982).

## Skin Infections

The integrity of the skin is one prerequisite to preventing infection among patients with cancer. When this barrier is breached, soft tissue and ultimately systemic infections may result. Skin breakdown related to poor tissue quality and decubiti during advanced disease may lead to sepsis. Extravasation of chemotherapeutic agents like vincristine and doxorubicin or the toxic effects of chemotherapy (e.g., mucositis), particularly when these coincide with conditions of neutropenia and immunosuppression, can result in cellulitis and bacteremia. Cellulitis and abscesses of the perirectal area are a frequent cause of sepsis in the immunosuppressed patient (Nadworny and Greene, 1984).

Intravenous catheters are the most significant skin source of sepsis in patients with malignancy. These catheters all serve as portals of entry for bacteria that colonize the skin. The incidence of vein sepsis and bacteremia related to peripheral access line increases with the duration of individual catheter use. Since complications related to infection increase markedly during the first 3 days of catheter use, peripheral intravenous lines should be changed every 48 to 72 hours.

Long-line venous access catheters used principally as central lines for support, medications, or nutrition are also associated with bacteremia and local skin sepsis.

However, the incidence of such infection can be markedly decreased if one uses meticulous aseptic technique during catheter insertion and care. The technique of tunnelling such devices as the Hickman and Broviac catheters under the skin before they enter the vein, followed by daily care with local Betadine gel plus occlusive dressings, has resulted in successful use of these intravenous catheters for prolonged periods of time (Nadworny and Greene, 1984).

The increase in gram-positive bacteremias noted on many oncology services has been ascribed to catheter-related infections, the majority of which are due to *S. aureus*. In patients with advanced disease, particularly those with neutropenia, an increase in bacteremias caused by normally nonpathogenic or opportunistic skin pathogens such as *Staphylococcus epidermidis*, *Bacillus* species, *Mimae* species, *Corynebacterium*, and diphtheroids is most often related to intravenous catheter sepsis and may rarely lead to endocarditis. Intravenous sites may also be the portal of entry for fungal species such as *Candida albicans* in the debilitated host.

It is not always necessary to remove an essential central intravenous catheter in cases of suspected sepsis of the catheter site. However, if there is persistent fever despite antibiotic therapy, removal and culture of long intravenous lines may be both diagnostic and therapeutic. There has been a suggestion that tunnel-site as opposed to exit-site infections may be more difficult to cure, especially if *Pseudomonas* is involved (Benezra et al, 1988). These infections should be followed carefully and certainly if positive cultures persist or if the clinical condition is unstable, the catheter should be removed. Conversely, in stable patients with minimal signs of infection, removal of a catheter will often result in cure without the need for antibiotic therapy.

## Pneumonias

Although the respiratory tract is a relatively infrequent site of infection in patients with gynecologic malignancy, it is always a potential source of sepsis. Sepsis associated with pneumonia is disproportionately associated with mortality. In patients with clinically significant pneumonia, there is almost always an underlying precipitating factor. Chief among these factors are preexisting respiratory compromise; general anesthetics and tracheostomies, which predispose to aspiration or colonization with virulent organisms; obstructive tumors metastatic to the lung; and neutropenia. Organisms of concern include *S. pneumoniae*, *K. pneumoniae*, and endogenously acquired organisms such as *P. aeruginosa* and *Serratia marcescens*. The high mortality associated with nosocomial infection necessitates aggressive attempts to identify and treat appropriately the causative organisms in cases of bacterial pneumonia.

Patients with advanced disease who are profoundly immunosuppressed will occasionally develop one of the progressive pneumonias more commonly seen in patients with prolonged neutropenia and suppressed cellular immunity. Although fungal and viral pneumonias must be considered when one is evaluating a nonbacterial pneumonia, the protozoon *Pneumocystis carinii* is emerging as a pathogen of particular importance among immunosuppressed patients with diffuse interstitial pneumonia (Bodey, 1975; Singer and Turnbull, 1979). The major signs associated with *Pneumocystis* are shortness of breath and tachypnea with hypoxemia and cyanosis, but often with few other findings on physical examination. *Pneumocystis* rarely disseminates. Respiratory infections may be either somewhat insidious or of acute onset, with a rapidly progressive course. Although early in the disease a chest x-ray may be unremarkable, diffuse bilateral interstitial infiltrates, most prominent in the hilar area, will develop.

When one encounters a patient with rapidly progressive, diffuse pneumonia or with an atypical pneumonia that does not respond to the usual antibacterial therapy, prompt, aggressive measures must be taken to establish a diagnosis. These may include transbronchial brushings and biopsy or open lung biopsy. It is important to differentiate pneumonia caused by *P. carinii* from other or concomitant diagnoses so that antimicrobial therapy and the respiratory support needed to improve survival in these patients can be instituted. In addition to intensive support, treatment of *Pneumocystis* pneumonia includes either pentamidine or trimethoprim-sulfamethoxazole.

## Fungal Infections

Invasive fungal disease with or without fungemia may occur in patients with advanced malignant disease after multiple courses of antimicrobial agents and hospitalizations have led to colonization of the gut and skin with fungi. *Candida* (particularly *C. albicans*) and *Aspergillus* are the most common causes of fungal disease in this population. The rate at which fungal infections are occurring in patients with solid tumors is increasing, and it is estimated that 0.5% of all such patients will eventually develop candidiasis (Bodey, 1986a). Fungal infections are responsible for approximately 5% of all fatal infections in this group.

Suppressed immunity, neutropenia, poor nutrition, and the long-term use of antibiotics, steroids, parenteral nutrition, and indwelling vascular catheters are all risk factors for invasive fungal infections. Approximately half the cases of disseminated candidiasis are associated with preceding bacterial infection, emphasizing the effects of both antibiotic use and underlying altered immunity on the development of invasive fungal infection.

Most fungal infections present initially as a fever of unknown origin. Organ involvement is determined by the organisms' site of origin. *Candida* colonizing the oral mucosa or gastrointestinal tract may spread to the esophagus or disseminate to the liver or spleen. *Aspergillus* colonizing the upper respiratory tract may spread to the lungs or sinuses. Fungi that colonize the skin near intravenous access sites may seed the heart, kidneys, or lungs.

Invasive candidiasis may be preceded by multiple sites of heavy and persistent colonization. However, such colonization is associated with invasive disease in less than 50% of cases (Bodey, 1986a). Also, more than

30% of the time, invasive infection is not preceded by detectable colonization (Meunier and Klastersky, 1988). Therefore, the use of "surveillance" cultures in an effort to predict the occurrence of invasive fungal infection has no proven value.

*Candidal infections* may present with localized manifestations or as disseminated disease, with or without fever. Candidal esophagitis causes pain and difficulty in swallowing as well as characteristic "cobblestone" lesions on barium swallow and esophagoscopy. Ulcerative candidal bowel disease is associated with abdominal discomfort, bloating, diarrhea, and rectal bleeding. Such superficial gastrointestinal disease can lead to dissemination. Primary pulmonary candidal involvement may present as diffuse, patchy infiltrates subsequent to bacterial pneumonia. More often, pulmonary disease associated with *Candida* is one manifestation of systemic candidiasis. Systemic infection with *C. albicans* may involve many systems, including the lungs, gastrointestinal tract, kidneys, liver, and central nervous system. It may present as a persistent fever, with steady deterioration following diagnosis or treatment of bacteremia, or as an acute, catastrophic infection with impressive fever and cardiovascular collapse. Fungal illness may be insidious and nonspecific; fungemia is often discovered coincidentally when a blood sample drawn to document presumed bacterial sepsis on culture becomes positive late in the incubation period. Invasive infection with *Candida* should be suspected when clinical deterioration occurs despite long-term, broad-spectrum antibiotic therapy or when a clinical illness is associated with colonization of multiple sites (e.g., urinary tract, pharynx, and skin). A key to the diagnosis of candidemia may be the presence of candidal endophthalmitis, characterized by fluffy white retinal exudates and a vitreous haze associated with visual changes.

The patient with candidemia must be evaluated thoroughly for multisystem involvement, including ophthalmologic, pulmonary, and cardiac assessments. Possible foci of colonization, such as intravenous or bladder catheters, may need to be removed. If candidemia is associated with an indwelling intravenous catheter and there are no signs of invasive disease, removing the catheter will eliminate most cases of fungemia without the need for concomitant antifungal therapy. Therefore, some clinicians choose not to treat a coincidentally discovered candidemia. However, since up to 20% of such patients have persistently positive blood cultures and some may even present later with deep-seated infection, other clinicians advocate amphotericin therapy for 2 weeks even when there is no evidence of invasive disease (Fainstein et al, 1987).

The majority of cases of invasive *aspergillosis* present as local infections with localizing signs and symptoms, often at a site of tissue damage, such as a preceding bacterial pneumonia. Local lesions are destructive, as in necrotizing bronchopneumonia or necrotizing rhinocerebral aspergillosis. Twenty to 30% of cases result from dissemination, with blood vessel invasion, thrombosis, and organ infarction such as hemorrhagic pulmonary infarction leading to lung abscesses. "Acute vascular events" in a febrile patient at risk for fungal disease should raise the suspicion of aspergillosis. Biopsy is often needed for diagnosis.

The early diagnosis of invasive fungal disease is difficult. Fifty percent of cultures may be persistently negative. Blood cultures that will eventually reveal fungi remain negative for at least 7 days after the onset of infection in 80% of cases (Bodey, 1986a). Antigen tests are not yet sensitive enough and specific antibody tests are not always available, so serologic diagnosis is not reliable.

When suspected or confirmed in a seriously ill patient, invasive fungal infection should be treated aggressively. Currently the treatment of choice for both candidiasis and aspergillosis is intravenous amphotericin B. Local lesions in aspergillosis often need to be surgically debrided. The ultimate success of therapy is most closely related to the stage of underlying malignancy and severity of neutropenia, with early, appropriate therapy also being a factor (EORTC, 1989).

## Viral Infections

There is no good evidence that the incidence or severity of common viral illnesses is increased in patients with cancer. In those with gynecologic malignancy, a limited number of viral infections are of importance. Latent viruses that become reactivated when cellular immunity is depressed (Pizzo and Schimpff, 1983) are not particularly problematic at present, although these are major causes of morbidity and mortality when aggressive chemotherapy leads to marked immunosuppression. As chemotherapy regimens are intensified, infections caused by members of the herpesvirus family—i.e., herpes simplex, cytomegalovirus, and varicella-zoster—may increase in incidence. The herpesviruses are capable of causing life-threatening multisystem disease or local infection that may be complicated by bacterial superinfection.

Most prevalent among patients with gynecologic cancer, particularly those who have undergone multiple or extensive surgical procedures, are those viral infections transmitted via transfusions of blood and blood products, i.e., hepatitis and cytomegalovirus (CMV) infection. The incidence of clinically apparent hepatitis after transfusion is 0.6 to 8.0 cases per 1,000 transfusions and increases with the number of transfusions received (Bodey, 1975). Since the advent of blood-bank screening for hepatitis B surface antigen, the major transfusion-related hepatitis is now non-A, non-B hepatitis. Non-A, non-B hepatitis has an incubation period of 14 to 180 days (average = 8 weeks). Most clinically apparent disease is mild, with mild liver function abnormalities, anorexia, and fatigue. Fifty percent of these patients are anicteric, and acute febrile disease sometimes occurs. As with hepatitis B, patients are probably at risk for chronic carriage of the associated antigen and chronic disease with atrophy. Currently, no antigenic markers have been identified to predict infectivity or the risk for long-term sequelae associated with non-A, non-B hepatitis.

CMV may also be transmitted by blood transfusion, with clinical manifestations usually apparent 2 to 4 weeks after the transfusion. The severity of CMV depends on the host's underlying condition and previous experience with this virus. CMV can be a cause of self-limited, diffuse interstitial pneumonia associated with hypoxemia and bilateral, reticular, ill-defined densities on chest x-ray. In addition, this virus can result in a systemic illness with fever, malaise, leukopenia or atypical lymphocytosis, and jaundice, which may rarely be fatal. It is not clear whether treatment with antiviral agents is efficacious for transfusion-related CMV.

Localized zoster may appear following chemotherapy in patients previously exposed to the varicella-zoster virus. This risk may be higher when active tumor is present. Patients with gynecologic malignancy present disproportionately with zoster lesions of the lumbar or sacral dermatomes (Rusthoven et al, 1988). Although the dissemination rate may be as high as 12%, varicella-zoster virus rarely causes death in the oncology patient.

## Noninfectious Causes of Fever

Virtually any noninfectious systemic illness, whether or not it is related to cancer and cancer therapy, may cause fever in patients with malignancy. A few of these illnesses are of particular concern to the gynecologic oncologist.

An important cause of fever to consider in the postoperative patient is anesthesia-related fever and hepatitis. Primarily halothane inhalation anesthesia and rarely methoxyflurane and enflurane anesthetics have been implicated in hepatic injury. This reaction is presumed to be idiosyncratic, resulting in centrilobular hepatic necrosis and giving rise to symptoms suggestive of hepatitis, including fever. Eosinophilia may be prominent. Multiple exposures to an implicated anesthetic agent, primarily halothane, appear to increase the risk of hepatotoxicity and to decrease the time interval between anesthetic exposure and onset of symptoms. The latent period may range from 24 hours to approximately 10 days. Anesthesia-related hepatonecrosis may be fatal; treatment should consist of supportive care until the time of hepatic recovery.

In the absence of demonstrable infection, fever may be related to the tumor itself. Most often, such "tumor fever" occurs in the earlier stages of the disease. Leiomyosarcoma, choriocarcinoma, and ovarian carcinoma have all been reported to present with fever of unknown origin (Holt and Nicholas, 1981; Hosang et al, 1982). Tumor fever may be either low-grade or characterized by daily spiking temperatures and occurs more commonly with necrotic or hemorrhagic lesions and tumors metastatic to the liver. It is not known whether tumor fever is a result of metabolic effects, hypersensitivity to tumor proteins, or a central effect of malignancy that modulates the patient's response to a pyrogen (Pennington, 1977). The etiology may be multifactorial. Treatment should be directed toward the primary disease process and is all too often delayed while other etiologies of fever are being sought.

## DIAGNOSIS AND TREATMENT OF INFECTION

### Diagnosis

The choice of initial therapy and evaluation of the therapeutic response in a patient with malignancy who presents with fever or other signs of infection must be guided by a thorough, well-organized diagnostic assessment. Any new fever or change in clinical condition, including alterations in mental status with or without fever, should prompt such an evaluation. The gynecologic oncologist should develop a uniform approach to patients suspected of having infection, investigating each in a comprehensive fashion in order to detect subtle clues that might influence management and outcome.

History, examination of the patient, and laboratory testing are aimed at eliciting predisposing factors for and current evidence of specific infection. At the outset, basic information relative to the patient's malignant disease should be clarified, including the type and extent of tumor plus all therapies received to date. All details of diagnostic and therapeutic procedures including dates performed and anesthetics, blood products, or antibiotics received should be summarized. The interview should concentrate on any history of contact with persons with infectious illnesses and a system-by-system review of the patient's symptoms.

Physical examination should be complete, focusing in particular on potential areas of and clues to infection. Skin, intravenous catheter sites, and mucous membranes must be examined closely for signs of breaks, localized infection, and stigmata of generalized infection. When neutropenia exists, characteristic signs of soft tissue infection are often not present. Even minimal erythema and tenderness of the skin, soft tissues, and bone may be a clue to a soft tissue source of sepsis. These signs should be sought at sites of recent and previous instrumentation and in the perianal and perineal areas. All lymph node areas should be examined. Signs of systemic infection should be sought in examination of the optic fundus and the peripheral extremities. Pelvic and rectal examinations should be performed unless specifically contraindicated. Signs of venous thrombophlebitis should be sought, as should any abnormalities of the heart, lungs, and abdomen (including the retroperitoneum). A brief neurologic evaluation should include an assessment of mental status, observation for signs of meningeal irritation, and determination of any gross lateralizing signs.

Laboratory evaluation of suspected sepsis should include, at a minimum, a complete blood count with differential counts, urinalysis, chest x-ray, and blood and urine cultures. At least two samples of blood for culture should be drawn, each from a different venipuncture site and preferably not at the same point in time. If any infected sites or secretions are exposed, specimens of the infected material should be obtained for culture and Gram stain. In cases of suspected urosepsis, the workup should also include a Gram stain of a drop of unspun urine.

If the source of sepsis remains unclear or if there are any particular risk factors for hepatic infection or damage, liver function tests including serum glutamic-pyruvic transaminase (SGPT), serum glutamic-oxaloacetic transaminase (SGOT), and bilirubin should be carried out. Baseline creatinine and blood urea nitrogen (BUN) determinations are helpful when one is choosing and assessing the therapeutic response. Serum should also be drawn and saved in case an evaluation of the antibody response is later indicated for a systemic infection such as CMV.

If an intraabdominal source of sepsis is suspected, the abdomen should be examined radiologically for obstruction, signs of perforation or of gas-producing organisms in soft tissues, or intraabdominal masses. A suspicion of complex upper UTI may prompt either intravenous pyelography or an ultrasound examination. If an intraabdominal abscess is suspected, ultrasound, computed tomography, and radionuclide scanning may aid in the diagnosis. However, in the neutropenic patient with a diminished inflammatory response, results of these tests may be less clear-cut.

Such a diligent initial evaluation when sepsis is suspected may reward the clinician with the ability to provide adequate, specific therapy at the time of presentation. At the least it should indicate the need for further diagnostic maneuvers and facilitate an evaluation of therapeutic response.

### Antimicrobial Therapy

Antimicrobial therapy for suspected sepsis is most often begun on an empiric basis, prior to documentation of an infecting organism by means of cultures. The choice of antimicrobial agent depends on the clinical presentation of the septic episode, the patient's general condition, specific toxicities (including allergies to potential drug regimens), and the general experience of the individual tumor service with specific types of infection (Table 21-6).

Guidelines for selecting antimicrobial agents for patients with malignancy take into account the multiple pathogens and numerous sites of infection that may be involved as well as the often nonspecific presentation, particularly when neutropenia is a factor. In most cases, parenteral antibiotics should be used. Bactericidal drugs are generally preferred to bacteriostatic drugs. The antibacterial or bactericidal effect of a drug on an organism in vitro can often be correlated with clinical response rates (Klastersky, 1977).

In general, multiple-drug regimens are preferable to single-drug therapies (Hathorn et al, 1987). When the exact cause of sepsis is unknown, multiple-drug regimens provide a sufficiently broad spectrum of coverage against most of the common pathogens. The use of two antibiotics has been found to achieve better cure rates in patients who present with bacteremia and in those with neutropenia, whereas the use of more than two antibiotics has not been shown to improve efficacy. Growth of resistant bacteria is reduced by the use of multiple-drug regimens, and superinfection, particularly in the neutropenic patient, is seen less often. If the

TABLE 21-6  Antimicrobial Therapy

| Antibiotic | Usual Dose | Major Toxicity | Major Use in Gynecologic Oncology |
|---|---|---|---|
| Penicillin G | 1.2–24 million units/day | Hypersensitivity | Pneumonia (pneumococcal, aspiration), clostridial sepsis |
| Semisynthetic penicillins<br>Oxacillin<br>Cloxacillin<br>Nafcillin | 6–12 gm/day<br>q4–6h | Hypersensitivity | Staphylococcal wound, soft tissue, or IV site infections |
| Ampicillin | 6–12 gm/day<br>q4–6h | Hypersensitivity, rash, diarrhea | Urinary tract sepsis<br>As part of combination therapy for pelvic or intraabdominal infection |
| Carbenicillin<br>Ticarcillin | 24–40 gm/day<br>18–24 gm/day q4h | Hypersensitivity, electrolytes, acid-base disturbances | As part of empiric combination therapy, particularly if *Pseudomonas* is of concern |
| Cephalothin<br>Cefazolin | 4–12 gm/day q6–8h<br>1–6 gm/day q6–8h | Hypersensitivity, possible additive renal toxicity with aminoglycosides | Urinary tract sepsis<br>As part of combination therapy for *Klebsiella* sepsis<br>Perioperative prophylaxis |
| Cefoxitin | 4–12 gm/day q4–8h | Hypersensitivity, thrombophlebitis | Urinary tract sepsis<br>Pelvic sepsis |
| Gentamicin<br>Tobramycin | 3–5 mg/kg day q8h | Nephrotoxicity, ototoxicity | As part of combination therapy for intraabdominal or pelvic infection or as empiric therapy for fever |
| Amikacin | 15 mg/kg/day<br>q8–12h | Ototoxicity, nephrotoxicity | Resistant Enterobacteriaceae or *Pseudomonas* |
| Clindamycin | 600 mg q6h | Pseudomembranous colitis, rash | Anaerobic coverge for intraabdominal pelvic and wound sepsis |
| Metronidazole | 30–60 mg/kg/day q6h IV<br>1.5–4 gm/day | Nausea and vomiting, reversible neutropenia, Antabuselike effect | Anaerobic coverage for intraabdominal pelvic and wound sepsis |
| Vancomycin | 2 gm/day q6–12h IV<br>0.5–2 gm/day | Ototoxicity, nephrotoxicity, hypersensitivity | Staphylococcal coverage in penicillin-allergic patients<br>Pseudomembranous colitis |
| Amphotericin B | Test dose = 1 mg; increase 5–10 mg/day to 1.0–1.5 mg/kg/day | Fever, chills, headache, nausea and vomiting, thrombophlebitis, nephrotoxicity | Sepsis due to *Candida, Aspergillus* |

infecting organism is documented on culture, if resistance is not a factor, and if the patient is not neutropenic, modifying therapy to single-drug coverage may be justified in individual cases.

Antimicrobial therapy should be initiated promptly in order to prevent septic shock and even death (Armstrong et al, 1971). Unless an episode of sepsis is clearly not of bacterial origin, treatment should be instituted as soon as proper cultures have been obtained.

No good comparative trials have been carried out to evaluate the antimicrobial treatment of sepsis in the patient with gynecologic cancer. Many broad-spectrum regimens have been tested in the general oncologic patient, and the results can be applied to some extent to those with gynecologic malignancy. However, in the latter group, it may be necessary to provide specific coverage against anaerobic organisms when there is concern about intraabdominal or tumor-related sepsis. Anaerobic coverage is rarely a concern in patients with other than gynecologic or gastrointestinal cancer. Combinations of antibiotics commonly include coverage against common and nosocomial skin flora as well as organisms that cause pneumonias. Whenever an intra-

venous catheter is present, coverage against *S. aureus* should be considered. A wide range of gram-negative enteric organisms, including *P. aeruginosa*, may also be of concern.

Whenever possible, synergistic combinations of antibiotics should be used preferentially (Bodey, 1975; Schimpff and Aisner, 1978; Klastersky and Zinner, 1982; EORTC, 1987). These have been shown to provide better clinical cure rates and to exhibit greater in vitro bactericidal activity than nonsynergistic combinations (Tables 21-7 and 21-8); these effects may be even greater in the neutropenic patient. Synergistic combinations of drugs are those with a combined efficacy that exceeds that which would be expected through a simple additive effect. One antimicrobial may enhance the efficacy of another by changing the surface permeability of bacteria to allow greater access of the second antibiotic, by inhibiting inactivating enzymes, by participating in a sequential block of metabolic pathways, or by other poorly elucidated mechanisms (Klastersky and Zinner, 1982). The efficacy of antibiotic combinations is even greater when the drugs are effective against the offending organism in vitro, although a synergistic

TABLE 21-7 Clinical Responses and Bactericidal Serum Activity in Patients with Cancer and Gram-Negative Bacillary Infections Who Received Synergistic or Nonsynergistic Combinations of Antibiotics

| Type of Combination (No. of Patients) | No. (%) with Favorable Clinical Response | Median Titer of Serum Bactericidal Activity | |
|---|---|---|---|
| | | Maximum | Minimum |
| Synergistic (100) | 80 (80)* | 1:16 | 1:8 |
| Nonsynergistic (105) | 52 (50)* | 1:4 | 1:2 |

Note: The studies were performed at the Institut Jules Bordet in Brussels.
*$p < 0.01$.
Source: Klastersky J: Empiric treatment of infections in neutropenic patients with cancer. Rev Infect Dis 5:S21, 1983.

effect can be demonstrated even when one drug in the combination regimen does not show in vitro activity.

Patterns of bacterial resistance to antimicrobial drugs in specific hospitals or as documented in previous cultures from a specific patient should play a major role in initial antibiotic therapy of the febrile oncology patient. It has been demonstrated that response rates to multiple-drug regimens are highest when the offending pathogen is sensitive to all the drugs used (Klastersky et al, 1986). Conversely, even if synergy can be demonstrated, response rates may be unacceptably low if the pathogenic organism is resistant to an empirically chosen antibiotic.

The toxicities of antibiotics and antibiotic combinations also influence one's choice of therapy. Particular attention must be directed to potential hematologic and renal toxicities of agents. For example, patients receiving myelosuppressive antitumor therapy may be at greater risk for hematologic side effects. Toxic renal effects of antimicrobial agents are also more common in patients receiving certain chemotherapeutic agents (e.g., cisplatin) and in patients whose renal function is even slightly impaired at the onset of therapy (Salem et al, 1982, Cimino et al, 1987).

It is more important for the gynecologic oncologist to be familiar with a limited number of appropriate antimicrobial agents and to use these well than to know about each new therapy as it is proposed. Salient features of some common antimicrobial agents that are particularly useful in patients with gynecologic malignancy will now be discussed.

TABLE 21-8 Results of 12 Controlled Clinical Trials of Single vs. Multiple and Synergistic vs. Nonsynergistic Combinations of Antibiotics in Neutropenic Patients Infected with Gram-Negative Bacilli

| Type of Therapy (No. of Patients) | No. (%) with Favorable Clinical Response |
|---|---|
| Single antibiotic (195) | 119 (61) |
| Multiple antibiotics (170) | 138 (81) |
| Nonsynergistic combinations (179) | 77 (43) |
| Synergistic combinations (208) | 158 (76) |

Source: Klastersky J: Empiric treatment of infections in neutropenic patients with cancer. Rev Infect Dis 5:S21, 1983.

***Ampicillin*** Ampicillin is a semisynthetic penicillin with a spectrum of action similar to that of penicillin, with the important addition of activity against some gram-negative enteric bacteria. It is not effective against penicillinase-producing S. aureus. Ampicillin is more effective that penicillin against the enterococcus and, when combined with gentamicin, acts synergistically against virtually all enterococci. This drug does provide coverage against E. coli, although the percentage of these organisms that are resistant to ampicillin increases with extent of antibiotic use and the number of hospitalizations. Ampicillin is also effective against Proteus mirabilis, Salmonella species, and Shigella species. Anaerobic cocci are sensitive to ampicillin; however, B. fragilis does not exhibit such sensitivity to any great extent.

The use of ampicillin and gentamicin in combination is particularly useful as empiric therapy for urinary tract sepsis. A sufficient number of gram-negative organisms are resistant to ampicillin to preclude its use as a single agent for UTI in this patient group. In addition, as part of combination therapy, ampicillin is frequently used to provide coverage against the enterococcus in cases of intraabdominal sepsis.

Two toxic effects of ampicillin therapy deserve mention. This drug tends to produce a maculopapular rash in patients with lymphoreticular malignancies and in those with viral infections, particularly infectious mononucleosis and CMV. This rash, which is believed to be mediated by the lymphocyte, is not considered a true allergy and does not preclude the use of penicillin-like antibiotics when these are indicated.

Five to 20% of adults who receive ampicillin will experience diarrhea as a side effect. For the most part, this diarrhea is idiosyncratic, although a toxin produced by *Clostridium difficile* may be a contributing factor (see below under Clindamycin).

***Antipseudomonal Penicillins (Carbenicillin, Ticarcillin, Azlocillin, Mezlocillin, Piperacillin)*** Antipseudomonal penicillins are semisynthetic penicillins that provide a range of coverage comparable to that of ampicillin, with some differences. In general, these drugs are not effective against penicillinase-producing S. aureus, and although they do provide coverage against other gram-positive aerobic organisms, ampicillin and penicillin provide better coverage, particularly against the enterococcus. As each successive drug in this class has been developed, expanded anaerobic spectrum and enhanced activity against gram-negative aerobic enteric bacilli have been provided. Most provide good coverage against anaerobes, including gram-positive cocci and *Bacteroides* species. They do provide increased coverage against *B. fragilis* but, except for piperacillin, are not the drugs of choice in this type of infection. These agents have been particularly useful in patients with malignancy because they are active against *P. aeruginosa* as well as many other gram-negative aerobic enteric bacilli. In addition, antipseudomonal penicillins act synergistically with aminoglycosides against many strains of *Pseudomonas*.

These agents are often used in combination with aminoglycosides to provide empiric broad-spectrum coverage against infection in the patient with malignancy, particularly when *Pseudomonas* is of concern. Over the years, the development of resistance to these agents has resulted in changing patterns of use (DeJace and Klastersky, 1986; Klastersky, 1988). For example, carbenicillin is now rarely an initial choice for empiric therapy in the febrile cancer patient. In some centers, resistance to the previously first-line agent ticarcillin has also become a factor mitigating against its use as standard empiric therapy.

These agents cross-react with penicillin and are therefore contraindicated in patients with true penicillin allergy. Both carbenicillin and ticarcillin can have important metabolic effects. One gram of carbenicillin, for example, provides 4.7 mEq of sodium, and this sodium load must be taken into consideration to avoid fluid imbalance. Both these drugs may produce hypokalemia, occasionally in association with a metabolic alkalosis. This is probably mediated by the loss of potassium in the renal tubules, although a redistribution of body potassium may also be a factor. Because both sodium loading and hypokalemia are dose-related effects, ticarcillin is generally preferable to carbenicillin, since the required dose of ticarcillin is about half that of carbenicillin. These metabolic effects are not major factors in the use of the other drugs in this class. Dose-related platelet dysfunction is also produced by an unknown mechanism and can lead to significant clinical bleeding.

Although the broad-spectrum coverage (including the major anaerobic effect) of piperacillin appears promising, its place in the treatment of the febrile patient with malignancy remains undefined. When combined with other agents, an increase in efficacy of piperacillin over less expensive regimens has not been shown. In addition, the emergence of resistant organisms has been documented and may be due in part to its enhanced anaerobic spectrum.

**Cephalosporins** First-generation cephalosporins such as cephalothin and cefazolin provide coverage against gram-positive aerobic cocci, including some strains of penicillinase-producing *S. aureus*. Most enterococci are resistant to cephalosporins. These drugs are also active against some gram-negative enteric bacilli, most notably some strains of *E. coli*, *P. mirabilis*, and *Klebsiella* species but not against strains of *Pseudomonas*. Although anaerobic cocci are usually sensitive to cephalosporins, *Bacteroides* species are not. Clinical therapeutic uses of the first-generation cephalosporins include broad-spectrum coverage when *staphylococci* may be of concern and a synergistic effect against *Klebsiella* when used along with aminoglycosides. Their limited activity against gram-negative organisms and lack of antipseudomonal activity reduce the usefulness of these agents. Their major application in the patient with gynecologic malignancy is as prophylaxis during surgical procedures.

Approximately 5% of patients who show an allergic reaction to penicillin will also be allergic to a first-generation cephalosporin. Although these drugs alone are not associated with major nephrotoxicity, their toxic effect on the kidney is increased when they are used in conjunction with aminoglycosides. For this reason, they are of limited usefulness in patients with malignancy.

Newer-generation cephalosporins and cephamycins offer expanded coverage against gram-negative bacilli and anaerobes, including *B. fragilis*. These agents are not effective against enterococci, and their activity against other gram-positive cocci is decreased, although this is not an important limitation in the doses commonly used. Individual agents have specific properties of note. For example, ceftazidime currently has a marked antipseudomonal effect. Other agents, such as cefperazone, and ceftriazone have long half-lives. It is tempting to use these newer agents as single-drug therapy to provide broad-spectrum coverage for infections in patients with malignancy; however, it appears that cure rates, at least in neutropenic patients with bacteremia are not comparable to those seen with multiple-drug regimens (Klastersky et al, 1986; EORTC, 1987). In terms of the efficacy of single-drug therapy, the limiting factor may well be the development of resistance, which tends to occur rapidly with these newer agents (Bolivar et al, 1983; Lagast et al, 1982).

The newer-generation cephalosporins and cephamycins are less cross-reactive with penicillin than are the first-generation cephalosporins, although they should be used with caution in patients with a history of immediate hypersensitivity to penicillin. Vitamin K–dependent prolongation of the prothrombin time, with clinical bleeding problems, has been described for some of these agents (Fainstein et al, 1983). This effect is particularly significant when the patient is predisposed to bleeding problems because of debility or concomitant therapies. The fact that these clinical bleeding problems were initially described in patients with malignancy underscores the dictum that all new drugs—including antibiotics—should be administered with caution to such patients (Levine et al, 1974).

**Aminoglycosides (Gentamicin, Tobramycin, Amikacin)** The aminoglycoside antibiotics are particularly useful for their wide gram-negative spectrum. They are effective against most Enterobacteriaceae and almost all strains of *P. aeruginosa*. In addition, they provide some antistaphylococcal activity. When combined with ampicillin, they display synergistic activity against group B beta-hemolytic streptococci, *S. viridans*, and enterococci. When combined with antipseudomonal penicillins or some cephalosporins, they display synergy for

*Pseudomonas.* Although aminoglycosides show little intrinsic activity against anaerobes, it is important to note that they do not interfere with the action of specific anaerobic antimicrobials. Aminoglycosides are rarely indicated as the sole therapeutic agent (Schimpff, 1985); often they are the drugs of choice in combination with other antibiotics when maximal gram-negative coverage is required. Even though gram-negative enteric bacteremia is sensitive to aminoglycosides, the low response rates are unacceptably low when treatment consists of aminoglycosides alone (EORTC, 1987).

Aminoglycosides cause two types of clinically significant toxicity. They are ototoxic, producing high-frequency hearing loss. Gentamicin and tobramycin are less ototoxic than other aminoglycosides, and ototoxicity is rare in the absence of renal problems. All aminoglycosides also cause dose-related, reversible nephrotoxicity, mainly of the renal cortical cells. This is usually manifest as nonoliguric renal failure with associated elevations in BUN and creatinine. Occasionally, acute tubular necrosis develops, necessitating temporary dialysis until recovery. Multiple courses of aminoglycosides, the administration of other renal toxic drugs, preexisting renal dysfunction, and hypovolemia all predispose to aminoglycoside-associated renal toxicity. When aminoglycosides are used along with certain cephalosporin antibiotics (such as cephalothin), this toxic effect may be additive (Wade et al, 1981; Schimpff and Aisner, 1978). Some minimal studies as well as limited clinical trials have suggested that tobramycin may cause less renal toxicity than compared with gentamicin (Smith et al, 1980). Although the significance of this potential decrease in renal toxicity is unclear, tobramycin may be used preferentially in patients who may be more susceptible to such effects.

Serum levels of aminoglycosides are useful guides to clinical care. Peak drug levels measured 30 minutes to 1 hour after administration correlate with therapeutic efficacy. Trough levels in samples drawn 30 minutes to 1 hour before the next dose can be used to monitor drug concentrations related to renal toxicity (Brown et al, 1982). Trough levels above 2 µg/ml have been associated with increased nephrotoxicity.

In general, gentamicin and tobramycin have similar antipseudomonal activity. Amikacin is usually reserved for infections caused by resistant strains of *Pseudomonas.* Over time, some institutions have observed increasing patterns of resistance of gram-negative enteric bacteria to a routinely used aminoglycoside of choice, necessitating a change to an alternate agent. Determining the aminoglycoside of choice for febrile oncology patients should be based on sensitivity patterns in local institutions.

**Clindamycin** Clindamycin is effective against most gram-positive aerobic cocci with the exception of the enterococci; furthermore, this drug excels against anaerobes, including penicillin-resistant *Bacteroides* species. However, it provides little or no gram-negative enteric coverage. It is used mainly in conjunction with aminoglycosides to provide broad-spectrum coverage, including that against gram-positive cocci in the patient allergic to penicillin or against resistant *Bacteroides* species when this is desired.

The major toxic effect of clindamycin is gastrointestinal. This drug is associated with diarrhea that is not related to the duration of antimicrobial use. To a disproportionate extent, this diarrhea is the result of pseudomembranous colitis, which is characterized by crampy diarrhea and sometimes by signs and symptoms similar to those in ulcerative colitis. It is associated with the presence of cytopathogenic toxin-producing C. *difficile* in the bowel. This type of diarrhea occurs 2 to 25 days after the onset of antimicrobial therapy and is probably more frequent with oral clindamycin and in patients receiving therapy for diarrhea (such as Lomotil). Pseudomembranous colitis is treated with oral vancomycin or metronidazole; however, despite treatment, this condition may recur. To date, it is still not clear whether patients who have undergone abdominal radiation therapy are any more likely to suffer from pseudomembranous colitis than are other patients.

**Metronidazole** In addition to its well-known trichomonacidal effect, metronidazole provides a broad spectrum of activity against anaerobic bacteria. *Bacteroides* species, including *B. fragilis*, *bivius*, and *melaninogenicus*, are particularly sensitive to this drug, and anaerobic gram-positive cocci are also sensitive to metronidazole, although anaerobic streptococci may be slightly less so. Metronidazole is useful in combination with coverage for gram-negative enteric bacilli when anaerobes are of particular concern, such as in cases of intraabdominal abscesses and tumor superinfections. In patients for whom clindamycin has been either ineffective or poorly tolerated, metronidazole has provided an effective substitute. In addition, therapeutic blood levels can often be achieved with oral administration of metronidazole.

Nausea, vomiting, and anorexia are the major toxic effects that limit the use of metronidazole, especially when these are exacerbated by concomitant chemotherapy. Metronidazole is also associated with a transient reversible neutropenia, possibly precluding its use in patients receiving myelosuppressive therapy.

**Chloromycin** Chloromycin is a broad-spectrum bacteriostatic agent effective against many strains of Enterobacteriaceae, gram-positive aerobes, and anaerobes (including *B. fragilis*). More strains of gram-negative bacilli are now becoming resistant to chloromycin, and this drug is not effective against *Pseudomonas.*

Although chloromycin is an excellent drug against anaerobic organisms, it is usually not used in patients with malignancy because of its bacteriostatic properties. Moreover, it causes both dose-related and reversible suppression of some or all hematopoietic precursors as well as idiosyncratic aplastic anemia. The latter is associated with over 50% mortality, and although it may become apparent after patients have been taking chloromycin for only 1 to 2 weeks, a latent period of weeks to months may elapse before the anemia develops. Since both these types of bone marrow depression are of concern in patients receiving myelosuppressive antitumor agents, the usefulness of chloromycin is limited in the cancer patient.

**Vancomycin** Vancomycin has a useful role in both penicillin-allergic patients and in combatting gram-positive penicillin-resistant organisms that are of increasing concern to the oncologist. The mechanism by which vancomycin inhibits cell-wall synthesis differs from that of the penicillins, so it is also effective against methicillin-resistant staphylococci. In the patient with sepsis, intravenous vancomycin would be the first choice agent as one drug in a multiple antibiotic regimen when there is a possibility of epidemic methicillin-resistant *S. aureus* or infection at the IV access site.

In addition, oral vancomycin is poorly absorbed. This fact plus its effectiveness against *Clostridia difficile* make it a first-line agents for treatment of antibiotic-associated pseudomembranous colitis.

Ototoxicity and nephrotoxicity are the major side effects of vancomycin, and both are directly related to serum levels. Concern about possible additive toxicity when vancomycin is given along with aminoglycosides mandates drug-level monitoring for both drugs (Cimino et al, 1987). Rapid administration of intravenous vancomycin may be associated with flushing, erythema, and other effects that are not true hypersensitivity reactions. Proper dilution and slow infusion can minimize these effects.

It is generally considered that initial empiric therapy maximizing coverage of gram-positive aerobic organisms provides no advantage in terms of response rates. Even though bacteremia with gram-positive organisms is a steady and perhaps increasing problem, mortality rates are low. The eventual response is the same whether specific coverage with an antibiotic such as vancomycin is provided initially or is added once culture results become available (Rubin et al, 1988; Hathorn et al, 1987). Under specific conditions, however, empiric therapy that includes vancomycin may be desirable. Such settings include severe sepsis coincident with obvious intravenous access site infection, local epidemics of methicillin-resistant *S. aureus*, and severe sepsis with underlying structural heart abnormalities.

**Amphotericin B** Amphotericin B, a parenteral antifungal agent, is mainly effective against pathogenic yeast and yeastlike fungi such as *Candida* species and *Aspergillus*. Amphotericin B is the major therapeutic agent used for systemic candidiasis and invasive aspergillosis. During intravenous administration, this drug shows significant toxicity consisting of fever, chills, headache, anorexia, nausea, vomiting, and hypokalemia. In addition, amphotericin B causes nephrotoxicity, which is manifested as increasing serum levels of BUN and creatinine with decreased creatinine clearance. This nephrotoxicity, although usually reversible, limits the maximal daily dose of the drug than can be given. Intravenous amphotericin B must be infused slowly, and the daily dose must be gradually built up to a level of tolerance. Therefore,

achieving an effective therapeutic level of amphotericin B may require 3 to 4 weeks.

**Antimicrobial Combinations** Multiple-drug regimens are commonly used to treat infection in patients with malignancy. Although combination antimicrobial therapy broadens the spectrum of activity and reduces the likelihood of drug resistance, it may also be more toxic. Current recommendations for empiric therapy in febrile cancer patients are based on the results of multiple, published comparative trials. Overall response rates to combination regimens, even in the severely neutropenic patient, are in the range of 55 to 80%. The patient at greatest risk for fatal sepsis is one who is severely and persistently neutropenic and who develops gram-negative aerobic bacteremia (Klastersky, 1988; Bodey, 1986b). Therefore, general recommendations for empiric therapy maximize its effectiveness in this group of patients but leave room for individualized management.

The current regimen of choice for empiric therapy of the febrile, neutropenic cancer patient is an aminoglycoside plus either an antipseudomonal penicillin or an antipseudomonal cephalosporin. Specific agents should be chosen based on the sensitivity patterns within institutions and results of previous cultures. The use of two beta-lactim broad-spectrum agents instead of an aminoglycoside has been studied. Despite theoretical concerns of antibiotic antagonism and some evidence for the development of dual resistance during ongoing therapy, this type of multiple-drug regimen has led to good response rates in some trials (DeJace and Klastersky, 1986). This may be the regimen of choice if particular concerns about nephrotoxicity preclude use of an aminoglycoside. Monotherapy with new broad-spectrum agents is not generally recommended because of concerns about bacterial resistance. However, in the febrile patient with an inherently good prognosis or at low risk for nosocomial, resistant bacteria—e.g., patients with no remaining tumor or no underlying morbidity who become febrile at home—monotherapy may occasionally be chosen. Although the above-mentioned combinations are often appropriate for the patient with gynecologic malignancy, one must also consider providing maximal anaerobic coverage when there is a possibility of intraabdominal infection with abscess formation or tumor superinfection.

## Response to Therapy

To some extent, the initial response to therapy among patients presumed to have sepsis can be predicted on the basis of bacteriologic evidence, the site of infection, and underlying diseases or conditions. Gram-negative bacillemias and polymicrobial bacteremias tend to respond poorly, whereas staphylococcal septicemia is associated with a good rate of response (EORTC, 1978; Inagaki et al, 1974). The prognosis is worse with intraabdominal infection and pneumonias than with simple urinary tract or soft tissue infections (Lau et al, 1977; Singer et al, 1977). A most important predictor of the response to therapy, however, is a change in the number of peripheral granulocytes, with severe neutropenia conferring a particularly bad prognosis (Klastersky, 1983; EORTC, 1978). In addition, the underlying condition of the patient is an extremely important prognostic factor. Infections that present with shock are associated with a higher mortality. Prognosis is poor in patients with persistent malignancy and older debilitated patients with baseline renal dysfunction who develop infection. The prompt initiation of appropriate antimicrobial therapy will improve response rates. However, this is only one aspect of the management of infection in patients with malignancy. Often, antibiotics are effective only in conjunction with other modalities, such as drainage or removal of a focus of infection (e.g., an intravenous or indwelling bladder catheter). If a patient does not appear to be responding to initial antibiotic therapy because fever persists or recurs during treatment, a thorough reevaluation is warranted. First, one must establish whether the therapy selected was appropriate. As soon as the site of infection becomes apparent or culture results are available, therapy must be tailored to the underlying infection and adjusted to match sensitivities exhibited in vitro. If antimicrobial sensitivities are in fact found to be appropriate, dosage schedules should be modified to maximize therapeutic drug levels. Consideration must also be given to whether delivery of the antibiotic to the site of infection is adequate. If obstruction is present, it must be relieved, just as abscesses must be drained or infected tumor resected.

If antibiotic therapy is deemed adequate but the patient is still not responding, one must consider the possibility of resistance and superinfection. Even while antibiotic therapy is continued, patients should be reevaluated, including a thorough microbiologic reassessment. Blood cultures in particular may be positive in cases of superinfection involving organisms such as fungi or resistant bacteria. Several trials have been carried out in which amphotericin B was given when fever persisted beyond 4 days despite antibiotic therapy. The results suggest that empiric antifungal therapy may be warranted in patients with a documented infection who are not responding and who remain persistently and severely neutropenic (EORTC, 1989). During the reevaluation, one should also consider noninfectious causes of fever such as systemic illnesses, drug fever, and tumor fever. Clinicians must be just as thorough in reassessing patients who are not responding to initial therapy as they were during the initial evaluation.

## Duration of Therapy

The duration of antibiotic therapy should be guided by the culture results and the therapeutic response. A decision to terminate antibiotic therapy can be made only after one weighs the risks of continuing therapy in terms of toxicity and superinfection against the risks of unmasking an incompletely treated infection by discontinuing the drug(s).

At 72 to 96 hours after antimicrobial therapy is begun, the therapeutic response should be evaluated. If a patient is clearly infected (as indicated by culture results or clinical signs) and fever has been reduced, antibiotics are generally continued for 7 to 10 days. Discontinuation of antibiotics before 7 days may be associated with a recurrence of fever in more than 25% of cases; more prolonged therapy invites superinfection and is therefore discouraged (Joshi et al, 1984; Bodey, 1986b).

If at the time of reevaluation infection has not been clearly documented based on culture results or the clinical course, and if the patient became afebrile immediately after antimicrobial therapy was instituted, the diagnosis of infection must be questioned. In this situation, antibiotics may be discontinued and the patient should be observed. In general, however, in the more debilitated host or in the presence of persistent neutropenia, it may be reasonable to complete the full antimicrobial course, although, as mentioned, there is no advantage to continuing therapy beyond 7 to 10 days.

If infection cannot be documented and the patient is still febrile, intensive efforts must be expended to establish a diagnosis. An infection will be documented in up to 50% of cases and the need for more antibiotics becomes apparent (Joshi et al, 1984). Whether or not antibiotics are continued in this situation depends upon the underlying clinical condition of the host. In the neutropenic patient, discontinuing antibiotics prior to 7 days, even if infection has not been documented, is associated with some excess mortality (Rodriguez et al, 1973). Continuing antibiotics beyond 7 days if no response is apparent results in greater infection rates with gram-positive cocci and fungi and is most often not warranted (Pennington, 1977). In the patient without neutropenia, if infection cannot be documented and the fever persists, one might reasonably discontinue the antibiotics, reevaluate the patient, and repeat cultures and sensitivity testing.

## Preventing Infection in the Patient with Malignancy

To prevent infection in patients with malignancy, the clinician must rely upon maintaining the integrity of mucocutaneous barriers and decreasing colonization of the host by virulent bacteria. Any unnecessary invasive procedures should be avoided in these patients, even if they are in good clinical condition, and the use of intravenous catheters and indwelling bladder catheters should be kept to a minimum. When such catheters are used, they should be inserted using aseptic techniques and should be meticulously maintained. All health-care personnel should observe proper handwashing technique between caring for different patients to minimize the spread of resistant bacteria among hospitalized patients. Whenever possible, attention should be directed to maximizing the patient's nutritional status.

Surveillance cultures or periodic assessments of colonizing organisms have not been shown to be helpful. This practice tends to be costly and relatively insensitive and rarely influences management because of the wide variety of potential pathogens that may be found at the multiple sites surveyed. Although some form of organism surveillance in a hospital setting is helpful in defining patterns of antimicrobial resistance, it is usually not of value with respect to the individual patient (Schimpff and Aisner, 1978; Gurwith et al, 1978*b*; Kramer et al, 1982).

It is appropriate to screen some populations for potential pathogens such as *N. gonorrhoeae* prior to any manipulations, since such a precaution may reduce the incidence of pelvic inflammatory disease after cervical biopsy or conization. However, general screening of the lower genital tract flora is of no value. Although rarely an issue in the patient with gynecologic malignancy, steroid therapy can reactivate tuberculosis. All patients who are likely to embark on immunosuppressive chemotherapy should therefore be screened using the tuberculin skin test; if the result is positive, they should be treated prophylactically with isoniazid (Armstrong et al, 1971; Levine et al, 1974). Patients at risk for pneumococcal sepsis, such as those with chronic lung disease or those who have undergone splenectomy, should receive the pneumococcal vaccine prior to chemotherapy and during the appropriate seasons (Bernard et al, 1981).

Major efforts have been directed toward controlling infection in patients with malignancy through manipulations of the environment. Attempts to decrease infection in immunosuppressed individuals through the use of totally protected environments and gastrointestinal decontamination are exceedingly complicated and expensive (Pizzo and Schimpff, 1983). Maximal protection includes the use of laminar-flow rooms; low-residue, sterilized diets; mucosal and skin antisepsis; and gastrointestinal decontamination with multiple antimicrobial and antifungal agents effective against all colonizing flora, from the pharynx to the perianal area. These radical measures have not proved to be efficacious in the general population of cancer patients. In addition, the side effects and cost severely limit their usefulness. For example, one side effect of decontamination is decreased absorption of nutrients and medications (Guiot and VanFurth, 1977). In addition, no combination of agents can totally suppress flora, and the development of resistance would remain a problem. As one would expect, compliance with such a regimen is a problem, and some have suggested consequences such as rebound overgrowth and superinfection in the noncompliant patient (Pizzo and Schimpff, 1983). There have been suggestions that oral antimicrobial prophylaxis may decrease the numbers of documented infections in neutropenic patients. However, with no clear-cut simultaneous decrease in the number of febrile episodes, this may simply reflect the influence of these agents on obtaining interpretable culture results.

Although protected environments and gastrointestinal decontamination may be effective in selected patients with prolonged neutropenia (Bodey, 1981), their usefulness in patients with gynecologic malignancy is limited by toxicity, costs, and lack of proof of their efficacy. Currently, the elimination of selected primary aerobic pathogens through antimicrobial modulation is being investigated (Pizzo and Schimpff, 1983). None of the recommended antimicrobial measures decreases infection in the patient with gynecologic malignancy, with the exception of perioperative antimicrobial prophy-

laxis (discussed earlier). Transfusion of pure white blood cell preparations may decrease mortality due to infection in patients with prolonged, severe granulocytopenia. However, the major risks of hepatitis and CMV infection plus the alloimmunization that compromises future transfusions or transplantation diminishes the usefulness of granulocyte transfusions in other, less severely immunocompromised patients (Young, 1981).

# INFECTION IN THE PATIENT WITH GRANULOCYTOPENIA

Granulocytopenia that occurs during the course of cancer therapy poses particular problems related to infection. Most often granulocytopenia is due to myelosuppression as a result of chemotherapy with cytotoxic agents, although occasionally it can occur as a complication of radiation therapy. Infectious complications due to granulocytopenia have not been a major concern in patients with gynecologic cancer, because until recently most of the chemotherapeutic regimens commonly used for this group of patients have not caused the profound granulocytopenia that accompanies the treatment of other cancers, such as hematologic malignancies and lymphomas. However, with more aggressive chemotherapy now being administered for gynecologic tumors, the incidence of granulocytopenia and its complications is increasing. It is therefore necessary for gynecologic oncologists to understand the particular problems associated with infection in the granulocytopenic patient and to develop a consistent approach to its evaluation and therapy. General principles outlined in the text have been summarized by Bodey (1986*b*) (Table 21-9).

---

**TABLE 21-9** General Management Principles for Fever in Neutropenic Patients

- Temperature of 101° F (38.5° C) persisting more than 2 hours and not unassociated with administration of pyrogenic substances indicates infection until proved otherwise.
- Characteristic signs and symptoms of infection are often absent.
- Nevertheless, a careful examination that includes the oral cavity, genitalia, and anus may reveal the site of infection.
- Untreated infection will rapidly disseminate and terminate fatally.
- Delays in administering appropriate antibiotic therapy result in suboptimal response rates.
- Consequently, antibiotic therapy with a broad-spectrum regimen must be instituted promptly.
- Most infections are caused by gram-negative bacilli.
- "Non-pathogenic" organisms can cause serious infections and must not be ignored.
- Despite in vitro activity, some antibiotics are ineffective.
- Initial antibiotic selection should be influenced by the prevalence and susceptibility patterns of organisms within the hospital.

Bodey GP: Infection in cancer patients. A continuing association. *Am J Med* 81(1A):11-26, 1986*b*.

## Level of Circulating Neutrophils

The incidence of fever is higher among cancer patients whose circulating neutrophil levels fall to less than $1,500/mm^3$. This complication increases the time spent in the hospital and may delay or prevent aggressive treatment of the primary disease. In these patients, fever is most often related to definite infection. As the number of granulocytes decreases, it becomes harder to localize and contain the infection. Not only do many granulocytopenic patients become infected, but their infections may be more severe and often require more aggressive antibiotic therapy; moreover, complications such as superinfections and death are more likely. In addition to a decrease in neutrophils, other factors may increase these patients' susceptibility to infection and compromise defense mechanisms.

Nevertheless, the single most important predictor of morbidity and mortality due to infection in patients with malignancy is the level of circulating neutrophils or granulocytes. Although any decrease in granulocytes to the subnormal level influences the risk for infection, incidence, severity, and associated mortality are directly related to the degree and duration of granulocytopenia (Bodey et al, 1966; Gurwith et al, 1978a; Schimpff, 1985). The risk for infection in patients with malignancy begins to rise when the absolute count of circulating neutrophils drops below $1,000/mm^3$, increases rapidly at levels below $500/mm^3$, and peaks at counts below $100/mm^3$. Infection is evident during more than half the time when neutrophil counts are below $100/mm^3$ (Gurwith et al, 1978b). Virtually all patients whose granulocyte counts are at such low levels for more than 3 weeks will become infected (Bodey et al, 1966).

More of the infections that occur when initial neutrophil counts are below $500/mm^3$ will be severe; when the initial neutrophil count is above $1,000/mm^3$, patients are much less likely to have severe infections; when counts exceed $1,500/mm^3$, it is difficult to document any increase in the number of days infection is present.

The outcome of infection is related to both the absolute level of circulating neutrophils and the change in this level during the first week of therapy. In general, an increase in this level is associated with a better prognosis for survival. Ninety percent of patients without neutropenia survive infection, but this rate decreases to 60% in patients with neutropenia at the onset of therapy (Grose et al, 1978). When the circulating levels remain below $100/mm^3$ during initial therapy, 50 to 70% of these neutropenic patients are likely to succumb to the infection, whereas recovery of the neutrophil count to above $500/mm^3$ is associated with survival rates approaching 90% (Grose et al, 1978; Klastersky, 1983; Kramer et al, 1982). In addition, an increase in the level of circulating granulocytes is associated with lower rates of recurrent sepsis after treatment for the initial episode (Hughes and Patterson, 1984). The absolute level of granulocytes in an infected neutropenic patient may be as important a predictor of response as proper antibiotic therapy, and the change in the level of circulating granulocytes during therapy may be more relevant to the patient's eventual response than is antibiotic therapy (Klastersky, 1983).

## Types of Infections

As with nonneutropenic patients, organisms that infect neutropenic patients are most often those which colonize body surfaces and cavities. Infections caused by endogenous flora tend to occur in areas where normal defense barriers may be compromised. Mucositis or ulceration that occurs as a side effect of chemotherapy may serve as a potential site for infection. In granulocytopenic patients, infection often originates at sites in the lungs, skin, pharynx, and perianal area (Wiernik, 1980; Nadworny and Greene, 1984). In addition, the tumor itself may provide a focus of infection in granulocytopenic patients who have gynecologic malignancies such as invasive cervical cancer and choriocarcinoma.

Granulocytopenic patients with infection more commonly present with systemic rather than local signs and symptoms. Bacteremia, a common feature of infection in granulocytopenic patients, may develop at any time but is most likely to occur early, concomitant with the onset of fever (Gurwith et al, 1978a) and when the neutrophil count is lowest (Schwartz et al, 1984). Fever and bacteremia may be the only presenting signs of infection in a patient with significant granulocytopenia.

The lack of local signs of infection in these patients is presumed to be due to the paucity of white blood cells and thus the absence of inflammation at the site of infection (Klastersky, 1983; Levine et al, 1974; Pizzo et al, 1979). While some patients may have erythema and pain, other signs such as exudates, fluctuation, swelling, and heat are often absent. Patients with UTI tend to present with fewer symptoms such as dysuria, frequency, and urgency, and those with pneumonias tend to present with less cough and sputum production. Intraabdominal abscess formation may be less discrete and therefore less definable by tests such as ultrasound or gallium scanning (Nadworny and Greene, 1984). All these factors should be taken into consideration when one is evaluating a granulocytopenic patient with fever. One example of clinical relevance is that the threshold for surgically exploring and debriding potential collections even if any subtle signs exist may be lowered in the neutropenic patient who is not responding to antibiotic therapy.

Bacteremias in neutropenic patients are caused by organisms similar to those seen in patients with malignancy who have normal numbers of circulating neutrophils, the major pathogens being *E. coli*, *K. pneumoniae*, *P. aeruginosa*, and *S. aureus*. However, polymicrobial bacteremias and bacteremias caused by organisms that normally have low pathogenic potential are seen more frequently in the granulocytopenic patient. Fungemias, particularly involving *Candida* species, are also seen much more often in granulocytopenic patients, especially those who are receiving or have received recent antibiotic therapy.

Patients with granulocytopenia who exhibit myelosuppression and possibly suppression of other cell lines may require transfusion of blood products. In light of this, the possibility that nonbacterial bloodborne infections, such as non-A, non-B hepatitis and CMV infection, may be the cause of the fever should be considered.

Broad-spectrum antimicrobial therapy to cover the major potential pathogens should be instituted as soon as initial evaluation of the febrile granulocytopenic patient has been completed. If therapy is withheld until an infectious site or causative organism has been determined, the mortality due to infection will increase dramatically.

Guidelines for therapy are similar to those discussed earlier. Antimicrobial therapy should be parenteral, bactericidal, and broad-spectrum and should involve combinations of synergistic agents whenever possible. The duration of therapy is rarely less than 7 days. Reevaluation of nonresponders should take into account the possibility of superinfection. In the neutropenic patient with persistent fever, empiric therapy with antifungal agents in addition to adequate antimicrobial coverage may prove lifesaving.

# REFERENCES

Alexander JW, Altemeier WA: Penicillin prophylaxis of experimental staphylococcal wound infections. *Surg Gynecol Obstet* 120:243-254, 1965.

Allen PJ, Downing JW: A prospective study of hepatocellular function after repeated exposures to halothane or enflurane in women undergoing radium therapy for cervical cancer. *Br J Anaesth* 49:1035-1039, 1977.

Armstrong D: Infectious complications of neoplastic disease: Their diagnosis and management (Part II). *Clin Bull* 7:13-20, 1977.

Armstrong D, Young LS, Meyer RD, Blevins AH: Infectious complications of neoplastic disease. *Med Clin NA* 55:729-745, 1971.

Bartlett JG, Moon NE, Goldstein PR, Goren B, Onderdonk AB, Polk BF: Cervical and vaginal bacterial flora: Ecological niches in the female lower genital tract. *Am J Obstet Gynecol* 130:658-661, 1978.

Bartlett JG, Onderdonk AB, Drude E, Goldstein D, Anderka M, Alpert S, McCormack WM: Quantitative bacteriology of the vaginal flora. *J Infect Dis* 136:271-277, 1977.

Benezra D, Kiehn TE, Gold JW, Brown AE, Turnbull AD, Armstrong D: Prospective study of infections in indwelling central venous catheters using quantitative blood cultures. *Am J Med* 85:495-8, 1988.

Bernard CH, Mombelli G, Klastersky J: Pneumococcal bacteremia in patients with neoplastic disease. *Eur J Cancer Clin Oncol* 17:1041-1046, 1981.

Blythe JG: Cervical bacterial flora in patients with gynecologic malignancies. *Am J Obstet Gynecol* 131:438-445, 1978.

Bodey GP: Infections in cancer patients. *Cancer Treat Rev* 2:89-128, 1975.

Bodey GP: Antibiotic prophylaxis in cancer patients: Regimens of oral, nonabsorbable antibiotics for prevention of infection during induction of remission. *Rev Infect Dis* 3(Suppl):S259-S268, 1981.

Bodey GP: Fungal infection and fever of unknown origin in neutropenic patients. *Am J Med* 80(Suppl 5C), 1986a.

Bodey GP: Infection in cancer patients. A continuing association. *Am J Med* 81(Suppl IA) 11-26, 1986b.

Bodey GP, Cuckley M, Sathe YS, Freireich EJ: Quantitative relationships between circulating leukocytes and infection in patients with acute leukemia. *Ann Intern Med* 64:328-340, 1966.

Bodey GP, Elting L, Kassamali H, Lim BD: *Escherichia coli* bacteremia in cancer patients. *Am J Med* 81(Supple IA):85-95, 1986.

Bolivar R, Fainstein V, Elting L, Bodey GP: Cefoterazone for the treatment of infections in patients with cancer. *Rev Infect Dis* 5(Suppl):5181-5187, 1983).

Borkowf HI: Bacterial gangrene associated with pelvic surgery. *Clin Obstet Gynecol* 16:40-65, 1973.

Brooker DC, Savage JE, Twiggs LB, Adcock LL, Prem KA, Sanders CC: Infectious morbidity in gynecologic cancer. *Am J Obstet Gynecol* 156:513-520, 1987.

Brown AE, Quesada O, Armstrong D: Minimal nephrotoxicity with cephalosporin-aminoglycoside combinations in patients with neoplastic disease. *Antimicrob Agents Chemother* 21:592-594, 1982.

Byron RL, Mishell DR, Yonemoto RH: The surgical treatment of invasive carcinoma of the vulva. *Surg Gynecol Obstet* 120:1243-1251, 1965.

Calame RJ, Wallach RC: An analysis of the complications of the radiologic treatment of carcinoma of the cervix. *Surg Gynecol Obstet* 124:39-44, 1967.

Carney DN, Fossieck BE, Parker RH, Minna JD: Bacteremia due to *Staphylococcus aureus* in patients with cancer: Report on 45 cases in adults and review of the literature. *Rev Infect Dis* 4:1-12, 1982a.

Carney DN, Parker RH, Fossieck BE: Staphylococcal bacteremia in cancer patients: Intravenous and oral antimicrobial therapy. *South Med J* 75:143-146, 1982b.

Cavanagh D, Rutledge F: The cervical cone biopsy-hysterectomy sequence and factors affecting febrile morbidity. *Am J Obstet Gynecol* 80:53-59, 1960.

Chambers SK, Schwartz PE: Neutropenia and fever in patients undergoing combination chemotherapy for malignant germ cell tumors of the ovary. *Obstet Gynecol* 68:842-846, 1986.

Chang TW: Antimicrobial-associated diarrhea and enterocolitis. *Drug Ther Hosp* May, 1981, pp 71-78.

Cho SY, Choi HY: Opportunistic fungal infection among cancer patients. *Am J Clin Pathol* 72:617-621, 1979.

Chou MY, Brown AE, Blevens A, Armstrong D: Severe pneumococcal infection in patients with neoplastic disease. *Cancer* 51:1546-1550, 1983.

Cimino MA, Rotstein C, Slaughter RL, Emrich LJ: Relationship of serum antibiotic concentrations to nephrotoxicity in cancer patients receiving concurrent aminoglycoside and vancomycin therapy. *Am J Med* 83:1091-1097, 1987.

Clarke JS, Conden RE, Bartlett JG, Gorbach SL, Michols RL, Ochi S: Preoperative oral antibiotics reduce septic complications of colon operations: Results of a prospective randomized, double-blind clinical study. *Ann Surg* 186:252-259, 1977.

Cone LA, Woodard D, Helm NA: Clinical experience in the diagnosis and treatment of infections in the compromised host. *Clin Ther* 4:45-54, 1981.

Creasman WT, Hill GB, Weed JC, Gall SA: A trial of prophylactic cefamandole in extended gynecologic surgery. *Obstet Gynecol* 59:309-314, 1982.

Daly JW, Pomerance AJ: Groin dissection with prevention of tissue loss and postoperative infection. *Obstet Gynecol* 53:359-399, 1979.

Daly JW, King R, Monif GRG: Progressive necrotizing wound infection in postirradiated patients. *Obstet Gynecol* 52(Suppl):5s-8s, 1978.

Davy M: The prognosis of cancer of the cervix with particular reference to infection. *Aust NZ J Obstet Gynaecol* 14:1-5, 1974.

DeCenzo JA, Malo T, Cavanagh D: Factors affecting cone-hysterectomy morbidity. *Am J Obstet Gynecol* 110:380-384, 1971.

DeJace P, Klastersky J: Comparative review of combination therapy: Two beta-lactams versus beta-lactam plus aminoglycoside. *Am J Med* 80(6B):29-38, 1986.

Dionigi R, Dominioni L, Campani M: Infections in cancer patients. *Surg Clin NA* 60:145-159, 1980.

Doran TA, Shier CB: Conization of the cervix. *Am J Obstet Gynecol* 89:367-374, 1964.

Dvoretsky PM, Richards KA, Angel C, Rabinowitz L, Beecham JB, Bonfiglio TA: Survival time, causes of death, and tumor/treatment-related morbidity in 100 women with ovarian cancer. *Hum Pathol* 19:1273-1279, 1988.

Elkins TE, Gallup DG, Slomka CV, Phelan JP: Postoperative morbidity in cases of cervical conization followed by vaginal hysterectomy. *South Med J* 75:264-266, 1982.

Elting LS, Bodey GP, Fainstain V: Polymicrobial septicemia in the cancer patient. *Medicine* 65:218-225, 1986.

EORTC International Antimicrobial Therapy Project Group: Three antibiotic regimens in the treatment of infection in febrile granulocytopenic patients with cancer. *J Infect Dis* 137:14-29, 1978.

EORTC International Antimicrobial Therapy Cooperative Group: Ceftazidime combined with a short or long course of amikacin for empirical therapy of gram-negative bacteremia in cancer patients with granulocytopenia. *N Engl J Med* 317:1692-1698, 1987.

————: Empiric antifungal therapy in febrile granulocytopenic patients. *Am J Med* 86:668-672, 1989.

Fainstein V, Bodey GP, Elting L, Masymiuk A, Keating MJ, McCredie KB: Amphotericin B or ketoconazole therapy of fungal infections in neutropenic cancer patients. *Antimicrob Agents Chemother* 31:11-15, 1987.

Fainstein V, Bodey GP, McCredie KB, Keating MJ, Estey EH, Bolivar R, Elting L: Coagulation abnormalities induced by beta-lactam antibiotics in cancer patients. *J Infect Dis* 148:745-751, 1983.

Folland D, Armstrong D, Seides S, Blevins A: Pneumococcal bacteremia in patients with neoplastic disease. *Cancer* 33:845-848, 1974.

Forney JP, Morrow CP, Townsend DE, DiSaia PJ: Impact of cephalosporin prophylaxis in conization-vaginal hysterectomy morbidity. *Am J Obstet Gynecol* 125:100-103, 1975.

Frick HC, Taylor HC, Guttmann RJ, Jacox HW, McKelway WP: A study of complications in the surgical and radiation therapy of cancer of the cervix. *Surg Gynecol Obstet* 11:493-506, 1960.

Galask RP, Larsen B, Ohm MJ: Vaginal flora and its role in disease entities. *Clin Obstet Gynecol* 19:61-81, 1976.

Gill FA, Robinson R, Maclowry JD, Levine AS: The relationship of fever, granulocytopenia and antimicrobial therapy to bacteremia in cancer patients. *Cancer* 39:1704-1709, 1977.

Grose WE, Rodriguez V, Norek G, Luna M, Bodey GP: *Escherichia coli* bacteremia in patients with malignant diseases. *Arch Intern Med* 138:1230-1233, 1978.

Guiot HFL, VanFurth R: Partial antibiotic decontamination. *Br Med J* 1:800-802, 1977.

Gurwith MJ, Brunton JL, Lank BA, Ronald AR, Harding GKM: Granulocytopenia in hospitalized patients. I. Prognostic factors and etiology of fever. *Am J Med* 64:121-126, 1978a.

Gurwith MJ, Brunton JL, Lank BA, Ronald AR, Harding GKM, McCullough DW: Granulocytopenia in hospitalized patients. II. A prospective comparison of two antibiotics. *Am J Med* 64:127-132, 1978b.

Hacker NF, Leuchter RS, Gastaldo TW, Lagasse L: Radical vulvectomy and bilateral inguinal lymphadenectomy through separate groin incisions. *Obstet Gynecol* 58:574-579, 1981.

Hathorn JW, Rubin M, Pizzo PA: Empirical antibiotic therapy in the febrile neutropenic cancer patient: Clinical efficacy and impact of monotherapy. *Antimicrob Agents Chemother* 31:971-977, 1987.

Heintz AP, Hacker NE, Berek JS, Rose TP, Munoz AK, Lagasse LD: Cytoreductive surgery in ovarian carcinoma: Feasibility and morbidity. *Obstet Gynecol* 67:783-788, 1986.

Holt P, Nicholas R: Recurrent bacteraemia: An unusual presentation of choriocarcinoma. *Br Med J* 282:1835-1836, 1981.

Hosang R, Bain BC, Denbow LE: Pyrexia of unknown origin: A case of uterine leiomyosarcoma. *Br J Obstet Gynaecol* 89:864-866, 1982.

Hughes WT, Patterson G: Post-sepsis prophylaxis in cancer patients. *Cancer* 53:137-141, 1984.

Husseinzadeh N, Nahhas WA, Manders EK, Whitney CW, Mortel R: Spontaneous occurrence of synergistic bacterial gangrene following external pelvic irradiation. *Obstet Gynecol* 63:859-862, 1984.

Inagaki J, Rodriguez V, Bodey GP: Causes of death in cancer patients. *Cancer* 33:568-573, 1974.

Jaszezak SE, Evans TN: Intrafascial abdominal and vaginal hysterectomy: A reappraisal. *Obstet Gynecol* 59:435-444, 1982.

Joshi JH, Schimpff SC, Tenney JH, Newman KA, DeJongh CA: Can antibacterial therapy be discontinued in persistently febrile granulocytopenic cancer patients? *Am J Med* 76:450-457, 1984.

Kaplan RA, Markman M, Lucas WE, Pfeifle C, Howell SB: Infectious peritonitis in patients receiving intraperitoneal chemotherapy. *Am J Med* 78(1):49-53, 1985.

Kilton LJ, Fossieck BE, Cohen MH, Parker RH: Bacteremia due to gram-positive cocci in patients with neoplastic disease. *Am J Med* 66:596-602, 1979.

Klainer AS, Beisel WR: Opportunistic infection: A review. *Am J Med Sci* 258:431, 1969.

Klastersky J: Use of combinations of antibiotics for severe infections in cancer patients. *Acta Clin Belg* 32:271-275, 1977.

Klastersky J: Treatment of severe infections in patients with cancer. *Arch Intern Med* 142:1984-1987, 1982.

Klastersky J: Empiric treatment of infections in neutropenic patients with cancer. *Rev Infect Dis* 5:S21, 1983.

Klastersky J: Empiric antimicrobial therapy for febrile granulocytopenic cancer patients. Lessons from four EORTC trials. *Acta Oncol* 27:497-502, 1988.

Klastersky J, Zinner SH: Synergistic combinations of antibiotics in gram-negative bacillary infections. *Rev Infect Dis* 4:294-301, 1982.

Klastersky J, Cappel R, Daneua D: Clinical significance of in-vitro synergism between antibiotics in gram-negative infections. *Antimicrob Agents Chemother* 2:470-475, 1972.

Klastersky J, Glauser MP, Schimpff SC, Zinner SH, Gaya H, and EORTC International Antimicrobial Therapy Cooperative Group: Prospective randomized comparison of three antibiotic regimens for empirical therapy of suspected bacteremic infection in febrile granulocytopenic patients. *Antimicrob Agents Chemother* 29:263-270, 1986.

Kottmeier HL: Complications following radiation therapy in carcinoma of the cervix and their treatment. *Am J Obstet Gynecol* 88:854-866, 1964.

Kramer BS, Carr DJ, Rand KH, Pizzo PA, Johnson A, Robichaud JK, Ychua JB: Prophylaxis of fever and infection in adult cancer patients: A placebo-controlled trial of oral trimethoprim-sulfamethoxazole plus erythromycin. *Cancer* 53:329-335, 1984.

Kramer BS, Pizzo PA, Robichaud JK, Witebsky F, Wesley R: Role of serial microbiologic surveillance and clinical evaluation in the management of cancer patients with fever and granulocytopenia. *Am J Med* 72:561-568, 1982.

Kucers A, Bennett NM: *The Use of Antibiotics*. London, William Heinemann, 1979.

Lacey CG, Futoran R, Morrow CP: *Clostridium perfringens* infection complicating chemotherapy for choriocarcinoma. *Obstet Gynecol* 47:337-341, 1976.

Lagast H, Meunier-Carpentier F, Klastersky J: Moxalactam treatment of anaerobic infections in cancer patients. *Antimicrob Agents Chemother* 22:604-610, 1982.

Larsen B, Galask RP: Vaginal microbial flora: Practical and theoretic relevance. *Obstet Gynecol* 55(Suppl):100s-113s, 1980.

Lau WK, Young LS, Black RE, Winston DJ, Linne SR, Weinstein RJ, Hewitt WL: Comparative efficacy and toxicity of amikacin/carbenicillin versus gentamicin/carbenicillin in leukopenic patients. *Am J Med* 62:959-966, 1977.

Laubach HB, McGanity WJ: Hysterectomy post-conization of the cervix. *Am J Obstet Gynecol* 91:437-442, 1965.

Lerner HM, Hones HW, Hill EC: Radical surgery for the treatment of early invasive cervical carcinoma (Stage IB): Review of 15 years' experience. *Obstet Gynecol* 56:413-418, 1980.

Levine AS, Schimpff SC, Graw RG Jr, Young RC: Hematologic malignancies and other marrow failure states: Progress in the management of complicating infections. *Semin Hematol* 11:141-202, 1974.

Lewis JH, Zimmerman JH, Ishak KG, Mullick FG: Enflurane hepatotoxicity. *Ann Intern Med* 98:984-992, 1983.

Linder JGEM, Plantema FHF, Hoogkamp-Korstanje JAA: Quantitative studies of the vaginal flora of healthy women and of obstetric gynaecological patients. *J. Med Microbiol* 11:233-241, 1978.

Love LJ, Schimpff SC, Schiffer CA, Wiernik PH: Improved prognosis for granulocytopenic patients with gram-negative bacteremia. *Am J Med* 68:643-648, 1980.

Mann WJ, Orr JW, Shingleton HM, Austin JM, Hatch KD, Taylor PT, Partridge E, Soony SJ: Perioperative influences on infectious morbidity in radical hysterectomy. *Gynecol Oncol* 11:207-212, 1981.

Mårdh PA, Weström L: Adherence of bacterial to vaginal epithelial cells. *Infect Immunol* 13:66-666, 1976.

Mayo JW, Wenzel RP: Rates of hospital-acquired blood stream infections in patients with specific malignancy. *Cancer* 50:187-190, 1982.

Mead PB: Cervical-vaginal flora of women with invasive cervical cancer. *Obstet Gynecol* 52:601-604, 1978.

Meleney FL: Bacterial synergism in disease processes. *Ann Surg* 94:961-981, 1931.

Meltzer RM: Necrotizing fasciitis and progressive bacterial synergistic gangrene of the vulva. *Obstet Gynecol* 61:757-760, 1983.

Meunier F, Klastersky J: Recent developments in prophylaxis and therapy of invasive fungal infections in granulocytopenic cancer patients. *Eur J Cancer Clin Oncol* 24:539-544, 1988.

Michal A, Torres JE, Schlosser JV: Complications of therapy for carcinoma of the cervix. *Am J Obstet Gynecol* 112:556-565, 1972.

Mikuta JJ, Giuntoli RL, Rubin EL, Mangan CE: The "problem" radical hysterectomy. *Am J Obstet Gynecol* 128:119-217, 1977.

Morgan LS, Daly JW, Monif GRG: Infectious morbidity associated with pelvic exenteration. *Gynecol Oncol* 10:318-328, 1980.

Nadworny HA, Greene WH: Surgical aspects of infection and supportive care in neutropenic patients. *Infect Surg* March, 1984, pp 182-188.

Onderdonk AB, Weinstein WM, Sullivan NM, Bartlett JG, Gorbach SL: Experimental intra-abdominal abscesses in rats: Quantitative bacteriology of infected animals. *Infect Immunol* 10:1256-1259, 1974.

Orr JW, Shingleton HM, Hatch KD, Mann WJ, Austin JM, Soong SJ: Correlation of perioperative morbidity and conization to radical hysterectomy interval. *Obstet Gynecol* 59:726-731, 1982.

Osoba D: Febrile morbidity in relation to cone biopsy followed by hysterectomy. *Can Med Assoc J* 79:805-809, 1958.

Oster MW, Vizel M, Edsall JR, Barron BA: *Pneumocystis* pneumonia in a patient with cervical carcinoma treated with combination chemotherapy. *Gynecol Oncol* 13:262-264, 1982.

Pennington JE: Fever, neutropenia and malignancy: A clinical syndrome in evaluation. *Cancer* 39:1345-1349, 1977.

Peterson BA: Opportunistic infections in patients with cancer. *Minnesota Med* 530-534, 1979.

Pizzo PA, Schimpff SC: Strategies for the prevention of infection in the myelosuppressed or immunosuppressed cancer patient. *Cancer Treat Rep* 67:223-234, 1983.

Pizzo PA, Hathorn JW, Hiemenez J, Browne M, Commers J, Cotton D, Gress J, Longo D, Marshall D, McKnight J, et al: A randomized trial comparing ceftazidime alone with combination antibiotic therapy in cancer patients with fever and neutropenia. *N Engl J Med* 315:552-558, 1986.

Pizzo PA, Ladisch S, Robichaud K: Treatment of gram-positive septicemia in cancer patients. *Cancer* 45:206-207, 1980.

Pizzo PA, Robichaud JK, Gill FA, Witebsky FG, Levine AS, Deisseroth AB, Glaubiger DL, Maclowry JD, Magrath IT, Poplack CG, Simon RM: Duration of empiric antibiotic therapy in granulocytopenic patients with cancer. *Am J Med* 67:194-200, 1979.

Platt R, Polk BF, Murdock B, et al: Mortality associated with nosocomial urinary-tract infection. *N Engl J Med* 307:637-642, 1982.

Polk BF: Antimicrobial prophylaxis to prevent mixed bacterial infection. *J Antimicrob Chemother* 8:115-129, 1981.

Rodriguez V, Burgess M, Bodey GP: Management of fever of unknown origin in patients with neoplasms and neutropenia. *Cancer* 32:1007-1012, 1973.

Rosenshein NB, Ruth JC, Villar J, Brumbine FB, Dillon MB, Spence MR: A prospective randomized study of doxycycline as a prophylactic antibiotic in patients undergoing radical hysterectomy. *Gynecol Oncol* 15:201-206, 1983.

Rubin RH: Empiric antibacterial therapy in granulocytopenia induced by cancer chemotherapy. *Ann Intern Med* 108:134-136, 1988.

Rubin M, Hathorn JW, Marshall D, Gress J, Steinberg SM, Pizzo PA: Gram-positive infections and the use of vancomycin in 550 episodes of fever and neutropenia. *Ann Intern Med* 108:30-35, 1988.

Rusthoven JJ, Ahlgren P, Elhakim T, Pinfold P, Stewart L, Feld R: Risk factors for varicella-zoster disseminated infection among adult cancer patients with localized zoster. *Cancer* 62:1641-1646, 1988.

Salem PA, Jabboury KW, Khalil MF: Severe nephrotoxicity: A probable complication of cis-dichlorodiammineplatinum (II) and cephalothin-gentamicin therapy. *Oncology* 39:31-32, 1982.

Savage JE, Philips B, Lifshitz S, Petzold CR, Buchsbaum HJ, Larsen B, Galask RP: Bacteriuria in closed bladder drainage undergoing intracavitary radium for treatment of gynecologic cancer. *Gynecol Oncol* 13:26-30, 1982.

Schiffer CA: Principles of granulocyte transfusion therapy. *Med Clin NA* 61:1119-1131, 1977.

Schimpff SC: Overview of empiric antibiotic therapy for the febrile neutropenic patient. *Rev Infect Dis* 7(Suppl 4):5734-5740, 1985.

Schimpff SC: Empiric antibiotic therapy for granulocytopenic cancer patients. *Am J Med* 80:(5C):13-20, 1986.

Schimpff SC, Aisner J: Empiric antibiotic therapy. *Cancer Treat Rep* 62:673-679, 1978.

Schwartz RS, Mackintosh FR, Schrier SK, Greenberg PL: Multivariate analysis of factors associated with invasive fungal disease during remission induction therapy for acute myelogenous leukemia. *Cancer* 53:411-419, 1984.

Sickles EA, Greene WH, Wiernik PH: Clinical presentation of infection in granulocytopenic patients. *Arch Intern Med* 135:715-719, 1975.

Singer C, Kaplan MH, Armstrong D: Bacteremia and fungemia complicating neoplastic disease. *Am J Med* 62:731-742, 1977.

Singer C, Turnbull AD: Diffuse interstitial pneumonia in immunocompromised hosts. *Curr Probl Cancer* 4:58-65, 1979.

Sinkovics JG, Smith JP: Septicemia with bacteroides in patients with malignant disease. *Cancer* 25:663-671, 1970.

Skaarup P, Berget A, Szczepanski K: The incidence of complications following hysterectomy in relation to the time interval between cone biopsy of the cervix and hysterectomy. *Acta Obstet Gynecol Scand* 50:321-324, 1971.

Smith CK, Lipsky JJ, Laskin OL, Hellmann DB, Mellits ED, Longstreth J, Lietman PS: Double-blind comparison of the nephrotoxicity and auditory toxicity of gentamicin and tobramycin. *N Engl J Med* 320:1106-1109, 1980.

Spiers ASD, Dias SF, Lopez JA: Infection prevention in patients with cancer: Microbiological evaluation of portable laminar air flow isolation, topical chlorhexidine, and oral non-absorbable antibiotics. *J Hyg Lond* 84:457-465, 1980.

Stone HH, Martin JD: Synergistic necrotizing cellulitis. *Ann Surg* 175:702-711, 1972.

Swartz WH, Tanaree P: Suction drainage as an alternative to prophylactic antibiotics for hysterectomy. *Obstet Gynecol* 45:305-310, 1975.

Symmonds RE: Morbidity and complications of radical hysterectomy with pelvic lymph node dissection. *Am J Obstet Gynecol* 94:663-678, 1966.

Talcott JA, Finberg R, Mayer RJ, Goldman L: The medical course of cancer patients with fever and neutropenia. Clinical identification of a low-risk subgroup at presentation. *Arch Intern Med* 148:2561-2568, 1988.

Thadepalli H, Savage EW, Rao B: Anaerobic bacteria associated with cervical neoplasia. *Gynecol Oncol* 14:307-312, 1982.

Tuomala RE, Berkowitz R, Polk BF, Cisneros R, Onderdonk A: A case-control study of cervical flora in women with invasive cervical cancer. Presented at the Meeting of Infectious Disease Society of Obstetrics and Gynecology, July, 1983.

VanHerik M: Fever as a complication of radiation therapy for carcinoma of the cervix. *Am J Roentgenol* 93:104-109, 1965.

Van Laethem Y, Lagast H, Klastersky J: Anaerobic infections in cancer patients: Comparison between therapy oriented strictly against anaerobes or both anaerobes and aerobes. *J Antimicrob Chemother* 10(Suppl A):137-144, 1982.

Wade JC, Schimpff SC, Wiernik PH: Antibiotic combination-associated nephrotoxicity in granulocytopenic patients with cancer. *Arch Intern Med* 141:1789-1793, 1981.

Wark HJ, Clifton B, Bookallil MJ: Halothane hepatitis revisited in women undergoing treatment of carcinoma of the cervix. *Br J Anaesth* 51:763-766, 1979.

Webb MJ, Symmonds RE: Radical hysterectomy: Influence of recent conization on morbidity and complications. *Obstet Gynecol* 53:290-292, 1979.

Weinstein WM, Onderdonk AB, Bartlett JG, Gorbach SL: Experimental intra-abdominal abscesses in rats: Development of an experimental model. *Infect Immunol* 10:1250, 1974.

Weinstein WM, Onderdonk AB, Bartlett JG, Louie TJ, Gorbach SL: Antimicrobial therapy of experimental intra-abdominal sepsis. *J Infect Dis* 132:282-286, 1975.

Wiernik PH: The management of infection in the cancer patient. *JAMA* 244:185-187, 1980.

Williams TJ, Johnson TR, Pratt JH: Time interval between cervical conization and hysterectomy. *Am J Obstet Gynecol* 107:790-796, 1970.

Wisborg T: The cone biopsy-hysterectomy time interval related to wound infection. *Acta Obstet Gynecol Scand* 51:1-4, 1972.

Wong KK, Hirsch MS: Herpes virus infections in patients with neoplastic disease. *Am J Med* 76:464-478, 1984.

Young LS: Nosocomial infections in the immunocompromised adult. *Am J Med* 70:398-404, 1981.

# Chapter 22 | Reconstructive Pelvic Surgery

### Jonathan S. Berek    Neville F. Hacker
### Leo D. Lagasse

With the use of more aggressive surgical treatment of gynecologic malignancy, as well as improved survival among patients with advanced disease, has come a greater need for postoperative reconstruction of the pelvic structures. Pelvic exenteration for recurrent tumors has resulted in 5-year survival rates as high as 50% (Morley and Lindenauer, 1976; Rutledge et al, 1977), and morbidity from this procedure has been significantly reduced since it was popularized by Brunschwig (1948). More creative attempts to preserve and reconstruct residual tissues have therefore become possible, and issues such as quality of life can be more directly addressed. In addition, reconstruction can improve both body image and function in patients who have undergone pelvic surgery for gynecologic cancer.

Extirpative surgery of the pelvic viscera and vulva can be mutilating and can severely damage the patient's self-esteem and perception of her body (Morley et al, 1973; Anderson and Hacker, 1983). Sexual function is commonly obliterated, and efforts to restore it are often neglected in the attempt to achieve a cure in patients with advanced disease. Frequently, extensive pelvic surgery results in pelvic floor defects that require a reconstructive procedure to prevent bowel herniation (Webb and Symmonds, 1977).

The major goals of reconstructive pelvic surgery are to restore the anatomy to as normal a configuration as possible, to replace the viscera so that their function can be preserved, and to conserve as much tissue as is necessary to close adequately all defects in exposed skin surfaces so as to preserve the patient's body image and provide support for the residual viscera (Berek et al, 1984). These goals may be attained through careful planning, good patient selection and preoperative preparation, a thorough knowledge of the types of grafts that can be employed, and meticulous operative technique. The surgeon must be innovative and creative in order to adapt to the patient's individual circumstance and to provide the best possible result. Although the need for reconstruction can be minimized by using modifications of extirpative surgery and combining radiation and surgery whenever possible, some functional restoration will be required in many patients treated for pelvic and vulvar cancer (Berek, 1989).

In this chapter, we will describe various methods of vaginal, vulvar, perineal, perianal, and pelvic floor reconstruction. Although reference is made to the important techniques of lower bowel and urinary tract reconstruction as they relate to the other procedures, more detailed descriptions of these specific techniques can be found in the chapters on urologic and gastrointestinal operations (Chapters 18 and 19).

## GENERAL PRINCIPLES

Pelvic reconstructive procedures should be adapted to the individual needs of the patient as dictated by the operative procedures required to cure her disease. All patients who undergo pelvic exenteration should have some degree of reconstruction of the pelvic floor and, whenever possible, reconstitution of the rectosigmoid colon and vagina and preservation of the bladder (Berek et al, 1984). Occasionally, vaginal reconstruction must be postponed because the patient's intraoperative condition is unstable, e.g., if there is excessive bleeding requiring a pelvic pack. Delayed vaginal reconstruction should be reserved for those individuals who intend to be sexually active, strongly desire such reconstruction, and are motivated to keep the graft patent (Berek et al, 1983).

Patients with vaginal stenosis, which typically occurs secondary to pelvic irradiation, can undergo vaginal reconstruction. Reconstruction should be offered to all patients who wish to be sexually active and who are motivated to use the neovagina (Berek et al, 1983).

Patients who undergo radical vulvectomy often have major defects in the vulva and groin that can be closed in a variety of ways. The selection of the type of graft to be employed should be individualized according to the nature of the defect. Whenever possible, primary closure of the vulvectomy skin incisions should be accomplished (Julian et al, 1971; Hacker et al, 1981). Split- and full-thickness skin grafts as well as cutaneous and myocutaneous pedicle grafts using the gracilis, gluteus maximus, and tensor fascia lata can also be employed in appropriate patients (Berek, 1989).

Anal reconstruction in patients who require sphincteroplasty or who have fecal incontinence can be accomplished in most cases by means of a primary sphincter plication. Patients in whom simple anal plications have failed, more often necessitating a colostomy, may be candidates for more elaborate muscle transposition procedures (Berek et al, 1982). Extensive pelvic exenterative surgery may increase the potential for bowel herniation if the defect is large. To a great extent, this complication can be prevented by careful reconstruction of the pelvic floor at the time of the exenterative procedure. When herniation does occur, it can be repaired by several techniques (see later).

### Harvesting of Skin Grafts

Skin grafts are harvested under sterile conditions. After the site of the donor graft has been selected (typically, either the anterior medial thigh or the buttock), the patient is positioned so that the graft can be harvested with a dermatome. Selection of the donor site must be made preoperatively after discussion with the patient. The buttock donor site offers the advantage that it may be more readily concealed, although during the postoperative recovery period, this is often more painful than a thigh donor site. When cosmesis is of no significant concern, the anterior or medial thigh offers a simpler donor site, because the patient does not need to be positioned prone and then moved into the lithotomy position for the grafting procedures—a maneuver that lengthens operating time.

The patient is prepared and draped in the usual fashion and positioned either prone or supine, with the legs abducted about 45 degrees so that the inner thigh is adequately exposed. The dermatome is selected, and a graft of the desired width and thickness is obtained by appropriately adjusting and setting the dermatome. Several different types of dermatomes are commonly available, including the Brown air-powered dermatome, the electrically generated dermatome, and the Padjett hand-held dermatome. The surgeon should select the dermatome with which he or she is most comfortable, since an equally good skin graft can be harvested using any one of these dermatomes. A split-thickness graft can be obtained by setting the thickness between about 14 and 16 one-thousandths of an inch; full-thickness grafts are about 20 to 24 one-thousandths of an inch thick. Prior to usage, the dermatome should be set for the appropriate thickness and checked to make sure that it is working properly. The surgeon should hold the dermatome up to a light to see that the thickness across its entire cutting edge is uniform.

When using the dermatome, the operator should apply firm, even pressure in order to harvest a graft of uniform thickness. Mineral oil is applied to the donor site so that the dermatome will move easily across the skin surface. The leading edge of the skin is stretched and flattened by the surgical assistant; typically, the edge of a tongue depressor is used for this purpose. The assistant picks up the leading edge of the graft as it is being harvested from the top of the dermatome. When the desired graft length is reached, a scissor or scalpel is used to cut the edge free from the donor site.

The harvested graft should be kept moist with saline and covered with a moist sterile gauze pad in the event that operating time is being expended to prepare the site on which the graft will be placed. Occasionally, two or more skin grafts are harvested and are sewn together, as for the creation of a neovagina. This is facilitated by using a wooden board to which the grafts apend or on which the operator can suture them together, for which purpose 3-0 or 4-0 absorbable sutures should be employed. It is useful to perforate or to "pie-crust" the graft by making small 0.5-cm incisions at 1- to 2-cm intervals along the length of the graft, which can be done by hand or by using an apparatus to "pie-crust" skin grafts. This permits the escape of free fluid that might collect under the graft and provides a means for expansion of the graft if this becomes necessary.

## Pedicle Grafts

The purpose of creating a pedicle graft is to cover the defect while preserving the blood supply to the pedicle. Full-thickness skin pedicle grafts are used on the vulva or groin (Julian et al, 1971; Barnhill et al, 1983; Berek, 1989). Adequate vascularity is preserved by making the length of the pedicle no greater than twice its base. Thus, when performing a V or Z plasty, the surgeon must carefully measure the grafts before the skin is incised. Prior to any incision, a skin marking pen should be utilized. In general, subcutaneous tissue is retained on any skin advancement flap in order to facilitate preservation of the blood supply.

When using myocutaneous pedicle grafts, the operator must carefully isolate and preserve the neurovascular bundle that supplies the muscle (Becker et al, 1979; Berek et al, 1984). Care must be taken to avoid placing undue tension on the neurovascular pedicle, which can compromise the blood supply to the donor pedicle. Prior to making the incision, the donor pedicle should be carefully examined to ensure that the desired length of graft is being isolated.

## Perioperative and Postoperative Management

In patients undergoing vaginal reconstruction with split-thickness grafts or delayed vaginal reconstruction in a fibrotic or previously irradiated pelvis, bed rest is prescribed for approximately 1 week while the graft is taking. For this reason, pneumatic calf compression or low-dose subcutaneous heparin is given for as long as the patient is immobilized. When a bladder is present, a transurethral Foley catheter is placed. Patients with a preserved or reconstructed rectosigmoid colon should undergo mechanical preoperative bowel preparation in order to minimize fecal soilage postoperatively. In addition, patients are typically placed on a clear liquid or low-residue diet and are given Lomotil, at least one tablet every 6 hours, to minimize colonic function. Prophylactic antibiotics may be administered perioperatively.

Donor sites are covered with either gentian violet- or scarlet red-impregnated gauze or a synthetic porous skin gauze such as Op-Site. This covering is left in place during the entire hospitalization period and should be changed if it becomes detached or contaminated. After about 5 days, the covering is removed, and the donor site is carefully irrigated and dried. Any necrotic areas should be carefully debrided, and a new dressing should be placed. Grafts are left uncovered so that their viability may be assessed during the postoperative period.

In a vaginal reconstruction using skin grafts, a vaginal stent or obturator must be inserted in order to keep the opposing walls of the neovagina separate. A gauze pack is placed at the time of surgery and is removed about 5 to 7 days later. Preferably, the graft is placed over a Heyer-Schulte stent inserted at the time of surgery. A soft vaginal stent, either a condom filled with packing gauze or a Heyer-Schulte stent, is then inserted into the neovagina. The patient is instructed about how to insert the stent and to keep it in place every day, removing it at least once daily for cleansing. Two to 3 months later, when the patient can initiate intercourse, the stent is retained within the neovagina during the night as needed. Thereafter, continued sexual activity may be sufficient to maintain the vaginal space and prevent vaginal stenosis (Berek et al, 1983).

In patients undergoing vulvar reconstruction, bed rest and relative immobilization for about 5 days may be necessary in order to avoid placing significant tension on pedicle grafts or disrupting the bed of the free skin graft. In patients undergoing vaginal reconstruction or low rectosigmoid colon anastomosis or sphincter reconstruction, bowel function should be minimized, as described previously.

## VAGINAL RECONSTRUCTION

Primary reconstruction of the vagina in cases of vaginal atresia can be readily performed using a split-thickness skin graft, as popularized by McIndoe and Banister (1938). Vaginal atresia is successfully treated in almost all patients using this technique. This operation can also be employed for patients who require vaginal reconstruction at the time of exenteration, who require delayed skin grafts following exenteration, or who develop vaginal stenosis after pelvic surgery or radiation therapy.

Several types of vaginal grafts are used in patients with gynecologic malignancies, including skin grafts, which are harvested from a donor site; cutaneous, subcutaneous pedicle, or "advancement" flaps for performing a V or Z plasty; and myocutaneous pedicle grafts (Magrina and Masterson, 1981).

### Vaginal Reconstruction With Pelvic Exenteration

Pevic exenteration has been a useful means of controlling recurrent pelvic malignancy, with as many as 50% of selected patients surviving for 5 years or longer. Until now, concern about restoring vaginal function has always been secondary to achieving a satisfactory postoperative course and potential cure. However, with improved perioperative management, the morbidity and mortality associated with the exenterative procedure have decreased considerably over the past several decades. Thus, in many cases, the surgeon may consider performing vaginal reconstruction simultaneously with an exenterative procedure.

Because exenteration often results in damage to the patient's body image and self-esteem, reconstructing the vagina might help to prevent these negative feelings as well as facilitate sexual rehabilitation in these patients.

Before performing exenteration and vaginal reconstruction, the physician must adequately counsel the patient so that she is aware of the nature of the reconstruction, its potential benefits, and the limitations of the neovagina. Some patients who are not sexually active or do not intend to become so may not desire vaginal reconstruction. However, in those women who require total pelvic exenteration, myocutaneous grafts

might contribute to the reconstruction of the pelvic floor, preventing herniation of the small bowel.

Pelvic reconstruction and exenteration should be performed simultaneously, preferably using a two-team approach. While the specimen is being resected from above, the surgeons below can be preparing the graft for positioning into the pelvis, and operative time can thus be considerably reduced.

### Vaginal Reconstruction Using Split-Thickness Skin Grafts

In patients undergoing anterior exenteration or in whom the rectosigmoid colon has been preserved or reconstructed, it is advisable to utilize split-thickness skin grafts to create a neovagina as opposed to bilteral myocutaneous gracilis or bulbocavernosus pedicle grafts, since the rectosigmoid may not accommodate placement of large myocutaneous grafts (Berek et al, 1984).

One or two split-thickness skin grafts are harvested from the buttock or medial thigh, as previously described. The skin grafts are sutured together over a Heyer-Schulte stent or a condom filled with gauze; whenever possible, an omental pedicle is placed into the pelvis to provide an additional vascular bed on which the skin graft can be placed. The omentum is mobilized by ligating and dividing the short gastric vessels along the greater curvature of the stomach, moving from the patient's right to left. The vascular pedicle is the left gastroepiploic artery (Fig. 22-1). The omentum can thus

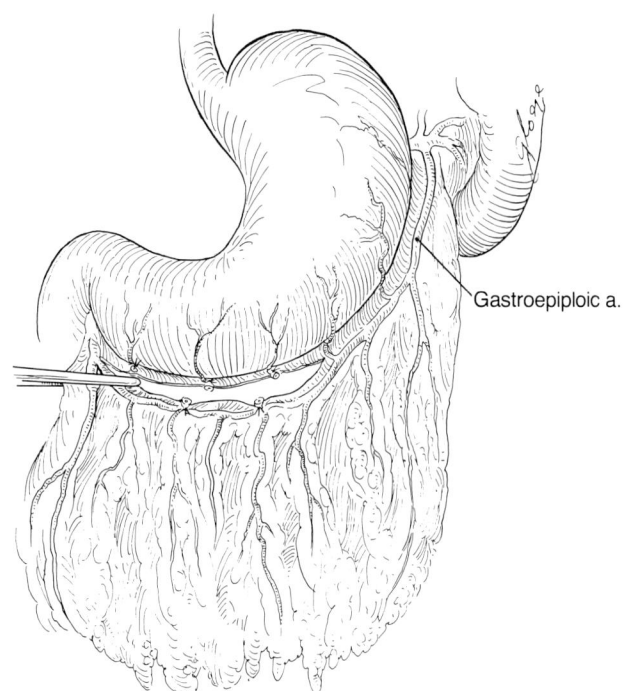

Gastroepiploic a.

**FIGURE 22-1** The omentum is mobilized by ligating and dividing the short gastric vessels along the greater curvature of the stomach. (From Berek JS: General surgical operations. In Berek JS, Hacker NF: *Practical Gynecologic Oncology.* Baltimore, Williams & Wilkins, 1989, pp 509-548.)

be positioned in the pelvis superior to the preserved or reconstructed rectosigmoid colon to provide adequate space for placing the graft (Fig. 22-2). The split-thickness grafts and stent are then inserted into the space so that the surfaces are well applied to the anterior rectosigmoid colon and omentum (Fig. 22-3). The omentum is positioned anteriorly and is sutured to the rectum. The final product will be a neovagina of satisfactory caliber (Fig. 22-4).

In a report by Berek et al (1984), seven patients received a neovagina at the time of pelvic enteration using split-thickness skin grafts. All the grafts took, since the omentum and bowel serosa served as a useful bed for the split-thickness skin grafts. Because two of these patients who were not having vaginal intercourse or regularly using a vaginal stent developed vaginal stenosis, we recommend this procedure only for sexually active patients.

## Bilateral Myocutaneous Gracilis Grafts

A number of researchers have reported on the use of bilateral myocutaneous gracilis grafts for the simultaneous creation of a neovagina and reconstruction of the pelvic floor in patients undergoing total pelvic exenteration (McGraw et al, 1976; Becker et al, 1979; Morrow et al, 1979; Berek et al, 1984; Cain et al, 1988; Lacey et al, 1988; Copeland et al, 1989). The advantage of these grafts is that they provide excellent support for the abdominal viscera, and as a neovagina, they only rarely become stenotic.

The technique for performing bilateral myocutaneous gracilis grafting is as follows. The patient is placed in a modified lithotomy position using stirrups

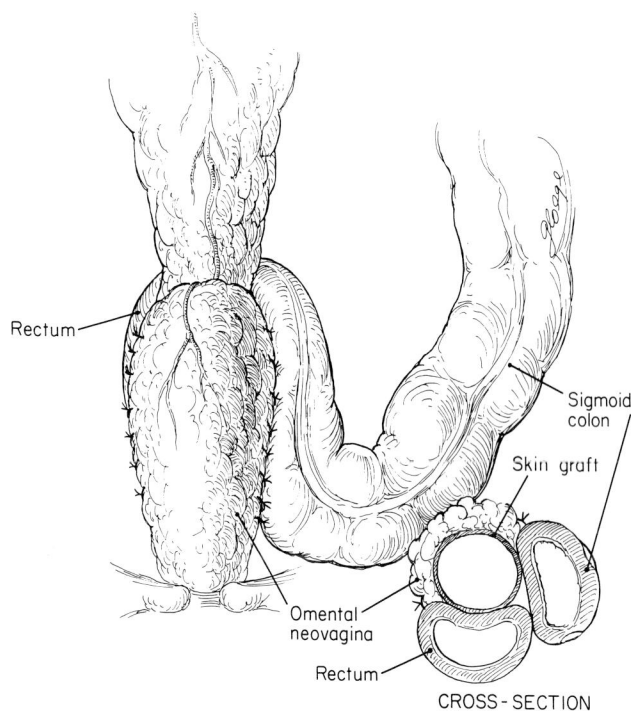

**FIGURE 22-3** Relationship of the preserved or reconstructed rectosigmoid colon to the omental pedicle and neovagina. (From Berek JS, et al: Vaginal reconstruction performed simultaneously with pelvic exenteration. *Obstet Gynecol* 63:322, 1984, by permission of The American College of Obstetricians and Gynecologists.)

that support the legs for their entire length. The hips are abducted to a 45-degree angle. The flap is outlined on the skin using a marking pencil (Fig. 22-5). The gracilis muscle is situated on the medial aspect of the thigh, posterior to a line drawn between the pubic tubercle and medial epicondyle of the knee, at the site of insertion of the semitendinosus tendon.

The flap is fusiform in shape and is taken from the

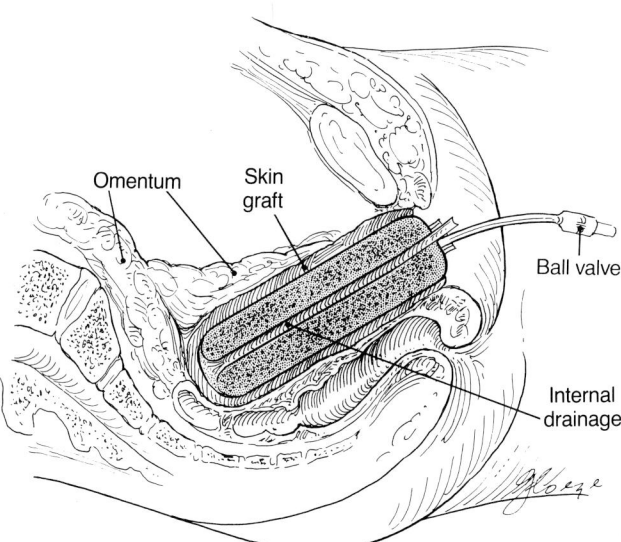

**FIGURE 22-2** The omentum is placed in the pelvis and sutured to the rectum posteriorly and the sigmoid colon laterally to create a "pocket" for the neovagina. Two split-thickness skin grafts are harvested, sutured together over a Heyer-Schulte stent, and inserted into the newly created pelvic space. (From Berek JS: General surgical operations. In Berek JS, Hacker NF: *Practical Gynecologic Oncology.* Baltimore, Williams & Wilkins, 1989, pp 509-548.)

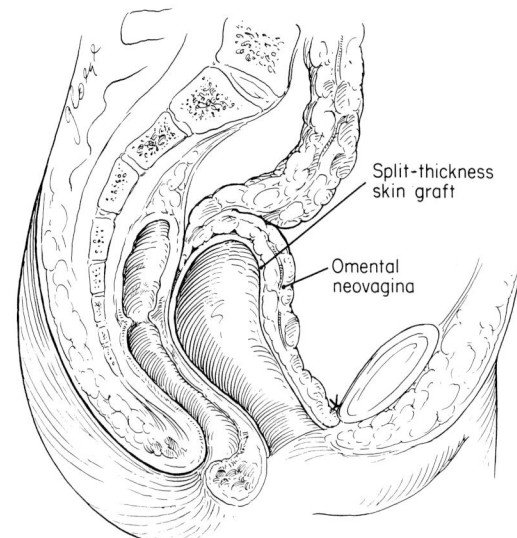

**FIGURE 22-4** A neovagina of satisfactory caliber is therefore achieved.

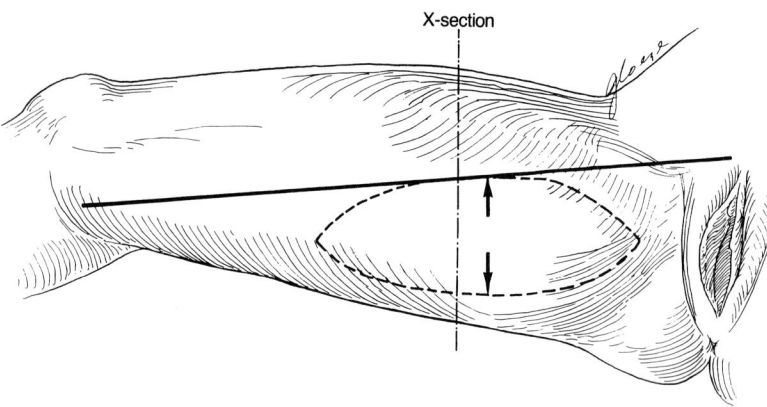

**FIGURE 22-5** The myocutaneous pedicle is drawn on the inner aspect of the thigh. Note the skin bridge that is to be preserved between the vulva and the pedicle. A line is drawn from the pubic tubercle to the medial epicondyle, delineating the anterior margin of the graft. (From Berek JS, et al: Vaginal reconstruction performed simultaneously with pelvic exenteration. *Obstet Gynecol* 63:319, 1984, by permission of The American College of Obstetricians and Gynecologists.)

proximal one-half to two-thirds of the upper inner thigh. A skin bridge is left from the apex of the incision to the vaginal introitus. The length of this bridge is about 6 cm. A "short" myocutaneous pedicle is preferable, with the length of the graft about 12 to 14 cm. We recommend a graft 6 cm in width, since wider grafts can create an overly capacious neovagina. After the graft is mobilized and sutured to the opposite side, the dimensions of the neovagina can be adjusted by trimming the distal end and edge of the graft to reduce its capacity.

The skin is incised with a scalpel and the flap is mobilized using electrocautery (Fig. 22-6), which minimizes operative time and maximizes hemostasis. The skin is resected en bloc with its subcutaneous tissue and the gracilis muscle. The gracilis muscle is transected distally and elevated from the underlying fascia of the vastus medialis muscle. This dissection is carried to the proximal thigh in order to identify the neurovascular pedicle, which is located 5 to 10 cm from proximal apex of the flap. The surgeon should be careful to avoid damaging this pedicle, since it provides the only significant blood supply to the muscle. Some authors have employed fluorescein dye to demonstrate the adequacy of blood flow to the pedicle, but we have not found this to be a reliable or necessary method.

When the pedicle has been isolated, the entire graft is brought under the skin bridge with gentle traction (Fig. 22-7). The gracilis muscle is not divided proximally but is mobilized to the tendons of origin, which provides sufficient mobility of the muscle.

The bilateral flaps are joined in the midline using interrupted sutures (Fig. 22-8). Hooks are positioned at the site where the proximal apex of the flaps is located prior to the dissection. Medial thigh incisions are closed using two layers of interrupted absorbable suture.

The neovagina is created by suturing both sides of the graft and the apex so that only one end of the tunnel is patent (Fig. 22-9). The operator's hand is inserted into the neovagina to assess the capacity of the structure. The open end is sutured to the patient's introitus. The muscular and subcutaneous tissues are thus positioned on the exterior of the graft to the thigh skin, forming the inner lining of the neovagina. The entire neovagina is then placed into the pelvis by rotating it posteriorly (Fig. 22-10) so that the side of the neovagina facing the operator becomes its posterior side. The graft is sutured to the introitus, and the apex of the neovagina is sutured to the sacral promontory. A vaginal pack is not necessary.

At the completion of the procedure, the omentum is mobilized from the greater curvature of the stomach in

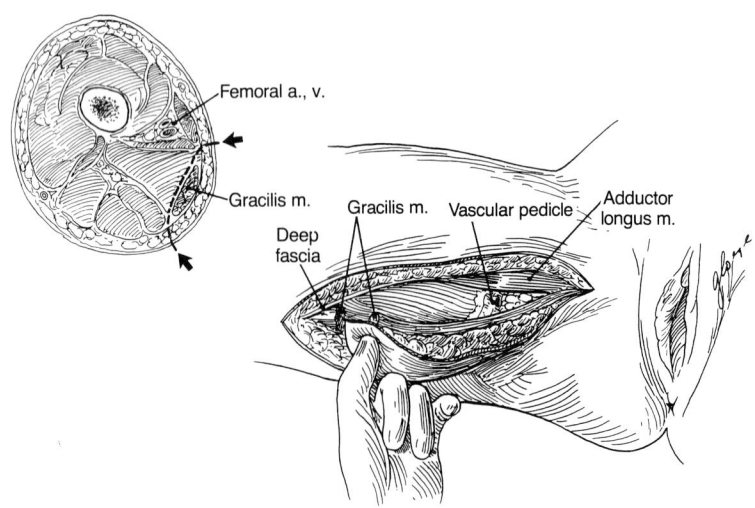

Femoral a., v.
Gracilis m.
Deep fascia
Gracilis m.    Vascular pedicle
Adductor longus m.

**FIGURE 22-6** The myocutaneous pedicle graft is mobilized by transecting the gracilis muscle distally in continuity with the skin and subcutaneous tissue. Note the vascular pedicle proximally, which must be carefully identified and preserved. A cross section across the thigh at the level of the pedicle reveals the relationship of the gracilis muscle to the femoral vessels. (From Berek JS, et al: Vaginal reconstruction performed simultaneously with pelvic exenteration. *Obstet Gynecol* 63:319, 1984, by permission of The American College of Obstetricians and Gynecologists.)

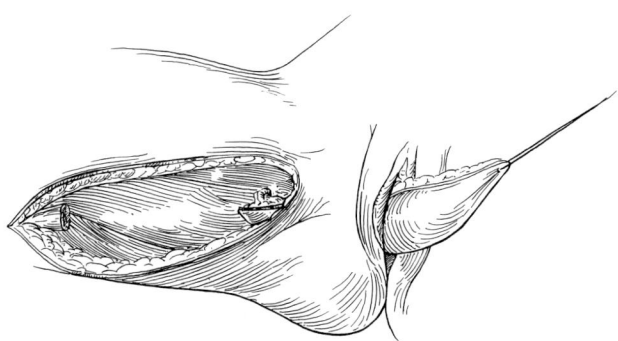

FIGURE 22-7 The entire pedicle is brought under the skin bridge with gentle traction and exteriorized through the introitus. (From Berek JS, et al: Vaginal reconstruction performed simultaneously with pelvic exenteration. *Obstet Gynecol* 63:319, 1984, by permission of The American College of Obstetricians and Gynecologists.)

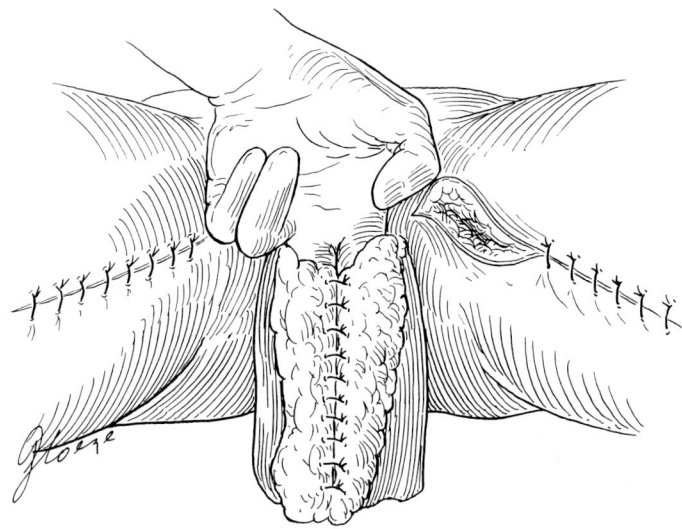

FIGURE 22-9 The neovagina is formed by suturing three sides of the skin and subcutaneous tissue together. The operator's two fingers are placed into the neovagina, demonstrating the desired size and caliber. (From Berek JS, et al: Vaginal reconstruction performed simultaneously with pelvic exenteration. *Obstet Gynecol* 63:320, 1984, by permission of The American College of Obstetricians and Gynecologists.)

the manner previously described. This covers the pelvic floor and separates the neovagina from the small bowel (Fig. 22-11).

Utilizing this technique, Becker et al (1979) reported a 95% success rate in 25 patients who underwent the procedure at the time of total pelvic exenteration. Berek et al (1983) indicated that in 86% of their patients (18 of 21), bilteral myocutaneous gracilis grafts were successful; 11 of these women (52%) had regular vaginal intercourse. In neither series did herniation of the bowel occur through the reconstructed pelvic floor, nor were there any fistulas in the absence of recurrent malignancies. Although patients who utilized the grafts for sexual intercourse reported altered and diminished vaginal sensation, many were gratified that they could remain sex-

ually active. Gracilis grafts are associated with a moderate to heavy, persistent vaginal discharge. In 3 of 21 patients (Berek et al, 1983) one side of the gracilis graft was lost, requiring resection and debridement.

## Bulbocavernosus Pedicle Grafts

Use of bilateral bulbocavernosus pedicle grafts has been reported by Hatch (1984). When compared with the gracilis myocutaneous graft, the bulbocavernosus graft was found to be easier to construct, with less operative blood loss and a shorter operating time. In addition,

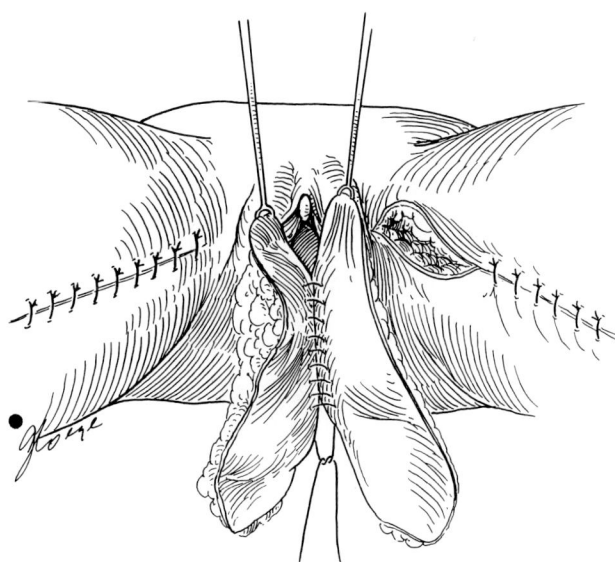

FIGURE 22-8 The bilateral pedicles are sutured together so that a neovagina can be created. The donor sites are closed in layers. Hooks are in position where the proximal apex of the flap is localized before its dissection. (From Berek JS, et al: Vaginal reconstruction performed simultaneously with pelvic exenteration. *Obstet Gynecol* 63:320, 1984, by permission of The American College of Obstetricians and Gynecologists.)

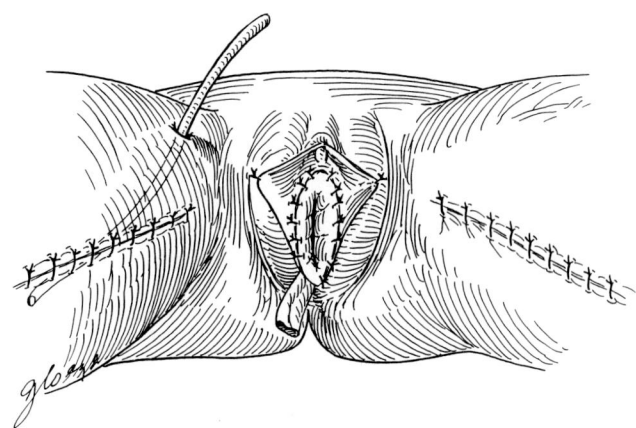

FIGURE 22-10 The neovagina is inserted into the pelvic space created by the exenteration by placing the closed end of the grafts up toward the sacral promontory, to which it is sutured. The open end of the neovagina is sutured to the preserved introitus. (From Berek JS, et al: Vaginal reconstruction performed simultaneously with pelvic exenteration. *Obstet Gynecol* 63:320, 1984, by permission of The American College of Obstetricians and Gynecologists.)

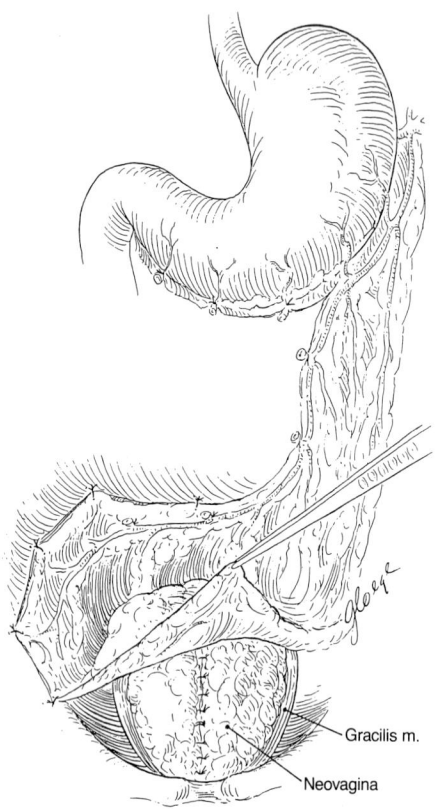

FIGURE 22-11 The omental pedicle is placed over the neovagina to interpose between the graft and the small bowel. (From Berek JS, et al: Vaginal reconstruction performed simultaneously with pelvic exenteration. *Obstet Gynecol* 63:320, 1984, by permission of The American College of Obstetricians and Gynecologists.)

cosmetic results were excellent and there were no complications. The procedure is initiated by making bilateral incisions over the labia majora. The bulbocavernosus muscle is isolated superiorly, carried to its origin, and mobilized on a posterior vulvar pedicle. These grafts are then tunneled under a skin bridge at the posterior introitus and are sutured together to create an anterior vaginal wall in patients with a preserved or reconstructed rectosigmoid colon.

## Reconstruction in the Fibrotic Pelvis

After extensive pelvic radiation or if the neovagina fails, the pelvis may become fibrotic, with marked scarring. This has often deterred surgeons from attempting to create a neovagina in patients who desire it for fear of injuring preserved bladder, rectosigmoid, or small bowel. Berek et al (1983) reported the results of 16 such procedures performed in 14 patients, all of whom had a successful graft.

Creation of the neovagina involves resection of the scarred vagina in order to provide a new bed on which the split-thickness skin grafts can be placed. The procedure is initiated with lateral incisions, and the scarred vagina is dissected to its apex. With the operator's finger inserted in the rectum to avoid rectal injury, a posterior dissection is performed to remove the vagina from the anterior rectal serosa (Fig. 22-12). The two lateral dissections are joined to the posterior dissection. After the scarred vagina has been resected on three sides, an anterior dissection is accomplished with much less risk. The entire scarred vagina can be removed.

After resection of the scar, a split-thickness skin graft is harvested in the usual fashion and sewn over a vaginal

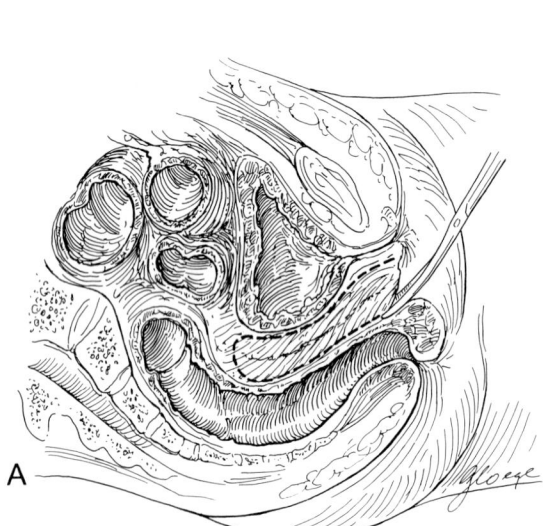

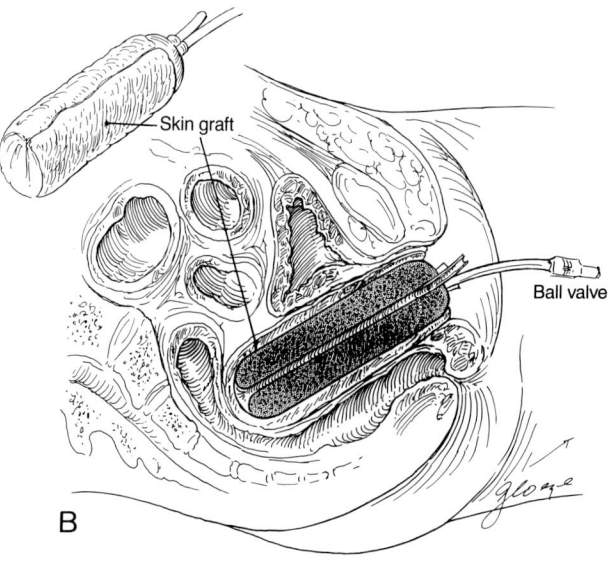

FIGURE 22-12 (A) Resection of the scarred vagina. After lateral planes are developed, the posterior plane is dissected carefully with Metzenbaum scissors, with a finger placed in the rectum. (From Berek JS: General surgical operations. In Berek JS, Hacker NF: *Practical Gynecologic Oncology.* Baltimore, Williams & Wilkins, 1989, pp 509-548.) (B) A Neyu-Schulte vaginal shunt has the slim graft placed around it, and this is inserted into the pelvic space to create a neovagina.

obturator. The operator then carefully and gently slides the graft off the obturator into the newly created vaginal space. A packing gauze is placed into the space as the obturator is removed. Prior to placing the graft, the operator must be sure to control any small-vessel bleeding.

## Pelvic Organ Transposition

Use of the transplanted bladder fundus or the sigmoid colon to create a neovagina has been found to be significantly less satisfactory than other techniques (Pratt and Smith, 1966; Watring et al, 1976; Lagasse et al, 1978). The transplanted bladder fundus technique results in a neovagina of limited dimensions that tends to stenose readily. The substituted sigmoid colon is also less practical and is associated with considerable discharge and a propensity for stenosis (Pratt and Smith, 1966). Therefore, we no longer employ or recommend these techniques.

Another technique reported by Bürger et al (1989) is the use of the ileocecal intestinal segment to create a neovagina. This procedure appears to be associated with fewer complications than use of the sigmoid colon, and the technique may prove useful in selected patients.

## Delayed Reconstruction

Several authors have advocated creation of a neovagina approximately 1 to 2 months after an exenterative procedure (Morley and Lindenauer, 1976; Watring et al, 1976). Morley and Lindenauer have recommended that vaginal reconstruction using split-thickness skin grafts be performed 3 to 5 weeks after the initial surgery. They feel that a satisfactory granulation bed must be established in the pelvic vault prior to creation of the neovagina. When this procedure was performed in 20 patients, no serious complications were encountered postoperatively, with the exception of some discomfort at the donor site. Sexual function following this procedure was not specifically reported.

The Williams procedure (Williams, 1964; Schellhas and Fidhar, 1975; Day and Stanhope, 1977), a vulvar perineorrhaphy, can be performed with minimal morbidity. It is performed by grasping the labia majora at their junction with the labia minora, and a U-shaped incision is made at the mucocutaneous junction and across the posterior fourchette. Beginning posteriorly, the medial edges of the mucocutaneous incision are sutured together, after which the lateral skin edges are approximated in a similar fashion to create a superficial pouch on the perineal body. This procedure is very simple, with minimal morbidity; however, the anatomic result is not as satisfactory as the one achieved with split-thickness skin grafts (Fig. 22-13).

The major problem associated with delayed vaginal reconstruction is that it requires a separate operative procedure. In our experience, a fresh bed is satisfactory for placement of a graft; one does not need to await the development of a granulation bed in the pelvis in order for a split-thickness graft to take. Furthermore,

delayed myocutaneous grafts are not practical because of the need to insert the graft to the level of the sacral promontory.

## VULVAR RECONSTRUCTION

The principal concept of vulvar surgery is that, whenever possible, primary closure the incision should be performed at the time of vulvectomy. After a radical vulvectomy of the Bassett type, with contiguous groin and vulvar dissections, a rather prominent defect will be present. Morbidity with an open groin and vulvar incision is significant, and the surgeon should make every effort to perform the primary closure.

Primary closure can often be accomplished by undermining the skin flaps and the outer vaginal mucosa, so that the remaining vulvar skin can be advanced over the underlying fascia (Julian et al, 1971). The vaginal mucosa is sutured to the skin flaps by means of horizontal mattress sutures of absorbable, braided 2-0 suture. The skin is also joined in the midline superior to the vulva. For appropriate closure of the anterior vulva and inguinal incisions, a vulvoplasty must occasionally be performed by creating relaxing incisions. This allows advancement of the skin medially, thus reducing the tension on the midline or apical closure. These skin flaps should be drained with rubber catheters placed subcutaneously and exteriorized laterally through separate stab incisions. We recommend that low, intermittent suction drainage be applied so that the advanced skin will remain adherent to the underlying fascia and no fluid will collect under the skin flaps.

It is important that this area be covered in patients undergoing an inguinal-femoral lymphadenectomy. We recommend transposition of the sartorius muscle, which is performed by dividing the muscle from its lateral attachment on the anterior-superior iliac spine. The muscle is then mobilized, brought over the femoral vessels, and sutured to the inguinal ligament medially. Suction drains should be placed beneath the skin flap, and the subcutaneous tissue should be approximated with interrupted sutures, using 2-0 or 3-0 absorbable material. The skin can be closed with interrupted sutures or skin clips.

In patients with early vulvar carcinoma, such as microinvasive carcinoma, or in patients with T1 or T2 primary lesions without evidence of palpably enlarged groin nodes, a more limited procedure should be considered. In a publication by Hacker et al (1981), 100 patients with carcinoma of the vulva underwent vulvectomy with bilateral inguinal-femoral lymphadenectomy performed through separate groin incisions. The morbidity of this procedure was significantly less than that seen with the Bassett operation, in that there was a very low incidence of major wound breakdown (14%); 14% of the patients had significant leg edema, and the average hospital stay was 19 days (range = 6 to 46 days). Using the separate incision technique, one can close the

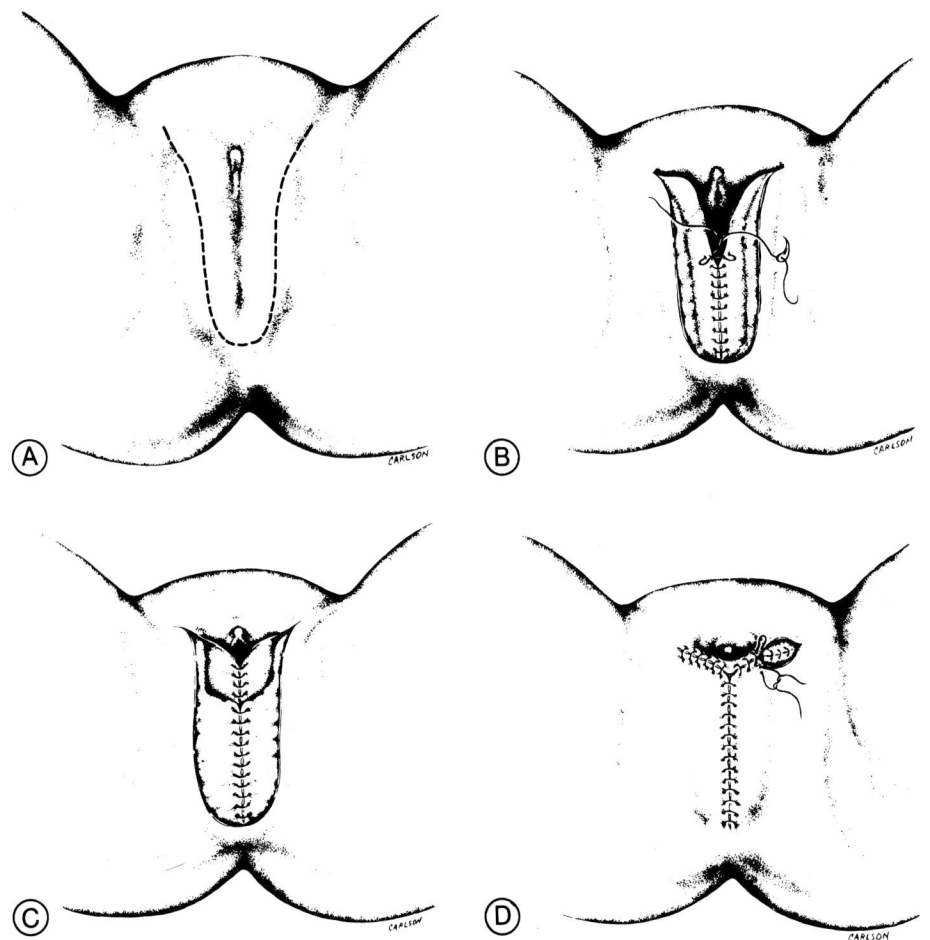

**FIGURE 22-13** A horseshoe-shaped incision is made (*A*), and the inner margins are closed with interrupted mattress sutures (*B*). Subcutaneous tissues are approximated in the midline (*C*). The outer margins are also approximated in the midline, and the diverging superior aspects of the incision are closed (*D*). (From Day TG Jr, Stanhope R: Vulvovaginoplasty in gynecologic oncology. *Obstet Gynecol* 50:362, 1977, by permission of The American College of Obstetricians and Gynecologists.)

incisions primarily, thus obviating a more extensive operation and minimizing the need for reconstructive surgery. In this group of selected patients, this technique did not compromise survival, and there were no recurrences in the intervening skin bridges.

## Cutaneous Pedicle Grafts

In patients with moderate-sized defects of the perineum or vulva (6 to 8 cm or less in width) after vulvectomy, cutaneous pedicle grafts can readily close the defect (Julian et al, 1971; Barnhill et al, 1983). A vulvoplasty is performed in a manner similar to that described for primary closure of incisions at the time of vulvectomy (Berek, 1989). Occasionally, only a unilateral procedure will need to be performed.

In cutaneous pedicle grafting, the skin and subcutaneous tissue are mobilized from the underlying fascia of the transversus perinei muscles and are rotated into position as indicated to close the defect (Berek, 1989) (Fig. 22-14). The incision is carried along the lateral thigh or buttock in order to obtain more extensive ped-

icle. The advantage of this technique is that it permits the surgeon to tailor the size of the skin pedicle graft to the size of the defect (Fig. 22-15).

## Myocutaneous Pedicle Grafts

For larger defects greater than 8 to 10 cm in size, a myocutaneous pedicle graft can be employed. The myocutaneous gracilis pedicle graft procedure has been described by Ballon et al (1979) and Wheeless et al (1979) and can be used to close a unilateral or bilateral defect. The myocutaneous gracilis pedicle is isolated in the manner described above and is rotated 90 degrees into position along the defect. The graft can be placed medial to a preserved skin bridge or can fill the entire space in the event that a skin bridge is absent.

Other pedicles that can be employed in a similar fashion include myocutaneous grafts from the gluteus maximus or, for very large defects, the tensor fascia lata pedicle graft. The tensor fascia lata is raised from the lateral aspect of the thigh, and the width of the graft is determined by the size of the defect. The length of the

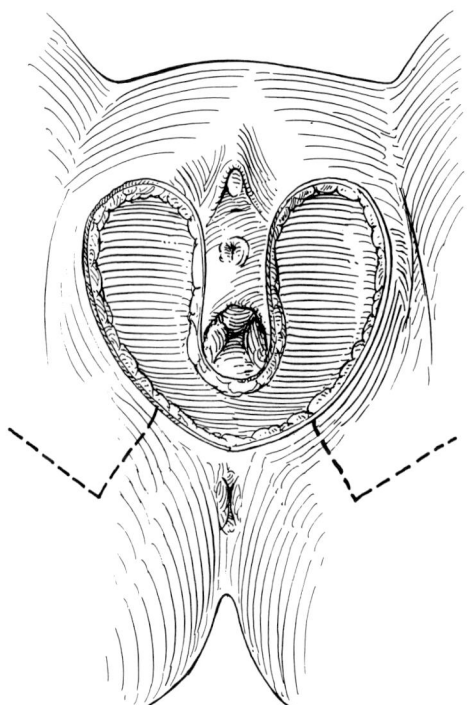

FIGURE 22-14 The rhomboid flap is used to close a posterior vulvar defect. (From Berek JS: General surgical operations. In Berek JS, Hacker NF: *Practical Gynecologic Oncology*. Baltimore, Williams & Wilkins, 1989, pp 509-548.)

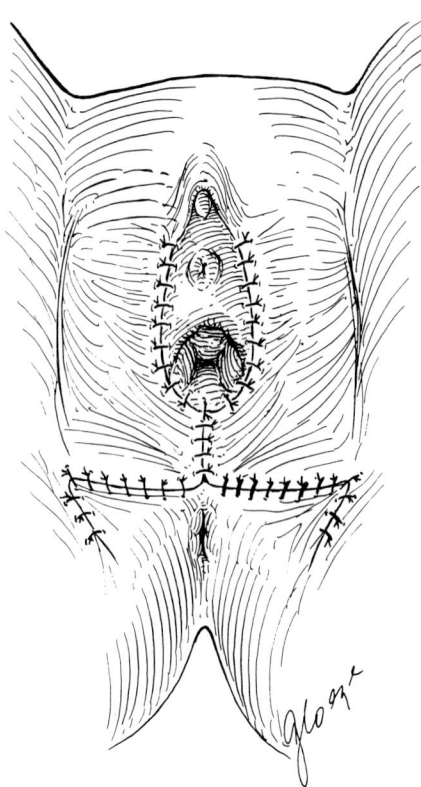

FIGURE 22-15 The pedicle grafts are bilateral "Z plasties" that are sutured together in the midline to close the vulvar defect completely. (From Berek JS: General surgical operations. In Berek JS, Hacker NF: *Practical Gynecologic Oncology*. Baltimore, Williams & Wilkins, 1989, pp 509-548.)

pedicle should not exceed three times the width of its base. The pedicle can be rotated 90 degrees to cover both an inguinal-femoral defect and a vulvar defect.

## PERIANAL RECONSTRUCTION

Anal sphincter incontinence can result from resection of a sizable portion of the sphincter muscle as part of radical surgery for extensive vulvar cancer or as a result of dysfunction secondary to scarring from multiple operations.

Primary surgical correction of sphincter incompetence consists of sphincter plication. This is performed using the uninjured portion of the sphincter or creating a purse-string type of sling around the muscles. The procedures is usually successful when there is sufficient muscular tissue remaining to permit primary reconstruction (Berek *et al*, 1982).

For anal sphincter plication, an incision is made across the anterior sphincter capsule at the level of the residual vaginal mucosa. A flap is then dissected, and the ends of the sphincter are mobilized and delivered. Individual interrupted sutures of absorbable material are placed in the sphincter. The remaining fascia of the sphincter capsule is brought together in a second layer using absorbable suture. This is reinforced by suturing the fascia of the levator ani together across the anterior sphincter. The vaginal incision is then closed with continuous or interrupted sutures.

If standard anal sphincter plication fails, or if there is insufficient muscular tissue to permit reconstruction,

muscle grafting operations might be necessary. Transposition of muscle strips from the gluteus maximus, gracilis, and levator ani has been reported; our preference is to use strips of the gracilis or levator ani muscle.

The levator ani is the broad, thin muscle situated on either side of the pelvis, and these muscles join to form the pelvic floor. The middle fibers of the levator ani insert into the side of the rectum, and the fibers blend with those of the residual anal sphincter and transversus perinei muscle. Thus, they are anatomically in an ideal position for muscle strip grafting. In addition, the nerve and blood supplies are derived from the same source as those of the anal sphincter, permitting a more anatomically suitable reconstruction.

The procedure is initiated by making an incision around the posterior introitus (Fig. 22-16). Using scissors and electrocautery for hemostasis, the vaginal mucosa and perianal skin are dissected bilaterally, and the skin flaps are raised to expose the underlying tissues.

The perirectal fascia is entered by blunt dissection at the level of the vagina, and the fascia overlying the levator ani is identified. Muscle flaps are isolated bluntly at their midportion and then dissected laterally to their origins. Levator ani muscles approximately 2 to 3 cm in width are isolated, and the flaps are mobilized to their origin at the pelvic sidewall to provide maximum length. Hemostasis is achieved using electrocautery to detach the muscles from their origin.

After mobilization, the muscles are brought together

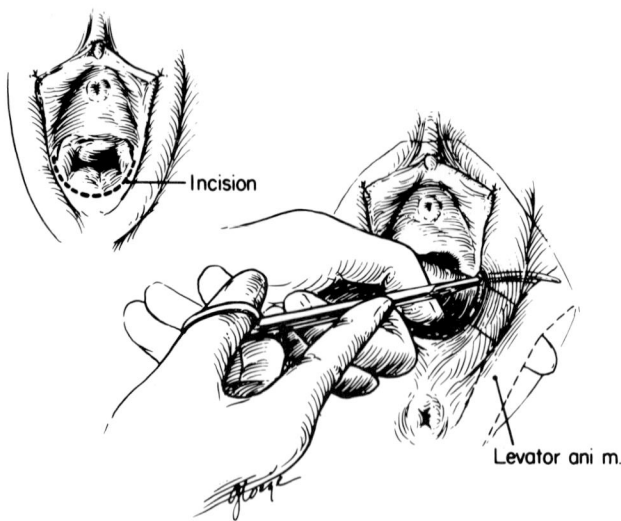

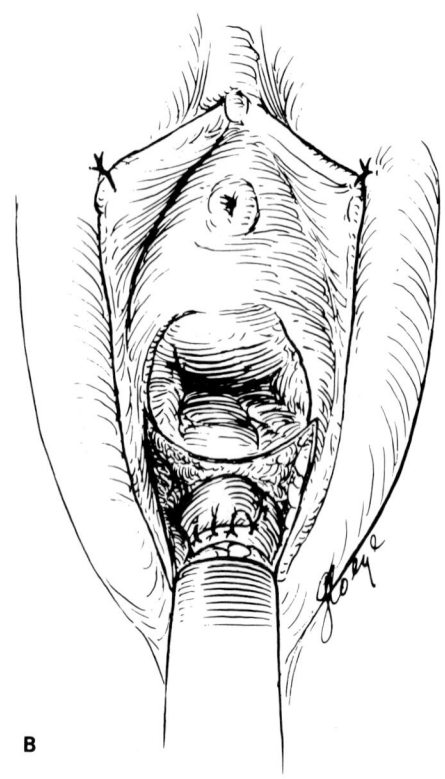

B

FIGURE 22-16  *Left*, the site of incision at the introitus. *Right*, A portion of the levator ani muscle is mobilized bilaterally using blunt and sharp dissection. (From Berek JS, et al: Levator ani transposition for anal incompetence secondary to sphincter damage. *Obstet Gynecol* 59:109, 1982, by permission of The American College of Obstetricians and Gynecologists.)

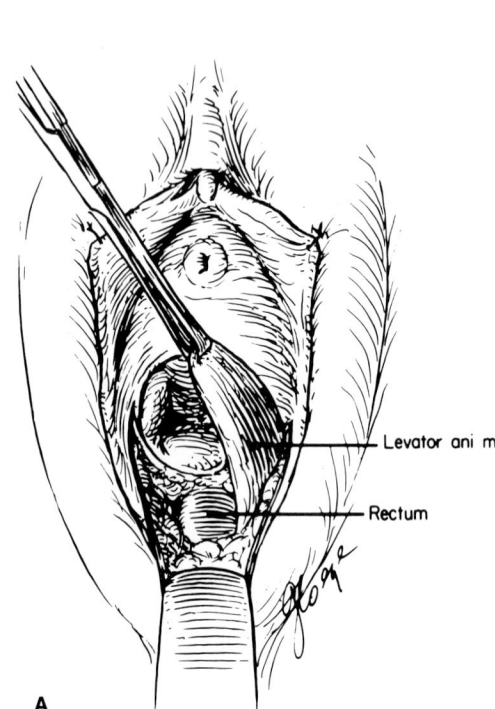

A

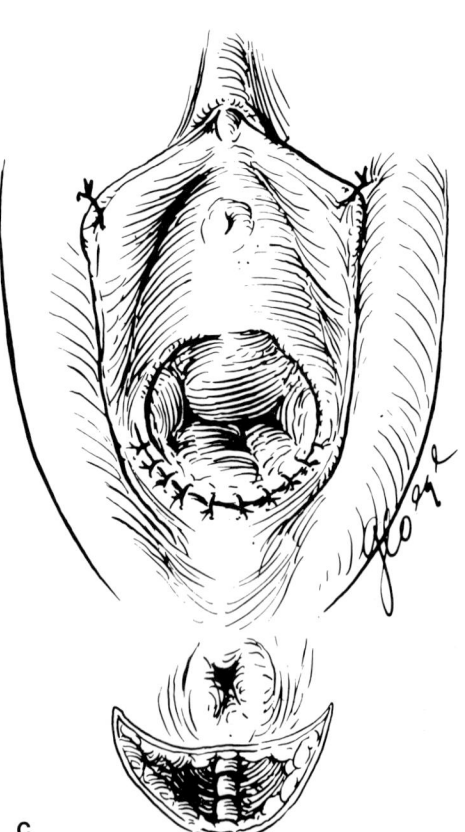

C

FIGURE 22-17  The levator ani muscles are brought together anterior to the rectum (*A*). The muscles and fascia are sutured together so they overlap (*B*). To complete the operation, several plication sutures are placed into the sphincter capsule posteriorly. (From Berek JS, et al: Levator ani transposition for anal incompetence secondary to sphincter damage. *Obstet Gynecol* 59:110, 1982, by permission of The American College of Obstetricians and Gynecologists.)

in the midline anterior to the defective anal sphincter (Fig. 22-17). They are then overlapped and sewn together with their fascia, using interrupted 2-0 braided, absorbable sutures. The plication sutures are placed posteriorly into the sphincter to strengthen and tighten the sphincter further. A finger inserted into the anus must fit snugly. The skin and vaginal mucosa are then approximated.

Postoperatively, patients are treated with a low-residue diet and fecal softeners, as well as with sitz baths two to three times a day for one week in order to minimize perineal discomfort and swelling.

## RECONSTRUCTION OF THE PELVIC FLOOR

At the completion of pelvic exenteration, attention must be paid to reconstruction of the pelvic floor. As outlined above, our preference is to use bilateral myocutaneous gracilis pedicle grafts whenever necessary because this operation simultaneously reconstructs the pelvic floor and provides a neovagina. None of our patients who have undergone this procedure has developed intestinal prolapse, and thus we have found it superior to other techniques described. Alternatively, a bulbocavernosus axial flap can be employed (Leuchter et al, 1982).

In addition, the omentum should be detached from the greater curvature of the stomach (as described earlier), brought inferiorly, and sutured to the pelvic peritoneum laterally to cover the floor of the pelvis or the neovagina (Valle and Ferraris, 1969; Rutledge et al, 1977).

Whenever possible, reperitonealization of as much of the pelvic defect as possible should be performed. Use of a peritoneal pedicle graft has been suggested by Morley and Lindenauer (1971). The pedicle is mobilized from the anterior abdominal wall and brought down into the pelvis to cover the defect. Because of the high incidence of bowel obstruction reported after peritoneal pedicle grafting, Symmonds et al (1975) have recommended using a free peritoneal patch dissected from the anterior abdominal wall. In patients in whom peritonealization is not possible or when the omentum is absent, the remaining contiguous pelvic structures must be approximated as much as possible. A pelvic lid can be created by suturing the residual or reconstructed sigmoid colon to the residual bladder and parietal peritoneum. Approximation of these structures decreases the space on which a free omental or peritoneal graft can be placed.

Synthetic meshes such as Marlex or Teflon have been associated with a high rate of infectious morbidity when utilized for pelvic reconstruction (Webb and Symmonds, 1977), and we therefore do not recommend their use. In addition, we avoid using pelvic packs, since they are not adequate substitutes for careful peritonealization, peritoneal pedicle or free peritoneal grafts, or omental grafts. Peritoneal packs have also been associated with considerable infectious morbidity and subsequent evisceration.

## SUMMARY

Pelvic reconstruction should be performed at the time of pelvic exenterative surgery so as to minimize the need for a secondary procedure and decrease the incidence of postoperative pelvic or vulvar defects. With primary closure of the incisions and operations modified to reduce the extent of radical surgery, the morbidity and permanent sequelae associated with large defects can be minimized.

## REFERENCES

Anderson RL, Hacker NF: Psychosexual adjustments following pelvic exenteration. *Obstet Gynecol* 61:331-338, 1983.

Ballon SC, Donaldson RC, Roberts JA, Lagasse LD: Reconstruction of the vulva using a myocutaneous graft. *Gynecol Oncol* 7:123-127, 1979.

Barnhill DR, Hoskins WJ, Metz P: Use of the rhomboid flap after partial vulvectomy. *Obstet Gynecol* 62:444-447, 1983.

Becker DW, Massey FM, McGraw JB: Musculocutaneous flaps in reconstructive pelvic surgery. *Obstet Gynecol* 54:178-183, 1979.

Berek JS: General surgical operations. In Berek JS, Hacker NF: *Practical Gynecologic Oncology.* Baltimore, Williams and Wilkins, 1989, pp 509-548.

Berek JS, Hacker NF, Lagasse LD: Vaginal reconstruction performed simultaneously with pelvic exenteration. *Obstet Gynecol* 63:318-323, 1984.

Berek JS, Hacker NF, Lagasse LD, Smith ML: Delayed vaginal reconstruction in the fibrotic pelvis following radiation or previous reconstruction. *Obstet Gynecol* 61:743-748, 1983.

Berek JS, Lagasse LD, Hacker NF, Leuchter RS: Levator ani transposition for anal incompetence secondary to sphincter damage. *Obstet Gynecol* 59:108-112, 1982.

Brunschwig A: Complete excision of the pelvic viscera for advanced carcinoma. *Cancer* 1:177-183, 1948.

Bürger RA, Riedmiller H, Knapstein PG, Friedberg V, Hohenfellner R: Ileocecal viginal construction. *Am J Obstet Gynecol* 161:162-167, 1989.

Cain JM, Diamond A, Tamimi HK, Greer BE, Figge DC: The morbidity and benefits of concurrent gracilis myocutaneous graft with pelvic exenteration. *Obstet Gynecol* 75:185-189, 1988.

Copeland LJ, Hancock KC, Gershenson DM, Stringer CA, Atkinson EN, Edwards CL: Gracilis myocutaneous vaginal reconstruction concurrent with total pelvic exenteration. *Am J Obstet Gynecol* 160:1095-1101, 1989.

Day TG, Stanhope R: Vulvovaginoplasty in gynecologic oncology. *Obstet Gynecol* 50:361-364, 1977.

Hacker NF, Leuchter RS, Berek JS, Moore JG, Lagasse LD: Radical vulvectomy and bilateral inguinal lymphadenectomy through separate groin incisions. *Obstet Gynecol* 58:574-579, 1981.

Hatch KD: Construction of a neovagina after exenteration using the vulvobulbocavernosus myocutaneous graft. *Obstet Gynecol* 63:110-114, 1984.

Julian CG, Callison J, Woodruff JD: Plastic management of extensive vulvar defects. *Obstet Gynecol* 38:193-198, 1971.

Karlen JR, Piver MS: Reduction of mortality and morbidity associated with pelvic exenteration. *Gynecol Oncol* 2:154-167, 1975.

Lacy C, Stern J, Feigenbaum S: Vaginal reconstruction after exenteration with use of gracilis myocutaneous flaps: The University of California San Francisco experience. *Am J Obstet Gynecol* 158:1278-1284, 1988.

Lagasse LD, Berman ML, Watring WG: The gynecologic oncology patient: Restoration of function and prevention of disability. In McGowan L (ed): *Gynecologic Oncology.* New York, Appleton-Century-Crofts, 1978, pp 398-400.

Leuchter RS, Lagasse LD, Hacker NF, Berek JS: Management of postexenteration perineal hernias by myocutaneous axial flaps. *Gynecol Oncol* 14:15-22, 1982.

Magrina JF, Masterson BJ: Vaginal reconstruction in gynecologic oncology: A review of techniques. *Obstet Gynecol Surv* 36:1-10, 1981.

McGraw JB, Massey FM, Shanklin KD, Horton CE: Vaginal reconstruction with gracilis myocutaneous flaps. *Plast Reconstr Surg* 58:176-183, 1976.

McIndoe AH, Banister JB: An operation for the care of congenital absence of the vagina. *J Obstet Gynaecol Br Emp* 45:490-498, 1938.

Morley GW, Lindenauer SM: Peritoneal grafts in total pelvic exenteration. *Am J Obstet Gynecol* 11:696-701, 1971.

Morley GW, Lindenauer SM: Pelvic exenterative therapy for gynecologic malignancy: An analysis of 70 cases. *Cancer* 38:581-586, 1976.

Morley GW, Lindenauer SM, Youngs D: Vaginal reconstruction following pelvic exenteration—surgical and psychological considerations. *Am J Obstet Gynecol* 116:996-1002, 1973.

Morrow CP, Lacey CG, Lucas WE: Reconstructive surgery in gynecologic oncology employing the gracilis myocutaneous pedicle graft. *Gynecol Oncol* 7:176-187, 1979.

Pratt JH, Smith GR: Vaginal reconstruction with a sigmoid loop. *Am J Obstet Gynecol* 96:31-40, 1966.

Rutledge FN, Smith JP, Wharton JT, O'Quinn AG: Pelvic exentertion: Analysis of 296 patients. *Am J Obstet Gynecol* 129:881-892, 1977.

Schellhas HF, Fidhar JP: Vaginal reconstruction after total pelvic exenteration using a modification of the Williams procedure. *Gynecol Oncol* 3:21-31, 1975.

Symmonds RE, Pratt JH, Webb MJ: Exenterative operations: Experience with 198 patients. *Am J Obstet Gynecol* 121:907-918, 1975.

Valle G, Ferraris G: Use of the omentum to contain the intestines in pelvic exenteration. *Obstet Gynecol* 33:772-775, 1989.

Watring WG, Lagasse LD, Smith ML, Johnson GH, Moore JG, Berman ML: Vaginal reconstruction following extensive treatment for pelvic cancer. *Am J Obstet Gynecol* 125:809-814, 1976.

Webb MJ, Symmonds RE: Management of the pelvic floor after pelvic exenteration. *Obstet Gynecol* 50:166-171, 1977.

Wheeless CR, McGibbon B, Dorsey JH, Maxwell GP: Gracilis myocutaneous flap in reconstruction of the vulva and female perineum. *Obstet Gynecol* 54:97-102, 1979.

Williams EA: Congenital absence of the vagina: A simple operation for its relief. *J Obstet Gynaecol Br Commonw* 71:511-512, 1964.

# Chapter 23 | Nutritional Support of the Patient with Cancer

*Maureen MacBurney*   *Donnamarie Maguire*

*Douglas W. Wilmore\**

In the perioperative period, the surgeon must prepare the patient to withstand the physiologic stresses imposed by the surgical procedure and take steps to minimize postoperative complications. Major perioperative risk factors include older age, obesity, associated chronic illness, cardiorespiratory dysfunction, and malnutrition.

In this chapter we will address the issue of nutritional care for patients with gynecologic cancer. In addition to perioperative nutritional support, specialized feedings are often needed for the patient with chronic bowel obstruction who requires operative treatment, chemotherapy, or radiation therapy or for those in the final stages of their disease who require intravenous support in the home setting.

## IMPORTANCE OF NUTRITIONAL STATUS

For patients with complex diseases such as gynecologic malignancies, optimal care requires multimodality ther-

apy. Not only are a variety of therapeutic approaches necessary to extirpate and control the cancer, but additional measures are required to treat complications such as concurrent infections or obstruction of the gastrointestinal or urinary tract. Multiple operations, recurring infections, and slow-growing intraabdominal tumors all contribute to the patient's nutritional debility, which may prolong recovery or impede survival.

For example, it has been observed that weight loss of approximately 30 to 40% of ideal body weight is usually lethal (Studley, 1936). In healthy individuals who have lost approximately 10% of their body weight, maximal physical performance is impaired (Keys and Brozek, 1950). Between these two extremes, progressive weight loss further debilitates a patient and affects normal immunologic and organ responses as well as impairing wound healing and tissue repair. In general, morbidity correlates closely with losses of body weight between the extremes of 10 and 30% (Studley, 1936).

A variety of *physiologic and biologic responses* are associated with nutritional status and are thus affected by malnutrition. For example, wound healing is prolonged during states of malnutrition. However, animal studies have shown that tissue repair is significantly altered only after nutritional deficits have become severe

\* Research supported by Trauma Grant #5 P50 GM36428-05.

(Irvin, 1978). This has generally been the impression among clinicians, although in one recent study postoperative nutritional support in well-nourished patients improved hydroxyproline deposition in an implanted Dacron tube compared with the response in conventionally treated patients (Haydock and Hill, 1987). In contrast to studies examining the effects of protein and calorie deficiency on wound healing, tissue responses are unequivocally impaired in patients with specific vitamin or trace element deficits. Selective deficiencies result in well-recognized syndromes that impair wound healing, such as scurvy.

The importance of nutrition in supporting *host defenses* against infection is also well known. The detrimental effects of generalized or specific dietary deficiencies on the development of acquired immunity in experimental animals have been adequately documented (Scrimshaw et al, 1959). Similar studies in humans are extremely difficult to interpret, since numerous factors exert immunosuppressive effects on host defense mechanisms. The patient with gynecologic cancer is a case in point; although immunosuppression may be associated with nutritional depletion, there is no assurance that correction of nutritional deficits will correct the immune dysfunction. Such immunosuppression may be related to the effects of the tumor burden or concomitant infection, or the impact of chemotherapy or radiotherapy.

However, it is well established that preoperative *anergy* is related to an increased incidence of postoperative septic complications. In a study of 60 patients admitted to a general surgical service, 26 showed normal skin test reactivity and 34 were anergic or relatively anergic (MacLean, 1979). The rate of sepsis in the 26 normal reactors was 15% and no deaths, whereas this rate was 25% in those with relative anergy and 59% in those with anergy, with mortality rates of 17% and 14%, respectively. Further studies by the same group demonstrated that some, but not all, of the anergic patients could be rendered immunologically responsive by means of preoperative nutritional support (Spanier et al, 1976).

In addition to immunologic defects associated with poor nutrition, *functional losses* also occur. The malnourished patient is less active, so that complications such as thrombophlebitis and pulmonary embolism occur more frequently. With the loss of strength, the ability to generate normal intrathoracic pressures and inspiratory volumes is decreased. In addition, the incidence of pneumonia is higher among malnourished patients compared with well-nourished control subjects. Among patients who require mechanical ventilation, weaning from the ventilator may be delayed (Driver and Lebrun, 1980).

Thus, malnutrition impairs a patient's ability to recover from surgical or other treatments. Immunosuppression, decreased wound healing, and decreased strength are common functional problems associated with nutritional deficits. However, in patients with advanced carcinoma, it may not be possible to correct these nutritional defects. Even when the defects have apparently been corrected, the associated problems may persist.

# RECOGNIZING MALNUTRITION

Nutritional assessment comprises a combination of techniques that measure body composition, secretory protein status, and immune function. Results are then compared with normal values, and a nutritional diagnosis is made (e.g., normal or mildly, moderately, or severely malnourished). The purpose of a nutritional assessment is to identify patients at "nutritional risk," to arrive at an appropriate nutrient prescription, and to evaluate the adequacy of the nutritional therapy. Based on this assessment, the physician should be able to determine the degree of protein-calorie depletion and accordingly prescribe the amount of calories and nitrogen needed for the patient to maintain weight or to replete body mass. Such an approach should also identify those patients at risk for increased morbidity and mortality due to nutritional deficiencies.

Since many of the measurements used to assess nutritional status are not specific to a patient's nutritional state, it is best to evaluate a combination of measurements rather than a single variable. Use of only one indicator, such as serum albumin, is likely to lead to a misdiagnosis of nutritional status and therefore inappropriate therapy.

## Body Composition

***Body Weight*** Body weight, a common, simple and readily available measurement, is used to assess changes in energy balance. Weight may be lost as a result of decreased food intake or increased energy requirements. Frequent, serial measurements of body weight—expressed in terms of percentage of usual weight, percentage of ideal body weight (IBW), and rate of weight loss (or gain)—provide the most useful information about how the energy balance is altered over time.

Height and weight should be measured, since the patient's recall may not be reliable. Body weight that is less than 80% of ideal body weight or a decrease in weight of 10% of the usual body weight within the past 6 months indicates that the patient is at risk for malnutrition, even when the patient is obese. When this degree of weight loss is identified, a nutrition history is taken to confirm the etiology of the weight loss (e.g., decreased food intake versus increased energy expenditure) (Table 23-1) and to determine the quality of the

| TABLE 23-1  Etiology of Weight Loss | |
| --- | --- |
| Decreased Intake | Increased Requirements |
| Depression | Infection/fever |
| Financial | Diarrhea/malabsorption |
| Dieting | Cancer |
| Poor dentition | Chronic bleeding |
| Anorexia | Steroids |
| Alcohol or drug abuse | Disease process |
| Nausea and/or vomiting | Hyperthyroidism |
| Tumor burden | |
| Chemotherapy and/or radiation therapy | |

patient's intake over the past month in terms of calories, protein, and other specific nutrients. The main problems with the reliability of body weight measurements, particularly in the hospitalized patient, are inconsistent measurement techniques and variations in the patient's hydration status (Table 23-2).

In the patient with gynecologic cancer, the assessment of weight is complicated by the tumor burden and ascites. Weight loss is a particularly ominous sign in women with breast cancer. Survival time is significantly reduced in women who lose even a small amount of weight (5%). Complete remission in response to chemotherapy is 2.5 times more frequent in patients who do not lose weight compared with those who show any degree of weight loss. Whether or not correcting weight loss will improve the outcome in this group of patients has not been determined, however (DeWys et al, 1981). Comparable data are not available in patients with ovarian or uterine malignancies.

**Anthropometrics** Anthropometric measurements other than height and weight are intended to provide additional information regarding body composition, i.e., the amount of body fat and skeletal muscle (Table 23-2).

*Measuring triceps skinfold (TSF)* thickness will determine the amount of subcutaneous fat present compared with "normal" values. Although TSF is relatively easy to measure, special skinfold calipers and an *experienced technician* are required to obtain accurate data. Approximately 4 to 6 months or practice involving repeated measurements are necessary before one is able to obtain reliable, reproducible measurements.

TSF measurements can be employed in certain equations to determine the degree of depletion (Table 23-2). These will provide information about the absolute amount of total body adipose mass, which can be compared with normal values. In addition, a person's loss of fat mass can be monitored by measuring TSF serially over time. The main variables associated with use of this measurement are inter- and intraobserver variations and differences due to sex, aging, hydration status, degree of obesity, and athletic activities.

*Mid-arm muscle circumference (MAMC)* provides a measure of skeletal mass by calculating muscle mass in the upper arm. It requires accurate measurement of the TSF (see above) and assumes symmetry of the upper arm. Although measurements of TSF and MAMC may be compared with standard values to assess the degree of depletion, they are most useful for detecting changes in an individual over time and are relatively insensitive to short-term changes.

**Techniques** Detailed explanations of the proper measurement techniques are available from many sources (Rombeau et al, 1989a; Krey and Murray, 1986).

**Standards** Ideally, the standards used for assessing a patient's status should reflect the population being examined. The results of the National Health and Nutrition Examination Survey (NHANES), conducted from 1971 to 1974, are fairly representative of the population of the United States. Tables 23-3 and 23-4 list average weights and TSF and MAMC values for women 18 to

**TABLE 23-2  Nutritional Assessment**

| Measurement | Indicators | Factors Affecting Variability |
|---|---|---|
| I. *Anthropometrics (Women)* | | |
| A.  Body weight | | Hydration status |
| Ideal body weight (IBW) = Standard of weight for height and age | | Ascites |
| | | Standards used |
| | | Measurement technique |
| % IBW = $\frac{\text{Actual weight}}{\text{IBW}} \times 100$ | < 80% IBW | |
| % Usual weight = $\frac{\text{Actual weight}}{\text{Usual weight}} \times 100$ | | |
| % Weight change = $\frac{(\text{Usual—Actual weight})}{\text{Usual weight}} \times 100$ | ≥ 10% decrease in usual body weight over the past 6 months | |
| B.  Triceps skinfold thickness (TSF) in mm: Assesses loss of fatty tissue  Standard = 16.5 | 90% standard = 14.9 mm  90 to 60% standard = 14.8 to 9.9 mm  < 60% standard = < 9.9 mm | For both TSF and MAMC:  Hydration status  Most useful as serial measurements over time; insensitive to short-term changes |
| C.  Mid-arm muscle circumference (MAMC) (in cm): Assesses loss of lean tissue  MAMC = Arm circumference (cm) − (0.314) × TSF (mm)  Standard = 23.2 cm | 90% standard = 20.9 cm  90 to 60% standard = 20.8 to 13.9 cm  < 60% standard = 13.9 cm | Difficult to obtain in obese and elderly  Age  Activity  Skill of observer |

*(continued)*

TABLE 23-2 Nutritional Assessment *(continued)*

| Measurement | Indicators | Factors Affecting Variability |
|---|---|---|
| II. *Biochemical Parameters* | | |
| A. Albumin (g/dl)<br>   Normal = 3.5 to 5.5<br>   Half-life 17 to 20 days | Moderate depletion 2.1 to 2.9<br>Severe depletion < 2.1 | Hydration status<br>Age<br>Disease state(s):<br>   —nephrotic syndrome<br>   —inflammation<br>   —trauma<br>   —protein-losing enteropathy<br>   —liver disease<br>   —diarrhea<br>   —fistula<br>   —infections |
| B. Transferrin (mg/dl)<br>   Normal = 170 to 250<br>   Half-life 8 to 10 days | Moderate depletion 150 to 170<br>Severe depletion < 150 | Chronic infection<br>Hydration status<br>Chronic liver disease<br>Iron status<br>Pregnancy or estrogen therapy |
| C. Blood urea nitrogen (BUN) mg/dl | Depletion < 5 mg/dl | Stress<br>Hydration<br>Hepatic and renal function |
| D. Total lymphocyte count (TLC)<br>   (in cu mm)<br>   Normal = 1,500 to 4,000<br>   TLC =<br>   $\dfrac{\text{WBC} \times \% \text{ Total lymphocytes}}{100}$ | Moderate depletion 800 to 1,499<br>Severe depletion < 800 | Decreased in<br>   —pneumonia<br>   —sepsis<br>   —malignancies<br>   —chemotherapy<br>   —uremia<br>Increased in<br>   —infectious hepatitis<br>   —tuberculosis<br>   —leukemia<br>   —fever<br>   —adrenal insufficiency |
| III. *Delayed cutaneous hypersensitivity*<br>   Normal = reactive | Depleted = anergic (no reaction)<br>Relatively anergic response to only 2<br>   antigens | Age<br>Malignant disease<br>Drugs<br>Zinc deficiency<br>Sepsis<br>Trauma<br>Infection<br>Radiation therapy |

*Source:* Adapted from Murray R: Interpreting the nutrition assessment. In Krey SH, Murray RL (eds): *Dynamics of Nutrition Support: Assessment, Implementation, Evaluation.* Norwalk, Connecticut, Appleton-Century-Crofts, 1986, p 171.

75 years of age taken from the NHANES (National Center for Health Statistics, 1987).

## Biochemical Measurements

Several proteins synthesized in the liver are sometimes measured to assess protein nutrition. These proteins include albumin, transferrin, pre-albumin, and retinol binding protein, with serum albumin and transferrin being most commonly used for this purpose (Table 23-2).

*Albumin* is often measured during routine blood screening and is therefore usually already noted on the patient's record. *Transferrin* may be measured directly from serum or calculated using serum iron and total iron-binding capacity (TIBC), although the direct measurement is the more accurate one.

Depressed concentrations of serum albumin and transferrin may reflect an inadequate intake of protein, as is found in primary malnutrition. However, in the acutely or chronically ill patient, many factors affect the interpretation of these measurements. For example, the distribution of albumin into ascitic fluid will lower its serum concentration, even though the total albumin mass may be increased. Although serum albumin levels may not be directly related to nutritional status, a low level is a fairly sensitive predictor of outcome (Hickman et al, 1980).

*Serum pre-albumin* and *retinol binding protein* are less frequently measured because they are not readily available in many laboratories. Because of their short half-life they may be more sensitive indicators of inadequate intake or nutritional repletion (Krey and Murray, 1986).

TABLE 23-3   Average Weight* for Height for Women Ages 18 to 74

| Height (in) | Age Group (yr) | | | | | |
|---|---|---|---|---|---|---|
| | 18-24 | 25-34 | 35-44 | 45-54 | 55-64 | 65-74 |
| 57 | 114 | 118 | 125 | 129 | 132 | 130 |
| 58 | 117 | 121 | 129 | 133 | 136 | 134 |
| 59 | 120 | 125 | 133 | 136 | 140 | 137 |
| 60 | 123 | 128 | 137 | 140 | 143 | 140 |
| 61 | 126 | 132 | 141 | 143 | 147 | 144 |
| 62 | 129 | 136 | 144 | 147 | 150 | 147 |
| 63 | 132 | 139 | 148 | 150 | 153 | 151 |
| 64 | 135 | 142 | 152 | 154 | 157 | 154 |
| 65 | 138 | 146 | 156 | 158 | 160 | 158 |
| 66 | 141 | 150 | 159 | 161 | 164 | 161 |
| 67 | 144 | 153 | 163 | 165 | 167 | 165 |
| 68 | 147 | 157 | 167 | 168 | 171 | 169 |

* Estimated values from regression equations of weight on height for specified age groups.
*Note:* Persons examined were measured without shoes; weight of clothing ranged from 0.20 to 0.62 pound, which was not deducted from weights shown.
*Source:* National Center for Health Statistics: Weight by height and age for adults 18-74 years. United States 1971-1974. Rockville, MD: National Center for Health Statistics, 1979. Vital and Health Statistics, Series II: Data from the National Health and Nutrition Examination Survey (NHANES), No 208. DHEW Publication No (PHS) 79-1656, 1979.

*Blood urea nitrogen* (BUN) decreases with low protein intakes and starvation. However, under conditions of stress, the BUN will increase as ureagenesis is accelerated or renal function altered.

### Assessment of Immunocompetence

*Delayed cutaneous hypersensitivity (DCH)* may be assessed to determine the impact of malnutrition on components of the immune system. The body's ability to respond to an antigen challenge can be assessed by means of the intradermal injection of multiple antigens. If induration exceeding 5 mm is seen at 24 or 48 hours, the patient is assumed to be immunocompetent. However, if there is little or no induration or a response to only one antigen, the patient is considered to be anergic or relatively anergic. Antigens commonly used for such

TABLE 23-4   Triceps Skinfold Thickness (TSF) and Mid-Arm Muscle Circumference (MAMC) in Women Ages 18 to 74

| Age Group | TSF (mm²)* | MAMC (mm²)* |
|---|---|---|
| 18 | 18 | 202 |
| 19-24 | 18 | 207 |
| 25-34 | 21 | 212 |
| 35-44 | 23 | 218 |
| 45-54 | 25 | 220 |
| 55-64 | 25 | 225 |
| 65-74.9 | 24 | 225 |

* 50th percentile.
*Source:* National Center for Health Statistics: Weight by height and age for adults 18-74 years. United States 1971-1974. Rockville, MD: National Center for Health Statistics, 1979. Vital and Health Statistics, Series II: Data from the National Health and Nutrition Examination Survey (NHANES), No 208. DHEW Publication No (PHS) 79-1656, 1979.

skin tests include *Candida*, tuberculin, mumps, *Trichophyton*, and dinitrochlorobenzene (DNCB) (Clark, 1986).

The usefulness of skin testing as a routine component of nutritional assessment was examined in a critical review by Twomey et al (1982). These authors concluded that its usefulness could not be proved in most of the studies owing to problems in experimental design and the low specificity of abnormal DCH responses. Recently Braga et al (1988) performed nutritional assessments using serum albumin, total iron-binding capacity, and weight loss and compared the presence of malnutrition with DCH responses as a prognostic indicator for postoperative septic complications in 405 patients. Among the malnourished patients, the incidence of postoperative sepsis was 37%. In patients who were anergic or relatively anergic, the incidence was 29.6%. He concluded that nutritional assessment and DCH responses contribute independently in predicting postoperative sepsis. However, it is important to note that among patients with DCH depression the incidence of postoperative sepsis was significantly higher in the malnourished group (37%) than in the normally nourished group (19%).

Some advocate determination of the *total lymphocyte count (TLC)* as an indicator of immune function. However, like skin testing, this measurement is relatively nonspecific and can be affected by many non-nutritional variables (Table 23-2).

## PATIENTS REQUIRING NUTRITIONAL ASSESSMENT

Anyone who presents with a history of recent weight loss or whose intake has been inadequate for more than 5 days because of physical symptoms, tests, medical therapies, surgery, or trauma should undergo a nutritional assessment. In addition, certain groups of patients are at high risk for malnutrition (Table 23-5). Early assessment and serial monitoring in these patients can provide useful information about possible nutritional changes as well as guidelines for nutritional intervention.

## MALNUTRITION AND GYNECOLOGIC CANCER

So far, there is little information regarding the incidence of malnutrition in women with gynecologic cancer. In 1983, Tunca examined the nutritional status of 97 women with cervical (35), endometrial (25), ovarian (28), and vulvar (9) cancer within 4 weeks of the initial diagnosis. Patients were assessed by determining weight loss, serum albumin and transferrin, total lymphocyte count, and DCH reaction. Only among those patients with Stage III and IV ovarian cancer was there a high prevalence of malnutrition (p < 0.01); for all other patients in all stages nutritional assessment parameters

| TABLE 23-5 Patients Likely to Become Malnourished | | |
|---|---|---|
| Chronic Disease | Gastrointestinal Abnormalities | Other |
| Malignancies | Pancreatic disease | Surgery |
| Kidney or liver disease | Inflammatory bowel disease | Chemotherapy |
| Peptic ulcer disease | Fistula | Radiation therapy |
| Diabetes mellitus | Diarrhea | |
| Congestive heart failure | Short bowel syndrome | |
| | Nausea and vomiting | |

were near-normal except for a slight recent weight loss (0.5 to 3.6 kg).

Orr et al (1985) prospectively assessed 78 patients within 24 hours of their being hospitalized to evaluate and treat cervical cancer. Although weight loss occurred in 35% of the patients, the mean weight-for-height ratio was still above the standards for normal (i.e., greater than 100%). Patients with Stage III and IV cancer were more likely to have sustained a 10 pound weight loss (p < 0.05) than were those with less extensive disease. Height/weight correlated directly with TSF (p < 0.001) and MAMC (p < 0.001). Abnormal anthropometrics were significantly more common in the patients with advanced cancer (Stages III and IV). Low albumin concentrations correlated positively with anergy, low total iron-binding capacity, and advancing stage of the disease. No patient had severe protein-calorie malnutrition, and approximately 12% showed evidence of moderate malnutrition that correlated with a history of recent weight loss. About one-third of the patients were anergic or hyporesponsive to all antigens, unrelated to the stage of disease; however, this response may have been related to the presence of tumor and not the presence of a nutritional deficit.

These studies indicate that, in general, women with newly diagnosed, untreated gynecologic cancer are not at high risk for nutritional deficits except in advanced stages of cervical and ovarian cancer. However, once the patient has been diagnosed, multimodality treatment is often initiated, which impacts on nutritional status.

## CAUSES OF MALNUTRITION

Changes in nutritional indicators observed in the late stages of ovarian cancer and some cervical cancer can be attributed to effects of the disease itself as well as its treatment. Patients frequently present with complaints of early satiety and dyspepsia. Fuller and Griffiths (1979) attribute the cachexia observed in ovarian cancer to its late diagnosis, which in turn is due to its silent spread and subtle, nonspecific symptoms. In its advanced stages, ovarian cancer is characterized by gastrointestinal debility. Recurrent symptoms of obstruction are caused by seromuscular infiltration of small bowel by tumor, which decreases intestinal motility and leads to stasis and segmental ileus. Adhesions of the

gastrointestinal tract may also develop. Delayed emptying of the stomach causes a decrease in appetite.

Gastrointestinal complications are associated with treatment throughout the duration of the disease. Radiation therapy affects the intestine because of its proximity to the radiation field and may cause symptoms ranging from mild enteritis to severe stenosis, perforation, and fistulization (Lavery et al, 1980). Repeated small bowel resections and fistula formation are not uncommon following operative intervention. Operative resection or bypass may result in the *short bowel syndrome*, which requires long-term specialized support. All forms of chemotherapy are associated with diminished food intake because of diarrhea and anorexia. Thus, a reduced food intake and/or altered bowel function are major reasons for the weight loss in these patients.

Another major cause of weight loss and depletion of lean body mass associated with cancer is the accelerated catabolism associated with various forms of treatment. Intraabdominal operations are often associated with negative nitrogen balance, with net protein catabolism occurring even when specialized nutritional support is provided during the perioperative period. Similarly, the effects of chemotherapy and radiation therapy enhance net protein breakdown even in the face of "adequate" nutrient intake. Finally, infection—the most frequent complication of multimodality cancer therapy—is known to be a major stimulus accelerating net protein breakdown and causing hypermetabolism. Feeding only attenuates the protein loss but does not totally abate the negative nitrogen balance associated with this complication

Finally, weight loss may be attributed to the metabolic effects of the tumor itself, since this rapidly growing mass of cells consumes nutrients and oxygen and may elaborate molecules that exert control over the host's metabolic response. One of the earliest effects of the cancer is anorexia, which results in initial weight loss. This response is probably due to the elaboration of cytokines, such as tumor necrosis factor or the interleukins, by host macrophages that are attempting to control or destroy the tumor cells. As the tumor progresses, additional changes are observed in the host metabolism; with progressive disease, changes in the metabolism of virtually all substrates have been reported (Douglas and Shaw, 1990).

Metastatic cancer has been associated with glucose intolerance and insulin resistance, accelerated nitrogen turnover and negative nitrogen balance, and increased mobilization and utilization of body lipid. Some of these effects may be attributed to diminished food intake or alterations that occur following therapy; however, these changes often persist or become manifest while parenteral or tube feeding is provided at a fixed rate over a prolonged period of time, thereby demonstrating the priming effect of the tumor. These metabolic changes must be kept in mind as specialized feeding is instituted, since the provision of substrate may not reverse the metabolic abnormalities in the tumor-bearing host. The catabolic response can be reversed only by removal of the tumor.

# NUTRITIONAL DEPLETION AND THE NEED FOR SPECIALIZED NUTRITIONAL INTERVENTION

There is little doubt that individuals who are malnourished (> 10% weight loss, albumin < 3.5 mg/dl, transferrin < 170 mg/dl, and anergy) have a greater incidence of postoperative complications and have decreased survival when complications do occur compared with normally nourished individuals.

The following issues should be addressed with regard to patients with gynecologic cancer:

1. Has poor nutrient intake altered the nutritional indicators?
2. Are indicators that are often thought to reflect nutritional changes simply indicators of patient prognosis and/or surgical risk?
3. Will improved nutritional intake normalize these indicators, or are they abnormal as a result of the cancer and its effect on the host (Krey and Murray, 1986)?
4. Will improved nutritional intake improve patient outcome from the disease process?
5. Will improved nutritional intake improve outcome from secondary complications (i.e., short bowel syndrome)?

Terada et al (1988) examined 88 patients with gynecologic disease who received 99 courses of parenteral nutrition: 92 courses in women with a variety of gynecologic malignancies and 7 courses in those with nonmalignant gynecologic conditions. All patients received adequate calories and protein for a mean of 14 days. Clinical outcome was poor for the women with poor nutritional indicators. However, the authors did not attempt to correlate improvement of nutritional parameters with improvement in clinical outcome.

Bozzetti et al (1987) were able to prevent further nutritional deterioration in 12 patients with cancer cachexia associated with a mean weight loss of 16.9% of usual body weight. After 20 days of nutritional intervention, five nutritional indicators improved—body weight, TSF, arm fat area, retinol binding protein, and nitrogen balance. The impact on survival was not examined. Bozzetti (1989) later reviewed the nutritional and metabolic effects of parenteral and enteral nutrition in adult cancer patients. Only studies that included data on tumor type, intake, and statistical analysis of the results were considered. Nutritional indicators that improved with parenteral or enteral nutrition were body weight, fat mass, nitrogen balance, and total body potassium; no indicators worsened during nutritional deterioration, but cachexia was rarely reversible.

Heber et al (1986) studied the metabolic response to hypercaloric feeding in six patients with nonmetastatic head and neck cancer who had significant weight loss (79% usual body weight, 77% ideal body weight). Patients were enterally fed at 125% basal requirements for 7 days; the feeding was then increased to 225% basal requirements for 19 days. During this time there were no significant changes in body weight or nitrogen balance despite supranormal calorie intake. However, serum urea increased significantly and in proportion to the protein intake. The authors interpreted this response to indicate that protein anabolism did not occur in response to increased calorie and protein intake.

Ovarian cancer is the leading cause of death due to gynecologic cancer and the fourth leading cause of cancer death in women (Clarke-Pearson et al, 1988). Gastrointestinal complications that interfere with the woman's ability to maintain a normal nutrient intake are also common. Ovarian cancer is the leading cause of bowel obstruction in gynecologic patients, and 50% of those women who die of this disease can be expected to develop obstruction at some time during their illness, most commonly of the small bowel (Krebs and Goplerud, 1987; Tunca et al, 1981). In the advanced stages, ovarian cancer may also cause intestinal dysmotility. These patients are often in terminal stages of their disease (Tunca et al, 1981).

Intestinal metastases and obstruction become more likely as the stage of cancer advances. In a study by Tunca et al (1981), the median time between diagnosis and intestinal obstruction was 181 days in patients with Stage III disease and 72.5 days in Stage IV. Mean survival after obstruction was 72 days for complete obstruction and 127 days for partial obstruction. Unfortunately, the majority of cases of ovarian cancer were diagnosed during the later stages of disease. To date, there is no evidence that aggressive nutritional intervention can alter the outcome in these cases (Tunca et al, 1981; Krebs and Goplerud, 1983; Clarke-Pearson et al, 1987). In a small series reviewed by Clarke-Pearson et al (1987), major postoperative complications, including wound infections, fistulas, and sepsis, occurred in 49% of patients with bowel obstruction due to ovarian cancer.

# INDICATIONS FOR NUTRITIONAL INTERVENTION

## Preoperative Feeding

As discussed earlier, many studies have described an association between malnutrition and an increased incidence of postoperative complications (Rombeau et al, 1989b). In some patients, preoperative feeding will improve the abnormal laboratory and anthropometric measurements associated with malnutrition (Mullen et al, 1980). However, the critical issue is *whether preoperative feedings can lower the incidence of postoperative complications and hence reduce the hospital stay and associated hospital costs.*

Two studies have compared the use of preoperative *enteral* feedings to no preoperative nutritional support and found that the former was beneficial (Shukla et al, 1984; Foschi et al, 1986). Patients supported for 10 to 21 days with tube feedings using a polymeric diet were compared with control patients who received an ad lib hospital diet. Those who received fixed enteral nutrition had a lower incidence of postoperative wound infections, anastomotic disruption, and other complications compared with control subjects. This shortened the hospital stay in a population that had a variety of clinical disorders, including both benign and malignant diseases.

Can these results be extrapolated to the use of preoperative *parenteral* nutrition? Prior to 1986, three randomized prospective trials reported benefit, whereas three others did not (Rombeau et al, 1989*b*). The largest of these studies involved patients with gastrointestinal cancer. Both incidence of major complications and mortality rate were reduced in the patients who received preoperative parenteral nutrition (Miller et al, 1982).

Since then, a larger study has been performed and can now be used as the basis for current recommendations. Sponsored by the Veterans Administration, this study compared the effects of standard care to preoperative feeding in 460 patients (Buzby, 1988). The study revealed no overall reduction in mortality but did indicate some benefit among the most severely malnourished patients. Patients who received preoperative parenteral nutrition appeared to have fewer major noninfectious complications, such as those related to prolonged immobility (venous thromboses or pulmonary emboli) and impaired wound healing (dehiscence and fistula formation). The infection rate among these patients was substantially higher than that among the control subjects; however, this could not be fully explained by the presence of the central venous catheter. Among the moderately malnourished patients, the increase in infectious complications offset any benefit from the reduction in noninfectious complications. In the severely malnourished group, however, the reduction in noninfectious complications was sufficient to significantly reduce the complication rate. In practical terms, this means that *patients with a weight loss of 15% or more of usual body weight will benefit from 10 to 15 days of preoperative nutritional support.*

### Perioperative Feeding

Enteral feedings are difficult after an abdominal operation, particularly if there is extensive and residual malignancy. Once gastrointestinal function has been restored, however, postoperative feedings should be instituted, using standard tube feeding techniques if required. In contrast, parenteral nutrition is possible in these patients shortly after the operation. A number of trials assessing perioperative parenteral nutrition have been performed with inconclusive results (Rombeau et al, 1989*b*).

Detsky et al (1987) performed a meta-analysis of 19 randomized or quasirandomized clinical trials assessing the efficacy of perioperative parenteral nutrition in reducing morbidity and mortality from major surgery. Four studies involved only postoperative feeding, five included preoperative feeding only, and 10 covered both periods. Fifteen of the trials involved patients with malignancy. The overall quality of the studies was considered fair to poor in terms of method of patient enrollment, assignment to treatment groups, and assessment of clinical outcomes. Many studies included both well-nourished and malnourished patients. However, the analysis demonstrated that perioperative feeding in unselected patients undergoing major surgery is not justi-

fied, particularly in patients who are well nourished preoperatively and who will resume oral intake within 10 days after the operation. No studies have assessed perioperative parenteral nutrition in subgroups who may be at high risk for postoperative complications, e.g., severely malnourished patients known to have a prolonged postoperative course without food intake.

Until more definitive data are available, it should be standard practice to restrict perioperative parenteral nutrition to malnourished patients whose operations are major, who cannot tolerate enteral nutrition, or in whom prolonged intestinal dysfunction is anticipated (more than 7 to 10 days after the operation).

### Long-Term Feeding

In some patients, long-term nutritional support may be necessary (see also Home Nutritional Support). These include individuals with short-bowel syndrome, pseudo-obstruction, radiation enteritis, carcinomatosis, intestinal fistulas, and possibly chronic intestinal obstruction. When acute problems such as infection and wound healing have been resolved, the patient's ability to take enteral fluids and nutrients should be evaluated. If maintenance by the enteral route would be inadequate or impossible, perioperative parenteral feedings should be continued until the problem resolves. In the absence of sepsis, postoperative resting energy expenditure may be similar to or only slightly higher than preoperative energy requirements. Chronic overfeeding may cause hepatic dysfunction, hyperglycemia, and increased carbon dioxide production. Glucose should be infused at a rate of 4 to 5 mg/kg/min (about 250 to 350 g/day), and amino acids should be administered at a rate no greater than 1.5 g/kg body weight. Lipid emulsions will provide approximately 30% of the resting energy requirements, reducing the potential for hyperglycemia, glycosuria, and abnormal fluid and electrolyte loss. More dilute solutions can be formulated to replace loss from drainage tubes, ostomies, or fistulas.

Realistic goals should be adopted, with end points that can be predictably achieved. For example, the majority of post-traumatic or postoperative fistulas in young, previously healthy individuals will frequently heal and close after 30 days of parenteral nutrition, whereas this success rate is not observed in patients with intraabdominal malignancy or those who have a fistulous tract in an area previously subjected to external radiation (Altomare et al, 1990). For stable patients requiring long-term parenteral feedings and other types of chronic care, transfer to a rehabilitation unit or chronic care facility should be considered. Individuals who require minimal care (other than feeding) should be evaluated for home care (see later). Table 23-6 provides an example of how to calculate energy (calorie) and protein requirements.

### Chemotherapy

The routine use of parenteral nutrition in patients undergoing chemotherapy is associated with a fourfold increase in the risk of significant infection. Intravenous feedings improve neither the response to chemotherapy

---

**TABLE 23-6** Estimating Calorie and Protein Requirements: An Example

A. Calories
1. Calculate *basal metabolic rate* (BMR) - using an accepted formula, such as the Harris-Benedict Equation*:
   (Women only)
   BMR = 655 + [9.6 x weight (kg)] + [1.85 × height (cm)] − [4.7 x age (yr)]
   If the woman is hypermetabolic due to disease or injury, multiply the BMR by a factor to reflect the increased BMR. For example,

   |   |   |
   |---|---|
   | Elective surgery | 1.2 |
   | Sepsis (minor) | 1.3 |

   This figure will give you the *adjusted BMR*.
2. Activity—An additional 25% should be added to the BMR to account for activity:
   BMR x 1.25 = MAINTENANCE CALORIE REQUIREMENTS
3. Weight gain—To achieve weight gain at a rate of 1 to 2 pounds per week, add 500 to 1,000 calories per day to MAINTENANCE calorie requirements:
   MAINTENANCE REQUIREMENTS + 1,000 KCAL = WEIGHT GAIN

B. Protein
1. Normal              0.8 to 1.0 g/kg body weight
2. Stressed            1.5 g/kg body weight

Example: The patient is a 56-year-old woman admitted with small bowel obstruction due to Stage III ovarian cancer. She is status post TAH, BSO, and radiation therapy. Over the past 3 months her intake has included a variety of foods but has been low in total calories.

| | | |
|---|---|---|
| Height = 5'6'' | | |
| Weight = 117 pounds (53 kg) | % weight loss = 22 | |
| Usual weight = 150 pounds (68 kg) | % usual weight = 78 | |
| Ideal weight = 130 pounds (59 kg) | % ideal weight = 90 | |
| Rate of weight loss = 16% over 3 months | | |
| Albumin = 3.0 mg/dl | | |

This patient sustained a significant weight loss (22%) over a short period of time and is therefore a candidate for preoperative feedings for a minimum of 7 days.

*Determining calorie requirements*:
   Goal: Weight gain
   BMR = 655 + (9.6 x 53 kg) + (1.85 x 167.6 cm)
         − (4.7 x 56 yr)
       = 1,211
   BMR + Activity = 1,211 x 1.25 = 1,514 cal/day required
                                   to maintain weight
Maintenance calories + 500 kcal/day = calories to gain weight
   = 1,514 + 500 = 2,014 calories
*Determining protein requirements*:
   Goal: I g protein/kg = 56 g/day

Caloric intake should be targeted to achieve weight maintenance or a steady rate of weight gain and to avoid complications of overfeeding associated with parenteral nutrition.

* Harris JA, Benedict FG: *A Biometric Study of Basal Metabolism in Man*. Washington DC, Carnegie Institute of Washington, Publ No 279, 1919.

---

nor survival. Again, there is the unresolved question of potential benefit in subgroups of patients who are malnourished (American College of Physicians, 1989).

## METHODS OF FEEDING

### Enteral Feeding

Enteral nutrition is the preferred feeding route for all patients in whom it may be used safely. When gastrointestinal output is below 600 ml/24 hr, it is generally considered safe to use the gastrointestinal tract. Intestinal obstruction, paralytic or segmental ileus, and enteric fistulas associated with excessively high output are contraindications to enteral feeding.

***Tube Feeding Sites*** *Nasogastric or nasoduodenal feeding tubes* may be used when intake is diminished because of anorexia or depression. Small (No 8 French) specially designed feeding tubes are well tolerated, with minimal discomfort. Long-term feeding or permanent access to the gastrointestinal tract may be achieved by means of a percutaneous endoscopic gastrostomy (PEG). The PEG technique of gastrostomy placement does not require an operative procedure, and the tube may be used for feeding within hours of being placed. Placement of a *gastrostomy or jejunostomy tube* at the time of operation may obviate prolonged intravenous support, with its associated risks and costs. This issue should be considered and discussed with the patient preoperatively.

***Formula Selection and Management of Feeding*** Patients with advanced gynecologic cancer may not tolerate enteral feedings for long-term support owing to progression of their disease. However, patients who are free of disease but who are left with intestinal compromise—

e.g., those with the short bowel syndrome or radiation enteritis—will benefit from appropriate enteral feedings.

Regardless of the location of the feeding tube, most patients will tolerate standard isotonic formulas that contain approximately 1 kcal/ml, administered at a constant rate. More concentrated formulas are available if fluid restriction is desired; however, patients who receive these more concentrated formulas require careful monitoring, since dehydration may occur insidiously over time (Table 23-7). Enteral feedings should be initiated slowly, with infusions begun at 20 to 30 ml/hr over 24 hours. If the patient experiences no abdominal discomfort or diarrhea, the feeding can be increased by 20 to 30 ml/hour. If signs of intolerance appear (cramping, diarrhea, nausea), the rate of infusion should be decreased to the next lowest level tolerable. In a day or two, the feeding can be advanced again.

Patients with *short bowel syndrome* due to extensive small bowel resection or bypass require special management. Initially, parenteral nutrition will be needed to meet calorie requirements. However, enteral feedings should begin as soon as total intestinal losses are below 600 ml/24 hr. Enteral feedings, even at very low intakes, will stimulate the remaining gastrointestinal tract to adapt and will accelerate the process of bowel adaptation. "Elemental" or "predigested" formulas that are low in fat, such as Vital®, Criticare® or TEN®, may be better tolerated initially; however, these formulas are hypertonic and must be diluted to isotonicity before they are administered. Adding sodium to a formula to a concentration of 60 to 90 mEq/L will enhance absorption (Jones, 1987), but isotonicity should be maintained. The infusion should be initiated slowly (i.e., 20

to 30 ml/hr), and fluid balance across the gastrointestinal (GI) tract monitored. Although total output may be high, the goal should be positive intestinal nutrient balance (total GI output less than total GI intake). Oral intake should consist of small volumes of isotonic liquids initially (i.e., half-strength juices, broth). Low-fat foods are also better tolerated in the beginning. As adaptation occurs over 6 to 18 months, high-calorie foods and frequent feedings will be needed to maintain weight. In the patient whose bowel has been subjected to radiation adaptation may be prolonged. Parenteral vitamin B$_{12}$ may be required as may additional calcium and zinc. Because patients with the short bowel syndrome require long-term management and monitoring for a variety of metabolic and nutritional disorders, consultation with a dietitian or specialist in long-term specialized feeding is recommended.

## Parenteral Nutrition

***Central Venous vs. Peripheral Venous Infusions*** Solutions prepared for infusion into central and peripheral veins consist of dextrose, amino acids, electrolytes, vitamins, and trace elements. The major distinction between these two types of solutions is the concentration of dextrose and amino acids, which will determine the osmolality and caloric concentration of the formula (Tables 23-8 and 23-9).

***Central Venous Infusions*** Central venous solutions are hypertonic solutions (> 1,900 mOsm/kg) that must be infused via a central venous catheter to avoid severe

TABLE 23-7   Composition of Balanced-Formula Diets

| Caloric Density (kcal ml) | Protein (g/L) | Carbohydrate (g/L) | Fat (g/L) | Products |
|---|---|---|---|---|
| 0.6 | 40 | 121 | 1.7 | Citrotein |
| 1.0 | 26-45 | 175-248 | 13-13.5 | Criticare HN Precision LR and High Nitrogen Diets, Vital High Nitrogen, Travasorb HN Peptide and Standard Diets |
| | 28-49 | 123-59 | 30-44 | Isocal, Ensure, Enrich,* Precision Isotonic Diet, Osmolite, Travasorb MCT Diet |
| | 60 | 130 | 23 | Sustacal |
| 1.5 | 55-61 | 190-200 | 53-57 | Ensure Plus, Sustacal HC |
| | 62-83 | 105-143 | 68-92 | Pulmocare, Traumacal |
| 2.0 | 70-75 | 225-250 | 80-91 | Magnacal, Isocal HCN |

* Based on product literature; includes as a fiber source 21 g soy polysaccharide/L.
*Source:* Rombeau JL, Rolandelli RH, Wilmore DW: Nutritional support. In Wilmore DW, et al (eds): *Care of the Surgical Patient*, Section II, Chapter 10. © 1989 Scientific American, Inc. All rights reserved.

TABLE 23-8 Indications for Central Venous and Peripheral Venous Nutrition

*Central Venous Infusions*
- To provide adequate nutrient intake to patients with a non-functional gastrointestinal tract who will require nutritional support for more than 10 days.

*Peripheral Venous Infusions*
- To provide initial feeding (< 10 days) before catheter insertion in patients who will require central venous nutrition.
- To satisfy energy requirements that are near basal (1,500 to 1,800 kcal/day) in a nondepleted patient who can tolerate a minimum of 2 liters of solution per day.
- To supplement enteral feedings that are inadequate because of gastrointestinal dysfunction.

thrombophlebitis and venous sclerosis, which would occur in peripheral veins. These solutions may contain concentrations of 10 to 25% dextrose and 3 to 5% amino acids and can provide up to 1,000 to 1,200 calories per liter (Table 23-9).

Central venous infusions containing 10% or higher concentrations of dextrose require placement of a central venous catheter dedicated to infusion of the nutrient solution. Oncology patients frequently have an established venous access for chemotherapy, and if this route is to be used for feeding as well, it is recommended that the parenteral nutrition solution contain dextrose in concentrations no higher than 10%. This precaution is intended to prevent fungal infections, which often occur when multipurpose venous lines are used in combination with high-dextrose concentrations. With this approach, the infusion can generally be initiated and completed without causing hyperglycemia or hypoglycemia.

***Peripheral Venous Infusions*** Peripheral venous solutions are also hypertonic (600 to 1,000 mOsm/kg) and may therefore be infused into peripheral veins for only a limited time, especially in patients whose peripheral veins have been used previously for intravenous therapy and/or chemotherapy. Formulas for peripheral venous

TABLE 23-9 Composition of Parenteral Nutrition Solution

| Contents | Central | Peripheral |
| --- | --- | --- |
| Dextrose | 250 g (25%) | 50 g (5%) |
| Amino acids | 50 g (5%) | 25 g (2.5%) |
| Nitrogen | 8.4 g/L | 4 g/L |
| Volume | 2,000 ml | 2,000 ml |
| Calories | 2,120 | 540 |
| Nitrogen-to-calorie ratio | 1:126 | 1:43* |
| . . . plus fat emulsion | | |
| Fat emulsion 20% | 500 kcal** | 1,000 kcal |
| Total calories | 2,620 kcal | 1,540 kcal |
| Nitrogen-to-calorie ratio | 1:156 | 1:193 |

\* Peripheral solutions require daily fat emulsion to provide adequate nonprotein calories.
\*\* May be administered as 1,000 cal/week to meet essential fatty acid requirements.

solutions are more dilute than those for central venous infusions and usually provide only 5% dextrose and 2.5 to 3.0% amino acids. Peripheral glucose and amino acid mixtures provide only 300 kcal/L; therefore, high fluid volumes (i.e., 2 to 3 liters) and the addition of fat emulsions (see below) to provide additional calories are required to meet calorie needs. Two liters of peripheral venous solutions with 1,000 calories of fat each day will provide 1,600 calories and 50 g of protein per day, which is usually sufficient in the nonstressed patient (Table 23-9). Patients who require high fluid volumes, such as those with small bowel obstruction and large nasogastric fluid losses, can receive an even higher calorie intake. In general, peripheral venous solutions are indicated for short-term feeding until enteral intake can be resumed or a central line can be placed (see Table 23-8).

***Fat Emulsions*** Fat emulsion is an isotonic solution available in concentrations of 10 and 20% (1.1 and 2.0 kcal/ml, respectively). There are two indications for the use of fat emulsion: (1) to prevent fatty acid deficiency in patients being supported solely by the parenteral route and (2) to provide a supplementary source of nonprotein calories when total requirements cannot be satisfied by administering solutions of carbohydrate and amino acids.

Fat emulsions may be administered via a separate peripheral vein or a central access port that is not being used for parenteral nutrition. Piggybacking (infusion of the fat through a Y-connector) into the central line port that delivers the dextrose/amino acid solution will increase the risk for infection; however, fat emulsion may be piggybacked with peripheral venous nutrition solutions. The infusion should be completed at least 2 hours before blood is drawn (i.e., by 3 am for 6 am blood drawing) to prevent distortion of blood chemistries e.g., triglycerides and sodium.

Alternatively, fat emulsion may be added directly to the dextrose/amino acid mixture. This is commonly called a triple-mix or 3-in-1 delivery and can be compounded in the intravenous pharmacy with all the nutrients required contained in a single delivery bag. With this method, it is not necessary to stop this infusion prior to blood drawing because the fat is considerably diluted by the other solutions.

***Electrolytes, Vitamins, and Minerals*** Electrolytes, vitamins, and minerals are required in the formulation of both peripheral and central infusions.

The addition of electrolytes to the dextrose/amino acid solution is routinely required in most patients. The elimination of any electrolyte warrants close monitoring of serum electrolyte levels, since ion shifts can occur rapidly. Sodium and potassium may be added as chloride and/or acetate salts. Acetate salts are used in lieu of sodium bicarbonate, when needed, since the latter is incompatible with the nutrient solution. Phosphate (administered as the potassium or sodium phosphate salt) and magnesium (administered as magnesium sulfate) are routinely added to provide intracellular electrolytes. Calcium is also required daily (Table 23-10).

| TABLE 23-10 Electrolytes Added to Parenteral Nutrition Solutions | | |
|---|---|---|
| | Typical Amount | Usual Allowable Range |
| Sodium (mEq/L) | 30 | 0-150 |
| Potassium (mEq/L) | 30 | 0-80 |
| Phosphate (mmol/L) | 15 | 0-20 |
| Magnesium (mEq/L) | 5 | 0-15 |
| Calcium (mEq/L)* | 4.7 | 0-10 |
| Chloride (mEq/L) | ** | 0-150 |
| Acetate (mEq/L) | ** | 70-200 |

\* As gluconate.
\*\* Total is based on use of chloride or acetate salts.
*Source:* Rombeau JL, Rolandelli RH, Wilmore DW: Nutritional support. In Wilmore DW, et al (eds): *Care of the Surgical Patient*, Section II, Chapter 10. © 1989 Scientific American, Inc. All rights reserved.

A *multivitamin* formulation containing both fat- and water-soluble vitamins should be added daily. Because vitamin K (phytonadione) is not commonly found in multivitamin preparations, 10 mg is administered once per week either as an additive to the parenteral nutrition solution or by separate injection.

*Trace elements* are administered daily. The usual requirements are satisfied by adding commercially available mixtures to the nutrient formulation. Zinc should be added in patients with malabsorption, massive small bowel resection with diarrhea, pancreatic insufficiency, renal failure with dialysis or nephrotic syndrome, or a history of alcoholism.

Table 23-11 provides examples of how to prescribe the solutions.

**Monitoring** All patients receiving parenteral nutrition should be weighed regularly, and weights should be recorded at least three times each week. Monitoring schedules for peripheral and central parenteral nutrient solutions differ slightly, since peripheral solutions are less likely to cause metabolic disorders such as hyperglycemia or hypophosphatemia (Table 23-12). Metabolic complications associated with parenteral nutrition are outlined in Table 23-13.

**Catheter Care and Catheter Sepsis** Proper catheter care is extremely important in preventing catheter sepsis. Central venous catheters that are to be used for parenteral nutrition should be inserted by physicians experienced in the procedure. Strict aseptic technique, including the wearing of a hat, mask, gown, and gloves, is essential to ensure sterility.

Once inserted, a lumen should be dedicated solely to infusion of the nutrient solution. The use and manipulation of the catheter should be governed by strict protocols and routines established regarding care and surveillance of the insertion site. Preferably, the catheter should be cared for by a nurse with expertise in parenteral nutrition or long-term intravenous access.

---

**TABLE 23-11   Prescribing Total Parenteral Nutrition**

*(For the patient described in Table 23-6)*

Generally, a central line is required to infuse hypertonic solutions in concentrations adequate to achieve weight gain and positive nitrogen balance. Peripheral parenteral nutrition may be used for short-term support or to supplement inadequate enteral intake.

A. *Glucose*—Total glucose infusion should not exceed 5 mg/kg/min.
Example: 56 kg × 5 mg = 280 mg/kg/min
280 mg × 1,440 min = 403 g glucose/24 hr
Calories: 403 g glucose × 3.4 cal/g = 1,370
B. *Amino Acids* (protein)
Example: 1 g protein × 56 kg = 56 g protein
Calories: 56 g × 4 cal = 224

**Total = 1,594**

1,594 calories will meet this patient's requirements for calories and protein. It can be provided in 2 liters of 20% dextrose, 2.8% amino acids.

C. *Fat emulsion*—Essential fatty acids are required at 4% of total calories. 1,000 calories of fat emulsion given weekly generally meets this requirement.
Example: This woman should receive 1,000 calories of fat emulsion weekly.
A fat emulsion may also be used to bring calorie intake up to estimated requirements.
Example: An additional 500 to 1,000 cal/day may be added to this patient's parenteral intake if weight gain is desired. Fat should never exceed 60% of total calories, and a total of no greater than 25 to 30% is generally recommended when fat is given regularly (i.e., daily).

Central venous solutions have been associated with an increased incidence of *catheter sepsis* (Maki et al, 1982). Primary catheter sepsis is defined as an episode of infection in which the catheter is thought to be the only focus, peripheral blood cultures are positive, and the catheter tip culture yields at least $10^3$ organisms (Maki, 1977, 1982). The central catheter lumen designated for the parenteral nutrition infusion should not be used for phlebotomy, including blood drawn for cultures. Secondary catheter sepsis occurs when the catheter is contaminated by an infection at another site.

Positive blood cultures or suspicion of a primary infection are indications for catheter removal. The catheter tip should be cultured to confirm the diagnosis. In primary catheter sepsis, the fever usually defervesces once the catheter has been removed.

If peripheral blood cultures are negative and a secondary source of infection is identified and treated, parenteral nutrition may continue through the original catheter. If symptoms persist despite appropriate treatment, the central catheter can be changed over a guidewire and the tip sent for culture. If the tip culture is negative, feedings may continue through the new catheter. However, if the culture is positive, the catheter should be removed and the infection treated. A catheter may be inserted into a new site when the septicemia has cleared.

TABLE 23-12  Suggested Monitoring During Initial Parenteral Nutrition

| Metabolic Variables | Central Access | Peripheral Access |
|---|---|---|
| *Blood* | | |
| Electrolytes | 3× weekly | 3× weekly |
| Blood urea nitrogen | 2× weekly | 2× weekly |
| Glucose | Daily, then 3× weekly | Weekly |
| Liver function tests | 2× weekly | Weekly |
| Total calcium and phosphorus | 2× weekly | Weekly |
| Magnesium | Weekly | Weekly |
| Triglycerides | Weekly | Weekly |
| Acid-base status | As indicated | As indicated |
| *Urine* | | |
| Glucose | 4 to 6× daily, then 2× daily | As indicated |
| *Intake* | | |
| Intravenous | Daily | Daily |
| Oral | Daily | Daily |
| *Output* | | |
| Urine | Daily | Daily |
| Other | As indicated | As indicated |
| Prevention and Detection of Infection | | |
| Clinical observations (activity, temperature symptoms) | Daily | * |
| WBC and differential counts | As indicated | * |
| Cultures | As indicated | * |

\* Applicable if central access is being used for the infusion.
*Source:* Modified, Wilmore DW: *Metabolic Management of the Critically Ill.* New York, Plenum Publishing Corp, 1977, p 231. *Care of the Surgical Patient,* Section II, Chapter 10. © 1989 Scientific American, Inc. All rights reserved.

# HOME NUTRITIONAL SUPPORT

## Candidates

Patients who require long-term nutritional support (i.e., longer than one month) may be candidates for home care. These include patients with short bowel syndrome, obstruction, and intestinal fistulas. Patients can generally be classified into two categories: (1) those presumed to be disease-free but who have treatment-induced intestinal dysfunction and (2) those with intestinal dysfunction related to advancing disease.

Home feedings are usually self-administered. This requires that the patient be physically and mentally capable of participating in the therapy. Therefore, the patient's medical condition and cognitive abilities must be evaluated before the decision is made for home discharge. If the patient is unable to participate in her own care, the assistance of another person must be enlisted. A daily commitment of long hours is required by the family or other care provider. Thus, a debilitated woman without support services is not a candidate for home feedings. These patients should then be considered for transfer from the acute care setting to a chronic care facility (Table 23-14).

## Goals of Home Therapy

Goals of patient care vary depending on the state of the disease. Repletion of body mass and restoration of normal activity are the goals for patients who are free of disease but have significant bowel dysfunction. Alternatively, maintaining body weight and adequate hydration may be realistic goals during periods of progressive disease.

## Appropriate Routes of Feeding

The ability to take enteral fluids and nutrients should be evaluated. Placement of a gastrostomy tube may allow gastric feeding in the absence of intestinal obstruction. For patients who have normal small bowel function but gastric ileus, a small feeding tube may be placed in the small bowel. When nutritional support and/or hydration cannot be maintained by the enteral route, long-term parenteral feedings should be considered.

Home parenteral feedings require a permanent access. Silastic right atrial catheters are the most common access devices. They are placed surgically by an experienced physician and are available with one or two lumens. The single-lumen catheter is appropriate for patients who require only parenteral nutrition, whereas the double-lumen catheter is useful for patients who require frequent phlebotomy, chemotherapy, or medications for pain management.

Tunneled catheters, such as the Hickman® or Broviac® catheter, exit the chest wall and should exit at a point low enough so that it is visible to the patient as she looks downward. This position enables the patient to perform the aseptic dressing changes every 48 to 72 hours (Maki, 1982) and facilitates inspection of the site for signs of infection.

The venous disk is another right atrial catheter that is completely subcutaneous. The patient must learn the sterile technique for accessing the disc using a specially designed noncoring needle. The disk is usually accessed daily; however, it may remain in place for a maximum of 5 days. Discussion with the patient prior to placement of the venous disk is essential, since many patients are reluctant to learn this technique and to perform the daily accessing procedure.

## Instructions for the Home-Care Patient

The patient is instructed about home care prior to discharge. This requires a minimum of 10 hours of instruction for intravenous feeding and 3 hours for enteral feeding. Teaching should be done by specially trained nurses from either a nutrition support team or a home-care vendor with established expertise in the area of home feedings. Many home-care vendors are able to provide teaching services and various levels of in-home support services; they can also prepare, deliver, and inventory formulas, supplies, and equipment.

Patients must be taught about how to care for and maintain the feeding access and to administer feedings, which include a sterile admixture of ingredients such as

TABLE 23-13  Metabolic Complications of Total Parenteral Nutrition

| Problems | Possible Etiologies | Solutions |
|---|---|---|
| 1. *Glucose* | | |
| Hyperglycemia, glycosuria, osmotic diuresis, hyperosmolar nonketonic dehydration and coma | Excessive total dose or rate of infusion of glucose; inadequate endogenous insulin; increased glucocorticoids; sepsis. | Limit total amount of glucose infused; increased insulin; administer a portion of calories as fat emulsion. |
| Postinfusion (rebound) hypoglycemia | Persistence of endogenous insulin production secondary to prolonged stimulation of islet cells by high carbohydrate infusion. | If dextrose concentration exceeds 10%, decrease TPN rate by ½ for last hour of TPN infusion. |
| Hypercarbia | High carbohydrate load. | Limit total carbohydrate dose to 5 mg carbohydrate/kg/min. |
| 2. *Fat* | | |
| Hypertriglyceridemia | Decreased clearance | Decrease or discontinue lipid infusion. |
| Essential fatty acid deficiency | Inadequate essential fatty acid administration. | Administer minimum of 1,000 kcal lipid every week to meet essential fatty acid needs. |
| 3. *Amino Acids* | | |
| Prerenal azotemia | Excessive amino acid infusion with inadequate caloric administration. | Reduce amino acid intake and increase nonprotein calories. |
| 4. *Miscellaneous* | | |
| Hypophosphatemia | Inadequate phosphorus administration, redistribution of serum phosphorus into cells, bone, or both. Malnourished patients are particularly at risk for this. | Administer phosphorus (15 mm phosphate/1,000 IV calories); evaluate antacid and calcium administration. |
| Hyperphosphatemia | Decreased clearance of phosphorus | Decrease or omit phosphorus. May need to decrease lipid as well (contains phospholipid). |
| Hypomagnesemia | Inadequate magnesium administration relative to increased requirements or increased losses (diarrhea, diuresis, medications). | Administer magnesium. |
| Hypermagnesemia | Excessive magnesium administration, renal failure. | Decrease or omit magnesium. |
| Elevations in liver function parameters | Overfeeding, particularly excess carbohydrate; cholestasis from NPO status. | Do not exceed caloric maintenance needs. Provide balanced substrate profile. |

*Source:* Adapted from Wilmore DW: Enteral and parenteral nutrition in hospital patients. In Rubenstein E, Federman DD (eds): *Scientific American Medicine,* Section 4, Subsection XIV. New York, Scientific American, Inc, 1990. © 1990, Scientific American, Inc. All rights reserved.

vitamins and other medications when intravenous feedings are used. In addition, they should understand the operation of a volumetric pump and how to "troubleshoot" and be alert for complications of both the feeding and the disease. Weight will be monitored and the patient should be alert to changes of 1 kg/day. The

patient must also know the signs of fluid overload or dehydration (Table 23-15).

Feedings, whether enteral or intravenous, may be infused over 12 to 24 hours. A cyclical infusion over 12 hours during the night allows the patient some autonomy and quality of life during the daytime hours. However, the circumstances for which the gynecologic oncology patient requires intravenous feedings often render them a complex home patient, since they frequently need other therapies such as gastric decompression or continuous pain management. Often this means 24 hours of supportive care and monitoring.

## Degree of Home-Care Monitoring (Table 23-16)

*Fluid Balance*  Careful measurements of intake and output must be taken daily if problems include diarrhea, losses from gastrostomy tubes, or ascites formation. The physician may need to evaluate fluid balance as often as two times a week to determine whether the intravenous fluid volume needs to be adjusted. This is best

---

TABLE 23-14  Procedures Prior to Discharge on Home Parenteral Nutrition

Contact home-care vendor
Contact nutrition support person
Determine insurance reimbursement
Place long-term central venous catheter
Evaluate cognitive and physical capabilities
Assess home and home support systems
Assess nutrient needs
Determine appropriate solution prescription
Educate patient/other responsible caregiver

TABLE 23-15   Considerations for Home Management of Parenteral Nutrition*

- Aseptic/clean technique
- Catheter care:
    - Dressing changes
    - Maintaining catheter patency
    - Appropriate response to or prevention of complications such as
        - —signs and symptoms of sepsis
        - —air emboli
        - —catheter breakage or occlusion
- Solution preparation and infusion:
    - Use of volumetric pump
    - Schedule and rates of infusion
    - Connection to and disconnection from long-term catheter
    - Dosage determination and admixing of ingredients
    - Signs of dehydration and fluid overload
    - Monitoring for glucose intolerance
    - Inspection of solution for
        - —leakage
        - —cloudiness
        - —oiling of fat emulsion
        - —expiration dates

* For patient or person responsible for patient's care.

done by fixing the volume of the nutritional solution that is administered and adjusting the fluid needed for hydration by varying the quantity of 5% dextrose in saline administered.

***Biochemical Monitoring***  Laboratory values should be monitored at least weekly until the patient is stable. When a period of stabilization has been reached, blood values may be determined every 2 to 3 weeks.

***Special Considerations***  The patient with a *short bowel* or *enteritis* will need to be instructed about the importance of oral fluid restriction. Initially, these patients should receive nothing by mouth so that the volume of intestinal losses can be determined. Once the daily stool output and electrolyte losses have been quantified, volume requirements can be determined. Only then can oral fluid intake be gradually liberalized. It is difficult for patients to understand that sometimes their increased thirst and diarrhea result from their large oral fluid intakes. Restricting oral fluid intake to 1,000 ml per day while supplementing additional intravenous fluid solutions may help control these massive gastrointestinal losses.

*Intestinal obstruction* as a result of advancing disease

TABLE 23-16   Routine Monitoring After Discharge

Catheter integrity
Nutrient intake
Weight changes
Nutritional deficiencies
Fluid and electrolyte status
Home environment and psychosocial changes

can cause prolonged nausea, vomiting, and abdominal pain. Prior to discharge it is imperative that gastric decompression be sufficient. For the short term, a nasogastric tube to drainage may expedite discharge, but if home decompression is expected to be longer than 2 to 3 weeks, a more permanent and less irritating drainage tube should be employed. With the technique of percutaneous endoscopic gastrostomy now available, a tube may be placed without requiring an operative procedure. Gastrostomy tubes can more easily be attached to gravity drainage, thus allowing more mobility. This is usually more comfortable for the patient and alleviates nasal and throat discomfort and avoids tissue damage to the mucous membranes of the nose and esophagus.

The patient with *end-stage disease* who has intestinal obstruction can also be supported with home therapy consisting of hydration fluid. The patient thus avoids the complexity and risks of feeding solutions. For these individuals, comfort measures are often decided on by the patient and physician, thus emphasizing pain management over all other therapies.

## REFERENCES

Altomare DF, Serio G, Pannarle OC, et al: Prediction of mortality by logistic regression analysis in patients with postoperative enterocutaneous fistulae. *Br J Surg* 77:450-453, 1990.

American College of Physicians: Position Paper: Parenteral nutrition in patients receiving cancer chemotherapy. *Ann Intern Med* 110:734-736, 1989.

Bozzetti F: Effects of artificial nutrition on the nutritional status of cancer patients. *JPEN* 13:406-420, 1989.

Bozzetti F, Migliavacca S, Pupa A, et al: Total parenteral nutrition prevents further nutritional deterioration in patients with cancer cachexia. *Ann Surg* 205:138-143, 1987.

Braga M, Baccari P, Scaccabarozzi S, et al: Prognostic role of preoperative nutritional and immunological assessment in the surgical patient. *JPEN* 12:138-142, 1988.

Buzby GP: The case for preoperative nutritional support. (Postgraduate course manual). American College of Surgeons Committee on Pre- and Post-operative Care, Chicago, October, 1988.

Clark N: Immune function tests. In Krey S, Murray RL (eds): *Dynamics of Nutrition Support.* Norwalk, Connecticut, Appleton-Century-Crofts, 1986, p 149.

Clarke-Pearson DL, Chin NO, DeLong ER, et al: Surgical management of intestinal obstruction in ovarian cancer. *Gynecol Oncol* 26:11-18, 1987.

Clarke-Pearson DL, DeLong ER, Chin NO, et al: Intestinal obstruction in patients with ovarian cancer. *Arch Surg* 123:42-45, 1988.

Detsky AS, Baker JP, O'Rourke K, et al: Perioperative parenteral nutrition: A meta-analysis. *Ann Intern Med* 107:195-203, 1987.

DeWys WD, Begg C, Band P, et al: The impact of malnutrition on treatment results in breast cancer. *Cancer Treat Rep* 65(Suppl):87-91, 1981.

Douglas RG, Shaw JHF: Metabolic effects of cancer. *Br J Surg* 77:246-254, 1990.

Driver AG, Lebrun M: Iatrogenic malnutrition in patients receiving ventilatory support. *JAMA* 244:2195-2196, 1980.

Foschi D, Cavagna G, Calloni F, et al: Hyperalimentation of jaundiced patients on percutaneous transhepatic biliary drainage. *Br J Surg* 73:716, 1986.

Fuller AF Jr, Griffiths CT: Ovarian cancer cachexia—Surgical interactions. *Gynecol Oncol* 8:301-310, 1979.

Haydock DA, Hill, GC: Improved wound healing response in surgical patients receiving intravenous nutrition. *Br J Surg* 74:320-323, 1987.

Heber D, Byerley L, Chi J, et al: Pathophysiology of malnutrition in the adult cancer patient. *Cancer* 58(Suppl):1867-1873, 1986.

Hickman DM, Miller RA, Rombeau JL, et al: Serum albumin and body weight as predictors of postoperative course in colorectal cancer. *JPEN* 4:314, 1980.

Irvin TT: Effects of malnutrition and hyperalimentation on wound healing. *Surg Gynecol Obstet* 146:33-37, 1978.

Jones BJM: Nutritional management of the short bowel syndrome. *J Clin Gastroenterol* 2:99-103, 1987.

Keys A, Brozek J, Henschel A, et al: *The Biology of Human Starvation*, Vol 1. Minneapolis, University of Minnesota Press, 1950, p 714.

Krebs HB, Goplerud DR: Surgical management of bowel obstruction in advanced ovarian carcinoma. *Obstet Gynecol* 61:327-330, 1983.

Krebs HB, Goplerud DR: Mechanical intestinal obstruction in patients with gynecologic disease: A review of 368 patients. *Am J Obstet Gynecol* 157:577-581, 1987.

Krey SH, Murray RL: *Dynamics of Nutrition Support: Assessment, Implementation, Evaluation*. Appleton-Century-Crofts, Norwalk, Connecticut, 1986.

Lavery IC, Steiger E, Fazio VW: Home parenteral nutrition in management of patients with severe radiation enteritis. *Dis Colon Rectum* 23:91-93, 1980.

MacLean LD: Host resistance in surgical patients. *J Trauma* 19:297-307, 1979.

Maki DG: Infections associated with intravascular lines. In Remington JS, Swartz MN (eds): In *Current Clinical Topics in Infectious Disease*, New York, McGraw-Hill Book Co, 1982, pp 309-363.

Maki DG, Wise CE, Saratin HW: A semiquantitative method for identifying intravenous catheter–related infection. *N Engl J Med* 296:1505-1509, 1977.

Miller JM, Brenner W, Dienist C, et al: Preoperative parenteral feedings in patients with gastrointestinal carcinoma. *Lancet* 1:68, 1982.

Mullen JL, Buzby GP, Matthews DC: Reduction of operative morbidity and mortality by combined preoperative and postoperative nutritional support. *Ann Surg* 192:604-613, 1980.

National Center for Health Statistics: Weight by height and age for adults 18-74 years. United States 1971-1974. Rockville, MD: National Center for Health Statistics, 1979. Vital and Health Statistics, Series II: Data from the National Health and Nutrition Examination Survey (NHANES), No 208. DHEW Publ No (PHS) 79-1656, 1979.

Orr JW Jr, Wilson K, Bodiford C, et al: Nutritional status of patients with untreated cervical cancer. *Am J Obstet Gynecol* 151:625-631, 1985.

Rombeau JL, Caldwell MD, Forlaw L, et al (eds): *Atlas of Nutritional Support Techniques*. Boston, Little, Brown and Co, 1989a.

Rombeau JL, Rolandelli RH, Wilmore DW: Nutritional support (Chap 10). In Wilmore DW, Brennan MF, Harken AH, et al (eds): *Care of the Surgical Patient*, Vol 1, Critical Care, Section II, Care in the ICU. New York, Scientific American, Inc, 1989b.

Scrimshaw NS, Taylor CE, Gordon JE: Interaction of nutrition and infection. *Am J Med Sci* 237:367-403, 1959.

Shukla HS, Rao RR, Banu W, et al: Enteral hyperalimentation in malnourished surgical patients. *Indian J Med Res* 8:339, 1984.

Spanier AH, Pictscit JB, Meakins JC, et al: The relationship between immune competence and nutrition. *Surg Forum* 27:332-333, 1976.

Studley HO: Percentage of weight loss. A basic indicator of surgical risk in patients with chronic peptic ulcer. *JAMA* 106:458, 1936.

Terada KY, Christen C, Roberts JA: Parenteral nutrition in gynecology. *J Reprod Med* 33:957-960, 1988.

Tunca JC: Nutritional evaluation of gynecologic cancer patients during initial diagnosis of their disease. *Am J Obstet Gynecol* 147:893-896, 1983.

Tunca JC, Buchler DA, Mack EA, et al: The management of ovarian-cancer-caused-bowel obstruction. *Gynecol Oncol* 12:186-192, 1981.

Twomey P, Ziegler D, Rombeau JL: Utility of skin testing in nutritional assessment: A critical review. *JPEN* 6:50-58, 1982.

# UNIT IV

## Supportive Care of the Cancer Patient

# *Chapter 24* | Pain in Gynecologic Malignancy

*David Borsook    Daniel B. Carr*

Pain related to cancer afflicts an estimated 20 million people around the world. Depending on the stage of the disease, pain has been reported in 60 to 70% of patients with cancer (Bonica, 1979, 1982; Twycross and Wald, 1976; Foley, 1979). This pain may be caused not only by the tumor itself but also by efforts to treat the disease and thereby extend life. Short of mortality, pain is often the prime issue that patients with cancer and their physicians must deal with. Some reports place the incidence of pain symptoms due to cancer therapy as high as 28% of total pain symptoms. As new or improved treatments are introduced and the life expectancy of patients with cancer continues to increase, it is possible that the prevalence of treatment-induced pain symptoms may increase as well.

Cancer pain has a significant psychosocial impact on the patient and usually interferes with her activities and lifestyle (Daut and Cleeland, 1977). Although some patients with cancer must cope with the abstract knowledge that they have a terminal illness, ongoing pain is an immediate practical problem that may hasten physical and emotional deterioration. For many of these patients, pain is the major liability of their illness. In 1953, Bonica reported that pain was not effectively relieved in a significant number of cancer patients. More recent studies have estimated that the proportion of this group of patient ranges from 45 to 100% (Cartwright et al, 1973; Parkes, 1978; Turnbull, 1979). According to Foley (1979), pain in gynecologic cancer is fairly prevalent, surpassed only by that in bone and oral cancer. Thus, some seven in 10 women with cancers involving the genitourinary system will have pain. In the United States, pain is present in 40 to 100% of cases of ovarian, uterine, or cervical tumors (Bonica, 1984).

Pain in patients with gynecologic cancer constitutes a significant problem that can and should be adequately dealt with in the majority of cases. Effective relief of the pain of malignancy requires not only identifying its underlying cause, but also allaying possible fears or misconceptions held by some patients and physicians concerning the use of narcotics or other modalities. Although complete pain relief is possible with appropriate therapy in the majority of patients, a few patients continue to have refractory pain despite the best care. This chapter examines the underlying physiologic basis for pain in gynecologic malignancies and presents an up-to-date approach to its treatment.

## PAIN ANATOMY AND PHYSIOLOGY

In this section, we present an overview of the mechanisms of gynecologic pain, taking special note of those visceral pathways mediating pain that originates from pelvic sites (Fig. 24-1). For the interested reader, some recent excellent monographs have provided broad, in-depth reviews of the anatomy and physiology of neural systems involved in the perception of pain (Willis, 1985; Fields, 1987; Wall and Melzack, 1989; Cousins and Bridenbaugh, 1988).

### Peripheral Nerves

Pain-sensitive regions include the skin, musculoskeletal and vascular systems, and viscera. Regardless of its site of origin, pain is transmitted from free nerve endings by unmyelinated C fibers and small myelinated A-delta fibers (Willis, 1985). Most if not all unmyelinated C fibers are nociceptive.

Afferent pain systems from the *skin and musculoskeletal system* have been thoroughly studied in animals and humans, leading to the characterization of three groups of pain receptors and their associated afferent nerve fibers. These respond directly to pressure (mechanoreceptors), to temperature (thermoreceptors), or to either of these stimuli (polymodal receptors). Pain-producing substances that activate nociceptor terminals or sensitize their response to thermal or mechanical stimuli include bradykinin, potassium, serotonin, histamine, prostaglandins, and leukotrienes (Hargreaves and Dionne, 1990). Nociceptors may be activated following the leakage of chemicals such as potassium from traumatized tissue; exposure to substances such as prostaglandins, bradykinin, and leukotrienes from damaged cells or from newly migrating lymphocytes; or elevated local concentrations of peptides, such as substance P, released from the receptor terminal itself.

Despite its clinical importance and particular relevance to gynecologic cancer, *visceral pain* or pain from deep structures is less well understood at a physiologic level. Clinically, this type of pain differs from that arising in the skin; it is not sharp and cannot be well localized (Cervero, 1983a). Visceral nociceptors have small myelinated or unmyelinated axons. Although deep nociceptive primary afferents have been characterized in animals (Cervero, 1982, 1983), there are no functional studies of deep receptors in humans. The viscera are relatively insensitive to heat, cutting, or pinching (Cervero, 1983a; Capps and Coleman, 1932) yet do respond to distention or torsion (Leek, 1977; Cervero, 1982; Paintal, 1954). Polymodal afferents from the testis carry noxious stimuli (Kumazawa and Mizurura, 1977), and presumably the same applies to the ovary, in view of its parallel embryologic origins.

Pain arising from viscera is often felt in regions distant from the site producing the pain. A classic example of such "referred pain" (Head, 1893; Lewis, 1942) is

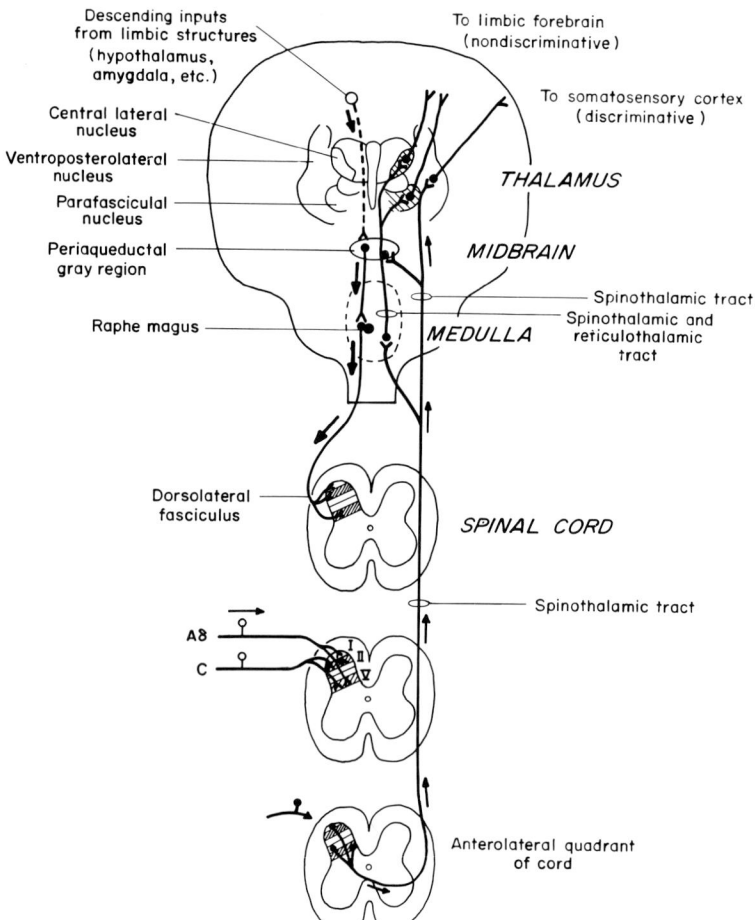

FIGURE 24-1 Principal ascending and descending pain pathways.

the pain felt along the left arm in association with myocardial infarction. Patterns of somatic referral are characteristic for each visceral structure; those sites corresponding to the female reproductive tract are listed below (see Pain Syndromes in Gynecologic Cancer). A number of explanations have been advanced for referred pain, the most convincing of which is the *convergence* of visceral and somatic afferents onto adjacent or identical convergence neurons (Ruch, 1946; Head, 1893; Mackenzie, 1893; Sinclair et al, 1948; Perl, 1984; Bahr et al, 1981; Pierau et al, 1982). Clinically, muscle tenderness and skin hypersensitivity may be noted in the referred myotome or dermatome, respectively.

Afferent pain fibers originating in pelvic viscera travel along sympathetic and parasympathetic pathways. The sympathetic system conveys afferent noxious information from the uterus, the medial fallopian tubes, and the upper third of the vagina to the paracervical plexus and then to the hypogastric plexus. Fibers from this plexus enter the lumbar and lower thoracic sympathetic chain and synapse within the spinal cord dorsal horn T1 to L2. Pain sensations from the ovary, the lateral fallopian tubes, and the peritoneum of the broad ligament pass along the ovarian vessels to the aortic plexus and into the sympathetic chain. The parasympathetic system is thought to convey noxious stimuli from pelvic

organs via the pudendal nerves that synapse in the spinal cord from S2 to S4. Figure 24-2 depicts the innervation of pelvic viscera (Brose and Cousins, 1990).

About 50% of visceral nerves consist of afferent fibers, and 80% of the latter are unmyelinated; 10% of dorsal roots are visceral fibers. A-delta– and C-fiber input from the splanchnic nerve has been shown to terminate in dorsal horn cells (Pomeranz et al, 1968; Hancock et al, 1975). After entering via the dorsal roots, primary afferent projections from the pelvic organs enter Lissauer's tract and course around the dorsal horn in two bundles, one medial and one lateral. The lateral and more prominent of the two bundles terminates in laminae V, VII, and X as well as in the contralateral cord, while the medial bundle sends collaterals to lamina X and branches to the dorsal columns. Somatic afferent projections carrying nociceptive information from the skin terminate principally in laminae I, II, and V. In contrast to somatic afferents from skin, visceral afferents do not have a direct projection to laminae II. A number of *neuropeptides* are present in visceral afferents. Vasoactive intestinal polypeptide (VIP), for example, is present in visceral afferents and at the sites of their termination within the cord (Kuo et al, 1985; Kawatani et al, 1983; Anand and Carr, 1989; Jessell and Dodd, 1989).

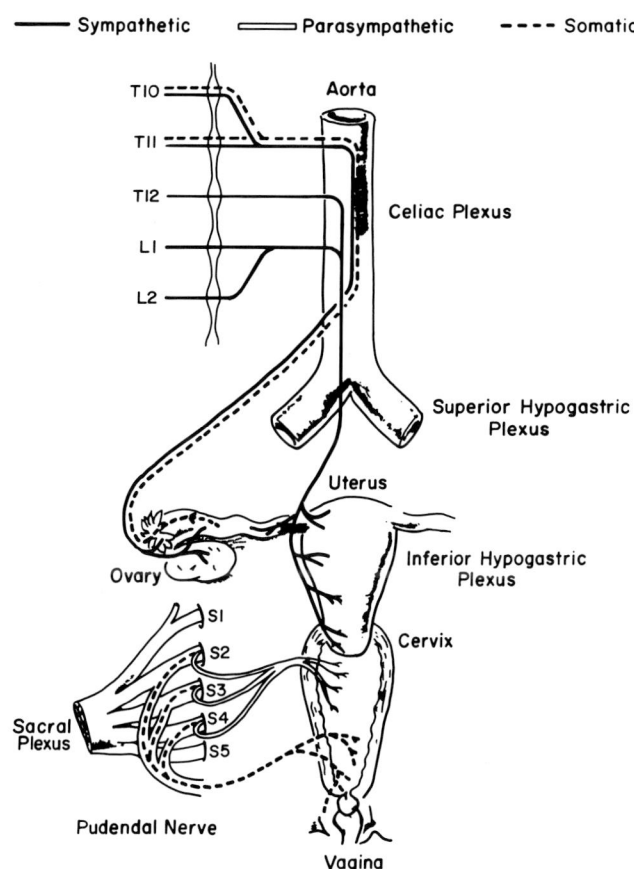

— Sympathetic    ⊏⊐ Parasympathetic    - - - Somatic

T10
Aorta
T11
T12
Celiac Plexus
L1
L2
Superior Hypogastric Plexus
Uterus
Inferior Hypogastric Plexus
Ovary
Cervix
S1
S2
S3
S4
S5
Sacral Plexus
Pudendal Nerve
Vagina

FIGURE 24-2 Innervation of the pelvic viscera. (Adapted from Brose WG, Cousins MJ: In Coppleson M (ed): *Gynecological Oncology*, 2nd ed. Edinburgh, Churchill Livingstone, 1991.

Several nonexclusive mechanisms are thought to underlie the chronic pain experienced after damage to peripheral nerves or the central nervous system. The nociceptor terminals may be sensitized; ectopic or abnormally frequent impulses may originate at the damaged site; or afferent nociceptive input may be "amplified" abnormally within a sensitized spinal segment or higher (Cook et al, 1987). *Ectopic impulses* may arise at sites of regenerating axons as in the case of neuroma formation, at sites affected by peripheral neuropathies, or from damaged dorsal root ganglion cells. Pharmacological therapies that are clinically useful in neuropathic pain syndromes are often directed against this ectopic activity. For example, the anticonvulsant phenytoin blocks sodium channels and decreases abnormal neural discharge. The use of drugs in the treatment of neuropathic pain as well as their mechanisms of action is discussed below.

## Central Nervous System

***Spinal Cord*** Primary afferent nociceptors project to dorsal horn cells in laminae I, II, and V (from skin) or in laminae I, V, VII, and X (from viscera) (Fitzgerald, 1989; Willis, 1985). Nociceptive information that reaches the spinal cord from skin proceeds through a number of pathways, including the *spinothalamic tract* and the spinoreticular tract. The spinothalamic tract, found on the ventrolateral quadrant of the spinal cord, receives most of its input from contralateral dorsal horn laminae (predominantly I, IV, and V). Axons from the dorsal laminae, after crossing the midline, join the spinothalamic tract one or two levels above their dorsal horn entry.

Although the spinothalamic tract is mainly a crossed pathway, an ipsilateral component is also present. Within the tract, fibers of caudal origin (e.g., from the leg) are found laterally and those from more cephalad sites (e.g., from the arm) are located medially. Based on the anatomy of its ascending projections, two divisions of this tract have been defined; paleospinothalamic (phylogenetically older) and neospinothalamic. The paleospinothalamic tract terminates within nuclei of the brainstem reticular formation and is thought to provoke nondiscriminative reactions to pain, including affective and autonomic changes; the neospinothalamic tract conveys discriminative information to the thalamus. Electrical stimulation at any level of the spinothalamic tract—from spinal cord to thalamus—will produce pain. Information about localizing visceral pain transmission pathways is meager.

***Thalamus*** The spinothalamic tract terminates within two broad areas of the thalamus: medial (centrolateral nucleus, lateral nucleus, intralaminar nucleus, and submedius) and lateral (posterior nuclei and ventrobasal nuclei). In general, pathways to the lateral thalamus are discriminative (conveying topographic information largely from laminae I and V), while pathways to the medial thalamus are nondiscriminative and receive projections mainly from deeper spinal laminae VI and VII. The medially located nucleus submedius, however, does not conform to this arrangement and receives topographic projections from lamina I.

Another major nociceptive pathway to the thalamus is the spinoreticular tract. This pathway is not important for discriminative sensory processing and is thought to play an important role in affective reactions to pain. It arises from laminae V to VIII and projects via the brainstem reticular formation to the intralaminar nucleus. The spinoreticular and paleospinothalamic tracts have been considered a single functional entity (Melzack and Casey, 1968).

The thalamic organization of nociceptive information into sensory discriminative (lateral) and nondiscriminative affective (medial) components allows selective medial thalamic lesions to be induced to relieve the affective/emotional components of pain with little loss of discriminative function (Mark and Ervin, 1965; Mark et al, 1961). Although Carstens and Yokota (1980) have identified neurons in the thalamus that respond to noxious visceral stimulation, little detailed information is available about their central connections. Nonetheless, in light of the general organization of the thalamus, one might speculate that in selected cases clinical visceral pain might be relieved by medial thalamic induced lesions but not by lateral induced lesions, which might be considered for refractory pain having a sensory-discriminative quality (White and Sweet, 1969).

***Sensory Cortex*** The role of the cerebral cortex in pain perception is still under investigation. Damage to large portions of the cortex usually does not result in any change in pain sensation, although there are reports that extensive lesions of the parietal cortex can result in deficits of pain perception (Marshall, 1951; Lewin and Phillips, 1952). Electrical stimulation or seizures of the somatosensory cortex rarely elicit pain (Young and Blume, 1983). However, electrophysiologic mapping of the somatosensory cortex has identified a population of pain-responsive neurons that appear to have a dual input from the medial and lateral thalamic groups (Kenshalo and Isensee, 1983). Thalamic nuclei involved in nociception have distinct cortical projections: lateral thalamic nuclei project densely to the primary somatosensory cortex, while medial thalamic nuclei receive bilateral input from the spinal cord and project widely without topographic information. The centrolateral nucleus, for example, has bilateral input from the spinal cord and projects to the basal ganglia and prefrontal, motor, somatosensory, and visual areas of cortex.

As proposed by Melzack and Casey (1968), "affective/emotional" pain has an ill-defined unpleasant character that may vary from individual to individual. Its anatomic substrate—much of which forms part of the limbic system—includes the paleospinothalamic and spinoreticular tracts, their connections with the reticular formation, and projections from the medial thalamic nuclei (e.g., intralaminar) to the frontal lobe. In patients after prefrontal lobotomy for pain relief, the perception of pain is unaltered but the attitude toward pain is improved (Freeman and Watts, 1950).

## Endogenous Processes That Inhibit Pain

Recognition of multiple short- and long-term adaptations within the pain system has expanded our concept of nociception from "hard-wired," passive transduction to a highly dynamic process in which living circuits are continuously transformed by the signals passing through them. In the past decade, inhibition of nociceptive messages by a highly organized descending system has been carefully studied and appears to form the basis for many clinically relevant responses and therapies. More recently, attention has returned to the phenomena of amplification and reverberation of neural signals, originally described over 50 years ago (Lorente de No, 1938). These phenomena deserve attention, since they have great clinical applicability (Wall, 1988).

***Analgesic Pathways*** There is no question that descending pathways, originating mainly in the forebrain and the brainstem, can modulate neuronal firing within the dorsal horn (Basbaum and Fields, 1984). The powerful inhibitory effects exerted by these descending analgesic pathways on afferent systems (mainly at the dorsal horn) may therefore alter the perception of pain, particularly during stress. For example, classic studies by Beecher (1959) described soldiers with extensive wounds reporting little or no pain.

Experiments using electrical stimulation have played a key role in defining the pathways mediating these effects. Reynolds (1969) showed that surgery without anesthetic could be performed on rats during electrical stimulation of the midbrain. Forebrain structures (including the hypothalamus, thalamus, amygdala, septal region, and preoptic region) or brainstem structures (the periaqueductal gray, raphe magnus of the medulla, and dorsolateral pontine tegmentum) can inhibit both nocifensive reflexes and activity of dorsal horn neurons responding to noxious stimuli (Dickenson, 1983; Gebhart et al, 1983; Carstens, 1982; Dostrovsky, 1988; Barbaro 1988). Stimulation of homologous midbrain sites in humans has significantly improved chronic pain without causing sensory changes (Richardson and Akil, 1977; Baskin et al, 1986).

From these brainstem structures (predominantly the periaqueductal gray and the raphe magnus), pathways descend in the dorsolateral funiculus (DLF) of the spinal cord to terminate on laminae I, II, and V. These layers have terminals of nociceptive afferents (II and V) and cell bodies of the spinothalamic tract (I). Lesions of the DLF reduce or abolish the analgesic effects of electrical stimulation of the periaqueductal gray or raphe magnus (Basbaum et al, 1977; Basbaum and Fields, 1984). Stimulation of the DLF can inhibit the response of spinothalamic neurons (Brown et al, 1973), while a cold block of the spinal cord selectively enhances the response to nociceptive input below the block (Hall et al, 1982; Handwerker et al, 1975).

The neurochemical basis for descending analgesia may be divided into two components: an opioid system and a non-opioid system dependent on biogenic amines. Both systems play a significant role in endogenous analgesia produced under physiologic conditions and both are everyday targets for the pharmacotherapy of pain.

*Opioid receptors* are widely distributed in the central nervous system (Carr, 1988) and tend to be most highly concentrated (like their endogenous peptide ligands) in structures involved in analgesia or related processes, such as cardiovascular control or stress hormone secretion (Carr and Murphy, 1988). Such structures include the amygdala, hypothalamus, raphe magnus, and dorsal horn of the spinal cord (laminae I, II, V, and X) (Atweh and Kuhar, 1983; Yaksh, 1987; Hokfelt et al, 1979). At these sites, most opioid neurons are inhibitory interneurons that diminish or "modulate" activity within underlying excitatory synapses. A now classic example of this is opioid inhibition of the release of substance P from primary afferent synapses in the superficial dorsal horn.

Opioid-containing projections from some nuclei (e.g., paragigantocellularis lateralis) to the spinal cord have been described (Hokfelt et al, 1979), and a number of types and subtypes of opioid receptors and families of endogenous opioid peptides are now recognized. The latter peptides, also termed *endorphins*, have been identified in other systems as well, including sympathetic nervous system, which is involved in visceral pain sensation, or the immune system. Administration of the opiate morphine systemically or locally (in minute quantities) at supraspinal sites such as the periaqueductal gray or spinally near the dorsal horn produces significant analgesia.

In the interest of brevity, interested clinicians are referred to recent reviews for more thorough discussions of the intricate, fascinating, and evolving neurobiology of opioids (Carr, 1988; Carr and Murphy, 1988; Carr et al, 1988; Carr et al, 1990; Lewis et al, 1987; Twycross and McQuay, 1989). However, several points have immediate clinical relevance and will be discussed here. First, not all the diverse areas of the dorsal horn and central nervous system that receive nociceptive afferents and their projections contain high concentrations of opioid receptors. This simple observation may help to explain the ineffectiveness of opioids in relieving certain types of clinical pain (e.g., bone pain). Second, certain clinically applied opioids are active at specific opioid receptor sites that in turn selectively process distinct nociceptive signals. Thus, even for pain that does respond to opioids, one type of opioid may prove more effective than another. For example, drugs such as morphine, which acts on mu receptors, are potent against pain due to local warmth, yet other opiates such as nalbuphine, which acts on kappa receptors, are potent in treating pain due to tissue disruption or pinching. Third, at a cellular level, opioids produce effects by altering the flow of ions across cell membranes, with the exact type of ion channel affected depending on the particular opioid given. This offers the clinician the opportunity to prescribe opioids concurrently with other drugs and thereby achieve analgesic synergy. For example, local anesthetics and opioids act on different ion channels, and mixtures of low concentrations of these two types of compounds can be quite effective when delivered epidurally near the dorsal horn.

*Non-opioid, nonaminergic systems* are important not only for their analgesic synergy with opioids but also in their own right as the second major neurochemical basis for descending analgesia. Many neurons that project within the DLF to the spinal cord originate in nuclei wherein biogenic amines, particularly serotonin (5-hydroxytryptamine [5-HT]) and norepinephrine, are concentrated. Chemical or ablative lesions of the serotonin system block the action of systemic opiates (Yaksh and Wilson, 1979; Vogt, 1974). Iontophoretic application of 5-HT onto dorsal horn neurons inhibits their response to noxious input (Jordan et al, 1979). The descending noradrenergic system arises in the dorsolateral pons (Westlund et al, 1984). When norepinephrine is injected into the spinal cord, it inhibits nociceptive neurons in the dorsal horn and blocks behavioral responses to painful stimuli (Duggan, 1985; Reddy and Yaksh, 1980). This inhibition appears to be mediated via an alpha-2 receptor. Agents such as clonidine or newer drugs that act upon the alpha-2 receptor not only augment opioid analgesia but also (if given alone) inhibit nociceptive dorsal horn neurons; such drugs have been shown to be effective analgesics in animals and in man when given spinally or systemically.

This brief description of descending inhibitory systems cannot do justice to the host of neuroactive substances including biogenic amines, substance P, calcitonin, and thyrotropin-releasing hormone that participate within them (Yaksh and Aimone, 1989; Akil and Lewis, 1987; Anand and Carr, 1989).

***Amplification of Neural Signals*** Endogenous inhibition of incoming nociceptive signals is balanced by an amplification process that may have equal or greater clinical importance. Brief noxious stimuli produce persistent changes in the dorsal horn. For example, stimulation of C-fiber afferents increases the basal discharge rate and lowers the threshold for subsequent activation by nociceptive stimuli in their dorsal horn projection cells (Cook et al, 1987). In addition, the receptive fields of such neurons enlarge after a noxious stimulus. These and related observations help to explain the clinical impression that it is more difficult to "bring pain under control" if it is allowed to become severe. Indeed, animal studies have demonstrated that the dose of morphine required to suppress the firing of a dorsal horn neuron after a noxious stimulus is 10 times higher than that needed for premedication (Woolf and Wall, 1986). As the dorsal horn becomes sensitized, the internal metabolism of the neurons within it, as reflected in neuropeptide content or corresponding gene expression, also shifts.

The practical benefits of assuring minimal nociceptive activation intraoperatively in terms of long-term quality of life (e.g., preventing phantom limb pain) are now being recognized (Bach et al, 1988). The simple expedient of providing opioid premedication for surgery that can then be carried out under local anesthesia exploits the phenomenon of drug synergy referred to above and greatly postpones the onset of postoperative pain (McQuay et al, 1988). Thus, in the patient with cancer, early diagnosis and aggressive treatment of pain—even pain surrounding infrequent events such as an operation—may forestall central sensitization and thereby simplify pain management over the long term. If this is accomplished, the patient's future quality of life (e.g., freedom from pain, mobility) will be improved. Survival may even be extended in patients with coexisting problems such as angina or emphysema who have difficulty tolerating the sympathetic activation or thoracic splinting that often occurs when pain is treated inadequately (see below).

## PAIN SYNDROMES IN GYNECOLOGIC CANCER

Nonetheless, even motivated physicians who are convinced of the benefits of aggressive diagnosis and treatment of pain may be frustrated in their efforts in the setting of gynecologic cancer. As outlined above, sensory innervation of the pelvic organs is diffuse, rendering the precise diagnosis of even "normal" causes of gynecologic pain difficult. Although in many series pelvic pain is the most common presenting complaint in gynecology clinics, the genesis of this symptom is often poorly understood (Morris and O'Neill, 1958; Henker, 1979). Pain-producing tumors of the female reproductive tract may cause an array of pain syndromes even in the absence of metastases. These pain syndromes may be classified in a number of ways (Table 24-1).

## Involvement of Primary Organ

Pain may be caused directly by tumors that invade the primary organ. Infiltration or expansion within an encapsulated organ may stretch the capsule or increase the intracapsular pressure, either of which may activate nociceptors that are otherwise silent, even during cutting or burning of the viscera. Estimates vary, but around 75% of cancer pain syndromes result from direct tumor involvement of the affected organs. When pelvic organs (uterus, ovary, vagina) are invaded by cancer, a visceral pain syndrome results in which the pain is diffuse and difficult to localize. Convergence of visceral and somatic sensory pathways at the level of the spinal cord (see earlier) often results in pain referred to the somatic segment (Table 24-2).

## Nervous System Involvement (Neuropathic Pain)

Neuropathic pain syndromes result from either peripheral or central damage (usually subclinical) of the somatosensory system. In discussions of neuropathic pain, the term "deafferentation" connotes a lesion of the pe-

**TABLE 24-2  Referred Pain Syndromes in Gynecologic Malignancies**

| Site | Referred Area and Dermatome |
|---|---|
| Ovary | Abdominal wall (T10-T11) |
| Uterus | Lower abdominal wall (T11-L1) for sympathetic |
| | Vagina, perineum (S2, 3, 4) for parasympathetic |
| Bladder and vagina | Vagina, perineum (S2, 3, 4) |

ripheral nervous system, while "central" indicates damage within somatosensory pathways at spinal or supraspinal levels of the central nervous system. Clinically, neuropathic pain is dull or burning and is referred to the area of altered sensation. "Causalgia" is another term for pain associated with a damaged peripheral nerve, although an obvious deficit may not be apparent in the early stages. Neuropathic pain may also be referred to the somatotopically equivalent area of central nervous system damage, for example, as in the hemibody pain syndrome seen in certain cases of thalamic stroke. The patient with neuropathic pain may complain of spontaneous shooting pains or pain evoked by touch, light pressure, or pinprick.

In the context of gynecologic cancer, neuropathic pain most commonly results from deafferentation (i.e., peripheral nerve involvement). This important cause of pain may occur alone or along with pain due to primary organ involvement. Gynecologic malignancies are the third most common cause of *lumbosacral plexopathy* among patients with cancer, accounting for 11% of such syndromes (Foley, 1979). The two major causes of this type of pain are direct spread of tumor along nerve sheaths and spread to nearby structures to produce extraneural compression. Animal studies have demonstrated that minimal pressure is required to produce a painful neuropathy (Bennett and Xie, 1988). Estimates of tumor involvement of other peripheral nerves or sympathetic nerves (see Pain Anatomy and Physiology above) are not available. Nonetheless, *phantom anal pain* due to sacral plexopathy is recognized as a difficult yet common problem in patients with tumors of this area or after operations such as pelvic exenteration. Pain is felt in the region of the anus or rectum and may be severely incapacitating.

*Compression of the spinal cord* due to epidural metastases occurs in about 5 to 10% of all cancers (Patchall and Posner, 1985; Gilbert and Grossman, 1986). Although infrequent as a manifestation of gynecologic malignancies, it is a medical emergency. Pain is nearly always the presenting symptom (Gilbert et al, 1978) and is typically described as a band around the abdomen or chest. Often, there is tenderness to percussion over the involved vertebra.

*Acute or post-herpetic neuralgias* are neuropathic pains that result from peripheral as well as central changes. Herpes zoster may befall up to 35% of patients within an immunosuppressed population. It may be present in any dermatome, the thoracic and cervical

**TABLE 24-1  Causes of Pain in Gynecologic Malignancies**

*Direct Effects of the Tumor*
1. Direct organ involvement by tumor
2. Metastatic spread
   a. Bone
   b. Nerve
      (1) External compression of nerve or plexus
      (2) Perineural spread
      (3) Spinal cord compression
   c. Blood vessels and lymphatics

*Indirect Effects of Tumor*
1. Infection (e.g., herpes zoster)
2. Paraneoplastic syndromes
   a. Affecting nerve (e.g., neuropathy)
   b. Affecting muscle (e.g., polymyositis)
   c. Affecting blood (e.g., hypercoagulable state)

*Treatment of the Tumor*
1. Surgery
   a. Phantom pain (e.g., phantom anal pain)
   b. Neuropathic pain (from lesions of nerves innervating pelvic viscera or somatic structures)
   c. Postoperative pain
2. Radiotherapy
   a. Fibrosis
   b. Lumbar plexopathy
3. Chemotherapy
   a. Neuritis
   b. Peripheral neuropathy

*Coincidental* (unrelated to tumor or treatment)

regions being the most commonly affected. The pain is steady and burning, with additional lancinating components. Certain aspects of the treatment of herpetic neuralgia (e.g., response to sympathetic blocks) are quite distinct from more general drug therapy of neuropathic pain and will be discussed separately below.

### Bone Involvement

Infiltration of bone by metastases is a leading cause of pain in cancer patients, although this is relatively uncommon with gynecologic tumors. Bone metastases are present in only 2 to 6% of patients with cancer of the ovary (Nystrom et al, 1977). Bone invasion or metastasis to the sacrum may be difficult to detect on plain films because of the normally irregular and variable contour of this bone, particularly if bowel gas is present. Furthermore, painful bone metastases may not be identified on radionuclide bone scans or plain films early in the course of the disease, sometimes for up to 6 months (Low, 1981; Kanner et al, 1982). Even then, such tests for metastases may be negative if radiotherapy has been given previously or the metastasis is osteoclastic (Thrupkaew et al, 1974).

***Iatrogenic Pain*** Pain as a complication of radiotherapy is present in 9 to 15% of patients with gynecologic tumors who receive this form of treatment (Borodon, 1982; Hogan et al, 1982; Perez and Camel, 1982). Most of these pain syndromes result from radiation injury to uninvolved organs producing fistulas, necrosis, cystitis, or stricture formation. Postirradiation neuritis is a further complication.

Chemotherapy of gynecologic cancers can also produce painful complications. For example, vincristine may produce a painful peripheral neuropathy, myalgias, or arthralgias; methotrexate may cause bone pain; and 5-fluorouracil may result in pain in the chest or eyes. Although these syndromes are relatively rare, the clinician should be aware of these painful side effects.

### Pain Syndromes Due to Secondary Causes

Gynecologic tumors can be responsible for an array of secondary causes of pain. These are usually clinically obvious and include infection (including abscess formation or superinfection of damaged mucous membranes or skin), fistula formation (due to primary disease or efforts to treat it by means of surgery or radiotherapy), venous obstruction or thrombosis, opiate-induced constipation, bed sores, and intestinal perforation or obstruction. Patients with cancer of the ovary seem to be susceptible to this last complication, which occurs in over 30% of cases.

Depression in response to the diagnosis and prognosis of malignancy, either as a primary psychiatric disorder or secondary to a cancer-related disorder (e.g., hypercalcemia), may be associated with an increase in pain complaints. Pain may be exacerbated by feelings of depression, as if such feelings lower the threshold for interpreting ongoing sensory input as pain and thus make such suffering more likely.

### "Normal" Pain Syndromes

The cancer patient may, of course, be afflicted with aches and pains similar to those affecting the general population, the most common being backache, headache, or muscle pain. However, such complaints should always be taken seriously and a cause sought by means of appropriate clinical tests.

## MEDICAL MANAGEMENT OF PAIN

The synergism between new motives and methods for treating pain aggressively has proved beneficial and will certainly continue to be so. Evidence for this trend can be found in the growing membership in and number of societies devoted to pain research or management, announcements of new journals in these areas, and the appearance of more reports in established journals concerning clinical investigations of pain. National and international organizations have already declared initiatives to eradicate "the tragedy of needless pain"—the title chosen by Melzack for his recent presidential address before the International Association for the Study of Pain (Melzack, 1988).

Beyond the traditional humane efforts to enhance patients' quality of life, the new motives for aggressive pain treatment are three-fold: First is the recognition that pain is a plastic and evolving process in which perceptual experience reflects not simply nociceptive stimuli but also the opposing dynamic actions of endogenous inhibitory and amplifying systems activated by such stimuli (see earlier discussion). Therefore, intervention at an early stage may greatly simplify subsequent pain management, such as administering preoperative epidural anesthesia to prevent postamputation phantom pain (Bach et al, 1988). Second, it is now clear that the perception of pain is simply one process amidst a host of autonomic, metabolic, and neuroendocrine responses to nociception (Carr, 1988). Thus, aggressive analgesia may avert cardiopulmonary or metabolic compromise that might result from unchecked nociceptive responses, such as after palliative abdominal surgery or in the diabetic. Third, it is not surprising in light of the above that studies of outcome after painful stressors such as surgery have demonstrated benefits (e.g., reductions in morbidity, mortality, and duration or expense of hospital stay) when newer methods of aggressive analgesia are applied, particularly in "high-risk" patient groups (Yeager et al, 1987).

New methods of pain control are also, broadly speaking, threefold. First, new drugs (or improved formulations of old drugs, such as sustained-release morphine) are now available. Second, "new" or previously unpopular routes of administration are being used to great effect, such as the delivery of opioids via intrathecal catheters or transdermal patches. Third, new devices such as rugged, portable, programmable pumps to infuse medications via new or old (e.g., subcutaneous) routes are changing conventional practice. Wide application of these new technologies has now blurred the distinction between techniques once considered suitable only for acute pain control in hospitalized patients and those deemed appropriate for chronic use in ambulatory outpatients. Many of the latter patients, for example, now receive continuous infusions of narcotics subcutaneously or intraspinally.

Given the increasing artificiality of restricting a particular method of pain control to either acute pain in hospitalized patients or chronic pain in outpatients as well as the fact that the acute and chronic components of pain typically coexist in both these settings, we will not "bisect" our survey of pain management. Instead, we will describe each type of treatment individually, without suggesting that their application be limited by the clinical setting or the duration of the targeted pain.

## Nonsteroidal Antiinflammatory Drugs (NSAIDs)

Most available NSAIDs inhibit cyclooxygenase, the enzyme responsible for the breakdown of arachidonic acid to prostaglandins in peripheral tissue. Recent evidence from both human and animal studies has implicated NSAIDs in central effects too, such as augmenting endogenous descending analgesic pathways. Except for an increase in gastrointestinal side effects with agents such as aspirin or indomethacin, there is no real advantage of one NSAID over another despite the fact that costs for these drugs vary enormously. Typical doses and intervals for commonly used NSAIDs are given in Table 24-3. Regardless of the particular choice of agent, NSAIDs must be titrated to an optimal dose; if relief is not obtained, a different NSAID should be tried.

When available intravenously or as a suppository, NSAIDs may reduce acute postoperative pain, particularly when coexisting conditions such as pulmonary disease constitute a relative contraindication to narcotic use. Indeed, it is possible to avoid postoperative opioids entirely in selected patients by combining NSAID therapy with the regional infusion of a local anesthetic (see below). NSAIDs are particularly effective against pain due to cancer-related inflammation or bone metastasis. Frequently, they provide relief when given alone, prompting the World Health Organization to recommend NSAID therapy (without opioids) as the initial step in treating cancer pain. Although longer-acting agents such as diclofenac acid are useful for cancer pain, a loading dose is required to obtain the same rapid analgesia as the short-acting agents. When given along with a narcotic, NSAIDs typically provide greater relief from cancer pain than when the opioid is given alone (Beaver, 1984).

## Opioids

Opioids are a mainstay of treatment for all cancer patients. Unfortunately, *undertreatment* with narcotics is a common problem in hospital practice. Ambivalence concerning opioid use is widespread among health professionals, reflecting what Melzack sees as society's tendency to confuse drug abuse by street addicts with the appropriate use of these agents for patients in pain (Melzack, 1988).

***Dosing Considerations*** Often the prescribed doses of narcotics are too small or the dosing interval is too long. Although dosage titration is a simple point, it is all too often overlooked and contributes unnecessarily to patients' suffering.

Conferring with the patient is the best way to determine the appropriate analgesic dose. Narcotic metabolism varies from individual to individual, so dosing intervals must often be adjusted. While the patient is on maintenance narcotics, a short-acting supplemental narcotic agent should available for "breakthrough" pain, which may ensue as a result of activity or unknown factors. For example, if a patient is taking 30 mg of long-acting morphine twice a day, a dose of 10 to 15 mg of oral immediate-release morphine elixir should be available whenever needed. By taking this approach and observing the frequency with which medications are used for breakthrough pain, one may easily assess the adequacy of the long-acting dose and alter it.

Another approach to overcoming dosing problems in patients with cancer, either in or out of the hospital, is *patient-controlled analgesia* (PCA). With PCA, a drug-delivery device is used to self-administer analgesics in patients who are specifically instructed about this technique. Morphine is most often selected as the opioid analgesic and is administered either intravenously (e.g., for inpatients) or subcutaneously (e.g., for outpatients). Different drugs or mixtures (e.g., fentanyl plus bupivacaine) and delivery routes (e.g., intraspinal or oral/transbuccal mucosa) are finding increasing application and, if their initial promise is borne out, may be more widely used for PCA. At present, intravenous PCA involves programming a small, computer-controlled pump to deliver a continuous, basal infusion of opioid

| TABLE 24-3   Non-Narcotic Analgesics | | | | |
|---|---|---|---|---|
| Drug | Trade Name(s) | Dose (mg) | Interval (hr) | Max Dose/Day (mg) |
| Acetaminophen | (many) | 500-1,000 | 4-6 | 4,000 |
| Acetylsalicylic acid | (many) | 500-1,000 | 4-6 | 4,000 |
| Diclofenac acid | Voltaren | 25-50 | 6-8 | 150 |
| Indomethacin | Indocin | 25 | 8-12 | 100 |
| Ibuprofen | Motrin | 200-400 | 4-6 | 2,400 |
| Magnesium trisilicate | Trilisate | 750 | 6-8 | 4,500 |
| Piroxicam | Feldene | 20 | 24 | 20 |

plus additional "demand" PCA bolus doses. Hourly limits on the total dose of opioid delivered along with lockout intervals to prevent continuous opioid dosing are also programmed. If pain is present at the time when PCA is applied, it is helpful to provide small, repeated doses of opioid to reduce pain intensity to minimal levels; subsequent pain control is thus simplified and may be accomplished using a very low continuous infusion rate plus small-bolus PCA doses (e.g., 1 mg of morphine sulfate). In studies of postoperative pain, the total daily amount of drug used during PCA has been found to be no greater—and in certain studies actually less—than that used in conventional methods, such as intramuscular injections as needed.

*Alternative routes* of opioid administration include sublingual, rectal, or continuous transdermal administration (Payne, 1989). The use of these methods in preference to oral or injectable dosing depends not only on the general ratio of desirable-to-undesirable side effects but also on the particular circumstance, such as providing a rectal morphine or oxymorphone suppository in patients who cannot take medications orally and for whom injections are a problem, as in cachexia. Spinal opioids deserve special mention and are discussed below.

**Tolerance and Addiction** Tolerance may develop during drug administration by any route. This means that the effect of a fixed dose of medication given over time begins to diminish, so that a larger dose of the drug is required to produce the same clinical effect. In vitro, the number of opioid receptors or postreceptor responses to opioids (e.g., cyclic nucleotide generation) have been found to be decreased after chronic opioid administration. Yet, the mechanisms of clinical tolerance are poorly understood and are likely to vary from patient to patient. For example, many patients with a slowly progressive malignancy enjoy good analgesia for weeks or more on a fixed dose of opioid. In the short term, total daily intravenous morphine doses given by PCA often remain constant (are not increased) for several days after operation, until oral agents are begun. Thus, it is possible that in vivo, steadily rising morphine requirements might reflect central sensitization (see above) rather than increased elimination or receptor downregulation.

When tolerance does occur to one type of opioid such as morphine, cross-tolerance to other morphine-like agents (e.g., meperidine or fentanyl) is normally present. Naturally, an abrupt rise in morphine requirement should raise the question of disease progression and trigger a prompt workup.

Tolerance should not be mistaken for addiction. The fear of addiction contributes to undertreatment with narcotics even though this problem is uncommon in the hospital setting, occurring in fewer than one in 3,000 patients newly treated with opioids (Porter and Jick, 1980).

**Equivalent Dosage** Inappropriate conversion between narcotics is another problem that needlessly contributes to undertreatment. Table 24-4 lists equivalent doses for those opioids frequently used to treat cancer pain. Although meperidine is included in this list, its long-term use is inadvisable in light of accumulation of its dysphorigenic and proconvulsant metabolite normeperidine (Kaiko et al, 1983). If meperidine is given during treatment with antidepressants of the monoamine oxidase inhibitor class (see below), a fatal hypertensive and hyperpyrexic crisis may ensue (Kaufman, 1976). It is worth noting that the time to peak analgesia for oral morphine is about 90 minutes, for intramuscular injections about 45 minutes, and for intravenous administration about 30 minutes.

**Spinal Narcotic Administration** In 1976, Yaksh and Rudy described analgesia due to the direct spinal effects of narcotics. Administration of opiates into the epidural or subarachnoid space activates opiate receptors within the spinal cord and produces significant analgesia. A "selective analgesia" is produced, in which a predominantly nociceptive blockade is established without loss of cutaneous sensation and with minimal motor effects (Bromage, 1978; Cousins et al, 1979; Cousins and Mather, 1984). Spinally administered narcotics will also affect more rostral sites, such as the periaqueductal gray, as a result of direct spread within the cerebrospinal fluid (CSF) or as a secondary phenomenon of redistribution within the vascular system. Highly lipid-soluble drugs (e.g., fentanyl) will be removed from the CSF faster than poorly lipid-soluble, hydrophilic drugs (e.g., morphine). Therefore, the latter agents will be carried rostrally by

---

TABLE 24-4 Opioids Used in Pain Therapy (Including Equivalent Doses)

| Drug | Trade Name | IM Dose (mg) | PO Dose (mg) | Interval (hr) |
|------|-----------|-------------|-------------|--------------|
| Morphine | | 10 | 20-30 | 4-5 |
| Methadone | Dolophine | 10 | 10-20 | 6-12 |
| Meperidine | Demerol | 75 | 50-100 | 3 |
| Hydromorphone | Dilaudid | 2 | 4 | 3-5 |
| Levorphanol | Levo-dromoran | 2 | 4 | 6-8 |
| Codeine | | 120 | 30-60 | 3-5 |
| Oxycodone | | | | |
| +ASA | Percodan | — | 10-15 | 3-5 |
| +ACET | Percocet | — | 10-15 | 3-5 |

the normal flow of CSF to produce a less segmental analgesia and rostral central nervous system depression. In such cases, bradycardia or respiratory depression may occur from 1 to 36 hours after the initial injection (Coombs et al, 1984a) and may also cause nausea, vomiting, urinary retention, or itching.

In selecting an epidural or intrathecal route for pain-relieving medications, one must first confirm that this will be effective (Waldman et al, 1986; Carr, 1987). Initially, a temporary percutaneous catheter is placed while the patient is observed in the hospital to determine whether the drug is effective or causes side effects. Correct placement of the catheter can be confirmed by fluoroscopic demonstration of radiopaque dye in the epidural space after injection through the catheter at the time of insertion, before any drugs are administered. If epidural analgesia is subtherapeutic, switching to a mixture containing a local anesthetic might be considered, or an intrathecal catheter might be placed.

A variety of options are available for catheterization. For a patient with a relatively short life-expectancy, a subcutaneous catheter tunneled under the skin with an external injection port or even a small subcutaneous reservoir is probably best, since it can be inserted rapidly without the need for surgery. Otherwise, a totally implanted system with a subcutaneous injection port or reservoir would be more appropriate. Factors such as the location of the pain, life expectancy, social environment, home support, and cost of the system will influence the decision to place a spinal catheter.

Intrathecal starting doses of 0.1 to 0.5 mg of preservative-free morphine have been used in patients with cancer who experience pain while taking oral opioids at high doses limited by side effects. The intrathecal dose is then doubled with each nonresponse. The starting doses of epidural morphine are five to ten times higher than intrathecal doses. Typically, for epidural administration, a daily morphine dose that is approximately 10% of the current systemic daily dose is given. With either route, it is possible to titrate dosage to achieve excellent analgesia with little drowsiness. Risks of the procedure include infection, neurologic dysfunction, hemorrhage, and gradual fibrosis and blockage of the catheter tip. However, reports of excellent long-term results are now numerous (Arner and Arner, 1985; Coombs et al, 1982; Poletti et al, 1981).

Several subpopulations of opioid receptors that may alter nociceptive processing are present in the dorsal laminae of the spinal cord (Castillo et al, 1986; Yaksh, 1984; Wood et al, 1981; Schmaus and Yaksh, 1984). Thus, selective opioid agonists of several types may produce analgesia (Carr et al, 1990). A peptide delta opioid agonist has been used successfully in a patient with rectal cancer who became tolerant of intrathecal morphine (Onofrio and Yaksh, 1983). Other opioid peptides look promising (Oyama et al, 1980; Wen et al, 1987), although controversy has arisen as a result of spinal neurotoxicity recently recognized in nonhuman species after direct intraspinal administration of pharmacologic doses of certain peptide analogs or fragments (Herman and Goldstein, 1985; Stevens et al, 1987; Long et al, 1988). The partial agonist-antagonist bu-

prenorphine may offer analgesic efficacy with fewer side effects for long-term use (Carl et al, 1986). Furthermore, the use of epinephrine or similar adrenergic agonists or local anesthetics in combination with narcotics may decrease side effects (Kepper et al, 1987) and provide improved analgesia. Additional clinical trials will be needed to determine whether the use of specific opioid agonists singly or in combination is advantageous.

## Local Anesthetics

Local anesthetic blocks are not usually feasible for treating cancer pain but are useful as diagnostic tools. In a few instances, these agents can be used therapeutically, as for examples in tumor-related sympathetic dystrophies or painful muscle spasms (Gerbeshagen, 1979). Topical application of local anesthetics has been shown to be useful in post-herpetic neuralgia (Rowbotham and Fields, 1989), while tocainide or mexilitene has been used for peripheral neuropathy (Dejgard et al, 1988).

Although single injections of local anesthetic agents are of limited value, these agents are very useful when given epidurally. Local anesthetics injected into the epidural or intrathecal sac can block pain by their action on axons of the nerve roots where they enter the spinal cord, on axons within the cord (Cousins and Mather, 1984), or on primary afferent nociceptors within the dorsal horn (Woolf and Wiesenfeld-Hallin, 1985).

Epidural local anesthetics usually provide complete relief from pain and are therefore useful for overcoming tolerance to spinal opioids. At higher concentrations the analgesia is nonselective, since other sensory or motor pathways are blocked. However, at lower concentrations (e.g., below 0.1% bupivacaine), some local anesthetics can provide analgesia with minimal motor effects. When local anesthetics are administered epidurally to treat the pain of gynecologic cancer, the catheter is usually placed in the lumbar region, and the patient is assisted during ambulation to watch for motor or sympathetic block that would result in weakness or orthostatic hypotension.

## Antidepressants (Table 24-5)

Pain may coexist with depression, or depression may be a consequence of chronic pain. These two clinical conditions involve changes in common neurotransmitters, namely, norepinephrine and serotonin. Whether or not there is a true common pathophysiologic pathway, antidepressants have been useful adjuvant medications in the treatment of cancer pain.

Antidepressants are thought to exert their analgesic effects by augmenting the synaptic action of biogenic amines. One mechanism that could account for their analgesic action is inhibition of serotonin and/or degradation of norepinephrine at the level of descending inputs from brainstem structures to the dorsal horn (see above). Commonly used tricyclic antidepressants inhibit serotonin and norepinephrine catabolism or synaptic reuptake, with the mechanism and amine selectivity depending on the agent. In animal studies, activation of the serotonergic system has been more efficacious than

TABLE 24-5  Antidepressants Used in Pain Therapy

| Drug | Trade Name | Side Effects | | | Usual Dose (mg/day) |
|---|---|---|---|---|---|
| | | Anticholinergic | Sedation | Hypotension | |
| *Tricyclics:* | | | | | |
| Amitriptyline* | Elavil | + + + + | + + + + | + + | 50-150 |
| Imipramine | Tofranil | + + | + + + | + + + | 100-200 |
| Nortriptyline | Pamelor | + + | + + + | + | 50-100 |
| Desipramine | Norpramin | + | + + | + | 50-150 |
| Doxepin | Sinequan | + + | + + + + | + + | 50-200 |
| Trazodone | Desyrel | + | + + + + | + + + | 150-200 |
| *Monoamine oxidase inhibitors:* | | | | | |
| Phenelzine | Nardil | + + | — | + + + + | 30-90 |
| Tranylcypromine | Parnate | + + | — | + + + | 10-40 |

\* Only agent shown in controlled clinical trials to relieve neuropathic pain (Max et al, 1987).
+ + + + = high; + + + = moderate; + + = low; + = lowest; — = none.

that of the adrenergic system. However, the few double-blind controlled clinical trials involving patients with chronic pain suggest a more significant role for norepinephrine systems (Max et al, 1987; Kishmore-Kumar et al, 1989).

Selective inhibitors of serotonin uptake have been disappointing in the treatment of chronic pain. There are no double-blind studies of the use of antidepressants in subjects with cancer pain. However, several authors have reported benefits from their use in that they provided a 50 to 90% decrease in cancer pain (Gebhart et al, 1969; Adjan, 1970; Deutschmann, 1971). These agents seem to be useful in certain neuropathic conditions, including post-herpetic neuralgia and radiation fibrosis or other conditions that cause symptoms of a dull, burning type of neuropathic pain.

The choice of a particular agent depends on the age of the patient and potential side effects, the most common of which are urinary retention and sedation. For example, trazodone (Desyrel) or desipramine (Norpramin) have fewer anticholinergic side effects than does amitriptyline (Elavil). It is important to emphasize that the use of meperidine with the monoamine oxidase inhibitors is potentially fatal and is absolutely contraindicated (Kaufman, 1976).

## Anticonvulsants

Useful anticonvulsants and related agents are listed in Table 24-6. These agents are primarily indicated for neuropathic pain and are thought to act by decreasing

TABLE 24-6  Anticonvulsants Used for Neuropathic Pain

| Drug | Trade Name | Usual Dose |
|---|---|---|
| Phenytoin | Dilantin | 100-200 mg tid |
| Carbamazepine | Tegretol | 100-200 mg tid |
| Baclofen | Lioresal | 10-30 mg tid |
| Clonazepam | Clonopine | 0.5-2.0 mg tid |

ectopic neuronal discharge. Clinically, symptoms of shooting or electric pains may respond to these agents. The usual side effects are nausea, dizziness, and somnolence. Tegretol can cause liver dysfunction and bone marrow suppression. Patients should be placed on anticonvulsants in slowly incremental doses; when the agent is withdrawn, it should be tapered over a minimum of 3 to 4 days. Plasma levels should be checked regularly and blood drawn weekly at the initiation of therapy and then monthly for complete blood count and liver function screening. For detailed reviews on the use of anticonvulsant agents in the treatment of chronic pain, see Swerdlow (1982) and Fields and Raskin (1976). Again, no controlled trials have examined the use of these agents for cancer pain.

## Other Adjuvant Pharmacologic Therapies

***Adrenergic Agonists***  As discussed earlier, descending noradrenergic pathways from the brainstem—notably the dorsolateral pons—act on dorsal horn neurons to inhibit nociceptive transmission (Hammond and Yaksh, 1984; Yaksh, 1985; Kuraishi et al, 1987). Norepinephrine administered into the dorsal horn suppresses activity of these neurons which are activated by painful afferent stimuli (Fleetwood-Walker et al, 1985). This effect is thought to be mediated by an alpha-2-adrenergic receptor, since specific alpha-2 agonists inhibit pain more effectively than do mixed agonists or beta agonists.

Clonidine, an alpha-2-receptor agonist, has been used successfully via the epidural route in patients with cancer (Coombs et al, 1984*b*; Tamsen and Gordh, 1984). This drug offers an alternative treatment for patients tolerant to morphine. Furthermore, since activation of the mu and alpha-2 receptors produces synergistic analgesia, the use of combination therapy permits effective analgesia with fewer side effects. Side effects from clonidine include mild sedation, dry mouth, and hypotension. The drug has also been used orally for neuropathic pain (Max et al, 1988; Petros and Wright, 1987).

***Neuroleptics*** The neuroleptics, such as haloperidol, may have direct analgesic effects. Methotrimeprazine has been shown to have specific analgesic effects (Lasagna and DeKornfeld, 1961; McGee and Alexander, 1979) and has been used effectively in postoperative, cancer, and chronic syndromes. Neuroleptics also potentiate narcotic analgesia and provide useful antiemetic properties. The main analgesic use of these agents is for patients whose pain is not treatable by other conservative means. Respiratory depression may occur when neuroleptics are administered along with opioids. The phenothiazines have significant side effects, including extrapyramidal syndromes, hypotension, and sedation.

***Stimulants*** Amphetamines markedly enhance the analgesic efficacy of narcotics and reduce the drowsiness produced by narcotics (Forrest et al, 1977). Accordingly, the addition of dextroamphetamine is frequently a useful therapeutic maneuver for patients in whom sedation limits the opioid dosage (Weintraub et al, 1986).

***Glucocorticoids ("Steroids")*** Unfortunately, no controlled studies have examined the use of glucocorticoids as primary treatment for cancer pain. Of course, these drugs are useful in settings in which edema and inflammation give rise to pain, as in the treatment of painful spinal or bony metastases or plexus lesions.

***Antihistamines*** Hydroxyzine given intramuscularly has some analgesic potency (Stambaugh and Lane, 1983) and also potentiates narcotic analgesia (Rumore and Schlichting, 1986). Given alone, it may be useful in patients in whom narcotics are contraindicated.

***Capsaicin*** Upon application to skin, capsaicin (derived from red peppers) depletes substance P and other neurotransmitters in both central and peripheral terminals of primary afferent neurons, particularly C fibers (Ainsworth et al, 1981; Nagy et al, 1981; Gamse et al, 1980). Furthermore, capsaicin can block axonal transport of substance P (Gamse et al, 1982) and electrical conduction in nerves (Petsche et al, 1983; Waddell and Lawsen, 1989). All these effects decrease sensitivity to pain. Only topical creams are currently applied in post-herpetic neuralgia and peripheral neuropathy. Recently, a higher concentration (0.075%) has become available. In animal models, capsaicin can inhibit visceral pain syndromes (Lembeck and Gamse, 1982), and studies are now evaluating its clinical application.

# NEUROSURGICAL MANAGEMENT OF PAIN

Despite major advances in the medical treatment of cancer pain, neurosurgery should always be considered when medical approaches no longer provide effective pain relief. It is only common sense—but often overlooked—that neurosurgical outcomes may be better and risks of operation lowered by operating early in the course of the disease rather than when the patient is preterminal. Indeed, recent reports of subtle, adverse neuropsychiatric effects of long-term opioid use suggest that quality of life might be enhanced by a neurosurgical procedure that permits chronic opioid therapy to be discontinued (Wood and Cousins, 1989).

In general, surgical ablation of nerves does not provide permanent pain relief. Yet, in carefully selected patients, neurosurgical techniques may be appropriate and useful, e.g., if life expectancy is limited and neurologic function is already compromised. Since this topic cannot be covered in depth here, the interested reader is referred to more complete reviews (Siegfried et al, 1984; Gybels and Sweet, 1989).

It should be noted that many neurosurgical techniques can be performed percutaneously, with minimal discomfort—an important consideration in patients with gynecologic cancer. Basically, two neurosurgical approaches are in use: ablative surgery to interrupt nociceptive pathways and electrical stimulation of neural structures to inhibit the passage of nociceptive information.

## Ablative Procedures

A number of ablative procedures can be performed to interrupt nociceptive pathways. Intrathecal injection of neurolytic agents such as absolute alcohol or phenol is a time-honored approach to central ablation (Cousins and Bridenbaugh, 1988). However, such techniques are imprecise compared with corresponding neurosurgical approaches and are ordinarily deferred when the latter are available. Some neurosurgical procedures, such as neurectomy, are of limited value in the patient with cancer, since selective ablation of pain fibers cannot be performed and sensorimotor function is abolished in the distribution of the nerve(s). Furthermore, rhizotomy, which usually involves a number of dermatomal levels, is often not successful in relieving pain even though it produces a loss of tactile and position sense (Loeser, 1972).

In 1979, use of the *dorsal root entry zone (DREZ) lesion* was introduced (Nashold and Ostahl, 1979). The DREZ lesion includes the central portion of the dorsal roots, Lissauer's tract, and laminae I to V of the dorsal horn. Proprioception and tactile sensation usually remain intact. In cancer patients with pain, a number of authors have reported good results in as many as 87% of patients treated in this way (Nashold and Ostdahl, 1979). The DREZ procedure should be reserved for patients with limited extension of the tumor and reasonable life expectancies. Patients suffering from deafferentation pain due to the primary tumor might be considered for DREZ lesions, although clinical experience in this area is still limited.

In gynecologic malignancies, midline pain in the perineal region is a frequent problem and one that is difficult to treat medically. *Myelotomy*, in which the spinal cord is divided along the midline in a rostrocaudal direction, starting three to four levels above the site of clinical pain, may be useful in patients with rectal, perineal, and sacral pain not responsive to more conventional forms of therapy. In one series, this approach provided pain relief in 86% of cases (Sindou and Daher, 1988).

In 1912, the first *anterolateral cordotomy* was performed (Spiller and Martin, 1912). This procedure (which may be performed percutaneously) interrupts the spinothalamic tract on the side opposite to the site of pain. Pain was relieved in 76 to 100% of patients immediately after operation, in 75% at 6 months postoperatively, and in 40% at 1 year (White and Sweet, 1979). Patients with more caudal pain syndromes, such as those with gynecologic malignancy, are good candidates, since caudal segments tend to be represented more superficially in the spinothalamic tract (Sweet and Poletti, 1989), and good results have been reported in patients with pain due to gynecologic cancer (Gildenberg and Hirchberg, 1984; Hogberg et al, 1989).

*Extralemniscal myelotomy* is a relatively new procedure in which radiofrequency lesions are placed at the center of the spinal cord (Hitchcock, 1970; Gildenberg and Hirshberg, 1984; Eiras et al, 1980). Good to excellent results (67 to 87%) have been reported, with few complications or side effects.

*Pituitary ablation* was initially devised as a hormonal treatment in patients with breast and prostate cancer. Yet, it has proved effective for pain relief in patients with widespread metastases, even when the growth of the tumor is not known to be dependent on pituitary hormones. An intranasal transsphenoidal approach is simplest; either cryoprobe or alcohol is used to ablate the gland. The mechanism of pain relief is not understood and various hypotheses have been advanced, including changes in as yet uncharacterized pituitary growth factors, central opioid peptide alterations, and damage to the hypothalamus or thalamus (Carr and Carr, 1983). In expert hands, the procedure is safe and often permits all analgesics to be withdrawn eventually.

### Electrical Stimulation of Brain Structures

Electrical stimulation of deep brain structures (periventricular gray of the caudal diencephalon, the internal capsule, or the parabrachial region) or the dorsal columns of the spinal cord has been used in cancer patients with some success and produces no systemic side effects. While dorsal column stimulator implantation and use is relatively benign, stimulation of central structures is significantly more complicated. For a review, readers are referred to the report by Gybels and Sweet (1989).

## CONCLUSIONS

Remarkable inroads have recently been made in our understanding of the biology of neoplasia, and the pace of discovery in this field is, if anything, quickening. Yet, until gynecologic cancer is uniformly curable and ways to prevent, detect, and treat it early are universally applied, pain will continue to be a potential source of suffering and disability. Happily, pain control now enjoys a high priority in settings where women are involved as mothers, such as pediatrics; as patients, such

as postoperatively; or in both roles, such as in childbirth. In each of these settings as well as in gynecologic cancer, pain control has emerged as a standard of care only in the last few years, having been previously overlooked.

Cancer pain may now be effectively treated and need not be helplessly tolerated. Knowing from the outset that pain relief is an attainable goal is most reassuring to the patient and her family. During followup, prompt and systematic efforts to keep pain well controlled will improve the patient's quality of life and strengthen her confidence in the health care network, which includes her family, primary physician, nurses, and consultants ranging from physical therapists to consultant physicians to clinical nurse specialists. The focal point for effective treatment is the shared awareness that ample resources are now available to control pain in most cases, that pain is neither inevitable nor acceptable, and that vigorous efforts to relieve pain are a right of every patient.

## ACKNOWLEDGMENTS

We thank the staff of the Pain Control Unit, Department of Anesthesia, Massachusetts General Hospital, for their formative role in shaping our collaborative practice approaches to the care of patients with pain. In particular, Elizabeth Ryder, R.N., M.S.N., provided helpful comments and a critical review of this manuscript.

## REFERENCES

Adjan M: Zur therapeutischen Beeinsflussung des Schmerzsymptoms bei unheilbaren Tumorkranken. *Ther Ggw* 109:1620-1627, 1970.

Ainsworth A, Hall P, Wall PD, Allt G, MacKenzie ML, Gibson S, Polack JM: Effects of capsaicin applied locally to adult peripheral nerve. II. Anatomy and enzyme and peptide chemistry of peripheral nerve and spinal cord. *Pain* 11:379-388, 1981.

Akil H, Lewis JW: Neurotransmitters and pain control. In Gildenberg PL (ed): *Pain and Headache.* Vol 9. Basel, Karger, 1987.

Anand KJS, Carr DB: The neuroanatomy, neurophysiology and neurochemistry of pain, stress and analgesia in newborns and children. In Schechter NL (ed): *Acute Pain in Children. Pediat Clin N Am* Vol 36. Philadelphia, WB Saunders Co, 1989, pp 795-822.

Arner S, Arner B: Differential effects of epidural morphine in the treatment of cancer-related pain. *Acta Anesth Scand* 29:32-36, 1985.

Atweh SF, Kuhar MJ: Distribution and physiological significance of opioid receptors in the brain. *Br Med Bull* 39:47-52, 1983.

Bach S, Noreng MF, Tjellden NU: Phantom limb pain in amputees during the first 12 months following limb amputation after preoperative lumbar epidural blockade. *Pain* 33:297-301, 1988.

Bahr R, Blumberg H, Janig W: Do dichotomizing afferent fibers exist which supply visceral organs as well as somatic structures? A contribution to the problem of referred pain. *Neurosci Lett* 24:25-28, 1981.

Barbaro NM: Studies of PAG/PVG stimulation for pain relief in humans. *Progr Brain Res* 77:165-173, 1988.

Basbaum AI, Fields HL : Endogenous pain control systems: Brainstem spinal pathways and endorphin circuitry. *Ann Rev Neurosci* 7:309-338, 1984.

Basbaum AI, Marley NJE, O'Keefe J, Clanton CH: Reversal of morphine and stimulus produced analgesia by subtotal spinal cord lesions. *Pain* 3:43-56, 1977.

Baskin DS, Mehler WR, Hosobuchi Y, Richardson DE, Adams JE,

Flitter MA: Autopsy analysis of the safety, efficacy and cartography of electrical stimulation of the central gray in humans. *Brain Res* 371:231-236, 1986.

Beaver WT: Combination analgesics. *Am J Med* 77:38-53, 1984.

Beecher HK: *The Measurement of Subjective Responses.* New York, Oxford University Press, 1959.

Bennett GJ, Xie YK: A peripheral mononeuropathy in rats that produces disorders of pain sensation like those in man. *Pain* 33:87-107, 1988.

Bonica JJ: *The Management of Pain.* Philadelphia, Lea and Febiger, 1953.

Bonica JJ, Greenwald H, Francis A, Bergner M: *Report on Epidemiology of Cancer Pain.* Meeting of National Cancer Institute, USA, 1979.

Bonica JJ: Cancer pain: Importance of the problem. In Bonica JJ, Ventafridda V (eds): Proceedings of the international Symposium on pain of advanced cancer. New York, Raven Press, 1979, pp 1-2.

Bonica JJ: Management of cancer pain. In Zimmerman M, Dings P, Wagner G (eds): *Recent Results in Cancer Research.* Vol 89. Berlin, Springer-Verlag, 1984, pp 13-27.

Borodon RC: Combined therapy as an alternative to exenteration for locally advanced vulvo-vaginal cancer: Rationale and results. *Cancer* 49:1085-1091, 1982.

Bromage PR: *Epidural Analgesia.* Philadelphia, WB Saunders Co, 1978.

Brose WG, Cousins MJ: In Coppleson M (ed): *Gynecological Oncology,* 2nd ed. New York, Churchill Livingstone, 1992, in press.

Brown AG, Kirk EJ, Martin HF: Descending and segmental inhibition of transmission through the spinocervical tract. *J Physiol* (Lond) 230:689-705, 1973.

Capps JA, Coleman GH: *An Experimental and Clinical Study of Pain in Pleura, Pericardium and Peritoneum.* New York, Macmillan, 1932.

Carl P, Crawford ME, Ravlo O, Bach V: Longterm treatment with epidural opioids: A retrospective study comprising 150 patients treated with morphine chloride and buprenorphine. *Anesthesia* 54:843-847, 1986.

Carr DB: Pain. In Firestone L, Cook CE, Lebowitz PW (eds): *Clinical Anesthesia Procedures of the Massachusetts General Hospital.* Boston, Little, Brown & Co, 1987, pp 571-585.

Carr DB: Opioids. In Firestone L (ed): *Molecular Basis of Drug Action in Anesthesia.* Boston, Little, Brown & Co, 1988, *Int Anesth Clin.* 26:273-287.

Carr DB, Carr JM: The role of brain opiates in pain relief. In Stoll BA, Parbhoo SP (eds): *Bone Metastasis and Its Treatment.* New York, Raven Press, 1983, pp. 375-393.

Carr DB, Murphy MR: Operation, anesthesia and the endorphin system. In Napolitano LM, Chernow B (eds): *Stress Responses During Anesthesia.* Boston, Little, Brown & Co, 1988, *Int Anesth Clin* 26:199-205.

Carr DB, Lipkowski AW, Silbert BS: Biochemistry of the opioid peptides. In Estafanous FG (ed): *Opioids in Anesthesia II.* New York, Butterworth, 1991, pp 3-16.

Carr DB, Saini V, Verrier RL: Opioids and cardiovascular function: Neuromodulation of ventricular ectopy. In Kulbertus HE, Franck G (eds): *Neurocardiology.* Mt Kisco, NY, Futura, 1988, pp. 223-245.

Carstens E: Inhibition of spinal dorsal horn neuronal responses to noxious skin heating by medial hypothalamic stimulation in the cat. *J Neurophysiol* 48:808-822, 1982.

Carstens E, Yokota T: Viscerosomatic convergence and responses to intestinal distention of neurons at the junction of the midbrain and posterior thalamus in the cat. *Exp Neurol* 70:392-402, 1980.

Cartwright A, Hockey L, Anderson ABM (eds): *Life Before Death.* London, Routledge and Kegan Paul, 1973.

Castillo R, Kissin I, Bradley EL: Selective kappa opioid agonist for spinal analgesia without risk of respiratory depression. *Anesth Analg* 65:350-354, 1986.

Cervero F: Afferent activity evoked by natural stimulation of the biliary system in the ferret. *Pain* 13:137-151, 1982.

Cervero F: Mechanisms of visceral pain. *Pain* 4:1-19, 1983a.

Cervero F: Somatic and visceral inputs to the thoracic spinal cord of the cat: Effects of noxious stimulation of the biliary system. *J Physiol* 337:51-67, 1983b.

Cervero F: Visceral nociception: Peripheral and central aspects of visceral nociceptive systems. *Trans R Soc Lond* 308:325-337, 1985.

Cleeland CS, Daut RL: *The Prevalence and Severity of Pain in Cancer.* Meeting of the National Cancer Institute, USA, 1982.

Cook AJ, Woolf CJ, Wall PD, McMahon SB: Dynamic receptive field plasticity in rat spinal cord dorsal horn following C-primary afferent input. *Nature* 325:151-153, 1987.

Coombs DW, Maurer LH, Saunders RL, Gaylor M: Outcomes and complications of continuous intraspinal narcotic analgesias for cancer pain control. *J Clin Oncol* 2:1414-1420, 1984a.

Coombs DW, Saunders RL, Gaylor M, Pageau MG: Epidural narcotic infusion reservoir: Implantation technique and efficacy. *Anesthesiology* 56:469-473, 1982.

Coombs DW, Saunders RL, Gaylor M, LaChance D, Jensen L: Clinical trial of intrathecal clonidine for cancer pain. *J Reg Anesth* 9:34-35, 1984b.

Cousins MJ, Bridenbaugh PO: *Neural Blockade in Clinical Anesthesia and Management of Pain,* 2nd ed. Philadelphia, JB Lippincott, 1988.

Cousins MJ, Mather LE: Intrathecal and epidural administration of opioids. *Anesthesiology* 61:276-310, 1984.

Cousins MJ, Wilson PR: Gynaecologic pain. In Coppleson M (ed): *Gynaecologic Oncology.* Edinburgh, Churchill Livingstone, 1981.

Cousins MJ, Mather LE, Glynn CJ, Wilson PR, Graham JR: Selective spinal analgesia. *Lancet* 1:1141, 1979.

Daut RL, Cleeland CS: The prevalence and severity of pain in cancer. *Cancer* 50:1913-1918, 1977.

Dejgard A, Petersen P, Kastrup J: Mexiletene for treatment of chronic painful neuropathy. *Lancet* 1:9-11, 1988.

Deutschmann W: Tofranil in der Schmerzbehandlung der Krebskranken. *Med Welt* 22:1346-1347, 1971.

Dickenson AH: A new approach to pain relief? *Nature* 320:681-682, 1983.

Dostrovsky JO: Stimulation produced antinociception. *Progr Brain Res* 77:159-164, 1988.

Duggan AW: Pharmacology of descending control systems. *Trans R Soc London* 308:375-391, 1985.

Eiras J, Garcia J, Gomez J, Carcavilla LI, Ucar S: First results with extralemniscal myelotomy. *Acta Neurochir Suppl* 30:377-381, 1980.

Fields HL: *Pain.* New York, McGraw-Hill, 1987.

Fields HL, Raskin NH: Anticonvulsants and pain. In Klawans HL (ed): *Clinical Neuropharmacology.* New York, Raven Press, 1976, pp 173-184.

Fitzgerald M: The course and termination of primary afferent fibres. In Wall PD, Melzack R (eds): *Textbook of Pain.* Edinburgh, Churchill Livingstone, 1989, pp 46-62.

Fleetwood-Walker SM, Mitchell R, Hope PJ, Molony V, Iggo A: An alpha 2 receptor mediates the selective inhibition of noradrenaline of nociceptive responses of identified dorsal horn neurones. *Brain Res* 334:243-254, 1985.

Foley KM: Pain syndromes in patients with cancer. In Bonica JJ, Ventafridda V (eds): *Advances in Pain Research and Therapy.* Vol 2. New York, Raven Press, 1979, pp 59-78.

Forrest WH: Dextroamphetamine with morphine for the treatment of postoperative pain. *N Engl J Med* 296:712-715, 1977.

Freeman W, Watts JW: *Psychosurgery—In the Treatment of Mental Orders and Intractable Pain,* 2nd ed. Springfield, IL, Charles C Thomas, 1950.

Gamse R, Holzer P, Lembeck F: Decrease of substance P in primary afferent neurones and impairment of neurogenic plasma extravasation by capsaicin. *Br J Pharmacol* 68:207-213, 1980.

Gamse R, Petche U, Lembeck F, Jancso G: Capsaicin applied to peripheral nerve inhibits axoplasmic transport of substance P and somatostatin. *Brain Res* 239:447-462, 1982.

Gebhart GF, Sandkuhler J, Thalhammer JG, Zimmerman M: Inhibition of spinal nociceptive information by stimulation of midbrain of the cat is blocked by lidocaine microinjected in the nucleus raphe magnus and medullary reticular formation. *J Neurophysiol* 50:1446-1459, 1983.

Gebhart KH, Beller J, Nischk R: Behandlung des Karzinomschmerzes mit Chlomipramin (Anafranil). *Med Klin* 64:751-756, 1969.

Gerbeshagen HU: Blocks with local anesthetics in the treatment of cancer pain. In Bonica JJ, Ventafridda V (eds): *Advances in Pain Research and Therapy,* Vol 2. New York, Raven Press, 1979, pp 311-323.

Gilbert MR, Grossman SA: Incidence and nature of neurologic problems. *Am J Med* 81:951-954, 1986.

Gilbert RW, Kim JH, Posner JB: Epidural spinal cord compression from metastatic tumor: Diagnosis and treatment. *Ann Neurol* 3:40-51, 1978.

Gildenberg PL: Myelotomy and percutaneous cervical cordotomy for the treatment of cancer pain. *Appl Neurophysiol* 47:208-215, 1984.

Gildenberg PL, Hirshberg RM: Limited myelotomy for the treatment of intractable cancer pain. *J Neurol Neurosurg Psychiat* 47:94-96, 1984.

Gybels JM, Sweet WH: Neurosurgical treatment of persistent pain. In Gildenberg PL (ed): *Pain and Headache*, Vol 11. Basel, S. Karger, 1989.

Hall JG, Duggan AW, Morton CR, Johnson SM: The location of brainstem neurons tonically inhibiting dorsal horn neurons of the cat. *Brain Res* 244:215-222, 1982.

Hammond DL, Yaksh TL: Antagonism of stimulation-produced antinociception by intrathecal administration of methysergide or phentolamine. *Brain Res* 298:329-337, 1984.

Hammond DL, Levy RA, Proudfit HK: Hypoalgesia following microinjection of noradrenergic antagonists in the nucleus raphe magnus. *Pain* 9:85-105, 1980.

Hancock MB, Foreman RD, Willis WD: Convergence of visceral and cutaneous input onto spinothalamic tract cells in the thoracic spinal cord of the cat. *Exp Neurol* 47:240-248, 1975.

Handwerker HO, Iggo A, Zimmermann M: Segmental and supraspinal actions on dorsal horn neurons responding to noxious and non-noxious skin stimuli. *Pain* 1:147-165, 1975.

Hargreaves KM, Dionne RA: Evaluating endogenous mediators of pain and analgesia in clinical studies. In Max MB, Portenoy RK, Laska EM (eds): *The Design of Analgesic Clinical Trials*. New York, Raven Press, 1991, pp 579-598.

Head H: On disturbances of sensation with especial reference to the pain of visceral disease. *Brain* 16:1-132, 1893.

Henker FO: Diagnosis and treatment of non-organic pelvic pain. *South Med J* 72:1132-1134, 1979.

Herman B, Goldstein A: Antinociception and paralysis induced by intrathecal dynorphin A. *J Pharmacol Exp Ther* 232:27-32, 1985.

Hitchcock E: Stereotaxic cervical myelotomy. *J Neurol Neurosurg Psychiat* 33:224-230, 1970.

Hogan WM, Littman P, Griner L, Miller CL, Mikuta JJ: Results of radiation therapy given after radical hysterectomy. *Cancer* 49:1278-1285, 1982.

Hogberg T, Rabow L, Rosenberg P, Simonsen E: The use of chordotomy to treat pain from gynecologic cancer. *Eur J Gynaecol Oncol* 10:337-340, 1989.

Hokfelt T, Terenius L, Kuypers HGJM, Dann O: Evidence for enkephalin immunoreactive neurons in the medulla oblongata projecting to the spinal cord. *Neurosci Lett* 14:55-60, 1979.

Jessell TM, Dodd J: Functional chemistry of primary afferent neurons. In Wall PD, Melzack R (eds): *Textbook of Pain*. Edinburgh, Churchill Livingstone, 1989, pp 82-99.

Jordan LM, Kenshalo DR, Martin RF, Haber LH, Willis WD: Depression of primate spinothalamic tract neurons by iontophoretic application of 5-hydroxytryptamine. *Pain* 5:135-142, 1979.

Kaiko RF, Foley KM, Grabinski PY, Heidrich G, Rogers AG, Inturrisi CE, Reidenberg MM: Central nervous system excitatory effects of meperidine in cancer patients. *Ann Neurol* 13:180-185, 1983.

Kanner RM, Martini N, Foley KM: Incidence of pain and other clinical manifestations of superior pulmonary sulcus (Pancoast) tumors. In Bonica JJ, et al (eds): *Advances in Pain Research and Therapy*, Vol 4. New York, Raven Press, 1982, pp 27-39.

Kaufman JS: Drug interactions involving psychotherapeutic agents. In Simpson LL (ed): *Drug Treatment of Mental Disorders*. New York, Raven Press, 1976, pp. 289-309.

Kawatani M, Lowe IP, Nadelhaft I, Morgan C, de Groat W: Vasoactive intestinal peptides in visceral afferent pathways to the sacral spinal cord of the cat. *Neurosci Lett* 42:311-316, 1983.

Kenshalo DR Jr, Isensee O: Response of primate SI cortical neurons to noxious stimuli. *J Neurophysiol* 50:1479-1496, 1983.

Kishmore-Kumar R, Schafer SC, Lawlor BA, Murphy DL, Max MB: Single doses of the serotonin agonists buspirone and m-chlorophenylpiperazine do not relieve neuropathic pain. *Pain* 37:223-227, 1989.

Klepper ID, Sherrill DL, Boetger CL, Bromage PR: The analgesic and respiratory effects of epidural sufentanil and the influence of adrenaline as an adjuvant. *Br J Anaesth* 59:1147-1159, 1987.

Kumazawa T, Mizurura K: The polymodal receptors in the testis of the dog. *Brain Res* 170:553-557, 1977.

Kuraishi Y, Satoh M, Takagai H: The descending noradrenergic system and analgesia. In Akil H, Lewis H (eds): *Pain and Headache*, Vol 9. Basel, S. Karger, 1987, pp 102-128.

Kuo DC, Kawatani M, de Groat WC: Vasoactive intestinal polypeptide identified in the thoracic dorsal root ganglia of the cat. *Brain Res* 330:178-182, 1985.

Lasagna L, DeKornfeld JJ: Methotrimeprazine. A new phenothiazine derivative with analgetic properties. *J Am Med Assoc* 178:887-890, 1961.

Leek BF: Abdominal and pelvic visceral receptors. *Brit Med Bull* 33:163-168, 1977.

Lembeck F, Gamse R: Substance P in peripheral sensory processes. In Ciba Foundation Symposium: *Substance P in the Nervous System*, Vol 16. Pitman Oncon, 1982, pp 35-48.

Lewin W, Phillips CG: Observations on partial removal of the post central gyrus for pain. *J Neurol Neurosurg Psychiat* 15:143-147, 1952.

Lewis J, Mansour A, Khachaturian H, Watson SJ, Akil H: Opioids and pain regulation. In Akil H, Lewis H (eds): *Pain and Headache*, Vol 9. Basel, S. Karger, 1987, pp 129-159.

Lewis T: *Pain*. New York, Macmillan, 1942.

Loeser JD: Dorsal rhizotomy for the relief of chronic pain. *J Neurosurg* 36:745-750, 1972.

Long JB, Petras JM, Mobley WC, Holaday JW: Neurological dysfunction after intrathecal injection of dynorphin A (1-13) in the rat. II. Nonopioid mechanisms mediate loss of motor, sensory and autonomic function. *J Pharmacol Exp Ther* 246:1167-1173, 1988.

Lorente de No R: Analysis of the activity of the chains of internuncial neurons. *J Neurophysiol* 1:207-244, 1938.

Low JC: The radionuclide scan in bone metastasis. In Weiss L, Gilbert HA (eds): *Bone Metastasis*. Boston, GK Hall, 1981, pp 231-244.

MacKenzie J: Some points bearing on the association of sensory disorders and visceral disease. *Brain* 16:321-354, 1893.

Mark VH, Ervin FR: Role of thalamotomy in treatment of chronic severe pain. *Postgrad Med* 37:563-571, 1965.

Mark VH, Ervin FR, Yakovlev PI: Correlation of pain relief, sensory loss, and anatomical lesion sites in pain patients treated by stereotaxic thalamotomy. *Trans Am Neurol Assoc* 86:86-90, 1961.

Marshall J: Sensory disturbances in cortical wounds with special reference to pain. *J Neurol Neurosurg Psychiat* 14:187-204, 1951.

Max MB, Culane M, Schafer SC, Gracely RH, Walther DJ, Smoller B, Dubner R: Amytriptyline relieves diabetic neuropathy pain in patients with normal or depressed mood. *Neurology* 37:589-596, 1987.

Max MB, Schafer SC, Culane M, Dubner R, Gracely RH: Association of pain relief with drug side effects: A single dose study of clonidine, codeine, ibuprofen and placebo. *Clin Pharmacol Ther* 43:363-371, 1988.

McGee JL, Alexander MR: Phenothiazine analgesia—Fact or fantasy? *Am J Hosp Pharm* 36:633-640, 1979.

McQuay HJ, Carroll D, Moore RA: Postoperative orthopedic pain—The effect of opiate premedication and local anesthetic blocks. *Pain* 33:291-295, 1988.

Melzack R: The tragedy of needless pain: A call for social action. In Dubner R, Gebhart GF, Bond MR (eds): *Proceedings of the Fifth World Congress on Pain*. New York, Elsevier-North Holland, 1988, pp 1-11.

Melzack R, Casey KL: Sensory, motivational, and central control determinants of pain. A new conceptual model. In Kenshalo DR Jr (ed): *The Skin Senses*. Springfield, IL, Charles C Thomas, 1968, pp 423-439.

Morris N, O'Neill D: Outpatient gynaecology. *Br Med J* 2:1038, 1958.

Moulin DE, Max MB, Kaiko RF, Inturrissi CE, Maggard J, Yaksh TL, Foley KM: The analgesic efficacy of intrathecal D-Ala-2-D-leu 5 enkephalin in cancer patients with chronic pain. *Pain* 23:213-221, 1985.

Nagy JI, Hunt SP, Iversen LL, Emson PC: Biochemical and anatomical observations on the degeneration of peptide-containing primary afferent neurones after neonatal capsaicin. *Neuroscience* 6:1923-1934, 1981.

Nashold BS, Ostahl RH: Dorsal root entry zone lesions for pain relief. *J Neurosurg* 51:59-69, 1979.

Nystrom JS, Weiner JM, Heffelfinger-Juttner J, Irwin LE, Bateman JR, Meshnik-Wolf R: Metastatic and histologic presentations in unknown primary cancer. *Semin Oncol* 4:53-58, 1977.

Onofrio BM, Yaksh TL: Intrathecal delta-receptor ligand produces analgesia in man. *Lancet* 1:1374-1375, 1983.

Oyama T, Jin T, Yamaya R, Ling N, Guillemin R: Profound analgesic effects of beta-endorphin in man. *Lancet* 1:122-124, 1980.

Paintal AS: The response of the gastric stretch receptors and certain other abdominal and thoracic vagal receptors to some drugs. *J Physiol* 126:255-270, 1954.

Parkes CM: Home or Hospital? Terminal care as seen by surviving spouse. *J Roy Coll Gen Pract* 28:19-30, 1978.

Patchall RA, Posner JA: Neurologic complications of systemic cancer. *Neurol Clin* 3:729-750, 1985.

Payne R: Novel routes of opioid administration. In Hill CS, Fields WS (eds): *Advances in Pain Research and Therapy*, Vol 11. New York, Raven Press, 1989, pp 319-338.

Perez CA, Camel HM: Long-term followup in radiation therapy of carcinoma of the vagina. *Cancer* 49:1308-1315, 1982.

Perl ER: Characterization of nociceptors and their activation of neurons in the superficial dorsal horn: First steps for the sensation of pain. *Adv Pain Res Ther* 6:23-51, 1984.

Petros AJ, Wright RM: Epidural and oral clonidine in domiciliary control of deafferentation pain. *Lancet* 1:1034, 1987.

Petsche U, Fleischer E, Lembeck F, Handwerker HO: The effect of capsaicin application to a peripheral nerve on impulse conduction in functionally identified afferent nerve fibers. *Brain Res* 265:233-240, 1983.

Pierau FK, Taylor DCM, Abel W, Friedrich B: Dichotomizing peripheral fibers revealed by intracellular recording from rat sensory neurones. *Neurosci Lett* 31:123-128, 1982.

Poletti CE, Cohen AM, Todd DP, Ojemann RG, Sweet W, Zervas NT: Cancer pain relieved by long-term epidural morphine with permanent indwelling systems for self-administration. *J Neurosurg* 55:581, 1981.

Pomeranz B, Wall PD, Weber WV: Cord cells responding to fine myelinated afferents from viscera, muscle and skin. *J Physiol* 199:511-532, 1968.

Porter J, Jick H: Addiction rare in patients treated with narcotics. *N Engl J Med* 302:123, 1980.

Reddy SVR, Yaksh TL: Spinal noradrenergic terminal system mediates antinociception. *Brain Res* 189:391-402, 1980.

Reynolds DV: Surgery in the rat during electrical analgesia induced by focal brain stimulation. *Science* 164:444-445, 1969.

Richardson DE, Akil H: Pain reduction by electrical brain stimulation in man. *J Neurosurg* 47:178-183, 1977.

Rowbotham MC, Fields HL: Topical lidocaine reduces pain in post herpetic neuralgia. *Pain* 38:297-301, 1989.

Ruch TC: Pathophysiology of pain. In Ruch TC, Patton HD (eds): *Physiology and Biophysics*. Philadelphia, WB Saunders, 1965, pp 345-363.

Rumore MM, Schlichting DA: Clinical efficacy of antihistaminics as analgesics. *Pain* 25:7-22, 1986.

Schmaus C, Yaksh TL: In vivo studies on spinal opiate receptor systems mediating antinociception. II. Pharmacological profiles suggesting a differential association of mu, delta, and kappa receptors with visceral chemical and cutaneous stimuli in the rat. *J Pharmacol Exp Ther* 228:1-12, 1984.

Siegfried J, Kuhner A, Sturm V: Neurosurgical treatment of cancer pain. In Zimmermann M, Drings P, Wagner G (eds): *Recent Results in Cancer Research*, Vol 89. Berlin, Springer-Verlag, pp 148-156.

Sinclair DC, Weddell G, Feindel WH: Referred pain and associated phenomena. *Brain* 71:184-211, 1948.

Sindou M, Daher A: Spinal cord ablation procedures for pain. In Dubner R, Gebhart GF, Bond MR (eds): *Proceedings of the Vth World Congress on Pain*. Amsterdam, Elsevier-North Holland, 1988, pp 477-495.

Spiller WG, Martin E: The treatment of persistent pain of organic origin in the lower part of the body by division of the anterolateral column of the spinal cord. *J Am Med Assoc* 58:1489-1490, 1912.

Stambaugh JE, Lane C: Analgesic efficacy and pharmacokinetic evaluation of meperidine and hydroxyzine alone and in combination. *Cancer Invest* 1:111-117, 1983.

Stevens CW, Weinger MB, Yaksh TL: Intrathecal dynorphins suppress hindlimb electromyographic activity in rats. *Eur J Pharm* 138:299-302, 1987.

Sweet WH, Poletti CE: Operations in the brainstem and spinal canal, with an appendix of open cordotomy. In Wall PD, Melzack R (eds): *Textbook of Pain*. Edinburgh, Churchill Livingstone, 1989, pp 811-831.

Swerdlow M: Anticonvulsant drugs and chronic pain. *Clin Neuropharm* 7:51-82, 1982.

Tamsen A, Gordh T: Epidural clonidine produces analgesia. *Lancet* 1:231, 1984.

Thrupkaew AK, Henkin RE, Quinn JL III: False negative bone scans in disseminated metastatic disease. *Radiology* 113:383-386, 1974.

Turnbull F: The nature of pain that may accompany cancer of the lung. *Pain* 7:371-375, 1979.

Twycross RG, McQuay HT: Opioid. In Wall PD, Melzack R (eds): *Textbook of Pain*, 2nd ed. Edinburgh, Churchill Livingstone, 1989, pp 686-701.

Twycross RG, Wald SJ: Long-term use of diamorphine in advanced cancer. In Bonica JJ, Albe-Fessard D (eds): *Advances in Pain Research and Therapy*, Vol 1. New York, Raven, 1976, pp 653-661.

Vogt M: The effect of lowering the 5-hydroxytryptamine content of the rat spinal cord on analgesia produced by morphine. *J Physiol* (Lond) 236:483-498, 1974.

Waddell PJ, Lawsen SN: C fibre conduction block caused by capsaicin on rat vagus nerve in vitro. *Pain* 39:237-242, 1989.

Waldman SD, Feldstein GS, Allen ML, Turnage G: Selection of patients for implantable intraspinal narcotic delivery systems. *Anesth Analg* 65:883-885, 1986.

Wall PD: The prevention of postoperative pain. *Pain* 33:289-290, 1988.

Wall PD, Melzack R: *Textbook of Pain*, 2nd ed. Edinburgh, Churchill Livingstone, 1989.

Wall PD, Woolf CJ: The brief and prolonged facilitatory effects of unmyelinated afferent input on the rat spinal cord are independently influenced by peripheral nerve injury. *Neurosci* 17:1199-1206, 1986.

Weintraub M, Valentine A, Steckel S: Cancer pain: A comparison of methadone, methadone-cocaine, and methadone-amphetamine. In Goldberg IK, Kutscher AH, Malitz S (eds): *Pain, Anxiety and Grief: Pharmacotherapeutic Care of the Dying Patient and the Bereaved*. New York, Columbia University Press, 1986, pp 128-141.

Wen HL, Mehal ZD, Ong BH, Ho WK: Treatment of pain in cancer patients by intrathecal administration of dynorphin. *Peptides* 8:191-193, 1987.

Westlund KN, Bowker RM, Ziegler MG, Coutler JD: Origins and terminations of descending noradrenergic projections to the spinal cord of monkey. *Brain Res* 291:1-16, 1984.

White JC, Sweet WH: *Pain and the Neurosurgeon*. Springfield, IL, Charles C Thomas, 1969.

White JC, Sweet WH: Anterolateral cordotomy: Open versus closed comparison of end results. *Adv Pain Res Ther* 3:911-919, 1979.

Willis WD: Control of nociceptive transmission in the spinal cord. In Auturum H, Ottoson D, Perl ER, et al (eds): *Progress in Sensory Physiology*. New York, Springer-Verlag, 1982, pp 1-159.

Willis WD: The pain system. In Gildenberg PL (ed): *Pain and Headache*, Vol 8. Basel, S. Karger, 1985.

Wood MM, Cousins MJ: Iatrogenic neurotoxicity in cancer patients. *Pain* 39:1-3, 1989.

Wood PL, Rackman A, Richard J: Spinal analgesia: Comparison of the mu agonist morphine and the kappa agonist ethylketazocine. *Life Sci* 28:2119-2125, 1981.

Woolf CJ, Wall PD: Morphine-sensitive and morphine-insensitive actions of C-fiber input on the rat spinal cord. *Neurosci Lett* 64:221-225, 1986.

Woolf CJ, Wiesenfeld-Hallin Z: The systemic administration of local anesthetics produces a selective depression of C afferent fiber evoked activity in the spinal cord. *Pain* 23:361-374, 1985.

Yaksh TL: Multiple spinal opiate receptor systems in analgesia. In Kruger L, Liebskind JC (eds): *Advances in Pain Research and Therapy*, Vol 6. New York, Raven Press, 1984.

Yaksh TL: Opioid receptors and the endorphins: A review of their spinal organization. *J Neurosurg* 39:47-52, 1987.

Yaksh TL: Pharmacology of spinal adrenergic systems which modulate spinal nociceptive processing. *Pharm Biochem Behav* 22:845-858, 1985.

Yaksh TL, Simone LD: The central pharmacology of pain transmission. In Wall PD, Melzack R (eds): *Textbook of Pain*, 2nd ed. Edinburgh, Churchill Livingstone, 1989, pp 181-205.

Yaksh TL, Rudy TA: Analgesia mediated by a direct spinal effect of narcotics. *Science* 192:1357, 1976.

Yaksh TL, Wilson PR: Spinal serotonin system mediates antinociception. *J Pharmacol Exp Ther* 208:446-453, 1979.

Yeager MP, Glass DD, Neff RK, Brinck-Johnsen T: Epidural anesthesia and analgesia in high risk surgical patients. *Anesthesiol* 66:729-736, 1987.

Young GB, Blume WT: Painful epileptic seizures. *Brain* 106:537-554, 1983.

Zollinger R: Observations following distention of the bladder and common bile duct in man. *Proc Soc Exp Biol Med* 30:1260-1261, 1933.

# *Chapter 25* | Psychological Aspects of Gynecologic Cancer

## *Edward J. Callahan*   *Robert E. Pawlicki*
## *Donald R. Nicholas*   *Sharon A. Hamilton*

With the exception of AIDS, cancer is undoubtedly the most dread disease known, threatening a person's survival and body image (Donahue and Knapp, 1977). Although treatment techniques and survival rates are improving, cancer strikes increasing numbers of people each year, and survivors must cope with the realization that they have a terminal disease (Sobel, 1981). Perhaps the most distressing forms of cancer are those involving the reproductive system and breasts.

In this chapter, we will consider the psychologic aspects of gynecologic cancer and how this disease affects both individual and family functioning. Our goal is to help the medical professional recognize these problems and provide counseling. Counseling should not be the sole province of the mental-health professional but rather the cooperative task of all health-care professionals. With this shared responsibility in mind, we will review research on the psychologic aspects of cancer, particularly gynecologic cancer.

In the past decade, the methodology used to study the psychosocial aspects of cancer has become much more sophisticated. Improvements in study design and psychologic tests have led to some surprising findings, often replacing long-held misconceptions, and have made it possible to document valid clinical observations of the past. Here, we will review some of the more sound methodologic contributions to the data base on the psychosocial aspects of gynecologic oncology and in other areas of psychologic research. This approach is intended to provide a basic understanding of some of these psychologic aspects as well as means for applying this knowledge in order to provide quality care.

After presenting a rationale for counseling gynecologic oncology patients, we will describe a model for counseling as well as a model for grief. These models will provide a structure for considering available data on the psychosocial adjustment of cancer patients, with a focus on psychopathology, depression, sexual adjustment, and pain. Finally, we will examine intensive psychosocial interventions and communication skills for medical personnel who work with these patients.

## COUNSELING THE CANCER PATIENT

As our efforts to treat the physical aspects of cancer have become more effective, so has the need to deal with the mental health of the cancer survivor become more evident. For the most part, such treatment is appropriately assigned to the specialist in mental health, i.e., the psychologist, psychiatrist, or social worker. Since the cancer patient does not require such specialized intervention frequently, she may be counseled more effectively by medical personnel with whom she has already established a trusting relationship. Given the current emphasis on treating the *whole* patient, it would be useful to consider a specific model that can be employed by those responsible for care of the cancer patient.

Recognizing a similar need in the area of sexual counseling, Annon (1976) proposed a model to help conceptualize how most counseling might be provided and by whom. Annon contended that most sexual counseling is not provided by trained therapists working in specialty clinics but by parents, teachers, and friends who do not consider their discussions formal counseling. To help persons other than trained sex counselors to conceptualize the levels of counseling possible for dealing with sexual problems and to recognize when a problem requires greater expertise, Annon developed the PLISSIT model (Fig. 25-1), in which several factors are arranged in the form of an inverted pyramid: the least expensive and most widely used counseling factor appears at the top, with each successive element in the pyramid requiring more time and expertise on the part of the

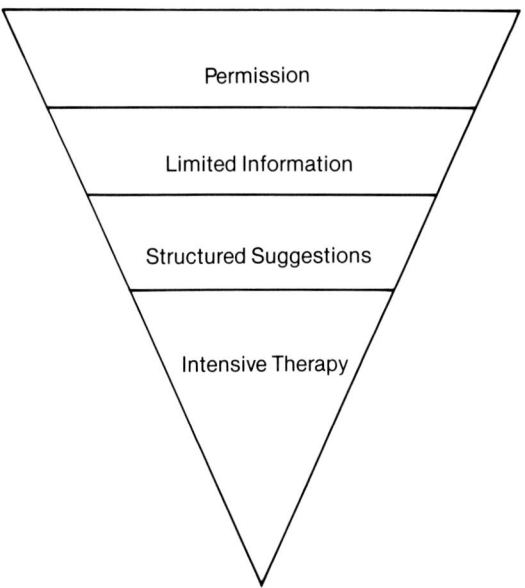

FIGURE 25-1    The PLISSIT model of the levels of sexual counseling. (From Annon JS: *Behavioral Treatment of Sexual Problems.* Hagerstown, MD, Harper and Row, 1976.)

counselor. When considering a patient's problem, the health professional can resort to the simplest interventions first. If the patient does not respond to these interventions, referral to a mental-health professional would be appropriate.

The simplest and most cost-effective element of counseling in the PLISSIT model is *permission*, which requires the least training and supervision. Permission involves giving the patient a verbal "okay" to feel or express an emotion. It may consist of reassuring the patient that her reaction to cancer is normal and does not mean that she is crazy. The next factor is *limited information*; this requires knowledge about the disease and its treatment, which the practitioner can teach the patient. Next, *structured suggestions* include those group and individual therapy techniques ordinarily considered to be the province of the mental-health specialist: cognitive restructuring, desensitization, communication-skills training, and the like. When a patient does not respond to these short-term therapeutic interventions, long-term *intensive therapy* may be necessary. Let us now consider each of these elements of counseling in turn.

## Factors to Consider

**Permission**    As mentioned, permission is the simplest of all forms of counseling and may consist of reassuring comments such as "It's all right to cry" or "It's normal to become angry under the circumstances." Medical personnel who acknowledge and accept a patient's emotional responses do that patient a valuable service. In many cases, the emotions reported can be predicted if we consider grief to be a normal response to the diagnosis and treatment of cancer. (Later in this chapter, we will briefly review the responses involved in grieving.)

Granting the patient permission to feel the natural emotions evoked by cancer is an important intervention for the distraught patient who may fear that she is going crazy. Permission may also help the patient in terms of feelings of sexuality and the search to fulfill sexual and nurturant needs even in the face of cancer. Most patients will not raise these issues themselves but wait for the staff to address them. In this case, giving permission can be a critical step toward helping the patient deal with these important issues.

**Limited Information**    Most often, the counseling technique that accompanies permission is the divulgence of limited information. One important reaction among patients newly diagnosed with cancer is confusion. Researchers studying the sexual adjustment of gynecologic cancer patients have consistently noted their desire for more information about the sexual impact of their disease on themselves and their partners (Anderson et al, 1988). For example, Vincent et al (1975) found that 70% of the patients with cervical cancer interviewed had been given no information about sexual adjustment. Limited information can be as simple as a statement that other patients have undergone the same procedures and have adjusted successfully or as complex as a technical description of chemotherapy and its side effects. Patients may be told that similar patients have continued to indulge in sexual activity or that medical interventions will not eliminate sexual needs. When the vagina has been shortened or removed, alternative forms of sexual interaction (i.e., oral sex or manual stimulation) may require an explanation as well as permission-giving.

Specific information might involve discussing successful sexual adjustments made by other patients with similar problems. However, even information-giving requires sensitivity on the part of the clinician. Andersen (1987) noted that some of the patients she studied were quite relieved that their disease had ended their sexual activity; promoting methods for sexual adjustment to such patients might therefore be offensive. While not all patients elect to continue sexual activity, all should have the right to continue to seek nurturance if they so choose. When information on diagnosis, treatment, or future adjustment is met by overwhelming anxiety, severe depression, or reports of intense marital or work strain, it may be appropriate to refer the patient for more specialized counseling. Referral to trained counselors can be explained as a normal event: "The mental-health specialists here work with normal people who are experiencing an unusually stressful event." Ordinarily, these will be the counselors who provide the next two levels of counseling, structured suggestions and intensive therapy.

**Structured Suggestions**    Some common treatments that constitute structured suggestions include systematic desensitization for anxiety, communication-skills training for marital problems, hypnosis or relaxation techniques to offset anticipatory nausea and vomiting during chemotherapy, and cognitive restructuring to relieve depression. In each of these treatment modalities, the therapist works closely with the patient to restructure her environment, her behavior in particular situations, or the payoffs for certain interactions in her world. Interventions are designed to facilitate the patient's adjustment to living with cancer and will be discussed in greater detail later in this chapter. These interventions differ from support groups in that they directly effect changes in the patient's life as opposed to being limited to nondirective support.

The following is an example of referral for this type of treatment:

> When a 40-year-old woman was diagnosed with vulvar cancer and radical vulvectomy was recommended, she became extremely angry (an appropriate grieving reaction) and refused to have the operation because it would interfere with her sexual attractiveness to her husband. However, when it became apparent that she and her husband were no longer sleeping together, she was referred for marital and supportive counseling. Encouraged to seek a second opinion concerning the need for radical vulvectomy, the patient was able to adjust to the operation and begin a productive course of individual psychotherapy and marital counseling.

Permission and information-giving were important counseling interventions in the early treatment of this patient. Without early permission to feel anger and to seek confirmation about therapy, the patient might have refused surgical treatment and might not have begun psychotherapy. Thus, the role of medical personnel in providing these early counseling interventions can be critical.

Although this level of counseling may be implemented by medical personnel, it is more often provided by the mental-health professional. Individual and group structured suggestions will sometimes fail; in these cases, intensive therapy should be undertaken by professionals with training in these techniques.

***Intensive Therapy*** Structured suggestion counseling may fail if the patient is afforded some secondary gain from her symptoms or is suffering from some life-long psychopathologic process or personality disorder. In such cases, short-term structured suggestion therapy is doomed. The patient may not comply with suggestions for changes at home or may even become psychotic and require longer-term intensive psychotherapy by trained mental-health professionals. A discussion of such a process is beyond the scope of this chapter.

In all the above interventions, it is necessary to distinguish between appropriate and inappropriate adjustment. Endicott (1984) points to a tendency to think of depression as a natural response to cancer: however, the data do not support this. Both Endicott (1984) and Derogatis and Spencer (1984) note that the traditional assessment of depression is confounded in the patient with cancer because the disease itself produces many of the somatic changes used to diagnose depression. Nonetheless, there is a high rate of adjustment disorder among cancer patients: Derogatis et al (1983) found psychiatric diagnoses in 47% of over 200 newly admitted cancer patients. Most of that sample had Axis I

disorders (44 to 47%), usually adjustment disorder (68%). Further, Andersen et al (1989*b*) found that both cancer patients and women with benign gynecologic disease showed acute depressive symptoms at the time of diagnosis that resolved after the conditions were treated. Thus, many patients experienced initial difficulties adjusting to their diagnosis, decision-making about treatment, and beginning treatment. However, because cancer produces somatic changes similar to those in depression, there may be a tendency to over-diagnose psychopathology in cancer patients.

Appropriate emotional responses to cancer are often the same as those seen in grieving; this makes sense, since cancer can involve *loss*: loss of organs; loss of work; loss of capabilities; and even loss of one's life, family or spouse. To distinguish between these two types of reactions, it is helpful to understand grieving as part of bereavement. We will briefly review the nature of grief and then examine the emotional components of grieving in the cancer patient's process of adjustment.

## Cancer and Grieving

Grief and mourning are the two interrelated components of bereavement (Averill, 1968). According to Averill, bereavement is "the total response pattern, psychologic and physiologic, displayed by an individual following the loss of a significant object or other." *Grief* refers to the biologic and affective components of that process. *Mourning*, on the other hand, refers to the culture's prescribed rituals (e.g., holding wakes, wearing black) in response to the loss of a loved one. Mourning behaviors most likely facilitate a healthy adjustment to loss; the fact that our culture lacks such rituals for losses experienced by the patient with cancer probably makes adjustment more difficult. Since American culture prescribes no mourning procedures for loss of a uterus or breast or of an individual's role as child bearer or nursing mother, our focus here will be on grieving.

Lindemann (1944) alerted professionals to the typical response pattern seen in grief. His five grief responses have been adapted in several ways by others into stage and component theories. *Stage theories* (Bowlby and Parkes, 1970; Engel, 1961, 1974; Kübler-Ross, 1969) suggest that the griever progresses through discrete periods; *component theories* (Bugen, 1977; Ramsay, 1979) describe a set of responses an individual must experience in order to cope with grief.

Let us review the stages in one well-known model of grief. According to Kübler-Ross (1969), grief occurs in five stages:

1. Denial
2. Rage and anger
3. Bargaining
4. Disorganization
5. Acceptance

These stages are valuable only for general reference; rarely do they occur in this order and many patients do not even experience all the phases. During the first stage, *denial*, the patient may not accept the reality of her loss and may hardly respond at all. On first hearing the diagnosis of cancer, the patient may be doubtful and seek a second opinion as a healthy manifestation of this stage; an unhealthy denial response would be withdrawal from all medical personnel, with the patient claiming that she knows she does not have cancer. It has now been documented that cancer patients tend to be confused soon after the diagnosis (Andersen et al, 1989*b*).

During the second stage of grief, the patient may direct feelings of *rage and anger* toward herself or the medical personnel involved in her case. In the third stage, *bargaining*, the patient may shift her efforts toward saving what she is losing. For example, a young woman may plead for radiation therapy instead of a hysterectomy or might try to strike a prayerful bargain with God for remission. The fourth stage is *disorganization*, a period of poor functioning and reduced activity that constitutes the longest adjustment phase in grieving. Presumably, failure to permit natural emotional responses as they arise will be disruptive to the patient.

Many people experience all these stages in their healthy adjustment to cancer. Often, unusual responses during the adjustment process can be predicted and understood if one refers to theories concerning grief. Such knowledge can help alleviate anxiety on the part of the patient, her family, the physician, and other medical personnel. As Small et al (1983) point out, professionals who work with the dying cancer patient are also subject to the experience of grief, and their own behavior may reflect the mood swings, anger, and distress that their patients are experiencing. In such cases, talking about these experiences with colleagues or mental-health professionals may be helpful.

With this awareness of grief as a natural and appropriate response to cancer, let us now examine the emotional components of grief as they affect the gynecologic cancer patient. Specifically, we will view her adjustment in terms of psychopathology, anxiety, depression, pain, and sexual functioning. Although it might seem that the healthiest response would be to achieve tranquility quickly and accept death, Lazarus (1989) warns that immediate resignation is not good from the perspective of either mental or physical health. Instead, patients should be encouraged to experience the full extent of their distress in order to make a healthy adjustment. Although no data are available to confirm either of these positions, one should probably attempt to balance the concept of passive adjustment with the concept of fighting for one's life (Cousins, 1989; Spiegel et al, 1986).

## ADJUSTMENT OF THE CANCER PATIENT

While the negative impact of cancer on a woman's psychologic and social well-being is logically apparent, the degree of disruption noted in previous studies may have been overestimated as a result of diagnostic and sampling factors. Studies reporting the prevalence of depression to be as high as 50% in cancer populations

have been based on psychiatric consultations (i.e., Hinton, 1972; Levine et al, 1978; Silberfarb and Greer, 1982) rather than on random samples of cancer patients. Lansky et al (1985) found that only 5.3% of a sample of 505 female cancer patients were clinically depressed when scored according to the Zung or the Hamilton rating scale. Thus, clinical depression is not as common among patients with gynecologic cancer as had been reported earlier. However, there is evidence to support some depressive reaction in their adjustment to cancer (Andersen et al, 1989*b*). Interestingly, disruptions in functioning within families of cancer patients are parallel but less severe (Cassileth et al, 1985).

Before elaborating upon this adjustment process, however, we should mention that much early information in this area is equivocal or requires qualification. For example, many of the initial studies were case reports and summaries of professional experiences that did not employ systematic methodology (Amias, 1975; Day, 1966; Donahue, 1978; Giacquinta, 1977; Weinberg, 1974; Wise, 1978). Although some researchers used structured or unstructured interviews and/or various self-report measures of adjustment, a review of these studies by Friedenbergs et al (1982) cites several problems with these methodologies. For example, the self-report measures had been developed initially to differentiate normal from psychiatric populations and therefore may not have been valid measures of psychosocial adjustment to cancer. Often the control groups were patients without cancer, thus precluding comparisons with healthy individuals. Finally, cancer patients were often considered as a single, homogeneous group with no distinctions made regarding site, stage, or medical treatment of the disease even though all these factors can influence adjustment. Polivy (1974) noted that studies on the psychologic effects of hysterectomy did not employ operationalized criteria to adjust for symptomatology, random selection of subjects, or experimental controls. Lewis and Bloom (1979) concluded that the negative psychosocial impact of breast cancer is apparent, but there is still a need for well-designed descriptive studies that include adequate experimental controls.

Given these limitations, we will present results of studies that are more methodologically sound. In several areas we can only summarize authors' ideas and their preliminary findings. In the following discussion of psychosocial adjustment on the part of the cancer patient, we will review information about psychopathology, depression, sexual adjustment, and pain.

### Overall Prevalence of Psychopathology

In a recent study on the prevalence of psychiatric disorders among 215 cancer patients, 47% of the patients were assigned diagnoses that are defined in the *Diagnostic and Statistical Manual of Mental Disorders* (3rd edition) (*DSM-III*) (Derogatis et al, 1983). Approximately 68% of these were adjustment disorders, 13% depression, 8% organic mental disorders, 7% personality disorders, and 4% anxiety disorders. These rates of prevalence are somewhat higher than those reported for medical populations in general, yet the problems are relatively mild. The majority of patients received no diagnosis, suggesting that clinically evident depression and anxiety do not necessarily affect patients with neoplastic disease but do occur frequently in treatable forms.

Anxiety and depression were reported in 18 to 50% of all patients in the studies reviewed by Friedenbergs et al (1982). Meyerowitz et al (1979) found that 62% of their patients reported unexplained anxiety, while 88% of their sample reported decreased levels of activity. Severely reduced activity is frequently a clinical sign of depression.

## Depression

Depression is the most serious and prevalent mental-health problem in the United States. Secunda et al (1973) reported that 15% of all adults between 18 and 74 years of age suffer significant depressive symptoms. In that context, the finding by Lansky et al (1985) that only 5.3% of the population show clinical depression is remarkable. Supporting this further, Schmale et al (1983) found no difference in mean Mental Health Index scores between a group of cancer survivors and a healthy control population. Nevertheless, a relationship between cancer and depressive symptoms can be documented, owing perhaps in part to their common link with pain.

Physical pain is frequently an important symptom of depression (Von Knorring, 1975). Von Knorring et al (1983) report that 57% of patients with a primary diagnosis of depression manifest pain as a secondary symptom. For the cancer patient, this relationship presents a particularly difficult problem. While the origin of cancer pain is organic, the disease itself is obviously a potential precursor of depression, which may increase the pain. How might this development occur?

Initially, distress and anxiety are associated with the diagnosis of malignant disease. Fears may relate to loss of social position, increasing medication, changes in interpersonal relations, and death. As the patient becomes increasingly disengaged from normal social functioning and dependent on medical providers, she begins to feel helpless. Depression is often then exacerbated by financial problems due to loss of employment and mounting medical costs. The ambiguities that parallel progression of the disease may also augment depression and anxiety: Will the pain get worse? Will I lose my dignity? Will the cancer metastasize? How will I be treated? How will I handle the treatment? Questions having no certain answers can reverberate, leading to debilitating depression. The fear of being unable to cope with the succession of intimate and intrusive problems often becomes manifest as denial, immobilization, and further depression. As treatment progresses and the prognosis becomes more clear, depression and anxiety wane (Andersen et al 1989*b*); group support can be of help in this process (Spiegel et al, 1989).

Another major depressive factor is the development of dependency. Interruption of an individual's lifestyle and daily patterns can have a devastating psychologic impact (Sawyer, 1977). The transition from perceiving oneself as a vital and productive member of one's family and of society to perceiving oneself as dependent may have a profoundly negative effect. Patients may not realistically recall their previous state of activity, and this contrast between their current state of immobilization, with an apparently dim future, and the memory of an idealized past serves to diminish the patient's self-image.

The patient with cancer must also deal with a general loss of reinforcement or gratification. For example, sexual intercourse may be painful or may fail to produce the usual feelings of relief (Andersen et al, 1989*a*). According to mental-health providers, a decline in pleasurable activity is the most prominent characteristic of depression. Whether necessary or not, most cancer patients report a lack of interest in sexual and other activities such as eating and socializing. The pleasure and satisfaction usually derived from such activity may be reduced, while fears about how others will respond to these changes may further aggravate the patient's sense of loss. If depression does occur, the pain of cancer is likely to increase, owing to the physiologic proximity of and interplay among centers in the brain that govern pain, depression, and sleep (Melzack, 1973). The patient's perception of pain increases with the decrease in her tolerance of pain, contributing further to depressive feelings. The cycle of diagnosis, anxiety, depression, and enhanced pain followed by a deeper depression is all too common among cancer patients.

Anxiety, depression, and anger are normal and appropriate reactions to the stresses imposed by a terminal disease. Andersen et al (1989*b*) have brought increased methodologic sophistication to the assessment of psychosocial function in the gynecologic cancer. These researchers studied 65 patients with gynecologic cancer, 22 with benign gynecologic disease, and 60 healthy women. Use of the control group with benign disease allowed them to study the effects of anticipating surgical intervention for a gynecologic problem. The authors documented the adjustment responses, particularly anxiety and depression, noted anecdotally around the time of diagnosis (before treatment). Thus they replicated the finding of Gottesman and Lewis (1982) who found that patients undergoing surgery for cancer and benign disease exhibited comparable levels of anxiety.

Andersen et al (1989*b*) also noted that these affective disturbances gradually resolved during followup of both the cancer patients and those with benign gynecologic disease. However, the cancer patients were significantly more confused following diagnosis than both the healthy women and those with benign disease. Quality of employment remained stable for all groups, with cancer patients differing only in that the total number of hours worked was reduced to a greater extent. Changes in marital relationships and loss of friendship occurred no more often among the cancer patients than among the other two groups. However, more husbands of cancer patients reported sexual difficulties during followup (usually difficulty in erectile dysfunction or reaching orgasm—problems perhaps complementary to the dyspareunia reported by their wives). Such results show the need for increased study of couple responses to health crises such as cancer.

Physicians who feel uncomfortable dealing with the natural psychologic outcome of progressive cancer tend to deny that the patient is having such problems or may respond to them inadequately. This is unfortunate, since the psychologic element of coping with cancer is probably as important as the physical progression of the disease.

Whether or not the depression will persist may hinge on the patient's interpretation of the problem, in other words, her perceptions of her world, her problem-solving abilities, her expectations, and how these processes affect the level of depression (Cobliner, 1977).

Cancer is not inevitably tied to depression. On the contrary, empiric evidence strongly supports the contention that most of these patients do not experience debilitating depression in dealing with malignancy. In a series of personal interviews with 300 women with gynecologic or breast cancer Cobliner (1977) found that the following factors correlated with positive adjustment: high self-esteem, a positive image of femininity, greater faith in doctors, a desire and opportunity to confide in others about worries, involvement in a satisfactory occupation or activity, congruence between life expectations and degree of attainment, and the nature and successful resolution of past crises.

Similarly, Weisman and colleagues found that "good copers" face facts, find something favorable, and then confidently comply with their doctor's recommendations (Weisman, 1976a, 1976b; Weisman and Sobel, 1979). That a patient's psychologic outlook is critical in predicting adjustment is supported by reports by Schonfeld (1972) and Morris et al (1977), who found that the presence of anxiety and depression predicted future psychosocial difficulties better than did medical data. In addition, Gordon et al (1980) found in a retrospective study of 136 cancer patients that medical data accounted for only 12% of the variance in patient-reported problems 6 months after hospital discharge. The most frequently reported dissatisfactions were with medical treatment, family problems, difficulties in social relations, and "activities of daily living."

These studies and other indicate that it is not the physical aspects of cancer itself but rather the patient's coping mechanisms, understanding, and expectations—and probably the response of others around them—that are critical in maximizing adjustment and minimizing depression. For patients with gynecologic and breast cancer, one of the most crucial factors is sexual adjustment.

## Sexual Adjustment

In terms of research, sexual adjustment to gynecologic cancer has received more attention than any other form of adjustment. Such attention is well deserved: Andersen (1985) reports significant sexual problems in 30 to 90% of all gynecologic oncology patients, depending on the

site of the disease and the nature of the treatment employed. However, it has not followed that this issue is always dealt with extensively during the medical education of these patients, who report that they would like more instruction in this area (Andersen et al, 1988; Vincent et al, 1975) but hesitate to bring up the issue themselves.

Interest in sexual adjustment to gynecologic cancer is logical, since the breasts, vagina, and/or uterus are often affected. All these organs are important in the physical aspects of sex and affect the woman's self-image (Derogatis and Melisaratos, 1979). One symptom of gynecologic cancer may be vaginal bleeding; because such bleeding can be triggered by intercourse, some patients will associate intercourse with their disease. Andersen et al (1986) found a surprisingly high frequency of sexual dysfunction in the months prior to the diagnosis of cervical and endometrial cancers. In these case, sexual disturbance secondary to abnormal bleeding was often the first sign of the presence of cancer. Furthermore, surgical treatment of these cancers may cause disfigurement and concomitant changes in body image. As Derogatis and Melisaratos (1979) have pointed out, persons who experience sexual dysfunction tend to have a negative body image, so that cancer patients are at high risk for such problems.

Sewell and Edwards (1980) agreed that it is appropriate to be concerned about the sexual adjustment of the patient with pelvic cancer. In their review of the literature on the psychologic adjustment of these patients, they found that adjustment tends to be good in all areas except sexuality. Since patients with pelvic cancer are rarely adequately consulted about sexual issues, this poor adjustment may reflect a lack of education; however, it may just as readily relate to the severity of the biologic and social changes that accompany this disease. Let us now look at the evidence indicating that cancer impairs sexual adjustment.

During the 1980s, studies of the psychosocial effects of gynecologic cancer have become increasingly sophisticated. Barbara Andersen and her colleagues have contributed significantly to our understanding of changes in sexual functioning related to cancer. Sexual functioning is a critical area of concern, with up to 90% of patients with gynecologic cancer reporting significant disturbances (Andersen, 1985), depending upon the site and treatment of the disease.

In one of their key studies, Andersen et al (1989a) prospectively followed three groups of sexually active women: 47 patients with early stage uterine or ovarian cancer (I or II), 18 women with benign gynecologic disease, and 57 healthy women as controls who were recruited at the time of a normal pelvic exam. Thus, it was possible to determine whether treatment of gynecologic disease had any impact on sexual function and whether that impact differed between the two patient groups. All cancer patients were treated with surgery, radiation therapy, or both.

Assessment of sexual function included not only the frequency of intercourse but also measure of desire, behavior, and self-reported physiology during the various phases of the sexual-response cycle. The authors noted a significant decrease in the frequency of sexual intercourse for both cancer patients and those with benign gynecologic disease, and this decreased rate remained stable through the 4-, 8-, and 12-month followup periods. Only cancer patients reported more difficulties during the excitement phase, possibly reflecting inadequate lubrication secondary to surgically induced menopause. Both women with cancer and women with benign disease had more difficulty with orgasm in contrast to the healthy controls. Closer analysis revealed that the decreases in arousability were specific to abbreviated foreplay and less frequent intercourse. Thus, desire was not directly affected.

Overall, these results led to the following recommendations for counseling the patient with gynecologic cancer: (1) couples should be advised about coital positions that allow the woman to control the depth of penetration, so that pain can be avoided; (2) since women frequently failed to feel the usual sense of relief from sexual intercourse after cancer surgery, support and information is probably needed; and (3) since sexual problems usually become evident soon after cancer treatment, preventive and education counseling are warranted.

These results are generally consistent with those reported by Kolodney et al (1979), who found that about one-third of all hysterectomy patients report a decrease in the frequency of intercourse, while another third report an increase; however, these experiences may reflect the patient's expectations. Zussman et al (1981) reported a greater decline in the frequency of intercourse (in 33 to 46% of patients) in their review of studies on sexual adjustment after hysterectomy and oophorectomy among women interviewed in the United Kingdom.

Although frequency of intercourse is an imperfect measure of sexual adjustment, results of studies on the sexual satisfaction of pelvic cancer patients parallel these findings. Harris et al (1982) found that 85% of their sample reported satisfaction with their sex lives before diagnosis and treatment, while only 48% felt satisfied afterward. Similarly, Dennerstein et al (1977) found that 37% of their patients reported a decrease in sexual satisfaction after hysterectomy and oophorectomy. Although estrogen replacement therapy was associated with a decrease in dyspareunia in this study, it was not associated with any increase in sexual satisfaction. Furthermore, patients about to undergo surgery who were anxious about later sexual adjustment had the poorest sexual adjustment on followup. Dennerstein et al recommend counseling for such patients.

Two further measures of sexual adjustment were reported by Harris et al (1982): frequency of orgasm and ability to communicate about sex. While 58% of their patients had orgasms regularly before surgery, only 33% reported regular orgasm after. The ability to communicate about sex showed a similar decline: 55% reported good communication about sex before surgery, while only 33% made the same report afterward. In addition, Harris et al reported that 50% of their patients stopped having intercourse altogether after surgery. Thus, the evidence is strong that sexual adjustment is

harmed by the diagnosis and treatment of pelvic cancer. What is also apparent is that the majority of these patients adjust to their illness and maintain a satisfying sexual life. While fewer patients stopped intercourse in the study by Andersen et al (1989a), these patients also commonly reported frustration due to sexual problems.

Several factors can influence sexual adjustment to cancer: the site of the cancer and stage of the disease, the treatment selected, the quality of the sexual relationship before cancer, and the counseling provided.

***Site of Disease*** Breast cancer may present special problems because the breast is the source of nourishment for the infant (a sign of motherhood), is a sign of sexual maturity and femininity, and is an erotic stimulus. Mastectomy resulted in serious sexual dysfunction in 20% of patients surveyed by Jamison et al (1978). However, when Morris et al (1977) compared the sexual adjustment of 69 breast cancer patients with that of 91 patients suffering from benign breast disease, there was no significant difference in the problems reported. Surveying other women across the same time period may be critical to determine the effects of disease versus the natural changes that may occur in a sexual relationship over time. There is some indication, too, that surgical interventions may help breast cancer patients to adjust. Gerard (1982) has found that patients who undergo breast reconstruction surgery after mastectomy rate themselves as more sexually aroused and sexually attractive than do those who undergo mastectomy without breast reconstruction. It is not clear whether counseling a patient about adjusting to a new body image after mastectomy can achieve equally positive results. Later in this chapter, we will discuss efforts of support groups (such as Reach to Recovery) for these patients.

Cancer of the pelvis may have unique sequelae as well. Cancer of the cervix, for example, may lead to a fear of cancer of the penis if intercourse occurs again. Often, cervical cancer is associated with bleeding after intercourse and may invoke fears about further sexual contact as well.

***Effects of Therapy*** The site of the cancer may interact with the type of treatment provided. For example, sexual adjustment after treatment for cervical cancer appears to differ depending on whether surgery or radiation is used. Seibel et al (1980) interviewed 46 women treated for cancer of the cervix. Those treated with radiation therapy reported a significant decrease in the frequency and enjoyment of intercourse, whereas those treated surgically reported that their sex lives did not change. Later, Seibel et al (1981) reported on women who underwent hysterectomy without oophorectomy, and this group reported no significant decrease in sexual enjoyment. The continued presence of estrogen may have been important in this regard.

Estrogen replacement therapy was found by Coppen et al (1981) to be no more effective than placebo in the long-term sexual adjustment of hysterectomy patients; however, results in both conditions were superior to those among untreated controls.

Pelvic exenteration is perhaps the most disfiguring of

the treatments for pelvic cancer. Not surprisingly, it also appears to be most damaging to sexual functioning. In a small study, Vera (1981) found that 12 of 15 patients undergoing pelvic exenteration reported no further sexual activity after surgery; the other 3 patients reported a loss of sexual desire and a decline in sexual activity. Only one patient reported this to be a major loss. Perhaps the magnitude of the threat to the patient's life allows a rational weighing of costs and benefits of surgery. Andersen and Hacker (1983) found similar levels of disruption in their study of 15 patients with vulvar cancer. Sewell and Edwards (1980) found similarly negative effects of pelvic exenteration, i.e., decline in body image and decreased frequency of sexual interaction.

**Previous Sex Life** Quality of the sexual relationship before the onset of cancer is probably also critical. Length of the relationship is also important; Jamison et al (1978) found that the younger patients in their sample reported the highest rate of marital disruption. Younger patients probably place a different value on the sexual aspect of their relationship. Regardless of the length or quality of the relationship, couples grappling with gynecologic cancer may be exposed to a variety of fears and misconceptions about the effects of cancer on their sex life, and they should be provided with accurate information. Andersen et al (1989a) noted that gynecologic patients do not need to be prompted to resume sexual behaviors already in their repertoire; rather, counseling is needed when those behaviors no longer produce comfort and pleasure.

**Counseling** Donahue and Knapp (1977) recommend that physicians assume primary responsibility for patient counseling, while Kreuger et al (1979) feel that this is an appropriate task for the nurse. Other programs assign this responsibility to physician's assistants or refer the patients to a mental-health specialist or a support group. Many programs probably fail to deal with sexual issues, perhaps rationalizing that the patients will ask if they want to know. Patients, on the other hand, report that they would like more information about sexual adjustment and hope that the medical personnel will initiate such discussions. The need for education and counseling on sexual adjustment should be apparent, and assigning the task to members of the treatment team is probably a critical step toward meeting this need.

## Pain and Cancer

Probably the most common and feared symptom associated with cancer is pain (see also Chapter 24). For many people, the terms *cancer* and *pain* are nearly synonymous. Ironically, there is much evidence to dispute this belief. Pain rarely occurs in the early stages of cancer and is not always present in its advanced stages. For example, Foley (1979) reports that while 75% of female patients with genitourinary cancer report pain, only 52% of breast cancer patients do so. According to Bonica's review of the literature (1979), only one-third of cancer patients experience moderate to severe pain during the intermediate stages of their disease. Ob-

viously, the stage and type of cancer play a pertinent role in the likelihood and severity of pain. Furthermore, while cancer patients generally fear dying in pain, few experience severe pain and most can be treated with minimal sedation (Houde, 1980; Lipman, 1980). Self-administered medication can be effective (Gallion et al, 1987).

Both the medical community and the general public have a bifurcated perception of pain. On the one hand, we assume that tissue damage has occurred and that pain is a direct manifestation of that underlying pathology. (In cancer, the physical basis for the presence of pain may take the form of bone destruction, infiltration or compression of nerves, luminal obstruction, and infiltration or distention of the integument or organ capsule [Turk et al, 1983]). On the other hand, to patients and those who attend to their needs, pain signifies more than a nociceptive event, more than a connection between a pain receptor or tissue damage and a pain response. To the patient, cancer and pain together are an emotional and physical response. This composite response represents the inability to cope physically, socially, and psychologically as well as the fears, ambiguities, and pejorative meaning associated with cancer (Sontag, 1979).

The tendency to move casually from one perception of cancer and pain to another has limited our effectiveness in pain management. How we conceive of pain will determine the strategies used to relieve it. Our position is that, clinically, cancer pain must be dealt with according to the patient's composite perception. Although this will require a range of potential interventions, such a multifaceted approach is likely to improve patient compliance. Since our professional training encourages a somewhat myopic focus upon one area of expertise, we are programmed to view the pain within a narrow perspective. However, if we recognize the complexity of cancer pain, we must consider the full range of physical and psychologic interventions in order to provide comprehensive treatment.

**Physical Pain** As early as 1946, Beecher noted the discrepancy between the magnitude of pain expression and the extent of tissue damage. While treating the wounds of soldiers fighting on Italy's Anzio Beach, Beecher was surprised to observe the minimal pain response of those suffering from severe trauma. The lack of response became even more noteworthy when Beecher returned to medical practice in the United States and observed patients' disproportionately strong response to significantly less trauma. This dramatic contrast led Beecher (1959) to conclude that "there is no simple direct relationship between the wounds per se and the pain experienced. The pain is in large part determined by other factors, and of great importance here is the significance of the wound."

That an isomorphic relationship does not exist between tissue damage and pain was well documented by Turk and Rennert (1981). They made two critical points: First, responses to identical procedures to eliminate pain are inconsistent. According to Toomey et al (1977), approximately 50% of patients with chronic pain fail to respond to organically oriented interventions. A procedure to interrupt or block pain pathways is effective in some but fails in others. Turk and Rennert (1981) also cite several studies in which 30 to 50% of patients in the terminal stage of cancer did not report pain even though at autopsy no differences were found in the extent of tissue damage between patients who had and had not experienced pain. Whether this difference was due to variations in training patients about how to report on their pain, some biochemical factor, or a combination of the two is not known. Second, Turk and Rennert cite a study by Byron and Yonemoto (1975) in which 77% of patients with advanced cancer reported 4 hours or more of complete relief with placebo medication. Given the varied pain responses to similar tissue changes and reports of pain relief with placebo intervention, one can obviously not characterize pain as a strictly physical entity.

***Psychologic Factors*** Sternbach (1974) has suggested that pain and chronic pain behavior are influenced by a variety of factors. Duration of illness; cultural and ethnic acceptance of pain behaviors; consequences of pain (Fordyce, 1976); and ambiguity and expectations regarding pain, anxiety, and depression all affect an individual's perception of pain. There is no reason to believe that cancer pain and its expression are any less influenced by these factors than is chronic pain. Moreover, for the cancer patient, pain has certain psychosocial implications, such as expectations concerning impending death, changing body image, grieving over one's own loss, fears about financial problems, and alterations in personal relationships, all of which can increase anxiety or depression and enhance pain.

***Analgesic Medication and Psychologic Factors*** Although the appropriate use of pain-relieving medications is covered extensively in Chapter 24, we will briefly discuss their effects on anxiety. Because narcotic analgesics are the most effective and widespread treatment for cancer pain, they play an important role in alleviating psychologic discomfort as well as in providing physical relief. By its very nature, pain is ominous and ambiguous. Its unpredictable and erratic course heightens anxiety and feeling of lack of control.

Anxiety and the accompanying fear, both potentiators of pain, can usually be dispelled, yet the full use of drugs for this purpose appears to be hindered by two factors. First, despite the special circumstances and reduced life span of most cancer patients, most physicians are reluctant to medicate the cancer patient fully. Guardedness about prescribing narcotics, the tendency to overestimate the duration of action of these drugs (Marks and Sachar, 1973), and concern about the development of tolerance and impairment of mental functioning have all resulted in the inappropriate underutilization of medication (Houde, 1979; Twycross, 1979). Second, a significant portion of patients, taught to "put on a brave face" and rewarded by nurses and family for their stoicism, endure unnecessary pain and anxiety (Bond, 1979; Lazarus, 1989). Since many studies indicate that anxiety, fear, and ambiguity may constitute a significant part of pain perception (Turk et al, 1983), these two factors can have a considerable debilitating and deleterious effect.

The research of Twycross and his colleagues (1979) at St. Christopher's Hospice in England is instructive. These authors contend that a pain-free state without sedation may be achieved in 85% of patients and can be raised to a remarkable 98% with the aid of immobilization techniques (Twycross, 1980). Two aspects of their program appear particularly relevant. First, a major component of the treatment was assuring patients that their pain would be controlled. When this was followed by a demonstration of immediate relief, the patient's confidence was increased while fear was reduced. Second, according to Twycross' observations, when narcotics were given according to a regular schedule, psychologic dependence did not occur. Adherence to such a schedule provided a means of combating pain before it reached its strongest level, gave patients a sense of control over their pain, and helped to prevent drug-seeking behavior.

This last point, in particular, is consistent with the principles of operant conditioning. The traditional approach of prescribing medication contingent upon a patient's complaints of pain appears to reinforce pain behaviors and to enhance the likelihood of psychologic dependence, whereas establishing a regular schedule of medication requires that the patient take the medication regardless of pain level or pain behavior and thus diminishes the occurrence of "learned pain" and psychologic dependence.

While we do not intend to provide recommendations regarding the complex topic of pharmacologic interventions for cancer pain, techniques that help reduce the psychologic component of pain should be investigated. Research by Twycross (1979) and Mount et al (1978) have provided significant information on this topic. Although drug therapy is the most common intervention for pain, its risks and benefits must both be considered. All pharmacologic interventions have some unintended side effects such as drowsiness or decreased alertness. Psychologic interventions have not been used frequently, but their potential is striking, with apparently minimal risk.

***Psychologic Interventions for Pain*** In the preceding sections, we dealt with the psychologic impact of cancer, the concomitant pain, and the potential for depression. For the cancer patient, the most immediate and pressing concerns are often how to cope with pain, the daily oppressive psychologic reactions leading to depression, and their own reaction to medical interventions—in other words, the day-to-day struggle of living with cancer and its treatment. What psychologic interventions are available to help patients face these difficulties?

As mentioned earlier, probably the most feared characteristic of cancer is pain, and psychologic factors play a significant role in an individual's perception of pain. Yet psychologic interventions are often not employed as a means of ameliorating pain. This is surprising given the positive effects of placebo therapy, the differential reports of pain among patients with comparable tissue damage, and the frequency of iatrogenic problems accompanying medication and invasive procedures. Given the risk involved in most medical interventions for relief of cancer pain and the relatively lower risk associated with psychologic interventions, the latter should certainly be considered as one therapeutic option in the health-care provider's armamentarium.

Unfortunately, most medical practitioners who deal with cancer patients probably think of psychologic interventions as being restricted to grief counseling and assisting the patient in working through the so-called stages of dying (Kübler-Ross, 1969). Although such counseling may be extremely valuable, it is not the only form of psychologic intervention, nor does it address the critical issue of pain management. As more cancer patients are being cured or are living longer, the need to enlist coping strategies has become increasingly important (USDHEW, 1975a, 1975b).

Psychologic interventions for pain management may be adjunctive to extensive medical intervention or may be prescriptive within a more general psychosocial framework.

## PSYCHOSOCIAL INTERVENTIONS

Much has been written about the psychosocial consequences of cancer (Friedenbergs et al, 1982), and a variety of intervention programs have been developed that differ in several respects: timing (at the time of diagnosis, after mastectomy, at the time of recurrence), treatment site (home, inpatient, outpatient), target population (all new patients, referred patients only), care provider (self-help, professional), and type of intervention (informational, emotional support, environmental manipulation, crisis intervention, brief psychotherapy). At present, intervention programs include self-help support groups (reviewed by Holland and Rowland, 1981) and inpatient programs (Winick and Robbins, 1976; Krant, 1976; Saunders, 1965; Sheldon et al, 1970). There are also several programs that combine these components to provide comprehensive support (Bloom et al, 1978; Gordon et al, 1980; Pfefferbaum et al, 1978; Wieder et al, 1978) as well as more focused specific psychologic interventions.

Some unexpected and intriguing findings have come from support groups in adjustment to breast cancer. While Morganstern et al (1984) presented interesting data suggesting that breast cancer patients in a support group survive longer than controls, methodologic problems made that result questionable. However, in a recent prospective trial by Spiegel et al (1989), 86 patients were assigned randomly to a year-long support group or to an untreated control group to study the psychosocial adjustment to metastasized breast cancer. More patients (50) were assigned to the support group and fewer (36) to the untreated control group in an effort to increase the chance of comparable numbers of completers and noncompleters. At 10-year followup, 3 of the 50 support group patients were still alive, while none of the 36 control subjects lived that long. There was a significant difference in survival rates between the groups using Cox's proportional hazards model beginning in the third year post randomization.

One methodologic concern is that randomization favored the intervention group in terms of stage of the disease, since more Stage II and III patients were assigned to the treatment group. However, stage of disease did not predict survival in the overall sample. (In fact, all patients in the study showed evidence of cancer metastasis as a criterion for admission to the study.) While further replication is needed, Spiegel's work suggests that psychosocial treatment in gynecologic cancer may have an exciting impact.

### Self-Help Support Groups

Self-help support groups for cancer patients have developed rapidly over the last 20 years, often generated by former patients who recognized the need for better emotional and social support (Holland and Rowland, 1981). Many are geared to patients with cancer at a specific site, such as Reach to Recovery for women who have had a mastectomy, while others are more generalized. Groups such as Living with Cancer, Project Living, and Cansurmount are all aimed at providing mutual support, information, personal visits, and—most importantly—successful role models; i.e., people who have adapted to living with cancer. Volunteers are typically veteran cancer patients who have undergone similar medical treatment and who visit patients in the hospital to offer them the opportunity to talk with someone who has made it through the diagnosis and the ongoing adaptation to living with cancer. The social support goals of self-help groups are similar to those sought in many inpatient interventions.

### Inpatient Interventions

Two examples of inpatient psychosocial intervention programs are as follows:

1. Winich and Robbins (1976) describe the Post-Mastectomy Rehabilitation Group (PMRG) program at the Memorial Sloan-Kettering Cancer Center. This program consists of a series of structured exercises, information-giving, and group therapy designed to help patients return to their previous level of activity and to adapt to the loss of a breast and the diagnosis of cancer. Patients are encouraged to participate on the first postoperative day. At first, they are seen individually. They then participate in four to five group sessions during their hospital stay. Information about their surgery, lymphedema, range-of-motion exercises, and bras and breast forms is provided by the nursing staff. In addition, a social worker leads a discussion centered on emotional and psychologic concerns. Self-report questionnaires showed that 84% of participants resumed their normal activities within 4 months postoperatively; 74% returned to full-time work within 3 months, and only 13% reported moderate to severe emotional distress. Ninety-eight percent reported that the program

was helpful. Obviously, these are not controlled data, but they do show that nearly all patients who participated received some benefit from the PMRG.

2. An inpatient, controlled investigation carried out by Ferlic et al (1979) consisted of a structured, interdisciplinary approach emphasizing patient education and supportive group counseling. Thirty recently diagnosed cancer patients with a wide variety of advanced malignancies were assigned to the treatment group, while a control group of 30 patients matched for age, sex, and education was also followed. All 60 patients were administered a battery of self-report questionnaires before and after the group sessions as well as at 6-month followup. The group counseling program consisted of six 90-minute sessions over a 2-week period during hospitalization. The content of each meeting was specified (e.g., nursing perspectives, psychologic aspects, sexuality, nutrition) and was led by both a social worker and a content expert (e.g., physician, dietitian, occupational therapist, chaplain). General group discussion and supportive counseling was also emphasized. At the end of the program, the treatment group reported better hospital adjustment, more comprehensive disease information, and more self-awareness and comfort about exploring death-related issues than the control group. Patients in the treatment group also had an improved self-concept compared with the controls. Thus, this structured educational and supportive group met some of the immediate in-hospital needs of the newly diagnosed cancer patient.

The results reported by Ferlic et al are encouraging in that they suggest that inpatient groups can have an immediate and positive effect on the adjustment of the cancer patient. Although more research is needed to define the most effective programs, it is difficult to conduct studies in this area because of staff discomfort about withholding treatment from some patients and about intruding on patients who may be dying. Such constraints are even more salient when one attempts to evaluate the effects of programs that deal with the dying patient.

## Interventions in Terminal Illness

Several systematic efforts have been made to improve the quality of life for the dying patient. The *hospice movement* is probably the best known of the intervention programs for the terminally ill (Holden, 1976). The hospice philosophy is that death should be allowed to occur in an environment that supports the spiritual and emotional needs of the patient, family, and staff while keeping the patient as physically comfortable as possible.

Krant (1981*a*) has proposed some principles for applying the hospice philosophy to the care of the terminally ill cancer patient. These include:

1. Sustained and meticulous medical and nursing care.
2. Psychologic and spiritual support for the patient, family, and involved staff.
3. Coordination of hospital and home-care programs.

4. An integrated service mode that allows ongoing support for patients and families, available on a 24-hour basis 7 days a week.
5. Patient and family participation in sharing information, making decisions, and discussing treatments.

Hospice units in the United States range from institutions geographically separate from any medical facility that care exclusively for terminal patients to loosely knit groups of professionals who use existing agencies to coordinate needed services to patients in their homes. Other hospices consist of designated units within existing inpatient settings or of a group of hospital-based personnel (physicians, nurses, social workers, chaplains, psychologists) who have no designated unit but who are available for consultation in other areas of the hospital (Krant, 1981*a*, 1981*b*).

Yalom and his colleagues (Spiegel and Yalom, 1978; Spiegel et al, 1981, 1989; Yalom and Greaves, 1977) report substantial experience with *outpatient group therapy* of terminally ill cancer patients. Most group members have been women with metastatic carcinoma of the breast. Support groups meet each week for 90 minutes and focus on the problems of terminal illness, including "improving relationships with family, friends, and physicians and living as fully as possible in the face of death."

These investigators have identified some of the "mechanisms of change" they find beneficial to the group of participants. These include altruism (being able to help others), catharsis, group cohesiveness, universality (learning that others share similar concerns and feelings), and death desensitization (a process whereby death is "detoxified" by being repeatedly approached, confronted, and discussed).

Spiegel et al (1981) presented early data on the efficacy of their approach. Fifty-eight patients were randomly assigned to either a no-treatment control group or one of three separate treatment groups. A battery of self-report questionnaires was administered before the start of treatment and again every 4 months for a period of 1 year. Results showed that patients in the treatment group were less anxious, less phobic, more vigorous, less fatigued, and less confused than the no-treatment controls. They also reported using fewer maladaptive coping mechanisms (e.g., alcohol, smoking, overeating) than did the control group. The authors concluded that "the cancer support group for women with terminal carcinoma of the breast was effective in preventing psychological deterioration and improving their capacity to master their predicament." Their later discovery of an impact on long-term survival may underline the importance of that adjustment (Spiegel et al, 1989).

## Comprehensive, Long-Term Psychosocial Interventions

There are several advantages associated with a comprehensive psychologic and psychosocial intervention:

1. By integrating psychologic and medical care dur-

ing the early stages of malignancy, one can attempt to offset or inhibit the patient's tendency to assume blame or fault for the disease. Often, emotional components or secondary reactions to any chronic disease are disregarded at first and are dealt with only after treatment for the organic illness has been instituted. This nonintegrated approach dichotomizes the disease into medical responsibility (organic) and patient responsibility (psychologic). Since the demands of dealing with cancer are so extensive and potentially depressive, patients have a propensity to accept personal blame for the emotional components of the disease. Use of a comprehensive psychosocial approach at all stages (particularly the early stages) makes it clear to the patient that psychologic and organic factors are intermingled, that psychologic pressures are a natural accompaniment to serious illness, and that the professional staff will help the patient cope with these new demands.

2. Comprehensive psychosocial programs can imbue the patient with a sense of control and hopefulness. By fully involving the patient in the treatment process, one can identify negative thought and behavior patterns, expectations, and fears before they develop into major debilitating factors. With this knowledge, the care provider and patient can plan responses to potential problems, thereby giving the patient a sense of control and reducing ambiguity. In addition, concerns that the patient cannot express to family members can be elicited and dealt with largely by professionals in order to prevent a breakdown in communication.

3. Several psychologic interventions, such as relaxation and imagery techniques (see later), can prevent or ameliorate pain and anxiety or loss of control, thereby minimizing distress. Just as identifying specific problems will increase the patient's control over them, providing psychologic tools for dealing with these problems will enhance her ability to master them.

4. If psychologic interventions are introduced early instead of in response to a symptom, their usefulness can be enhanced. Any intervention is more effective before the problem is maximized. Often, psychologic interventions are implemented only as a response to pain or the side effects of invasive pharmacologic interventions, whereas, if provided early, these interventions could help to reduce such complications with minimal risk to the patient.

Despite the obvious advantages of intensive, ongoing psychologic intervention, most programs for the cancer patient focus on death and dying. Less attention has been directed to the major problem of living with cancer, and most reports have been descriptive and have lacked adequate controls. Recently, however, two psychosocial programs have been reported that used control groups and analyzed specific procedures (Gordon et al, 1980; Weisman et al, 1980), one of which will be examined here in some detail.

Gordon et al (1980) designed a study to (1) develop a means for adequately assessing the psychosocial problems of cancer patients, (2) develop and implement appropriate interventions for these problems, and (3) evaluate the effectiveness of these interventions. Three different types of cancer were assessed: breast, lung,

and melanoma. Data were collected on 151 control and 157 intervention-group subjects on four different occasions: on admission, at discharge, and at 3 and 6 months after discharge. Medical, demographic, psychosocial, and behavioral data were drawn from patients' medical records, self-reports, and structured interviews in order to identify systemically specific day-to-day difficulties experienced by cancer patients. The intervention program was developed on the basis of a thorough literature review, a pilot study, and consultation with oncology personnel. It involved three basic types of intervention: (1) education, (2) counseling, and (3) environmental manipulation.

The *educational component* consisted of providing the patient with information about the medical system, the patient's own disease, and living with cancer. As emphasized previously, loss of control, ambiguity, and inappropriate expectations play a major role in the development of anxiety and depression. A comprehensive educational program helps to prevent these difficulties and can have significant palliative potential. *Counseling* focused on patients' reactions to their malignancy. Patients were permitted to express and interpret their thoughts, feelings, and behavior and were encouraged to develop positive coping mechanisms to overcome their fear and loss of control and thus inhibit depression and anxiety. *Environmental manipulation* involved decisions made by health-care personnel regarding formal health-service referral for individual patients. The various interventions were provided by an *oncology counselor* (psychologist, social worker, psychiatric nurse), a term developed by these investigators to emphasize that each patient should be served by one health-care provider who could develop a close and accepting relationship with the patient. Individual treatment plans were developed and periodically reviewed by the entire team.

Complete data were collected for 102 patients in the intervention group and 95 patients in the control group, and results were analyzed for the three sites individually. Results in the psychosocial intervention group included a more rapid decline of negative affect scores (i.e., anxiety and hostility), a more realistic outlook on life, a greater number of patients returning to work, and a behavior pattern suggesting more active use of time. Although each of the three types of cancer was associated with different clinical and recovery issues, all patients responded favorably to treatment.

Despite certain shortcomings (e.g., lack of a placebo control group), this study and the research done by Weisman et al (1980) can serve as an empiric basis for determining the efficacy of comprehensive psychosocial interventions. Any medical specialist wishing to address the full needs of the cancer patient would do well to examine these two reports in detail.

## Adjunctive Psychologic Interventions

Health-care providers who specialize in the psychologic care of cancer patients are usually consulted for management of the patient's general distress or anxiety. Often, the request stems from the physician's fear of dealing with the emotional components of her illness. The interventions themselves tend to fall into three categories: (1) ways of coping within the terminal or dying process, (2) responses to various adjustment problems, and (3) strategies for coping with pain. Since the literature is replete with material on death and dying (e.g., Kübler-Ross, 1969; Spiegel and Yalom, 1978), attention will be focused on the latter two categories.

**Adjustment Problems** Problems of adjustment for the cancer patient may be extensive and varied. Yet many of the issues dealt with and the skills utilized are similar to, if not the same as, those implemented in therapy for other diseases. Comments such as "Things are getting out of control," "I don't know why this is happening to me," "I feel boxed in with no options," "This is awful," and "I can't stand this" are frequent comments made by patients with cancer or some other disease.

Although psychotherapies differ in emphasis, therapists commonly use two techniques to obtain their objectives: (1) teaching patients a set of new terms and models to help them understand their difficulties and (2) providing patients with some feedback or data so that they can evaluate the usefulness of their thinking and behavioral styles (Turk et al, 1983). This approach is applicable to both cancer and noncancer patients. Cancer patients are repeatedly exposed to unfamiliar and often frightening problems for which previous experience or models have not prepared them. A good health-care provider can be invaluable in guiding these patients through their new dilemmas.

**Strategies for Coping with Pain** There are numerous approaches to pain, and the three most prominent—relaxation, imagery, and activity management—will be described here. (See the earlier discussion of limited information.)

*Relaxation* has been found to reduce pain directly or to minimize it by reducing muscle tension. Anxiety tends to exacerbate pain, while relaxation tends to diminish it. In addition, relaxation facilitates sleep, thus allowing the patient's own recuperative powers to take over. With relaxation, other pain relief methods have proved to be more effective (McCaffery, 1979). Training the patient in relaxation techniques may involve special breathing patterns, evoking passive imagery, alternate tensing and relaxing of particular muscle groups to become aware of fine discriminations, and so forth. Although such techniques are relatively easy to learn, they should be taught by trained personnel who are sensitive to issues of compliance, are knowledgeable about multiple relaxation techniques, and can use the techniques appropriately.

The concept of *imagery* has much in common with relaxation. Simply put, it is very similar to daydreaming but probably requires more individual input than does relaxation. Patients are systematically encouraged to see, touch, feel, hear, and even taste images that will distract and relax them and decrease their anxiety. Images are designed specifically to reduce pain and may take the form of cutting the nerve fibers that transmit the pain, turning off pain switches, or building a wall of ice around a burning pain. A skillful therapist can help the patient turn a seemingly mild diversion into a truly effective analgesic.

*Activity and exercise management* is another area in which a therapist may intervene. The diagnosis of cancer frequently results in unnecessary as well as necessary physical limitations. Obviously, the individual's activity and normal routine will be changed to some degree owing to physical alterations, the presence of pain, and debilitating side effects of treatment. However, the degree of limitation and the ability to cope with these changes are psychologic in nature. Lack of exercise and activity and disruption of normal functioning can have detrimental effects, such as the onset of depression, whereas the opposite occurs when patients maintain a high level of activity or maximize the potential resources available to them. Patients will feel better, depression will be less likely, pain will be minimized, and others will respond more positively to the patient.

Because patients may tend to focus on what they are unable to do and may idealize their previous level of activity, the therapist's task becomes one of assisting the patient in overcoming despair and accurately perceiving which activities are still feasible. Transforming a vague feeling of inadequacy into a desire to meet specific, measurable goals and motivating a patient to initiate new activities can have a strong positive impact. A skilled therapist can frequently accomplish this by focusing on those areas of the patient's life which have been *unaffected* by the pain (Karol and Anderson, 1980) or by breaking down a difficult task into a series of manageable steps. Once again, sensitivity and listening skills are essential for the therapist.

It is important to note that these approaches represent only a sample of the psychologic interventions available. The well-trained health therapist can offer a vast repertoire of tools for dealing with the cancer patient. For a more comprehensive discussion of psychologic interventions, the interested reader should consult the work of Turk et al (1983).

## Summary and Critique of Psychosocial Interventions

A wide variety of interventions have been presented, including self-help support groups; inpatient educational and supportive programs; interventions for terminal illness; and comprehensive, long-term psychosocial interventions. To date, most studies have been descriptive or anecdotal; well-controlled evaluations of program effectiveness are rare (Morganstern et al, 1984; Spiegel et al, 1989; Gordon et al, 1980; Weisman et al, 1980). As more experimentally trained behavioral scientists enter the field of psychosocial oncology, more rigorous scientific study design is being called for (Meyerowitz et al, 1983; Silberfarb, 1982). One major criticism has been the lack of specificity in previous attempts to study the psychosocial problems of living with cancer, strategies for coping, possible interventions, and program effectiveness (Meyerowitz et al, 1983). Most studies of patients' adaptation to cancer fail to take into account crucial disease-related variables such as primary tumor site, time since diagnosis, and prognosis. Many personal variables such as age, social support, and pre-morbid coping style are also ignored in studies of coping and treatment intervention. Consequently, many questions remain regarding the most effective type of intervention, its effects, which patients should be treated and by whom, and the appropriate setting for such interventions.

## COMMUNICATION SKILLS

Greater involvement of mental-health agents in the training of medical students and personnel has shown the importance of teaching interviewing skills. If one accepts the notion that some topics are more difficult to discuss than others, communication-skills training for medical students might profitably focus on these subjects. Three particularly difficult topics are death (Callahan et al, 1983), sexuality (Lief and Karlen, 1976), and cancer (Wortman and Dunkel-Schetter, 1979). Indeed, the greater the extent of the cancer, the greater the reported barriers to communication.

What are the payoffs for good communication skills? There appear to be many. Physicians who receive high ratings on their communication skills are perceived by patients as being the most technically competent (DiMatteo and Hays, 1980). Furthermore, when Di-Matteo (1979) interviewed patients to find out why they continued to see a certain doctor, it was found that the patient's decision was based on the doctor's ability to communicate a feeling of caring and concern. Good communication skills have also been linked to increased compliance with treatment (Freeman et al, 1971). Finally, malpractice suits are reportedly filed most often when patients are disturbed by the way the physician communicates. Better communication will enhance positive feelings between doctor and patient, making a difficult job more rewarding.

Delivering health care in a supportive manner is not always easy, particularly when health-care providers have their own fears and misconceptions about how to talk to the patient who has cancer (Wortman and Dunkel-Schetter, 1979). Cassileth and Cassileth (1979) list nine fears students have when learning to care for cancer patients: (1) telling patients the diagnosis, (2) responding to questions, (3) dealing with family members, (4) helping the terminally ill, (5) sensing an unending responsibility, (6) experiencing death, (7) dealing with patients' experiences of the side effects of treatment, (8) facing the limitations of medical competence, and (9) excessive emotional involvement. The authors responded to these concerns by encouraging physicians to be honest while conveying as much information as the patient can incorporate as well as a sense of hope.

Reynolds et al (1981) compared two ways in which physicians could communicate information to their patients: (1) using the normal communication practices of oncologists or (2) asking patients if they want to know about specific categories such as diagnosis, treatment, and symptoms. Interactions of both groups were tape-recorded so that patients could refer to them at home.

Patients in the second group remembered more of the information about which they had asked; however, there were no differences between the groups in terms of patients' satisfaction with the amount of information they received. The authors suggest that the latter result may be due to patients' general reluctance to express dissatisfaction with their physicians.

Further support for the patient's need for information comes from a report by Alexy (1982). In this study, patients in the oncology unit wanted to know about day-to-day activities, such as medical tests and unit rules. Also, Jackson (1979) found that an informative pamphlet aided women's sexual adjustment after a hysterectomy; some of these women suggested that even more information about postoperative problems be included. Wortman and Dunkel-Schetter (1979) observed that family members also need information and suggested that health-care providers inquire at early stages of treatment about the social support network of the patient in order to provide relevant information to such individuals. Advising family members about possible consequences of treatment can help them be more tolerant of the patient's illness.

Donahue and Knapp (1977) highlight several ways in which physicians can communicate with gynecologic patients to enhance their sexual rehabilitation. First, it is important to dispel myths and correct misinformation through prompt explanations of tests and results. Physicians are encouraged to address fears about disfigurement and defeminization by describing the functional and anatomic changes that will follow treatment. One must consider the patient's sexual attitudes and include the partner and family in sexual counseling while accentuating the positive aspects of treatment, such as the end of pelvic pain.

Good communication skills are only part of the physician's interaction with the cancer patient; the professional must also know when and how to intervene. Certain basic questions need to be addressed concerning communication. Specifically, should patients be told that they have cancer, and what should be the patient's role in decision-making? After reviewing what is known about successful interviews with cancer patients, we will discuss model training programs. Let us turn first to the issue of whether patients want to know that they have cancer.

### Communicating the Diagnosis of Cancer

It has long been the conventional wisdom that many patients with cancer do not want to know their diagnosis. The question of how much to tell the cancer patient is also a controversial issue (McIntosh, 1974). Hardy et al (1980) concluded from their review of the literature that 98% of patients preferred to be told their diagnosis. They also found that 98% of physicians who were questioned responded that they always or usually told patients when they found cancer; however, this self-reporting should be accepted with some reservation. A physician may feel he or she has divulged the diagnosis to the patient, yet the patient may not understand the terms used ("You have a malignancy") or the implication may not be clear ("You have a tumor that we must remove"). Hamilton et al (1983) recently found that patients who were referred to an oncology center from outlying clinics felt that their physician had not informed them at that they had cancer. The patient's emotional response at the time of diagnosis (especially if considered as part of the denial stage of grieving) may preclude her "hearing" accurately.

It is possible that people will work to avoid hearing the diagnosis of cancer. When Jones (1981) told patients with inoperable bronchial carcinoma that they could ask any questions that they wanted, only half asked their diagnosis. Does this mean that half the patients studied did not want to know? Perhaps patients withhold questions because they do not wish to take up the doctor's time or because they fear bridging the social gap between the physician and themselves. In gynecology, there is often a male doctor–female patient relationship in which the patient may assume a subservient and powerless role. Furthermore, patients who ask questions are sometimes labeled as troublemakers. In addition, the physician may inadvertently communicate an unwillingness to answer the patient's questions (McIntosh, 1974).

Do patients accept the diagnosis of cancer over time? Mitchell and Glickman (1977) report that most patients used the terms *cancer* or *malignant tumor* when discussing their disease, implying that they have adjusted to the diagnosis. Slavin et al (1982) explored the effects of informing the patient that he or she has cancer in a longitudinal study of pediatric clients. Informed patients made a better long-term adjustment than did uninformed patients; in fact, the latter showed more common and intense signs of maladjustment. If it is agreed that informing the patient of the diagnosis is the best course, it is critical that the information be delivered in a way that will not destroy a patient's hope (Cassileth and Cassileth, 1979). At this point, let us turn to a related issue: Should the patient participate in decision-making about treatment?

## Patient Involvement in Decision-Making

Schain (1980) emphasizes that it is important to acknowledge the patient's rights in decision-making by keeping the patient informed. Since cancer patients tend to experience a loss of control and power (Silberfarb and Greer, 1982), Schain suggests that physicians can help patients regain control by including them in decision-making and by providing information about what they can expect in the future. She relates five responsibilities of the physician: (1) to encourage the patient to ask questions; (2) to provide relevant information in a language and manner the patient can understand; (3) to consider the psychological needs of the patient; (4) to determine the patient's mode of information-seeking; and (5) to use strategies to enhance patient compliance, such as written instructions.

Most patients do want to know and discuss the facts of their illness and its medical management (Mitchell and Glickman, 1977). However, even Schain recognized the difficulties with the concept of completely involving

the patient in decision-making, and she points out that the physician must take into account a patient's knowledge, social background, interest, and needs. Any of these factors may affect the patient's ability or willingness to make treatment decisions. Usually the patient is not equipped to evaluate treatment options (Wortman and Dunkel-Schetter, 1979) and prefers to know what therapy the physician recommends.

To summarize, it appears that the physician should involve the patient in the decision-making process to the extent that the patient wishes to do so and is capable of doing so. Let us now turn to research concerning physician (or medical student) and patient input in identifying communication skills.

## Previous Psychologic Research

Communication with the cancer patient is difficult and may become more difficult as the disease becomes more severe (Wortman and Dunkel-Schetter, 1979). In fact, talking about cancer may be conceptualized as a fear in order to understand the development of a training program. In order to overcome a fear, one must practice gradually responding to the feared stimulus, with positive reinforcement provided for success (Leitenberg and Callahan, 1973).

It can be argued that for many people fear is not the cause of their communication problem; the problem is lack of skill. However, regardless of its cause, the same programs used for dealing with fears can be used to teach communication skills. We will now review some of the programs that have been developed to teach interviewing skills to physicians or medical students who care for cancer patients. (For the interested reader, Cormier and Cormier [1979] have written an excellent text on teaching interviewing skills.)

## Teaching Communication Skills

Winefield (1982) designed a low-cost, low-technology approach to teaching communication skills that involved eight contact hours with 137 medical students. Using Egan's model of the helping process, in which four skills are progressively developed, she looked specifically at the first two: attending and communicating accurate empathy. An independent judge rated the students' empathy based on videotapes made before and after these sessions, and two-thirds of the students were said to have improved their empathy skills on the later observation.

Another attempt to develop a low-cost method for teaching communication skills focused specifically on dealing with cancer patients (Anderson, 1982). Students were given a brief case history of a terminal cancer patient who had not been told his diagnosis or prognosis. They were asked to write down individually what they would tell the patient, how they would tell him, and who should do so. They then discussed their answers in pairs, groups of four, and groups of eight and were required to arrive at a consensus at each of these steps. The consensus of each large group was presented, followed by the viewing and discussion of a videotape showing a simulation of a patient being told by a doctor in a sensitive and nonjudgmental way that he had terminal cancer. The results of the study were that 38% of the students changed their minds about at least one aspect of the problem; 90% had talked with someone with a different point of view; and 79% learned something from the experience. Although the outcome measures were weak, this study provided some interesting ideas about how to teach communication.

Another strategy was reported by Thompson and Anderson (1982), who conducted a seminar with fourth-year medical students to discuss research on medical interviewing. After the seminar, student-patient interviews were videotaped, and following discussion and feedback, students were again videotaped in another patient interview. After each interview, patients rated the students on whether they were easy to talk to, sympathetic, irritating, warm, easy to confide in about personal problems, and competent. A blind independent assessor also randomly rated the interview tapes. Students were rated higher after the second interviews, although more differences showed up in the rater's assessment than in the patients' ratings. Whether this indicates patient reluctance to criticize physicians or whether communication skills are more important to researchers than to patients is not clear.

## CONCLUSION

In this chapter, we have presented an overview of the psychologic aspects of gynecologic cancer. Specific topics covered have included the rationale for the use of counseling as part of the oncologic service, a model for counseling by medical personnel, ways of helping cancer patients adjust to their illness, reviews of single and comprehensive treatment programs, and a brief discussion of models used for communications-skills training. It is our hope that some of this information will be useful to practitioners and that some will spur further research in this critical and complex area.

## REFERENCES

Aitken-Swan J: Nursing the later cancer patient at home: The family's impression. *Practitioner* 183:64-69, 1959.
Alexy W: Perception of ward atmosphere on an oncology unit. *Int J Psychiat Med* 11:331-340, 1981-1982.
Amias AS: Sexual life after gynecological operations. *Br Med J* 2:608-609, 1975.
Andersen BL: Sexual functioning complications in women with gynecologic cancer—Outcomes and directions for prevention. *Cancer* 60:2123-2128, 1987.
Andersen BL: *Women with Cancer: Psychological Perspectives.* New York, Springer-Verlag, 1985.
Andersen BL, Anderson B, de Prosse C: Controlled prospective longitudinal study of women with cancer. I. Sexual functioning outcomes. *J Consult Clin Psychol* 57:683-691, 1989a.
Andersen BL, Anderson B, de Prosse C: Controlled prospective longitudinal study of women with cancer. II. Psychological outcomes. *J Consult Clin Psychol* 57:692-697, 1989b.
Andersen BL, Hacker NF: Psychosexual adjustment after vulvar surgery. *Obstet Gynecol* 62(4):457-462, 1983.
Andersen BL, Lackenbush PA, Anderson B, et al: Sexual dysfunction and signs of gynecologic cancer. *Cancer* 57:1880-1886, 1986.
Andersen BL, Turnquist D, La Polla J, et al: Sexual functioning after treatment of in situ vulvar cancer: Preliminary report. *Obstet Gynecol* 71(1):15-19, 1988.
Anderson, J: Evaluation of a practical approach to teaching about communication with terminal cancer patients. *Med Educ* 16:202-207, 1982.
Annon JS: *Behavioral Treatment of Sexual Problems.* Hagerstown, Maryland, Harper & Row, 1976.
Averill JR: Grief: Its nature and significance. *Psychol Bull* 70:721-748, 1968.
Beecher H: *Measurement of Subjective Responses.* New York, Oxford University Press, 1959.
Bem SL: The measurement of psychological androgyny. *J Consult Clin Psychol* 42:155-162, 1974.
Bloom JR, Ross RD, Burnell G: The effect of social support on patient adjustment after breast surgery. *Patient Counsel Health Educ* 1:50-59, 1978.
Bond MR: Psychological and emotional aspects of cancer pain. In Bonica JJ, Ventafridda V (eds): *Advances in Pain Research and Therapy*, Vol. 2. New York, Raven Press, 1979, pp. 215-222.
Bonica JJ: Importance of the problem. In Bonica JJ, Ventafridda V (eds): *Advances in Pain Research and Therapy*, Vol. 2. New York, Raven Press, 1979, pp. 115-130.
Bowlby J, Parkes CN: Separation and loss. In Anthony EJ, Koupernik C (eds): *The Child and His Family.* New York, John Wiley & Sons, 1970, pp. 197-216.
Bugen LA: Human grief: A model for prediction and intervention. *Am J Orthopsychiatry* 47:196-206, 1977.
Byron R, Yonemoto R: Pain associated with malignancy. In Crue B Jr (ed): *Pain Research and Treatment.* New York, Academic Press, 1975, pp. 319-321.
Cain EN, Kohorn EI, Quinlan DM, et al: Psychosocial benefits of a cancer support group. *Cancer* 57:183-189, 1986.
Callahan EJ, Brasted WS, Granados J: Fetal loss and sudden infant death: Grieving and adjustment for families. In Callahan EJ, McCluskey KA (eds): *Life-Span Developmental Psychology: Non-Normative Life Events.* New York, Academic Press, 1983, pp. 148-166.
Capone MA, Good RS, Westie KS, et al: Psychosocial rehabilitation of gynecologic oncology patients. *Arch Phys Med Rehabil* 61:128-132, 1980.
Carkuff R: *Helping and Human Relations, Vol. I: Selection and Training.* New York, Holt, Rinehart and Winston, 1969.
Cassileth B: Cancer, a biopsychosocial model. In Cassileth B (ed): *The Cancer Patient: Social and Medical Aspects of Care.* Philadelphia, Lea & Febiger, 1979, pp. 17-31.
Cassileth BR, Lusk EJ, Strouse TB, et al: Psychosocial status in chronic illness. *N Engl J Med* 311:506-511, 1984.
Cassileth BR, Lusk EJ, Strouse TB, et al: A psychosocial analysis of cancer patients and their next-of-kin. *Cancer* 55:72-76, 1985.
Cassileth P, Cassileth B: Learning to care for cancer patients: The student's dilemma. In Cassileth B (ed): *The Cancer Patient: Social and Medical Aspects of Care.* Philadelphia, Lea & Febiger, 1979, pp. 301-318.
Cobliner WG: Psychosocial factors in gynecological or breast malignancies. *Hosp Phys* 4:38-40, 1977.
Coppen A, Bishop M, Bernard E, Collins W: Hysterectomy, hormone and behavior: A prospective study. *Lancet* 1:126-128, 1981.
Cormier WH, Cormier LS: *Interviewing Strategies for Helpers: A Guide to Assessment, Treatment and Evaluation.* Belmont, California, Wadsworth, 1979.
Cousins N: *Head First: The Biology of Hope.* New York, E.P. Dutton, 1989.
Day E: The patient with cancer and the family. *N Engl J Med* 274:883-886, 1966.
Dennerstein L, Wood C, Burrows GD: Sexual response following hysterectomy and oophorectomy. *Obstet Gynecol* 49:92-96, 1977.
Derogatis LR: Breast and gynecologic cancers. Their impact on body image and sexual identity in women. *Frontiers Radiat Ther Oncol* 14:1-11, 1979.
Derogatis LR, Melisaratos N: The DSFI: A multidimensional measure of sexual functioning. *Sex Marital* 5:244-281, 1979.
Derogatis LR, Spencer PM: Psychometric issues in the psychological assessment of the cancer patient. *Cancer* 53:2228-2234, 1984.

Derogatis L, Morrow G, Fetting J, Penman D, Paisetsky S, Schmale A, Henricks M, Carnicke C: The prevalence of psychiatric disorders among cancer patients. *JAMA* 249:751-757, 1983.

DiMatteo MR: A social-psychological analysis of physician-patient rapport: Toward a science of the art of medicine. *J Soc Issues* 35:12-33, 1979.

DiMatteo MR, Hays R: The significance of patients' perception of physician conduct. *J Commun Health* 6:18-34, 1980.

Donahue VC: Sexual rehabilitation of gynecologic cancer patients. *Med Aspects Human Sexuality* 12:51-52, 1978.

Donahue VC, Knapp RC: Sexual rehabilitation of gynecological patients. *Obstet Gynecol* 49:1118-1121, 1977.

Endicott J: Measurement of depression in patients with cancer. *Cancer* 53(Suppl):2243-2248, 1984.

Engel GL: Is grief a disease? *Psychosom Med* 23:18-22, 1961.

Engel GL: *Psychological Development in Health and Disease.* Philadelphia, WB Saunders Co, 1974.

Ferlic M, Goldman A, Kennedy BJ: Group counseling in adult patients with cancer. *Cancer* 43:760-766, 1979.

Foley KM: Pain syndromes. In Bonica JJ, Ventafridda V (eds): *Advances in Pain Research and Therapy*, Vol. 2. New York, Raven Press, 1979, pp. 59-75.

Fordyce WE: *Behavioral Methods for Chronic Pain and Illness.* St. Louis, C.V. Mosby Co, 1976.

Freeman B, Negrete V, Davis M, Korsch B: Gaps in doctor-patient communication: Doctor-patient intervention analysis. *Pediatr Res* 5:298-311, 1971.

Friedenbergs I, Gordon W, Hibbard M, et al: Psychosocial aspects of living with cancer: A review of the literature. *Int J Psychiatry Med* 11:303-329, 1981-1982.

Gallion HH, Wermeling DP, Foster TS, et al: Patient-controlled analgesia in gynecologic oncology. *Gynec Oncol* 27:247-252, 1987.

Gerard D: Sexual functioning after mastectomy: Life vs. lab. *J Sex Marital Ther* 8:305-315, 1982.

Giacquinta B: Helping families face the crises of cancer. *Am J Nurs* 77:1585-1588, 1977.

Gordon WA, Friedenbergs L, Diller L, Hibbard M, Wolfe C, Levine L, Lipkins R, Ezrachi D, Lucido D: Efficacy of psychosocial intervention with cancer patients. *J Consult Clin Psychol* 48:743-759, 1980.

Gottesman D, Lewis M: Difference in crisis reactions among cancer and surgery patients. *J Cons Clin Psychol* 50:381-388, 1982.

Gustafson J, Whitman H: Toward a balanced social environment on the oncology service: The cancer patients' group. *Soc Psychol* 13:147-152, 1978.

Hamilton SA, Callahan EJ, Ashraf M, Kincaid C: An assessment of physician communication and patient satisfaction. Paper presented to the 8th World Congress of Behavior Therapy, Washington, D.C., 1983.

Hardy R, Green D, Jordan H: Communication between cancer patients with physicians. *South Med J* 73:755-757, 1980.

Harris R, Good RS, Pollack L: Sexual behavior of gynecologic patients. *Arch Sex Behav* 11:503-510, 1982.

Hinton J: Psychiatric consultation in fatal illness. *Proc Roy Soc Med* 65:29-32, 1972.

Holden C: Hospices: For the dying, relief from pain and fear. *Science* 193:389-391, 1976.

Holland JC, Rowland JH: Psychiatric, psychosocial and behavioral interventions in the treatment of cancer: An historical review. In Weiss SM, Herd A, Fox B (eds): *Perspectives on Behavioral Medicine.* New York, Academic Press, 1981.

Houde RW: Systemic analgesics and related drugs: Narcotic analgesics. In Bonica JJ, Ventafridda V (eds): *Advances in Pain Research and Therapy*, Vol. 2. New York, Raven Press, 1979, pp. 263-273.

Houde RW: The rational use of narcotic analgesics for controlling cancer pain. *Drug Ther* 10:63-68, 1980.

Izsak FV, Engel J, Medalie JH: Comprehensive rehabilitation of the patient with cancer: Five year experience of a home care unit. *J Chron Dis* 26:363-367, 1973.

Jackson P: Sexual adjustment to hysterectomy and the benefits of a pamphlet for patients. *NZ Med J* 90:471-472, 1979.

Jamison KR, Wellisch DK, Pasnau RO: Psychosocial aspects of mastectomy. *Am J Psychiatry* 135:432-436, 1978.

Jones S: Telling the right patient. *Br Med J* 283:291-292, 1981.

Karol JB, Anderson RU: Neuropharmacologic evaluation in spinal cord injury patients using membrane catheter cystosphincterometry. *J Urol* 124:395-396, 1980.

Kolodney RC, Masters WH, Johnson VE: *Textbook of Sexual Medicine.* Boston, Little, Brown, 1979.

Krant MJ: Problems of the physician in presenting the patient with the diagnosis. In Cullen JW, Box BH, Isom PN (eds): *Cancer: The Behavioral Dimensions.* New York, Raven Press, 1976, pp. 269-274.

Krant MJ: Hospice philosophy in late-stage cancer care. *JAMA* 245:1061-1062, 1981*a*.

Krant MJ: Psychosocial impact of gynecologic cancer. *Cancer* 48:608-712, 1981*b*.

Kreuger J, Hassell J, Goggins D, Ishimatsu T, Pablico M, Tuttle E: Relationship between nurse counseling and sexual adjustment after hysterectomy. *Nurs Res* 28:145-150, 1979.

Kübler-Ross E: *On Death and Dying.* New York, Macmillan, 1969.

Lansky SB, List MA, Herrmann CA, et al: Absence of major depressive disorder in female cancer patients. *Oncology* 3(11):1553-1560, 1985.

Lazarus R: The trivialization of distress. In Rosen J, Solomon L (eds): *Primary Prevention of Psychopathology in Health Care.* Hanover, New Hampshire, University of New England Press, 1989.

Leitenberg H, Callahan EJ: Reinforced practice and reduction of different kinds of fears of adults and children. *Behav Res Ther* 11:19-30, 1973.

Levine P, Silberfarb PM, Lipowski ZJ: Mental disorders in cancer patients: A study of 100 psychiatric referrals. *Cancer* 42:1385-1391, 1978.

Lewis F, Bloom J: Psychosocial adjustment to breast cancer: A review of selected literature. *Int J Psychiatry Med* 9:1-17, 1978-1979.

Lief HI, Karlen A: *Sex Education in Medicine.* New York, Spectrum Press, 1976.

Lindemann E: Symptomatology and management of acute grief. *Am J Psychiatry* 101:141-148, 1944.

Lipman AG: Drug therapy in cancer pain. *Cancer Nursing* 3:39-46, 1980.

Marks RM, Sachar EJ: Undertreatment of medical inpatients with narcotic analgesics. *Ann Intern Med* 78:173-181, 1973.

McCaffery M: Sociological effects of cancer pain. In Bonica JJ, Ventafridda V (eds): *Advances in Pain Research and Therapy*, Vol. 2. New York, Raven Press, 1979, pp. 99-112.

McCartney CF, Larson DB: Quality of life in patients with gynecologic oncology. *Cancer* 60:2129-2136, 1987.

McIntosh J: Processes of communication, information seeking and control associated with cancer: A selected review of the literature. *Soc Sci Med* 8:167-187, 1974.

Medio FJ: Teaching interpersonal communication skills to medical students: A comparison of four methods. Unpublished doctoral dissertation, West Virginia University, 1980.

Melzack R: *The Puzzle of Pain.* New York, Basic Books, 1973.

Meyerowitz BE, Sparks F, Spears I: Adjuvant chemotherapy for breast carcinoma: Psychological implications. *Cancer* 43:1613-1618, 1979.

Meyerowitz BE, Heinrich RL, Coscarelli Schag C: A competency-based approach to coping with cancer. In Burish TG, Bradley LA (eds): *Coping with Chronic Disease: Research and Applications.* New York, Academic Press, 1983, pp. 137-158.

Mitchell G, Glickman A: Cancer patients: Knowledge and attitudes. *Cancer* 40:60-61, 1977.

Morganstern H, Gellert GA, Walter SD, et al: The impact of a psychosocial support program on survival with breast cancer: The importance of selection bias in program evaluation. *J Chron Dis* 37:273, 1984.

Morris T, Greer HS, White PW: Psychological and social adjustments to mastectomy. *Cancer* 40:2381-2387, 1977.

Mount BM, Melzack R, MacKinnon KJ: The management of intractable pain in patients with advanced malignant disease. *J Urol* 120:720-725, 1978.

Pfefferbaum B, Pasnau RO, Jamison K, Weylisch DK: A comprehensive program of psychosocial care for mastectomy patients. *Int J Psychiatry Med* 8:63-72, 1977-1978.

Plumb MM, Holland J: Comparative studies of psychological function in patients with advanced cancer. I. Self-reported depressive symptoms. *Psychosom Med* 39:264-276, 1977.

Polivy J: Psychological reactions to hysterectomy: A critical review. *Am J Obstet Gynecol* 118:417-426, 1974.

Ramsay RW: Bereavement: A behavioral treatment of pathological grief. In Sjoden PO, Bates S, Dockin WS (eds): *Stress and Anxiety*, Vol. 4. New York, John Wiley & Sons, 1979, pp. 217-248.

Reynolds P, Sanson-Fisher R, Poole A, Harkir J, Byrne M: Cancer and communication: Information giving in an oncology clinic. *Br Med J* 282:1449-1451, 1981.

Saunders C: The last stages of life. *Am J Nurs* 65:70-75, 1965.

Sawyer MM: Pain associated with cancer. In Jacox AK (ed): *Pain: A Source Book for Nurses and Other Health Professionals*. Boston, Little, Brown, 1977, pp. 373-389.

Schain W: Patient's rights in decision making: The case for personalism vs. paternalism in health care. *Cancer* 46:1035-1041, 1980.

Schmale AH, Morrow GR, Schmitt MH, et al: Well-being of cancer survivors. *Psychosom Med* 45:163-169, 1983.

Schonfeld J: Psychological factors related to delayed return to earlier life-style in successfully treated cancer patients. *J Psychosom Res* 16:41-46, 1972.

Secunda JK, Katz MM, Friedman RJ, Schuler D: *Special Report: 1973—The Depressive Disorders*. Washington D.C., U.S. Government Printing Office, 1973.

Seibel M, Freeman MG, Graves WL: Carcinoma of the cervix and sexual function. *Obstet Gynecol* 55:484-487, 1980.

Seibel M, Freeman MG, Graves WL: Hysterectomy for carcinoma *in situ* and sexual function. *Oncology* 11:195-199, 1981.

Sewell H, Edwards D: Pelvic genital cancer: Body image and sexuality. *Front Radiat Ther Oncol* 14:35-41, 1980.

Sheldon A, Ryser CP, Krant MJ: An integrated family-oriented cancer case program. *J Chron Disease* 22:743-755, 1970.

Silberfarb PM: Psychiatric problems in breast cancer. *Cancer* 53:820-824, 1984.

Silberfarb PM: Research in adaptation to illness and psychosocial intervention: An overview. *Cancer* 50:1921-1925, 1982.

Silberfarb PM, Greer S: Psychological concomitants of cancer: Clinical aspects. *Am J Psychother* 36:470-478, 1982.

Slavin LA, O'Malley JE, Koocher GP, Foster DJ: Communication of the cancer diagnosis to pediatric patients: Impact on long term adjustment. *Am J Psychiatry* 139:2, 1982.

Small EC, Anderson B, Watring WF, et al: Ovarian carcinoma—Management of stress in patients and physicians. *Gynecol Oncol* 15:160-165, 1983.

Sobel W: Depression and dying in the cancer patient. In Sobel HJ (ed): *Behavior Therapy in Terminal Care: A Humanistic Approach*. Cambridge, Mass, Ballinger Press, 1981, pp. 69-94.

Sontag S: *Illness as Metaphor*. New York, Vintage Books, 1979.

Spiegel BS: *Love, Medicine and Miracles*. New York, Harper and Row, 1986.

Spiegel D, Yalom I: A support group for dying patients. *Int J Group Psychother* 28:233-245, 1978.

Spiegel D, Bloom JR, Kraemer JC, et al: Effects of psychosocial treatment on survival of patients with metastatic breast cancer. *Lancet* 2:888-891, 1989.

Spiegel D, Bloom JR, Yalom I: Group support for patients with metastatic cancer: A randomized prospective outcome study. *Arch Gen Psychiatry* 38:527-533, 1981.

Sternbach R: *Pain Patients: Traits and Treatment*. New York, Academic Press, 1974.

Swensen C: *An Approach to Case Conceptualization*. New York, Houghton-Mifflin, 1968.

Thompson J, Anderson J: Patient preference and the bedside manner. *Med Educ* 16:17-21, 1982.

Toomey T, Ghia J, Mao W, Gregg J: Acupuncture and chronic pain mechanisms: The moderating effects of affect, personality, and stress on response to treatment. *Pain* 3:137-145, 1977.

Turk DC, Rennert K: Pain and the terminally ill cancer patient. In Sobel HJ (ed): *Behavior Therapy in Terminal Care: A Humanistic Approach*. Cambridge, Mass, Ballinger Press, 1981, pp. 95-124.

Turk DC, Meichenbaum D, Genest M: *Pain and Behavioral Medicine: A Cognitive Behavioral Perspective*. New York, Guilford Press, 1983.

Turnbull F: Pain and suffering in cancer. *Can Nurse* 67:28-30, 1971.

Twycross RG: Overview of analgesia. In Bonica JJ, Ventafridda V (eds): *Advances in Pain Research and Therapy*, Vol. 2. New York, Raven Press, 1979, pp. 617-633.

Twycross RG: The relief of pain in far-advanced cancer. *Reg Anaesth* 5:2-11, 1980.

U.S. Department of Health, Education, and Welfare: *Recent Trends in Survival of Cancer Patients* (U.S. Public Health Service Publication No. 75-767). Washington D.C., U.S. Government Printing Office, 1975a.

U.S. Department of Health, Education and Welfare: *Third National Cancer Survey: Incidence Data* (National Cancer Institute Monograph No. 41, U.S. Public Health Service Publication No. 75-787). Washington D.C., U.S. Government Printing Office, 1975b.

Vera M: Quality of life following pelvic exenteration. *Gynecol Oncol* 12:355-366, 1981.

Vincent CE, Vincent B, Greiss FC, et al: Some marital-sexual concomitants of carcinoma of the cervix. *South Med J* 68:552-558, 1975.

Von Knorring L: The experience of pain in depressed patients. *Neuropsychobiology* 1:155-165, 1975.

Von Knorring L, Perris C, Eisenmann M, Erikson U, Perris H: Pain as a symptom in depressive disorders. I. Relationship to diagnosis, subgroup and depressive symptomatology. *Pain* 15:19-26, 1983.

Wieder S, Schwarzfeld J, Fromewick J, Holland J: Psychosocial support program for patients with breast cancer at Montefiore Hospital. *QRB* 4:10-18, 1978.

Weinberg P: Psychosexual impact of treatment in female genital cancer. *J Sex Marital Ther* 1:155-157, 1974.

Weisman AD: Coping behavior and suicide in cancer. In Cullen JW, Fox BH, Isom RN (eds): *Cancer: The Behavioral Dimensions*. New York, Raven Press, 1976a.

Weisman AD: *Coping with Cancer*. New York, McGraw-Hill, 1979.

Weisman AD: The existential plight in cancer: Significance of the first 100 days. *Psychiatr Med* 7:1-15, 1976b.

Weisman AD, Sobel HJ: Coping with cancer through self-instruction: A hypothesis. *J Human Stress* 5(1):3-8, 1979.

Weisman AD, Worden JW, Sobel HJ: *Psychosocial Screening and Intervention with Cancer Patients*. Massachusetts General Hospital, Cambridge, Mass, 1980.

Werner A, Schieder J: Teaching medical students interactional skills: A research-based course in doctor-patient relationships. *N Engl J Med* 290:1232-1237, 1974.

Winefield H: Subjective and objective outcomes of communication skills training of the first year medical students. *Med Educ* 16:192-196, 1982.

Winick L, Robbins G: The Post-Mastectomy Rehabilitation Group. *Am J Surg* 132:599-602, 1976.

Wise TN: Effects of cancer on sexual activity. *Psychosomatics* 19:769-775, 1978.

Wortman C, Dunkel-Schetter C: Interpersonal relationship and cancer: A theoretical analysis. *J Soc Issues* 35:120-155, 1979.

Yalom I, Greaves C: Group therapy with the terminally ill. *Am J Psychiatry* 134:396-400, 1977.

Zussman L, Zussman S, Sunley R, Bjornsen E: Sexual response after hysterectomy-oophorectomy: Recent studies and reconsideration of psychogenesis. *Am J Obstet Gynecol* 140:725-729, 1981.

# Index